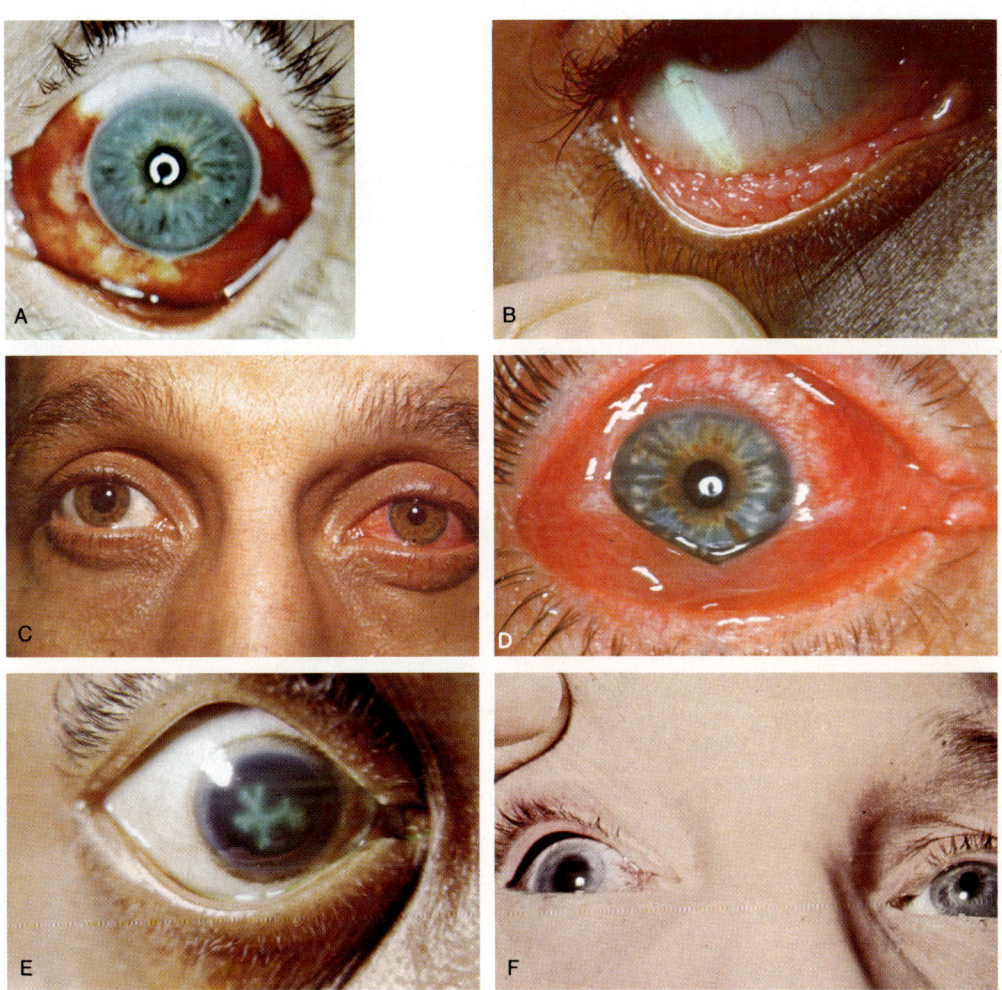

COLOR PLATE 1. *External signs of eye pathology. (A) Subconjunctival hemorrhage. (B) Ocular allergy, enlarged lid follicles. (C) Acute iritis. (D) Acute epidemic keratoconjunctivitis showing corneal infiltrates and chemosis. (E) Herpes simplex (dendritic keratitis). (F) Narrow angle-closure glaucoma showing dilated pupil, loss of corneal luster, and red eye. (From Scheie, HG, and Albert, DM: Textbook of Ophthalmology, 9th ed. Philadelphia, W. B. Saunders, 1977.)*

EMERGENCY MEDICINE

AN APPROACH TO
CLINICAL PROBLEM SOLVING

EDITED BY

GLENN C. HAMILTON, M.D.
Professor and Chair
Department of Emergency Medicine
Program Director
Integrated Residency in Emergency Medicine
Wright State University School of Medicine
Dayton, Ohio

ARTHUR B. SANDERS, M.D.
Professor of Emergency Medicine
University of Arizona College of Medicine
Tucson, Arizona

GARY R. STRANGE, M.D.
Chairman and Residency Director
Dean's Program in Emergency Medicine
University of Illinois College of Medicine
Chief of Emergency Service
University of Illinois Hospital
Chicago, Illinois

ALEXANDER T. TROTT, M.D.
Associate Professor of Emergency Medicine
University of Cincinnati College of Medicine
Director for Clinical Affairs
Center for Emergency Care
University of Cincinnati Medical Center
Cincinnati, Ohio

EMERGENCY MEDICINE

AN APPROACH TO CLINICAL PROBLEM-SOLVING

W.B. SAUNDERS COMPANY
A Division of Harcourt Brace & Company
Philadelphia   London   Toronto   Montreal   Sydney   Tokyo

W.B. SAUNDERS COMPANY
A Division of
Harcourt Brace & Company

The Curtis Center
Independence Square West
Philadelphia, Pennsylvania 19106

Library of Congress Cataloging-in-Publication Data

Emergency medicine : an approach to clinical problem-solving /
edited by Glenn C. Hamilton . . . [et al.].   p.   cm.
ISBN 0-7216-4487-2

   1. Emergency medicine.   I. Hamilton, Glenn C.
[DNLM: 1. Emergencies.   WB 105 E553]
RC86.7.E5783   1991   616.02'5—dc20
DNLM/DLC   90-9061

Editor: Darlene D. Pedersen
Developmental Editor: Rosanne Hallowell
Designer: Dorothy Chattin
Production Manager: Bill Preston
Manuscript Editor: Ruth Low
Illustration Coordinator: Brett MacNaughton
Indexer: Helene Taylor
Cover Designer: Anita Curry

EMERGENCY MEDICINE: AN APPROACH TO CLINICAL   ISBN 0-7216-4487-2
PROBLEM-SOLVING

Copyright © 1991 by W. B. Saunders Company

All rights reserved. No part of this publication may be reproduced or transmitted in any form or by any means, electronic, mechanical, including photocopy, recording, or any information storage and retrieval system, without written permission from the publisher.

Printed in the United States of America

Last digit is the print number: 9   8   7   6   5   4   3   2

DEDICATION

This book is written as a tribute to the memory of Harold Jayne, M.D. (1943–1986), an innovative educator and talented teacher. We miss him greatly.

The editors also make the following dedications:

To George and Maxine for their 60th anniversary. A small gift after a lifetime of love and support. To Lynda, James, and Kate for encouraging a dream and tolerating its fulfillment.

G. C. H.

To Katie for being. To Doug Lindsey for demonstrating that love, sweat, and the spirit of inquiry are the essence of teaching; the process is more important to the student than the information conveyed.

A. B. S.

To my wife, Sarah, and daughters, Jackie and Betsy, who soon forbade me to ever mention the word "chapter" in their presence but nevertheless remained patient and understanding.

G. R. S.

To Jennifer who always guides me with her unfailing wisdom and support.

A. T. T.

CONTRIBUTORS

MARK G. ANGELOS, M.D.

Assistant Professor, Department of Emergency Medicine, Wright State University School of Medicine, Dayton, Ohio
Cardiopulmonary Cerebral Resuscitation

RONALD S. BARRECA, M.D., FACEP

Assistant Professor of Clinical Emergency Medicine, University of Illinois College of Medicine; Chairman, Department of Emergency Medicine, Lutheran General Hospital, Chicago, Illinois
Heat Illness

NICHOLAS BENSON, M.D.

Associate Professor and Vice Chairman, Department of Emergency Medicine, East Carolina University School of Medicine; Medical Director and Program Director, Pitt County Memorial Hospital, Greenville, North Carolina
Earache

LOUIS S. BINDER, M.D.

Assistant Professor, Department of Emergency Medicine, Texas Tech University Health Sciences Center at El Paso; Attending Physician, R. E. Thomason General Hospital, El Paso, Texas
Stroke

ROBERT A. BITTERMAN, M.D., FACEP

Clinical Instructor, Emergency Medicine, Department of Surgery, University of Michigan Medical School, Ann Arbor; Director of Emergency Services, Samaritan Health Center, Detroit, Michigan
Acute Diarrhea

JUDITH C. BRILLMAN, M.D., FACEP

Assistant Professor, Family, Community and Emergency Medicine, University of New Mexico; Clinical Director, Emergency Department, University Hospital, University of New Mexico Medical Center, Albuquerque, New Mexico
Headache

SAMUEL T. COLERIDGE, D.O., FACEP

Clinical Assistant Professor of Emergency Medical Services, University of Texas Health Science Center at San Antonio, San Antonio, Texas; Clinical Assistant Professor of Military Medicine, Uniformed Services University of the Health Sciences, F. Edward Hebert School of Medicine, Bethesda, Maryland; Clinical Associate Professor, Division of Emergency Medicine, Department of General and Family Practice, Texas College of Osteopathic Medicine, Ft. Worth, Texas; Chief, Department of Emergency Medicine, Brooke Army Medical Center, San Antonio, Texas
Pelvic Pain in Women

HELENE CONNOLLY, M.D., FACEP

Assistant Professor of Clinical Emergency Medicine, University of Illinois College of Medicine; Medical Director, Department of Emergency Medicine, Mercy Hospital and Medical Center, Chicago, Illinois
Stridor

MARY ANN COOPER, M.D., FACEP

Research Director and Assistant Professor of Emergency Medicine, University of Illinois College of Medicine; Attending Physician, University of Illinois Hospital, Chicago, Illinois
Hypothermia

WILLIAM C. DALSEY, M.D., FACEP

Chief of Emergency Medical Services, Wilford Hall U.S. Air Force Medical Center, and Residency Director, Joint Military Medical Command Emergency Medicine Program, Lackland Air Force Base, Texas
Abdominal Trauma

DANIEL F. DANZL, M.D., FACEP

Professor of Emergency Medicine, University of Louisville School of Medicine; Acting Chairman, Department of Emergency Medicine, Humana Hospital–University Medical Center, Louisville, Kentucky
Hypothermia

JAMES DOUGHERTY, M.D.

Assistant Professor, Emergency Medicine, Northeastern Ohio Universities College of Medicine; Senior Staff Physician and Research Director, Department of Emergency Medicine, Akron General Medical Center, Akron, Ohio
Cocaine

MICHAEL EARL, M.D.

Senior Resident, Department of Emergency Medicine, University of Cincinnati College of Medicine, Cincinnati, Ohio
Dysuria

MARK A. EILERS, M.D., FACEP

Assistant Professor and Education Coordinator, Department of Emergency Medicine, Wright State University School of Medicine, Dayton, Ohio
The Potentially Suicidal Patient

TIMOTHY C. EVANS, M.D.

Assistant Professor of Emergency Medicine and Assistant Emergency Medicine Residency Director, Medical College of Pennsylvania, Allegheny Campus; Attending Staff, Emergency Department, Allegheny General Hospital, Pittsburgh, Pennsylvania
Hyperkalemia

RICHARD FELDMAN, M.D.

Assistant Professor of Clinical Emergency Medicine, University of Illinois College of Medicine; Attending Physician and Chairman, Department of Emergency Medicine, Illinois Masonic Medical Center, Chicago, Illinois
Medicolegal

CARL M. FERRARO, M.D.

Assistant Professor of Clinical Emergency Medicine, University of Illinois College of Medicine; Program Director, Emergency Medicine, Mercy Hospital and Medical Center, Chicago, Illinois
Metabolic Complications of Diabetes Mellitus

DENISE J. FLIGNER, M.D.

Assistant Professor of Emergency Medicine, Department of Family Practice, Rush Medical College, Chicago; Research Director, Department of Emergency Medicine, Christ Hospital and Medical Center, Oak Lawn, Illinois
Febrile Infants

CLOYD GATRELL, M.D.

Lieutenant Colonel, United States Army Medical Corps; Clinical Assistant Professor, Section on Emergency Medicine, Department of Military Medicine, Uniformed Services University of the Health Sciences; Chief, Department of Emergency Medicine, Madigan Army Medical Center, Tacoma, Washington
Suspected Sepsis

GARY GELESH, D.O., FACEP

Associate Professor of Emergency Medicine, Northeastern Ohio Universities College of Medicine; Attending Physician, Emergency Department, Akron General Hospital, Akron, Ohio
Alcohol Intoxication

KILBOURN GORDON III, M.D.

Assistant Clinical Professor, Division of Emergency Medicine, Department of Medicine, University of California, Irvine, College of Medicine; Attending Physician, University of California, Irvine, Medical Center, Orange, California
Head and Neck Trauma

SUCHINTA N. HAKIM, M.D., FAAP, FACEP
Clinical Assistant Professor, Department of Medicine, Loyola University Stritch School of Medicine, Maywood; Staff Physician, Department of Emergency Medicine, Hinsdale Hospital, Hinsdale, Illinois
Febrile Infants

GLENN C. HAMILTON, M.D., M.S., FACEP, FACP, FACEM (Hon.)
Professor and Chair, Department of Emergency Medicine; Program Director, Integrated Residency in Emergency Medicine; and Associate Professor, Department of Internal Medicine, Wright State University School of Medicine, Dayton, Ohio
Introduction to Emergency Medicine; Acute Chest Pain; Sickle Cell Disease; Behavioral Disorders

FRED HARCHELROAD, M.D.
Assistant Professor of Emergency Medicine, Medical College of Pennsylvania, Allegheny Campus, Pittsburgh, Pennsylvania
Acute Metabolic Acidosis and Metabolic Alkalosis

JAMES W. HOEKSTRA, M.D.
Assistant Professor of Emergency Medicine, Ohio State University College of Medicine, Columbus, Ohio
Acute Abdominal Pain

GEORGE HOSSFELD, M.D.
Assistant Professor of Clinical Emergency Medicine, University of Illinois College of Medicine; Director of Research and Academic Affairs, Department of Emergency Medicine, St. Francis Hospital, Evanston; Education Director, Department of Emergency Medicine, Riverside Medical Center, Kankakee, Illinois
Upper Extremity Injury: Closed Injuries

DAVID S. HOWES, M.D., FACEP
Assistant Professor of Medicine, University of Chicago; Residency Director, University of Chicago Emergency Medicine Program, University of Chicago Hospitals, Chicago, Illinois
The Red Painful Eye

RICHARD HUNT, M.D.
Assistant Professor, Department of Emergency Medicine, East Carolina University School of Medicine; Attending Physician, Department of Emergency Medicine, Pitt County Memorial Hospital, Greenville, North Carolina
Emergency Medical Services and Prehospital Personnel

KENNETH V. ISERSON, M.D., M.B.A., FACEP
Associate Professor of Surgery and Residency Director in Emergency Medicine, University of Arizona College of Medicine; Chairman, Bioethics Committee, University Medical Center, Tucson, Arizona
The Problem Patient

TIMOTHY G. JANZ, M.D.

Assistant Professor, Departments of Emergency Medicine and Internal Medicine, Wright State University School of Medicine, Dayton, Ohio
 Cardiopulmonary Cerebral Resuscitation

DIETRICH JEHLE, M.D.

Assistant Professor of Emergency Medicine, Medical College of Pennsylvania, Allegheny Campus; Director of Emergency Medicine Research, Allegheny General Hospital, Pittsburgh, Pennsylvania
 Acute Metabolic Acidosis and Metabolic Alkalosis

STEVEN M. JOYCE, M.D., FACEP

Associate Clinical Professor of Surgery and Emergency Medicine, University of Utah School of Medicine; Emergency Physician, University of Utah Hospital, Salt Lake City, Utah
 Epistaxis; Acute Sore Throat

THOMAS KRISANDA, M.D.

Attending Physician, Department of Emergency Medicine, York Hospital, York, Pennsylvania
 Vaginal Bleeding

JON R. KROHMER, M.D.

Assistant Professor, Section of Emergency Medicine, College of Human Medicine, Michigan State University, East Lansing; Assistant Program Director, Emergency Medicine Residency Program, Butterworth Hospital, and Emergency Medical Services Medical Director, Kent County Emergency Medical Services, Grand Rapids, Michigan
 Emergency Medical Services and Prehospital Personnel

EUGENE L. KWONG, M.D., FACEP

Clinical Director, Department of Emergency Medicine, San Bernardino County Medical Center, San Bernardino, California
 Acute Gastrointestinal Bleeding: Hematemesis, Hematochezia, and Melena

M. ANDREW LEVITT, D.O., FACEP

Assistant Professor of Medicine and Director of Research, Division of Emergency Medicine, University of California, San Francisco; Attending Physician, Department of Emergency Medicine, Highland General Hospital, Oakland, California
 Palpitations

ROBERT LINDBLAD, M.D., FACEP

Instructor in Emergency Medicine, Northeastern Ohio Universities College of Medicine, Akron; Attending Staff, Emergency Medicine, Aultman Hospital, Canton, Ohio
 Alcohol Intoxication

JOELLEN LINDER, M.D.
Assistant Clinical Professor; University of California, San Francisco/Fresno–Central San Joaquin Valley Medical Education Program, Fresno; Emergency Medicine Staff Physician, St. Agnes Medical Center, Fresno, California
  Sexual Assault

RONALD B. LOW, M.D., M.S., FACEP
Assistant Professor, Department of Medicine, Section of Emergency Medicine, University of Chicago; Attending Physician, University of Chicago Hospitals, Chicago, Illinois
  Hypertension

ROBERT A. LOWE, M.D., FACEP, FACP
Assistant Clinical Professor, Division of Emergency Medicine, University of California, San Francisco, School of Medicine; Attending Physician, Emergency Department, University of California, San Francisco, Medical Center, San Francisco, California
  Airway Management

STEPHEN LUDWIG, M.D.
Professor of Pediatrics, University of Pennsylvania School of Medicine; Director, General Pediatric Division, Children's Hospital of Philadelphia, Philadelphia, Pennsylvania
  Suspected Child Abuse

MICHAEL G. MANSKE, M.D.
Attending Physician, St. Mary's Medical Center, Racine, Wisconsin
  Behavioral Disorders

MARCUS L. MARTIN, M.D., FACEP
Associate Professor, Emergency Medicine, and Emergency Medicine Residency Director, Medical College of Pennsylvania, Allegheny Campus; Senior Attending Staff and Associate Director, Emergency Department, Allegheny General Hospital, Pittsburgh, Pennsylvania
  Hyperkalemia

MYRON L. MILLS, M.D., FACEP
Assistant Professor of Surgery and Medicine, Vanderbilt University School of Medicine; Attending Physician, Emergency Department, Vanderbilt University Medical Center, Nashville, Tennessee
  Suspected Meningitis

MARC S. NELSON, M.D., M.A., FACEP
Associate Professor of Surgery, Division of Emergency Medicine, Stanford University School of Medicine; Associate Medical Director, Emergency Services, and Medical Director, Life Support Training Center, Stanford University Hospital, Stanford, California
  Seizures

ROBERT L. NORRIS, M.D., FACEP

Attending Staff, Department of Emergency Medicine, Brooke Army Medical Center, Fort Sam Houston, Texas
Wheezing

EVE NORTON, M.D.

Assistant Clinical Instructor of Emergency Medicine, University of North Carolina, Chapel Hill; Teaching Faculty, Department of Emergency Medicine, Charlotte Memorial Hospital and Medical Center, Charlotte, North Carolina
Rash

GREGG A. PANE, M.D., FACEP

Associate Adjunct Professor and Assistant Chief and Residency Director, Division of Emergency Medicine, University of California, Irvine, College of Medicine; Attending Physician, University of California, Irvine, Medical Center, Orange, California
Nausea and Vomiting

PETER T. PONS, M.D.

Assistant Professor of Emergency Medicine, Department of Surgery, University of Colorado Health Sciences Center; Associate Director, Emergency Department, Denver General Hospital, Denver, Colorado
Multiple Trauma

T. J. RITTENBERRY, M.D., FACEP

Assistant Professor of Clinical Emergency Medicine, University of Illinois College of Medicine; Director of Emergency Medicine Education, Illinois Masonic Medical Center, Chicago, Illinois
Upper Extremity Injury: Closed Injuries; Lower Extremity Injury

JOHN P. RUDZINSKI, M.D., FACEP

Clinical Assistant Professor of Surgery, University of Illinois College of Medicine at Rockford; Associate Director, Emergency Department, Rockford Memorial Hospital, Rockford, Illinois
Hypercalcemia

KYM A. SALNESS, M.D., FACEP

Clinical Professor of Medicine, University of California, Irvine, College of Medicine; Chief, Division of Emergency Medicine, and Director of Emergency Department, University of California, Irvine, Medical Center, Orange, California
Syncope

ARTHUR B. SANDERS, M.D., FACEP, FACP

Professor of Emergency Medicine, University of Arizona College of Medicine; Attending Physician, University Medical Center, Tucson, Arizona
Syncope; Dizziness

CLIFTON A. SHEETS, M.D.
Assistant Clinical Professor, Wright State University School of Medicine; Attending Physician, Emergency Department, Miami Valley Hospital, Dayton, Ohio
The Patient with Abnormal Bleeding

JONATHAN SINGER, M.D.
Professor of Emergency Medicine and Associate Professor of Pediatrics, Wright State University School of Medicine; Staff Physician, Children's Medical Center, Dayton, Ohio
Dehydration

EDWARD P. SLOAN, M.D.
Assistant Professor of Emergency Medicine and Director of Emergency Medicine Research Development, University of Illinois College of Medicine; Attending Physician, University of Illinois Hospital, Chicago, Illinois
Lower Extremity Injury

MARTIN J. SMILKSTEIN, M.D.
Assistant Professor, Section of Emergency Medicine and Trauma, Department of Surgery, University of Colorado; Attending Physician, Emergency Department, University of Colorado Health Sciences Center, Denver, Colorado
The Poisoned Patient

REBECCA R. S. SOCOLAR, M.D.
Fellow, General Pediatrics, Albert Einstein College of Medicine, New York, New York
Suspected Child Abuse

MICHAEL SPADAFORA, M.D.
Assistant Professor, Department of Emergency Medicine, and Director, Center for Hyperbaric Medicine, University of Cincinnati Medical Center, Cincinnati, Ohio
Chest Trauma

J. STEPHAN STAPCZYNSKI, M.D.
Chairman, Department of Emergency Medicine, University of Kentucky Medical Center, Lexington, Kentucky
The Swollen and Painful Joint

SIDNEY STARKMAN, M.D.
Assistant Professor of Medicine/Emergency Medicine and Neurology, University of California, Los Angeles, School of Medicine; Director, UCLA Emergency Medicine Residency Program, UCLA Medical Center, Los Angeles, California
Altered Mental Status

GARY R. STRANGE, M.D., FACEP

Chairman and Residency Director, Dean's Program in Emergency Medicine, University of Illinois College of Medicine; Chief of Emergency Service, University of Illinois Hospital, Chicago, Illinois
Metabolic Complications of Diabetes Mellitus; Hyponatremia; Stridor; Low Back Pain

HERBERT N. SUTHERLAND, D.O., FACEP

Director of Emergency Services, Central Dupage Hospital, Winfield, Illinois
Low Back Pain

RAYMOND P. TEN EYCK, M.D., FACEP

Associate Professor, Department of Military Medicine, Section of Emergency Medicine, Uniformed Services University of the Health Sciences, Bethesda, Maryland; Chairman, Department of Emergency Medicine, United States Air Force Medical Center, Wright-Patterson Air Force Base, Ohio
Accidental Exposure to Biologic Agents

ALEXANDER T. TROTT, M.D.

Associate Professor of Emergency Medicine, University of Cincinnati College of Medicine; Director for Clinical Affairs, Center for Emergency Care, University of Cincinnati Medical Center, Cincinnati, Ohio
Chest Trauma; Dysuria

TIMOTHY L. TURNBULL, M.D.

Assistant Professor of Emergency Medicine, University of Illinois College of Medicine; Director of Operation, University of Illinois Hospital, Chicago, Illinois
The Poisoned Patient

DENNIS T. UEHARA, M.D., FACEP

Clinical Assistant Professor, Department of Surgery, Division of Emergency Medicine, University of Illinois College of Medicine at Rockford; Chairman, Department of Emergency Medicine, Rockford Memorial Hospital, Rockford, Illinois
Open Injuries to the Hand and Wrist

WARREN J. VENTRIGLIA, M.D., FACEP

Assistant Medical Director, Emergency Department, Burdette Tomlin Memorial Hospital, Cape May Court House, New Jersey
Eye Trauma

FRANK G. WALTER, M.D.

Clinical Instructor, Department of Family and Community Medicine, University of California, San Francisco, School of Medicine, San Francisco; Assistant Chief of Emergency Medicine, Valley Medical Center, Fresno, California
Airway Management

SETH W. WRIGHT, M.D.
Instructor of Surgery and Medicine, Division of Emergency Medicine, Vanderbilt University School of Medicine; Attending Physician, Vanderbilt University Hospital, Nashville, Tennessee
> *Acute Dyspnea; Penile and Vaginal Discharge*

BRIAN ZINK, M.D.
Assistant Professor of Emergency Medicine, Albany Medical College; Attending Physician, Albany Medical Center Hospital, Albany, New York
> *Wound Care*

DAVID N. ZULL, M.D., FACEP
Assistant Professor of Clinical Medicine and Residency Director, Combined Emergency Medicine/Internal Medicine Training Program, Northwestern University Medical School; Associate Chief of Medicine, Northwestern Memorial Hospital, Chicago, Illinois
> *Anaphylaxis*

ROBERT L. ZURCHER, M.D.
Attending Physician, Holy Family Hospital, Spokane, Washington
> *Sickle Cell Disease*

PREFACE

As is usually the case, this prologue is an epilogue. When we first met in early 1986 to discuss this book, our binding interest was to create a unique "course of study" in emergency medicine for medical students, residents, and practicing physicians. We agreed that the clinical approach in emergency medicine was different from other specialties, and traditional textbook formats did not capture its essence. We wanted to lay out the thought process of the practicing emergency physician when confronted with an undifferentiated patient complaint or presentation. We were aware of the fact that emergency physicians think in parallel. Thoughts on stabilization, evaluation, diagnosis, management, disposition, time limits, and the next patient run concurrently. We believed the unique aspects of our specialty could be communicated despite the sequential structure of the printed word. As educators, we wanted to convey the process as well as the content. In addition, each of us hoped to give something back to the specialty that has given us so much opportunity and satisfaction.

Though consuming our youth, emergency medicine has allowed us the chance to contribute to the real needs of many people, to share in creating a much needed discipline, and to work with a group of talented and dedicated academicians and clinicians who over the years have become friends and compatriots in our quest for quality in and recognition of our specialty. We hope this personal debt can be partially repaid by our writing a thoughtful delineation of guiding principles and supplying a framework for solving the many clinical problems that confront us daily.

As time and words have flowed, the motives for this book have remained the same, although the format and depth of coverage have evolved. The book has grown considerably in size since we first conceived of the project. Instructors of four- to eight-week clerkships and rotations in emergency medicine may find it useful to select key chapters rather than assign the entire text.

Though we have moved close to the "comprehensive textbook" size, much more could be written. We chose the topics representing those problems most often seen in the emergency department, thereby generating the greatest interest for the broadest readership. Many of the topics in this text have well-established management principles applicable to emergency medicine. In others we sailed uncharted waters to discover the "key" questions that drive our decisions.

Two purposes remained steadfast throughout. First, we wanted to systematically establish a workable approach to pursue an undifferentiated patient complaint from the prehospital setting to disposition. To do so, we struck a balance between redundancy to maintain each chapter as free-standing as possible and integration to illustrate the core concepts of the specialty. For example, common activities are repeated in the Prehospital and Initial Approach sections of many chapters. In the Diagnostic and Management sections, there is considerable cross-referencing to other chapters, and the emphasis is on principles rather than details of care. Second, we have sought to answer the difficult questions facing emergency physicians in their clinical practice: What information is important to gather and how valuable is it in differentiating specific clinical possibilities? How much assessment is necessary before consultation or disposition? Which patients go home and which are admitted to the hospital? If admitted, when is a critical care unit appropriate? If discharged, what information, cautions, and plans for follow-up are given? Importantly, what information is necessary to document on the patient's chart? In offering at least one set of answers we tried to give the reader an understanding of the information and the thought processes necessary to make these decisions. As is appropriate, we take full responsibility for our recommendations, and we invite the readership to communicate their concerns, corrections, and comments.

GLENN C. HAMILTON, M.D.
ARTHUR B. SANDERS, M.D.
GARY R. STRANGE, M.D.
ALEXANDER T. TROTT, M.D.
June, 1990

ACKNOWLEDGMENTS

We are pleased to acknowledge the many contributions of the following individuals. Without their considerable assistance, this book would simply be an unpublished sheaf of papers yellowing in one of our files.

At the W.B. Saunders Company: William Lamsback, who encouraged our effort, set sail with us, but was unable to finish the voyage; and Darlene Pedersen, Rosanne Hallowell, Tina Rebane, Bill Preston, and Ruth Low, who dedicatedly worked with us to finish the task. Their advice and patience were greatly appreciated.

In Dayton: Great indebtedness to and sighs of relief from Sheila Maston, Shirley Foreman, and Linda Crook from the Department of Emergency Medicine. Also sincere gratitude to Carol Enigk, Director, and to the staff of the Word Processing Center at the Wright State University School of Medicine for maintaining and revising the entire text during its many stages.

In Tucson: Special thanks to Glenda King for her patience, dedication, and support in completing this project.

In Chicago: Special thanks to Karlene Montgomery for her ever-present support and unfailing good cheer through seemingly endless revisions. Thanks to Janet DeJanovich and Rose Sturgill-Bradford for secretarial support beyond the call of duty.

In Cincinnati: Many thanks to Laverne Young, who cheerfully and competently undertook the numerous and varied tasks necessary to complete the manuscript.

In general: Thanks to Jerris Hedges, M.D., and Thomas Matthews, M.D., who took the time to review several manuscripts for format, content, and accuracy. Finally, our deepest appreciation to the 60-plus authors who created the substance of this text. In the face of multiple commitments they accepted our many communiques, adapted as we matured the format, and worked as hard as we did to codify and communicate the reality of our specialty.

CONTENTS

SECTION ONE
ORIENTATION TO EMERGENCY MEDICINE

Chapter 1
Introduction to Emergency Medicine   **3**
Glenn C. Hamilton, M.D.

Chapter 2
Airway Management   **19**
Frank G. Walter, M.D., and Robert A. Lowe, M.D.

Chapter 3
Cardiopulmonary Cerebral Resuscitation   **39**
Mark G. Angelos, M.D., and Timothy G. Janz, M.D.

Chapter 4
Multiple Trauma   **60**
Peter T. Pons, M.D.

SECTION TWO
ABDOMINAL AND GASTROINTESTINAL DISORDERS

Chapter 5
Acute Abdominal Pain   **83**
James W. Hoekstra, M.D.

Chapter 6
Acute Gastrointestinal Bleeding: Hematemesis, Hematochezia, and Melena   **104**
Eugene L. Kwong, M.D.

Chapter 7
Acute Diarrhea   **122**
Robert A. Bitterman, M.D.

Chapter 8
Nausea and Vomiting   **136**
Gregg A. Pane, M.D.

Chapter 9
Abdominal Trauma **152**
William C. Dalsey, M.D.

SECTION THREE
CARDIOVASCULAR DISORDERS

Chapter 10
Acute Chest Pain **173**
Glenn C. Hamilton, M.D.

Chapter 11
Palpitations **196**
M. Andrew Levitt, D.O.

Chapter 12
Syncope **214**
Kym A. Salness, M.D., and Arthur B. Sanders, M.D.

Chapter 13
Hypertension **231**
Ronald B. Low, M.D.

SECTION FOUR
CUTANEOUS DISORDERS

Chapter 14
Rash **251**
Eve Norton, M.D.

Chapter 15
Wound Care **271**
Brian Zink, M.D.

SECTION FIVE
IMMUNOLOGIC DISORDERS

Chapter 16
Anaphylaxis **299**
David N. Zull, M.D.

SECTION SIX
INFECTIOUS DISORDERS

Chapter 17
Suspected Sepsis **315**
Cloyd Gatrell, M.D.

Chapter 18
Accidental Exposure to Biologic Agents **333**
Raymond P. Ten Eyck, M.D.

SECTION SEVEN
TOXICOLOGIC/ENVIRONMENTAL DISORDERS

Chapter 19
The Poisoned Patient 347
Timothy L. Turnbull, M.D., and Martin J. Smilkstein, M.D.

Chapter 20
Alcohol Intoxication 378
Robert Lindblad, M.D., and Gary Gelesh, D.O.

Chapter 21
Heat Illness 394
Ronald S. Barreca, M.D.

Chapter 22
Hypothermia 409
Mary Ann Cooper, M.D., and Daniel F. Danzl, M.D.

Chapter 23
Cocaine 424
James Dougherty, M.D.

SECTION EIGHT
HEMATOLOGIC DISORDERS

Chapter 24
The Patient with Abnormal Bleeding 439
Clifton A. Sheets, M.D.

Chapter 25
Sickle Cell Disease 455
Robert L. Zurcher, M.D., and Glenn C. Hamilton, M.D.

SECTION NINE
HORMONAL, METABOLIC, AND NUTRITIONAL DISORDERS

Chapter 26
Metabolic Complications of Diabetes Mellitus 471
Carl M. Ferraro, M.D., and Gary R. Strange, M.D.

Chapter 27
Hyponatremia 486
Gary R. Strange, M.D.

Chapter 28
Hyperkalemia 499
Marcus L. Martin, M.D., and Timothy C. Evans, M.D.

Chapter 29
Hypercalcemia 508
John P. Rudzinski, M.D.

Chapter 30
Acute Metabolic Acidosis and Metabolic Alkalosis **516**
Dietrich Jehle, M.D., and Fred Harchelroad, M.D.

SECTION TEN
DISORDERS OF THE HEAD AND NECK

Chapter 31
Epistaxis **537**
Steven M. Joyce, M.D.

Chapter 32
Acute Sore Throat **547**
Steven M. Joyce, M.D.

Chapter 33
Earache **561**
Nicholas Benson, M.D.

Chapter 34
The Red Painful Eye **575**
David S. Howes, M.D.

Chapter 35
Eye Trauma **595**
Warren J. Ventriglia, M.D.

SECTION ELEVEN
DISORDERS PRIMARILY PRESENTING IN INFANCY AND CHILDHOOD

Chapter 36
Febrile Infants **619**
Suchinta N. Hakim, M.D., and Denise J. Fligner, M.D.

Chapter 37
Stridor **636**
Helene Connolly, M.D., and Gary R. Strange, M.D.

Chapter 38
Suspected Child Abuse **652**
Stephen Ludwig, M.D., and Rebecca R. S. Socolar, M.D.

Chapter 39
Dehydration **669**
Jonathan Singer, M.D.

SECTION TWELVE
MUSCULOSKELETAL DISORDERS

Chapter 40
The Swollen and Painful Joint **687**
J. Stephan Stapczynski, M.D.

Chapter 41
Upper Extremity Injury: Closed Injuries   **703**
George Hossfeld, M.D., and T. J. Rittenberry, M.D.

Chapter 42
Open Injuries to the Hand and Wrist   **727**
Dennis T. Uehara, M.D.

Chapter 43
Lower Extremity Injury   **748**
T. J. Rittenberry, M.D., and Edward P. Sloan, M.D.

Chapter 44
Low Back Pain   **783**
Herbert N. Sutherland, D.O., and Gary R. Strange, M.D.

SECTION THIRTEEN
NERVOUS SYSTEM DISORDERS

Chapter 45
Altered Mental Status   **807**
Sidney Starkman, M.D.

Chapter 46
Headache   **830**
Judith C. Brillman, M.D.

Chapter 47
Suspected Meningitis   **848**
Myron L. Mills, M.D.

Chapter 48
Seizures   **862**
Marc S. Nelson, M.D.

Chapter 49
Stroke   **877**
Louis S. Binder, M.D.

Chapter 50
Head and Neck Trauma   **894**
Kilbourn Gordon III, M.D.

Chapter 51
Dizziness   **924**
Arthur B. Sanders, M.D.

SECTION FOURTEEN
PSYCHO-BEHAVIORAL DISORDERS

Chapter 52
Behavioral Disorders   **937**
Michael G. Manske, M.D., and Glenn C. Hamilton, M.D.

Chapter 53
The Potentially Suicidal Patient   **951**
Mark A. Eilers, M.D.

Chapter 54
Sexual Assault   **964**
JoEllen Linder, M.D.

SECTION FIFTEEN
THORACO-RESPIRATORY DISORDERS

Chapter 55
Acute Dyspnea   **981**
Seth W. Wright, M.D.

Chapter 56
Wheezing   **1000**
Robert L. Norris, M.D.

Chapter 57
Chest Trauma   **1020**
Michael Spadafora, M.D., and Alexander T. Trott, M.D.

SECTION SIXTEEN
UROGENITAL DISORDERS

Chapter 58
Dysuria   **1043**
Michael Earl, M.D., and Alexander T. Trott, M.D.

Chapter 59
Pelvic Pain in Women   **1058**
Samuel T. Coleridge, D.O.

Chapter 60
Vaginal Bleeding   **1075**
Thomas Krisanda, M.D.

Chapter 61
Penile and Vaginal Discharge   **1091**
Seth W. Wright, M.D.

SECTION SEVENTEEN
ADMINISTRATION

Chapter 62
Medicolegal   **1105**
Richard Feldman, M.D.

SECTION EIGHTEEN
EMERGENCY MEDICAL SERVICES

Chapter 63
Emergency Medical Services and Prehospital Personnel **1117**
Jon R. Krohmer, M.D., and Richard Hunt, M.D.

SECTION NINETEEN
PHYSICIAN INTERPERSONAL SKILLS

Chapter 64
The Problem Patient **1133**
Kenneth V. Iserson, M.D., M.B.A.

Index **1141**

# SECTION ONE

ORIENTATION TO EMERGENCY MEDICINE

CHAPTER 1

INTRODUCTION TO EMERGENCY MEDICINE

GLENN C. HAMILTON, M.D.

As a third-year medical student entering the emergency department for the first time in 1971, my first impression was, "Here is a place that can make a difference in patients' lives, but I don't think I would want to live here!" Surely, thousands of students, residents, and attending physicians had similar thoughts. The emergency department was at the bottom of the medical prestige ladder. The students, interns, and residents supervised themselves, and patients were delivered by modified hearses run by the mortuary. Two decades later, the emergency department still "makes a difference." What has changed is that physicians *have* chosen to "live" in the emergency department, and to make it their place of specialty practice, thereby influencing the quality of care and often the quality of life of the millions of patients who are brought or who present themselves 24 hours a day, 365 days a year.

Beginning in 1968 with the formation of the American College of Emergency Physicians, emergency medicine has grown as a clinical specialty and academic discipline in concert with the increasing public demand for competent and compassionate emergency care. This growth has had several milestones:

1970: The first emergency medicine residency program was established at the University of Cincinnati.

1973: The Emergency Medical Services Act authorized the establishment and expansion of emergency medical services system and research.

1975: American Medical Association House of Delegates approved a permanent Section on Emergency Medicine and accepted standards for emergency medicine residencies.

1979: Emergency medicine was recognized as the twenty-third medical specialty by the American Medical Association and the American Board of Medical Specialties. Certification examinations began the following year.

1982: Special requirements for emergency medicine residency training programs were approved by the Accreditation Council for Graduate Medical Education.

1989: Primary board status was granted by the American Board of Medical Specialties.

Each of these steps has contributed to establishing the credentials and rewarding the commitment of the thousands of individuals who make up the "emergency medical care team" serving in the United States and throughout the world.

Table 1–1 lists the vital statistics of the specialty as it existed in the United States in early 1990. As a critical factor in the health care of this country, emergency medicine continues to be an essential subject in the training of medical students, a highly sought residency training experience, and a valuable and satisfying career for thousands of physicians.

This chapter is written to introduce the reader to the scope of emergency medicine practice, the principles of care behind the practice, and the basis for the problem-solving approach used in this book. In addition, a number of "pearls from practice" supplied by the authors are listed. Sharing the lessons learned by the practitioners is hopefully another way of conveying the character of emergency physicians and their speciality.

TABLE 1–1. U.S. Emergency Medicine Statistical and Historical Profile—1990

Emergency Physicians	
Total emergency physicians (approximate)[a]	23,000
Members of American College of Emergency Physicians	13,360
Diplomats of American Board of Emergency Medicine	8,332
Members of Society for Academic Emergency Medicine	1,600
Emergency Medicine Residencies	
Emergency medicine residency programs approved by Residency Review Committee/Emergency Medicine (RRC/EM)	80
Total residency graduates	3,293
Average annual number of graduates (approximate)	450
Total residents currently in training in RRC/EM-approved programs	1,629
Emergency Nurses	
Total emergency nurses (approximate)[b]	85,000
Nurses certified by the Board of Certification for Emergency Nurses	17,180
Emergency Medical Technicians[c]	
Basic	434,498
Intermediate	35,971
Paramedics	51,265
Emergency Departments[d]	
Hospital-based emergency departments (approximate)	5,600
Emergency department visits (1988)	86,641,305
EMS Air Ambulance Service[e]	
Air ambulance services	332
Total air ambulances	616
Ground ambulance services	12,116
Ground ambulance vehicles	34,917

[a] Figure reflects total number of full-time equivalent physicians practicing in emergency medicine, not just board-certified emergency physicians.
[b] McGraw-Hill 1989 Research Survey of the Nurse Universe.
[c] Training and Certification of EMS Personnel, The National EMS Clearinghouse, 1989.
[d] American Hospital Association: Hospital Statistics. American Hospital Association, 1989.
[e] Emergency Medical Services Transportation Systems and Available Facilities, The National EMS Clearinghouse, 1988.
Table modified from American College of Emergency Physicians, ACEP News, Dallas, Texas, February, 1990, with permission.

SCOPE OF PRACTICE IN EMERGENCY MEDICINE

In 1975, the House of Delegates of the American Medical Association defined the emergency physician as a physician trained to engage in:

1. The immediate initial recognition, evaluation, care, and disposition of patients with acute illness and injury.
2. The administration, research, and teaching of all aspects of emergency medical care.
3. The direction of the patient to sources of follow-up care, in or out of the hospital as may be required.
4. The provision when requested of emergency, but not continuing, care to in-hospital patients.
5. The management of the emergency medical system for the provision of prehospital emergency care.

Six years later, as part of a "Definition of Emergency Medicine" developed by the American College of Emergency Physicians and endorsed by the three other organizations representing residents in training and academic emergency physicians, a paragraph was published that summarized the practice of the specialty:

Emergency medicine encompasses the immediate decision making and action necessary to prevent death or any further disability for patients in health crises. Emergency medicine is practiced as a patient-demanded and continuously accessible care. It is the time-dependent process of initial recognition, stabilization, evaluation, treatment, and disposition. The patient population is unrestricted and presents with a full spectrum of episodic, undifferentiated physical and behavioral conditions. Emergency medicine is primarily hospital-based, but with extensive prehospital responsibilities.

Despite growth and changes brought by the intervening years, the essence of this clinical specialty remains captured in those words.

One critical word in the paragraph needs to be clarified. *Emergency* is defined by the perception of the patient who comes or the people who bring the patient to the emergency department. Over 70% of emergency patients believe they need medical care within 2 hours of their decision to seek help. Therefore, the patient defines the "emergency" regardless of the ultimate nature of the illness or injury. Although discrepancies may exist between what the patient feels is emergent and how that concern is perceived by the emergency physician, many problems need 24 to 48 hours or more of evaluation and treatment before they are retrospectively determined to be "emergent." This gap between the patient's perception, the emergency physician's perception, and the time delay before the reality of the hazard is revealed is often a source of frustration and anger. This difficult situation may affect the emergency physician's relationship with the patient, the admitting physician, family members of the patient, and the insurance system involved in reimbursing the transaction. Accepting the contextual nature of the term *emergency* will help the reader to understand the specialty more fully.

In addition to the acute care of the ill or injured patient, the specialty has evolved to accept new responsibilities in the following areas:

1. Administration. Management of the medical and administrative aspects of the emergency medical services system is included in this category—e.g., public education about services, 911 telephone access, and emergency department categorization.

2. Disaster planning and management for both natural and manmade events.

3. Toxicology. This includes poison center development and improved means of recognition of environmental hazards.

4. Health care services research. Problems in society and in our health care delivery system are often noted first in the emergency department. For example, problems of the homeless, hospital closures, and the drug "war" have manifested themselves as increasing numbers of patients with higher acuity of illness crowding into the emergency department—with no place else to go. Emergency medicine is the front line of medicine. It has a special obligation to ensure access to quality health care for all patients and communicate problems in this access to the rest of organized medicine when they occur.

5. Education. The emergency department has always been a popular training site. The recent emphasis on ambulatory care education has made it an even more valuable asset.

6. Preventive medicine. Only a brief exposure to the practice of emergency medicine will generate an interest in improving and enforcing the laws regarding seat belt use, driving while intoxicated, or job-related safety.

7. Basic and clinical research. The scientific rationale for the efficacy of resuscitative interventions is an essential element in expanding the academic base of the specialty.

The future holds bright promise for the scope of practice available in emergency medicine. Pediatric emergency care, trauma care, aerospace medicine, critical care medicine, industrial medicine, clinical epidemiology, and quality assurance have benefitted and will continue to gain from the ideas and energy of emergency physicians.

Emergency medicine is a specialty that was created to fulfill the needs of ill and injured people. It arrived at a time when both the general population and a select group of physicians recognized its importance. It remains a clinical specialty serving all those who find themselves seeking its care, competence, and advocacy.

PRINCIPLES OF EMERGENCY CARE

The nature of clinical emergency medicine has been briefly described. In this section, twelve principles guiding the decisions made in practice are examined. "Guiding principles" is a carefully chosen phrase. Emergency medicine should not be identified with or practiced by "cook-book" or algorithmic thinking. The patients rarely follow the recipe, and often don't cooperate at the branch points. Emergency medicine is best practiced by following *heuristics*, that is, incomplete guidelines that lead to new knowledge or discovery.

1. *Is a life-threatening process causing the patient's complaint?*

   This is always the first question asked by the emergency physician. Emergency medicine is primarily a *complaint-oriented* rather than *disease-specific* speciality. Its emphasis rests on anticipating and recognizing a life-threatening *process*, rather than seeking the diagnosis. This is an important difference between emergency medicine and other specialties. A patient with severe substernal chest pain is first considered as having a life-threatening problem with hypoxia, hypoperfusion, or potential dysrhythmia rather than as having a myocardial infarction. Anticipation of life-threatening problems focuses the physician's attention on both the underlying pathophysiology and the influence of time on the presentations and outcome of dynamic disease processes. The goal is simply to think about and plan to prevent "bad things" from happening or progressing in the patient.

2. *What must be done to stabilize the patient?*

   Stabilizing a patient may require the direct intervention in a life-threatening process, or an intervention that *anticipates* a critical problem developing. In a patient with chest pain, a cardiac monitor and an intravenous line are placed in anticipation of a dysrhythmia and the need for medications or volume repletion. These steps demonstrate the emergency physician's awareness of the hazards of the processes associated with the presenting symptoms, not the diagnosis. They represent actions performed to monitor the course of the process while preparations are made to intervene quickly, if necessary.

3. *Beyond the life-threatening process, what are the most serious disorders (highest potential morbidity) that are consistent with the patient's presentation?*

   The emergency physician approaches a problem by considering the most serious disease consistent with the patient complaint and working to exclude it. "Thinking the worst" is a reversal of the assessment sequence in many specialties. In emergency medicine, the "worst comes first." Only after it has been ruled out are the more benign processes considered.

   This principle is even more important when it is placed in the context of the patient population seen in the emergency department. The majority of patients are strangers to the physician, many have an altered sensorium owing to intoxication or anxiety, and many are brought by others rather than come of their own volition. Confronted with an array of fragmented histories, masked physical findings, and emotional overlay, it is imperative for the emergency physician to maintain the highest level of suspicion for serious disease.

4. *Is more than one active pathologic process present?*

   A single diagnosis is not always possible or appropriate. The emergency physician must maintain an open and continually probing approach that is the hallmark of the effective clinician. Always thinking "Is that all there is?" encourages the physician to consider alternative diagnoses and seek additional information from the patient, other sources, or response to therapy. The time for assessment is usually brief, and it is essential to resist the tendency to rapidly narrow the underlying possibilities. An example is the driver involved in a motor vehicle accident who is hypotensive. The hypotension may be the result of the trauma, but it may also have been the cause. Hypotension after a motor vehicle accident is very likely to be secondary to blood loss, but the possibilities of anaphylaxis, myocardial failure, or distributive shock from a drug overdose must be considered.

5. *Would a diagnostic-therapeutic trial serve in this case?*
   One of the emergency physician's important tools is a stabilizing therapy that also gives diagnostic information. This information may be precise or may just help differentiate the seriously ill patient from others. Glucose, thiamine, and naloxone given to the unconscious patient are examples of this "diagnostic-therapeutic" concept. Judicious fluid boluses to improve a patient's hemodynamic status are another. Integrating therapy and diagnosis is especially valuable in the time-dependent setting that usually begins with undifferentiated illness. Seeking new *diagnostic-therapeutic* tests or maneuvers and determining where they can be applied is an important role of the emergency physician.
6. *Is a diagnosis possible or even necessary?*
   One of the most difficult aspects of emergency medicine is becoming comfortable with uncertainty regarding an exact diagnosis before important decisions are made. This principle has been discussed in terms of stabilization. It also applies throughout the steps of care in the emergency department, especially during disposition decisions. Knowing when to stop an assessment or treatment is as important as knowing when to persist. Many common complaints such as chest or abdominal pain remain undiagnosed by the time the patient leaves the emergency department. Other serious problems may require early disposition to sites outside of the department without a diagnosis being made; e.g., obvious penetrating trauma to the abdomen.
7. *Is hospitalization appropriate?*
   The "bottom line" decision for the emergency physician is whether the patient is admitted to the hospital or discharged from the emergency department. In many cases, once the patient's condition has been recognized as requiring hospitalization and stabilization has begun, much of the emergency physician's clinical work is accomplished. Still, there are other reasons for continued care. It may be necessary to benefit the admitting physician, to maintain one's clinical acumen, or because the hospital staff do not have an available inpatient bed.
8. *If the patient is to be discharged, is the disposition adequate?*
   The most difficult patients cared for by the emergency physician are the ones who are discharged. This is doubly true for those who leave without a clear diagnosis. Unfortunately, in a limited and often first-time assessment, the data available may be insufficient for a disease process to be identified or understood. Despite their wishes, both patients and physicians must recognize that all important information is not available immediately. To ensure optimal care, an appropriate discharge disposition should include the patient's basic understanding of (1) the underlying problem that caused him or her to seek emergency care, (2) the evaluation and treatment given in the emergency department, (3) when and with whom follow-up is planned, and (4) criteria by which the patient can judge whether a return for further assessment is necessary.
9. *In working with admitting or primary physicians, has the concept of "our" patient been well established?*
   Emergency physicians have a unique relationship with other physicians. They serve as the "always available" consultant and specialist in common and catastrophic diseases. Combining the historical knowledge of the primary physician with the emergency physician's information obtained from the patient's bedside can offer the best of acute care. Emergency physicians are the gatekeepers of one of the major access routes into the medical system. Their relationship with other physicians is always based on the concept of "our" patient. It must be a healthy relationship—one based on mutual trust and respect.
10. *Does the chart reflect the full extent of evaluation and treatment given in the emergency department?*
    The medicolegal cliché, "If it isn't charted, it didn't happen," is true. Part of the experience in emergency medicine is learning to write or dictate accurate,

useful information in limited time and space. The importance of developing patterns of recording the right information efficiently cannot be overstated.

11. *Have the patient's expectations, voiced and unvoiced, been met?*
    The emergency physician must often look beyond the words of a complaint to sense the patient's fears and concerns about being in the emergency department. "Am I going to die?" "Is it cancer?" "Will there be a scar?" and "Can you relieve my pain?" are questions to be anticipated and answered. The hidden potential for suicide or the reality of child abuse must also be uncovered during a brief interview within an often harried environment. This skill demands a sensitivity, awareness, and ability to concentrate on many clues during the physician–patient exchange. Only training and a commitment to clinical excellence in this setting allow these skills to develop fully.

    Every patient assessed in the emergency department is given something. It may be an explanation, a referral, or a specific therapeutic regimen. Each patient has a requirement, and the emergency physician makes an attempt to fulfill it if it is legitimate and reasonable. If the requirement cannot be met, an explanation in layman's terms is necessary. For example, parents may ask for a skull radiograph for their asymptomatic child's head contusion. This expectation is addressed by discussing the lack of indications, the hazards of radiation, and the expense. On occasion, when reason fails, obtaining the films may be appropriate. The key is to ensure the cooperation of the parents so that they will comply with the more important follow-up observation.

12. *Are the resources available to allow the full range of emergency services to be efficiently administered?*
    The emergency physician has a role in maintaining the equipment and staffing of the department at the highest level of quality. Trends and breakthroughs are monitored in the literature. Equipment and supplies representing real advances in patient care are purchased. The education and skills development of the staff are maintained. Developing a viable and continuous quality assurance program for physicians and staff, maintaining a relationship with attending physicians to facilitate patient care, and actively participating in the affairs of the hospital and medical services in the community are all necessary to contribute to the overall quality of medicine.

    An important correlate of this principle is the recognition of what the emergency department team cannot do. It cannot be all things to all people. It should not be thought of as a walk-in clinic when other facilities are nearby and available, a storage depot for patients waiting to be admitted, or an extended critical care unit on demand. To serve its purpose, the emergency department must be dedicated first to the critically ill and injured patient. Since this degree of severity is not always realized immediately, no one is turned away without an appropriate assessment. This service is essential to the community, and it must not be abused.

These twelve principles are valued guides for the practice of this specialty. By accepting and practicing them, the emergency physician can deliver high-quality and humane care while enjoying a satisfying and respected career.

THE APPROACH TO CLINICAL PROBLEM SOLVING IN THE TEXT

The process of clinical problem solving begins with the acquisition of a fundamental body of knowledge including anatomy and physiology as well as the pathology and epidemiology of disease patterns. The clinician uses this knowledge base to address specific patient complaints. The emergency physician is particularly concerned with conditions that may result in morbidity or mortality if not immediately addressed. The secondary concern is the common or serious diseases that may be the cause of the patient's complaint.

In the typical sequence of care, anticipating the emergent condition is the focus of emergency medicine in the prehospital and initial stabilization period. After initial stabilization, the emergency physician applies the knowledge of disease processes to direct specific data gathering from the patient and other sources. This complaint-directed assessment in a time-limited framework is not a simple task. The data gathered are added to the understanding of the pathophysiology of diseases to develop a rational set of guidelines regarding the further assessment, treatment, and disposition of each patient. These decisions are made in the context of the inexact science of clinical medicine. It is not improbable for the same patient to present in different emergency departments with the same history and physical findings and be treated differently at each hospital. There are few totally right answers in clinical medicine. There *are* wrong interpretations, priorities, and actions that violate the scientific basis of practice or the accepted principle of "do no harm."

An element of problem solving is the discipline of decision analysis. This quantitative science attempts to attach actual probabilities to the various options available at decision points. When given the probabilities of various alternatives, the clinician can then choose the most likely alternative. Unfortunately, this discipline is relatively new in medicine. At present, the emergency physician does not have sufficient information to reliably calculate probabilities at every decision point for each disease process. The specialty therefore continues to rely on judgments about the probabilities of various decision alternatives based on experience, the scientific literature, and data gathered from the patient. In situations where probability analysis is available and valuable, the information is included in this text.

Another element in clinical problem solving involves the subjective factors of the patient, the setting, and treating physician. The patient who is particularly uncooperative or has poor social support may need a more extensive evaluation than the responsible patient who will follow up with his or her primary physician. The new "alternative health care delivery" setting can make a difference in how a problem is solved. A "managed care" plan physician may refuse admission for a patient that the emergency physician believes may benefit from inpatient care. This may result in other dispositions, such as home health care, being sought. Although not always acknowledged, the emergency physician's personality and experience can influence the approach to clinical problem solving. A physician who has been affected by the malpractice environment may practice more defensive and expensive medicine than the physician who is more comfortable with uncertainty. One clinician believes that if a 1% chance exists that the patient with a headache has a subarachnoid hemorrhage, a diagnostic computed tomographic head scan is indicated. Another physician may accept a 5% or 0.5% probability before ordering the same test.

Despite all these influences, in emergency medicine a decision about a particular problem still must be made in a timely manner. These decisions are often made with incomplete information and a changing clinical pattern. For example, a beta agonist aerosol treatment may be ordered to relieve a patient's symptoms of severe dyspnea and wheezing. Later in the assessment, it is determined that the patient does not have a pulmonary source of the symptoms, but has congestive heart failure from an acute myocardial infarction. Was the aerosol order a wrong decision? The emergency physician must accept the fact that many decisions made in emergent or urgent circumstances are not optimal. Each patient is different and presents with unique diagnostic challenges. Decisions must be accepted and integrated into the next decision. Understanding the approach to problem solving and how decisions are reached is one element in the maturation of a specialist in emergency care.

This textbook is designed to reflect the thinking process of the emergency physician confronted by a patient with an undifferentiated clinical complaint. It represents the most common sequence of events followed in caring for emergency patients. Although the chapters are written in a sequential format, it is assumed that in many situations stabilization, evaluation, diagnosis, and thoughts about disposition must proceed simultaneously. The organization of the book's major headings is the same as that used in the Emergency Medicine Core Content published by the American Board of Emergency Medicine and the American College of Emergency Physicians. This listing covers the full range of subjects included in the specialty, and it is classified into 20 major systems. This text is not an exhaustive listing of all these presentations but represents the complaints encountered in the great majority of clinical practices.

Most chapters begin with a specific complaint or presentation, and most have a similar structure. A few chapters present laboratory findings, e.g., hyponatremia, hyperkalemia. In these chapters the format is modified to give the laboratory values before the preliminary differential diagnosis. The final three chapters include topics important to emergency medicine practice: medicolegal issues, emergency medical services (EMS) and prehospital personnel, and the problem patient. They are presented in a manner that is consistent with the other chapters but does not follow their format.

To facilitate the reader's understanding of the chapter format used, each chapter heading is explained briefly. Statements made in these paragraphs are applicable to all designated chapter sections in the book.

Problem-Solving Scenarios

Problem cases are integrated throughout the chapters as a means of reinforcing the material that precedes them. The author's comments on the case management are presented at various points in the problem. These cases are supplemental to the text.

Questions to Consider

These important questions are answered by the information presented in each chapter. They are objectives for the reader to attain by reading the material. The goal is to list the valuable questions that a physician needs to ask when confronted by a specific complaint. Some of them are repetitive for a number of presenting complaints.

Introduction

The introductory paragraphs are written to supply the basic information necessary to help solve the clinical problem. First, the important basic scientific data necessary to make a set of decisions are given. These include pertinent anatomy, physiology, and pathophysiology. Second, the importance of the presenting complaint to emergency medicine is discussed. Clinical epidemiologic data are useful to provide context for the incidence, significance, and outcome of the patient's complaint and some of the diseases that cause it.

Prehospital Care

Prehospital care personnel are the extension of emergency services into the community. They serve an essential role in the assessment and stabilization of emergency patients. Though not every patient concern warrants the involvement of a rescue squad, the majority of patients they bring to the emergency department are appropriate for their skills and can benefit from their care. In emergency medicine, the clinical problem is often first encountered and addressed by prehospital personnel. The section is written to establish the actions and skills the emergency physician should expect from personnel at the Advanced Emergency Medical Technician or Paramedic level of training. Chapter 63 describes the content of this training. This section details the data to be given to the physician by the prehospital care providers. By knowing what to anticipate, the emergency physician can facilitate a rapid and complete exchange. The interventions listed are the actions the rescue squad is expected to take using "standing" orders or after a set of radio orders from the physician. Many of the interventions are repeated in each chapter. This allows each chapter to stand on its own.

Initial Approach in the Emergency Department

During the first 5 to 15 minutes of care, many of the most important decisions for the patient are made. This section describes the initial or primary survey directed toward the vital areas of airway, breathing, circulation, and others. The first stabilizing actions are also discussed. This care is often closely integrated with the activities pursued during the prehospital care period, and the two are considered complementary to one another.

As part of this initial approach, the emergency physician first determines whether the patient is "sick" and rapidly confirms or excludes the presence of catastrophic disease. Second, the physician must stabilize the patient's vital signs, while anticipating the complications the underlying disease process may manifest. Third, the physician needs to address relief of the patient's acute symptoms. Although this is not always possible or advisable at this stage, the relief of suffering is central to the values of medical practice. To do so, medication is not always necessary. A brief commentary about early clinical impressions, especially thoughts on serious problems that are *not* present, can do much to lessen the patient's fears. The simple phrase, "We are here to help you feel better," can help build trust and decrease anxiety. It also helps establish the patient's confidence regarding the competency of the entire department team.

Data Gathering

The history is a directed exploration of the presenting complaint. A full history and physical examination are generally not warranted in the emergency department. Each chapter supplies the reader with the elements of data gathering appropriate to the specific complaint, and why they are pertinent.

Certain historical elements appear repeatedly to maintain chapter autonomy and to stress their importance. These include allergies, medications, and pertinent past medical history. The need to obtain information from many sources is emphasized in a number of chapters. It is easy to allow one's data-gathering efforts to remain trapped behind the automatic doors of the emergency department. Information is always gained and the patient's statements corroborated by discussions with friends, family, witnesses, and primary physicians. Communicating with contacts in the waiting room can provide information while alleviating their often escalating concerns.

The physical examination commonly begins with a reassessment of the primary survey. This is followed by a more thorough, but often directed, examination emphasizing the organ systems involved in the chief complaint. Selected diagnostic maneuvers, such as orthostatic vital signs and oculovestibular testing (cold caloric tests), may be included in this section. When possible, the value of specific findings in determining serious problems and data on the limits of a variety of physical findings are given.

As in most clinical presentations, the combination of the history and physical examination results in a reasonable diagnosis or recognition of serious disease in the vast majority of patients.

Decision Priorities and the Preliminary Differential Diagnosis

After data gathering, the emergency physician usually has sufficient information to answer specific questions that will prioritize management decisions and establish a preliminary differential diagnosis. In this section the bridge between emergency medicine and the more traditional specialties is established. The focus is first on life-threatening disease: How has the patient progressed with stabilizing efforts? Are any unrecognized life-threatening processes present? If so, what organ system do they involve? What is the major diagnostic possibility within this organ system? Second, attention is directed toward identifying the less urgent and common causes of the patient's signs or symptoms. Again, the findings are weighed against a series of differential diagnostic categories, and a preliminary list of possible causes is developed.

Each question is asked, answered, and repeated throughout the remainder of the patient's stay. This serial and comparative analysis is the core of the problem-solving process in the emergency department.

In the text the common and catastrophic causes of the condition are discussed in either a table or a paragraph. This information is given to more clearly define the characteristics of specific diseases, thereby allowing better comparisons with the patient's findings.

Diagnostic Adjuncts

The preliminary differential diagnosis guides the selection of diagnostic studies. In most cases, the tests are chosen as confirmatory evidence of a specific disease or to rule out a serious process. Occasionally, the test makes the diagnosis or at least must be available before a differential pathway is rational. This section covers the topics of laboratory studies, radiologic imaging, electrocardiography, and other tests. These are the "tools of the trade" that support the initial clinical impressions. Suggestions are made about when to order diagnostic adjuncts, how they may be interpreted, and, once interpreted, how valuable this information is in identifying a specific disease process.

The emergency physician plays an important role in cost control through test selection. Knowing when a battery versus a single test is indicated is an important skill. Since clinical judgment is influenced by a variety of factors, including cost, the physician must be aware of the relative costs of the commonly ordered tests in the emergency department. These are listed in Table 1–2. A conscious effort to limit the number of ancillary tests ordered, within the constraints of high-quality medicine, is the responsibility of all physicians. Unfortunately, this positive goal is often offset by the present medicolegal environment in this country, summarized by the phrase, "When things go wrong, no one thanks you for saving them money." Cost awareness remains an important area to be mastered in clinical emergency medicine.

Refined Differential Diagnosis

After ancillary testing, additional or more specific diagnoses may be made. A definitive diagnosis may not be available or necessary, but an improved "working" diagnosis can guide management and disposition decisions. It is common not to have a precise diagnosis at the time of disposition. For example, in up to 40% of patients presenting with undifferentiated abdominal pain, the cause remains undiagnosed when the patient leaves the emergency department. In many cases it is more important to have a clear idea of what is *not* going on than it is to have a precise diagnosis. Overattention to seeking the definitive cause can promote inefficiency and divert effectiveness in the emergency department.

Principles of Management

This text assumes that treatment is the natural outcome of the problem-solving process that includes all the information preceding it. Its emphasis is on the general principles of assessment and management for a presenting complaint. A secondary listing of specific therapies is given for specific diseases. The purpose is to give the reader an overview of what needs to be done and a limited number of details about selected problems.

Special Considerations

In most complaints, age, pregnancy, or an immunosuppressed condition is a complicating factor. This section gives additional information about pediatric, geriatric, and other at-risk populations that may influence the evaluation, diagnosis, and treatment of the patient. This material is considered supplemental to the problem-solving process up to the disposition. It is a means of including important "risk factors" not always viewed as contributing to the patient's illness or injury.

Disposition and Follow-up

Disposition and follow-up plans are often the most difficult components of problem resolution. Even when admission is obviously needed, decisions remain about the appropriateness of critical care monitoring, the need for surgical intervention, and other problems. Discharge from the emergency department has its own set of risks for both the patient and the physician. Because of this difficulty, useful guidelines for admission to the hospital, admission to the critical care unit, continued observation, obtaining consultation, and discharge are not often found in the emergency medicine literature. Each chapter lists guidelines intended to aid these decisions.

Patients admitted to the hospital are under the care of their attending or primary physician. No recommendations for admitting orders are given because, with rare exceptions, this is not the task of the emergency physician. Writing these orders extends liability, assumes more complete knowledge of the patient than may be correct, and may create a sense of complacency on the part of the admitting physician.

Discharging patients is a complex process often overlooked by the emergency physician. It is a time when the most important influence on following care instructions is established. All discharge procedures are initiated by the physician and reinforced by

TABLE 1–2. Cost Ranges for Diagnostic Adjuncts Commonly Ordered in the Emergency Department—1990

	Range (in $)
Laboratory Tests[a]	
Chemistry	
Alkaline phosphatase	6.00– 8.00
Amylase	8.00– 12.00
Arterial blood gas	50.00– 75.00
Aspartate aminotransferase	6.00– 8.00
Bilirubin, total	5.00– 10.00
Blood urea nitrogen	6.00– 10.00
Calcium	5.00– 7.00
Creatinine phosphokinase (CPK)	6.00– 13.00
CPK MB fraction	25.00– 35.00
Creatinine	9.00– 12.00
Electrolyte panel (sodium, potassium, chloride, bicarbonate)	25.00– 35.00
Glucose	9.00– 12.00
Human chorionic gonadotropin, beta subunit	14.00– 18.00
Lactate dehydrogenase (LDH)	6.00– 8.50
LDH isoenzymes	25.00– 40.00
Lactic acid	18.00– 22.00
Hepatitis B surface antigen	13.00– 22.00
Heterophil antibody, monospot	8.50– 10.50
Human immunodeficiency virus	15.00– 30.00
Osmolality, serum	15.00– 20.00
Osmolality, urine	15.00– 20.00
Potassium	4.50– 9.00
Sodium	7.00– 10.00
Toxicology	
Screen (EMIT)	45.00– 60.00
Comprehensive (routine)	80.00–100.00
VDRL	5.50– 14.00
Urinalysis (dipstick and microscopic)	10.00– 15.00
Urine chemistry (sodium/potassium)	9.00– 12.00 each
Hematology	
Complete blood count and differential	25.00– 30.00
Hemoglobin/hematocrit	12.00– 15.00
Platelet count	5.00– 8.00
Partial thromboplastin time	8.00– 14.00
Prothrombin time	6.50– 8.00
Peripheral smear	15.00– 20.00
Bacteriology	
Blood culture	40.00– 50.00
Gonococcus culture	25.00– 35.00
Gram stain	8.00– 12.00
Chlamydial culture	45.00– 55.00
Streptococcus screen	20.00– 25.00
Throat culture	40.00– 50.00
Urine culture	40.00– 50.00
Radiologic Imaging[b, c]	
Plain Films	
Skull series	80.00– 90.00
Cervical spine series	75.00– 85.00
Lateral only	35.00– 45.00
PA and lateral chest	60.00– 70.00
Portable AP chest	110.00–120.00
Abdominal series (four views)	90.00–100.00
AP pelvis	50.00– 60.00
Lumbosacral spine series	90.00–100.00

Table continued on following page

TABLE 1–2. Cost Ranges for Diagnostic Adjuncts Commonly Ordered in the Emergency Department—1990 *Continued*

	Range (in $)
Radiologic Imaging[b,c] *(Continued)*	
Plain Films (Continued)	
Upper extremity	
Shoulder	55.00– 65.00
Humerus	45.00– 55.00
Elbow	45.00– 55.00
Forearm	45.00– 55.00
Wrist	45.00– 55.00
Hand	45.00– 55.00
Lower extremity	
Hip (with pelvis)	80.00– 90.00
Femur	70.00– 80.00
Knee	45.00– 55.00
Tibia/fibula	65.00– 75.00
Ankle	45.00– 55.00
Foot	45.00– 55.00
Soft tissue of neck	45.00– 55.00
Foreign body, soft tissue	55.00– 65.00
Facial series	65.00– 80.00
Contrast	
Esophagus (barium swallow)	80.00– 90.00
Urethrogram	90.00–100.00
Cystogram	150.00–165.00
Intravenous pyelogram	140.00–160.00
Computerized Tomography	
Head (noncontrast)	250.00–300.00
Chest	260.00–280.00
Abdomen (noncontrast)	250.00–300.00
Cervical spine	265.00–285.00
Nuclear Medicine	
Lung scan	260.00–280.00
Testicular scan	75.00–100.00
Angiography	
Aortic Arch	475.00–530.00
Ultrasound	
Pelvis	120.00–140.00
Abdomen (visceral)	140.00–160.00
Electrocardiography[b]	
12-lead ECG	40.00– 60.00

[a]Many hospital laboratories add a $4–6 STAT surcharge because the tests are ordered from the emergency department.
[b]The charge for interpretation is not included.
[c]Portable radiographs have a $50–70 added charge.

the nursing staff. The information is given to the patient and to individuals responsible for further care. The discharge instructions include:

1. A summary of findings.
2. A brief description of the problem from the physician's perspective. This is linked to the reason for the patient's coming to the emergency department.
3. Treatment plans, including medications, possible hazards, and, optimally, their approximate cost.
4. Queries of the patient or family members as to whether they have other questions, and a brief quiz to make sure they understand the instructions.
5. Plans for follow-up care after leaving the emergency department. Reasons for returning to the department are also given.

All of this information is supported in writing. Preprinted materials written in the lay puplic's terminology are very helpful.

Discharged patients should contact their primary physician within 24 to 48 hours of being seen in the emergency department. They may not need an appointment, but all are instructed to call their physician's office to give notice of their emergency care and a statement of their present condition.

In high-risk situations or by the patient's own request, the primary physician is contacted near the time of discharge and the responsibility for ensuring follow-up is shared between the physician and patient. In these situations, a specific appointment date and time increase the patient's compliance by 40% to 50%.

Documentation

Adequate documentation is essential for communicating with other physicians, satisfying certain medicolegal expectations, fulfilling quality assurance requirements, and as an aid to organizing the physician's problem-solving thoughts and approach. Listed in each chapter are the important elements recommended for inclusion on the chart. They do not define absolute standards but may serve as a template for sharing adequate information. At a minimum, the physician should consider why an item of information suggested in this section is not to be included. Some general guidelines include addressing all questions or complaints raised in the prehospital run report and nursing notes and asking if the chart as completed can support the ruling in or out of serious disease. The continued acceptance of transcribed over written charts will benefit the quality of documentation in the emergency department.

Summary and Final Points

This section lists the important points made in each chapter. These points are not directly related to the Questions to Consider, but many supply the answers to these questions. This section is a means of quick review or a way of presenting the "highlights" of problem solving given in the chapter. Each of these sections is well worth remembering.

Bibliography

Emergency medicine remains a maturing academic science. The student of the specialty should have a familiarity with the literature that contributes to its growth. Each chapter has a list of useful texts and papers pertinent to the subject. In addition, the following texts are considered standard references for the specialty:

1. Roberts JR, Hedges JR: Clinical Procedures in Emergency Medicine. Philadelphia, Saunders, 1985.

2. Rosen P, Baker FJ, Barkin RM, et al: Emergency Medicine: Concepts and Clinical Practice (2nd ed). St. Louis, Mosby, 1988.

3. Tintinalli JE, Krome RL, Ruiz E: Emergency Medicine: A Comprehensive Study Guide (2nd ed). New York, McGraw-Hill, 1988.

4. Fleischer FR, Ludwig S: Textbook of Pediatric Emergency Medicine (2nd ed). Baltimore, Williams & Wilkins, 1988.

CLINICAL PEARLS

The practice and art of this specialty is like that of any other medical specialty. It is learned over time, patient by patient. The "sixth sense" used to identify serious illness is an acquired skill. The patient who manifests seizures as a sign of hemodynamic collapse from a ruptured ectopic pregnancy, the child abuser who brings his infant to the emergency department and then attempts to sign out quickly, the surviving accident victim who was trying to commit suicide but now fears and desires discovery—all these patients and thousands more demand the learned patience, perception, and understanding that a trained, experienced emergency physician can offer.

The following is a list of selected clinical pearls gathered from the authors of this text. Many apply every day to care in the emergency department. Many will stand the test of time, others will be forgotten as research proves them obsolete. At the present time, they offer an insight into the hazards and rewards of the specialty. Reviewing them before each tour of duty is a worthwhile exercise. Though many others are worth learning, these are some of the best.

A. The New Job
 1. Respect is earned.
 2. Befriend, through a show of respect, your nursing staff.

B. Maximizing Patient Satisfaction with Your Care
 1. Avoid medical jargon.
 2. Learn how to tell a patient you don't know what's wrong.
 3. Let the patient know he or she is always welcome to return.

C. Minimizing Patient Dissatisfaction
 1. One hour feels like three behind a curtain.
 2. A companion makes the wait less unbearable.
 3. Give the patient an estimate of the time needed to complete the evaluation. Significant delays require an honest accounting.

D. You Are the Patient's Advocate
 1. If you must err, err on the side of helping the patient.
 2. Respect the patient's need for privacy.
 3. Always consider the "costs" of your interventions.
 4. Don't negotiate any medically important decision with a patient with an altered sensorium, particularly if it is due to alcohol or other substance abuse.
 5. If a patient is a source of potential harm to himself or others, or cannot take care of himself, he must stay for observation or admission.
 6. Physical restraint may be necessary and appropriate to protect the patient or emergency department staff.
 7. Do not discharge a now "sobered" patient who has recovered from acute alcoholism without performing a repeat history and physical examination.
 8. Anxiety and hysteria are diagnoses of exclusion.

E. Clinical Judgment
 1. When the clinical impression does not fit with the history, physical examination results, or laboratory evaluation, STOP! Rethink and expand the differential diagnosis.
 2. If the patient can't walk, he can't go home.
 3. If the ancillary data do not fit the clinical picture, reconfirm the accuracy of the data before making treatment and disposition decisions.
 4. If you seriously consider a specific diagnosis when working through a differential diagnosis, then you should rule it out with the appropriate tests.
 5. "If you don't know what to do—do nothing." Observe the patient *closely* for the evolution of the disease process instead of gambling on a marginally indicated therapeutic intervention.
 6. *Always* assume that females of childbearing age might be pregnant, and act accordingly.
 7. The patient who returns to the emergency department on an unscheduled basis is first asssumed to be at high risk for a serious illness.
 8. Abnormal vital signs must be repeated and explained.
 9. A patient who won't look at you during the history and physical examination is usually either depressed or manipulative. Almost never is such a person shy.
 10. Patients usually have one major medical problem for each decade of life after the age of 60.
 11. Never completely trust a young child, a geriatric patient, an alcoholic, or a drug abuser. That is, corroborate the history and carefully interpret the physical findings in each of these patients.
 12. Listen closely to the suggestions of patients and their families about what is wrong and how they should be treated.

F. Specific Clinical Situations
1. During the winter months, if the whole family has "the flu," be sure to consider carbon monoxide poisoning.
2. Ask what *caused* the trauma in the patient you are treating. Trauma is often considered the *only* problem and not potentially the *result* of another problem.
3. Consider the diagnosis of ruptured (or expanding) abdominal aortic aneurysm in all patients over 60 years old who appear to have renal colic.
4. Since the eye is to see, record its acuity!
5. Always confirm a field or bedside glucose oxidase strip reading in the emergency department with a blood glucose level.
6. Multiple drug allergies often correlate highly with functional or psychogenic complaints.
7. Chest pain radiating below the umbilicus or above the maxilla is seldom cardiac in origin.

G. The Pediatric Encounter
1. Speak to children in language they can understand.
2. Allow the parent(s) to stay in the room. Observing the child's interaction with his parents is an important part of the evaluation.
3. Children are rarely hypochondriacs.
4. Examine neurovascular and motor integrity before focusing on the injured area.

H. Communicating with the Attending or Consulting Physician
1. Confirm admission or discharge with the primary physician before committing yourself to the patient.
2. When in doubt, a second opinion to confirm a clinical impression is always appropriate.

I. Avoid Supporting the Legal Profession
1. Don't think you are going to win just because you are in the "right."
2. Protect yourself by protecting the patient.
3. A printed form never saved anyone.
4. One of the most hazardous moments in emergency medicine is "signing out" patients to a colleague at the end of one's shift. A complete and accurate exchange of information and impressions is necessary.

J. Destroying Your Credibility
1. Subvert the call schedule or be chronically late.
2. Yell at someone.
3. Give an opinion before looking at the patient.
4. Treat a number, not the patient.

K. Your Mental Health
1. Every physician has moments of self-doubt.
2. There is always a disposition.
3. When you find yourself becoming angry with a patient ("positive personal hypertension sign") during history taking, you must step away momentarily. The patient may be malingering and withholding or providing misleading information or you may be fatigued or have lost your perspective on your role. In any case, the emotion and its origin must not be allowed to influence or impair your judgment.
4. If possible, take a break, e.g., lunch, during each shift.

L. Do's
1. Meet every patient turned over to you at the change of shift.
2. Order soft tissue radiographs to rule out suspected soft tissue foreign bodies.
3. Respond to complaints by private attendings immediately to avoid irreparable damage.
4. Always see and interpret the diagnostic studies you have ordered.

M. Don'ts
1. Never say: "There is nothing wrong with you."

2. Do not expect patients to remember verbal information.
3. Do not try to weasel out of accepting responsibility when you blew it—admit the error, apologize, and get on with life.

BIBLIOGRAPHY

1. Definition of emergency medicine. Ann Emerg Med 10:385–388, 1981.
2. Rosen P: The biology of emergency medicine. J Am Coll Emerg Phys 8:58–61, 1979.
3. American College of Physicians: Standards for Residency Training Programs in Emergency Medicine, as approved by the American Medical Association House of Delegates on June 17, 1975.
4. Gifford MJ, Franaszek JB, Gibson G: Emergency physicians' and patients' assessments: Urgency of need for medical care. Ann Emerg Med 9:502–507, 1980.
5. Hamilton GC, Lumpkin JR, Tomlanovich MC, et al: Special Committee on the Core Content Revision, "Emergency Medicine Core Content." Ann Emerg Med 15(7):853–862, 1986.

CHAPTER 2

AIRWAY MANAGEMENT

FRANK G. WALTER, M.D.
ROBERT A. LOWE, M.D.

PROBLEM 1 A rescue squad responds to a call from a private home after receiving a report that an elderly man had "passed out." They find him apneic and pulseless. Their attempts at cardiopulmonary resuscitation (CPR) with mouth-to-mask ventilations produce little chest wall motion.

PROBLEM 2 A 20 year old male who ingested 50 amitriptyline tablets about 30 minutes ago is becoming somnolent. The emergency physician is concerned about intubating the patient prior to gastric lavage because the patient will certainly resist the attempt.

PROBLEM 3 A 45 year old man shot himself in the mouth with a pistol. The primary survey reveals an apneic, hypotensive patient with an oral cavity full of blood, tissue, and teeth.

QUESTIONS TO CONSIDER

1. Which patients have the highest risk of airway compromise?
2. How are airway and breathing assessed during the primary survey?
3. What are the indications for airway management?
4. What questions must be answered before proceeding with airway management?
5. How can supplemental oxygen be delivered? What is the percentage of inspired oxygen delivered by each method?
6. What are the proper techniques for orotracheal intubation? For nasotracheal intubation?
7. What maneuvers help ensure that an endotracheal tube is properly positioned?
8. What pharmacologic adjuncts can aid in airway management? What are their indications and hazards?
9. When is a cricothyrotomy indicated?

INTRODUCTION

Airway assessment and management have priority over all other aspects of resuscitation in critically ill and injured patients. Airway management is the *A* in the ABC mnemonic (*a*irway, *b*reathing, *c*irculation) used to prioritize the care of critically ill or injured patients.

The most common error in airway management is failure to anticipate the need for active intervention in patients at high risk for airway obstruction or respiratory insufficiency. This group includes patients with decreased levels of consciousness, cardiorespiratory disease, head and neck pathology, and major traumatic injury.

Despite the importance of anticipating the need for airway management, there are a few important exceptions to the rule that airway management has first priority. (1) The patient with ventricular fibrillation or pulseless ventricular tachycardia should be immediately defibrillated prior to CPR or intubation if the rescuer is alone and has immediate access to a monitor-defibrillator. (2) An immediate solitary precordial thump is recommended in the pulseless patient with a witnessed cardiac arrest prior to CPR and intubation if a monitor-defibrillator is not immediately available. (3) Immediate defibrillation prior to CPR and intubation is recommended in a pulseless patient if a defibrillator is available without a monitor.

First aid, including the Heimlich maneuver (subdiaphragmatic abdominal thrusts), chest thrusts, and finger sweeps, will not be covered in this chapter. They are discussed in the *Standards and Guidelines for Cardiopulmonary Resuscitation (CPR) and Emergency Cardiac Care (ECC)*, which is part of the Advanced Cardiac Life Support course published by the American Heart Association (see Bibliography [texts, reference 1, and journal articles, reference 12]).

Airway Anatomy

An understanding of basic airway anatomy is essential for successful airway management. This section reviews the pertinent structures.

The nasal cavity is often used to provide access to the upper airway. Its inferomedial aspect is the safest route for passage of an endotracheal tube. The nasal turbinates and paranasal sinus ostia occupy lateral positions in the nasal cavities and are sites of potential complications. During intubation, the turbinates can be lacerated or fractured, and once the endotracheal tube is in place, the paranasal sinus ostia may be occluded, resulting in sinus blockage and infection.

The oropharynx begins below the posterior opening of the nasal passage just beyond the soft palate. Entry into this area may stimulate the protective gag reflex mediated by the glossopharyngeal nerve (cranial nerve IX). The laryngopharynx (hypopharynx) extends from the vallecula to the true vocal cords and includes the piriform recesses (piriform sinuses) just superolateral to the thyroid cartilage (Fig. 2–1A). The epiglottis serves to cover and protect the glottic opening. The thyroid cartilage forms the laryngeal prominence and thyroid notch. Between the thyroid and cricoid cartilages is the cricothyroid membrane (Fig. 2–1B). It is an important site in emergency surgical airway management. The cricoid cartilage is the only circumferential cartilage of the airway and provides structural stability. If the cartilage is cut or fractured, that stability can be endangered. Below the cricoid cartilage, the cervical trachea is deep and is partially covered by the

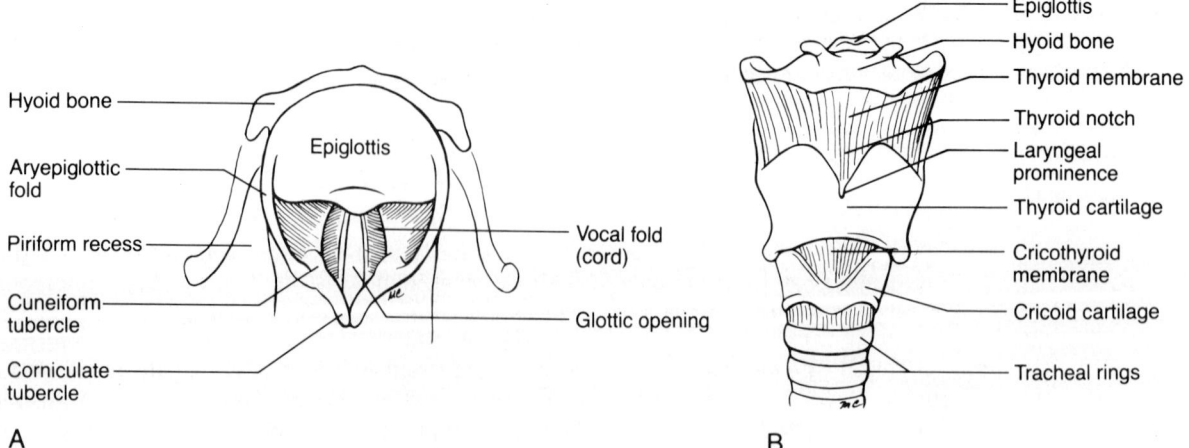

FIGURE 2–1. A, *Larynx, from above.* B, *Larynx, anterior view.*

thyroid gland and other vascular structures. It is near the cupola of the lungs, and its posterior membranous portion is adjacent to the esophagus.

Indications for Airway Management

The six general indications for airway management are as follows:

- Establish and maintain patency
- Protection from aspiration
- Oxygenation
- Ventilation
- Secretion control
- Administration of resuscitative drugs

Patency is mandated when there is impending or existing airway obstruction. Protection of the airway from aspiration is mandatory in the patient who cannot guard his own airway; such a situation is clinically evident by the absence of a gag reflex. Adequate oxygenation and ventilation are fundamental and are part of every patient's clinical care. Secretion control is necessary if secretions are voluminous or cannot be raised. Administration of the following drugs through an endotracheal tube is effective when an intravenous line is not available: naloxone, atropine, Versed (midazolam), epinephrine, and lidocaine. A useful mnemonic for remembering the list of endotracheal drugs is NAVEL.

PREHOSPITAL CARE AND INITIAL APPROACH IN THE EMERGENCY DEPARTMENT

The fundamentals of airway assessment and management are the same in the prehospital setting and in the emergency department. The practice of each rescue squad will vary with their level of training and local policies. An assessment of the airway and breathing status is performed in every patient. Failure to secure the airway in a timely manner is the most common fatal error in airway management. The goal is to determine whether the airway is patent and protected and whether breathing is present and adequate. A standardized approach will allow the care provider to recognize the patient with a subtle deficit and avoid being diverted by more "dramatic" problems.

Assessment of Airway and Breathing

The primary survey of airway and breathing is completed in 10 to 15 seconds and consists of inspection, palpation, and auscultation. *Inspection* includes observing the patient's mental status, respiratory rate, and effort. If the patient is responsive, talking spontaneously, and speaking clearly and comfortably, there is seldom a need for airway management beyond supplemental oxygen. If there is uncertainty about the protection or patency of the upper airway, a tongue depressor is used to test the gag reflex and examine the mouth for blood, vomitus, or foreign bodies. If doubt persists about the patient's ability to protect the airway and there is no possibility of cervical spine injury, a direct laryngoscopic examination is attempted. If the patient allows the vocal cords to be visualized without a struggle, he requires intubation. This last statement may be tempered by special circumstances, e.g., respiratory depression and loss of the gag reflex due to an opiate ingestion that is rapidly reversed by naloxone. Still, it remains a valuable guideline.

Palpation includes feeling for tracheal deviation and for chest deformities, bony crepitance, or subcutaneous emphysema. Placing a hand or ear near the patient's mouth and nares provides a crude assessment of air motion.

Auscultation begins with listening to the patient speak and assessing the voice quality. Noisy breathing suggests partial airway obstruction and mandates further inspection. Hoarseness signifies laryngeal pathology. Both hemithoraces are auscultated in the midaxillary lines for symmetry of breath sounds and adventitious sounds.

Based on the 10- to 15-second primary survey of the airway and breathing, the airway should be classified as:

- intact: patent and protected
- in jeopardy: unprotected or questionable status
- partially obstructed
- completely obstructed

If the airway and breathing are intact, supplemental oxygen is supplied to any critically ill patient. If the airway is in jeopardy, partially obstructed, or completely obstructed, the rescue squad or emergency physician must intervene immediately.

A simplified schematic guideline for decision making in airway management is illustrated in Figure 2–2. It emphasizes patency of the airway, the patient's ability to protect the airway, the adequacy of ventilation, and the importance of integrity of the cervical spine. The oxygenation status of the patient is initially less important in choosing airway management procedures, since supplemental oxygen is routinely given.

Manual Airway Opening Maneuvers

The most common cause of airway obstruction is laxity of the genioglossus (tongue) and other supporting muscles accompanying decreased levels of consciousness. This allows the tongue to fall posteriorly and obstruct the oropharynx, or the epiglottis to fall posteroinferiorly and obstruct the glottic opening. Regardless of the cause, a manual airway opening maneuver is indicated in any patient with partial or complete airway obstruction.

The most effective manual airway opening maneuver is the head-tilt–*chin*-lift (Fig. 2–3A). However, in the trauma setting, the neck must not be moved because of the possibility of a cervical spine injury. In this case, the jaw-thrust maneuver is used (Fig. 2–3B). The American Heart Association no longer recommends the head-tilt–*neck*-lift maneuver, which has been found to be less effective.

Suction

A functioning large-bore, large-volume suction device is important in any airway management procedure. There are three main types of suction tips: the dental suction tip, the tonsil suction tip, and the catheter suction tip. The dental suction tip is usually the best choice until definitive airway management is achieved because it has the largest bore and allows rapid clearance of fluids and particulate matter, e.g., vomitus.

Basic Airway Devices

Although manual airway opening maneuvers require no equipment, they do require the constant involvement of one rescuer. To overcome this disadvantage, an oropharyngeal airway or nasopharyngeal airway can be used to hold the tongue away from the posterior wall of the pharynx (Fig. 2–4).

The oropharyngeal airway is inserted with the concave side down, with a tongue blade depressing the tongue during insertion of the airway, or concave side up, followed by 180-degree rotation when the flange is at the lips. The latter method is not recommended in children owing to their relatively larger tongues and the potential for further obstruction of the pharynx by pushing the tongue posteriorly. Contraindications to insertion of the oropharyngeal airway include tightly clenched teeth and intolerance of the airway as evidenced by gagging. Almost all patients who can tolerate an oropha-

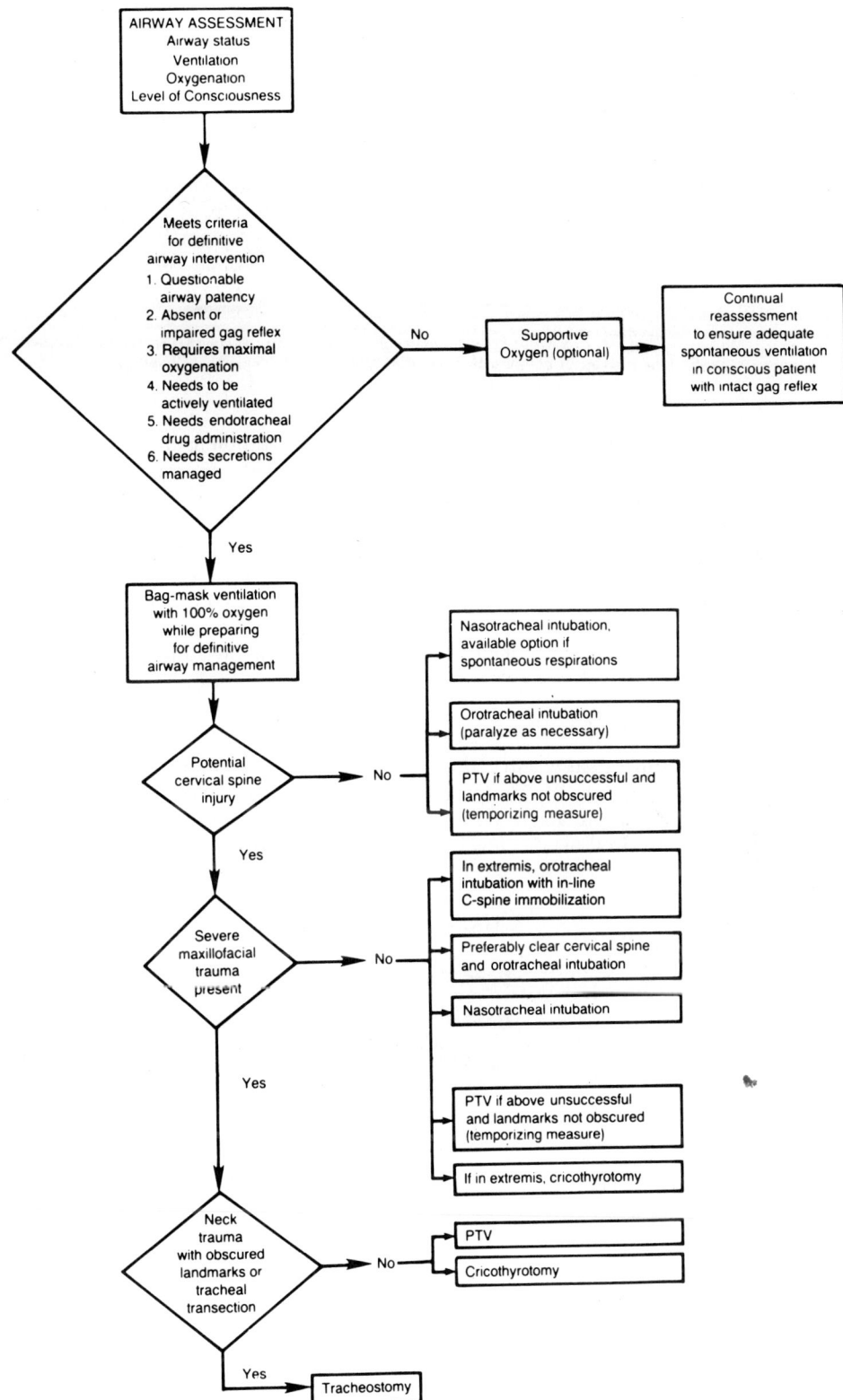

FIGURE 2–2. Simplified algorithm for definitive airway management. (Reproduced with permission from Kastendieck JG: Airway management. In Rosen P, et al. [eds]: Emergency Medicine: Concepts and Practice, ed 2. St. Louis, 1988, The CV Mosby Co.)

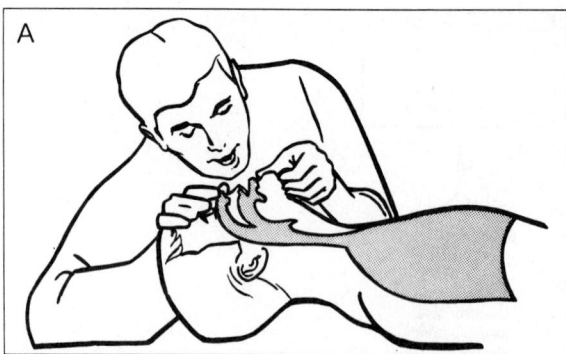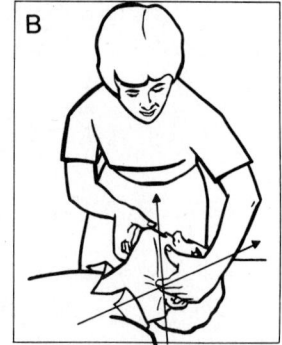

FIGURE 2–3. Chin-lift maneuver: (A) Chin lift and (B) jaw thrust. (From Guildner CW: Resuscitation—opening the airway: A comparative study of techniques for opening an airway obstructed by the tongue. JACEP 5:588, 1976. Used by permission.)

ryngeal airway without gagging have a problem in protecting their airway and require more definitive airway management. After orotracheal intubation, the oropharyngeal airway is used to prevent biting and occlusion of the endotracheal tube.

Insertion of a nasopharyngeal airway is indicated in patients who "snore" because of a partial airway obstruction in patients with tightly clenched teeth. This device bypasses the soft palate but does not always reach a level in the oropharynx that ensures protection from blockage by the tongue. It is relatively contraindicated in patients with nasal polyps because it can produce epistaxis and tissue damage. Its major usefulness is to establish an opening through the nasal passage to allow administration of supplemental oxygen.

Oxygen

Immediately after the airway is opened and the oropharynx suctioned, supplemental oxygen is administered. Table 2–1 lists the most common oxygen delivery systems and the approximate percentages of oxygen they can deliver. More precise measurements of inspired oxygen levels are made by oximetry testing.

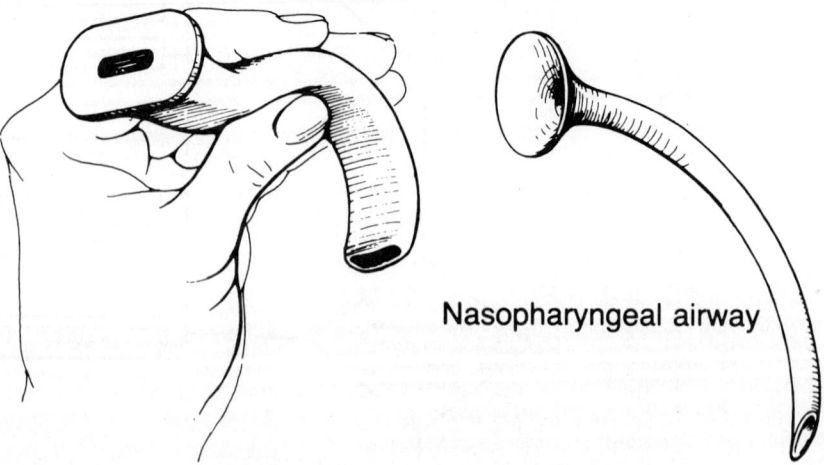

FIGURE 2–4. Simple artificial airways: oropharyngeal and nasopharyngeal. (From Clinton JE, Ruiz E: Emergency airway management procedures. In Roberts JR, Hedges JR [eds]: Clinical Procedures in Emergency Medicine. Philadelphia, Saunders, 1985, p. 6.)

TABLE 2-1. Supplemental Oxygen Delivery Systems

System	O_2 Percentage	Advantages	Disadvantages
Nasal cannula	Additional 2–4%/liter/min	Comfortable at ≤6–8 liters/min	Intolerable and impractical at >6–8 liters/min. Exact FIO_2 uncertain because it varies with respiratory rate and depth
Simple and partial rebreather masks	60% at 10 liters/min	Higher FIO_2	May promote CO_2 retention at lower flow rates
Venturi mask, Ventimask	24% or 28% at 4 liters/min; 31% at 6 liters/min; 35% or 40% at 8 liters/min; 50% at 10 liters/min	Fairly exact FIO_2 control. Excellent for COPD with chronic CO_2 retention	Poorly humidified
Reservoir nonrebreathing mask	90% at 15 liters/min	High FIO_2 for severe hypoxia and CO poisoning	Oxygen toxicity a small concern in emergency department
Bag-valve-mask	Almost 100% at 15 liters/min	High FIO_2 for severe hypoxia and CO poisoning. Ventilatory assistance	Mechanical device between patient and physician. Variable operator skill needed
Manually triggered oxygen-powered breathing device (OPBD)	100% with 40 liters/min	Highest FIO_2. Ventilatory assistance	Contraindicated in children due to barotrauma. Can be "too much of a good thing" in inexperienced hands

FIO_2 = fraction of inspired oxygen

Ventilation

The patient having inadequate respiration after the airway is opened needs positive pressure ventilation. This can be started with mouth-to-mouth or mouth-to-mask ventilation, but when the equipment is available, bag-valve-mask ventilation with supplemental oxygen is preferable. The mask should be the proper size for the patient's face and should have an inflatable rim to facilitate a tight seal. Because it is difficult for one person to hold the mask tightly on the face, perform a jaw-thrust maneuver, and squeeze the bag, two rescuers are often needed to use the bag-valve-mask method. In adult patients rescuers can use a mask incorporating an oxygen-powered breathing device (OPBD), which releases oxygen under pressure when a button on the mask is pushed. Oxygen is always administered prior to more definitive airway management procedures.

Esophageal Obturator Airway

The esophageal obturator airway (EOA) is a temporizing airway management tool used almost exclusively in the prehospital setting. Because of its questionable ventilatory efficacy and significant hazards in use, it is becoming less popular, but it still may be encountered in the emergency department. It combines a mask with a tube incorporating a balloon, which is placed in the esophagus. When pressurized oxygen or air is delivered through the mask, the balloon occluding the esophagus allows ventilation only through the trachea (Fig. 2–5).

The EOA is indicated for temporary oxygenation and ventilation in the field in patients with cardiac arrest or in deeply comatose, hypoventilating patients without a gag reflex who tolerate its insertion. It can be placed with minimal neck movement in trauma victims with suspected cervical spine injuries. It does not protect the trachea from aspiration of secretions or blood, and regurgitation frequently occurs when it is removed.

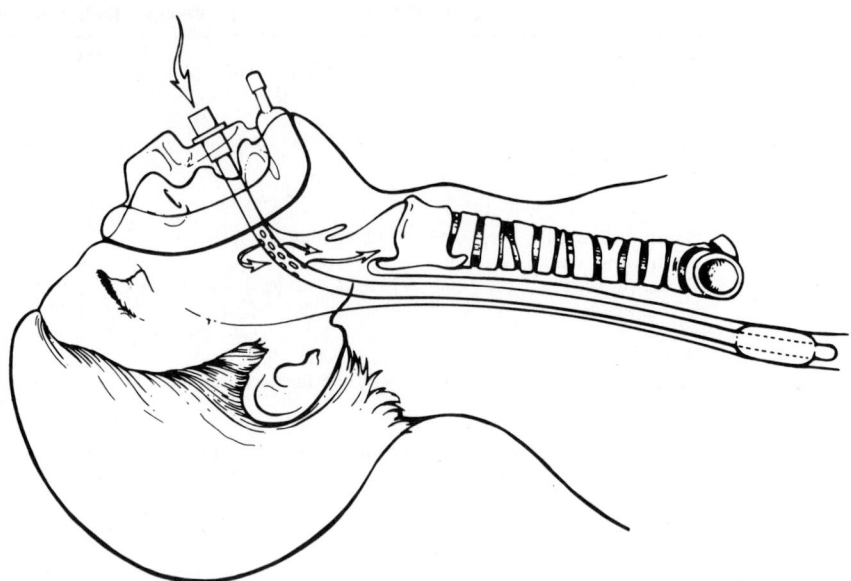

FIGURE 2–5. *Esophageal obturator airway: correct placement of the esophageal airway with the cuff inflated in the esophagus caudad to the bifurcation of the trachea. (From Clinton JE, Ruiz E: Emergency airway management procedures. In Roberts JR, Hedges JR [eds]: Clinical Procedures in Emergency Medicine. Philadelphia, Saunders, 1985, p. 7.)*

Therefore, unless the patient has regained consciousness, *an endotracheal tube must be placed prior to EOA removal.*

Contraindications to EOA placement include patients too small for the EOA to lie properly in the esophagus (height less than 5 feet or age less than 16 years), known esophageal disease (varices, esophageal cancer, or caustic ingestions), intact gag reflex, and any other intolerance of the device. Complications of EOA use include emesis, regurgitation, aspiration, tracheal intubation with the esophageal tube causing asphyxia or tracheal rupture, esophageal rupture, gastric rupture, esophageal mucosal damage if the tube is left in place longer than 2 hours, and death. Modifications of the EOA include the esophageal gastric tube airway (EGTA), the pharyngotracheal lumen airway (PTLA), and the esophageal tracheal combitube (ETC). All have benefits and drawbacks, and have not gained universal acceptance.

PROBLEM 1 The rescue squad performs a head-tilt–chin-lift maneuver but is still unable to ventilate the patient. The patient's mouth is opened, and some emesis and a large piece of steak is suctioned out. The steak was obstructing the oropharynx, and its removal allowed good mouth-to-mask ventilations with the head-tilt–chin-lift maneuver. An oral airway is inserted, and the patient is ventilated with a bag-valve-mask device with 100% oxygen. Breath sounds are symmetric, and the patient is transported to the emergency department with an estimated arrival time (ETA) of 5 minutes.

Most airway problems can be managed for the first few minutes with the temporizing techniques described above and listed in Table 2–2. However, the paramedic or emergency physician must provide more definitive stabilization of the airway.

PRINCIPLES OF DEFINITIVE AIRWAY MANAGEMENT

Definitive airway management techniques are listed in Table 2–2. They are divided into nonsurgical techniques, consisting of endotracheal intubation by either oral or nasal

TABLE 2–2. Temporizing Versus Definitive Airway Management Techniques

Temporizing Airway Management	Definitive Airway Management
Nonsurgical	**Nonsurgical**
Head-tilt–neck-lift maneuver	Orotracheal intubation with direct laryngoscopy
Chin-lift maneuver	Nasotracheal intubation (blind)
Jaw-thrust maneuver	Retrograde orotracheal intubation
Oropharyngeal airway	Fiberoptic bronchoscopic endotracheal intubation
Nasopharyngeal airway	Tactile orotracheal intubation
Esophageal obturator airway (EOA)	Lighted stylet endotracheal intubation
Esophageal gastric tube airway (EGTA)	**Surgical**
Pharyngotracheal lumen airway (PTLA)	Cricothyroidotomy
Esophageal tracheal combitube (ETC)	Tracheostomy
Surgical	
Percutaneous transcricothyroid or transtracheal catheter ventilation	

routes, and surgical techniques, which require placement of an endotracheal tube through the cricothyroid membrane or trachea.

Deciding which of these approaches to use can often be difficult and usually involves answering these questions (see Fig. 2–2):

1. *Is the patient breathing?*
   A nasotracheal tube cannot be placed without spontaneous respiration.
2. *How urgent is the patient's respiratory difficulty?*
   Orotracheal intubation is usually the fastest method.
3. *Is there a high possibility of a basilar skull fracture or central facial fracture?*
   Nasotracheal intubation is to be avoided in these conditions because of the risk of violating the cranial vault.
4. *What is the risk of cervical spine injury?*
   Although most patients at risk are still managed with orotracheal intubation and in-line immobilization of the head and cervical spine, the nasotracheal and surgical approaches are very appropriate alternatives.
5. *What is the operator's level of comfort with the procedure?*
   In emergent circumstances, the practitioner should always use the most familiar appropriate procedure.

General Preparation

The first step and key to success in endotracheal intubation is proper preparation. The following equipment is available in the proper sizes and should be checked for proper function at the beginning of each shift:

1. Adjunctive items
   a. Intravenous access
   b. Cardiac monitor-defibrillator
2. Procedure-specific items
   a. Oxygen source with bag-valve-mask setup
   b. Suction unit with dental suction tip
   c. Pharyngeal airways
   d. Laryngoscope and blades
   e. Endotracheal tubes and stylets
   f. Cricothyroidotomy tray
3. Intubation drugs
   a. Analgesics (opioids and lidocaine)
   b. Sedative hypnotics
   c. Neuromuscular blocking agents

This list of equipment is part of the optimal setup. Obviously, intubation of the apneic patient *must not be delayed* for these items. The patient is placed on a cardiac monitor, and an intravenous line is placed to anticipate dysrhythmias that may be associated with intubation. Skilled personnel should ventilate the patient with 100% oxygen by bag-valve-mask or OPBD for at least 30 seconds. This serves to increase the patient's PaO_2, allowing better tolerance of apnea during the intubation attempt. Dentures, if present, are removed just prior to the intubation attempt.

Orotracheal Approach

Orotracheal intubation is the most common procedure in definitive airway management. Its only absolute contraindication is a documented unstable cervical spine injury, as shown by cervical radiographs or clinical findings of acute spinal cord injury. Strong relative contraindications are suspected cervical spine injury or severe degenerative changes of the cervical spine, e.g., ankylosing spondylitis, rheumatoid arthritis. Other limiting situations include patients who need intubation but are not deeply comatose and bite or gag on the laryngoscope, and patients with trismus.

If the physician has prepared the airway and provided bag-valve-mask ventilation with 100% oxygen as described above, orotracheal intubation can be performed in a calm, orderly manner, as outlined in Table 2–3.

Step No. 9 in Table 2–3 is the most common source of error if the tube is "inserted" without complete visualization of the glottic opening. This is not the time for a "blind effort." Less time is lost by removing the laryngoscope, reventilating the patient, and

TABLE 2–3. Technique of Orotracheal Intubation

1. The two main types of blades are straight (e.g., Miller) and curved (e.g., MacIntosh). Most adults can be intubated using a size 3 blade, although some physicians prefer the guideline "the larger the better." Assemble the laryngoscope and blade, checking the light and making sure that the bulb is screwed in tightly and will not fall off during the intubation.
2. Select an endotracheal tube of the proper size. Average sizes are 8.0–8.5 mm for men and 7.0–8.0 mm for women.
3. Using a syringe, inflate the cuff on the tube until it is taut and palpate it to check for leaks. Then deflate it completely. The ventilator adaptor on the proximal end of the tube is twisted and pressed firmly onto the tube.
4. It is best to use a malleable wire stylet, placed so that the distal end of the stylet is 2–3 cm proximal to the tip of the endotracheal tube. The stylet adds rigidity and allows the tube to be curved to facilitate passage.
5. Unless there is a concern about cervical spine injury, the patient's head is extended on the neck, and the neck is slightly flexed in relation to the trunk. The "sniffing position" allows optimal visualization of the vocal cords.
6. Preferably, an assistant stands to the physician's right, holding suction and endotracheal tubes in one hand and using the other hand to depress the cricoid cartilage posteriorly, thereby occluding the esophagus to decrease the risk of regurgitation and aspiration and positioning the glottis for easier viewing during laryngoscopy.
7. The laryngoscope is held in the left hand and the patient's mouth is opened with the right hand by pushing the superior teeth rostrally with the index finger and the inferior teeth caudally with the thumb. The laryngoscope blade is inserted on the far right side of the patient's mouth, and the blade is used to sweep the tongue to the left, out of the field of view. Suction is used as necessary to clear the oropharynx.
8. The tip of the blade is advanced along the dorsal surface of the tongue, looking for the epiglottis. When a curved blade is used, the tip is positioned in the vallecula anterior to the epiglottis and lifted, thus lifting the epiglottis and exposing the glottic opening (Fig. 2–6A). The blade is not used as a lever, which can damage teeth. With a straight blade, the tip of the blade is placed posterior to the epiglottis and lifted to expose the vocal cords (Fig. 2–6B).
9. When the vocal cords are clearly seen, the endotracheal tube tip is passed through the vocal cords until the proximal end of the cuff is 2 cm beyond the cords. The laryngoscope and stylet are removed, and the balloon cuff is inflated with 5–10 ml of air.
10. In most adults, the tube will be properly positioned when the 22-cm mark is at the patient's teeth, yielding the TT–TT mnemonic (tip-to-teeth, twenty-two).
    a. The tube should be fixed to the upper lip with tape or tied with a ribbon, using tape or a ribbon that completely encircles the head. It should never be secured to the lower lip because the mobility of the mandible allows too much motion.
    b. Tube placement should be confirmed with a chest radiograph as soon as possible.

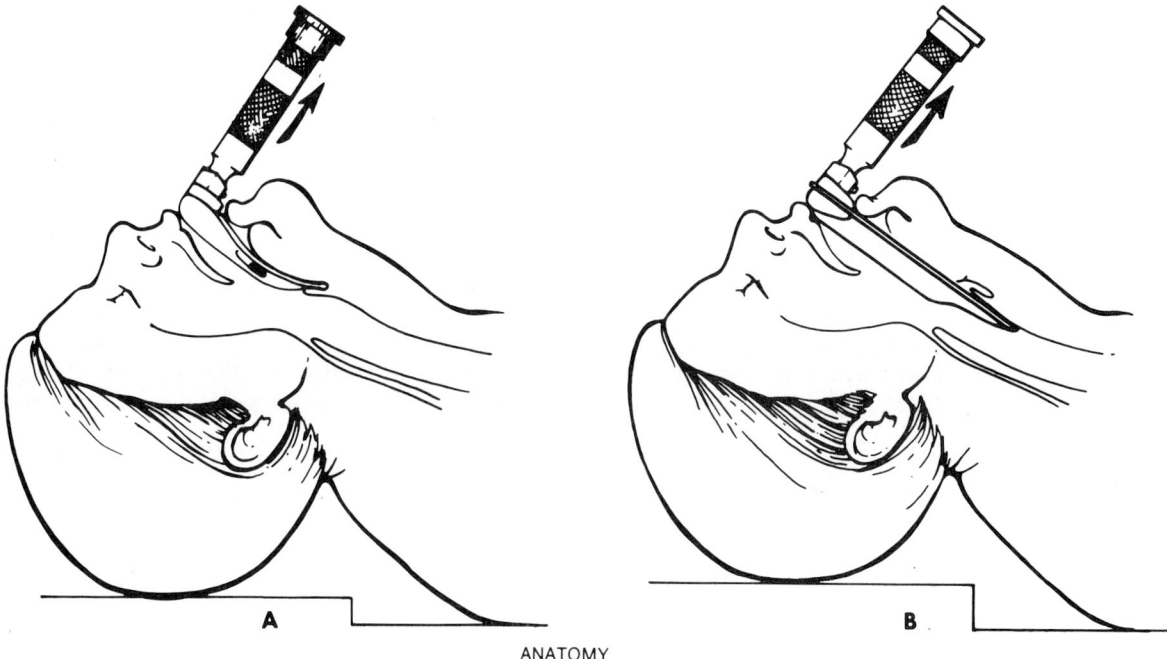

ANATOMY

FIGURE 2–6. Orotracheal intubation. (A) *Use of the curved laryngoscope blade.* (B) *Use of the straight laryngoscope blade.* (From Clinton JE, Ruiz E: Emergency airway management procedures. In Roberts JR, Hedges JR [eds]: Clinical Procedures in Emergency Medicine. Philadelphia, Saunders, 1985, p. 11.)

trying again. To roughly gauge the amount of time taken for intubation, the physician should take a deep breath and hold it while intubating. If the feeling of needing a breath occurs, assume the patient needs one too. The tube and laryngoscope are removed, the patient ventilated and reoxygenated, and another attempt is made.

PROBLEM 1 After being notified of the patient's 5-minute ETA in the emergency department, the emergency team assembles and checks the suction and intubation equipment. On arrival, a bag-valve-mask connected to 100% oxygen is used to continue ventilation during the primary survey. The patient's gag reflex is decreased, and breath sounds are equal. The patient has a palpable carotid pulse and decreased sensorium. The patient is intubated orotracheally.

This is a relatively straightforward intubation case. In this patient there are at least four of six reasons for airway management (lack of patency, protection, oxygenation, and ventilation), and definitive care is required. The most important factor driving this process is lack of protection with aspiration risk and an indeterminate time for patient recovery. With preparation and skill, orotracheal intubation can be rapid and atraumatic. Since there will be other patients to care for, make the decision and get it done.

Blind Nasotracheal Intubation

Blind nasotracheal intubation is the preferred method of airway management for patients who are breathing and need definitive airway management but have proven or potential cervical spine injuries or tightly clenched teeth.

Since air movement is required to guide the tube, it cannot be performed on apneic patients. It is not used in patients with fractures of the upper midface or anterior cranial fossa because the tube could pass through the fracture into the cranium. Other contraindications include cerebral spinal fluid rhinorrhea, choanal atresia, known bleeding diatheses or immunosuppressed states, upper airway foreign bodies, acute epiglottitis, parapharyngeal and retropharyngeal abscesses, and bilateral large nasal polyps. The nasotracheal approach requires a smaller endotracheal tube and may be suboptimal for patients who need large minute ventilation or who may be difficult to wean from a respirator after admission to the hospital. The steps for nasotracheal intubation are outlined in Table 2–4. The physician should be limited to two or three attempts before trying tube placement maneuvers. After five to six total attempts it is reasonable to consider other methods.

Potential complications include significant epistaxis with aspiration of blood, airway obstruction from blood clots or avulsed turbinates, and bacteremia from disruption of the nasal mucosa. After several days, obstruction of the paranasal sinus ostia can cause sinusitis with complications including meningitis and septicemia. Pharyngeal perforation with retropharyngeal dissection can occur, or a tube can be pushed through a skull

TABLE 2–4. Technique of Nasotracheal Intubation

1. As with oral intubation, proper preparation is crucial. There are important differences between oral and nasotracheal intubation.
    a. A stylet is not used in nasotracheal intubation.
    b. The endotracheal tube is 0.5–1.0 mm smaller in diameter.
    c. The tube may be tied into a loose knot and left for a minute to increase its curvature.
    d. Optimally, both nares are sprayed with a topical anesthetic and a vasoconstrictor such as cocaine or a mixture of phenylephrine and lidocaine.
    e. The outside of the tube is lubricated lightly with water-soluble lubricant.
    f. The most patent nostril is selected after inspection.
2. During the intubation attempt, an oxygen mask or other source of high-flow oxygen is held near the mouth.
3. Intubation is begun by rotating the tube so that the distal bevel is flat against the nasal septum. The tube is gently slid posteriorly along the inferomedial aspect of the nasal cavity. It is during this part of the procedure that massive epistaxis can be produced. Therefore, advance the tube slowly and gently past any resistance. If resistance is firm against slight pressure, pull out and try the other naris. When the tip of the tube passes the posterior choana into the oropharynx, the resistance will decrease.
4. After the tube passes the posterior choana, the physician should position his ear directly over the endotracheal tube adaptor so that air passing through the tube can be heard and felt. Breath sounds become louder as the tip of the tube approaches the glottic opening. Advance the tube to the loudest point.
5. When the patient inspires move the tube gently forward 2–4 cm. The glottis and vocal cords are open during inspiration, and the tube should advance without significant resistance. As the tube passes into the trachea, the patient will often cough, and a rush of air will come out of the tube. Other material may come out with it, so one must be aware which way the proximal end is directed.
6. If the tip of the endotracheal tube has not entered the trachea, it will usually be in one of four places: in the esophagus, just above the cords, in a piriform sinus, or in the vallecula. If the patient is not intubated successfully on the initial attempt, the physician should continue to supply oxygen, assess the location of the endotracheal tip, and take corrective measures.
    a. Esophagus: All air motion through the tube will cease. Withdraw the tube until loud breath sounds are heard. Apply more cricoid pressure to occlude the esophagus and displace the larynx posteriorly. If neck motion is not contraindicated, the neck can be extended. The tube is then readvanced.
    b. Rostral to the cords: Laryngospasm may be blocking passage of the tube. Position the tube just on the cords and maintain very gentle pressure until the patient takes a deep breath. If the patient's ventilation is compromised by the laryngospasm, the tube should be removed and the patient ventilated with bag-valve-mask. Intravenous and transcricothyroid lidocaine may be necessary if laryngospasm is severe.
    c. Piriform sinus: Location of the tube in the piriform sinus often causes a visible or palpable bulge superolateral to the thyroid cartilage. This condition can be corrected by slightly withdrawing and rotating the tube tip away from the bulge. If neck motion is not prohibited the patient's head can also be rotated toward the side of the bulge. The tube is readvanced.
    d. Vallecula: This location is rare. It causes a visible or palpable bulge superior to the hyoid bone. Gentle anterior traction is applied on the larynx. If neck motion is not contraindicated, the neck is flexed. The tube is advanced. If these measures fail, a tube with less curvature can be used.
7. After the tube enters the trachea, the cuff should be inflated and tube placement confirmed. Because of the increased risk of esophageal intubation in the blind technique, it is crucial to auscultate over the stomach to be sure that gurgles are not heard during ventilation.

PROBLEM 2 The patient, who had ingested a potentially lethal dose of amitriptyline, is placed on oxygen by nasal cannula. As a large-bore nasogastric tube for gastric lavage is being prepared, he rapidly becomes more somnolent, groaning only to painful stimuli. The gag reflex is weak, and the patient clenches his teeth when oral intubation is attempted.

Nasotracheal intubation is an essential skill for the emergency physician. It should be practiced selectively in patients with adequate respirations and a need for definite airway care. This case is a classic example of nasotracheal intubation being indicated.

Confirmation of Endotracheal Tube Placement

Unrecognized intubation of the esophagus is rapidly fatal. Intubation of a mainstem bronchus can cause pneumothorax, atelectasis of the unventilated lung, and hypoxia. Therefore, it is crucial to confirm correct endotracheal tube position by a variety of methods:

Auscultation. If the tube is below the vocal cords, the patient is unable to speak. Breath sounds are checked in the midaxillary line in both hemithoraces. If the tube has been inserted too far, it usually goes into the right mainstem bronchus, resulting in decreased breath sounds on the left. If the tube has been placed in the esophagus, "breath" sounds may still be heard over the chest, but ventilation results in loud gurgles heard at the epigastrium.

Observation. If the tube is in the trachea, condensation usually appears inside the tube with each exhalation. Bilateral symmetric chest wall movement is seen with ventilation.

Palpation. The resistance of the ventilation bag to compression is usually less if the tube is in the trachea. Any significant resistance represents a problem to be addressed. If the patient is breathing spontaneously, air is exhaled with each breath and can be detected when the hand or ear is placed over the endotracheal tube adapter. Using this method to guess the tidal volume as "adequate" is subject to significant error, and a standard measuring device is recommended.

Imaging. Soon after the endotracheal tube is in place, a chest radiograph is taken. The tip of the endotracheal tube should lie at the level of the aortic knob, 3 to 4 cm above the carina, with *no* aspect of the tube outside of the tracheal shadow.

Measurement. A more recent development is the end-tidal carbon dioxide detector. It can verify endotracheal placement and assist in monitoring the course of care.

PROBLEM 2 The physician attempts nasotracheal intubation but fails even with basic endotracheal tube and laryngeal maneuvers. The patient is sufficiently conscious to become agitated, struggle, and hold his breath whenever the tube approaches his epiglottis. When efforts to intubate him are interrupted, he becomes somnolent and slightly cyanotic.

This patient is a candidate for nasotracheal intubation, but attempts at intubation have not succeeded. One or two advanced techniques may assist in definitive management of this patient's airway.

Supplemental Techniques to Endotracheal Intubation

Magill Forceps

The Magill forceps is an instrument that facilitates nasotracheal intubation under direct laryngoscopy. The patient must have no contraindications to orotracheal intubation, and two people are necessary. Once the nasotracheal tube passes into the oropharynx, direct laryngoscopy is done to illuminate the tube and expose the tracheal opening. The Magill forceps is used to grasp the distal tube proximal to the balloon and insert it between the vocal cords under direct vision. The forceps and laryngoscope are removed, and tube placement is assessed in the standard manner.

Neuromuscular Blockade

Patients with no contraindications to orotracheal intubation who cannot be nasotracheally intubated due to combativeness, severe laryngospasm, or bradypnea may need orotracheal intubation assisted by paralyzing agents. Neuromuscular blocking drugs give the physician control of the patient and *complete responsibility* for the patient's airway *and* breathing. It is a procedure for the experienced physician only.

There are two general classes of neuromuscular blocking drugs. Succinylcholine is the only depolarizing, noncompetitive, neuromuscular blocking drug in clinical use for emergency orotracheal intubation. Intravenous succinylcholine induces complete paralysis in under 1 minute and usually lasts less than 10 minutes. There are three commonly used nondepolarizing, competitive, neuromuscular blocking drugs: pancuronium bromide, vecuronium bromide, and atracurium besylate. Because these three nondepolarizing drugs have a slower onset and a longer duration of action than succinylcholine, they are not used for emergent intubations.

Before considering the use of succinylcholine, a few criteria must be met. The patient must have an intact facial structure and mandible to allow bag-valve-mask ventilation. If the physician is unable to intubate the paralyzed patient, bag-valve-mask ventilation is a necessity. Other absolute contraindications to succinylcholine include known hypersensitivity to succinylcholine, major burns or crush injuries more than 5 to 7 days old (due to the increased risk of acute hyperkalemia), unstable cervical spine injuries, and a history of malignant hyperthermia. The presence of surgical airway management equipment such as a cricothyroidotomy kit or a transcricothyroid catheter ventilation device is part of the preparation for the use of neuromuscular blockers.

Once the materials are ready, succinylcholine is given slowly in a dose of 1.0 to 1.5 mg/kg intravenously. An assistant applies posterior pressure on the cricoid cartilage to occlude the esophagus (Sellick's maneuver). The abdominal muscle contractions that occur during succinylcholine induction can predispose the patient to regurgitation. After succinylcholine is given, the patient is ventilated until the masseter muscles relax. This occurs at about the same time as fluttering of the eyelids. The patient is orotracheally intubated at this time. Children are premedicated with intravenous atropine, 0.01 mg/kg (minimum dosage, 0.1 mg), to prevent bradycardia or asystole. Paralysis in an awake alert patient is terrifying. If the patient has a normal mental status, an intravenous sedative, e.g., diazepam, is given immediately prior to succinylcholine administration.

Complications of succinylcholine include aspiration, dysrhythmias, muscle aches, myoglobinuria, malignant hyperthermia, masseter spasm, increased intracranial pressure, increased intraocular pressure, and prolonged paralysis in patients with decreased pseudocholinesterase levels.

Other Drugs that Facilitate Intubation

Lidocaine, 1.5 mg/kg intravenously, given 1 to 3 minutes prior to intubation, helps to limit the increases in blood pressure, heart rate, and intracranial pressure that occur as a physiologic response to intubation. Lidocaine also decreases cardiac dysrhythmias associated with intubation. Preintubation lidocaine is used in patients with heart disease or intracranial disease and perhaps in most other patients as well unless a contraindication exists.

The benzodiazepines diazepam (Valium) and midazolam (Versed) are commonly used for sedation and amnesia during intubation, but further respiratory depression and hypotension are common complications of these agents. Opioids are often used to provide analgesia and reversible sedation in airway management. The selection and dosage of these drugs depend on the physician's experience and preference.

PROBLEM 2 The patient remains on high-flow oxygen by mask. A second physician is summoned to prepare for cricothyroidotomy if necessary. All the equipment for orotracheal intubation is readied. While cricoid pressure is applied, the patient is given succinylcholine 75 mg intravenously. The patient is ventilated until the masseters relax and respirations slow about 30 seconds later. Orotracheal intubation is successful. Cricoid pressure is maintained until the endotracheal tube balloon cuff is inflated, the endotracheal position of the tube is confirmed, and the tube is secured.

Some authorities believe that paralysis and oral intubation are safer than blind nasotracheal intubation. However, the experience of the individual physician with the two techniques is a crucial factor in selecting an approach. Unless the physician is expert in the use of the bag-valve-mask and oral intubation, succinylcholine can convert a breathing patient with a poor airway into an apneic patient with no airway.

Surgical Airway Management

Surgical airway management in the emergency department consists of percutaneous transcricothyroid (or transtracheal) catheter ventilation or cricothyroidotomy. Percutaneous transcricothyroid or transtracheal catheter ventilation is indicated when nonsurgical airway management procedures have failed or are contraindicated (Fig. 2–7). This procedure is a temporizing one. It does not protect the airway from aspiration, requires constant attention, and may lead to hypercapnia after 30 to 45 minutes. It is relatively contraindicated in patients with bleeding diatheses. Complications include pneumothorax, infection at the puncture site, massive soft tissue emphysema, puncture into the retrotracheal space, mediastinal emphysema, mediastinitis, esophageal perforation, bleeding, and air embolism.

Cricothyroidotomy is indicated for definitive airway control when all nonsurgical methods have failed or are contraindicated (Fig. 2–8). Cricothyroidotomy is relatively contraindicated in patients with bleeding diatheses, infectious laryngeal pathology, and laryngotracheal or cervical tracheal disruption. Only relative contraindications exist because it is usually the airway procedure of last resort. Immediate complications include bleeding, subcutaneous emphysema, esophageal laceration, laceration of the neurovascular structures in the carotid sheath, tube misplacement (anterior to the trachea), fracture or dislocation of the thyroid or cricoid cartilages, asphyxia, and death. Problems developing later include cellulitis, subglottic granulations, cuff site granulomas, and cuff site strictures. It is not done in children under 6 years old because of the small size of the cricothyroid membrane and a high incidence of complications.

Emergency tracheostomy is technically difficult and time-consuming and is best performed by a surgeon experienced in the procedure. Its only indication in the emergency department is a disrupted larynx or cervical trachea, in which an orotracheal tube cannot be passed across the injured segment.

PROBLEM 3 A 45 year old male with a gunshot wound of the mouth is initially placed on percutaneous ventilation through a 14-gauge catheter puncture of the cricothyroid membrane. The cricothyroidotomy kit is obtained, and the cricothyroid membrane is incised and then spread with a trousseau dilator. A cuffed tracheostomy tube is successfully placed.

This patient has apnea, near-obliteration of the upper airway, and a high probability of cervical spine injury. Oral and nasal intubation are precluded. The patient needs definitive airway management with an immediate cricothyroidotomy. Percutaneous transcricothyroid catheter venti-

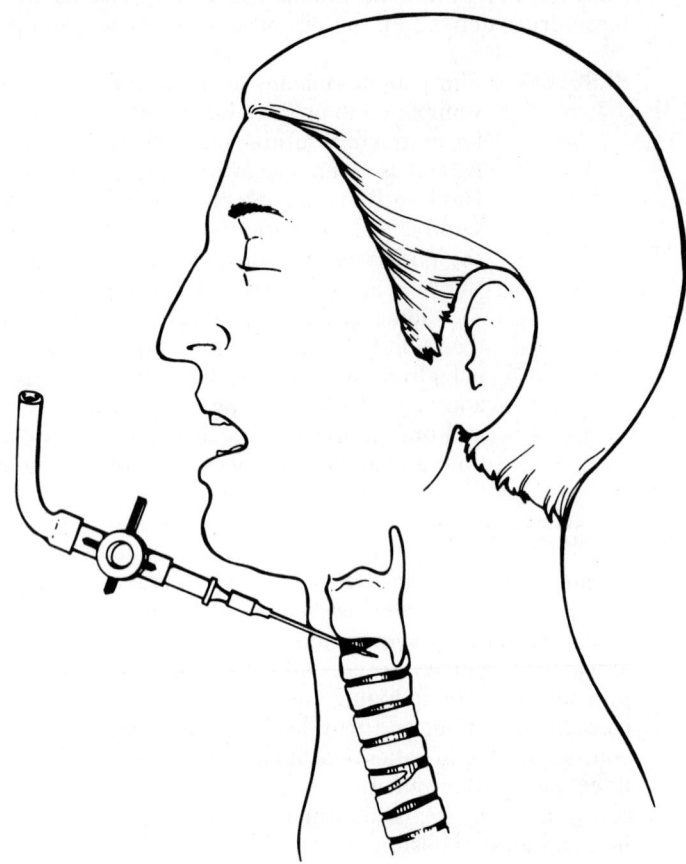

FIGURE 2–7. Percutaneous transcricothyroid catheter ventilation. (From Clinton JE, Ruiz E: Emergency airway management procedures. In Roberts JR, Hedges JR [eds]: Clinical Procedures in Emergency Medicine. Philadelphia, Saunders, 1985, p. 25.)

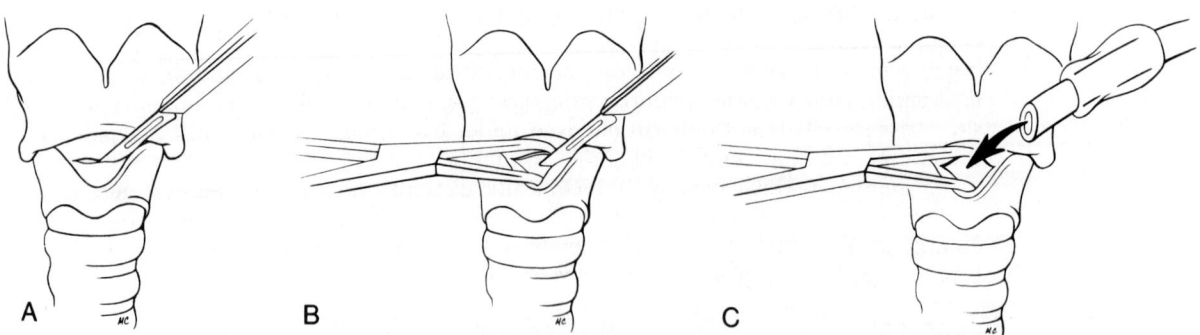

FIGURE 2–8. Cricothyroidotomy.

lation is a useful temporizing alternative, but it does not protect against aspiration and does not allow for potentially therapeutic hyperventilation.

DIFFERENTIAL DIAGNOSIS

Although an understanding of the pathophysiologic cause of respiratory distress is important in the management of the critically ill patient, initial assessment and stabilization do not depend on the differential diagnosis. Contemplating the cause of respiratory failure rather than intervening immediately can be a fatal error.

A differential diagnosis based on familiarity with the causes of upper airway obstruction, either partial or complete, is still very helpful in airway management. Altered anatomy and other findings during intubation may be anticipated from causes listed in Table 2-5.

Last, if definitive management of the upper airway does not result in clinical improvement, the physician must be able to review and explore rapidly the many other causes of respiratory failure (see Chap. 55):

1. Malfunction of central nervous system regulation of ventilation, e.g., central hypoventilation
2. Ventilation (bellows) inadequacy, altered thoracic cage structure, neuromuscular or muscular weakness
3. Loss of negative intrapleural pressure, e.g., pneumothorax
4. Inadequate airway, e.g., endotracheal tube failure or obstruction, large or small airway obstruction
5. Ventilation-perfusion mismatch, e.g., pneumonia, pulmonary embolism
6. Decreased lung compliance, e.g., adult respiratory distress syndrome
7. Decreased oxygen-carrying capacity of the blood, e.g., anemia, hemoglobin abnormality
8. Increased tissue extraction of oxygen, e.g., hypermetabolism, decreased perfusion

DIAGNOSTIC ADJUNCTS

In the emergency department most indications for airway management appear during the primary survey. The airway must be stabilized immediately, prior to determining arterial blood gas levels, taking radiographs, or performing other diagnostic adjuncts. These studies are often ordered after the fact and are an important part of the patient's respiratory management. Occasionally information obtained by these means is part of the decision process during which definitive management of a patient's airway in a "semi-

TABLE 2-5. Causes of Upper Airway Obstruction

Decreased level of consciousness	Foreign bodies
Inflammation	Trauma
Angioedema	Soft tissue edema
Cricoarytenoiditis	Hemorrhage
Inhalational injury due to closed	Fractures of the mandible and larynx
space burns or volatile toxins	Massive soft tissue emphysema
Caustic ingestions	Penetrating airway injuries
Infection	Tracheal and laryngotracheal disruption
Epiglottitis	Tumors
Croup	Benign
Bacterial tracheitis	Malignant
Diphtheria	Reflex
Ludwig's angina	Laryngospasm
Peritonsillar abscess	
Retropharyngeal abscess	

elective" manner is chosen. This situation most commonly occurs in patients with reversible airways disease (asthma) or chronic obstructive pulmonary disease (COPD). Guidelines for ordering these tests and using them to make airway management decisions are given in Chapters 55 and 56.

SPECIAL CONSIDERATIONS

Airway Management in Trauma Patients

Any blunt trauma victim is at risk for cervical spine injury. There is substantial controversy between advocates of oral intubation with cervical in-line immobilization and proponents of immediate cricothyroidotomy for the management of patients in whom blind nasotracheal intubation has failed or is contraindicated for other reasons, such as apnea or major facial trauma. Since any method of oral intubation involves some neck movement, the need for immediate airway management must be balanced against the risk of injuring the spinal cord. If oral intubation is selected, the head and neck are *immobilized* manually by an assistant. Axial *traction* should *not* be applied because traction may increase displacement of cervical fractures. Other alternatives for airway management in the blunt trauma victim include percutaneous transcricothyroid catheter ventilation, intubation using a fiberoptic bronchoscope, blind oral intubation guided by intraoral palpation, intubation over a lighted stylet placed through the mouth, or retrograde intubation over a wire placed through the cricothyroid membrane and threaded out the mouth.

Pediatric Airway Management

The pediatric airway is more prone to obstruction because it has a smaller caliber, its opening is surrounded by aggregates of lymphoid tissue, and a child has a relatively large tongue. Table 2–6 outlines the major differences between the adult and pediatric airways. Children tend to have bradycardia during intubation, so premedication with atropine

TABLE 2–6. Pediatric Versus Adult Airway Anatomy and Management

Category	Adult	Pediatric
Airway caliber	Larger	Smaller
Airway resistance	Lesser	Greater
Mucosa and submucosa	More adherent and less fragile	Looser and more fragile
Lymphoid tissue	Less prominent	Prominent
Hyoid bone	Far from larynx	Close to larynx
Epiglottis	More pliable, less prominent	Stiffer, more prominent, U-shaped
Pharyngolaryngeal angle	Less acute	More acute
Larynx	Relatively caudal and posterior	Relatively rostral and anterior
Laryngeal prominence	Apparent or palpable	More obscure
Cricothyroid membrane	Palpable	More obscure (not palpable in infants)
Narrowest portion of airway	Glottis	Subglottic (cricoid cartilage)
Lung cupola	Less rostral	More rostral
Blind finger sweeps to clear airway	OK if unconscious	Contraindicated because of high risk of foreign body and small orifice
Flexion at the cervicothoracic junction used in the sniffing position	Requires flat object under occiput	Naturally present in infants due to relatively large heads
Laryngoscope blade	Curved or straight	Straight in infants less than 2 years old; straight or curved in infants more than 2 years old
Endotracheal tube	Cuffed	Uncuffed if child is less than 8 to 12 years old
Cricothyroidotomy	Appropriate	Very difficult and relatively contraindicated

(0.01 mg/kg body weight, with a minimum dose of 0.1 mg) is recommended if an intravenous line has been established.

The appropriate size of endotracheal (ET) tube can be estimated by matching it to the size of the little finger or using the formula:

$$\text{ET tube diameter (millimeters)} = 4 + \frac{\text{age (years)}}{4}$$

Premature newborns need a 2.5- to 3.0-mm endotracheal tube; term newborns need a 3.0- to 3.5-mm endotracheal tube; and infants (less than 1 year) need a 3.5- to 4.0-mm endotracheal tube. There is great individual variability.

Laryngoscope blade types and sizes vary with age. A size 0 straight blade is used for premature newborns, and a size 1 straight blade is used with term newborns and infants through approximately 2 years of age. After age 2 a size 2 straight or curved blade may be used, and after age 12 a size 3 straight or curved blade is appropriate.

Blind nasotracheal intubation is not recommended in infants or children because of its low success rate due to the relatively anterosuperior position of the larynx and the sharp pharyngolaryngeal angle. There is also a greater risk of bleeding and avulsion of the large, friable adenoids and the loose fragile mucosa with nasotracheal intubation in infants and children.

Percutaneous transcricothyroid catheter ventilation is preferred in children because cricothyroidotomy is extremely difficult and carries an increased incidence of short- and long-term complications in pediatric patients.

DISPOSITION

Patients who require definitive airway management in the prehospital setting or the emergency department usually need admission to the intensive care unit. A possible exception is the patient who presents with decreased mental status due to alcohol or another short-acting CNS depressant, is intubated for gastric lavage, and awakens in the emergency department. If the emergency department is staffed to allow prolonged observation, such a patient may be extubated and then watched for at least 6 to 8 hours for deterioration of mental status or signs of airway complications such as laryngeal edema or aspiration. It is extremely rare to discharge a patient who has required active airway management. Any thoughts about this possibility are best shared and discussed with another physician.

All intubated patients must have their airway reassessed prior to transfer out of the emergency department. Because endotracheal tubes frequently move during transport, tube position must be confirmed before and after moving the patient.

DOCUMENTATION

The medical record of a critically ill patient should describe airway patency, airway protection, and quality of spontaneous ventilation. For patients requiring airway intervention, a procedure note should mention the following items:
1. Indications and contraindications
2. Equipment: ET tube size
3. Technique used
4. Complications or lack thereof
5. Medications used
6. Laboratory results, e.g., arterial blood gas measurements

For patients undergoing intubation and cricothyroidotomy, the medical record should show that the tube was placed appropriately, symmetric breath sounds were documented, the tube secured at an appropriate distance from the tip, and the chest radiograph interpreted as showing proper tube placement.

SUMMARY

- Patients at highest risk for airway compromise are those with a decreased level of consciousness, cardiorespiratory disease, head and neck pathology, and major traumatic injury.
- Airway and breathing are assessed in the primary survey through combined inspection, palpation, and auscultation. Listening to the patient speak and testing the gag reflex are essential elements in this assessment.
- Indications for airway management include loss of patency, loss of protection, oxygenation, ventilation, difficulty in handling secretions, and endotracheal drug dosing.
- Major decisions in airway management are based on the answers to these questions: Is the patient breathing? How urgent is the situation? What is the stability of the cervical spine? Is the facial bony structure intact? What is the experience and comfort of the physician with the procedure being considered?
- The key to endotracheal intubation is proper preparation, including preoxygenation of the patient.
- Endotracheal tube placement must be assessed by inspection, palpation, and auscultation.
- Neuromuscular blockers have an important role in definitive airway management. They are to be used with caution by trained and experienced physicians only.
- Surgical airway management can be lifesaving in circumstances of severe laryngospasm, cervical spine injury, laryngotracheal injury, or massive facial trauma.

BIBLIOGRAPHY

Texts

1. Adjuncts for airway control, ventilation, and supplemental oxygen. In American Heart Association: Textbook of Advanced Cardiac Life Support (3rd ed). Dallas, American Heart Association, 1987, pp. 27–39.
2. Campbell WH (ed): Airway Management and Anesthesia in the Emergency Department. Emerg Med Clin North Am 6(4):1988.
3. Clinton JE, Ruiz E: Emergency airway management procedures. In Roberts JR, Hedges JR (eds): Clinical Procedures in Emergency Medicine. Philadelphia, W.B. Saunders, 1985, pp. 2–29.
4. Danzl DF: Principles of airway management. In Callaham ML (ed): Current Therapy in Emergency Medicine. Toronto, B.C. Decker, 1987, pp. 1–38.

Journal Articles

1. Birmingham PK, Cheney FW, Ward RJ: Esophageal intubation: A review of detection techniques. Anesth Analg 65:886–891, 1986.
2. Bivins HG, Ford S, Bezmalinovic Z, et al: The effect of axial traction during orotracheal intubation of the trauma victim with an unstable cervical spine. Ann Emerg Med 17:25–29, 1988.
3. Blanc VF, Tremblay NAG: The complications of tracheal intubation: A new classification with a review of the literature. Anesth Analg 53:202–213, 1974.
4. Dronen SC, Merigian KS, Hedges JR, et al: A comparison of blind nasotracheal and succinylcholine-assisted intubation in the poisoned patient. Ann Emerg Med 16:650–652, 1987.
5. Flancbaum L, Wright J, Trooskin SZ, et al: Orotracheal intubation in suspected laryngeal injuries. Am J Emerg Med 4:167–169, 1986.
6. Gaddis GM, Sheets CA, Gaddis ML, et al: Endotracheal midazolam pharmacokinetics in dogs (abstract). Ann Emerg Med 17:879, 1988.
7. Hamill JF, Bedford RF, Weaver DC, et al: Lidocaine before endotracheal intubation: Intravenous or laryngotracheal? Anesthesiology 55:578–581, 1981.
8. Hammargren Y, Clinton JE, Ruiz E: A standard comparison of esophageal obturator airway and endotracheal tube ventilation in cardiac arrest. Ann Emerg Med 14:953–958, 1985.
9. McGill J, Clinton JE, Ruiz E: Cricothyrotomy in the emergency department. Ann Emerg Med 11:361–364, 1982.
10. Roberts DJ, Clinton JE, Ruiz E: Neuromuscular blockade for critical patients in the emergency department. Ann Emerg Med 15:152–156, 1986.
11. Steward RD, Paris PM: Signs of endotracheal intubation in a field setting. Ann Emerg Med 14:276–277, 1985.
12. 1985 National Conference on Standards and Guidelines for Cardiopulmonary Resuscitation and Emergency Cardiac Care: Standards and guidelines for cardiopulmonary resuscitation (CPR) and emergency cardiac care (ECC). JAMA 255:2905–2989, 1986.

CHAPTER 3

CARDIOPULMONARY CEREBRAL RESUSCITATION

MARK G. ANGELOS, M.D.
TIMOTHY G. JANZ, M.D.

PROBLEM 1 A 60 year old male with a past history of angina developed severe substernal chest pain associated with dyspnea and diaphoresis. He asked his wife to call the rescue squad. When the paramedics arrived 10 minutes later he was unresponsive, pulseless, and apneic.

PROBLEM 2 A 48 year old male collapsed in a physician's office. He was apneic and pulseless. Cardiopulmonary resuscitation (CPR) and bag ventilation were started. The paramedics arrived a few minutes later.

QUESTIONS TO CONSIDER

1. What information is exchanged when an emergency medical service (EMS) radio report of a cardiac arrest victim is called to the emergency department?
2. How is the emergency department prepared for the arrival of a patient in cardiac arrest?
3. What items in the history are critical for initial management?
4. What elements of the physical examination must be repeatedly assessed?
5. What are the treatable causes of cardiac arrest?
6. What laboratory studies are necessary to facilitate care?
7. How are the following cardiac dysrhythmias managed: asystole, electromechanical dissociation (EMD), ventricular fibrillation, ventricular tachycardia, and bradycardia?
8. What myocardial and cerebral resuscitation techniques are clinically useful to prevent complications in the postresuscitation period?

INTRODUCTION

The emergency physician must be prepared to treat cardiac arrest in an organized manner. Well accepted principles have been established through the Basic and Advanced Cardiac Life Support (BLS and ACLS) programs developed by the American Heart Association. Their goal is to save hearts and minds "too good to die."

Cardiopulmonary arrest is the preterminal event in over 600,000 "out-of-hospital" deaths in the United States. Although cardiopulmonary cerebral resuscitation (CPCR) of all cardiac arrest patients is not possible or ethical, there are many patients who may return to a normal life if they are treated quickly and correctly. Most cardiac arrest patients seen in the emergency department are victims of "sudden cardiac death." This is usually an ischemia- or dysrhythmia-based event that occurs with little or no prodrome. Prior to the widespread use of external CPR and the development of emergency medical services, such an event frequently resulted in death. Currently, 15% to 30% of all sudden cardiac death patients are resuscitated in the field or the emergency department. Approximately 15% of these patients are discharged from the hospital functionally intact. Following initial resuscitation, central nervous system impairment remains the greatest cause of morbidity and mortality. The most important factor determining the chance of survival to discharge is the time that elapses from cardiac arrest until restoration of adequate perfusion. Basic CPR started within 4 minutes can result in a survival rate of up to 43% as opposed to a 6% survival rate if it is delayed to 8 minutes. Early advanced cardiac life support, particularly the ability to defibrillate, has a similar influence on outcome.

The many pathophysiologic causes of cardiac arrest can be divided into three general categories. Each should be considered while CPCR is being initiated:
1. Electrical or conduction failure
    a. Primary dysrhythmia
    b. Electrocution
2. Decrease in myocardial oxygen delivery
    a. Decreased flow, e.g., coronary artery thrombosis, cardiac tamponade, tension pneumothorax, pulmonary embolus
    b. Decreased oxygen content, e.g., low hemoglobin, hypoxemia, drowning, asphyxia, airway obstruction
3. Myocardial toxicity
    a. Electrolyte abnormalities, e.g., hyperkalemia or hypokalemia, hypocalcemia
    b. Drug-induced, e.g., tricyclic antidepressant, propranolol, digitalis

The most common dysrhythmia presenting as prehospital cardiac arrest is ventricular fibrillation. It occurs in two-thirds of the cases, followed in frequency by bradyasystole, electromechanical dissociation, and ventricular tachycardia. Ventricular tachycardia has the best prognosis (Table 3–1).

Neurologic sequelae in cardiac arrest survivors also correlate with the length of arrest. Recovery of good neurologic function becomes increasingly less likely with longer arrest time (more than 6 minutes) and CPR time (more than 30 minutes).

A major problem in treatment is the marginal cerebral and coronary blood flow provided by standard external CPR techniques. It averages 15 to 20% of normal cardiac output. Even under optimal conditions, cardiac output and cerebral blood flow are usually less than 30% of normal. With prolonged CPR, this flow may decrease to near zero.

PREHOSPITAL CARE

Since the opportunity for successful resuscitation is time dependent, intervening at the scene may be lifesaving. The extent of therapy depends on the training level of responders. Defibrillation, endotracheal airway management, intravenous access, and use of cardiac drugs are part of the paramedic (EMT-P) on-scene capability. When ventricular fibrillation is discovered, early defibrillation by prehospital care responders at the scene is the most important priority. Emergency medical technicians having the ability to defibrillate (EMT-D) and nonparamedic personnel using automatic defibrillators may allow the widespread use of early defibrillation. In field trials, automatic external defibrillators have been as effective as standard defibrillators.

Beyond the initial therapy, field care is limited by the need for rapid transport to

TABLE 3–1. Prognosis of Presenting Cardiac Arrest Rhythms

Rhythm	Survival to Hospital Discharge
Ventricular tachycardia	66–76%
Ventricular fibrillation	10–25%
Asystole and EMD	0–2%

the hospital. The emergency physician should expect the following information to be given during the initial radio contact:
1. Status of the airway—intubated or not
2. Vital signs including presence of pulse or blood pressure
3. Cardiac rhythm—from cardiac monitor or "quick look" paddles
4. Therapy given and response to therapy
5. Other significant findings: skin color, pupillary size and reflexes, mental or motor status
6. Briefly, events preceding arrest that may give a clue to the etiology
7. Estimated time since arrest—"down time"
8. Estimated time of arrival

Treatment orders are given depending on this information. Prehospital personnel are encouraged to follow BLS or ACLS protocols for cardiac arrest while rapidly transporting the patient to the emergency department. The emergency department staff is notified of the anticipated arrival.

PROBLEM 1 Basic life support was initiated, and a "quick look" with the monitor paddles showed ventricular fibrillation. Three successive countershocks with 200, 300, and 360 joules failed to defibrillate the heart. The patient was orotracheally intubated. Bag ventilation with oxygen and chest compressions were continued. Repeated attempts to establish an intravenous line were unsuccessful. Radio contact was made with the base hospital. The paramedics were instructed to give 1 mg of 1:10,000 epinephrine (10 ml) through the endotracheal tube, continue CPR, and transport the patient to the hospital as rapidly as possible.

Once ventricular fibrillation is noted, immediate defibrillation becomes the top priority. As was done in this case, three successive shocks with increasing joules is recommended. Endotracheal drug administration is relatively unique to emergency medical care. Absorption of selected drugs is rapid, without pulmonary sequelae. In the right circumstances, use of this route may be lifesaving. Other drugs that may be administered by this route are naloxone, atropine, lidocaine, and isoproterenol.

PROBLEM 2 The paramedics noted narrow regular QRS complexes at a rate of 120 per minute. The patient was intubated and ventilated with oxygen, and an intravenous line was started en route to the hospital.

The paramedics correctly noted a sinus tachycardia rhythm on the monitor in the absence of palpable pulses. This constitutes electromechanical dissociation.

INITIAL APPROACH IN THE EMERGENCY DEPARTMENT

The cardiac arrest patient within the emergency department is initially managed as a team approach. The team may include physicians, nurses, electrocardiography (ECG) and radiology technicians, and respiratory therapy personnel. Members of the team and supplies are mobilized to provide immediate and continued ACLS therapy upon the patient's arrival.

Preparation

Once notified of an incoming cardiac arrest patient, the staff prepares immediately. Equipment and supplies for (1) airway management, (2) defibrillation, (3) cardiac drugs, and (4) intravenous access are readied in the resuscitation area.

Airway. Airway management equipment is made available at the bedside. Oxygen tubing is attached to the oxygen wall outlet on one end, and the Ambu bag is attached on the other end. The endotracheal tube is prepared, the balloon tested, a stylet placed in the tube, and the laryngoscope checked. The Ambu bag and mask are placed at the head of the bed with high-flow oxygen turned on. Suction equipment is turned on and the dental suction tip placed at the head of the bed.

Defibrillation. The defibrillator is turned on at the bedside; contact pads or paste is made readily available. Cardiac monitoring with the defibrillator display monitor allows rapid selection of defibrillation, cardioversion, or external pacing. Special large pads (8 to 10 cm) are applied on the anterior and posterior thorax if external pacing is necessary.

Cardiac Drugs. Selected emergency and cardiac drugs are placed at the bedside. Drug dosing including concentrations for mixing continuous intravenous infusions must be memorized or readily available.

Intravenous Access. Peripheral and central intravenous lines and materials are prepared. Optimally, during cardiac arrest, drugs are given centrally. Animal studies have demonstrated that drugs make a more rapid central appearance and reach higher peak levels when they are administered through a central line compared to a peripheral line. This advantage is tempered by the time delay and difficulties often encountered in obtaining central access.

A "code" or "crash" cart containing most drugs and supplies is brought to the bedside (Table 3–2). In addition to airway equipment and emergency drugs, this cart contains intravenous catheters and supplies, needles, syringes, blood gas kits, pericardiocentesis needles, and ECG and transcutaneous pacer pads.

TABLE 3–2. Standard Elements in Crash Cart Airway Equipment at Bedside

Endotracheal tubes—multiple sizes from 6.0 to 9.0 mm internal diameter	
Laryngoscope with curved and straight blades	
Stylet	
Oxygen—high-flow	
Ambu bag and mask	
Suction with dental tip	
Lubricating gel	
Tape for securing tube	
Lidocaine (both topical and parenteral)	
Oral and nasal airways	
Needle cricothyrotomy set-up	
Cricothyrotomy set-up	
Emergency Drugs (standard packaging)	
Epinephrine	1 mg/10 ml (1:10,000 sol)
Sodium bicarbonate	(50 mEq/50 ml)
Atropine	1 mg/10 ml
Isoproterenol	1 mg/5 ml
Lidocaine	20–40 mg/ml
Procainamide	100 mg/ml
Bretylium	600 mg/10 ml
Dopamine	200 mg/5 ml
Dobutamine	250 mg/vial
Naloxone	0.4 mg/ml
Phenytoin	50 mg/ml (2 and 5 ml)
Diazepam	10 mg/2 ml
Succinylcholine	200 mg/10 ml
Morphine sulfate	10 mg/ml
Calcium chloride	1 gm/10 ml
Magnesium sulfate	1 gm/2 ml (50% sol)
Furosemide	10 mg/ml
Aminophylline	250 mg/10 ml
Verapamil	5 mg/2 ml
Nitroprusside	50 mg/vial
Nitroglycerin	Multiple concentrations, 50 mg/10 ml
50% dextrose in water	25 mg/50 ml

Radiology, ECG, and respiratory therapy personnel are notified. In a trauma-related cardiac arrest, the surgery department and the blood bank are also notified. Individual assignments are made before the patient's arrival, i.e., airway management, chest compression. One physician is designated as the team leader to direct, monitor, and oversee therapy.

On Arrival

First, the cardiac rhythm is determined from the cardiac monitor or the "quick-look" option through the defibrillator paddles. If the patient's rhythm is ventricular fibrillation or ventricular tachycardia without a palpable carotid or femoral pulse, immediate defibrillation is performed. If the patient is pulseless, external cardiac massage is begun. If a spontaneous pulse is palpable, a blood pressure measurement is obtained. The pulse is continuously checked, and chest compressions are reinstituted if a spontaneous pulse is lost. A spontaneously pumping heart generating a palpable pulse supplies better perfusion than external CPR.

If the patient is not intubated, the oropharynx is suctioned of debris, the airway is opened using a jaw-thrust maneuver, and the lungs are ventilated with 100% oxygen by bag-mask or mouth-to-mask techniques. The effectiveness of the ventilatory effort is checked by noting the anterior chest wall rise and listening for symmetric breath sounds.

The patient is orotracheally intubated if initial defibrillation attempts fail or if the patient has an unprotected airway. If an esophageal obturator airway (EOA) or esophageal gastric tracheal airway (EGTA) is in place, the esophageal balloon is left inflated while the endotracheal tube (ET) is inserted in the trachea. The EOA or EGTA is removed only after successful endotracheal intubation.

If the patient was intubated in the field, location of the endotracheal tube must be confirmed. The endotracheal tube can dislodge into the esophagus or right mainstem bronchus during transport. To confirm, breath sounds are auscultated over both lung fields and the stomach. The chest wall is observed for symmetric expansion during ventilation. If proper endotracheal tube placement is in question, the vocal cords are visualized with the laryngoscope. Adequacy of the airway and ventilation is assessed serially throughout the resuscitation. The physician should be familiar with the known pitfalls of field resuscitation, e.g., right mainstem bronchial intubation, esophageal intubation, and rib fractures. Checking for these complications is an important part of the initial assessment after ACLS has been initiated in the field.

PROBLEM 1 The squad arrived in the emergency department 6 minutes after their last radio contact. The patient was noted to have symmetric chest expansion and bilateral breath sounds during ventilation. No palpable carotid or femoral pulse was noted. Chest compressions were continued. The cardiac monitor showed ventricular fibrillation. The patient was successfully defibrillated after two 360-joule countershocks. The postdefibrillation rhythm was complete third-degree heart block at a rate of 40 beats/minute. The systolic blood pressure was 70 mm Hg. An IV line was established.

In both the emergency department and the prehospital setting, defibrillation is *not delayed* until after intravenous access is established. Placement of the endotracheal tube was correctly done. A well-functioning resuscitation team will accomplish all of the early essential elements almost simultaneously.

DATA GATHERING

Once the airway, pulse, blood pressure, and cardiac rhythm are addressed, a brief history is taken, and a physical examination is completed.

History

The initial source of the history is usually the rescue personnel. The following questions are asked:

1. What were the *events surrounding* the *cardiac arrest?*
2. What was the *estimated time since* the *arrest* and initiating *CPR?*
3. What was the *estimated duration* of *CPR?*
4. What was the *initial rhythm?*
5. What *airway intervention* was performed?
6. Was *defibrillation* performed? If so, how many times, and at what energy level?
7. What *drug therapy* was given?
8. Was *restoration* of *blood pressure* or *pulse* achieved? Even temporarily?
9. What has been the *mental status* of the patient *throughout* the resuscitation?
10. What is the *past medical history* including medical problems, medications, and allergies?

Answers to these questions will assist in determining any reversible etiologies and the need for additional therapy.

The physician is notified when the family arrives. Family members need to have their fears addressed, and they can supply valuable information concerning the patient's past problems and the events preceding the cardiac arrest. If it is not possible for the senior physician to leave the bedside, another physician should talk briefly with the family. During this first contact it is necessary to communicate the critical nature of the patient's problem and establish the basis for the next visit after the resuscitative effort.

PROBLEM 2 On arrival in the emergency department, the rescue squad provided the following history obtained at the physician's office: The patient went to his primary physician with complaints of intermittent indigestion and episodes of dizziness when standing upright. The rescue squad was called when the patient got up from the doctor's examining table and collapsed. The physician initiated BLS protocols immediately.

The history suggests hypovolemia as a possible reason for the patient's cardiac arrest and EMD. This is potentially reversible with rapid appropriate treatment. Obviously, there are a number of other potential causes. It is important to first consider the "reversible" causes in the cardiac arrest patient.

Physical Examination

Once CPR is begun, the physical examination is brief and has two objectives. The first is to determine the cause of the cardiac arrest. A close look at the patient may provide additional clues to the patient's prearrest medical problems. For example, the presence of an arteriovenous fistula may suggest renal failure with complicating hyperkalemia. The second objective is to assess the effectiveness of cardiac arrest therapy and possible complications. Table 3–3 outlines the directed physical examination during cardiac arrest. This examination is repeated every 5 to 10 minutes throughout the resuscitation effort, or as indicated by a change in patient status or a new intervention.

PROBLEM 1 Paramedics related that the 60 year old patient had a prior history of myocardial infarction. His medications included furosemide, digoxin, potassium replacement, and nitroglycerin. Reassessment of the patient's physical condition revealed absent breath sounds on the left side with asymmetric chest expansion. The ET tube was pulled back 2 to 3 cm, and equal breath sounds were heard.

Right mainstem bronchus intubation is the most common cause of asymmetric breath sounds during cardiac arrest. It can easily evolve during

TABLE 3–3. Directed Physical Examination During Cardiac Arrest

Physical Examination	Abnormalities	Possible Diagnoses/Comments
General appearance	Pallor, evidence of trauma or blood loss, emaciation or tumor masses	Hypovolemic arrest; possible cancer patient
Airway	Secretions, vomitus or blood, stridor, resistance to ventilation	Airway obstruction leading to respiratory arrest or hypoxia, tension pneumothorax
Neck	Distended neck veins, deviated trachea	Cardiac tamponade, tension pneumothorax
Lungs	Unilateral breath sounds, rales, bronchi, wheezing	Pneumothorax, main stem intubation, significant bronchospasm, aspiration, pulmonary edema
Heart	Muffled or absent heart tones, irregular rhythm	No functional cardiac output, cardiac tamponade, COPD, dysrhythmias
Abdomen	Distention, tympanitic or dull on percussion, palpable or pulsating mass; include rectal examination on first assessment	Stomach inflated with air, ruptured viscus, ruptured or pulsating aortic aneurysm; gross blood sought
Extremities	Asymmetric pulses	Arterial occlusion, aortic dissection, very low perfusion state
Neurologic signs	Dilated pupils, no pupillary light response	Cerebral hypoxia

the resuscitation effort despite the endotracheal tube being "secured." The history and use of medications support a cardiac origin for this arrest.

DEVELOPMENT OF THE PRELIMINARY DIFFERENTIAL DIAGNOSIS

Two questions need to be addressed in any cardiopulmonary arrest situation:

1. What is the immediate rhythm disturbance associated with the cardiopulmonary arrest?

Establishing the rhythm disturbance is critical for administering appropriate care. Although basic life support is instituted in all arrests, definitive treatment differs according to the rhythm disturbance present. An excellent example is the classic "sine wave" ECG pattern associated with significant hyperkalemia. This pattern requires specific treatment (calcium) that would usually not be given if the rhythm were not recognized. Knowledge of the rhythm may also be helpful in determining the origin of the arrest. For instance, electromechanical dissociation has different causes than bradydysrhythmias.

2. What is the most likely underlying cause of the cardiopulmonary arrest?

Of the estimated 1000 cardiac arrests that occur per day in the United States, approximately half (48%) are cardiac in origin. Underlying ischemic heart disease accounts for two-thirds of these arrests. Another major cause of cardiopulmonary arrest is hypoxia, which results in dysrhythmias, myocardial ischemia, and eventual infarction. Hypoxia may be the result of alveolar hypoventilation, upper airway obstruction, or any severe parenchymal lung disease. Lethal dysrhythmias are also associated with severe acid-base disorders, electrolyte abnormalities, and drugs or toxins (Table 3–4).

PROBLEM 1 Applying the above questions to this case shows that ventricular fibrillation was the immediate rhythm disturbance responsible for the arrest state. From the limited history available, the immediate cause of the arrest was probably a cardiac disturbance secondary to ischemic heart disease; however, noncardiac etiologies should remain in the differential diagnosis.

The use of quick-look paddle electrodes allowed the paramedics to identify the presence of ventricular fibrillation rapidly and institute treatment immediately. The history, physical examination, and ECG rhythm

TABLE 3–4. Common Causes of Cardiopulmonary Arrest

Immediate Cause	Associated Disease	Comments
Cardiac etiology	Ischemic heart disease, cardiomyopathies, hypertensive heart disease, valvular heart disease, intrinsic rhythm disturbances, circulatory shock or hypovolemia	Two-thirds of cardiopulmonary arrests from primary cardiac disorders are due to ischemic heart disease; acute myocardial infarction accounts for only 25% of cardiac-related arrests; 20% of ischemic heart disease patients will have cardiac arrest as their initial presentation; circulatory shock and hypovolemia are always included in the differential diagnosis of EMD (see Table 3–6)
Respiratory etiology		
1. Alveolar hypoventilation	CNS disease, head trauma, neuromuscular disease (e.g., Guillain Barré syndrome, myasthenia gravis), drugs (narcotics, sedatives), metabolic encephalopathies (e.g., hepatic, uremic)	Any pulmonary disease is capable of causing a cardiopulmonary arrest; however, the common denominator is severe hypoxemia
2. Upper airway obstruction (UAO)	Foreign body, infection, trauma, neoplasm	The most common causes of upper airway obstruction in adults are foreign body aspiration and neoplasms; in children, foreign body aspiration and infection (epiglottitis/croup) are the most common causes
3. Lung disease	Asthma, COPD, pneumonia, pulmonary edema, pulmonary embolus, others	Primary lung disease, COPD, and pneumonia are the most common causes of pulmonary origin cardiac arrest
Electrolyte abnormalities	Hypokalemia, hyperkalemia, hypomagnesemia, hypocalcemia	Ventricular dysrhythmias are the most frequent rhythm disturbances associated with electrolyte abnormalities; renal failure is often associated with hyperkalemia or hypocalcemia and is prone to ventricular dysrhythmias
Drugs and toxins	Digitalis, antiarrhythmics (such as quinidine, procainamide, encainide, flecainide); tricyclic antidepressants, cocaine, carbon monoxide	The most common drugs associated with lethal dysrhythmias are cardiovascular agents. Especially common are digitalis toxicity and quinidine. Currently, cocaine is the drug most commonly associated with life-threatening rhythm disorders
Other	Lightning or electrical injuries, drowning or near-drowning, autonomic dysfunction, hypothermia	These are unusual causes of cardiopulmonary arrest. The clinical setting often suggests their involvement

monitoring are the most useful evaluative tools during cardiopulmonary arrest.

PROBLEM 2 The immediate rhythm disturbance in this 48 year old patient appeared to be sinus tachycardia; however, the patient had no palpable pulse. Therefore, EMD was the dysrhythmia associated with the arrest. Although EMD is often the result of irreversible cardiac damage, reversible causes should always be considered. The differential diagnosis includes problems that may cause the arrest or result from the resuscitation, i.e., hypoxemia, acidosis, volume depletion, cardiac tamponade, or tension pneumothorax.

DIAGNOSTIC ADJUNCTS

Electrocardiogram and Cardiac Monitoring

The ECG and cardiac monitoring are the most useful tests performed in cardiac arrest patients. Continuous electrocardiographic monitoring is maintained during the resuscitation. Lead II or a modified V_1 lead is usually used to identify the underlying rhythm disturbance. A 12-lead ECG is mandatory after all successful resuscitations.

Acute myocardial infarction occurs in an estimated 20% of patients with cardiac arrest and may manifest as ST-segment elevation, inverted T waves, or Q waves. The ECG can be useful in patients with noncardiac causes of cardiac arrest as well. For example, prominent U waves are often associated with hypokalemia, and large peaked T waves, prolonged P–R and QRS complexes, loss of P waves, and a sine wave configuration of the QRS complex are associated with significant hyperkalemia. Findings compatible with hyperkalemia should suggest a presumptive diagnosis of renal failure.

At times ventricular fibrillation can present in some leads with small undulations or may even masquerade as asystole. In apparent asystole, more than one lead is interpreted to exclude the presence of fine ventricular fibrillation.

Laboratory Studies

Arterial Blood Gases. Arterial blood gas (ABG) measurements are obtained as quickly as possible in an arrest situation and are used to monitor the patient's oxygenation and acid-base status. Although arterial blood gases are preferred, venous blood gases obtained during external cardiac compression can also be useful as a rough approximation of acid-base balance but not oxygenation. Recent research has questioned the role of arterial pH determination because it does not seem to predict the degree of tissue acidosis or the success of resuscitation efforts. In addition, arterial P_{CO_2} may not be a good representation of tissue or cellular carbon dioxide levels. Central venous or mixed venous blood samples may correlate better with tissue pH and carbon dioxide levels and may be better predictors of the resuscitation outcome. At present, ABGs continue to be part of the serial monitoring of resuscitation efforts during a cardiac arrest situation.

Serum Electrolytes. The serum potassium level is valuable to measure early in the arrest. Although it is usually determined from serum, it can be measured from plasma. Plasma levels do not require clot formation, and if the determination is prearranged with the laboratory, the turnaround time is less than 5 minutes. A plasma potassium level requires a heparinized blood sample. It is 0.35 to 0.5 mEq/liter lower than a serum potassium level and is more accurate. Plasma potassium is not affected by potassium release during platelet activation and clot formation and is most useful in the setting of severe thrombocytosis. A serum potassium level can also be determined from arterial blood samples; however, it may be as much as 1.1 mEq/liter lower than that from a venous sample. The presence of hyperkalemia and presumptive renal failure warrants specific therapy and determining serum creatinine and blood urea nitrogen (BUN) levels.

Toxicology Studies and Drug Levels. If the situation dictates, toxicology studies or serum concentrations of therapeutic agents may be useful in making a presumptive diagnosis. Results may take hours to days to complete and cannot be relied on during the arrest.

Radiographs

Chest radiographs can be useful in establishing a definitive diagnosis in a patient with cardiac arrest associated with a respiratory disease, and in confirming the placement of endotracheal tubes and central venous catheters. Because of the time involved in acquiring chest radiographs, they are not useful in the immediate resuscitation period and are not used to diagnose tension pneumothorax or cardiac tamponade before instituting treatment. Optimally, these diagnoses are based on physical assessment rather than radiographic studies.

REFINED DIFFERENTIAL DIAGNOSIS

After the initial rhythm disturbance is identified and the history, physical assessment, and basic diagnostic studies are completed, a more definitive diagnosis can be determined. The history is often very useful in establishing a presumptive cause. The past medical history and a listing of current medications from the family or paramedics can support or suggest an underlying disease process (Table 3–5). For instance, a past history of hypertension, diabetes mellitus, and hypercholesterolemia or the use of nitrates, beta blockers, or calcium channel blockers should raise the suspicion of ischemic heart disease as the underlying cause of the arrest. Hypoxia of pulmonary origin significant enough to result in cardiac arrest is associated with serious or advanced lung disease. Hypokalemia,

TABLE 3–5. Expanded Differential Diagnosis of Cardiopulmonary Arrest

Cardiovascular Causes	**Toxins**
Intrinsic dysrhythmias	Cardiac medications
Ventricular	Digitalis
Bradydysrhythmias	Antiarrhythmics
Sinus arrest	Quinidine
Second- or third-degree atrioventricular block	Procainamide
Ischemic heart disease	Encainide
Angina	Flecainide
Myocardial infarction	Beta blockers
Silent ischemia	Calcium channel blockers
Cardiomyopathies or congestive heart failure	Beta agonists or inotropic agents
Valvular heart disease	Catecholamines (natural or synthetic)
Hypertensive heart disease	Amrinone
Congenital heart disease	Drug overdose
Circulatory shock	Tricyclic antidepressants
Hypovolemic (hemorrhagic)	Stimulants
Gastrointestinal bleeeding	Cocaine
Trauma	PCP (phencyclidine)
Anaphylactic	Amphetamines
Septic	Antihistamines
Cardiogenic	CNS depressants
Cardiac tamponade	Others
Respiratory Causes	**Other Causes**
Tension pneumothorax	Lightning or electrical injuries
Pulmonary embolism	Drowning or near-drowning
Hypoxia	Trauma
Upper airway obstruction	Autonomic dysfunction
Any serious parenchymal lung disease	Hypothermia
Cor pulmonale	
Metabolic Causes	
Electrolyte abnormality	
Hypokalemia	
Hyperkalemia	
Hypomagnesemia	
Hypocalcemia	
Severe acid-base abnormality	
Acidosis	
Alkalosis	
Thyroid disease	
Thyroid storm	
Myxedema coma	

hyperkalemia, hypomagnesemia, and hypocalcemia can each result in ventricular dysrhythmias. A clinical situation in which ventricular dysrhythmias are particularly likely to occur is renal failure associated with hyperkalemia and hypocalcemia.

Nontraumatic cardiac arrest in a young or middle-aged individual always raises the suspicion of drug ingestion until another cause has been proved. The most common drug is cocaine. It can induce hypertension, acute myocardial ischemia or infarction, and various cardiac dysrhythmias, including ventricular tachycardia, ventricular fibrillation, and asystole (see Chap. 23).

PRINCIPLES OF MANAGEMENT

Management of cardiac arrest is centered around four principles. A fifth principle comes into play if the resuscitation attempt is successful.

Principle I: The Underlying Cardiac Arrest Rhythm Determines the Initial Therapy

The 1985 National Conference on Cardiopulmonary Resuscitation (CPR) and Emergency Cardiac Care (ECC) updated the suggested guidelines and algorithms for the therapy of cardiac arrest rhythms. Initial drug therapy is dependent on the underlying cardiac rhythm.

Ventricular fibrillation remains the most common underlying rhythm of cardiac arrest. The goal of therapy is to convert ventricular fibrillation (or pulseless ventricular tachycardia) rapidly to a stable and perfusing cardiac rhythm. The conversion is done with electrical defibrillation because ventricular fibrillation rarely if ever spontaneously converts. Only after initial defibrillation attempts fail is epinephrine administered and the patient's airway definitively managed (Fig. 3–1).

Ventricular tachycardia may be a hemodynamically perfusing rhythm or a nonperfusing "cardiac arrest" rhythm. The urgency of treatment is established based on the patient's mental status, pulse, and blood pressure (Fig. 3–2).

Bradydysrhythmias leading to asystole have a uniformly poor prognosis. Efforts to reestablish a spontaneous rhythm focus on the use of epinephrine, atropine, and adequate oxygenation. Atropine may enhance sinus node automaticity and atrioventricular conduction through its vagolytic activity. Attempts to electrically pace these patients have had uniformly dismal results. With the availability of external pacers, early pacing of patients with bradydysrhythmias can be accomplished in the prehospital setting. To date, they are rarely successful (Fig. 3–3).

Many disease processes present as electromechanical dissociation (EMD). This rhythm has cardiac electrical activity without mechanical pumping, i.e., a rhythm without a pulse (Table 3–6). Hemorrhagic shock due to gastrointestinal bleeding or trauma is the

TABLE 3–6. Differential Diagnosis of Electromechanical Dissociation

Hypovolemic shock	Obstructive shock
Hemorrhagic causes	Pericardial tamponade
Adrenal crisis	Massive pulmonary embolus
Severe dehydration	Tension pneumothorax
Distributive shock	Dissecting thoracic aneurysm
Septic factors	Thoracic or abdominal aneurysm rupture
Anaphylactic factors	
Toxigenic factors	Severe hypoxia or acidosis
Cardiogenic shock	
Severe left ventricular dysfunction	
Left ventricular rupture	
Papillary muscle rupture	

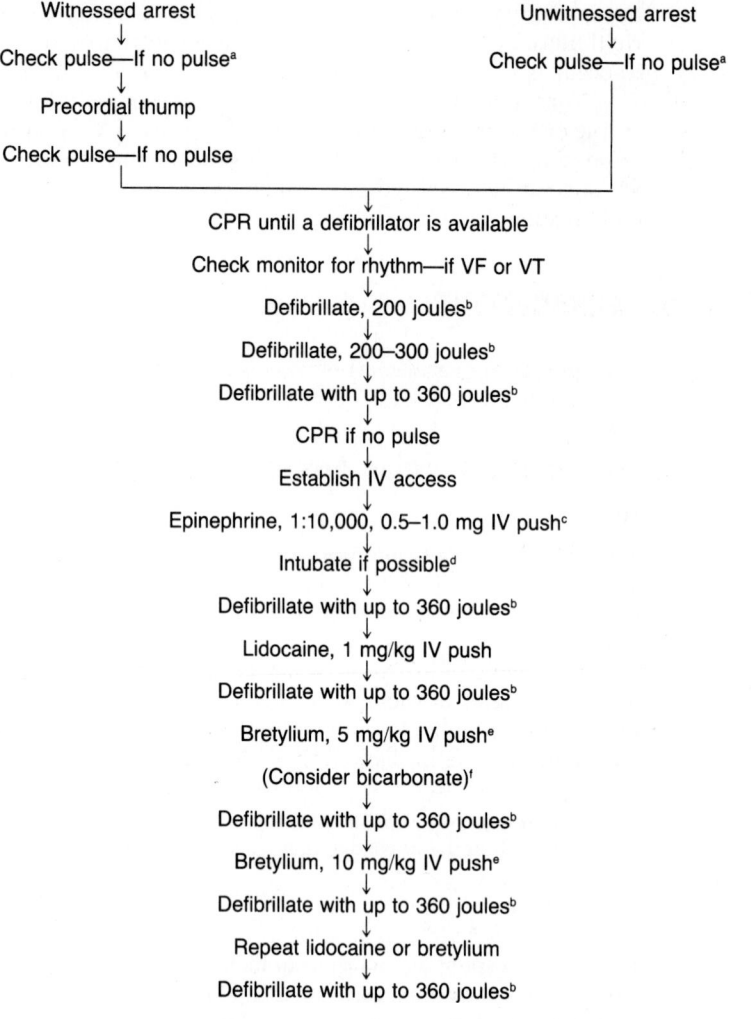

FIGURE 3–1. *Ventricular fibrillation (and pulseless ventricular tachycardia).*[a] *This sequence was developed to assist in teaching how to treat a broad range of patients with ventricular fibrillation (VF) or pulseless ventricular tachycardia (VT). Some patients may require care not specified herein. This algorithm should not be construed as prohibiting such flexibility. Flow of algorithm presumes that VF is continuing. CPR indicates cardiopulmonary resuscitation.*

[a]*Pulseless VT should be treated identically to VF.*

[b]*Check pulse and rhythm after each shock. If VF recurs after transiently converting (rather than persists without ever converting), use whatever energy level has previously been successful for defibrillation.*

[c]*Epinephrine should be repeated every 5 minutes.*

[d]*Intubation is preferable. If it can be accompanied simultaneously with other techniques, then the earlier the better. However, defibrillation and epinephrine are more important initially if the patient can be ventilated without intubation.*

[e]*Some may prefer repeated doses of lidocaine, which may be given in 0.5–mg/kg boluses every 8 minutes to a total dose of 3 mg/kg.*

[f]*Value of sodium bicarbonate is questionable during cardiac arrest, and it is not recommended for routine cardiac arrest sequence. Consideration of its use in a dose of 1 mEq/kg is appropriate at this point. Half of original dose may be repeated every 10 minutes if it is used. (From 1985 National Conference Committee on Standards and Guidelines for Cardiopulmonary Resuscitation and Emergency Cardiac Care: Standards and guidelines for cardiopulmonary resuscitation (CPR) and emergency cardiac care (ECC). JAMA 255(21):2946, 1986. Copyright 1986, American Medical Association.)*

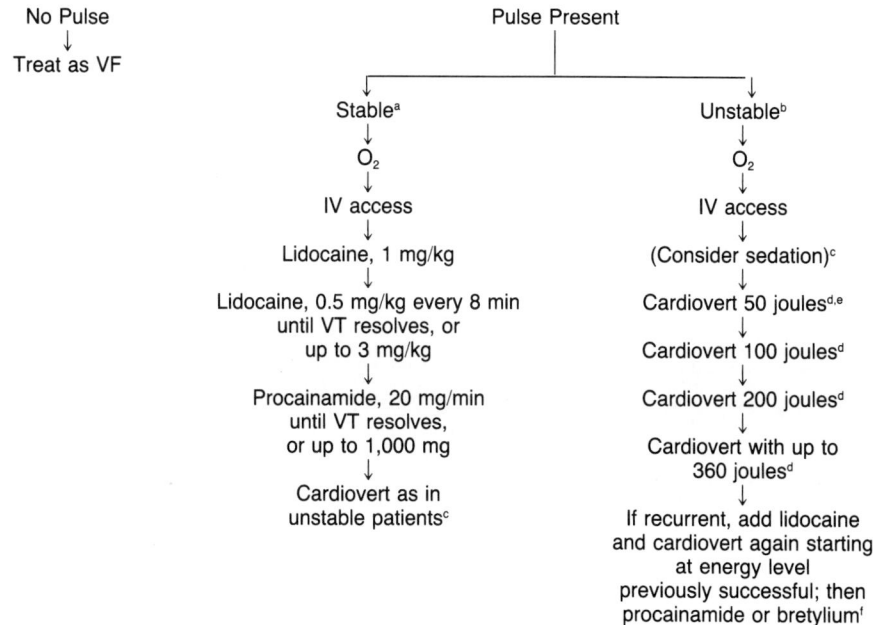

FIGURE 3–2. Sustained ventricular tachycardia (VT). This sequence was developed to assist in teaching how to treat a broad range of patients with sustained VT. Some patients may require care not specified herein. This algorithm should not be construed as prohibiting such flexibility. Flow of algorithm presumes that VT is continuing. VF indicates ventricular fibrillation.
[a] If patient becomes unstable (see footnote b for definition) at any time, move to "Unstable" arm of algorithm.
[b] Unstable indicates symptoms (e.g., chest pain or dyspnea), hypotension (systolic blood pressure <90 mm Hg), congestive heart failure, ischemia, or infarction.
[c] Sedation should be considered for all patients, including those defined in footnote b as unstable, except those who are hemodynamically unstable (e.g., hypotensive, in pulmonary edema, or unconscious).
[d] If hypotension, pulmonary edema, or unconsciousness is present, unsynchronized cardioversion should be done to avoid delay associated with synchronization.
[e] In the absence of hypotension, pulmonary edema, or unconsciousness, a precordial thump may be employed prior to cardioversion.
[f] Once VT has resolved, begin intravenous (IV) infusion of antiarrhythmic agent that has aided resolution of VT. If hypotension, pulmonary edema, or unconsciousness is present, use lidocaine if cardioversion alone is unsuccessful, followed by bretylium. In all other patients, recommended order of therapy is lidocaine, procainamide, and then bretylium. (From 1985 National Conference Committee on Standards and Guidelines for Cardiopulmonary Resuscitation and Emergency Cardiac Care: Standards and guidelines for cardiopulmonary resuscitation (CPR) and emergency cardiac care (ECC). JAMA 255(21):2947, 1986. Copyright 1986, American Medical Association.)

most common form of hypovolemic shock presenting as cardiac arrest. Cardiac tamponade is most commonly associated with hemorrhagic pericardial effusions related to trauma, neoplasms, uremia, or blood dyscrasias. Although it may occur spontaneously, tension pneumothorax is typically traumatic or iatrogenic (e.g., central line insertion, thoracocentesis) in origin. A large pulmonary embolus obstructing more than 50 to 60% of the pulmonary blood flow may present as EMD; however, cardiopulmonary arrest is more commonly related to severe hypoxemia and subsequent lethal dysrhythmias. In the setting of EMD, some therapeutic maneuvers may be diagnostic. Tension pneumothorax can be treated and diagnosed by a needle thoracostomy followed by insertion of a chest tube. A 16- or 18-gauge needle is inserted into the anterior second or third intercostal space of the involved hemithorax. A rush of air from the needle on insertion is diagnostic of tension pneumothorax. The immediate treatment of cardiac tamponade is pericardiocentesis. If blood is aspirated from the pericardial space, it usually is defibrinated and clots poorly. In addition, the removal of 10 to 20 ml of pericardial fluid may be associated with significant improvement in the cardiovascular status. This improved cardiac function

> If rhythm is unclear and possibly ventricular
> fibrillation, defibrillate as for VF. If asystole is present[a]
> ↓
> Continue CPR
> ↓
> Establish IV access
> ↓
> Epinephrine, 1:10,000, 0.5–1.0 mg IV push[b]
> ↓
> Intubate when possible[c]
> ↓
> Atropine, 1.0 mg IV push (repeated in 5 min)
> ↓
> (Consider bicarbonate)[d]
> ↓
> Consider pacing

FIGURE 3–3. Asystole (cardiac standstill). This sequence was developed to assist in teaching how to treat a broad range of patients with asystole. Some patients may require care not specified herein. This algorithm should not be construed to prohibit such flexibility. Flow of algorithm presumes asystole is continuing. VF indicates ventricular fibrillation; VI, intravenous.
[a]Asystole should be confirmed in two leads.
[b]Epinephrine should be repeated every 5 minutes.
[c]Intubation is preferable; if it can be accomplished simultaneously with other techniques, then the earler the better. However, cardiopulmonary resuscitation (CPR) and use of epinephrine are more important initially if patient can be ventilated without intubation. (Endotracheal epinephrine may be used.)
[d]Value of sodium bicarbonate is questionable during cardiac arrest, and it is not recommended for the routine cardiac arrest sequence. Consideration of its use in a dose of 1 mEq/kg is appropriate at this point. Half of original dose may be repeated every 10 minutes if it is used. (From 1985 National Conference Committee on Standards and Guidelines for Cardiopulmonary Resuscitation and Emergency Cardiac Care: Standards and guidelines for cardiopulmonary resuscitation (CPR) and emergency cardiac care (ECC). JAMA 255(21):2947, 1986. Copyright 1986, American Medical Association.)

directly related to pericardiocentesis is very suggestive of cardiac tamponade. A fluid challenge, e.g., with 300 to 500 ml of normal saline, is also warranted in EMD. The development of palpable pulses after fluid administration strongly suggests hypovolemia as the underlying cause.

PROBLEM 2 The patient was immediately intubated and ventilated with 100% oxygen. Because of the suspicion of hypovolemia, two large-bore peripheral IV lines were started, and 500 ml of lactated Ringer's solution were rapidly infused. A nasogastric tube was placed, and a large amount of bright red blood was aspirated. Melena was noted on rectal examination. Two units of type O blood were immediately infused. At this point a palpable pulse was obtained. External chest compressions were stopped, and the patient continued to receive volume resuscitation.

This patient with EMD needed rapid volume expansion. The underlying disease was gastrointestinal hemorrhage. CPR and drugs alone would not have succeeded in resuscitating this patient.

Principle II: Adequate Ventilation Rather than Bicarbonate Is Critical for Early Acid-Base Management

Measurement of mixed venous gases probably reflects the tissue and cellular acid-base state better than arterial blood gases. Typically, they show a respiratory acidosis rather than a metabolic acidosis as the primary acid/base disorder early in cardiac arrest. Elevated Pco_2 levels may worsen intracellular acidosis and cause further depression of myocardial and cerebral function. The administration of sodium bicarbonate may exacerbate the problem owing to additional carbon dioxide being liberated when the hydrogen ions are buffered. Sodium bicarbonate administration may cause other detrimental effects including hyperosmolality, hypernatremia, and a left shift of the oxyhemoglobin dissociation curve. Consequently, current recommendations place their emphasis on alveolar ventilation to control acidemia. Sodium bicarbonate administration may be indicated in hyperkalemia, prolonged arrest states, preexisting metabolic acidosis, and certain toxic states, i.e., tricyclic antidepressant overdose.

Principle III: In Order to Perfuse the Heart, an Arteriovenous Pressure Gradient Must Exist Across the Heart

Perfusion of the heart depends on the coronary perfusion pressure. Experimentally, this pressure has been approximated as the mean arterial diastolic pressure minus the mean right atrial pressure. Animal studies suggest that a certain minimal coronary perfusion pressure is necessary to successfully resuscitate the fibrillating heart.

During cardiac arrest, perfusion is obtained by external CPR and the use of alpha-adrenergic agents, primarily epinephrine. It is the alpha effects of epinephrine that account for the improved perfusion seen during CPR. During CPR the alpha-agonist activity seems to prevent vascular collapse, particularly of the intrathoracic vessels. In addition, vasoconstriction causes shunting of blood flow from less essential vascular beds.

Principle IV: The Cardiac Rhythm Can Frequently Change During Resuscitation

Throughout the resuscitation attempt there may be numerous dysrhythmias requiring intervention. Following initial therapy, the cardiac rhythm must be continuously observed. After successful defibrillation, the patient's rhythm may degenerate back into ventricular fibrillation. If the patient is closely monitored, immediate repeat defibrillation has an improved chance of conversion. Bradydysrhythmias and heart blocks often occur during CPR. Again, close cardiac monitoring is essential to guide therapy to prevent further ischemic injury. Degeneration of the cardiac rhythm to asystole is an ominous sign associated with a very poor recovery rate.

PROBLEM 1 When the cardiac monitor was rechecked, the patient was found to be in complete heart block with a heart rate of 40 beats/minute. Blood pressure was 60 mm Hg palpable. A total of 2 mg atropine was administered IV without any change in heart rate or rhythm. A transcutaneous external pacemaker was applied. The patient was paced at a rate of 70 beats/minute. Blood pressure improved to 100/60.

Following defibrillation, various dysrhythmias may occur and require therapy. Cardiac monitoring is usually the best means of recognizing these changes in rhythm. The use of a transcutaneous external pacer, as in this case, is indicated for patients with hemodynamically significant bradydysrhythmias.

Principle V: An Organized Approach to Postresuscitative Care Is Indicated in All Cardiac Arrest Patients Who Are Successfully Resuscitated

The ideal resuscitation attempt results in an awake, responsive, and spontaneously breathing patient. More often, the patient is hemodynamically unstable, requires ventilatory support, and has an altered mental status. Correctly managing the immediate postresuscitative period is critical to the patient's survival.

Initial Assessment

All successfully resuscitated patients require a thorough repeat physical examination. In addition, ancillary studies usually include a 12-lead ECG, chest radiograph, arterial blood gases, cardiac enzymes, electrolyte and renal panel, complete blood count, and determination of drug levels if appropriate. Particular attention is directed toward adequate oxygenation and ventilation, correcting existing acid-base and electrolyte abnormalities, and careful cardiovascular monitoring. Endotracheal tube placement is reconfirmed by physical examination and chest radiograph. Mechanical ventilation is initiated, if required. Adequacy of oxygenation and ventilation is best assessed with frequent arterial blood gas determinations.

Dysrhythmia Management

Because dysrhythmias are a major cause of recurring cardiac arrest, continuous ECG monitoring and the standard 12-lead ECG are critical elements in postresuscitative care. All patients resuscitated from cardiac arrest due to ventricular tachycardia or ventricular fibrillation are maintained on continuous antidysrhythmic therapy, usually lidocaine, for a minimum of 24 to 36 hours.

Hemodynamic Monitoring

Special attention is given to closely monitoring the status and stability of the cardiovascular system. Close attention to the patient's blood pressure and pulse rate is essential. Hypotension in the postresuscitation period is common and often requires the use of vasopressors, e.g., dopamine or norepinephrine. Although blood pressure control is very important, blood pressure is not necessarily a good indicator of cardiac function. Patients who remain cardiovascularly unstable or vasopressor dependent may require invasive hemodynamic monitoring, i.e., intra-arterial catheterization and a pulmonary artery flow-directed catheter. Invasive hemodynamic monitoring can precisely and continuously assess the intravascular fluid status and cardiac function. The ability to accurately determine the pulmonary artery pressure, pulmonary artery wedge pressure, cardiac output, and systemic vascular resistance offers the physician more precise guidance in fluid administration as well as diuretic, vasopressor, inotropic, and vasodilator therapies.

Cerebral Resuscitation

Current research suggests that some neuronal function may be preserved after 30 to 60 minutes of total anoxia. Unfortunately, a significant amount of brain damage may occur as blood flow is *reestablished* after resuscitation. This effect is called *reperfusion injury* and involves complex pathophysiologic processes combining hypoperfusion, local tissue acidosis, cytotoxic cerebral edema, mitochondrial dysfunction, and toxic oxygen free radical generation. In addition to the complex biochemical milieu established with anoxia and reperfusion, the immediate postresuscitation period is associated with reduced cerebral blood flow despite adequate systemic blood pressure. This response appears to be related to the vasoconstriction of the cerebral vasculature. Evidence suggests that abnormal calcium ion influx into the neuron may play a major role in reperfusion injury. A variety of therapeutic modalities have been suggested to reduce cerebral damage in the postresuscitation period. These include barbiturates, calcium channel blockers, oxygen free radical scavengers, phenytoin, prostaglandin inhibitors, hemodilution, hypothermia, and chelating agents. Much of this work remains experimental, but some basic principles to apply are included in Table 3–7.

The most clinically relevant therapy is maintenance of an adequate systemic blood pressure and oxygenation. Cerebral anoxia is associated with loss of cerebral autoregulation, and cerebral blood flow is directly dependent on mean arterial pressure (MAP). Therefore, maintenance of adequate blood pressure and oxygenation is paramount during the postresuscitative period.

TABLE 3–7. Guidelines for Cerebral Stabilization During the Postresuscitation Period

Cardiovascular Stabilization
Maintain normotension (MAP = 80–100 mm Hg)
Normalize blood volume
Use invasive hemodynamic monitoring in unstable states
Maintain adequate oxygen-carrying capacity (Hgb = 10–12 gm/dl)
Elevate head of bed 10–30 degrees
*Induce brief mild hypertension (MAP = 110–130 mm Hg)
*Normovolemic hemodilution with phlebotomy and crystalloids/colloids (Hct = 25–30%)

Metabolic Stabilization
Maintain:
 PaO_2 ≥ 80–100 mm Hg (avoid pulmonary end-expiratory pressure [PEEP])
 $PaCO_2$ = 35–45 mm Hg
 pH = 7.35–7.45
 Glucose = 100–250 mg/dl
 Serum osmolality = 280–320 mOsm/kg H_2O
Avoid hypoproteinemia (albumin < 3.0 gm/dl)
Avoid hyperthermia (temperature > 100° F or 38° C)
Control or avoid seizures (diazepam, phenytoin, barbiturates)

Cellular or Neuronal Stabilization
*Calcium channel blockers (lidoflazine, nimodipine, flunarizine)
*Toxic oxygen radical scavengers (superoxide dismutase, dimethyl sulfoxide)
*Chelating agents (deferoxamine)
*Prostaglandin inhibition (indomethacin)
*Suppression of lactic acid production (dichloroacetate)
*Phenytoin

Diagnostic Considerations
CT scan
 Mass lesions
 Intracerebral hemorrhage
 Subarachnoid hemorrhage
Lumbar puncture
 Meningitis
 Subarachnoid hemorrhage
Electroencephalogram
 Subclinical seizure activity
 Certify brain death
Cerebral perfusion scan
 Certify brain death

* = Experimental treatment.

SPECIAL CONSIDERATIONS

Pediatric Cardiac Arrest Patients

Adult cardiopulmonary arrest is most commonly due to cardiac disease. Pediatric arrest is more often the result of acute respiratory failure. Attention to airway control and breathing is paramount in resuscitating the child. The approach to airway control and artificial ventilation is the same as that used in adults; however, pediatric endotracheal intubation requires experience with the smaller, uncuffed endotracheal tubes. Many methods of estimating endotracheal tube size in children have been developed. One standard is to match the size of the little finger.

Another major difference in pediatric resuscitation concerns defibrillation and drug dosage based upon the patient's weight. In the unusual circumstance that pediatric cardiopulmonary arrest requires defibrillation, the initial setting of the defibrillator is 2 joules/kg and 4 joules/kg if the initial defibrillation attempt is unsuccessful. Epinephrine, sodium bicarbonate, lidocaine, and bretylium are given in the same weight-adjusted doses as those used for adults. However, atropine is given as 0.02 mg/kg/dose and is repeated, but the dose must not exceed a total of 1 mg in the child (Table 3–8).

TABLE 3–8. Drug Dosing for Pediatric CPR

Drug	How Supplied or Prepared	Dose
$NaHCO_3$	1 mEq/ml	1–2 mEq (1–2 ml)/kg
Epinephrine	0.1 mg/ml (1:10,000 solution)	0.01 mg (0.1 ml)/kg
Atropine	0.1 mg/ml	0.02 mg (0.2 ml)/kg
Isoproterenol	1.5 mg/250 ml D_5W (6 μg/ml)	0.1–1.0 μg (1–10 ml)/kg/min
Calcium chloride	100 mg/ml (10% solution)	20 mg (0.2 ml)/kg
Lidocaine	10–20 mg/ml (1–2% solution)	1 mg (0.1 ml)/kg
Lidocaine infusion	300 mg (15 ml of 2% solution)/ 250 ml D_5W (1200 μg/ml)	20 μg (1 ml)/kg/hr
Dopamine	150 mg (3.75 ml)/250 ml D_5W (600 μg/ml)	10 μg (1 ml)/kg/min

Trauma Patients

The most common sources of traumatic arrest are hypovolemia, tension pneumothorax, and cardiac tamponade. Trauma patients who are unresponsive to vigorous fluid resuscitation require open thoracotomy, cardiac massage, and surgical intervention. Cardiac arrests due to blunt chest or abdominal trauma continue to have a dismal outcome despite early and appropriate intervention (see Chap. 4).

Pregnant Patients

Prior to 24 weeks' gestation, survival of the fetus in a pregnant woman with cardiac arrest is unlikely, and resuscitative measures are directed toward the mother. Resuscitation from cardiopulmonary arrest in a pregnant woman occurring after 24 weeks' gestation is directed to both the mother and the fetus. Standard resuscitation techniques are applied in the pregnant patient without modification, including pharmacologic therapy. In the more than 24 weeks setting, if standard resuscitative therapy is not successful after 10 to 15 minutes of cardiac arrest, immediate cesarean section is considered.

Electrocution Patients

Cardiopulmonary arrest secondary to electric shock, especially from alternating current, is most commonly due to ventricular fibrillation. Arrest secondary to lightning injury is often caused by asystole or accompanying respiratory arrest. Resuscitation is initiated with these etiologies in mind.

Do Not Resuscitate Orders

Considerable controversy surrounds the legal and ethical aspects of deciding when not to resuscitate a patient. Not all patients who suffer a cardiopulmonary arrest need resuscitative care. Severely debilitated patients or those with known terminal disease (e.g., metastatic cancer, severe dementia, end-stage cardiac disease) may not be candidates for resuscitation. Patients have a right to die with dignity; therefore, patients who request no life-sustaining measures should not be resuscitated. A thin line often separates the legal ramifications of no resuscitation from the patient's right to die with dignity. A "living will" or a written physician order that is available at the time of cardiopulmonary arrest may represent adequate documentation not to resuscitate. However, since the issue is far from resolved, the emergency physician should always err on the side of active resuscitation if any doubt exists about the patient's "do not resuscitate" status.

DISPOSITION

Prior to transfer to the intensive care unit, the patient should be as stable as possible. Orders may be written for maintenance of intravenous infusions (e.g., lidocaine, dopamine), for ventilator settings (e.g., rate, mode, tidal volume), and for supplemental oxygen. The physician who will be caring for the patient in the coronary care unit is contacted and the case discussed in as much detail as possible. The patient's family is briefed in detail about the progress and continued critical status of the patient. One or two family members may accompany the patient to the intensive care unit, depending on the patient's condition and hospital policy.

> **PROBLEM 1** The patient was maintained on the lidocaine drip and the external transcutaneous pacemaker. Once in the coronary care unit, the transcutaneous pacemaker was discontinued. Results of laboratory studies including arterial blood gases, electrolytes, glucose, and complete blood count were within

normal limits. The patient's blood pressure and mental status normalized over several hours. The patient required a permanent pacemaker and had an otherwise uneventful hospital course.

PROBLEM 2 The patient was admitted to the intensive care unit. He underwent emergency endoscopy and a bleeding ulcer was located and cauterized. The patient's course was complicated by renal failure and a residual neurologic deficit.

Death in the Emergency Department

Approximately 70 to 80% of cardiopulmonary arrest patients will not be successfully resuscitated. One of the most difficult responsibilities of a physician is informing the family and relatives of the death of a loved one. Even though no standard approach works in every case, a few guidelines are worth remembering (Table 3–9). Informing the family is best done in a private room with the assistance of a clergyman or social worker. After introducing oneself to the family, the physician should sit with the family and address the member closest to the patient. A brief summary of the events that have taken place can be a good introduction, preparing the family for the fatal outcome. When

TABLE 3–9. Guidelines for Informing the Family of an Unexpected Death

Step into the room and gain control of the scene. Do not respond to quick questioning such as "Is he dead?" Introduce yourself, and determine who is present. Address the closest relative or the one who looks the most composed.

Sit down, if possible. Unless the situation is a hostile circumstance, move away from the door and physically join the group.

Briefly, in less than 30 seconds, relate the circumstance as you know it. Give the status of activity in the Emergency Department up until the cessation of resuscitative efforts. Then describe the present situation, i.e., the patient is dead. If you use other terminology, it may need to be repeated or clarified.

Anticipate a grief response and give physical comfort if you are comfortable in doing so, but do not move away.

After the initial response has lasted 30 to 60 seconds, ask the least emotional or closest person to the deceased a question about their knowledge of the events preceding the arrest. This usually stops or lessens the grieving in the group.

Talk with them about the history. Reassure them there was no pain involved (unless this is obviously not so); support the emergency medical services and other physicians. If major problems in the quality of care exist, do not address them at this time. If asked, simply state more information must be gathered. If appropriate, reassure family and friends that they did everything they could. This is important to decrease their potential guilt.

At this time, enlist the aid of the clergy or the social service, if present. You should be preparing to leave.

Once completely standing, explain your tasks of notifying the coroner, private physician, etc. This introduces the work you must leave to do. Also, direct questions concerning burial arrangements to the clergy or social service.

As part of your closure to the first visit, inquire about the potential for an autopsy and transplantation. Don't press this issue at this juncture. Ask if they want to view the body and make sure all arrangements are made before they do.

Let them know you will return to answer any questions after your discussions with the coroner and the private physician.

Express your sorrow for their loss, and scan the group for those who might need further support.

Make every effort to speak with them again after talking with the coroner or private physician. Discuss the autopsy and transplantation request in more depth. Know the law and the hospital procedures, e.g., who pays for the autopsy if not requested by the coroner. Have the appropriate paperwork readily available and know how to complete it.

Again, express your sympathy and allow the interested individuals to view the body, no more than two at a time.

Direct the social service personnel to follow-up on individuals who seem to need further support and with the person closest to the deceased. Make sure this person has a reasonable support system.

Do not prescribe sedatives or sleeping medications to group members without having them register.

At some point, arrange a debriefing session both medically and emotionally with the emergency department nursing staff and others involved. This is difficult to arrange but worthwhile.

Modified from Hamilton GC: Sudden death in the ED: Telling the living. Ann Emerg Med 17(4):382, 1988.

informing the family, one should be as direct as possible and should use terms such as *died* and *dead*, avoiding vague terms such as *passed on* or *no longer with us*. It is also important to allow a brief period of immediate grieving and to answer any questions that the family may have. If the family wishes to view the deceased, one should inform the nurses and allow time for preparation of the body.

DOCUMENTATION

1. Any and all *predisposing factors* that led to the cardiac arrest.
2. *Current medications* and past medical history, especially *risk factors* associated with cardiac disease.
3. *Physical examination* of the patient on presentation in the emergency room, findings during the resuscitation attempt, and successful postresuscitation assessment.
4. *Therapies administered* during the resuscitation effort as well as the response to therapy. This item includes medications used during the resuscitation, e.g., epinephrine, atropine, lidocaine.
5. Any *procedures* performed during or after the resuscitation attempt, including airway control maneuvers, central line insertion, needle or tube thoracostomy, and pericardiocentesis.
6. *Laboratory* results, including ECG findings on both continuous monitoring and 12-lead electrocardiogram.
7. *Presumptive diagnosis* of the disease process leading to the cardiac arrest.
8. In successfully resuscitated patients admitted to the critical care unit, *dosages* of administered drugs as well as continuous infusions at the time of transport and ventilator settings, if appropriate. In unsuccessful resuscitation cases, the *time of death*, any discussions with family members or the patient's private physician and final disposition of the body.

The purpose of documentation is not only to inform other health professionals of the events that occurred during the immediate preresuscitation, resuscitation, and postresuscitation time periods but also to allow the emergency physician to review what was done and the effectiveness of treatment.

SUMMARY

- Cardiopulmonary resuscitation is the true life or death emergency. Successful resuscitation depends on rapidly identifying the cardiac arrest victim and promptly instituting basic life support maneuvers. Once basic life support has been established, recognition of the rhythm disturbance is necessary, and advanced cardiac life support is begun.
- The best survival results in cardiac arrest victims occur with early recognition and defibrillation of patients with ventricular fibrillation or pulseless ventricular tachycardia.
- Prognosis in patients with EMD is very poor unless a reversible cause can be identified and corrected.
- The best preparation for treating cardiopulmonary arrest is familiarity with and ability to recognize and treat lethal cardiac rhythms. This subject is best summarized in the American Heart Association's Standards for Advanced Cardiac Life Support (see references 1 [texts] and 10 [journals]).

- Although all patients in cardiopulmonary arrest are candidates for resuscitation, not all need to be resuscitated. The patient who is "dead on arrival," one who does not desire life-support measures, or the patient with documented "terminal" disease should not be resuscitated.

BIBLIOGRAPHY

Texts

1. Albarran Sotelo R, Atkins JM, Bloom RS, et al: Textbook of Advanced Cardiac Life Support. American Heart Association, 1987.
2. Braunwald E: Heart Disease. A Textbook of Cardiovascular Medicine (3rd ed). Philadelphia, W.B. Saunders, 1988.
3. Rippe JM, Irwin RS, Alpert JS, et al: Intensive Care Medicine, Boston, Little, Brown, 1985.
4. Safar P, Bircher NG: Cardiopulmonary Cerebral Resuscitation (3rd ed). Philadelphia, W.B. Saunders, 1988.

Journals

1. Bass E: Cardiopulmonary arrest. Pathophysiology and neurologic complications. Ann Intern Med 103:920–927, 1985.
2. Buxton AE: Sudden cardiac death—1986. Ann Intern Med 104:716–718, 1986.
3. Criley JM, Niemann JT, Rosborough JP: Cardiopulmonary resuscitation research 1960–1984: Discoveries and advances. Ann Emerg Med 13:756–758, 1984.
4. Cummins RO, Eisenberg MS: Pre-hospital cardiopulmonary resuscitation. Is it effective? JAMA 253:2408–2412, 1985.
5. Ewy GA: Alternative approaches to external cardiac compression. Circulation 74 (Suppl IV):98–107, 1986.
6. Hamilton GC: Sudden death in the ED: Telling the living. Ann Emerg Med 17:382, 1988.
7. Hanashiro PK, Wilson JR: Cardiopulmonary resuscitation. A current perspective. Med Clin North Am 70:729–747, 1986.
8. Kirsch JR, Dean JM, Rogers MC: Current concepts in brain resuscitation. Arch Intern Med 146:1413–1419, 1986.
9. Krischer JP, Fine EG, Davis JH, et al: Complications of cardiac resuscitation. Chest 92:287–291, 1987.
10. Rogers MC, Kirsch JR: Current concepts in brain resuscitation. JAMA 261:3143–3147, 1989.
11. Standards and Guidelines for Cardiopulmonary Resuscitation (CPR) and Emergency Cardiac Care (ECC). JAMA 255:2905–2985, 1986.
12. Steuven HA, Waite EM, Philip T, et al: Prehospital cardiac arrest—a critical analysis of factors affecting survival. Resuscitation 17:251–259, 1989.

CHAPTER 4

MULTIPLE TRAUMA

PETER T. PONS, M.D.

PROBLEM 1 A 45 year old male was found unresponsive in his automobile after the car had struck a tree. His lap and shoulder restraints were in place. There was no interior damage to the vehicle. Rapid evaluation revealed a small bruise on the left side of the head and decerebrate posturing.

PROBLEM 2 A 23 year old male was pushed out of a car at the entrance to the emergency department. He was awake, intoxicated, and hostile. A gunshot wound in his left chest was readily apparent.

QUESTIONS TO CONSIDER

1. How is multiple trauma defined?
2. Once notified of the arrival of a patient with multiple injuries, how does the emergency physician prepare?
3. What is meant by the term *mechanism of injury* and what is its importance?
4. What is the primary survey?
5. How is the secondary survey defined?
6. What is a trauma scale or score and how is it used?
7. What are the common pitfalls and problems in multiple trauma management?
8. When is a consultant contacted in multiple trauma cases?

INTRODUCTION

Trauma is the number one cause of death in the United States for persons under 39 years of age. Approximately 150,000 patients die annually in the United States from trauma. For all age groups only atherosclerotic disease and cancer result in greater mortality. Fifty million injuries occur each year, and about 20% of these result in permanent disability. The cost to society is billions of dollars.

Caring for patients with multiple injuries is a challenging task. The physician's knowledge of the mechanism of injury is used to anticipate specific patterns of inquiry. A standard evaluation procedure is followed to avoid overlooking important findings in the time-limited and stressful setting of trauma care. Optimal care of the trauma victim is delivered by a coordinated team effort led by a trained and experienced physician.

Management of the trauma patient requires an institutional commitment of personnel and resources to provide rapid diagnosis and intervention. This commitment involves the staff in the emergency department with a hospital-wide system that includes blood banking, laboratory support, diagnostic imaging capability, operating space, and medical talent: emergency physicians, surgeons, anesthesiologists, and others.

The American College of Surgeons Committee on Trauma has created criteria for categorizing hospitals as Trauma Centers. The Level I center is a large teaching and research institution that has comprehensive capabilities and resources. The Level II center has made the commitment to trauma care but does not have the teaching and research role of the Level I center. The Level III center is a community hospital committed to trauma care but lacking the resources or personnel of the Level I or II centers. Though only 1% to 5% of all trauma victims sustain major life-threatening injuries, these patients benefit most if they are transported to a trauma center directly from the scene, even if it means bypassing a closer hospital. Several studies have shown that patient outcome is improved if the trauma victim is treated at a trauma center.

Trauma is generally classified into two broad categories: penetrating injury and blunt injury. As a general rule, penetrating trauma, e.g., from gunshot or stab wounds, produces injury involving one or at the most two organ systems located in proximity to the wound site. Blunt trauma, e.g., from falls or auto accidents, often leads to damage of multiple organ systems and sites. As the name implies, multiple trauma represents injury to two or more organ systems.

Mechanism of Injury

Knowledge of the mechanism of injury and the pattern of injuries that may result is important in managing the trauma victim. Information from the scene assists the physician in estimating the amount of physical force applied to the body. General mechanisms of injury and the injury patterns they can produce are listed in Table 4–1.

Certain mechanisms of injury produce particular patterns. Falls, car accidents, and other deceleration mechanisms commonly produce cervical spine injury and may cause aortic rupture. Jumping from a height and landing on one's feet often causes both calcaneus and lumbar spine fractures. A pedestrian struck by a moving vehicle may have a triad of injuries comprising a leg fracture where the bumper hit first, a chest injury from falling over the hood, and head trauma from striking the windshield.

Anticipating the pattern of injury linked to a specific injury mechanism is important to alert the physician's suspicion regarding the potential impact of trauma on the entire body. Since trauma care can be fraught with surprises, knowledge of the mechanism or pattern of injury does not preclude a complete physical examination but serves as an initial guide for concern. Significant force usually begets significant injury despite a possible lack of initial or impressive findings. Mechanisms of injury with potential for severe damage have been tabulated. They are an important component in field and hospital triage decisions (Table 4–2). If the physical findings are inconsistent with the

TABLE 4–1. Mechanisms of Injury in Trauma

Type of Trauma	Mechanics of Injury	Types of Injury
Penetrating	Direct injury	The penetrating object usually follows a straight path; therefore, the direction of travel is determined and the potential organ injuries are visualized. Missiles (bullets) may ricochet, fragment, or create bone fragments, leading to additional injury
	Indirect injury	Missiles have an associated shock wave that may damage structures that are proximate to but not directly in the pathway. The denser the structure (e.g., bone), the greater the damage
Blunt	Direct injury	Injury may occur either when an object strikes the body (i.e., assault with a baseball bat) or when the body strikes an object (i.e., fall from a height, striking the steering wheel or windshield during a car accident)
	Indirect injury	Organs may be injured indirectly by means of sudden deceleration of the body. For example, a moving auto hits a tree, the car stops, but the driver's inertia keeps him moving forward until his chest strikes the steering wheel and his head hits the windshield. Inside the body, the heart and aorta keep moving until the heart strikes the sternum and the aorta shears. Inside the skull, the brain continues its forward motion until it strikes the skull.

TABLE 4–2. Mechanisms of Injury with a High Potential for Serious Injury

Motor vehicle accidents
  High-speed traffic accident (>30 mph)
  Vehicle space invaded ≥1 foot
  Pedestrian accident (age <12 years or >65 years)
  Pedestrian accident (vehicle moving >20 mph)
  Pedestrian thrown >15 feet by car
  Ejection from vehicle
  Death of other persons in vehicle
  Prolonged extrication time (>20 minutes)

Anatomic factors in injuries
  Penetrating trauma to head, neck, torso, or groin to mid-thigh
  Major burn (covering >20% partial-thickness or full-thickness skin area)
  Major amputation above ankle or wrist
  Paralysis

Falls of more than 15 feet

Environment
  Drowning
  Hostile environment, e.g., desert, swamp

---

known mechanisms of injury, the physician must search for other causes that will explain the findings. For example, the patient who took an overdose of a drug before shooting himself may present in shock despite a superficial wound.

PROBLEM 1 When the automobile hit the tree, there was a sudden deceleration. The patient's head may have hit the windshield, producing a head injury or cervical spine fracture. He may have broken ribs or a fractured sternum due to striking the steering wheel as well as a contusion of the heart or tear of the aorta. Also, he may have an intra-abdominal injury such as a ruptured spleen caused by the seat belt or steering wheel. A fractured pelvis or long bone may result from striking the dashboard. A physician who is aware of the injury mechanism has an idea of the possibilities of injury even before examining the patient.

PROBLEM 2 After a gunshot wound to the left chest, the injury to the lung will most likely cause a hemo-pneumothorax. Other involved organs can include the heart and great vessels, spinal cord, and perhaps the upper abdomen if the bullet traversed the diaphragm. The damage is generally limited to the path of the penetrating object, but ricocheting fragments and the effect of the "shock wave" must be anticipated.

Hemorrhagic Shock

Prior to any discussion of patient care, it is necessary to review the pathophysiology of blood loss and the production of shock. External or internal hemorrhage is a potentially lethal combination of intravascular volume loss and decreased oxygen-carrying capacity. The body responds with volume shifts from interstitial and intracellular fluid, increases in the respiratory and cardiac rates, an increase in cardiac contractility, and constriction of capacitance vessels. As hemorrhage continues, more fluid shifts occur, blood is shunted toward the heart and brain, and inadequately perfused cells shift toward an anaerobic mode of metabolism, producing lactic acid. If this situation is uncorrected, cardiac output falls, and the patient loses consciousness owing to inadequate cerebral perfusion. At some point in the interaction among blood loss, time, and the physiologic capability of the body, the process reaches an irreversible stage. Early death from cardiopulmonary arrest or, depending on resuscitative efforts and timing, late death from multisystem failure ensues. In all cases of trauma, whether it is of blunt or penetrating etiology, the usual problem to be addressed in the emergency department is blood loss leading to circulatory compromise, hypoxia, and vital organ dysfunction. Other problems such as actual disruption of tissue parenchyma or organ dysfunction are usually managed later in the course of care.

The Advanced Trauma Life Support course describes four classes of shock based on the amount of blood loss (see reference 1 [text]): class I, up to 15% blood loss; class II, 15% to 30% blood loss; class III, 30% to 40% blood loss; class IV, more than 40% blood loss.

To reverse this process, class I and II types of hemorrhage require crystalloid to replace volume shifts and loss, and class III and IV hemorrhages additionally need blood as part of the fluid resuscitation. A method for estimating these needs follows in the section on Initial Approach in the Emergency Department.

Other causes of shock may also be present in the trauma patient. Obstructive shock is seen in patients with pericardial tamponade and tension pneumothorax. Distributive shock due to dilated capacitance or resistance vessels may result from the insult that may have caused the accident, e.g., anaphylaxis, or may occur after the injury, e.g., spinal shock. Cardiogenic shock is rarely a major concern in trauma cases but may occur in patients with severe myocardial contusion or after myocardial infarction from an intimal tear of the coronary artery. Patients in shock due to each of these causes may initially respond to volume replacement, but developing a differential diagnosis of shock states other than hemorrhagic shock is necessary if the patient is not responding as anticipated.

PREHOSPITAL CARE

The prehospital and emergency department phases of care are generally evaluative and resuscitative in nature. These actions usually progress simultaneously. In most serious trauma cases, definitive care is provided in the operating room by surgical control of hemorrhage, debridement of devitalized tissue, and anatomic reconstruction. Prehospital and emergency department care are aimed at rapid assessment of the type and scope of injury, measuring the physiologic impact and tolerance of injury, and intervention to avoid further morbidity and mortality.

Field stabilization of the trauma victim is a controversial issue. Definitive care is often surgical and available only at the hospital. Some physicians advocate minimal intervention on scene (scoop and run) with any procedures performed en route. Others believe that field intervention is appropriate. The decision depends on the nature of the patient's injuries, the technical abilities of the personnel, the documented speed with which procedures can be performed, the distance to a location providing definitive care, and the medical control of the system. In most urban settings, the goal of on-scene management is to provide the necessary care in an on-scene time of 10 minutes or less.

The scene assessment by field personnel is crucial in initiating preparations in the hospital. Optimally, the following information is transmitted by field personnel:

History
1. If the patient is conscious, what complaints are voiced?
2. What was the "mechanism of injury"?
3. If the patient fell, from what height did he fall and onto what surface (deceleration information)?
4. If patient was in an auto accident, what was the estimated speed of the vehicle? The stopping distance? (The more deceleration, the more damage results.) Was the patient restrained? Were the steering wheel and windshield intact? Was the patient found inside or outside the car? What was the status of other victims?
5. If penetrating trauma occurred, what type of weapon was used?

Physical examination
1. What was the general appearance of the patient when the ambulance arrived on scene?

2. What are the vital signs?
3. How has the patient changed over time?

Interventions

The following procedures, based on the mechanism of injury and patient assessment, are usually performed by prehospital personnel.

1. Airway and oxygen. A patent and protected airway is established. Blood and vomitus, if present, are suctioned. Supplemental oxygen is provided to all trauma patients at high flow rates (10 to 12 liters/min) if no other contraindication exists.

2. Spinal immobilization. If the mechanism of injury is compatible with producing a spine injury, the patient is immobilized. Generally, immobilization is accomplished by placing the patient on a backboard, taping the head to the board, and using a blanket roll or "hard" type of collar.

3. Intravenous (IV) access. Preferably, a large-bore (14 to 16 gauge) cannula is used. The issue of whether insertion of an IV line should be performed on the scene, in the ambulance, or at all is central to the prehospital trauma care controversy. The IV fluid is an isotonic crystalloid solution.

4. Splinting of extremity fractures is performed en route.

5. Analgesia. In most cases pain medication is not administered until the patient is transported to the hospital and is examined. Exceptions to this rule include patients with isolated extremity injuries and burns.

6. The pneumatic antishock garment (PASG) is commonly used but is of unproven efficacy. For victims of penetrating trauma in an urban environment, it is ineffective in altering patient outcome. For persons with blunt injuries or in rural areas, further evaluation is needed.

At the close of discussions with the prehospital personnel, the emergency physician should have a clear understanding of what happened at the scene, what was found, what treatment was given, and how the patient responded.

Trauma or Injury Severity Scores

Trauma scores or injury severity scores were developed to identify and prioritize (triage) trauma victims requiring transport to a trauma center. They are also used to evaluate patient outcome, compare epidemiologic data, and provide a means of documenting quality of care. There are two types of scoring systems: One is based on the anatomic injury sustained, and the other is based on physiologic observations and parameters. The Abbreviated Injury Scale and Injury Severity Score (ISS) are anatomic injury scores that are applied only after the complete diagnosis has been made. Anatomic injury criteria have evolved for the field triage setting. The Glasgow Coma Scale, Trauma Score, and CRAMS (*c*irculation, *r*espiration, *a*bdomen, *m*otor, and *s*peech) scale are physiologic parameter scores (Table 4–3). These scales have the advantage of being dynamic, that is, the score may be determined in the prehospital setting and reassessed during the course of care, thus documenting improvement or deterioration. They have been linked to a number of predictive indexes that are of use in determining prognoses. The most commonly used outcome is the probability of survival (Table 4–4). Years of validation have made these scores an important tool in evaluating trauma and communicating data about trauma. All have limitations and are used adjunctively, not as a mainstay of decision making in trauma care and disposition. The combination of physiologic parameter scores, mechanism of injury information, and on-scene anatomic injury criteria are important advances in making triage and treatment decisions. They are important areas of continued research.

PROBLEM 1 The field personnel extricated the patient while maintaining spine immobilization. He remained unconscious. They placed him on a backboard and immobilized his head. His vital signs were BP 98/56, pulse 104, respirations 18. The physical examination was grossly unremarkable except for the

TABLE 4–3. Physiologic Status Based Trauma Scoring Systems

	Score
I. Glasgow Coma Scale (GCS)	
Eye opening	
Spontaneous	4
To voice	3
To pain	2
None	1
Verbal Response	
Oriented	5
Confused	4
Inappropriate words	3
Incomprehensible	2
None	1
Motor Response	
Obeys commands	6
Localizes pain	5
Withdraws to pain	4
Flexion to pain	3
Extension to pain	2
None	1
Best score 15; coma defined as ≤8	
II. CRAMS Scale	
Circulation	
BP >100 mm Hg systolic, capillary refill normal	2
BP <85–100 mm Hg systolic, capillary refill delayed	1
BP <85 mm Hg systolic, capillary refill absent	0
Respirations	
Normal	2
Abnormal	1
Absent	0
Abdomen	
Abdomen, thorax not tender	2
Abdomen or thorax tender	1
Abdomen rigid or flail chest	0
Motor	
Normal	2
Responds to pain	1
No response or decerebrate	0
Speech	
Normal	2
Confused	1
Unintelligible	0
Score: ≤8 = major trauma; ≥9 = minor trauma	
III. Trauma Score (TS)	
Glasgow Coma Scale	
14–15	5
11–13	4
8–10	3
5–7	2
3–4	1
Systolic blood pressure	
>90 mm Hg	4
70–90 mm Hg	3
50–69 mm Hg	2
<50 mm Hg	1
No carotid pulse	0
Capillary refill	
Normal	2
Delayed	1
Absent	0
Respiratory rate/min	
10–24	4
25–35	3
>35	2
1–9	1
None	0
Respiratory effort	
Normal	1
Shallow, retractive	0

Score: sliding scale, higher numbers better, but tends to underestimate serious trauma.

TABLE 4–4. Probability of Survival for Commonly Used Physiologic Trauma Scoring Systems

Score	% Probability of Survival
Glascow Coma Scale (GCS)	
15	99
14	97
13	88
12	83
11	83
10	83
9	79
8	77
7	77
6	75
5	50
4	50
3	16
Trauma Score	
16	99
15	98
14	95
13	91
12	83
11	71
10	55
9	37
8	22
7	12
6	7
5	4
4	2
3	1
2	0
1	0

Adapted from Champion HR, Sacco WJ: Measurement of injury severity and its practical application. Trauma Q 1(4):25–36, 1984. With permission of Aspen Publishers, Inc., © 1984.

patient's mental status. The gag reflex was intact, and oxygen at 5 L/min by nasal cannula was begun. Field personnel transported him to the nearest trauma center and initiated an IV line with normal saline en route.

The mechanism of injury was compatible with possible spine injury, so the patient was immobilized. The assessment was rapidly performed, and total on-scene time was 9 minutes. The patient's trauma score was about 10 because the Glasgow Coma Scale had to be estimated. This score placed the patient in the moderately injured category.

INITIAL APPROACH IN THE EMERGENCY DEPARTMENT

Once notified by the rescue squad that a multiple trauma patient is en route, the emergency physician prepares for the patient's arrival. Members of the trauma team are notified. Based on the radio report, equipment for anticipated procedures is readied. One physician member of the team is designated the trauma team captain. Direction for the resuscitation effort comes from the captain. Procedures are preferably delegated to others because many tasks are accomplished simultaneously rather than sequentially. *It is important to always assume that the worst possible injury exists, to intervene aggressively until the "worst injury" is proved to be not present, and then to decrease or redirect the resuscitative effort.*

When the patient arrives, a "primary survey" is performed quickly to identify the immediate, life-threatening problems. A structured approach provides the most information in the shortest amount of time. Simultaneously, the field personnel give a formal report on the patient's condition, treatment, and response to care. An expanded description of the scene is often useful; for example, in reviewing a motor vehicle accident, an account of the damage done to the windshield, steering wheel, and dash, seat belt use, estimated speed of the vehicle, and the status of the other passengers is helpful.

Precautions are needed to protect emergency personnel from human immunodeficiency virus transmission, i.e., gloves, gowns, and goggles. Procedures not accomplished in the field are performed by team members during the survey.

The primary survey focuses attention upon the ABCs: patency of the airway, adequacy of breathing and circulation, the integrity of the cervical spine, and the status of the central nervous system. It is a focused, screening examination that takes no more than 30 to 60 seconds. Initial treatment (e.g., intravenous access) is not delayed by the assessment.

1. **Airway.** As in the prehospital setting, securing the patency and protection of the airway is the top priority of airway management (Chapter 2). The gag reflex is tested in patients with altered mental status. If the mechanism of injury does not suggest an injury to the spine, and either patency or protection is in jeopardy, orotracheal intubation is the choice for active airway management. If the cervical spine may be damaged and airway intervention is necessary, nasotracheal intubation or cricothyroidotomy is indicated.

2. **Breathing.** After the airway is assessed and secured, ventilatory status is checked. The structural integrity of the chest and ventilatory adequacy are determined. The chest is visually examined for evidence of equal excursion of the ribs and for paradoxical motion of any segment of the chest wall, i.e., flail chest. The thorax is palpated for bony crepitus or subcutaneous emphysema. Last, the lungs are percussed and auscultated for the presence, absence, equality, and abnormal quality of lung sounds. Symptoms and signs suggesting tension pneumothorax warrant immediate decompression. Significant pneumothorax or hemothorax requires a tube thoracostomy.

3. **Vital signs.** Accurate measurements of the pulse, blood pressure, respiratory rate, and temperature are essential. Beware of complacency if the vital signs are normal. Many young patients maintain "normal" vital signs until their compensatory mechanisms fail all at once. Older patients may be taking medications that block the normal responses to hypovolemia. Vital signs are continuously reassessed and are considered stable only after several hours of normal values.

4. **Unclothe the patient.** Immediately on arrival, the patient is completely undressed. The clothing is cut off if necessary. The patient's temperature and modesty are maintained by covering with a sheet. A diagnosis of serious injury can be missed or delayed without full exposure.

5. **Circulation.** Pulse rate and quality, blood pressure, capillary refill, and sites of obvious external hemorrhage are evaluated. Active bleeding is immediately controlled by local pressure. A palpable radial pulse is estimated as representing a systolic blood pressure (BP) of 80 mm Hg, a femoral pulse indicates a BP of 70 mm Hg, and a carotid pulse indicates a BP of 60 mm Hg.

6. **Cervical spine.** If the patient has altered consciousness or is uncooperative, and the mechanism of injury is consistent with cervical spine trauma, the patient's head and neck are immobilized. This is usually accomplished in the prehospital setting. Conscious and cooperative patients are asked about neck pain, and the neck is palpated for tenderness. If pain or tenderness is absent, they are asked to slowly raise the head. Patients who are pain free are unlikely to have a serious cervical spine injury. Immobilization is continued if warranted by the mechanism of injury.

7. **Neurologic examination.** Neurologic function is rapidly evaluated by checking the level of consciousness (eye opening and verbalizing) and gross movement of the extremities. The response of the patient to simple commands or painful stimuli is assessed.

Verbal contact may be made and brief reassurance given. Observation of extremity movement, either spontaneous or stimulated by verbal command or pain, provides information about spinal cord function.

Primary Resuscitation

Resuscitation of the patient proceeds in concert with the primary survey. In patients with hemorrhagic shock, estimating the amount of blood loss allows the physician to anticipate volume needs and whether blood is required. The information obtained from the primary survey is translated by a classification scheme used in the Advanced Trauma Life Support course (Table 4–5) to allow an estimate of blood loss.

Patients in all classes of shock require crystalloid replacement, usually an isotonic crystalloid solution. The amount necessary is estimated by these calculations:

Equation 1. Calculate the patient's blood volume by multiplying the estimated weight in kilograms by 70 ml blood/kg in adults (80 ml/kg in children).

Equation 2. Multiply the estimated percentage of blood loss (from the class the patient best represents) by the blood volume to get the estimated blood loss.

Equation 3. Multiply the estimated blood loss by 3 to get the estimated crystalloid replacement need.

The last equation uses the 3:1 replacement rule as a guide to crystalloid volume. The additional fluid is thought to replenish the volume shifted from the interstitial and intracellular space. Controversy continues about this rule, but it is a useful first guide. In class III or class IV hemorrhage, blood replacement is necessary. The amount of blood needed is estimated directly from equation 2. It is given in addition to the crystalloid volume from equation 3.

These data give an estimate only of the volume replacement requirements of the patient during the first several hours of care. The calculations assume that the hemorrhage has slowed or stopped. The physician should not over-rely on these numbers; they are only a starting point to gauge the degree of resuscitative effort needed. Serial measurements of the patient's vital signs, mental status, urine output, and other parameters are necessary for appropriate volume replacement. Often a lower replacement volume than that calculated is necessary, but it is influenced by patient condition, actual blood loss,

TABLE 4–5. Estimated Fluid and Blood Requirements for Acute Blood Loss*
(Based on Initial Presentation of the Patient)

	Class I	Class II	Class III	Class IV
Blood loss (ml)	Up to 750	750–1500	1500–2000	2000 or more
Blood loss (% blood volume)	Up to 15%	15%–30%	30%–40%	40% or more
Pulse rate	<100 beats/min	>100 beats/min	>120 beats/min	140 beats/min or higher
Blood pressure	Normal	Normal	Decreased	Decreased
Pulse pressure (mm Hg)	Normal or increased	Decreased	Decreased	Decreased
Capillary blanch test	Normal	Positive	Positive	Positive
Respiratory rate	14–20	20–30	30–40	>35
Urine output (ml/hr)	30 or more	20–30	5–15	Negligible
CNS-mental status	Slightly anxious	Mildly anxious	Anxious and confused	Confused, lethargic
Fluid replacement (3:1 rule)	Crystalloid	Crystalloid	Crystalloid + blood	Crystalloid + blood

*For a 70-kg male.
Adapted from American College of Surgeons Committee on Trauma: Advanced Trauma Life Support—Instructors' Manual. Chicago, American College of Surgeons, 1988.

other causes of shock, time to definitive care, and severity of injury. When in doubt, anticipate the worst.

Other early resuscitative efforts include:

1. **Oxygen supplementation.** High-flow oxygen, 10 to 12 liters/min, is given if no contraindications exist. It has been suggested that as many as 50% of trauma victims are hypoxic.

2. **Intravenous access.** A minimum of two large-bore catheters, at least 14 to 16 gauge, are needed. These lines are placed percutaneously in any easily accessible vein or by venous cutdown using the saphenous vein at the ankle. Central venous catheterization can be used for volume restoration, but unless the catheter is large, the additional length can cause increased resistance to flow. Measurement of central venous pressure (CVP) is not reliable, although low values (less than 3 cm water) are suggestive of decreased intravascular blood volume, and high values (more than 15 cm water) can be an early finding in cardiac tamponade or tension pneumothorax.

3. **Cardiac monitoring.** Monitoring of cardiac rhythm is important for those patients who may have sustained a cardiac contusion and are prone to dysrhythmias. The monitor "beep" provides auditory information about the heart rate.

4. **Volume resuscitation.** If the patient is in shock, fluid is infused as rapidly as possible (wide open IV lines) to return and maintain the mean arterial pressure (MAP) to 100 ± 10 mm Hg. The volume requirements are estimated from the calculations given above. Other indicators of perfusion are also utilized to determine the adequacy of volume restoration, such as improved color, decreasing diaphoresis, and improved mentation. If the patient is not easily classified or if hemorrhage continues and the vital signs are still abnormal after 2000 ml of crystalloid have been given, blood replacement is usually necessary and is administered. Patients presenting with normal vital signs are started on IV fluid at a rate of 150 ml/hr. The physician should be prepared to increase the amount of fluid if the patient's condition deteriorates. A central venous pressure (CVP) line may provide additional information if there is a risk of cardiac tamponade or cardiovascular compromise from fluid resuscitation due to an underlying problem, e.g., old age, diabetes, renal failure, cardiac insufficiency.

5. **Hematocrit.** The hematocrit provides a baseline value only, even in patients with major blood loss. Most trauma victims have a normal first hematocrit reading because too little time has elapsed for fluid shifts to occur. An initial low hematocrit means that the blood volume and oxygen-carrying capacity are at great risk. It may represent an anemia predating the trauma or time after injury sufficient for compensatory fluid shifts. Rapid crystalloid infusion can also decrease the hematocrit.

6. **Blood sample for type and cross-match.** A clotted blood sample is sent to the laboratory as soon as possible because the full cross-matching process may take up to 1 hour. Type-specific blood with ABO and Rh systems checked can be ready in 15 minutes. Notifying the laboratory of the situation and the patient's estimated needs often facilitates the process. Two units (500 ml) more than the estimated blood loss is a reasonable starting point.

7. **Blood administration.** Typed and cross-matched blood is preferred. However, if massive hemorrhage is obvious, type-specific (if ready) or type O blood is substituted. This category includes patients who do not respond to crystalloid infusion, deteriorate in spite of resuscitative efforts, or present with significant ongoing hemorrhage. The complication rate with either of these blood choices is extremely low.

8. **Vital signs.** Frequent repetition of measurement of vital signs and patient assessment is crucial to monitor and detect any change in condition. An accurate temperature (usually rectal) must be obtained early in the patient's care. Hypothermia is a common complication in multiple trauma.

9. **Pneumatic antishock garment.** The patient may have the PASG in place on arrival. These garments have a potential temporary use in hypotensive patients while volume replacement is established. They can tamponade abdominal, pelvic, and lower extremity hemorrhage and can serve as a pneumatic splint. Before removing the PASG,

the pressure should be released compartment by compartment while the vital signs are checked.

10. **Early radiographs.** A portable AP chest film and cross-table lateral view of the cervical spine are often ordered during the initial assessment. Appropriate management is not delayed or limited by waiting for these films.

PROBLEM 1 The patient was still unconscious on arrival in the emergency department. The vital signs were BP 100/60 mm Hg, pulse 104/min, and respirations 16/min. The patient was immediately intubated nasotracheally. His breath sounds were equal, and no obvious chest trauma was identified.

Although there were no secretions in the pharynx, intubation was indicated to protect the airway. The nasotracheal route was chosen because he may have a cervical spine injury. At least the vital signs had not deteriorated.

PROBLEM 2 (Note to reader: The comments in this case may point out areas of concern as a teaching method.) The shooting victim was carried into the emergency department. The entrance wound was found in the left chest at the third intercostal space in the midclavicular line; there was no exit wound. Vital signs were BP 100/64 mm Hg, pulse 112/min, and respirations 24/min. The skin felt moist, and the patient was confused. He was undressed and placed on oxygen; two IV lines were started, and a chest radiograph was ordered. While the film was being developed, cardiac arrest occurred.

The vital signs were clearly abnormal for a young patient, reflecting hypovolemia. The patient should have had an immediate chest tube inserted, not a chest radiograph. This would have permitted reexpansion of the collapsed lung and stopped the bleeding from the injured pulmonary parenchyma. Instead, the patient continued to hemorrhage to the point of cardiac arrest. Obstructive shock from cardiac tamponade or tension pneumothorax could also cause this result. The status of the patient's neck veins needed to be checked.

Although the cardiac arrest modified priorities, the patient's initial survey placed him in class IV shock. Blood and crystalloid were necessary. His estimated weight was 70 kg. Calculation of his estimated fluid needs proceeded as follows:
1. Seventy kg × 70 ml/kg equals 4900 ml blood volume. This is rounded to 5 liters.
2. Five thousand ml blood volume × 40% to 50% loss equals a blood loss of 2000 to 2500 ml.
3. A blood loss of 2000 to 2500 ml × 3 equals 6000 to 7500 ml crystalloid needed for replacement.

If the hemorrhage were stopped at the time of admission, this patient would have needed 2000 to 2500 ml of blood (four to five units) and 6000 to 7500 ml of crystalloid (six to eight 1-liter bags). Although an estimate, the calculation lets the physician gauge the severity of the hemorrhage and realize just how far behind he is in volume restoration. This is another reason for not delaying treatment to process a chest radiograph.

DATA GATHERING

Once the immediate life-threatening injuries have been found and managed, a complete history and a head-to-toe secondary survey are necessary.

History

The history as related by the prehospital caregivers or other observers can be explored at this point for other important information. If possible, the patient is questioned about the event and recall assessed. Amnesia for the traumatic incident suggests at least momentary loss of consciousness and probable concussion. Other useful data include:

1. Events preceding the trauma. These may be valuable in indicating other problems (e.g., a suicide attempt)
2. Ethanol or drug use
3. Past medical history
4. Medications
5. Allergies
6. Last meal, in anticipation of anesthesia risk
7. Tetanus status

Physical Examination

Since multiple trauma involves injury to two or more organ systems, a complete, careful examination (secondary survey) is needed to avoid overlooking significant injuries not discovered during the primary survey (Table 4–6). It is also a time to reassess the effectiveness of the procedures and therapies given thus far, e.g., the vital signs and position of the endotracheal tube are rechecked.

DECISION PRIORITIES AND PRELIMINARY DIFFERENTIAL DIAGNOSIS

As the initial resuscitation effort and data gathering progress, the physician must form a preliminary impression of the severity of the injuries by answering the following questions:

1. *What are the immediate life-threatening problems and have they been addressed?*
   Immediate threats to life should be managed during the primary survey; however, they may appear at any point in the patient's course. They include:
   a. Loss of airway patency or protection
   b. Inadequacy of oxygenation or ventilation
   c. Inadequate volume restoration
   d. Cardiac tamponade or tension pneumothorax
   e. Uncontrolled hemorrhage
2. *Does the patient require immediate surgical intervention?*
   Once the immediate threats to life have been addressed, the next decision is whether the patient needs immediate surgery. Patients with obvious major hemorrhage (i.e., shock with increasing abdominal distention), with unexplained, persistent shock, or with obvious injury necessitating repair such as a gunshot wound of the abdomen should be taken directly to the operating room. Patients not requiring emergency surgery can undergo more extensive evaluation and diagnostic efforts.

DIAGNOSTIC ADJUNCTS

Radiologic Imaging—Plain Films

For victims of blunt trauma, portable radiographs are obtained first, including an anteroposterior (AP) view of the chest, a lateral view of the cervical spine, and an AP view of the pelvis.

1. Anteroposterior chest radiograph. This screening film is used to assess pulmonary, cardiac, mediastinal, and diaphragmatic injury and the placement of tubes and catheters. If possible, the chest series should be completed in the radiology department.

TABLE 4–6. Secondary Survey: Physical Examination in the Multiple Trauma Patient

Area of Examination	Specific Component	Comments
Vital signs	Heart rate/pulse	Tachycardia suggests hypovolemia, possible myocardial contusion; assess symmetry, presence or absence of pulses
	Blood pressure	Hypotension suggests hypovolemia, tension pneumothorax, or cardiac tamponade
	Respiratory rate	Tachypnea is an early sign of shock, pulmonary contusion, or inadequate ventilation or oxygenation from other causes, especially tension pneumothorax
	Rectal temperature	Hypothermia is easily missed in patients exposed to outside environment, air-conditioned emergency department, and unwarmed resuscitation fluids
General appearance	Observe position, movement, diaphoresis, color, smell of clothes and breath	Rough gauge of distress; ethanol adds to complications and worsens prognosis; a speaking patient allows a quick assessment of CNS, airway, voice, and respiratory status
Head	Scalp/skull	Palpate for hematomas, depressed fracture, mastoid hematoma (Battle's sign)
	Eyes	Altered pupil size and reactivity suggest intracranial injury or complicating ingestant; palpate orbital rims; assess visual acuity
	Ears	Blood behind tympanic membrane (TM) is consistent with basilar skull fracture; blood in ear canal may be from outside, canal laceration, or ruptured TM
	Nose	Palpate for fracture; check cerebrospinal fluid (CSF) leak (because patient must sit up, this is usually assessed later in the course of care)
	Mouth	Check teeth, bite—if misaligned or pain, mandibular fracture may be present. Check for mobility of maxilla
Neck	Observation	Neck vein distention, position of trachea, shape of larynx
	Palpation	Tenderness, crepitus, or anatomic abnormality (e.g., step-off cervical spine anteriorly or posteriorly)
Chest (repeated)	Observation	Symmetric expansion of chest, paradoxical motion suggests flail chest
	Palpation	Feel for subcutaneous emphysema, bony crepitus; percuss for hyperresonance (air) or dullness (fluid)
	Auscultation	Equality, presence, or absence of breath sounds
Abdomen (repeated)	Observation	Look for increasing distention
	Palpation	Feel for tenderness, rebound, masses
	Auscultation	Generally not useful because trauma may induce ileus; bruits may be heard
Genitalia	Observation	Blood at urethral meatus in males suggests urethral tear, possible pelvic or prostatic disruption
Rectum	Observation, digital examination	Check for sphincter tone, sensation, gross blood, and position of prostate in males (potential of urethral tear, associated pelvic fracture)
Extremities	Observation	Note position, obvious deformities, source of blood loss
	Palpation	Feel for tenderness, deformities, bony crepitus, distal pulses
Neurologic (repeated)	Central and peripheral	Note altered sensorium, symmetric motor function/strength, sensory levels; repeat coma scale

2. Cross-table lateral view of cervical spine. This film is often examined first because it influences the decision on airway management and patient immobilization. It has a diagnostic accuracy of 90% to 95% in demonstrating significant findings consistent with risk to the spinal cord. Still, anyone with a highly suspicious history, neck pain, or neurologic finding should remain immobilized until the other standard views of the cervical spine are cleared. If suspicion of injury remains, tomography, computed tomography, or magnetic resonance imaging are ordered as necessary. In patients with suspicious findings, a conservative approach and consultation with a radiologist are recommended. A normal cervical spine series does not preclude an adequate neurologic examination. Spinal injury and spinal cord syndromes can occur with a normal bony alignment.

3. Anteroposterior pelvis radiograph. This high-yield film is taken to determine possible fractures and the potential source of major blood loss. Additional portable films, e.g., of the long bones or joints, may be ordered if the patient's condition is unstable.

Patients who have sustained penetrating wounds generally undergo radiologic evaluation of the organs near the involved site only. One exception exists in cases in which there is a possibility of a ricocheted or embolic projectile. Because of symptoms or an inability to find a missile that has not exited the body, a plain film series is done, surveying adjacent sites first and, if necessary, the entire body until the projectile is located.

Radiologic Imaging—Special Studies

Specialized radiologic studies such as intravenous pyelograms, angiograms, and computed tomograms may also be necessary in patients with hematuria, suspected arterial injury, or head or abdominal trauma. *Patients are never sent to the radiology department until it has been demonstrated that they are stable. That is, vital signs remain within normal range after two to three measurements and sources of major injury have been found. All films are taken as "portable" up to that time.*

Laboratory Studies

Laboratory studies include a complete blood count, electrolytes, blood urea nitrogen, glucose, creatinine, blood type and cross-match (if not already done), and other studies as indicated, such as amylase level, ethanol level, toxicology screens, arterial blood gases, and coagulation studies. Urinalysis is performed, and a dipstick test for blood is done early in the patient's care. Results will influence the need for contrast studies of the urinary tract. Many institutions have the results of several of these studies predefined and identified as a trauma panel (Table 4–7). It must be remembered that none of these studies help in the acute management and decision-making phase of patient care.

TABLE 4–7. Laboratory Trauma Panel

Test	Comment
Complete blood count	Hemoglobin–hematocrit often normal. Lower levels represent patient's previous condition or significant blood loss. Baseline needed in advance of volume resuscitation
Electrolytes	Baseline needed in advance of volume resuscitation
Blood urea nitrogen	Shows baseline renal function. May be elevated in patients with shock or increased protein load, e.g., gastrointestinal absorbed RBCs
Blood glucose	Usually elevated; if low, it may be the cause of trauma; hypoglycemia is corrected rapidly
Creatinine	Shows baseline renal function
Type and cross-match	Amount derived from estimated blood loss plus two units to anticipate needs. Complete cross-match can be interrupted at any time after "typing" for emergent transfusion

Electrocardiogram (ECG)

An electrocardiogram is indicated in multiple trauma patients. A myocardial infarction may have caused the trauma or may result from the physiologic stress. The patient may have a myocardial contusion secondary to blunt trauma to the anterior chest wall. The mechanism of injury, e.g., abrupt deceleration, can assist in this decision.

Diagnostic-Therapeutic Procedures—Nasogastric Tube and Foley Catheter

A nasogastric tube and Foley catheter are indicated in the multiple trauma victim. They often supply clinical information while providing treatment at the same time. The nasogastric tube can empty the stomach as well as determine the presence of blood in the upper gastrointestinal tract. Prior to insertion of the Foley catheter, rectal examination should confirm the normal position of the prostate, and the urethral meatus is checked for blood. If the prostate is "floating" or high riding or if blood is noted at the meatus, urethral injury is strongly suggested, and catheterization is deferred in favor of urethrography. The urine should be immediately tested for blood. Monitoring of urine flow is a rough guide to whether the patient's central perfusion is responding to the resuscitation attempt.

Special Studies—Evaluation of Abdomen: Diagnostic Peritoneal Lavage/Computed Tomography

Evaluation of the abdominal cavity for visceral injury is often difficult. Patients with altered levels of consciousness due to drugs, alcohol, head injury, or other major injury often do not perceive abdominal pain or tenderness. Diagnostic peritoneal lavage (DPL) and computed tomography are important procedures in evaluating the abdomen.

Diagnostic Peritoneal Lavage. DPL involves the insertion of a peritoneal dialysis catheter into the abdomen just below the umbilicus and aspirating the peritoneal space for blood. A nasogastric tube and Foley catheter must be in place in order to decompress the stomach and bladder prior to inserting the dialysis catheter. The catheter may be inserted percutaneously but is often placed as a surgical procedure with direct visualization of the peritoneal membrane. The test results are positive if 10 ml of gross blood are aspirated. If the test results are negative, 1 liter in adults and 10 ml/kg in children of isotonic crystalloid are infused and then drained. An aliquot of the sample is tested for red and white blood cell counts, amylase, and alkaline phosphatase. Positive results are red blood cell counts of more than 50,000 to 100,000/mm^3 after lavage for blunt trauma or more than 5000/mm^3 for suspected penetrating gunshot wound. White blood cell counts of more than 500/mm^3 are abnormal. Gross bacterial contamination is considered a positive finding. Amylase (more than 200 μ/dl) is a late finding that may be useful in discriminating between equivocal results. Alkaline phosphatase (more than 25 μ) has been found as a marker in small bowel injuries. With these combined data, positive results on DPL can determine the need for surgical exploration in 90% of blunt trauma cases. Patients with negative results on DPL are admitted for observation. The physical examination may be confusing after DPL because of the pain and distention caused by the procedure. There is a 5% chance of a false-negative interpretation.

Computed Tomography. CT may noninvasively evaluate the abdomen for possible injury. It can localize blood and identify sites of injury and does not change the physical examination. The patient's condition must be sufficiently stable to allow him to go to the radiology area, and this is a major differentiating factor in choosing it over DPL. The timing and selection of DPL versus CT are currently under debate and depend on local practice.

During all of these diagnostic efforts it is important to reassess continually the patient's status, vital signs, and neurologic signs and to note any changes that occur with time.

PROBLEM 1 The evaluation of the patient who hit the tree with his car has progressed. Cervical spine and pelvis radiographs were normal. The chest radiograph was interpreted as showing a widened mediastinum suggesting possible aortic disruption. DPL was performed and proved to be grossly negative for blood.

Although the patient may have an aortic tear, he had survived long enough for other potentially life-threatening problems to be diagnosed. Therefore, he underwent peritoneal lavage before going to angiography. The DPL was performed because the patient could not cooperate with the physical examination. The finding of additional injuries in a patient presenting primarily with head trauma is typical of blunt trauma.

PRINCIPLES OF MANAGEMENT

Optimal management of the trauma victim depends on careful orchestration of the evaluation and resuscitation efforts. Although many elements have been discussed in the initial approach, some repetition is necessary. The emergency physician must proceed rapidly, thoroughly, and in an orderly fashion to evaluate the patient and the potential injuries. As with any emergency patient, the guiding principle is always to assume the presence of the worst possible injury consistent with the mechanism of injury and then to prove that it is not there. Findings inconsistent with the mechanism of injury require further exploration of the history, physical examination, and possible causes of trauma.

The following outline summarizes the general sequence:
1. **Anticipation.** Based on the information provided by the rescue squad, the emergency physician anticipates the likely injuries based on the mechanism of injury and makes the appropriate preparations.
2. **Initial evaluation.** A primary survey is performed to identify the immediate life-threatening injuries. Blood loss is estimated.
3. **Stabilization.** Life-threatening processes found during the primary survey are corrected.
   a. Oxygen is given to prevent *hypoxemia* after the airway and ventilation are ensured.
   b. Intravenous access is established, and fluid is administered to correct *hypovolemia*.
   c. *Hemorrhage* is *controlled*.
   d. The spinal column *is immobilized*.
4. **Secondary survey.** This survey comprises a complete head-to-toe examination.
5. **Diagnostic measures.** Appropriate radiologic and laboratory studies are ordered.

Up to this point, no mention has been made of consultations. Ideally, an organized trauma team or service exists and is mobilized for these patients. The trauma surgeon and team are notified as soon as the emergency physician is informed of the imminent arrival of a trauma victim. The emergency physician and surgeon work side by side during the resuscitative effort. Additional consultants such as orthopedists and neurosurgeons are contacted as additional needs are defined.

As mentioned before, the orchestration and timing of the resuscitation effort and procedures are crucial components in successful management. When multiple injuries are present, prioritization of the numerous diagnostic measures needed becomes crucial.

Tetanus prophylaxis is easily overlooked in the concerns and urgency of treating the patient with multiple injuries, yet it must not be forgotten. If the patient can provide a history of having an up-to-date tetanus immunization, the injection is not given; however, if the patient is unsure or is unable to provide the information, tetanus prophylaxis should be administered. All too often, if it is not given in the emergency department, it is never given.

Antibiotic administration is indicated for such injuries as open fractures and suspected bowel wounds, but in general, antibiotic prophylaxis is not routinely warranted.

SPECIAL CONSIDERATIONS

Pediatric Patients

Blunt trauma accounts for 80% to 90% of pediatric trauma. Head injury is the most common finding in these patients. The major causes of trauma are motor vehicle accidents (50%), child abuse (15%), accidental falls (15%), drowning (10%), and burns (5% to 10%). Most emergency physicians have limited experience with pediatric trauma. The development of the Pediatric Trauma Score as a valid instrument of predicting injury severity and outcome is an important advance because it focuses attention on the critical areas in pediatric trauma assessment and offers a guide to interpreting the findings (Table 4–8).

The general principles of management and evaluation of pediatric patients are the same as those used for adults. A number of special considerations apply:

1. Vital signs in children differ from those in adults and must be interpreted based on the normal values for a specific age (Table 4–9).

2. Fluid resuscitation is begun carefully with a bolus infusion of 20 ml/kg. Because of the patients' smaller size and smaller blood volume, uncontrolled fluid administration can lead to significant complications. Venous access is often difficult in young children. Interosseous infusion is an alternative method for fluid delivery. In this method a special or spinal needle is inserted into the marrow space of the distal femur or proximal tibia, and crystalloid is given through it.

TABLE 4–8. The Pediatric Trauma Score and Prediction of Mortality

Component	Pediatric Trauma Score Severity Category		
	+2	+1	−1
Body size	>20 kg	10–20 kg	<10 kg
Airway	Normal	Maintainable	Unmaintainable
CNS	Awake	Obtunded	Comatose
Systolic BP	>90 mm Hg	90–50 mm Hg	<50 mm Hg
Open wounds	None	Minor	Major or penetrating
Skeletal injury	None	Closed fracture	Open/multiple fracture

[a]If proper sized BP cuff not available, BP can be assessed by assigning: +2 = pulse palpable at wrist; +1 = pulse palpable at groin; −1 = no pulse palpable.

Mortality Associated with Individual Pediatric Trauma Scores

Pediatric Trauma Score	Mortality (%)[b]
−1 to −6	100
0	99
+1	88
+2	76
+3	61
+4	51
+5	37
+6	24
+7	10
+8	2
>+9	0

[b]National Pediatric Trauma Registry

Modified from Ramenofsky ML, Ramenofsky MB, Jurkovich GJ, et al: The predictive validity of the pediatric trauma score. J Trauma 28(7):1038–1042, © by Williams & Wilkins, 1988.

TABLE 4–9. Pediatric Vital Signs

Age	Respirations (per min)	Pulse (beats/min)
Newborn–1 year	20–30	120–130
2 years–4 years	16–24	120
4 years–8 years	12–18	100
>10 years	10–14	70–80

3. Heat loss is a greater problem in children because of the proportionately larger body surface area.

4. Cervical spine injuries are less common, but when they are present radiographs of the neck are more commonly interpreted as negative.

5. Patterns of automobile versus pedestrian or bicycle injury include the same femur, chest, and head injuries seen in adults. Neck, head, and chest injuries occur from inappropriate car seat (in seat but unrestrained) or shoulder harness use.

6. Suspected child abuse is discussed in Chapter 38.

Burns

Burns represent a specialized type of trauma involving the skin, subcutaneous structures, and occasionally deeper organs such as muscle.

1. Numerous formulas exist for calculating the fluid requirements for a burn victim. A general guideline is 2 to 4 ml of isotonic crystalloid solution times the percentage of body surface area burned up to 50% times the weight in kilograms. Subsequent fluid replacement volumes are guided by central hemodynamic monitoring, vital signs, and urinary output.

2. Systemic prophylactic antibiotics are not indicated.

3. Exposure to smoke increases the possibility of carbon monoxide or other toxic poisoning.

4. Direct referral or transport to a burn center is recommended.

Trauma Arrest

The management of the trauma victim who arrives in or rapidly deteriorates into cardiac arrest represents a special challenge. The injuries that are most amenable to treatment involve major vascular hemorrhage or cardiac tamponade. These wounds occur most often after penetrating injury that causes relatively isolated trauma. Thus, victims of stab or gunshot wounds are most likely to benefit from aggressive and invasive resuscitation. These patients should undergo immediate thoracotomy in the emergency department. Victims of blunt trauma usually have sustained injuries to multiple organ systems and are unlikely to respond. Except in rare circumstances, patients with blunt injury who suffer cardiac arrest should generally be pronounced dead and not undergo heroic resuscitative efforts.

Emergency thoracotomy is performed by making an incision in the left fourth intercostal space from the sternal border to the midaxillary line. The chest is entered through this incision, and the following procedures are performed:

1. Cross-clamp of the aorta to preserve blood flow above the diaphragm.

2. Opening of the pericardium to determine the presence of and relieve tamponade.

3. Control of hemorrhage and repair of cardiac or vascular wounds. Cross-clamping of the pulmonary hilum may be necessary.

PROBLEM 2 Because of the rapidity of deterioration of the patient's condition and the penetrating injury, an emergency thoracotomy was performed. Instead of 2000 to 3000 ml of blood in the hemithorax as anticipated, there was only 200 ml. A tense pericardium was noted and opened with a gush of 100 ml of blood. The patient regained a pulse. On inspection, a small hole in the left auricle was noted. It was gently clamped to await definitive surgical care.

The outcome in this case is more the exception than the rule. A tremendous amount of work remains to be done in this patient's care. Continued volume resuscitation, ventilation, cardiac repair, and sedation are necessary. The emergency physician must maintain skills in a variety of procedures that may be used infrequently, e.g., thoracotomy, skull trephination.

DISPOSITION AND FOLLOW-UP

The disposition of the trauma victim depends on the response to the initial resuscitation effort, the primary survey, and the subsequent complete diagnostic evaluation. At any point in the sequence, if the patient manifests unstable vital signs and a site of significant hemorrhage has been identified, the patient is taken to the operating room for surgical control of the bleeding site.

If the physical examination reveals multiple injuries but no obvious need for surgery, the patient is admitted to the hospital. The choice of intensive care versus floor admission depends on the injuries diagnosed and the need for close observation and monitoring.

PROBLEM 1 The patient was given a full evaluation. All plain films were negative. The DPL results were negative, and the head CT was normal, yet the patient was still comatose. The laboratory called and informed the physician that the patient had a blood sugar level of 22 mg/dl. After 50 ml of dextrose 50% had been given, the patient awakened and told the physician that he was a diabetic on insulin, had taken today's dose but hadn't eaten because he was late for work.

Accidents frequently occur as a result of underlying medical illnesses such as diabetes mellitus, epilepsy, myocardial infarction, dysrhythmias, or cerebrovascular accident. Careful evaluation for associated disease must be performed as an integral part of the trauma assessment.

DOCUMENTATION

1. History
   Mechanism of injury
   Medications and allergies
   Past medical history
2. Prehospital care
   Findings at the scene
   Treatment rendered
   Response to treatment
3. Emergency department physical examination
   Complete examination findings (including pertinent negatives)
4. Laboratory and radiologic studies
   Documentation of tests ordered and results
5. Emergency department course
   Record of response to treatment, consultation, and disposition

SUMMARY AND FINAL POINTS

- The care of the victim of trauma requires an organized and disciplined approach to identifying and treating injuries and to making decisions.

- The recommended approach evaluates the potential immediate life-threatening problems first and avoids focusing on obvious, visible soft tissue and extremity injuries.
- The reasons for the traumatic incident, e.g., other diseases or patient intent, are always explored.
- Serial examination is central to success in trauma care.
- Physiologic parameters, mechanism of injury, and actual anatomic injury all play a role in the field and hospital triage and treatment decision-making process.
- Volume resuscitation efforts are based on an estimate of present blood loss and a projection of ongoing losses plus compensatory fluid shifts.
- Multiple trauma deaths continue to occur because of too little anticipation, too little intervention, and too late implementation.

BIBLIOGRAPHY

Texts

1. American College of Surgeons Committee on Trauma: Advanced Trauma Life Support. Chicago, American College of Surgeons, 1988.
2. Jorden RC, Rosen P: Airway management in the acutely injured. In Moore EE, Eiseman B, Van Way CW, III (eds): Critical Decisions in Trauma. St. Louis, C.V. Mosby, 1984.
3. Martinez R: Injuries: Patterns and Prevention. Dallas, American College of Emergency Physicians, 1988.
4. Moore EE: Resuscitation and evaluation of the injured patient. In Zuidema GD, Rutherford RB, Ballinger WF (eds): The Management of Trauma (4th ed). Philadelphia, W.B. Saunders, 1985.

Journal Articles

1. Blumberg M, Bove JR: Un-cross-matched blood for emergency transfusion. JAMA 240:2057, 1978.
2. Charlton OP, Gehweiler JA, Martinez S: Roentgenographic evaluation of cervical spine trauma. JAMA 243:1073, 1979.
3. Champion HR, Sacco WJ: Measurement of injury severity and its practical application. Trauma Q 1(4):25–36, 1984.
4. Cwinn AA, Pons PT, Moore EE, et al: Prehospital advanced life support for critically injured victims of blunt trauma. Ann Emerg Med 16:399, 1987.
5. Federle MP, Crass RA, Jeffrey RB, et al: Computed tomography in blunt abdominal trauma. Arch Surg 117:645, 1982.
6. Kreis DJ, Fine EG, Gomez GA, et al: A prospective evaluation of field categorization of trauma patients. J Trauma 28(7):995–1000, 1988.
7. Majernick TG, Bieniek R, Houston JB, et al: Cervical spine movement during orotracheal intubation. Ann Emerg Med 15:417, 1986.
8. Mattox KL, Bickell WH, Pepe PE, et al: Prospective randomized evaluation of antishock M.A.S.T. in post-traumatic hypotension. J Trauma 26:779, 1986.
9. Pons PT, Honigman B, Moore EE, et al: Prehospital advanced trauma life support for critical penetrating wounds to the thorax and abdomen. J Trauma 25:828, 1985.
10. Shaffer MA, Doris PE: Limitations of the cross table lateral view in detecting cervical spine injuries: A retrospective analysis. Ann Emerg Med 10:508, 1981.
11. Smith JP, Bodai BI, Hill AS, et al: Prehospital stabilization of critically injured patients: A failed concept. J Trauma 25:65, 1985.

SECTION TWO

ABDOMINAL AND GASTROINTESTINAL DISORDERS

CHAPTER 5

ACUTE ABDOMINAL PAIN

JAMES W. HOEKSTRA, M.D.

PROBLEM 1 A 70 year old female presents to the emergency department with severe low back pain and lightheadedness of 6 hours' duration. She had passed out once at home.

PROBLEM 2 A 20 year old male presents to the emergency department with fever, burning epigastric pain, and vomiting of 8 hours' duration. He now complains of pain in the right lower quadrant as well.

QUESTIONS TO CONSIDER

1. What are the mechanisms of pain transmission in the abdomen, and how do they help define a differential diagnosis?
2. What are the potentially life-threatening causes of acute abdominal pain?
3. What is nonspecific abdominal pain?
4. What constitutes an acute surgical condition of the abdomen?
5. What are the basic steps in the stabilization and initial management of abdominal emergencies?
6. What are the life-threatening extra-abdominal causes of abdominal pain?
7. What laboratory studies, radiographs, and other tests are helpful in the evaluation of abdominal pain?
8. When is pain relief appropriate for patients with abdominal pain?
9. Which patients with abdominal pain can be safely sent home after evaluation?

INTRODUCTION

Acute abdominal pain is the presenting complaint in approximately 5% of emergency department visits. It comprises about one-third of the surgical problems seen. Of patients presenting with abdominal pain, approximately 15% to 30% will require a surgical procedure. In selected patient populations such as the elderly, this percentage is even higher.

The most common diagnosis made in patients with acute abdominal pain presenting to the emergency department is nonspecific abdominal pain. It is found in 40% to 60% of patients. Nonspecific pain is defined as abdominal pain for which no organic disease can be found after an extensive work-up. Gastroenteritis is the second most common diagnosis, followed by pelvic inflammatory disease, urinary tract disease, appendicitis, cholecystitis, and bowel obstruction. Appendicitis is the most common surgical diagnosis and is present in 4% to 24% of patients with acute abdominal pain presenting to emergency departments. Cholecystitis, bowel obstruction, perforated ulcer, and pancreatitis are common causes of surgical abdominal pain in descending order of frequency (Table 5–1).

TABLE 5–1. Common Causes of Abdominal Pain in the Emergency Department for All Age Groups

Cause	Percentage
Abdominal pain of unknown cause	41.3
Gastroenteritis	6.9
Pelvic inflammatory disease	6.7
Urinary tract infection	5.2
Ureteral stone	4.3
Appendicitis	4.3
Acute cholecystitis	2.5
Intestinal obstruction	2.5
Constipation	2.3
Duodenal ulcer	2.0
Dysmenorrhea	1.8
Pregnancy	1.8
Pyelonephritis	1.7
Gastritis	1.4
Other causes	15.3

Modified from Brewer RJ, et al: Abdominal pain: An analysis of 1000 consecutive cases in a university hospital emergency room. Am J Surg 131:219–223, 1976.

Neuroanatomy of Pain Transmission

The diagnosis of abdominal pain is aided by an understanding of the anatomy and physiology of the peritoneum, the intra-abdominal viscera, and the neural pain pathways.

Visceral pain is generated by stretch receptors located in the visceral peritoneum surrounding hollow organs and the capsules of solid organs. Distention or ischemia of the abdominal organs stimulates these receptors. Because these organs are simultaneously innervated from both sides of the spinal column, most visceral pain is midline in nature. Because visceral pain fibers are bilateral and unmyelinated and enter the spinal cord at multiple levels, visceral pain tends to be dull, achy, crampy, and poorly localized. It is often associated with "visceral" symptoms such as nausea, vomiting, and diaphoresis. It usually cannot be localized to a certain organ, but, given the neural pathways, certain organ groups can be implicated based on the location of the discomfort. Visceral pain from the liver, stomach, gallbladder, and duodenum is generally felt in the epigastrium. Pain from the small intestine, appendix, and cecum is felt in the periumbilical area, and pain from the colon, kidneys, bladder, and pelvic organs is felt in the hypogastrium. Ischemia and inflammation lower the threshold for the perception of this type of pain.

Somatic pain is initiated by pain receptors located in the parietal peritoneum and the roots of the mesentery. Pain produced by ischemia, inflammation, or stretch of the parietal peritoneum is transmitted through myelinated afferent fibers to specific dorsal root ganglia on the same side and at the same dermatomal level as the origin of the pain. This type of pain is more sharp, discrete, and localized. It is responsible for the physical findings of tenderness to palpation, guarding, and rebound. The finding of somatic pain often allows anatomic localization of pain to a specific organ. Given somatic tenderness in a certain quadrant, the differential diagnosis can be narrowed down solely by anatomic elimination as shown in Figure 5–1.

Referred pain is pain that is felt at a cutaneous site distant from the diseased organ. These cutaneous areas are supplied by the same or adjacent dermatomes as the diseased organ. For instance, visceral afferents from the diaphragm enter the spinal cord at C3–C5. Pain from the diaphragm is thus referred to the cutaneous distribution of C3–C5, the lateral neck and posterior shoulder. Knowledge of the visceral pain pathways allows one to predict the common referred pain pathways as shown in Figure 5–2. It is important to note that extra-abdominal organs can cause referred pain to the abdomen by a similar mechanism. Because the lungs and abdomen share the T9 dermatome distribution, pulmonic processes such as pneumonia and pulmonary embolus can be perceived as abdominal pain. Pelvic and inguinal structures innervated by T11 and T12 can cause

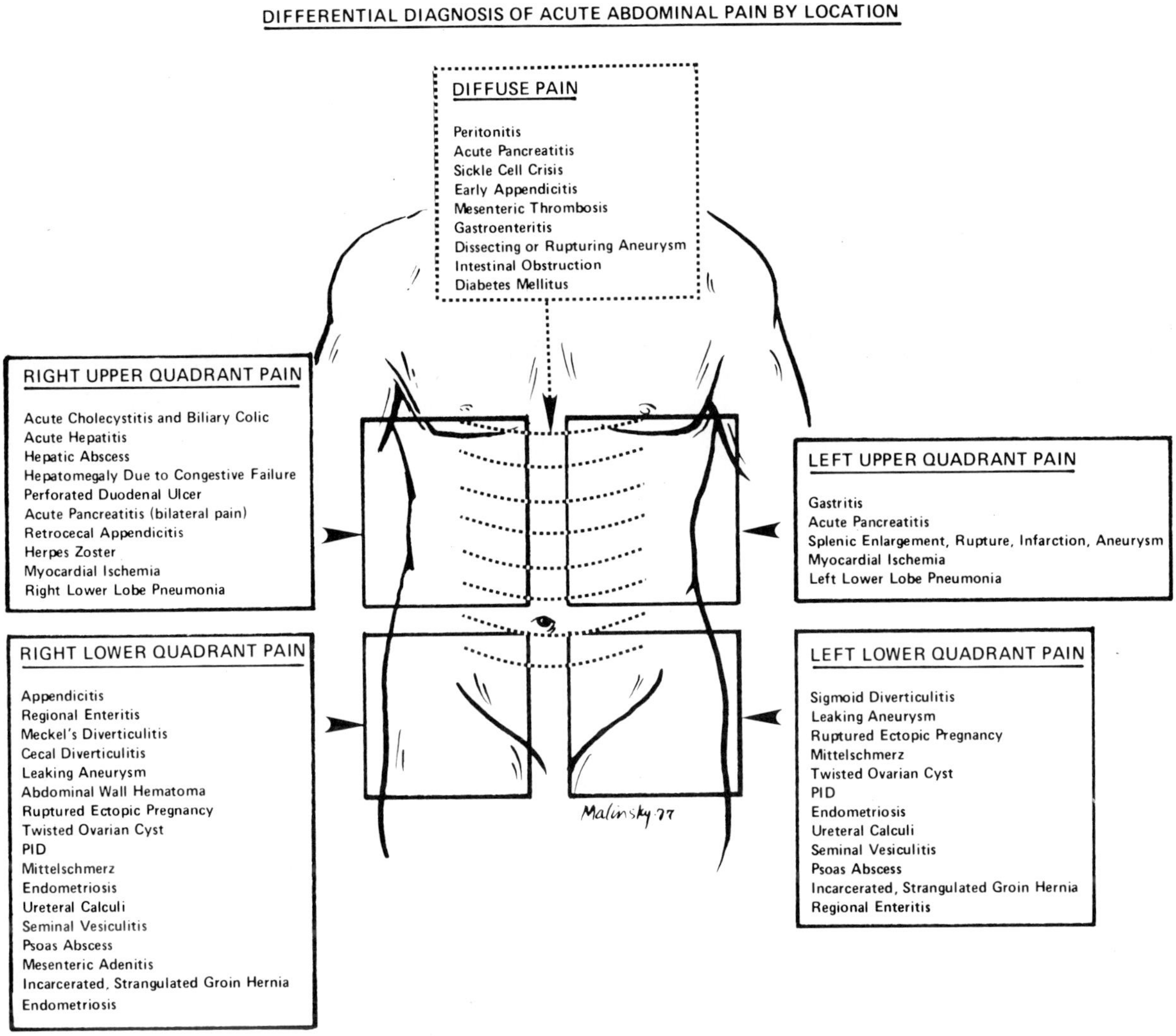

DIFFERENTIAL DIAGNOSIS OF ACUTE ABDOMINAL PAIN BY LOCATION

DIFFUSE PAIN

- Peritonitis
- Acute Pancreatitis
- Sickle Cell Crisis
- Early Appendicitis
- Mesenteric Thrombosis
- Gastroenteritis
- Dissecting or Rupturing Aneurysm
- Intestinal Obstruction
- Diabetes Mellitus

RIGHT UPPER QUADRANT PAIN

- Acute Cholecystitis and Biliary Colic
- Acute Hepatitis
- Hepatic Abscess
- Hepatomegaly Due to Congestive Failure
- Perforated Duodenal Ulcer
- Acute Pancreatitis (bilateral pain)
- Retrocecal Appendicitis
- Herpes Zoster
- Myocardial Ischemia
- Right Lower Lobe Pneumonia

LEFT UPPER QUADRANT PAIN

- Gastritis
- Acute Pancreatitis
- Splenic Enlargement, Rupture, Infarction, Aneurysm
- Myocardial Ischemia
- Left Lower Lobe Pneumonia

RIGHT LOWER QUADRANT PAIN

- Appendicitis
- Regional Enteritis
- Meckel's Diverticulitis
- Cecal Diverticulitis
- Leaking Aneurysm
- Abdominal Wall Hematoma
- Ruptured Ectopic Pregnancy
- Twisted Ovarian Cyst
- PID
- Mittelschmerz
- Endometriosis
- Ureteral Calculi
- Seminal Vesiculitis
- Psoas Abscess
- Mesenteric Adenitis
- Incarcerated, Strangulated Groin Hernia
- Endometriosis

LEFT LOWER QUADRANT PAIN

- Sigmoid Diverticulitis
- Leaking Aneurysm
- Ruptured Ectopic Pregnancy
- Mittelschmerz
- Twisted Ovarian Cyst
- PID
- Endometriosis
- Ureteral Calculi
- Seminal Vesiculitis
- Psoas Abscess
- Incarcerated, Strangulated Groin Hernia
- Regional Enteritis

FIGURE 5–1. Differential diagnosis of acute abdominal pain by location. (From Wagner DK: Approaches to the patient with acute abdominal pain. Current Topics *(a program of the Medical College of Pennsylvania), 1:3, 1978. Used by permission.)*

referred pain to the lower abdomen. Most notable is the perception of epigastric abdominal pain in association with myocardial infarction. Interestingly, a preexisting disease process can influence the perceived site of origin of a new process. For example, epigastric discomfort as a symptom of cardiac ischemia can occur more often if there is prior gallbladder or peptic ulcer disease.

PREHOSPITAL CARE

After arriving on the scene, the rescue squad can initiate several evaluation and stabilization measures. The basic data to be obtained include:

History

Pain History. Onset, duration, and location of the pain are important. Any associated symptoms, e.g., nausea, vomiting, diarrhea, bleeding, or syncope, are determined.

86 — ABDOMINAL AND GASTROINTESTINAL DISORDERS

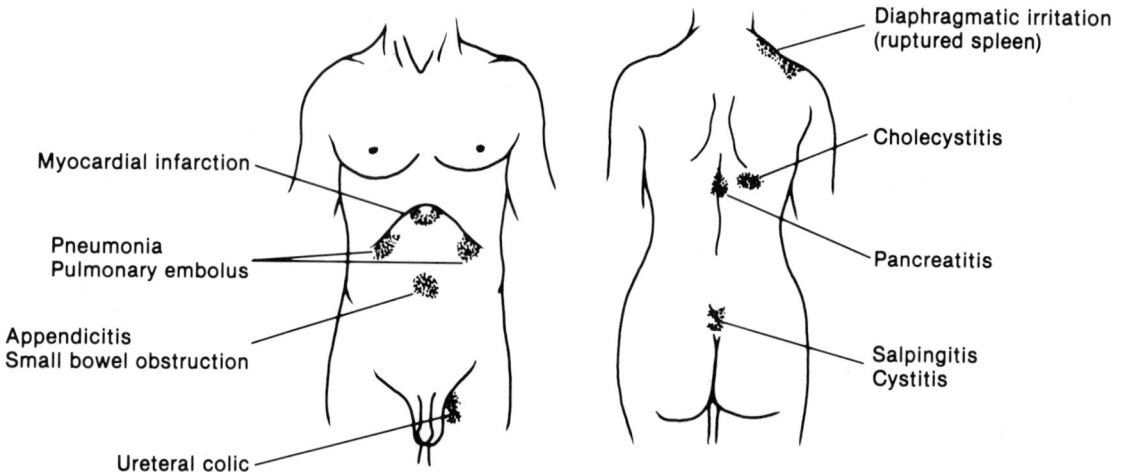

FIGURE 5–2. Referred pain patterns. Pain or discomfort in these areas often provides clues to underlying disease process. (From Trott AT: Acute abdominal pain. In Rosen P, et al [eds]: Emergency Medicine: Concepts and Clinical Practice. St. Louis, CV Mosby, 1988.)

Past Medical History. The pertinent related medical history and medications are obtained. These include a history of myocardial infarction, hypertension, vascular disease, or kidney stones.

Physical Examination

Vital Signs. Blood pressure, pulse, and respiratory rate are essential in patients with abdominal pain because they help gauge the severity of illness. Level of consciousness and patient's tolerance of the pain are important.

Brief Examination. The prehospital personnel can perform a brief abdominal examination to assess the location and severity of tenderness, presence of abdominal distention, discoloration, or bruising. Breath sounds are important in patients in whom extra-abdominal causes of abdominal pain are being considered.

Intervention

Intravenous Access. At least one peripheral IV line, 14 or 16 gauge, is recommended. Another is added when hypovolemia, bleeding, or sepsis is suspected. An isotonic crystalloid such as lactated Ringer's solution or normal saline is the solution of choice. Vigor of fluid resuscitation is dictated by the vital signs, physical findings, and medical history (see Chap. 4).

Pneumatic Antishock Garment. A PASG can be applied in selected circumstances in which hypovolemic shock is a complication, e.g., suspected rupture of an abdominal aortic aneurysm.

Analgesia. Pain medication is not given, except in very extenuating circumstances, e.g., recurrent kidney stones.

PROBLEM 1 The patient had an acute onset of pain while watching TV that evening. The pain was sharp and severe and was located in the lumbar spine area with radiation to the umbilicus. The patient reportedly fainted on getting out of the chair. She was pale and diaphoretic. Her vital signs were blood pressure (BP) 100/60 mm Hg, pulse 110 beats/min, respirations 20/min. Her abdomen was mildly distended and diffusely tender. She was known to have hypertension and a "heart condition." The rescue squad placed the patient on 4 liters of oxygen by nasal cannula and started an intravenous line with normal saline run at 500 ml/hr.

This patient has the potential for becoming critically ill in a very short period of time. Sudden onset of back pain in an elderly person is always significant. Her blood pressure of 100/60 mm Hg is even more worrisome in a patient with longstanding hypertension. In her case, transport to the emergency department should occur without delay.

INITIAL APPROACH IN THE EMERGENCY DEPARTMENT

The majority of patients that present with acute abdominal pain do not arrive by rescue squad but are ambulatory. Ambulatory patients may have an occult catastrophic disease, and skillful triage is necessary to recognize these patients.

Risk factors that can identify the more acutely ill patients are as follows:

- Extremes of age. Causes of abdominal pain in elderly patients are more likely to be surgical disease, vascular catastrophes, myocardial disease, or sepsis. Infants become dehydrated more easily, become septic sooner, and cannot communicate their history or degree of pain well. Vital signs in these groups often do not accurately reflect their degree of illness.
- Any abnormal vital sign
- Severe pain of rapid onset
- Signs of dehydration
- Skin pallor and diaphoresis
- Once triage is accomplished, the following steps are performed in advance of or coincidentally with the arrival of the physician:

1. *Nursing intervention.* The nurse confirms the patient's history, paying special attention to medical problems, medications, hospitalizations, and allergies.

2. *Vital signs.* Vital signs are obtained and compared with those taken by the rescue squad or during triage.

3. *Initial examination.* A rapid overview assessment is performed while the patient is being completely undressed. Attention is given to the level of consciousness, general appearance including skin color, signs of dehydration, external discoloration or bruising, and peripheral pulses. Breath sounds are assessed. A rapid assessment of the abdomen is carried out including palpation to localize tenderness and estimate the degree of discomfort.

4. *Orthostatic vital signs.* In patients with syncope, lightheadedness, significant vomiting, diarrhea, signs of dehydration, or a history of gastrointestinal or vaginal bleeding, orthostatic vital signs are a necessity. Testing for orthostatic changes is done selectively using clinical judgment and an understanding of the risk for the patient. Blood pressure and pulse are recorded with the patient in the supine position for at least 3 minutes. The patient is asked to stand for 1 minute and then the blood pressure and pulse are recorded again. The test is considered positive if the pulse rate rises more than 20 beats per minute or the systolic blood pressure drops more than 20 mm Hg. The patient is carefully watched for syncope or complaints of dizziness while standing and returned to the supine position if symptoms occur. Palpating the radial pulse during this assessment can give useful information about the heart rate and character of the pulse during the time the patient is symptomatic.

5. *Oxygen administration.* If the patient is short of breath (respiratory rate of more than 20), shows signs of peripheral or central cyanosis, or has a history compatible with myocardial infarction, supplemental oxygen is continued or administered.

6. *Cardiac monitoring.* If myocardial ischemia is suspected or if there is a possibility

of any serious illness, the patient is placed on a cardiac monitor and observed for dysrhythmias.

7. *Intravenous access.* Establishment of intravenous access and drawing of initial blood for testing are often done by nurses prior to the physician's arrival. If the IV line was started in the field, it is rechecked, and an estimate is made of the fluid volume given the patient prior to entering the emergency department. In general, if significant vomiting, diarrhea, bleeding, signs of dehydration, hypotension, or abnormal orthostatic vital signs are present, a second large-bore IV is started. Isotonic crystalloid is used, and boluses of 200 to 300 ml are initially given to assess the patient's response. Blood and urine samples are collected when the IV is started and held pending physician orders.

8. *Analgesia.* Despite the patient's major complaint of pain, analgesia is seldom given at this point. A caring manner and a brief explanation of the hazards of analgesia in covering important pain symptoms can usually help gain the patient's cooperation for a short time period.

9. *Nasogastric tube* and *bladder catheterization.* Depending on the severity of the illness, a nasogastric tube is placed as part of the early care. The tube has therapeutic potential to relieve distention and serve as a conduit for gastric lavage. A urinary catheter may be therapeutic in relieving bladder obstruction but is more often a diagnostic aid used to obtain urine for analysis and monitor the patient's response to fluid therapy.

PROBLEM 1 The patient was brought quickly by the squad into the resuscitation room. A brief history and rapid physical examination confirmed the squad's findings. Repeat vital signs were BP 100/60 mm Hg, pulse 110 beats/min, respirations 20/min, temperature 97.6°F (36.4°C). The patient was placed on oxygen and a continuous cardiac monitor. An electrocardiogram (ECG) was ordered. A second 16-gauge IV line of normal saline was established while simultaneously drawing blood samples for laboratory evaluation. Two 300-ml fluid challenges were given rapidly. Her BP rose to 120/90 and pulse dropped to 100 beats/min. An indwelling catheter was placed to collect urine and monitor urine output. The emergency physician was present throughout the assessment and stabilization effort. Appropriate laboratory and radiographic studies were ordered.

In situations requiring multiple procedures in a short period of time, organization is important. Each member of the team should have a specific job to do while the physician assesses the patient. It is necessary to act quickly and thoroughly to prevent more serious problems. Anticipating the possibility of the patient's "crashing" and doing something to prevent it is central to the basis of emergency medicine. Because of her acute onset of pain, syncopal episode, and BP of 100/60 mm Hg with tachycardia, this patient required an aggressive assessment and volume replacement to improve her circulatory status.

PROBLEM 2 During the initial triage by the nurse, the patient was noted to be uncomfortable and appeared slightly pale. His vital signs were BP 130/80 mm Hg, pulse 80 beats/min, respirations 14/min, and temperature 100.6°F (38.1°C). Because of the patient's appearance and the fever, the nurse drew initial blood samples and started an IV line of normal saline. The patient was placed in a regular examination room and the physician was notified of his presence.

Although this patient appeared ill, there was no evidence during the triage examination that he was hemodynamically unstable. The nurse made an appropriate decision to place the patient in a regular examination room and notify the physician right away. The physician, having been notified properly, can then prioritize the care of this patient with regard to that of other patients in the emergency department.

DATA GATHERING

After or during the initial stabilization of the patient with abdominal pain, a thorough history is obtained. Only 50% of patients with acute abdominal pain are specifically diagnosed in the emergency department, despite physical examination and laboratory testing. Therefore, the history must be as complete as possible in the often limited time that is available. A chronology of events is often useful in obtaining a complex or extended history—"and then what happened?" It is important to make sure descriptive terms are mutually understood. Unclear language can be a significant source of error.

History

Pain History

Onset. Rapid onset of severe pain is more consistent with a vascular catastrophe, passage of a stone, or rupture of a viscus, cyst, or ectopic pregnancy. Slower, insidious onset is more typical of an inflammatory process such as appendicitis or cholecystitis.

Duration and Pattern of Change. Pain that is less than 24 hours in duration or is steadily increasing in intensity is more likely to need surgical intervention.

Character of Pain. The patient's description of the pain can vary significantly given cultural and educational background, levels of anxiety, and motives for coming to the emergency department. Pain that is dull, achy, or burning is more likely to be visceral than somatic. Pain that is sharp or stabbing is more likely to be peritoneal or somatic in nature. Crampy pain is classically associated with obstruction of a viscus, whereas tearing pain is classic for a dissecting aneurysm.

Severity. The patient's quantification of pain is notoriously unreliable. In general, nonspecific abdominal pain is less severe than pain from surgical causes, but there is considerable individual variation. Severe pain out of proportion to physical findings is classic for mesenteric ischemia or pancreatitis.

Location. The location of abdominal pain can vary with time, especially as the pain progresses from a visceral to a somatic origin. Periumbilical pain that migrates to the right lower quadrant is classic for appendicitis. Epigastric pain that eventually localizes during a period of several hours to the right upper quadrant is characteristic of cholecystitis.

Radiation. Given the pain patterns already discussed, involvement of certain organs can be implicated based on the radiating pattern of the pain (see Fig. 5–2).

Aggravating or Alleviating Factors. What makes the pain better or worse? Parietal peritoneal pain is aggravated by movement, such as hitting bumps on the ride to the hospital or even walking. This finding is particularly supportive of the diagnosis of appendicitis, when it is part of the differential diagnosis. Ulcer pain is usually relieved by eating, whereas biliary colic is made worse by eating fatty foods. The pain of pancreatitis is alleviated somewhat by assuming a curled-up posture.

Prior Pain History. The easiest question to ask is, "Have you ever had this pain before?" The majority of patients with cholecystitis have had similar pain with eating prior to presentation. Ulcers tend to be recurrent, as do pancreatitis and diverticulitis.

Pain Treatment. What has the patient done to relieve the pain? What has the response been? The treatment gives some insight into the medical sophistication of the patient. The response can help measure the severity and evolution of the pain.

Associated Symptoms

Nausea and Vomiting. Almost any kind of visceral abdominal pain will elicit nausea and vomiting (Chapter 8). The presence of vomiting is less useful for diagnosis than for determining the severity of dehydration or the eventual ability of the patient to manage care at home. Excessive vomiting should raise the suspicion of bowel obstruction or pancreatitis, whereas lack of vomiting is common in uterine or ovarian pathology. How was the onset of pain related to the onset of vomiting? Pain that is present before vomiting is more likely to have a surgical cause, whereas vomiting that precedes pain is more likely to occur in patients with nonspecific abdominal pain or gastroenteritis.

Anorexia. Is the patient hungry? If his favorite food were here, would he eat it? Anorexia can be a significant symptom of an intra-abdominal inflammation. It is a consistent historical finding in patients with appendicitis.

Change in Bowel Habits. Are the stools loose or watery? How many bowel movements has the patient had in the last 24 hours? The presence of diarrhea with vomiting is almost always associated with gastroenteritis, but diarrhea also occurs with pancreatitis, diverticulitis, and, less commonly, appendicitis (15%). Is the patient unable to pass gas or stool? Ileus from inflammation and blockage from mechanical obstruction are common causes of this complaint.

Genitourinary Causes. Has there been a change in the number of times the patient urinates? Any change in the amount, color, or odor? Dysuria, urgency, and frequency are seen not only with cystitis but also with inflammatory conditions at or around the bladder wall such as salpingitis, diverticulitis, or appendicitis. Hematuria can be an indicator of renal colic or cystitis.

Cardiopulmonary Causes. Cough, dyspnea, and chest pain are not symptoms one would expect to find with a purely abdominal process. Still, referred pain does occur and the presence of these symptoms is investigated.

Past Medical History

Medical Illness. Patients with diabetes, heart disease, lung disease, liver disease, hypertension, or renal disease are not only at increased risk for certain abdominal disorders but may also require significantly different methods of stabilization, treatment, and surgical preparation.

Medications. Steroids and other immunosuppressants can significantly alter the patient's response to infection. Many antibiotics, e.g., erythromycin and tetracycline, cause gastrointestinal upset and diarrhea. Laxatives, narcotics, and psychotropic medications can alter gut motility and cause abdominal pain. Aspirin and nonsteroidal anti-inflammatory agents are frequent causes of gastritis and peptic ulcer disease.

Past Surgery. Prior surgery not only can eliminate many diagnoses but can increase the risk of others. For instance, abdominal surgery with secondary adhesions is the most common cause of bowel obstruction in adults.

Menstrual History. A complete menstrual history is essential, especially in the evaluation of lower abdominal pain in young females. A history of salpingitis, intrauterine devices, or tubal ligation all increase the risk of ectopic pregnancy.

Habits. The potential for alcohol and laxative abuse requires specific questioning. Alcohol abuse predisposes the patient to ulcers, gastritis, and pancreatitis. Laxative abuse is associated with diverticular disease and cecal volvulus.

PROBLEM 2 The patient reported a gradual onset over 12 hours of epigastric and periumbilical burning pain. The pain had intensified during the past 4 hours. He had vomited twice but denied diarrhea. When he noticed the onset of right lower quadrant pain, he drove to the emergency department. The ride was very uncomfortable. He denied any medications, allergies, or hospitalizations.

Remembering the neuroanatomy of pain transmission, it is evident that this patient is describing the classic progression of visceral to somatic abdominal pain. Coupled with a relatively short duration, this history should cause concern for a potentially serious and evolving surgical process.

Physical Examination

A reliable physical examination requires not only a thorough, systematic inspection of the abdomen but also considerable patient cooperation. An intoxicated or uncooperative patient will significantly diminish the accuracy of the examination. A calm, reassuring approach on the part of the physician will often alleviate patient anxiety and make the examination more meaningful.

The major purpose of this assessment is to localize the disease process to a certain area of the abdomen by defining the maximal area of tenderness. Other goals are to assess the patient's general medical condition and to evaluate how closely the physical examination, specifically tenderness, matches the subjective reporting of pain by the patient.

The major components of the physical examination in a patient with acute abdominal pain include:

General Appearance. The patient's color and attitude in bed are important. Patients who are pale and diaphoretic and are lying perfectly still in bed are generally more acutely ill and are more likely to have local or diffuse peritonitis. Patients who are agitated or writhing in pain are more likely to have visceral causes of abdominal pain, nonspecific abdominal pain, renal or biliary colic, or mesenteric ischemia.

Vital Signs

Temperature. The patient's temperature has been used as a general indicator of the presence or absence of infection, but it can be deceiving. Appendicitis and cholecystitis, for instance, usually first appear with a temperature of less than 100.2°F (37.9°C), and only 40% to 70% of patients will have an elevated temperature at all. A temperature higher than 101° to 102°F (38.3° to 38.9°C) should raise the suspicion of salpingitis, pyelonephritis, bacterial enteritis or a ruptured viscus. In elderly or immunosuppressed patients, a normal temperature does not rule out an infectious process, whereas in children and young people, the temperature is often elevated with infection.

Blood Pressure and Pulse. These vital signs are helpful in gauging the severity of the disease process and the potential for blood or fluid loss.

Respiratory Rate. Pneumonia, pulmonary embolism, and myocardial infarction can raise the respiratory rate. Acidosis due to sepsis or hypoperfusion can do the same thing.

Extra-abdominal Examination. Before examining the abdomen, the physician should listen quickly to the heart and lungs to avoid missing an extra-abdominal cause of abdominal pain. This first contact in an "unconcerned" area can help put the patient at ease. The peripheral pulses are quickly palpated and the skin and mucous membranes assessed for signs of jaundice, hypoperfusion, or dehydration.

Abdominal Examination

Inspection. Signs of distention, asymmetry, prior surgery, large masses, bruises, or pregnancy or the cutaneous signs of portal hypertension may quickly narrow the differential diagnosis.

Auscultation. Auscultation prior to palpation avoids a false increase in bowel sounds. Decreased bowel sounds are heard in peritonitis and other inflammatory processes that cause an adynamic ileus. Increased bowel sounds are heard in patients with nonspecific abdominal pain and gastroenteritis, whereas high-pitched sounds and rushes are classic for bowel obstruction. In reality, bowel sounds are unreliable and of limited value in the problem-solving process.

Percussion. Gentle percussion of all four abdominal quadrants can localize the site of pain initially. Percussing the abdomen can often provide information about the size of certain organs and the origin of abdominal distention, gaseous or solid. It is also useful for determining bladder size from urinary retention.

Palpation. Most of the time and effort in the abdominal examination is spent on palpation. At this point, the patient needs to be most cooperative and at ease. Asking the patient to flex the legs at the hip and knee may relax the abdominal musculature. It is important to note the patient's facial expressions during palpation. A grimace is usually more significant than the statement, "it hurts." At times, distraction of the patient by asking historical questions during palpation is necessary to overcome factitious or hysterical false-positive findings.

Palpation is begun as far as possible from the perceived location of the pain. The epigastrium, hypogastrium, and all four quadrants are slowly and gently palpated systematically, ending at the perceived pain location. Palpation is gentle but firm, not jerky. The fingertips are pressed fairly deep to reach the posterior structures such as the kidneys, pancreas, and retrocecal appendix. Gradual increases of pressure while palpating are better tolerated than a single movement. Deep palpation is often limited by the patient's pain tolerance. In pain of visceral origin, localization of tenderness is usually not possible. With somatic tenderness, localization is more likely, and the following associated findings are assessed:

1. *Muscular Signs.* Guarding is the reflex spasm of the abdominal wall musculature in response to palpation or underlying peritoneal irritation. Voluntary guarding is less significant than involuntary guarding. Involuntary guarding is elicited by asking the patient to take a deep breath while firm pressure is held on the tender area. If the spasm is not relieved, involuntary guarding is present. If the muscles relax, voluntary guarding is present, and deeper palpation is made possible.

2. *Rebound Tenderness.* Rebound is classically the hallmark of peritoneal irritation, although it may be present in up to 25% of patients with nonspecific abdominal pain and absent in up to 50% of patients with appendicitis. It is elicited by slow, gentle, deep palpation of the tender area followed by abrupt but discreet withdrawal of the examiner's hand. Optimally, the patient is distracted by conversation. Often this procedure is not necessary because rebound can be discovered more gently by asking the patient to cough, shaking the bed, or gently percussing the area of tenderness. When rebound is tested for in a nontender area of the abdomen and pain is caused in the distant area of perceived subjective pain, true peritoneal involvement is more likely at the site of disease. It is important to differentiate this superficial finding from tenderness of the abdominal wall.

Special Techniques

Psoas and Obturator Signs. Flexion and internal rotation of the hip against resistance will cause pain from inflammatory processes (like appendicitis and salpingitis) in the retrocecal area and pelvis.

Murphy's Sign. While the physician palpates deeply in the right upper quadrant, the patient is asked to take a deep breath. Abrupt cessation of inspiration because of pain is consistent with cholecystitis, hepatitis, or other right upper quadrant abnormalities.

Fist Percussion. Gently percussing the costovertebral angles of the back with a fist elicits pain in patients with pyelonephritis or obstructive uropathy.

Related Examinations

Vascular. Both femoral pulses and the aorta are palpated. Gently approaching the aorta from both sides with the fingers in the nonobese patient can estimate the aortic diameter. Auscultation of bruits is done over the upper and lower abdomen and the inguinal areas.

Hernias and Genitals. The groin areas are inspected and palpated for direct and indirect hernias. Unrecognized hernias can progress to bowel obstruction. External genitals are examined and the scrotal contents carefully palpated.

Rectal. This examination is needed to search for occult blood, masses, and prostate tenderness. It is important in diagnosis and is not to be deferred. Rectal tenderness is an important sign of appendicitis, salpingitis, or any process that allows inflammatory fluid to collect in the pelvic cul-de-sac.

Pelvic. All women of childbearing age with abdominal pain require a pelvic examination. Cervical appearance, cervical motion tenderness, uterine size, adnexal size and tenderness, and status of the cul-de-sac are all assessed.

DECISION PRIORITIES AND PRELIMINARY DIFFERENTIAL DIAGNOSIS

After completing the history and physical examination, the preliminary differential diagnosis for the patient's abdominal pain is developed according to the following principles:

1. *Is there a threat to life?*

   Even though life-threatening causes of abdominal pain do not occur as frequently as common causes, they always take the highest priority. Table 5–2 summarizes the important life-threatening intra-abdominal causes of acute abdominal pain. Extra-abdominal life-threatening diseases presenting as acute abdominal pain include myocardial infarction, pulmonary embolus, and lobar pneumonia.

TABLE 5–2. Potential Life-Threatening Causes of Abdominal Pain

	Epidemiology	Etiology	Presentation	Physical Findings	Useful Tests
Ruptured leaking abdominal aortic aneurysm	Incidence increases with advancing age. Men outnumber women. HTN, DM, smoking, COPD and CAD are risk factors	Atherosclerosis in over 95%. Intimal dissection causes aortic dilatation and creation of a false lumen. Leakage or rupture causes hypovolemia	Patient often asymptomatic until rupture. Acute epigastric and back pain often associated with or followed by syncope or signs of shock. Pain may radiate to back, groin, or testes	Vital signs may be initally normal (in 70% of patients) to severely hypotensive. Palpation of pulsatile abdominal mass is usually possible. Bruits or inequality of femoral pulses may be evident	Abdominal plain films abnormal in 80% of cases. Ultrasound can define length and diameter of aneurysm. CT can detect retroperitoneal rupture
Perforated viscus	Incidence increases with advancing age. History of peptic ulcer disease or diverticular disease common	Most often a duodenal ulcer that erodes through the serosa. Colonic diverticula, large bowel, small bowel, and gallbladder perforations are more rare. Spillage of bowel contents causes local or generalized peritonitis	Acute onset of epigastric pain is common. Vomiting in 50%. Fever may be present later. Pain may localize with omental walling off of peritonitis	Fever, usually low-grade, is common; higher fever occurs with time. Tachycardia is common. Shock may be present with bleeding or sepsis. Abdominal examination reveals diffuse guarding and rebound. A "boardlike" abdomen in later stages. Bowel sounds decreased	WBC count usually elevated due to peritonitis. Amylase may be elevated as well. LFT results are variable. Upright view radiographs reveal free air in 70%–80% of cases with perforated ulcers
Acute pancreatitis	Peak age in adulthood, rare in children and elderly. Male preponderance. Alcohol abuse and biliary tract pathology	Alcohol, gallstones, hyperlipidemia, hypercalcemia, or endoscopic retrograde pancreatography causes pancreatic damage, saponification, and necrosis. ARDS, sepsis, hemorrhage, and renal failure are secondary	Acute onset of epigastric pain radiating to the back. Nausea and vomiting common	Low-grade fever common. Patient may be hypotensive or tachypneic. Some epigastric tenderness usually present. Since retro-peritoneal organ, guarding or rebound not present unless severe	Amylase remains test of choice. CT scan may show abscesses, bleeding, or pseudocysts
Intestinal obstruction	Peaks in infancy and with advancing age. More common with history of abdominal surgery	Adhesions, carcinoma, hernias, abscesses, volvulus, and infarction. Obstruction leads to vomiting, third spacing of fluid, strangulation, and necrosis of bowel	Crampy diffuse abdominal pain associated with vomiting	Vital signs usually normal unless dehydration or bowel strangulation has occurred. Abdominal distention, hyperactive bowel sounds, and diffuse tenderness. Local peritoneal signs indicate strangulation	WBC count may indicate strangulation if elevated. Electrolytes will indicate degree of dehydration. Abdominal plain films are very useful for identifying level of obstruction

Table continued on following page

TABLE 5–2. Potential Life-Threatening Causes of Abdominal Pain *Continued*

	Epidemiology	Etiology	Presentation	Physical Findings	Useful Tests
Mesenteric ischemia	Occurs most commonly in elderly people. Responsible for 1 of 1000 hospital admissions. Mortality 70%	30%–50% of lesions are nonocclusive, and the causes of ischemia are multifactorial, including transient hypotension in the presence of a preexisting atherosclerotic lesion. The remainder are secondary to emboli or acute arterial thrombosis	Severe pain, often colicky, that starts in periumbilical region and then becomes diffuse. Vomiting and diarrhea are often associated	Early examination results can be remarkably benign in presence of severe infarction. Bowel sounds often still present. Rectal examination important because mild bleeding with positive guaic stools can be present	Often a pronounced leukocytosis is present. Elevations of amylase and creatine phosphokinase levels are seen. If infarction present, metabolic acidosis due to lactic acidemia is often seen. Abnormal laboratory findings herald a poor prognosis; therefore, early angiography based on suspicion is often warranted

HTN = hypertension, DM = diabetes mellitus, COPD = chronic obstructive pulmonary disease, CAD = coronary artery disease, ARDS = adult respiratory distress syndrome, WBC = white blood cell, LFT = liver function tests.

2. *Is the pain acute and is there a potential surgical cause for the pain?*
Severe pain accompanied by localized tenderness with peritoneal findings are the hallmarks of serious and possibly surgical disease. Usually the pain will have been acute in onset, and there will be accompanying abnormal vital signs or laboratory test results to support the suspicion of surgical disease. Table 5–3 summarizes other causes of acute abdominal pain. All have the potential for requiring surgical intervention.

While formulating the preliminary differential diagnosis, it is important to recall that up to one third of patients will present with atypical features of their underlying disease process.

PROBLEM 1 The patient appeared pale while lying in bed. Decreased bowel sounds were heard on auscultation, and on palpation there was diffuse abdominal tenderness with rebound and some involuntary guarding. Aortic pulsations were also palpable, but because of the obesity of the patient, it was difficult to estimate the size of the aorta.

Because of the finding of a palpable pulsating aorta, this patient clearly was a true emergency. Every effort should be made to expedite her care, and in particular, to obtain an appropriate diagnostic study of the abdomen to assess the possibility of a leaking aortic aneurysm.

PROBLEM 2 As the history suggested, this patient had not only pain localized to the right lower quadrant but also specific tenderness with rebound and involuntary guarding in the same area. A rectal examination revealed no specific abnormality or tenderness.

In spite of the normal rectal examination, the physical findings of right lower quadrant tenderness and the peritoneal signs were highly suspicious for appendicitis. In all likelihood, the laboratory and radiologic examinations will offer little more to confirm or deny the suspicions of the clinician. Still, in most similar situations, diagnostic adjuncts are included in the assessment.

TABLE 5–3. Common Causes of Abdominal Pain

	Epidemiology	Etiology	Presentation	Physical Findings	Useful Tests
Acute appendicitis	Peak age adolescence and young adulthood. Less common in children and elderly. Higher perforation rate in women, children, and geriatric patients	Appendiceal lumen obstruction leads to swelling, ischemia, infection, perforation	Epigastric pain migrates to right lower quadrant over 8–12 hr. Later presentations associated with higher perforation rates. Pain and anorexia very common, vomiting and fever less common	Mean temperature 100.5° F (38° C); higher temperature with perforation. Temperature may be normal, especially in geriatric patients. Right lower quadrant tenderness with rebound in majority of cases. Rectal tenderness also common	Leukocyte count usually elevated or may show left shift. Urine may show sterile pyuria
Biliary tract disease	Peak age 35–60, rare in persons less than 20. Females-to-males ratio of 3:1. Multiparity, obesity, alcohol intake, and birth control pills are risk factors	Passage of gallstones causes biliary colic. Impaction of stone in cystic duct or common duct causes cholecystitis or cholangitis	Crampy right upper quadrant pain radiates to right flank. Prior history of pain is common. Longer duration of pain favors diagnosis of cholecystitis or cholangitis	Temperature normal in biliary colic, elevated in cholecystitis and cholangitis. Right upper quadrant tenderness, rebound, and, less commonly, jaundice may be present	WBC count elevated in cholecystitis and cholangitis. Amylase and liver function tests may help differentiate this entity from gastritis or ulcer disease. Ultrasound shows stones or duct dilatation. Hepatobiliary scintigraphy can diagnose cholecystitis
Ureteral colic	Average age 30–40, mostly in men. Family history or prior history of kidney stones is common	Family history, gout, *Proteus* sp. infections, RTA, and cystinuria lead to stone formation. Stones cause pain, hematuria, and ureteral obstruction	Acute onset of flank pain radiating to groin. Nausea, vomiting, and pallor are common. Patient usually writhing in pain	Vital signs usually normal. Tenderness on CVA percussion but normal results on abdominal examination are characteristic	Urinalysis usually shows hematuria. Abdominal plain films show stones in up to 80% of cases. Intravenous pyelography is mainstay of diagnosis
Diverticulitis	Incidence increases with advancing age; occurs in males more than females. Recurrences are common	Colonic diverticula become infected or perforated or cause local colitis. Obstruction, peritonitis, abscesses, fistulas result from infection or swelling	There is commonly a change in stool frequency or character. Rectal bleeding may be evident. Left lower quadrant pain is common. Fever, nausea, vomiting may be seen	Fever is usually low grade unless perforation and peritonitis have occurred. Other vital signs usually normal. Abdominal examination shows left lower quadrant tenderness with or without rebound. Stools may be heme positive	WBC count usually elevated, although not extremely so. LFTs and amylase usually normal. Plain films may show obstruction or mass effect. Barium enema is often diagnostic

Table continued on following page

TABLE 5–3. Common Causes of Abdominal Pain *Continued*

	Epidemiology	Etiology	Presentation	Physical Findings	Useful Tests
Peptic ulcer	Peptic ulcers occur in all age groups but peak at age 50. Men affected twice as often as women. Perforation or severe bleeding occurs in less than 1% of patients per year	Cause of peptic ulcer disease still unknown. Abnormal secretion of acid and pepsin occurs in only one-third of patients. Risk factors include relatives with ulcers, cigarette smoking, alcohol intake, and chronic obstructive pulmonary disease	The cardinal symptom is nonradiating epigastric pain that starts 1–3 hours after eating and is relieved by food or antacids. Pain frequently awakens patient at night	Physical examination is of limited value in diagnosis of uncomplicated ulcer. Often only epigastric tenderness is present without peritoneal findings. Perforation or bleeding leads to more severe clinical findings	Barium contrast studies can identify ulcers in 70–80% of cases. Duodenoscopy is valuable in recognizing smaller ulcers or identifying sites of hemorrhage. Uncomplicated cases seen in the emergency department are usually treated with antacids or H_2 blockers before invasive studies are contemplated
Nonspecific abdominal pain	More common in persons of young and middle age, women of childbearing years, or low social class and in those with psychiatric disorders. Up to 10% of patients over 50 years of age prove to have intra-abdominal cancer	Unknown at time of presentation	Variable but tends to be chronic or recurrent	Variable, but peritoneal signs should not be present	Variable, and can often be done on an outpatient basis

RTA = renal tubular acidosis; LFT = liver function tests; CVA = costovertebral angle

DIAGNOSTIC ADJUNCTS

Laboratory Studies

Laboratory testing is often ordered in patients with acute abdominal pain. Although occasionally pinpointing a specific diagnosis, most laboratory results either support the emergency physician's concern about "serious disease" or set a direction for further studies.

White Blood Cell Count and Differential. The white blood cell (WBC) count is a relatively useful test in evaluating acute abdominal pain. An elevated WBC count or a left-shifted differential occurs in acute appendicitis in more than 80% of cases. In most cases of appendicitis, pelvic inflammatory disease, and cholecystitis, WBC counts average 12,000 to 15,000/mm^3, and left shifts are common. WBC counts are often higher in patients with perforation, peritonitis, fulminant pancreatitis, or sepsis. Unfortunately, leukocytosis is found in up to 40% of patients with gastroenteritis and 30% of patients with abdominal pain of unknown etiology. In geriatric or immunosuppressed patients, the WBC may be normal or low. At no time is the WBC count or differential the single deciding factor as to whether or not an acute surgical condition of the abdomen is present.

Hemoglobin-Hematocrit. The hemoglobin-hematocrit is important in patients who have suspected hemorrhage, dehydration, or anemia. If an acute hemorrhage is suspected, as in a patient with a ruptured ectopic pregnancy or leaking aortic aneurysm, the initial hemoglobin-hematocrit level will usually be unchanged but will provide a baseline from which to estimate blood loss over time. If chronic bleeding from a gastrointestinal or genitourinary source is suspected, the initial hemoglobin-hematocrit reading will help estimate the degree of blood loss.

Amylase. The serum amylase level is often considered the laboratory cornerstone in the diagnosis of pancreatitis. The test is not specific for pancreatic disease, and small elevations in the serum amylase may also be caused by peptic ulcer disease, small bowel obstruction or ischemia, common duct stones, ectopic pregnancy, renal failure, alcohol intoxication, or facial trauma (salivary amylase). As many as 20% of patients with proven pancreatitis may present with normal serum amylase values. In general, the amylase concentration has remained a good test in the diagnosis of pancreatitis despite these shortcomings. An elevated amylase level, despite its lack of specificity, often is indicative of serious abdominal pathology. Occasionally, a urine amylase concentration will be elevated in spite of a normal serum level. It can serve as a more sensitive indicator of elevated amylase, but it is often not available in a timely manner.

Urinalysis. As a general rule, the presence of more than 10 WBC per high-power field, a positive nitrite level, or a positive leukocyte esterase determination in a clean-catch urine sample is consistent with a diagnosis of urinary tract infection. Red cells in the urine are consistent with infection, tumor, trauma, or stone. The urinalysis is interpreted with caution in patients with abdominal pain. For instance, appendicitis, retroperitoneal abscesses, and endocarditis can cause pyuria in up to 10% to 15% of patients without actual urinary tract infection.

Tests for Pregnancy. Any woman of childbearing age who presents with acute abdominal pain, especially if located in the lower abdomen, deserves a pregnancy test. The most important gynecologic emergency that causes abdominal pain is a ruptured ectopic pregnancy. The probability of this problem being present is significantly lessened by negative results from a reliable pregnancy test. Testing for pregnancy is discussed in more detail in Chapter 60.

Serum Electrolytes. Potassium levels are measured in patients with associated vomiting or diarrhea. A low bicarbonate level may be found in an anion gap acidosis, as seen in sepsis, mesenteric ischemia, or diabetic ketoacidosis. An abnormal bicarbonate level is a reason to order arterial blood gas analysis in these patients.

Liver Function Tests. Alkaline phosphatase, bilirubin, and liver enzyme measurements have recently become available on a stat basis in most emergency departments. Elevations in the alkaline phosphatase and bilirubin levels are consistent with biliary tract disease or common bile duct obstruction. Elevations of the aminotransferases (AST and ALT) are consistent with hepatitis. There is a significant amount of overlap between conditions that cause elevations in liver function test results, and such tests are not to be overinterpreted.

Radiologic Imaging

Chest Radiograph. An upright chest radiograph can help diagnose pneumonia, pleural effusion, and other pulmonary causes of abdominal pain. It is also the best view for detecting free intraperitoneal air from a perforated viscus, and is capable of detecting as little as 2 to 5 cc of air.

Abdominal Radiograph. An abdominal film series usually consists of flat and erect views of the abdomen as well as a chest view. Abdominal films are usually of low yield in patients with abdominal pain. Radiographic findings that either confirm or reveal the cause of the pain occur in only 10% to 38% of cases. Of these radiographs, only 10% will actually alter the diagnosis or management plan. Radiographic signs that are most commonly looked for are dilated loops of small or large bowel, air fluid levels, abnormal calcifications in the urinary tract system or vascular calcifications outside of their usual anatomic location (aortic aneurysm), free air under the diaphragm, and gallstones.

Contrast Imaging. Barium or water-soluble iodinated agents can aid diagnosis in selected cases. Barium is contraindicated in patients with suspected perforation. A contrast enema can differentiate ileus from mechanical obstruction.

Ultrasound Imaging. Ultrasound imaging is now available on an emergency basis in most emergency departments. It can show multiple organ systems including the biliary tract, gallbladder, pancreas, kidneys, aorta, and uterus. The sensitivity of ultrasound in the detection of gallstones approaches 94% to 100%. Other conditions commonly detected by ultrasound include biliary obstruction, aortic aneurysms, pancreatic pseudocysts, ureteral obstruction, and intrauterine versus ectopic pregnancies.

Computed Tomography. CT is in general less available than ultrasound and is more expensive. It is used in a goal-directed manner, not as a screening test. The advantages of CT over ultrasound are most notable in viewing the pancreas, retroperitoneal space, and spleen. It is particularly useful for visualizing pancreatic hemorrhage, retroperitoneal abscesses, and leaking abdominal aortic aneurysms.

Nuclear Medicine. Hepatobiliary scintigraphy with technetium-99m radiolabeled imaging agents is particularly useful in the diagnosis of cholecystitis, especially when ultrasound cannot confirm a diagnosis of gallstones or inflammation. Nonfilling of the gallbladder is consistent with a stone obstructing the cystic duct. The tests is not affected by the level of bilirubin.

Angiography. This diagnostic procedure is usually reserved for patients with a suspected aortic aneurysm, gastrointestinal hemorrhage, or mesenteric ischemia. It is time consuming and by necessity is performed outside the emergency department.

Electrocardiogram

Because myocardial ischemia can cause abdominal pain, most patients over 40 years old with abdominal pain deserve an ECG, particularly if the pain is located in the upper abdomen.

PROBLEM 1 The laboratory examination of the patient revealed a hematocrit of 38% and a WBC count of 16,300/mm^3. Differential count, urinalysis, and electrolytes were all normal. Chest films showed an ectatic aorta. Abdominal films revealed aortic calcifications in the general shape of an abdominal aortic aneurysm. Ultrasound showed a 7-cm aortic aneurysm.

This patient was taken immediately to surgery. The aneurysm was found to be leaking. The repair was carried out, and the patient was transferred to the surgical intensive care unit.

PROBLEM 2 Results of the patient's laboratory studies revealed a WBC count of 10,300/mm^3 with 76% neutrophils and 20% band forms. The urinalysis showed 3 to 5 WBCs but no bacteria. Amylase and liver function test results were normal. Abdominal films were unremarkable.

This patient's laboratory examination served only to confirm the physician's suspicion that an inflammatory process of acute duration was evolving in the right lower quadrant. The physician still suspected appendicitis as the most likely diagnosis. The appearance of white blood cells in the urine is consistent with the diagnosis of an inflammatory process adjacent to the bladder and should not lead the physician away from suspecting a more serious cause for the abdominal pain.

PRINCIPLES OF MANAGEMENT

The main goals of the emergency physician in managing patients with acute abdominal disorders are to reverse the systemic effects of the underlying disorder and to prepare the patient for surgical intervention, if necessary. Principles of management include: volume repletion, gastric emptying, control of emesis, and pain relief.

Volume Repletion

Not all patients with abdominal pain require intravenous access or hydration. However, many will have accompanying anorexia or vomiting and will be in a relatively volume-depleted state. Intravenous access with volume repletion is clearly indicated in patients who have demonstrable orthostatic changes in vital signs, dry mucous membranes, or a history consistent with significant vomiting or diarrhea. An intravenous line is also indicated in patients who need to avoid oral intake prior to possible surgical intervention. The usual choice of intravenous solution is an isotonic crystalloid, either lactated Ringer's solution or normal saline. The rate of volume repletion is determined by the degree of hypovolemia, the cardiovascular status of the patient, and the response of the vital signs to initial therapy.

Gastric Emptying

Nasogastric suction is indicated in patients in whom a surgical cause of disease is suspected, and gastric emptying needs to be achieved prior to transfer to the surgical suite. It is also indicated in a patient with persistent vomiting, suspected ileus, or bowel obstruction. This measure has long been used in patients with pancreatitis, but recent clinical studies indicate that nasogastric emptying has little effect on the clinical outcome of patients with pancreatitis.

Control of Emesis

In general, antiemetics are used with caution in any patient with abdominal pain (see Chap. 8). They can be useful in patients with gastroenteritis, gastritis, renal colic, or other conditions in which nausea and vomiting are prominent. It is generally felt that antiemetics do not alter pain sensation but can make a patient lethargic, drowsy, and confused. This effect is seen especially in very young and very old patients. Commonly used antiemetics include promethazine (Phenergan) and prochlorperazine (Compazine).

Pain Relief

Narcotic analgesias can give true pain relief but, like antiemetics, can alter the sensorium. Most consulting surgeons prefer that a narcotic analgesic not be used prior to a surgical consultation in order to avoid masking potentially important peritoneal findings. It remains controversial whether narcotics in small doses can actually alter the physical findings of the abdomen in any significant manner. An alternative strategy is to give 25 to 50 mg of hydroxyzine (Vistaril) intramuscularly. It will relieve some of the anxiety surrounding the pain yet not directly interfere with the perception of pain during the examination.

PROBLEM 2 After the evaluation was completed, the emergency physician telephoned to discuss the care of the patient with a consulting surgeon. The surgeon felt that appendicitis was the most reasonable diagnosis but wanted to examine the patient prior to giving narcotic analgesia. Hydroxyzine 25 mg was administered to the patient and provided some relief from his discomfort. On arrival in the emergency department, the surgeon confirmed the findings, and arrangements were made to transfer the patient to surgery.

It can be very distressing to emergency physicians and staff who have to care for patients awaiting consultation or disposition to another floor while they are in pain. The acceptable alternative is to use a mild sedative drug such as hydroxyzine. In some cases when the wait is prolonged and the pain is severe, narcotic analgesics can be used judiciously. It has been suggested by some observers that, if narcotic analgesia may mask pain, then narcotic antagonists may be used to reverse the effect of the narcotic prior to the examination by the consulting surgeon.

SPECIAL CONSIDERATIONS

Pediatric Patients

As has been mentioned previously in this chapter, the etiologies, physical findings, and laboratory analysis in children with abdominal pain are different from those of adults. Children are not always able to articulate their complaints. The physician must take particular care in eliciting the history from the child *and* the parent. On the other hand, children also can localize to the abdomen pain originating from extra-abdominal disease such as pharyngitis or pneumonia. The physician has to be gentle, reassuring, and thorough to make an appropriate diagnosis in children with abdominal pain.

In children, about 57% of pain is of medically related origin, 35% of unknown source, and 8% of surgical etiology. The probable cause of acute abdominal pain differs from that in adults. Gastroenteritis, mesenteric adenitis, and appendicitis are relatively more common in children, while biliary tract disease, pancreatitis, gynecologic disease, and vascular disease are relatively rare.

In a child with a bowel obstruction, intussusception, hernias, and volvulus are more likely than adhesions to be the cause of obstruction. Other obstructive diseases unique to children include pyloric stenosis, midgut volvulus, and Hirschsprung's disease.

In younger children with appendicitis, the chances of perforation are significantly increased compared with adults. A WBC count of over 13,000 or a temperature of over 102°F (38.8°C) is consistent with a perforated appendix in children. It is useful to remember that the peak age incidence for appendicitis is 12 years.

Geriatric Patients

Like pediatric patients, geriatric patients with acute abdominal pain have their own unique etiologies, physical findings, and laboratory results. Elderly patients tend to have a higher pain tolerance and stay away from health care facilities longer than young adults. They have lower WBC counts and temperatures than young adults given the same disease processes. The addition of diabetes or other immunosuppressing diseases enhances these differences, making the diagnosis difficult. Some special considerations with regard to the elderly are listed below:

- The etiology of abdominal pain changes with increasing age. Surgical causes of abdominal pain such as cholecystitis and diverticulitis increase in incidence with age, whereas nonspecific abdominal pain becomes less common (see Table 5–4). The cause of pain is a surgical condition in 33% of elderly patients as opposed to 16% in young adults. Vascular catastrophes such as aneurysms and mesenteric ischemia are more common with advancing age.
- Malignancy is a much more common cause of abdominal pain in elderly patients. In patients over 50 with nonspecific abdominal pain, a malignancy will be found as the cause of the pain in 3% to 15%.
- Geriatric patients with appendicitis are more likely to seek medical care late in the course, have a normal or low WBC count, and have a normal temperature. Elderly patients present with a perforated appendix in 57% to 92% of cases.
- In patients with abdominal pathology, two-thirds will have at least one complicating diagnosis that will significantly alter their prognosis.
- Postoperative complications are more frequent, hospital stays are longer, and mortality is higher in elderly patients.

TABLE 5–4. Causes of Abdominal Pain in Patients Over 70 Years Old

Cause	Percentage
Acute cholecystitis	26.0
Malignant disease	13.2
Ileus	10.7
Nonspecific abdominal pain	9.6
Gastroduodenal ulcer	8.4
Acute diverticular disease of colon	7.0
Incarcerated hernia	4.8
Acute pancreatitis	4.1
Acute appendicitis	3.5
Other causes	12.7

From Fenyo G: Acute abdominal disease in the elderly. Am J Surg 143:751, 1982.

DISPOSITION AND FOLLOW-UP

There are three possible dispositions available to an emergency physician for patients with acute abdominal pain. It is important to emphasize, however, that each patient must be treated individually, and no recommendations for disposition are highly specific or concrete.

Immediate Surgical Consultation

Localized or diffuse peritoneal signs accompanied by historical and laboratory findings consistent with a surgical disease require an urgent surgical consultation. Evidence of bowel obstruction, clinically and radiographically, is also obviously an indication. Acute appendicitis, intestinal obstruction, perforated ulcer, and acute cholecystitis are the four most common surgical causes of abdominal pain.

Emergency Department Observation

Patients who have mild or equivocal abdominal tenderness on examination and who have no supportive laboratory findings indicative of a potential surgical cause of disease are often observed in the emergency department for a period of up to 6 hours. It is during this observation period that multiple examinations of the patient are carried out, preferably by the *same* physician. This sequential assessment is very important in monitoring the evaluation of the process and the patient's pain tolerance. A repeat white blood cell count may also be performed. This strategy of observation often allows the clinical situation to clarify as either the patient's condition worsens or more information is gained to allow a decision on disposition. Occasionally these patients will have complete resolution of the complaints and can be discharged home.

Discharge

Patients with the subjective complaint of abdominal pain but no accompanying abdominal tenderness or other abnormality may also be observed for a period of time in the emergency department. If their condition does not become worse and selected laboratory testing is not supportive of serious disease, they can be discharged home.

It is recommended that any patient discharged to the home environment from the emergency department be put on a clear liquid diet and have follow-up arranged within a 24-hour period. The patient is also instructed to call his or her primary physician or return to the emergency department at any time should the clinical course change for the worse. In one large clinical series of 732 patients sent home from an emergency department following a work-up for abdominal pain, 11 returned within 24 hours. The most common diagnosis on return was acute appendicitis. In that study, only one patient was judged to have a worse outcome because of the decision to discharge home. In another study, appendicitis and intestinal obstruction were the most common findings in patients found to be incorrectly discharged. All the patients with obstruction had prior intra-abdominal surgery and all had abdominal plain films interpreted as normal.

DOCUMENTATION

1. History. The history of the pain is documented. Location, onset, duration, and associated symptoms should be listed. Risk factors are noted.
2. Past history. Past surgeries especially are documented.
3. Medications
4. Last meal. If surgery is imminent, the anesthesiologist will want to know the time of the last meal.
5. Vital signs
6. Physical examination. The extra-abdominal examination is documented. The abdominal examination should include bowel sounds, location of tenderness, presence or absence of peritoneal findings, and presence or absence of masses. Pelvic and rectal examinations are documented.
7. Key laboratory and radiographic findings
8. Disposition. This is most important. A statement of the physician's impression and plan is most crucial. Whatever consultations were made, whatever follow-up arrangements were made, and conditions under which the patient was instructed to return are listed.

FINAL POINTS AND SUMMARY

- Abdominal pain is one of the most challenging complaints that can face an emergency physician. Despite the best and most intense diagnostic efforts, only 50% of patients presenting with this complaint will eventually be assigned a diagnosis.
- It is the responsibility of the emergency physician to be able to recognize the 10% to 20% of patients who have a surgical cause of their pain.
- Abdominal pain is a common symptom of the large number of varied organs that reside within the abdominal cavity. Often the pain will remain visceral in nature and therefore will not progress to a more somatic component, which would allow the examiner to elicit specific tenderness over an inflamed organ.
- The physician's most important diagnostic tools are the history and physical examination. Particular emphasis is placed on palpation to elicit specific tenderness.
- Laboratory and other ancillary diagnostic procedures are of limited value in the patient with abdominal pain. The management and disposition of the patient will depend on the clinical skill of the emergency physician.
- One of the most significant factors on the side of the physician in caring for the patient with abdominal pain is time and repeated examinations.
- Patients who do not have an obvious diagnosis are observed for a period of several hours. This management strategy will allow the physician to observe any significant changes in the patient's pain pattern and overall medical condition.

BIBLIOGRAPHY

Texts

1. Beal JM, Raffensperger JG: Diagnosis of Acute Abdominal Disease. Philadelphia, Lea & Febiger, 1979.
2. Silen W: Cope's Early Diagnosis of the Acute Abdomen (15th ed). New York, Oxford University Press, 1979.
3. Way LW: Abdominal pain. In Sleisenger MH, Fordtran JS (eds): Gastrointestinal Disease: Pathophysiology, Diagnosis, and Management (4th ed). Philadelphia, W. B. Saunders, 1989.

Journal Articles

1. Brewer RJ, Golden GT, Hitch DC, et al: Abdominal pain: An analysis of 1000 consecutive cases in a university hospital emergency room. Am J Surg 131:219, 1976.
2. de Dombal FT: Acute abdominal pain—an OMGE survey. Scand J Gastroenterol 14:29, 1979.
3. Eisenberg RL, Heineken P, Hedgecock MW, et al: Evaluations of abdominal radiographs in the diagnosis of abdominal pain. Ann Surg 197:464, 1983.
4. Fenyo G: Acute abdominal disease in the elderly. Am J Surg 143:751, 1982.
5. Hickey MS, Kiernan GJ, Weaver KE: Evaluation of abdominal pain. Emerg Clin North Am 7(3):437–542, 1989.
6. Jehle D, Davis E, Evans T, et al: Emergency department sonography by emergency physicians. Am J Emerg Med 7(6):605–611, 1989.
7. Jess P, Bjerregaard B, Brynitz S, et al: Prognosis of acute nonspecific abdominal pain. Am J Surg 144:338, 1982.
8. Lewis FR, Holcroft JW, Boey J, et al: Appendicitis, a critical review of 1000 cases. Arch Surg 110:667, 1975.
9. Marchand A, Van Lente F, Galen RS: The assessment of laboratory tests in the diagnosis of appendicitis. Am J Clin Pathol 80:369, 1983.
10. Moossa RA: Diagnostic tests and procedures in acute pancreatitis. N Engl J Med 311:639, 1984.
11. Rang EH, Fairbairn AS, Acheson ED: An inquiry into the incidence and prognosis of undiagnosed abdominal pain treated in hospitals. Br J Prev Soc Med 24:47, 1970.
12. Ranson JHC, Rifkind KM, Roses DF: Diagnostic signs and the role of operative management in acute pancreatitis. Surg Gynecol Obstet 139:69, 1974.

CHAPTER 6

ACUTE GASTROINTESTINAL BLEEDING: HEMATEMESIS, HEMATOCHEZIA, AND MELENA

EUGENE L. KWONG, M.D.

PROBLEM 1 The rescue squad was called to the home of a 50 year old male 10 minutes after he vomited a large amount of bright red blood. He complained of nausea and persistent epigastric pains.

PROBLEM 2 A 69 year old female was brought to the emergency department by anxious family members. She complained of 2 days of lower abdominal pains and recent passage of black tarry stools. She also reported a decrease in appetite and recent weight loss.

QUESTIONS TO CONSIDER

1. What clinical findings help distinguish between patients with life-threatening gastrointestinal hemorrhage and less serious bleeding?
2. How can the patient's history of present illness and the past medical history suggest possible causes of gastrointestinal bleeding?
3. Can upper gastrointestinal bleeding be differentiated clinically from lower gastrointestinal bleeding? Is the distinction important?
4. Which laboratory tests can help assess the degree of blood loss and possible cause of bleeding? Are there other useful diagnostic procedures?
5. What emergency therapy is appropriate in patients with severe upper and lower gastrointestinal bleeding?
6. When is a gastroenterologist or a general surgeon consulted?
7. Do all patients with acute gastrointestinal bleeding require admission? Which ones are admitted to a critical care unit?

INTRODUCTION

Two percent of all hospital admissions in the United States are related to acute gastrointestinal bleeding. Of these, about 10% require surgical intervention to control hemorrhage. In spite of modern diagnostic and therapeutic efforts, the overall mortality remains 6% to 8%. Most cases of acute gastrointestinal bleeding are first encountered in the emergency department, where the knowledge and expertise of the care provider can mean the difference between life and death. The term *acute* in this chapter is an imprecise description of severity that accounts for both the rapidity of hemorrhage and the speed of its onset.

Hematemesis is the vomiting of blood, "bright red" or otherwise. The "coffee grounds" material often seen with upper gastrointestinal bleeding is partially digested whole blood. Hematochezia is the passage of obviously bloody stools as opposed to the black tarry stools of melena. Maroon, burgundy, or currant jelly stools are simply descriptive terms for stools that contain partially metabolized hemoglobin. The color of the stool, whether bright red or densely black, is dependent on the rate of bleeding and the time the blood has spent passing through the intestines. Therefore, color alone does not help to localize the site of hemorrhage. A common cause of frank hematochezia is still an upper gastrointestinal hemorrhage.

Upper gastrointestinal bleeding presenting as hematemesis is usually due to a breakdown of the mucosal and vascular integrity of the esophagus, stomach, or duodenum. Anatomically, it is defined as occurring proximal to the ligament of Treitz, which separates the relatively fixed duodenum from the mobile jejunum. Clinically, this anatomic site is important in that bleeding distal to the ligament of Treitz rarely regurgitates back into the duodenum or stomach. Exceptions are seen in patients with bowel obstruction. Melena is the usual result in nonmassive upper gastrointestinal hemorrhage. The blood is digested during its transit through the gut.

Lower gastrointestinal tract bleeding that manifests as hematochezia or nonmelenic stool is commonly due to hemorrhoids, diverticula, carcinoma, upper gastrointestinal hemorrhage, and infectious or inflammatory bowel conditions. Its origin is similar to that of upper gastrointestinal bleeding, although vascular causes are more common than mucosal damage.

PREHOSPITAL CARE

The information from the field is directed toward gauging the severity of hemorrhage and the patient's physiologic tolerance to the blood loss.

History

A brief description is elicited regarding the circumstances of the bleed itself, e.g., estimated blood loss, time of onset, concurrent vomiting. The presence of associated postural dizziness or syncope is noted. Symptoms of chest or abdominal pain, nausea, or dyspnea are recorded.

Physical Examination

During the general physical examination vital signs are obtained, and the patient's appearance and mental status are noted. Pallor, diaphoresis, or cyanosis is reported. The patient's circulatory and intravascular volume status is assessed by the quality and strength of the pulses and capillary refill time. In specific examinations the patency and protection of the airway are established, and the symmetry and quality of breath sounds are reported. Obvious abdominal tenderness, rigidity, distention, or masses are noted.

Interventions

The basic precepts of field stabilization are to initiate volume replacement and supplemental oxygen while readying the patient for transport. It is preferable to perform procedures while in transit.

Airway. The patient may be obtunded owing to drugs, alcohol, or hypovolemic shock. The airway is established, protected, and maintained. Suction devices are readily available to clear the airway in the event of vomiting. If vomiting is severe, the patient can be placed in the left lateral decubitus position.

Oxygen. Loss of red cell mass means oxygen-carrying capacity is decreasing as well. Oxygen by nasal cannula is begun at a flow of 4 to 6 liters/minute initially.

Intravenous Access. One or two large-bore, 14- to 16-gauge, peripheral intravenous (IV) catheters are inserted but not at the expense of delay in transport. Isotonic crystalloid solution is given at infusion rates dictated by the clinical circumstances and the estimate of blood loss (see Chap. 4). If there is hemodynamic instability, at least two lines are started, and the crystalloid solution is infused under pressure. The amount of fluid given in the prehospital care phase is recorded for the emergency staff.

Cardiac Monitoring. Knowledge of the cardiac rhythm can help the rescue squad indirectly assess the patient's hemodynamic status and monitor dysrhythmias induced by the combination of hypovolemia and increased sympathetic nervous system response.

Pneumatic Antishock Garment (PASG). Application of the garment may be suitable for the hemodynamically unstable patient if intravenous lines cannot be established, and the expected transport time is more than 10 to 15 minutes. The device preferentially redistributes blood flow to the central core circulation by increasing the peripheral vascular resistance (afterload) in the lower extremities. It is only a temporizing measure until adequate crystalloid and blood can be delivered. Its influence on the actual outcome of patient survival is questionable. The use of PASG is contraindicated if the patient has pulmonary edema or congestive heart failure.

Patient Comfort. A brief discussion of what is happening can allay the fears and anxiety of the patient, family, or friends. The loss of blood of an undeterminable amount plus the urgency of starting IV lines, monitoring, giving oxygen, and a blaring siren can be very frightening.

PROBLEM 1 On arrival at the patient's home, the rescue squad found him lying on the bathroom floor. He was alert but pale and diaphoretic. There was obviously bloody vomitus in the toilet bowel. His blood pressure was 80/50 mm Hg, pulse 130 beats/min, and respirations 24/min. The patient stated that the episode came on suddenly after 1 to 2 days of persistent abdominal pain. The patient was placed supine on a stretcher; his airway was noted to be patent and protected, breath sounds were equal, and the abdomen was tender but soft. Oxygen at 4 liters/min was given by nasal cannula. He was transported to the ambulance, IV equipment was readied, and a radio call was placed to the hospital.

The squad acted quickly to assess the patient while simultaneously initiating stabilization. Only the essential historical information was collected, and the physical examination was limited to examination of the airway, chest, heart, and abdomen. Transport was the first priority, and IV access procedures were completed while in transit.

INITIAL APPROACH IN THE EMERGENCY DEPARTMENT

Patients with acute gastrointestinal hemorrhage who arrive by ambulance are taken immediately to a monitored bed for assessment. Ambulatory patients who give a history of gastrointestinal bleeding are rapidly triaged and assigned to an area appropriate for their clinical status.

History

The prehospital history is confirmed, and questions are asked about possible etiologies of the bleed, e.g., alcohol, medications. A brief overview of previous gastrointestinal disorders or other complicating conditions (e.g., heart disease, pulmonary disorders) is obtained.

Physical Examination

The vital signs are repeated and compared to the prehospital findings. The patient is undressed. If the patient is not hypotensive, orthostatic vital signs ("tilt test") are taken.

The blood pressure and pulse are recorded after the patient has been supine for at least 3 minutes. The patient is then asked to stand for a minimum of 1 minute, and the blood pressure and pulse are recorded again. The test results are considered positive if the pulse rate rises more than 20 beats/min or the systolic blood pressure drops more than 20 mm Hg. The patient is warned to mention the onset of dizziness and is watched for syncope. If symptoms occur, the patient is quickly returned to the supine position. The pulse is taken while the patient is standing to determine if any significant change in pulse rate or quality coincides with the patient's symptoms. A "positive" test result is reasonably predictive of intravascular volume loss of 20% to 30% or greater. It may be influenced by a number of factors including age and medications, e.g., beta-blocking agents.

The initial physical examination focuses on the level of consciousness, the adequacy of respirations, and the cardiovascular status. Skin color and presence of sweating are noted. The patient is observed for the stigmata of chronic alcohol use or advanced cirrhosis. The abdomen is examined for distention, tenderness and organomegaly. A rectal examination is performed, and any stool is tested for blood.

Intervention

Oxygen. Oxygen through the nasal cannula is continued. The airway is protected by whatever interventions are required. Suction may be necessary depending on the patient's ability to protect the airway. Vomiting is common in patients with upper gastrointestinal bleeding and the possibility of aspiration is high.

Cardiac Monitor. Monitoring is continued, and an electrocardiogram is taken early if there is associated chest pain or if acute myocardial ischemia is suspected.

Initial Volume Resuscitation. If the patient is hypotensive or in shock, additional large-bore IV lines are started, and isotonic crystalloid is infused rapidly. The degree of acute hemorrhage is estimated by simple clinical parameters and the volume replacement amount adjusted accordingly (see Table 6–1 and Chap. 4).

Blood Transfusion. Blood transfusion therapy is directed toward the restoration of diminished oxygen-carrying capacity, coagulation factors, or platelet function. Since patients bleed whole blood, it would seem logical to transfuse whole blood. However, there are flaws with this approach. Whole blood has a storage time of up to 6 weeks, but coagulation factors, granulocytes, and platelets are physiologically impaired in 1 week. In addition, the plasma from a whole blood transfusion exposes the recipient to a greater risk of immunologic reaction. Separated blood component therapy helps obviate these

TABLE 6–1. Estimated Fluid and Blood Requirements for Acute Blood Loss*
(Based on Initial Presentation of the Patient)

	Class I	Class II	Class III	Class IV
Blood loss (ml)	Up to 750	750–1500	1500–2000	2000 or more
Blood loss (% blood volume)	Up to 15%	15%–30%	30%–40%	40% or more
Pulse rate	<100 beats/min	>100 beats/min	>120 beats/min	140 beats/min or higher
Blood pressure	Normal	Normal	Decreased	Decreased
Pulse pressure (mm Hg)	Normal or increased	Decreased	Decreased	Decreased
Capillary blanch test	Normal	Positive	Positive	Positive
Respiratory rate	14–20	20–30	30–40	>35
Urine output (ml/hr)	30 or more	20–30	5–15	Negligible
CNS-mental status	Slightly anxious	Mildly anxious	Anxious and confused	Confused, lethargic
Fluid replacement (3:1 rule)†	Crystalloid	Crystalloid	Crystalloid + blood	Crystalloid + blood

*For a 70-kg male.
†Multiply estimated blood loss by 3 to get estimated crystalloid replacement.
Adapted from American College of Surgeons Committee on Trauma: Advanced Trauma Life Support. American College of Surgeons, 1988.

clinical problems and treats the specific hematologic deficit. Packed red blood cells (PRBCs) help restore the body's need for oxygen transport while reducing the risk of a plasma-related mismatch reaction. Fresh frozen plasma (FFP) can be stored for a year without appreciable loss of coagulative function. The acutely hemorrhaging patient needs red cells most. PRBCs can easily be reconstituted with crystalloid and infused rapidly through a large-bore IV line. FFP may be given later if the prothrombin or partial thromboplastin time (PT/PTT) values are prolonged, indicating possible depletion of coagulative factors. Platelet transfusion may be indicated in patients with thrombocytopenia or if there is suspected platelet dysfunction, e.g., with recent aspirin or nonsteroidal anti-inflammatory drug (NSAID) use. A reasonable clinical guideline in the emergent situation is to give 1 unit of FFP and 5 to 10 platelet packs for every 8 to 10 units of PRBCs given during a massive transfusion. A massive transfusion is defined as half the patient's blood volume (70 to 80 ml/kg) given in 6 hours or less, or the replacement of the patient's entire blood volume in a 24-hour period.

The completeness of cross-match of red cells is varied depending on the urgency of need for blood replacement. Type O− blood is considered a "universal donor" and can be administered immediately without cross-match. The Rh factor is important for women of childbearing age but not for men. Therefore, O+ blood can be given to males. In type-specific blood, which can be available in 10 to 15 minutes, the ABO and Rh groups are matched. It has a very low incidence of major transfusion reactions. The full cross-match takes 30 to 45 minutes. The hematology laboratory may be contacted in advance of or on the patient's arrival to discuss the type and timing of the blood product needed. Type and cross-match are requested for at least four units of packed red cells.

Initial Laboratory Studies. Most emergency departments have a capillary tube centrifuge, and a spun hematocrit can be a valuable initial parameter. The hematocrit is the ratio of red blood cells to plasma. A normal value tells nothing about the severity of blood loss, because early in a severe bleed essentially whole blood is lost. Assuming that the patient's hematocrit was normal before the hemorrhage, a lower hematocrit alerts the physician to the presence of blood loss and the fact that sufficient time has passed for the body to begin to compensate by shifting fluid into the intravascular space. Patients with previous anemia can confuse the interpretation.

Gastric Intubation. If upper gastrointestinal bleeding is suspected, a nasogastric tube is placed, and the gastric aspirate is tested for hemoglobin. The lavage aspirate is considered normal if the fluid is blood-free (Gastroccult negative) and bile-tinged. This finding implies that the stomach and duodenum contain no intraluminal blood and assumes that bleeding distal to the ligament of Treitz does not move retrograde. If these test results are slightly positive, the stomach is lavaged with water or isotonic crystalloid in 50- to 100-ml aliquots until the aspirate returns clear. One hundred milliliters of fluid is left in the stomach, and the patient is observed for 10 to 20 minutes. The fluid is aspirated again and reassessed for blood. This method can help determine the presence of persistent slow bleeding. If upper gastrointestinal bleeding is active or if the patient is vomiting blood, a larger gastric tube is passed. A large-caliber (30-Fr) orogastric tube is preferred to a nasogastric tube because it is large enough to evacuate blood clots and obviates possible nasal trauma.

PROBLEM 1 After arrival in the emergency department, the patient's repeat vital signs were blood pressure of 90/60 mm Hg, pulse 120 beats/min, and respirations of 20/min. He was less confused and anxious but still pale and diaphoretic. His capillary blanch test was clearly abnormal. The rescue squad had established one large-bore intravenous line and had infused 1 liter of Ringer's lactate. The PASG garment was in place, and the leg compartments were inflated.

Based on the vital signs, appearance, and signs of poor peripheral perfusion, the patient had a class III (30% to 40%) blood loss and required further crystalloid as well as blood infusion (see Table 6–1). A second large-bore IV line was established, and Ringer's lactate was maintained at high flow until blood was available. Chapter 4 reviews the calculations needed to estimate the patient's blood loss and volume replacement needs.

PROBLEM 2 During the triage assessment by the nurse, the patient was noted to be somewhat pale and complained of slight dizziness. Her vital signs were pulse 90 beats/min, blood pressure 140/90 mm Hg, and respirations 18/min. Postural vital signs were taken. On standing, the pulse rose to 120 beats/min and the blood pressure dropped to 100/70 mm Hg. She complained that the dizziness was worse.

Clearly, this patient has significant orthostatic changes. Based on her history of black stools, the origin is probably blood loss. She was now a higher priority case. The nurse notified the doctor, transferred the patient to a higher acuity area, established intravenous access for fluid administration, and drew appropriate blood samples for laboratory testing.

DATA GATHERING

The source and extent of gastrointestinal bleeding are often defined by a careful history and physical examination. If the patient is unable to give a detailed history, useful information is frequently available from the accompanying friends or family, rescue squad, available old records, or primary physician.

History

Onset of Bleeding. *When* did the *bleeding begin?* Because of the dramatic presentation of most acute gastrointestinal bleeding, the time of onset is easily noted by the patient. Did the onset occur before or after vomiting? Was it of gradual or rapid onset?

Blood Loss. Can the *amount* of blood loss be *estimated?* Patients usually overestimate the amount of loss, but a gross estimate is helpful.

Syncope. Is there a *history* of *syncope* or *near syncope?* Obviously, this is a serious symptom. It is a useful predictor of abnormal orthostatic vital signs.

Related Past History. Has there been a past history of *similar events?* Many patients with upper gastrointestinal bleeding have an easily identified cause, e.g., liver disease, peptic ulcer disease, the use of nonsteroidal anti-inflammatory drugs, salicylates, or ethanol. The causes of lower gastrointestinal bleeding are not as easy to discern.

Extra-gastrointestinal Sources. Has there been *bleeding* in or from the *mouth* or *nose?* An occult posterior nosebleed can present as an acute gastrointestinal bleed.

Abdominal Pain. Is there *abdominal pain?* What is its *character?* Bleeding can be either painless or associated with the pain of the underlying condition. Peptic ulcer disease ranging from gastritis to penetrating ulcer is typically painful in advance of the hemorrhage. Symptoms that occur during defecation can point toward the cause of lower gastrointestinal bleeding.

Extra-abdominal Symptoms. Are there *associated symptoms* such as chest pain or shortness of breath? Hemodynamic compromise can result in poor myocardial perfusion causing ischemia. One to two percent of upper gastrointestinal bleeds are associated with myocardial infarction, often "silent" in nature.

Family History. Is there a *family history* of bleeding disorders or a gastrointestinal problem? Patients with peptic ulcer disease are more likely to have relatives with the same condition.

Physical Examination

Just as the history of the present illness is stimulated by the chief complaint, the physical examination is guided by clues from the history. Its goal is to assess the severity of bleeding and search for clues to the source.

General Appearance. How does the patient present initially? What is the patient's mental status? How is the patient tolerating the event? Is there diaphoresis, pallor, cyanosis, or jaundice? Are there any stigmata of liver disease such as spider and cherry angiomas, or purpura and petechiae such as occur with a blood dyscrasia?

Vital Signs. In the nonhypovolemic patient, the blood pressure and pulse in the upright position closely approximate the values occurring when the patient is supine. However, an intravascular volume loss of up to 20% to 30% can occur without causing a measurable difference in the comparative blood pressures, particularly in younger patients. Clinicians may be falsely reassured by misleading vital signs that the blood volume is adequate. Since pulse rate changes occur before blood pressure declines, hypovolemia may be heralded by a persistent tachycardia or a significant increase in pulse rate with orthostatic testing. The value of orthostatic vital signs is discussed in the section Initial Approach in the Emergency Department. The patient is watched carefully for postural hypotension during the process of data gathering. Patients presenting with "hypotensive" vital signs do not require orthostatic testing for confirmation.

Head and Neck. The nose and mouth are examined for sources of recent or active bleeding. Is there evidence of recent trauma or surgery? Is there an infectious or inflammatory condition in the oropharynx? The conjunctiva should be checked for pallor or jaundice.

Chest and Cardiac Examination. The male chest is inspected for gynecomastia, which can occur in liver disease. The lungs are examined for signs of possible aspiration. The heart is examined to assess any dysrhythmia that might be induced by hypoxemia or ischemia.

Abdomen. The abdomen is inspected for distention and the presence of any abnormal skin findings. Bowel sounds are auscultated, although both hyperactive and hypoactive sounds are common. The presence of arterial bruits is actively sought. The abdomen is palpated for hepatosplenomegaly, possible abdominal aneurysms or thrills, hernias, or other masses. Tenderness on palpation is localized, and the presence of guarding or rebound is noted. The latter may indicate increased risk of a surgical emergency. Percussion techniques can help to identify the presence of ascites.

Rectum. The perianal area and rectum are examined to check for local anal, perianal, or rectal pathology as well as the presence of blood in the stool.

Special Tests

Examination for Occult Blood. Testing for occult blood in the stool or vomitus is based on the peroxidase activity of hemoglobin (Hgb). It results in a reagent changing to a blue color where present. Normal blood loss in the alimentary tract is 2 to 2.5 ml of blood/day. The Hemoccult card (Smith Kline Diagnostics) is a guaiac-impregnated filter paper that tests positive if there is a gastrointestinal blood loss of 5 to 10 ml/day. This amount corresponds to 5 to 10 mg Hgb/gm of stool. The Hemoccult card is 95% sensitive if there is 20 mg Hgb/gm of stool. False-negative results can occur if the bleeding is intermittent. False-positive results occur in up to 12% of samples. Peroxidase-containing foods such as bananas, turnips, and broccoli can cause false-positive test results. Iodine also causes a false-positive result. Ingested iron and bismuth may darken the stool color but will not cause a positive result in the Hemoccult test.

Nasogastric Aspirate and Lavage. Although a nasogastric tube is more often part of the management process, it can also be an excellent diagnostic aid. In patients without obvious gastrointestinal hemorrhage, the nasogastric aspirate and lavage fluid are tested for hemoglobin (Gastroccult test). This is a quick and reasonably accurate test for blood in the upper gastrointestinal tract. If blood is present, gastric lavage may serve as a rough gauge of the rate of bleeding. The stomach is lavaged until 100 to 200 ml of clear fluid are left in the stomach. Then an aspirate sample is examined and tested for hemoglobin 10 to 20 minutes later. A positive test result correlates with active hemorrhage.

PROBLEM 2 A careful examination of the woman's abdomen revealed an enlarged, irregular, hard liver. On closer questioning she recalled experiencing anorexia and weight loss over a several week period. She did not think the symptoms were significant until the onset of postural dizziness. Her stool test for hemoglobin showed very positive results. During evaluation, she received 500 ml of normal saline. Her pulse rate slowed to 90, and her symptoms resolved.

It is not uncommon for older people to ignore medical symptoms. Often there is fear that a fatal disease might be diagnosed. As a consequence, a crisis is reached, and the emergency department becomes the place where not only the immediate threat to life is reversed but also the initial diagnosis of underlying disease is made.

DECISION PRIORITIES AND PRELIMINARY DIFFERENTIAL DIAGNOSIS

The initial clinical information guides management decisions by establishing the condition of the patient and allowing a preliminary formulation of a differential diagnosis. Key questions influencing these decisions are:

1. *What is the severity of blood loss and how is the patient tolerating it? Is there clinical evidence of hypoperfusion of vital organs, i.e., "shock"?*
   The initial estimates of blood loss (Table 6–1) are reassessed in the context of more information and the patient's response to treatment.
2. *Is true gastrointestinal bleeding occurring?*
   Food or medication may be mistaken for blood in vomitus or stool (e.g., black stools from a recent ingestion of iron supplement tablets). Swallowed blood from epistaxis or oropharyngeal bleeding can be mistaken for gastrointestinal bleeding. A careful ear, nose, and throat history and examination should resolve the issue.
3. *If gastrointestinal blood is present, is it upper or lower in origin?*
   The gastric aspirate and lavage is the initial screening tool used to locate the site of the bleeding. Bleeding below the ligament of Treitz rarely appears in the stomach. Localizing the bleeding site is important in terms of immediate and subsequent therapy, possible causes, and prognosis. Tables 6–2 and 6–3 list the more frequent causes of upper and lower gastrointestinal hemorrhage. Brisk upper gastrointestinal bleeding is a very common cause of lower gastrointestinal hematochezia.
4. *How rapid is the blood loss?*
   Rate of blood loss can be estimated by the time of onset and the clinical status of the patient. Aspirate from a nasogastric tube can assist in monitoring slow to moderate bleeding rates. Brisk upper gastrointestinal bleeding usually does not clear with lavage. Esophageal varices and a rapidly bleeding duodenal or gastric ulcer are the most common causes of massive upper gastrointestinal bleeds. A bleeding colonic diverticulum is the most common lower gastrointestinal source.

TABLE 6–2. Causes of Upper Gastrointestinal Bleeding

Common	Uncommon
Epistaxis and oral bleeding	Aortoenteric fistula
Duodenitis	Boerhaave's syndrome
Duodenal ulcer	Blood dyscrasias
Esophageal varices	Carcinoma, leiomyoma
Esophagitis	Mallory-Weiss lesions
Gastric ulcer	Vascular anomalies
Gastritis	Arteriovenous malformations
	Hereditary telangiectasia
	Angiodysplasia

TABLE 6–3. Causes of Lower Gastrointestinal Bleeding

Common	Uncommon
Angiodysplasia	Aortoenteric fistulas
Anal fissures	Blood dyscrasias
Carcinoma	Meckel's diverticulum
Colonic diverticula	Mesenteric ischemia
Hemorrhoids	
Infectious diarrhea with invasive agents	
Inflammatory bowel disease	
Inflammatory proctitis	

5. *Is there the possibility of a hemostatic disorder?*

It is important to consider the integrity of the hemostatic system as well as the mucosa while gathering data from the patient. Mucosal bleeding is primarily associated with disorders of platelets. A history of aspirin or NSAID use or thrombocytopenia may explain persistent hemorrhage.

PROBLEM 1 After a careful history and physical examination, it was apparent that this patient had several risk factors for severe gastrointestinal bleeding. He was a heavy alcohol abuser and took aspirin regularly for his "hangovers." He had some stigmata of advanced liver disease including spider angiomas, splenomegaly, and enlarged abdominal veins. An orogastric tube was placed and yielded 300 ml of bright red blood.

Although no definitive diagnosis could be reached at this point, it was evident that this patient had active blood loss, was tolerating the loss poorly, and had at least an upper gastrointestinal source of blood loss. Considering his underlying ethanol abuse, the likely causes of hemorrhage include bleeding esophageal varices, erosive gastritis, and duodenal ulcer. All are capable of causing life-threatening hemorrhage. His aspirin use, especially within the last week, increased his risk for serious mucosal bleeding because of induced platelet dysfunction.

DIAGNOSTIC ADJUNCTS

Laboratory Studies

Laboratory testing can assist in assessing the severity of hemorrhage, the physiologic tolerance and compensation for the hemorrhage, and the general metabolic condition of the patient. Tests are usually ordered early in the course of evaluating a patient with an acute gastrointestinal bleed. In patients with severe bleeding, all of the tests listed below are requested.

Hemoglobin/Hematocrit. Acute recent hemorrhage may not present as anemia. The hemoglobin level or hematocrit alone is a poor estimate of blood volume because it takes a few hours for the body to mobilize extravascular fluid to compensate for an acute blood loss. The test establishes a "baseline" of red cell volume and, indirectly, oxygen-carrying capacity.

White Blood Cell Count and Differential. A mild leukocytosis may be evident during active bleeding. A very high count, more than 25,000 cells/mm^3 with a "leukemoid" reaction on peripheral smear, may be seen in patients with cancer of gastrointestinal origin.

Electrolytes. The most useful value is the bicarbonate (HCO_3^-) concentration. It may decrease secondary to lactic acidosis from tissue ischemia or to another cause of metabolic acidosis, e.g., salicylism. The sodium, potassium, and chloride concentrations are not significantly changed with hemorrhage but may reflect medication use or underlying disease states.

Blood Urea Nitrogen and Creatinine. The blood urea nitrogen (BUN) and creatinine are indirect measures of renal function. A high BUN–creatinine ratio (normal, 10:1) may signify severe dehydration. Digested blood protein absorbed through the gastrointestinal tract may also contribute to a high BUN level. A low BUN may occur with hepatic failure.

Blood Glucose. Blood glucose levels tend to be higher than normal during massive bleeding due to glycogen breakdown secondary to the increased circulating levels of the "stress hormones" epinephrine and glucagon.

Coagulation Studies. The prothrombin and partial thromboplastin times can suggest severe or advanced liver disease or a primary coagulation disorder. Both values begin to increase when the coagulation factor levels fall below 40% of normal. This occurs after the liver loses 85% to 90% of its functional ability to produce coagulation factors.

Platelets. A platelet count is not a measure of platelet function. The count may be decreased because of the effects of ethanol, splenomegaly, or diffuse intravascular coagulopathy. The most common drugs that impair platelet function are aspirin and the nonsteroidal anti-inflammatory drugs, e.g., ibuprofen.

Arterial Blood Gas. Measurement of arterial blood gases is useful indirectly in evaluating the efficacy of cardiac output in hypovolemic shock and the metabolic acidemia that occurs secondary to hypoperfusion. The PaO_2 measures the dissolved oxygen in the blood rather than the oxygen content. Oxygen content more accurately represents the patient's oxygenation status.

Liver Function Tests. These tests are helpful in recognizing the patient with preexisting hepatic disease. Hypovolemic shock can also cause a rise in liver enzyme levels due to centrilobular necrosis.

Ammonia. The ammonia level may be indicative of hepatic encephalopathy secondary to severe acute or chronic liver disease.

Radiologic Imaging

Chest Radiograph. A chest radiograph is part of the assessment of patients being considered for admission to the hospital. Aspiration of blood is possible, and other sources of pulmonary pathology are sought. Free air in the peritoneum is best seen on this view.

Abdominal Radiograph. Plain abdominal radiographs in the supine and upright positions are only indicated if perforation with free peritoneal air is suspected.

Barium Contrast Radiographs. This study was once the mainstay for the detection of peptic ulcer disease and colonic lesions such as neoplasms and diverticula. However, barium studies are not indicated during acute bleeding. They do not detect mucosal lesions as well as upper and lower gastrointestinal endoscopy, and prior use of barium may obscure the endoscopic view. Only 70% to 80% of duodenal ulcers detectable through an endoscope are localized by barium studies.

Electrocardiogram

An ECG is indicated in any patient with hemorrhage resulting in unstable vital signs. As noted previously, an acute myocardial infarction occurs in about 1% to 2% of all patients with upper gastrointestinal bleeds, often without symptoms.

Other Tests

Anoscopy and Sigmoidoscopy. Lower gastrointestinal bleeding is much less common than bleeding from the upper alimentary tract. Direct visualization techniques are more readily available and useful in finding many common sources of bleeding. Anal and distal rectal lesions may be seen with an anoscope. It is a simple tool to master, and its use is a valuable addition to the skills of the emergency physician. Sigmoidoscopy is used to detect rectal and sigmoid colon lesions. It is a procedure performed by a consultant, usually outside of the emergency department.

Upper Gastrointestinal Endoscopy. Endoscopy of the esophagus, stomach, and duodenum is usually performed in an endoscopy suite. In patients with severe bleeding, it can be done by a consultant in the emergency department. Though not a procedure done by the emergency physician, one must be familiar with its indications in patients with upper gastrointestinal hemorrhage. Most patients with persistent bleeding or with volume losses sufficient to cause hematemesis or melena are candidates for eventual endoscopy.

PROBLEM 1 The laboratory results showed a hemoglobin–hematocrit of 8.0 gm and 24%. The electrolyte measurements were normal except for a bicarbonate level of 20 mEq/liter and potassium level of 5.5 mEq/liter. The platelet count was 92,000/mm^3, and the PT was 3 seconds over control.

The patient had a major loss of blood. The metabolic acidemia was probably related to hypoperfusion. Other possible causes for the acidemia e.g., salicylism, should be considered. The platelet count and PT may have been abnormal because of severe liver disease or early diffuse intravascular coagulation (DIC). A peripheral smear looking for broken cells (schizocytes) might point to DIC (see Chap. 24).

REFINED DIFFERENTIAL DIAGNOSIS

The actual anatomic site of gastrointestinal bleeding may not be determined in the emergency department, but the differential diagnosis is often narrowed to a few choices. Table 6–2 lists the common and uncommon causes of upper gastrointestinal bleeding. Ninety percent of all cases of upper gastrointestinal bleeding result from peptic ulceration, erosive gastritis, and esophagogastric varices. The causes of lower gastrointestinal bleeding are given in Table 6–3.

Upper Gastrointestinal Bleeding
Peptic Ulceration

Peptic ulceration is the most common cause of upper gastrointestinal bleeding, accounting for 25% to 40% of cases. Approximately 20% to 30% of patients with documented ulcers will have significant bleeding at some point during the disease. The characteristic history of persistent aching or burning pain usually precedes the bleeding episode. Occasionally, hemorrhage is the initial manifestation of the disease. This is often seen in elderly patients. Duodenal ulcers are two to three times more common in males than females and have a prevalence in the population estimated to be 6% to 15%. Most of these ulcers are located in the upper and mid-duodenum. Predisposing factors for peptic ulcer disease include heredity (it is three times more common in first-degree relatives), blood group O, and cigarette smoking. The importance of stress and other psychologic factors remains controversial.

The majority of patients with duodenal ulcer present with burning or gnawing epigastric pain that occurs 1 to 3 hours after eating. This pain is usually accompanied by tenderness in the epigastrium or just to the right of that location. Changes in the character of the pain can herald the onset of complications. Acute onset and persistent pain suggest perforation, particularly if peritoneal signs develop.

Erosive gastritis is responsible for 10% to 15% of cases of gastrointestinal bleeding. Predisposing factors include indiscretionary use of ethanol, nonsteroidal anti-inflammatory drugs, prolonged steroid use, and severe underlying disease with associated stress, e.g., major trauma, burns, and head injury. The clinical presentation of gastritis is often indistinguishable from that of duodenal ulcer, although consumption of food tends to make the pain better in patients with gastritis and worse in those with peptic ulcer disease. The diagnosis of this disease is based on the clinical setting, characteristic predisposing factors, and confirmation by endoscopy.

Esophageal Varices

Some of the most catastrophic and difficult-to-manage upper gastrointestinal hemorrhages are seen in patients with esophagogastric varices. These dilated veins occur with elevated portal venous system pressure, most often in the esophagus and proximal stomach. Bleeding from varices is often abrupt and massive. One-third of all cases of massive upper gastrointestinal bleeding are due to varices. Bleeding has been reported to occur in 30% of patients with varices secondary to cirrhosis. Clinical clues supporting varices as the source of bleeding include the stigmata of advanced liver disease with portal hypertension, e.g., ascites, enlarged abdominal wall veins, splenomegaly, and hemorrhoids. Unfortunately, up to 50% of patients with known varices have bleeding episodes from gastritis or peptic ulcer disease, and endoscopy is necessary to confirm the source of hemorrhage. The mortality rate within 1 year of the first bleeding episode is 70%.

Mallory-Weiss Tear

A relatively uncommon but dramatic cause of upper gastrointestinal bleeding is a Mallory-Weiss tear of the esophagus. This is a partial-thickness longitudinal laceration of the gastroesophageal junction that is usually caused by violent vomiting, coughing, or retching. The abrupt onset of significant hemorrhage soon after such an episode is characteristic. The bleeding can be life-threatening in degree. Occasionally after vomiting or retching a complete rupture of the esophagus (Boerhaave's syndrome) can occur with leakage of gastric contents into the mediastinum and chest. This is a catastrophic event with a very poor prognosis.

Lower Gastrointestinal Bleeding
Anorectal Sources

Anorectal problems, most commonly internal and external hemorrhoids, are the most common cause of lower gastrointestinal bleeding. Other sources include fissures, fistulas, foreign bodies, and infectious proctitis. Hemorrhoids result from increased hydrostatic pressure in the portal venous system. Straining at stool is by far the most common cause of such increased pressure, followed by pregnancy and systemic venous hypertension. The bleeding of hemorrhoids presents as bright red blood on toilet paper or red streaking of stool. If present at all, pain symptoms range from mild anal discomfort to the severe pain of thrombosis. The diagnosis of hemorrhoids can be made by inspection and digital examination. Anoscopy is confirmatory for internal hemorrhoids. Even in patients who have known hemorrhoids, new-onset lower gastrointestinal bleeding often is caused by other lesions.

Diverticulosis

Diverticular disease is generally seen in older patients and is the most common cause of massive lower gastrointestinal bleeding. Diverticula are found in 20% to 50% of Americans over the age of 50, and in 70% of patients aged 75 to 80 years. They occur most commonly in the sigmoid and descending colon. Bleeding is much less common than irritation and inflammation (diverticulitis) and results from the erosion of a small vessel in the diverticular sac by a fecalith. The bleeding is usually painless and self-limited. Significant bleeding requires angiography for diagnosis and localization of the bleeding site.

Mesenteric Ischemia

Mesenteric ischemia is seen in patients, often elderly, who have peripheral atherosclerotic vascular disease, cardiac dysrhythmia, or any condition predisposing to thrombus formation and embolization, e.g., congestive heart failure, atrial fibrillation, or even oral contraceptive use. The ischemia evolves from a low-flow state or frank occlusion of a mesenteric artery secondary to thrombus or emboli. Clinically, patients with mesenteric ischemia often have severe abdominal pain and a high white count out of proportion to their relatively benign examination. A typical laboratory finding is a significant anion-gap metabolic acidosis secondary to lactic acid metabolism. This may be the only finding in the elderly or obtunded patient. Bleeding occurs from ischemic-necrotic sloughing of intestinal mucosa. The mortality in mesenteric ischemia is high, up to 70%, regardless of the exact cause.

Angiodysplasia

Angiodysplasia is a lesion that occurs predominantly in the cecum and right colon. Like diverticular disease, it is common and affects people over the age of 50. Hypertension and aortic stenosis are associated conditions. Angiodysplasia usually does not cause massive bleeding but can cause a large blood loss over a period of time.

Cancer

Cancer of the large bowel is the second most common site of carcinoma in both males and females in their sixth decade. Seventy-five percent of these carcinomas occur in the descending colon and rectosigmoid area. Early symptoms are often vague and include malaise, change in bowel habits, weight loss, and anemia. Rectal bleeding is likely to be noticed by 70% of patients who have left-sided lesions, whereas fewer than 25% of patients with right-sided lesions have that complaint. Pain is an unusual symptom of colonic cancer. Diagnosis is made by barium enema or colonoscopy.

Other Causes of Bleeding

There are many other causes of lower gastrointestinal bleeding. Inflammatory bowel disease has its peak incidence in the second and third decades of life. It presents with abdominal cramping, weight loss, and a varying degree of bloody diarrhea. Infectious diarrheas can cause lower gastrointestinal bleeding. A history of travel to endemic areas, eating suspect foods, or variant sexual practices is explored as appropriate.

> **PROBLEM 2** The laboratory values of the patient included a hematocrit of 28%. Her liver profile showed an abnormal elevation of liver enzymes. The remainder of the laboratory studies were normal. Abdominal films were unremarkable. After limited volume resuscitation, she was hemodynamically stable and no longer orthostatic. She was transferred to an inpatient bed.
> Based on the available clinical and laboratory data, it seemed probable that this patient had a malignant process. It was likely to be a colon carcinoma with metastases to the liver. Because her condition had become stable, plans for transfusion could be completed as an inpatient. With a hematocrit level of below 30%, she was a candidate for packed red cells. It was unlikely that she would respond to iron supplement alone.

PRINCIPLES OF MANAGEMENT

The main objectives of emergency department management are to replace lost volume and prevent hemodynamic instability. Eighty to ninety percent of gastrointestinal hemorrhage is self-limited and ceases spontaneously within 24 to 48 hours. General support includes oxygen, volume replacement with isotonic crystalloid, and blood component transfusions as indicated. The goal is always to anticipate the possible needs of the patient rather than to react to a series of acute problems or complications. Most bleeding will not require advanced treatment techniques in the emergency department.

If the gastrointestinal hemorrhage is persistently active or associated with hemodynamic instability, it is essential to seek early consultation with a gastroenterologist. If the patient's status does not rapidly stabilize, a general surgeon is also asked to consult.

Specific Therapy
Upper Gastrointestinal Bleeding

Gastric Lavage. Lavage is performed to clear the stomach of blood and clots, to roughly quantify the bleeding, and to shrink the stomach, an action that may be helpful in aiding hemostasis. The short-term goal of lavage is to clear the stomach in order to permit good visualization for subsequent endoscopy. Lavage is carried out by introducing 50- to 100-ml aliquots of fluid down the orogastric tube and gently aspirating the fluid with a large syringe. This procedure is continued until the return fluid is clear. There is no significant difference in efficacy between normal saline versus tap water or iced versus room temperature solutions. Plain tap water is a plentiful and economical lavage fluid. Some evidence suggests that a cold environment inhibits fibrin deposition and the coagulation cascade. The risk of water intoxication is minimal in the adult.

Esophageal Tamponade. If there is a strong suspicion of massively bleeding esophageal varices, a Sengstaken-Blakemore tube can be passed orogastrically and the two balloons inflated to provide a pressure tamponade of the varices. There is a large intragastric balloon and another esophageal balloon, with a single suction port at the distal tip in the stomach. It is usually left in place 12 to 24 hours. Complications include esophageal rupture and pharyngeal blockage with asphyxiation from the esophageal portion of the balloon. The Edlich-Minnesota modification of the Sengstaken-Blakemore tube provides proximal esophageal suction, thereby minimizing the risk of aspiration. With improved endoscopic diagnostic techniques and other modes of therapy, balloon tamponade is not used as often as previously.

Esophagogastroduodenoscopy. Once the bleeding has been stabilized or abated by lavage, endoscopy can be performed to visualize the bleeding source. If the bleeding is located, a variety of transendoscopic therapies can be used to treat it. These include needle sclerotherapy for esophageal varices, direct application of medication to the bleeding site, and laser photocoagulation. Laser therapy is a powerful addition to the endoscopic technique. It is available in two forms: argon and Nd-YAG (neodynium-yttrium-aluminum-garnet). The Nd-YAG beam is stronger and can penetrate tissues to 2 to 4 mm. Laser therapy has proved effective in treatment of angiodysplasias and peptic ulcer disease. Another recent development in endoscopy involves thermocoagulation devices and heat probes. Early studies suggest that thermocoagulation rivals or exceeds laser therapy and may become a low-cost alternative. However, more clinical evaluation of this method is necessary.

Vasopressin Infusion. Infusion of vasopressin following the angiographic demonstration of the upper gastrointestinal bleeding site has been successful in controlling bleeding from esophageal varices, severe erosive gastritis, and uncontrolled stress ulcers. Adjunctive therapy with beta-blockers is thought to decrease cardiac output and hence portal venous flow to esophageal varices.

H_2 Histamine Antagonists. Histamine antagonists are thought to decrease bleeding by blocking acidity in the stomach and constricting vessels at the bleeding site, thereby decreasing the "force" of bleeding. H_2 histamine antagonists and antacids are used more for prevention than for stopping active bleeding. Their benefit in acute upper gastrointestinal bleeding has not been substantiated.

Arteriography. Selective abdominal angiography may be useful in patients with brisk bleeding (more than 1.0 ml/min) that does not allow either blood to be cleared from the stomach or accurate endoscopic assessment. If the bleeding vessel is located, the catheter is left in place and vasopressin infused through it. Though the technique is less popular today, the use of autologous clot to embolize the bleeding vessel occasionally can give dramatic results. The patient must be in a reasonably stable condition before being transported to the radiology department.

Surgical Intervention. Surgical intervention is the final option in treating upper gastrointestinal hemorrhage. Most esophageal bleeding episodes are treated nonoperatively. In other sites (stomach and duodenum), massive bleeding, continued bleeding, or rebleeding are the usual indications for surgery. In patients with a gastric ulcer, a visible bleeding vessel is associated with a rebleeding rate of over 50%. The need for operative intervention is also about 50%. Emergent surgical indications include free perforation into the peritoneal cavity and massive bleeding unresponsive to medical or endoscopic treatment.

PROBLEM 1 Gastric lavage was successful, and bleeding ceased after 30 minutes. The patient was given 4 liters of Ringer's lactate and three units of type-specific packed red cells to reverse the hypovolemia and hypoperfusion. The blood pressure returned to 110/80 mm Hg, pulse to 90 beats/min, and respirations to 18/min. After stabilization, the PASGs were successfully removed without causing hemodynamic deterioration.

After lavage and stabilization, the patient was ready for esophagogastroduodenoscopy. This procedure is usually not carried out in the emergency department, and the patient was readied for transfer to the endoscopy suite. The laboratory tests were repeated to be sure that the coagulation and platelet values had improved. Because of the patient's history of alcoholism and probable liver disease, he may benefit from a vitamin supplement including vitamin K.

Lower Gastrointestinal Bleeding

Arteriography. If a bleeding lower gastrointestinal tract lesion cannot be identified by anoscopy, sigmoidoscopy, or colonic endoscopy, or if endoscopy is prevented by continuous bleeding, selective arteriography is used to detect the bleeding site. For this procedure to be used, the bleeding rate from the site must exceed 0.5 to 1 ml/min; if bleeding is intermittent, the test may be falsely negative. Arteriography is necessary for the evaluation of areas not amenable to endoscopy or in the difficult circumstance of a suspected aortoenteric fistula. Selected vessel angiography can also be used for the infusion of vasopressin.

Vasopressin Infusion. Vasopressin is used for its vasoconstrictor action. Direct vasopressin infusion by selective catheterization of the mesenteric arteries has not been shown to be more effective in reducing hemorrhage than IV systemic vasopressin alone. It is rarely initiated in the emergency department, and consultation is necessary.

Surgical Intervention. The indications for urgent interventional surgery in cases of lower gastrointestinal bleeding are similar to those for upper gastrointestinal causes. If medical support does not stabilize the patient's condition, operative control of the bleeding site is the only recourse. Of sources of lower gastrointestinal bleeding, diverticular disease is the most likely to bleed heavily and to rebleed. Severe bleeding requiring a transfusion of more than four units of PRBCs is associated with an operative rate of close to 60%. In patients with other lesions, such as an aortoenteric fistula, the need for early surgical control of hemorrhage is clear if the diagnosis is made in time.

SPECIAL CONSIDERATIONS

Pediatric Patients

The evaluation of gastrointestinal bleeding in the pediatric population is often complicated by communication limitations between the physician and the patient. The history given by the parent or guardian and the physical examination assume primary importance. Associated symptoms such as pain, irritability, changes in normal activity and feeding, vomiting, diarrhea, or altered stools can accompany a wide range of potential diagnoses. Information about a term or premature birth, any perinatal complications, or a history of similar familial disorders must be known. True pediatric emergencies are described below.

1. Vomiting with evidence of upper or lower gastrointestinal bleeding suggests a bowel obstruction with possible hemorrhage from injured or ischemic intestinal mucosa.

2. Lower gastrointestinal bleeding can be due to a colonic polyp, intussusception, or Meckel's diverticulum. Intestinal polyposis may be an inherited familial condition. Intussusception is characterized by progressively more frequent episodes of abdominal colic with apparently normal intervals. Older infants and young children are most affected. The classic finding of "currant jelly stool" with intussusception is a late finding that implies bowel mucosal damage. A Meckel's diverticulum is a remnant of the omphalomesenteric duct found near the terminal ileum. It can contain ectopic rests of acid-producing gastric mucosa in about 50% of cases. These can erode the intestinal mucosa and induce bleeding. It also can mimic the presentation of appendicitis and is associated with a higher risk of intestinal obstruction.

3. In the neonatal or young infant period, congenital malrotation of the gut with a midgut volvulus can present as acute hemorrhage. Emergent surgery is needed to prevent massive intestinal gangrene. Another neonatal condition, although very rare, is portal hypertension with bleeding esophageal varices secondary to congenital hepatobiliary disease or extrahepatic portal vein thrombosis.

4. Noncongenital causes of pediatric gastrointestinal bleeding must always be considered as well, such as the possibility of nonaccidental trauma or sexual abuse, foreign body ingestions, or toxic ingestion, e.g., massive iron overdose.

Management of pediatric patients generally follows adult guidelines except for the amount of fluid used in volume resuscitation. Isotonic crystalloid is the initial fluid of choice, preferably delivered through a volume control IV device. Early consultation with the appropriate specialists in pediatrics, pediatric surgery, and radiology is vital for appropriate diagnostic testing and definitive treatment.

DISPOSITION AND FOLLOW-UP

Almost all patients with upper or lower gastrointestinal bleeding are admitted to the hospital. Patients are admitted to critical care units if their condition remains unstable in the emergency department, their bleeding persists, or the hemorrhage is massive.

Admission

Any person who has bleeding with abnormal orthostatic vital signs or a new-onset anemia is admitted for observation and diagnosis even if he or she is young and otherwise healthy. If the patient has a preexisting anemia, a new bleed may compromise an already reduced hemodynamic reserve. Any patient with a significant degree of blood loss demonstrable by vomiting, gastric lavage, or stool analysis in the emergency department is admitted. In addition, recurrent bleeding for any gastrointestinal source except hemorrhoids is an indication for admission.

Discharge

Patients who can safely be discharged home with self-care instructions include (1) those with minimal upper gastrointestinal bleeding that has ceased, for example, following an episode of gastritis; (2) those with simple uncomplicated fissures and hemorrhoids; and (3) elderly people with occult blood in the stool without discernible disease requiring admission. These patients should all have normal, stable vital signs, no orthostatic changes, no anemia or blood dyscrasias, and no other serious complicating associated conditions. Follow-up with a primary care physician is arranged within 1 to 3 days.

DOCUMENTATION

1. Identity and age of patient and current medications
2. Site of bleeding and estimate of amount
3. Risk factors for hemorrhage, including alcohol use
4. History of past bleeds, other pertinent facts in medical and surgical history
5. Vital signs (including orthostatic measurements and serial responses to volume resuscitation)
6. Hemoglobin/hematocrit and hemostasis studies
7. Assessment and disposition
8. Outpatient care instructions and follow-up appointment if arranged

SUMMARY AND FINAL POINTS

- In spite of the fact that most patients ultimately do well after a gastrointestinal bleed, mortality still approaches 8%. Any patient with historical or physical findings suggestive of gastrointestinal bleeding must be cared for as if a crisis could occur. These patients are triaged to higher level care areas of the emergency department and given priority by both physician and nurse.
- The first responsibility of the emergency team is to determine the hemodynamic stability of the patient. In addition to assessing the patient for peripheral signs of hypoperfusion and vital signs, particular attention is paid to any orthostatic changes. Patients can lose up to 20% to 30% of their blood volume and still maintain a normal blood pressure in the supine position.
- Patients who appear stable and do not initially show evidence of a major bleed require placement of an intravenous line as a security measure until a thorough assessment can be carried out.
- Once emergency department stabilization has been carried out, patients are usually transferred to other diagnostic or care areas for definitive diagnostic and treatment measures.
- Only patients with the most insignificant bleeds, such as those caused by mild gastritis or hemorrhoids, can be considered for outpatient management.

BIBLIOGRAPHY

Texts

1. Bongiovanni G (ed): The Essentials of Clinical Gastroenterology (2nd ed). New York, McGraw-Hill, 1988.
2. Sleisenger MH, Fordtran JS (eds): Gastrointestinal Disease: Pathophysiology, Diagnosis, and Management (4th ed). Philadelphia, Saunders, 1989.

Journal Articles

1. Consensus Conference: Therapeutic endoscopy and bleeding ulcers. JAMA 262(10):1369–1372, 1989.
2. Gilbert DA, Saunders DR: Ice saline lavage does not slow bleeding from experimental canine gastric ulcers. Dig Dis Sci 26:1065–1068, 1981.
3. Gostout CJ: Acute gastrointestinal bleeding—A common problem revisited. Mayo Clin Proc 63:596–604, 1988.
4. Kinard HB, Powell DW, Sandler RS, et al: A current approach

to acute upper gastrointestinal bleeding. J Clin Gastroenterol 3:231–240, 1981.
5. Lebred C, Poynard T, Bernuau J, et al: A randomized controlled study of propranolol for prevention of recurrent gastrointestinal bleeding in patients with cirrhosis; a final report. Hepatology 4:355, 1984.
6. Letter: Lower gastrointestinal bleeding. Br J Surg 76(5):526–527, 1989.
7. Lower gastrointestinal bleeding. Br J Surg 76(1):3–4, 1989.
8. Ostro MJ, Russell JA, Soldin SJ, et al: Control of gastric pH with cimetidine: Boluses vs primed infusions. Gastroenterology 89:532, 1985.
9. Silverstein FE, Feld AD, Gilbert DA: Upper gastrointestinal tract bleeding: Predisposing factors, diagnosis, and therapy. Arch Intern Med 141:322, 1981.
10. Silverstein FE, Gilbert DA, Tedesco FJ, et al: The national ASGE survey on upper gastrointestinal bleeding. Gastrointest Endosc 27:80–93, 1981.
11. Swain CP, Kirkham JS, Salmon PR, et al: Controlled trial of Nd-YAG laser photocoagulation in bleeding peptic ulcers. Lancet 1:1113, 1986.
12. Terés J: Balloon tamponade vs. endoscopic sclerotherapy in the management of active variceal hemorrhage. Hepatology 10(3):393–394, 1989.
13. Zuckerman G, Welch R, Douglas A, et al: Controlled trial of medical therapy for active upper gastrointestinal bleeding and prevention of rebleeding. Am J Med 76:361–366, 1984.

CHAPTER 7

ACUTE DIARRHEA

ROBERT A. BITTERMAN, M.D.

PROBLEM A 20 year old male came to the emergency department complaining that for the last 18 hours he had had frequent loose stools associated with cramps, abdominal pain, chills, and fever.

QUESTIONS TO CONSIDER

1. Which patients with diarrhea are at high risk for serious problems?
2. What are the common causes of diarrhea and which serious illnesses may present as diarrhea?
3. What diagnostic adjuncts are useful in determining the etiology of diarrhea?
4. When should stool cultures be obtained or tests for parasitic disease performed?
5. Which patients need intravenous rehydration? When is oral hydration appropriate?
6. When are antidiarrheal medications prescribed?
7. What public health issues need to be considered?

INTRODUCTION

Diarrhea is defined as the rapid passage of excessively fluid stool. It accounts for 5% to 7% of outpatient visits to physicians. It is second only to the common cold as a cause of days lost from work, and it continues to be a significant cause of morbidity and mortality around the world.

Some of the more common causes of diarrhea include infection, inflammation, toxins, foods, medications, malabsorption syndrome, and acute psychosocial stress. Viruses, such as rotaviruses and the Norwalk virus, cause 50% to 80% of cases of infectious diarrhea. These agents are more common in children and in family outbreaks during the winter months. Bacterial agents account for about 10% to 15% of cases, and parasites for another 6% to 10%. Toxin-induced diarrhea can occur in sporadic epidemics when the source is contaminated food or water. Most of the other causes of diarrhea produce only mild, short-lived disease or are chronic in nature. Most patients who come to the emergency department suffering from diarrhea are symptomatic owing to the prolonged duration of frequent stools, fever, abdominal pain, vomiting, bloody stools, or dehydration.

Although an enormous number of stimuli result in diarrhea, there are three basic pathophysiologic mechanisms: an increase in gastrointestinal volume load, a decrease in the absorptive capacity of the bowel, and an increase in gut motility. Frequently all three elements combine in producing diarrhea. Normally the gastrointestinal tract is presented with 8 to 9 liters of secretions and ingested fluids per day. Absorption by the small intestine reduces this to 500 to 600 ml, and further absorption in the colon results in about 100 ml of fluid lost in stool per day. Water is absorbed passively following the osmotic gradient created by the active absorption of sodium.

The editors wish to recognize the special contributions made to this chapter by Douglas Propp, M.D.

The small intestine may contribute to the production of diarrhea either by exposing the colon to a volume of intestinal contents at a rate that exceeds its absorptive capacity or by allowing the entry of substances into the colon that stimulate rapid emptying. Cholera is the classic example of volume overload of the colon resulting in frequent stools. Cholera toxin disrupts the sodium secretion–regulating system in the small intestinal mucosa. Massive influx of sodium and fluid into the bowel lumen exceeds the resorptive capacity of the small intestine and the colon. The colon simply fills to capacity, and watery diarrhea follows. More common examples of toxin-induced secretory diarrhea include the enterotoxigenic *Escherichia coli* infection common in travelers, viral gastroenteritis, toxigenic food poisoning syndromes, cryptosporidiosis, and some *Shigella* infections.

Invasive or inflammatory diseases induce mucosal erosion, ulceration, and bleeding of the bowel. The epithelial barrier is destroyed, leaving a raw exuding surface with poor absorptive properties. Deeper involvement of the bowel wall further diminishes absorptive capacity and may stimulate bowel motility. Infectious diseases, such as those due to *Salmonella*, *Shigella*, and *Campylobacter*, and inflammatory bowel diseases such as ulcerative colitis predominantly involve the colon, leading to diarrheal disease.

Psychologic stress can increase gut motility in certain patients. This predisposition can result in the irritable bowel syndrome. Chronic or situational stress can induce episodes of diarrhea that are often separated by periods of constipation.

The precise cause of the patient's diarrhea is not usually determined in the emergency department. The goals of patient care are to differentiate serious illness from benign disease, relieve patient discomfort, and initiate appropriate diagnostic, treatment, and follow-up plans.

INITIAL APPROACH IN THE EMERGENCY DEPARTMENT

The initial evaluation focuses on quickly identifying which patients need immediate fluid and electrolyte resuscitation or sepsis evaluation. Initial data gathering is directed toward these primary concerns.

History

1. What is the duration of the illness?
2. What is the frequency and amount of fluid loss due to diarrhea or associated vomiting?
3. Are fever and chills present?
4. Is any postural dizziness present?
5. Is there blood or mucus in the stool?
6. Are there any underlying medical conditions that leave the patient intolerant of small changes in electrolyte alterations?

Physical Examination

1. Vital signs are measured, including orthostatic vital signs if the patient's condition allows it. A rise in pulse rate of 20/min and a drop in mean blood pressure of 20 mm Hg after 1 minute in a standing position suggest significant hypovolemia.
2. Dry mucous membranes, decreased mentation, poor skin turgor, sunken eyes, and poor capillary refill are signs of poor hydration status.
3. Signs of shock are pallor, diaphoresis, or diminished mental status.
4. A brief abdominal examination is performed to identify localized findings or peritoneal signs.

Intervention

In any potentially unstable patient, the following interventions are performed:

1. Supplementary oxygen is administered at a rate of 2 to 4 liters/min through a nasal cannula.
2. The patient is placed in a recumbent position.
3. Cardiac monitoring is established.
4. Two large-bore catheters are inserted for intravenous access. Isotonic crystalloid is the fluid of choice. The rate is dependent on the severity of findings.

DATA GATHERING

History

The history is the most important part of the evaluation of patients with acute diarrhea. Generally, a thorough, detailed history will give the examiner a good idea about the type and severity of the diarrhea that is present. There are five areas of questioning that need to be covered:

1. *What is the character of the stools?* Copious, watery diarrhea suggests abnormal small bowel secretion, which is usually due to enterotoxic food poisoning or viral infection. Blood, mucus, and pus in the stool have a high correlation with bacterial infections or inflammatory colon disease. Foul-smelling, floating stools suggest malabsorption, which is consistent with parasitic infection.
2. *What are the temporal characteristics of the diarrhea?* Diarrhea of abrupt onset and short duration is most characteristic of a toxigenic etiology. Acute but persistent diarrhea suggests an invasive cause. Recurrent or chronic diarrhea suggests an underlying intestinal disease. A hallmark of "stress-related" diarrhea is that it usually occurs during the day, and the patient is remarkably free of symptoms during sleep.
3. *Are there contributing exogenous factors?* Five exogenous factors must be considered in all patients with acute diarrhea: medications, foods, travel, sexual practice, and exposure to known infections or epidemics.
    a. *Medications.* Many medications can produce diarrhea. Any newly prescribed medication should be suspected if its administration precedes the onset of diarrhea. Antibiotics are the most common offenders. Antacids containing magnesium may also cause diarrhea.
    b. *Food.* Food poisoning—gastroenteritis secondary to food-borne organisms and toxins—is suggested when two or more persons become similarly ill after eating at the same restaurant, attending the same social function, or sharing a common meal. Large epidemics of Norwalk virus–induced gastroenteritis have resulted from ingestion of inadequately cooked or raw shellfish. Food poisoning should also be considered when symptoms begin 1 to 6 hours after eating foods such as seafood, fried rice, or rewarmed meat dishes.
    c. *Travel.* Persons traveling to warm weather climates with poor sanitation and water systems often acquire "traveler's diarrhea." The most common etiologic agent is toxigenic *E. coli*. In the United States outdoor enthusiasts may pick up *Giardia lamblia* from drinking stream or lake water. Some infections, especially those due to parasitic agents, have a 1 to 3-week incubation period, so the patient may not realize that a history of travel is connected with the diarrhea. It is important to ask patients "where have you been?"
    d. *Sexual practice.* Homosexual men frequently acquire infectious diarrhea. Multiple infecting organisms may be present simultaneously. A work-up that includes *Neisseria gonorrhea, Chlamydia, Cryptosporidium,* and hepatitis as well as the more common infectious agents is appropriate.
    e. *Exposure and environment.* What is the patient's job? Does he or she work with animals, in a day-care center, or in a closed institution such as a prison? Does

anyone else at home have the same problem? All these questions address the possibility of bacterial or parasitic infections spread by close contact through the fecal-oral route.
4. *Are there associated symptoms?* Diarrhea generally occurs as part of a constellation of symptoms rather than as an isolated event.
   a. *Fever.* Significant fever suggests bacterial infection. It is unusual for fever to occur with the toxigenic diarrheas.
   b. *Vomiting.* Nausea and vomiting are nonspecific; however, sudden and violent vomiting usually indicates a toxin-mediated event.
   c. *Abdominal pain.* Abdominal pain is also nonspecific, but when severe and persistent it tends to be associated with inflammatory bowel disease or invasive infections. Although patients with viral gastroenteritis often have cramping pain, there is little associated localized tenderness on examination.
   d. *Weight loss.* Weight loss suggests prolonged disease or malabsorption. If the patient's symptoms are prolonged, gastrointestinal carcinoma is considered in the assessment.
   e. *Constipation.* Diarrhea alternating with constipation suggests an obstructing colonic mass lesion, often cancer, but may be due to the irritable bowel syndrome.
   f. *Flatulence.* Flatulence and bloating are common in patients with malabsorption syndromes or parasitic infections.
5. *Is there a related history?*
   a. Does the patient have a known gastrointestinal disease such as ulcerative colitis or regional enteritis?
   b. Is there an infection of another organ system? Otitis media in children is associated with concomitant diarrhea.
   c. Is there an underlying chronic medical illness? Immunodeficiency syndromes, especially acquired immunodeficiency syndrome (AIDS), suggests *Cryptosporidium* infection.

Physical Examination

The physical examination is a search for the cause of the diarrhea and an assessment of its effects on the patient. After cardiovascular status, the status of the abdomen and mental faculties is of primary importance.

General. Is there any evidence of "toxicity" or dehydration? Poor skin turgor, dry mucous membranes, and, in infants, a depressed fontanelle are signs of dehydration. Muscle strength and stretch reflexes may be decreased, suggesting hypokalemia.

Vital Signs. Is the patient febrile, tachycardic, hypotensive, or orthostatic?

Abdomen. Is there distention, focal tenderness, rebound, or guarding? True localized tenderness is unusual in patients with viral or toxin-induced diarrhea. Tenderness can be present in bacterial diarrheas, particularly in those induced by *Campylobacter jejuni*. The discovery of peritoneal signs raises the suspicion of other diseases such as appendicitis. Bowel sounds are typically hyperactive in patients with diarrhea.

Rectum. Look for perianal inflammation and redness consistent with severe or prolonged diarrhea. Fissures or a fistula suggest Crohn's disease. The rectal examination may reveal blood, mucus, pus, or mucosal tenderness indicative of invasive bacterial infection, amebiasis, or inflammatory bowel disease. It is not rare for a patient presenting with a complaint of "diarrhea" to actually have upper gastrointestinal bleeding with frequent melanotic stools. Elderly or bedridden patients who have a fecal impaction may have "overflow" diarrhea. These diagnoses can be missed if the rectal examination is omitted.

PROBLEM The patient stated his illness progressed rapidly. He passed 15 to 20 watery stools containing flecks of blood and mucus and vomited four times in the last 3 hours. He appeared uncomfortable and moderately dehydrated. His vital signs were, blood pressure 110/70 mm Hg, pulse 115 beats/min, respiratory rate 22/min, and temperature 102.4°F (39.1°C). Orthostatic vital signs revealed a rise in pulse rate to 145/min and a drop in blood pressure to 90/50. The abdomen showed mild diffuse tenderness, and on rectal examination there was liquid stool that showed positive results when tested for blood.

This patient appears ill with fever, chills, pain, vomiting, diarrhea, and dehydration that is progressively worse over 18 hours. The blood in the stool confirms the impression of an invasive process. The severity of this patient's illness requires emergency rehydration and a more extensive evaluation.

DECISION PRIORITIES AND PRELIMINARY DIFFERENTIAL DIAGNOSIS

On completion of the history and physical examination, the physician addresses two important questions. Based on the answers to these questions, initial stabilization is begun, and decisions are made about appropriate diagnostic testing.

1. *Does the patient's underlying problem or current clinical condition represent a life-threatening state?*
   If the patient is hemodynamically unstable or significantly dehydrated, fluid resuscitation is started as outlined under Initial Approach in the Emergency Department. Fluid loss can rapidly result in hypovolemic shock at the extremes of age. Both pediatric and geriatric patients require aggressive resuscitation and careful monitoring. In some cases, diarrhea may be the presenting complaint when an underlying problem is truly life-threatening. Gastrointestinal bleeding, as from a peptic ulcer, diverticular disease, or ischemic bowel disease resulting in melena, may be described by the patient as diarrhea. Patients, especially children, with high fever, chills, and severe abdominal pain accompanying diarrhea, are potentially infected with *Salmonella typhi*, the agent causing typhoid fever. The patient with toxic megacolon due to ulcerative colitis may present with diarrhea, and surgical intervention may be necessary.

2. *Is the diarrhea most likely to be of invasive or toxic origin?*
   Table 7–1 outlines the clinical parameters needed to classify a patient's diarrhea as either invasive or toxic in origin. This categorization is very helpful in determining the likely cause and in deciding on the appropriate diagnostic evaluations. Diarrhea of invasive origin includes diseases caused by mucosal invasion and resulting inflammation. This group includes the invasive bacterial pathogens and the inflammatory bowel diseases, which, although not "invasive," do destroy the mucosa by an inflammatory process. Toxic diarrhea compromises diseases caused by toxins that induce mucosal hypersecretion but cause no mucosal destruction.

   Patients with invasive bacterial disease typically become ill gradually, and the diarrhea is associated with fever and significant abdominal pain and tenderness. Systemic symptoms such as headache, nausea, vomiting, malaise, and myalgias are often present, and blood and white blood cells are present in the stools.

   Diarrhea caused by toxigenic agents is characterized by the absence of fever and systemic constitutional symptoms. Onset is prompt, but the duration is brief, and the physical findings are generally scant. These patients may complain of severe watery diarrhea, but they do not appear overtly ill.

PROBLEM This patient's history of frequent stools and vomiting as well as the significant orthostatic blood pressure changes dictated aggressive intravenous fluid resuscitation. Two large-bore intravenous (IV) catheters were inserted for access. An isotonic crystalloid solution was given at 20 ml/kg/hr until the patient's

TABLE 7-1. Clinical Categorization of Acute Diarrhea of Infectious Origin

Characteristics	Invasive	Toxigenic
Incubation period	1-3 days	2-12 hr
Onset	Gradual	Sudden
Duration	1-7 days	10-24 hr
Abdominal pain	Common; tends to be severe, persistent, and associated with tenesmus	Less common and generally mild, intermittent, and crampy
Systemic symptoms	Common; nausea, vomiting, headache, malaise, myalgias, etc.	Uncommon
Physical findings	Fever, "toxic" appearance, abdominal tenderness prominent	No fever; minimal, if any abdominal tenderness
Stool blood, mucous, inflammatory cells (fecal leukocytes)	Present	Absent
Etiology		
Viruses		Rotaviruses, Norwalk virus, many other viruses
Bacteria	Salmonella	Vibrio cholera
	Campylobacter	Escherichia coli (enterotoxigenic)
	Shigella	
	Vibrio parahemolyticus	
	Yersinia	
	Clostridium difficile	
Parasites	Entamoeba histolytica	Giardia lamblia
	Others, rare	Cryptosporidium
Toxins		Staphylococcal
		Bacillus cereus
		Clostridium perfringens
		Scrombroid fish

vital signs began to improve. Fluid replacement needs were estimated to be 2 to 4 liters, using the methods given in Chapter 4.

The 18-hour history associated with fever and chills as well as the guaiac-positive stool examination results supports the probability that an invasive bacterial agent is responsible for this illness. *Salmonella, Shigella, Campylobacter,* and *Yersinia* are considered as well as other, less common offenders. Although volume deficit estimates are notoriously inaccurate, it is important to have an approximate goal for fluid repletion (see Chapter 4). At a minimum, these goals are a reminder to reassess the patient and reestimate their volume requirements.

DIAGNOSTIC ADJUNCTS

Since most acute diarrheal illness is self-limited and benign, diagnostic testing may not be necessary or may be very limited in scope. Each patient is approached individually based on the clinical setting and the judgment of the physician. For example, patients with acute noninvasive diarrhea who are hemodynamically stable and have no significant findings do not need diagnostic assessment.

Diagnostic studies and basic clinical criteria for their use include the following:

Laboratory Studies

Complete Blood Count and Differential. A complete blood count (CBC) and differential are obtained when the history or physical examination findings suggest significant blood loss or systemic toxicity.

Serum Electrolytes. Measurements of serum electrolytes are ordered in patients with significant dehydration or those manifesting symptoms suggestive of electrolyte abnormalities. In almost all forms of diarrhea, the abnormally formed stools result from small bowel hyperexcretion of fluid and electrolytes. Sodium and chloride concentrations in diarrheal stool are slightly less than those in plasma. Bicarbonate concentration is two times that of plasma, and potassium loss is invariably substantial. Children generally produce stools with a sodium concentration significantly less than that in plasma. Serum electrolyte measurements are indicated in cases of significant fluid loss. The most common abnormality is hypokalemia, but hypernatremia due to excessive fluid loss may also be found.

Blood Urea Nitrogen/Creatinine. Due to dehydration, the BUN level is frequently elevated out of proportion to the creatinine level. In patients with severe dehydration leading to hypovolemic shock, acute tubular necrosis may occur, leading to marked elevation of both the BUN and creatinine levels.

Microbial Studies

Fecal Leukocyte Stain. Normally white blood cells are not present in the stool. The presence of fecal leukocytes indicates a break in integrity of the intestinal mucosa due to infection or inflammation, and strongly suggests invasive bacterial or parasitic enteric infection. The sensitivity and specificity of a stain positive for fecal leukocytes for the presence of a bacterial or parasitic pathogen is about 85%. The fecal leukocyte test is best used when there is clinical uncertainty about whether the patient has diarrhea due to an invasive or toxigenic cause (Fig. 7-1).

When testing for fecal leukocytes, a fresh stool specimen is placed on a clean glass slide and mixed with a drop of Loeffler's methylene blue. Microscopic examination after 2 minutes will demonstrate nuclear staining of leukocytes if they are present. If fecal leukocytes are identified, stool culture for invasive pathogens is indicated.

Stool Culture. For optimum results, a fresh stool specimen collected in a cup is recommended. A rectal swab does not provide an adequate specimen. A culture is

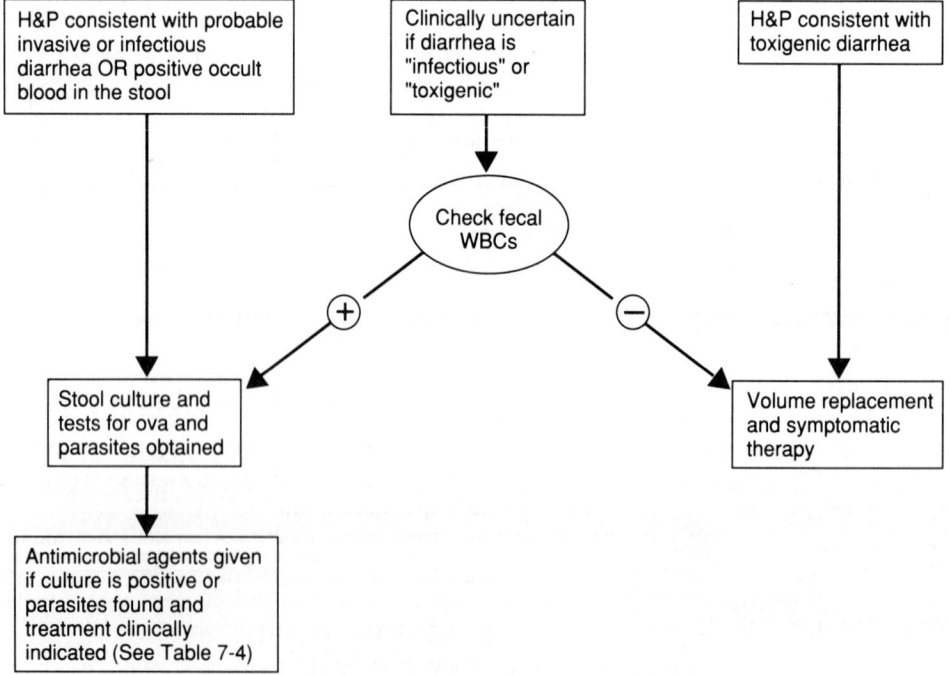

FIGURE 7-1. *Evaluation of acute diarrhea. H&P = history and physical examination.*

appropriate when the history and physical examination suggest invasive-type diarrhea or when the results of the fecal leukocyte test are positive.

Stool Test for Ova and Parasites. It is essential not to use cotton swabs for collection or transfer of specimens intended for ova and parasite testing. Some agents, such as amoebae, adhere to the cotton and are lost. A glass or metal rod is used instead. Ova and parasite testing is indicated when symptoms are chronic, when there is an epidemic of parasitic disease, when the patient has recently traveled in underdeveloped areas or has had contact with a high-risk environment such as a day care center or hospital for the mentally handicapped, or when he indulges in high-risk sexual activities.

Radiologic Imaging

Radiographs of the abdomen are usually unnecessary in patients with diarrhea. They are ordered if there are peritoneal findings, if obstruction is suspected, or if abdominal pain is present and the diagnosis is unclear.

PROBLEM Because of the patient's degree of illness, a full set of laboratory tests was ordered. The values were reported as follows: CBC, white blood cells 14,000/mm^3; hemoglobin, 16 gm; hematocrit, 48%; differential, 78 neutrophils, 15 bands; BUN, 30 mg/dl; creatinine, 1.2 mg/dl; electrolytes, within normal limits (WNL). Since there were no indications for radiographs, none were ordered. Fecal leukocyte testing was not done because of the high suspicion for invasive disease.

The laboratory results represent moderate dehydration (a slight increase in hematocrit, although it was within normal range, and an elevated BUN (more than 10:1) in proportion to creatinine). The normal electrolyte values are not uncommon.

REFINED DIFFERENTIAL DIAGNOSIS

A specific etiologic diagnosis is not usually reached in the emergency department. However, it is important for emergency physicians to be familiar with the important causes of diarrheal disease and the characteristics of the syndromes that they produce. The bacterial, viral, and parasitic agents commonly encountered and the characteristics of illness due to them are outlined in Table 7–2.

Inflammatory bowel disease frequently presents as diarrhea. Undiagnosed ulcerative colitis can present in one of two forms. About half of these patients will have acute onset of fever, crampy abdominal pain, tenesmus, urgency, and frequent painful passage of grossly bloody mucoid stools. The other half will give a history of an insidious, recurrent course of fever, abdominal pain, anorexia, weight loss, and mild diarrhea that is usually but not always bloody. Crohn's disease presents like a typical invasive enteritis or acute appendicitis, and the diagnosis is made only after an exhaustive work-up or at operating table.

PRINCIPLES OF MANAGEMENT

Management of the patient with diarrhea has four objectives: (1) rehydration and prevention of future dehydration, (2) increasing patient comfort with symptomatic therapy, (3) preventing spread of the illness, if it is infectious, and (4) specific treatment, if possible, of the underlying cause.

Rehydration and Prevention of Dehydration

For most patients with diarrhea, the most important aspect of therapy is replacement of fluid and electrolytes lost in the stool and prevention of dehydration. It is well established

TABLE 7-2. Characteristics of Diarrhea Caused by Infectious Agents

	Agent	Features
Invasive agents		
	Campylobacter jejuni	Fecal-oral spread
		Occurs in wet, warm months
	Shigella	Highly infectious
		Person-to-person spread
		>50 WBC/high-power field
	Salmonella	Common source of epidemic
		Antibiotics can be used rarely in those with septicemia, or those who are immunocompromised or young
	Invasive *Escherichia coli*	Rare in United States
		Mimics *Shigella* infection clinically
	Yersinia enterocolitica	Mimics appendicitis
		Antibiotics can be used selectively in those with septicemia, immunocompromised status, or focal extraintestinal infection
	Vibrio parahemolyticus	Common in Japan
		Shellfish contaminant
	Clostridium difficile	Associated with antibiotic use
		Severe illness
		Work-up may include sigmoidoscopy, cytotoxin assay
Toxin producers		
	Staphylococcus	2–6 hr incubation period
		Self-limited
		Emesis predominant
		Toxin in food is identified
	Clostridium perfringens	12–16 hr incubation period
		Self-limited (24–48 hr)
		Incriminated food is cultured
	Vibrio cholera	Occurs in near, middle, and far East
		Raw oysters
	Toxigenic *E. coli*	Common in travelers
		Self-limited (1 wk)
	Bacillus cereus	Emetic and diarrheal forms
		Culture foods
		Self-limited (12–24 hr)
Virus		
	Rotavirus	Occurs in young children or winter months
		Lasts less than 5 days
		Diagnose with rotazyme
	Norwalk agent	Family outbreaks
		Lasts less than 36 hr
Parasites		
	Giardia lamblia	2–3 wk incubation period
		Malabsorption, flatulence, prolonged symptoms
	Entamoeba histolytica	Low-grade fever
		Bloody stool
		Up to 3-wk incubation period
	Cryptosporidium	Immunocompromised status
		Special request needed for laboratory stain

that sodium transport and glucose are coupled in the small intestine through the phenomenon of "solvent drag." The presence of glucose stimulates the absorption of solutes and water. This transport mechanism remains largely intact even in the most severe acute diarrhea. Thus, diarrheal fluid losses can usually be replaced by the oral intake of fluids that contain glucose.

Patients who are dehydrated but not ill enough to be hospitalized should be rehydrated in the emergency department prior to discharge. Usually it is easier, faster, and more effective to rehydrate patients with intravenous (IV) fluids. Indications for the use of IV fluids include moderate or severe dehydration, orthostatic vital sign abnormalities, and inability to tolerate oral fluids. Adult patients with moderate to severe dehydration may require 2 to 3 or more liters of IV fluids. Even patients with mild diarrhea will benefit from 1 to 2 liters of intravenous fluid replacement. Patients will feel subjectively better, and the rate of vomiting and diarrhea may be slowed. Table 7–3 outlines the recommended fluid formulas. Remember that patients with significant vomiting lose acid, offsetting the bicarbonate lost in the stool. In these cases, bicarbonate should not be added to the formula, but more potassium chloride will be required.

For more specific guidelines concerning fluid replacement in children, refer to Chapter 39. Adults with a healthy cardiovascular system can be rehydrated rapidly at fluid rates of up to 500 to 1000 ml/hr for the first 2 or 3 liters. The goal is a patient who is comfortable, is not vomiting, and can stand without orthostatic symptoms or vital sign changes.

Rehydrating patients in the emergency department by the oral route alone is indicated only in patients with mild dehydration who are not actively vomiting and are willing and able to drink large amounts of fluids. Ideally, rehydration is best done with solutions containing 60 to 90 mEq Na^+/liter (Table 7–3). The recommended World Health Organization (WHO) solution can be formulated easily by a pharmacy, and the others are ready-to-use, commercially available preparations.

Symptomatic Therapy

Rehydration alone often makes the patient feel much better. Patients who are vomiting can be given an antiemetic such as prochloperazine (Compazine) or promethazine (Phenergan). If the patient has severe cramps or pain and the diagnosis of gastroenteritis is certain, meperidine (Demerol) can be added to the injection. These medications will help patients rest comfortably while hydration is carried out.

Traditional outpatient symptomatic therapy of diarrhea has been bed rest and the use of either kaolin-pectin adsorbents or antiperistaltic agents such as diphenoxylate-atropine (Lotomil), loperamide (Imodium), and paregoric. The kaolin-pectins are inert adsorbent compounds. They may reduce the fluidity of the diarrheal stools in mild cases but will not influence the course of the patient's disease in any meaningful way.

TABLE 7–3. Fluids Used to Treat Diarrhea

Intravenous Fluids
To: 1 liter of 5% dextrose and half normal saline (adult)
or
1 liter of 5% dextrose and 25% normal saline NS (child)
Add: 50 mEq NaHCO (1 amp)
    and
10 to 20 mEq KCl*
This provides per liter:

	Adult	Child
Na (mEq)	125	87
Cl (mEq)	85–95	47–57
HCO_3^- (mEq)	50	50
K (mEq)	10–20	10–20
Dextrose (gm)	50	50

Oral Fluids

	World Health Organization Solution	Rehydralyte	Pedialyte RS	Lytren	Pedialyte	Infalyte	Gatorade
Na^+ (mEq/liter)	90	75	75	50	45	50	21
K^+ (mEq/liter)	20	20	20	25	20	20	2.5
Cl^- (mEq/liter)	80	65	50	45	35	40	11
HCO_3^- (mEq/liter)	30	30	30	30	30	30	0
Sugar (gm/liter)	20 (2%)	25 (2.5%)	25 (2.5%)	20 (2%)	25 (2.5%)	20 (2%)	60 (6%)

*If significant vomiting is present, NaHCO should not be added and more KCl may be required.

Antiperistaltic drugs should not be used in invasive diarrhea. It has been clearly shown that these drugs increase the duration of fever, diarrhea, secretion of organisms, and the incidence of bacteremia. They may also precipitate toxic megacolon. Diarrhea is a host-defense mechanism whereby the body rids itself of pathogens or toxins. Slowing intestinal transit time allows more time for infectious invasion of the gut mucosa. These antimotility agents may be used judiciously in patients felt to have toxigenic diarrhea.

Bismuth subsalicylate (Pepto Bismol) can significantly cut down the number of stools passed without making an infectious diarrhea worse. Bismuth subsalicylate works as an antisecretory agent by blocking the small bowel hypersecretion of fluids and electrolytes. The recommended dose for adults is 1 ounce every half hour for a total of eight doses. If this dose is exceeded, salicylism may result. One ounce of bismuth subsalicylate contains approximately the same amount of salicylate as that found in one 5-gr aspirin tablet.

Prevention of Spread

Osler once said, "Soap and water and common sense are the best disinfectants." All infectious diarrheas can be spread by the fecal-oral route. Preventing spread begins in the emergency department with proper handwashing by the staff between patients. Patients and family are instructed in basic good personal household hygiene. Children with infectious enteritis should be kept home from school and out of day care centers until the episode resolves. Food handlers are kept off the job until it is determined that they are incapable of passing disease. Health care personnel with diarrhea should not be intimately involved in the care of patients.

Specific Treatment

Specific antimicrobial therapy for the infectious diarrheas is outlined in Table 7–4. Patients are not usually treated with antibiotics empirically at the time of their initial visit. A definitive diagnosis is not possible at that time, and the treatment may be detrimental. For example, in patients with uncomplicated *Salmonella enteritis*, a carrier state can be induced by giving antibiotics, and these are recommended only for the few patients who are severely ill with *Salmonella* enteritis.

Specific treatment for inflammatory bowel disease is generally not started in the emergency department. Consultation with the primary physician or a gastroenterologist is recommended.

PROBLEM After the first liter of normal saline was administered over a half hour, the second liter was given at a slower rate of 300 ml/hr as the patient's vital signs improved. The third liter of intravenous fluid was changed to 5% dextrose in normal saline with 50 mEq of sodium bicarbonate and 10 mEq of potassium chloride added. Prochlorperazine (50 mg intramuscularly) was given to decrease the nausea and control the vomiting. The patient remained at bed rest, and the family was notified of the patient's improving condition.

The combination of fluid replacement and prochlorperazine alleviates the patient's symptoms and allows him to rest. The switch in fluids reflects the predicted fluid losses in a patient with severe diarrhea. The patient's improvement with therapy is a good indicator of recovery. Because his emergency department stay is likely to be several hours, this plan and a status report are communicated to the family.

DISPOSITION AND FOLLOW-UP

Most episodes of acute diarrhea resolve spontaneously without specific therapy or sequelae. There are occasions, however, when admission to the hospital is advisable. The following are guidelines to selection of the appropriate patient management plan.

TABLE 7–4. Antibiotic Therapy for Infectious Diarrhea

Pathogen	Antibiotic*
Shigella dysenteriae†	Trimethoprim-sulfamethoxazole (TMP/SMX) or Norfloxacin
Shigella sonnei or *S. flexneri*†	Same treatment, but decision to administer antibiotic is based on clinical situation.
Salmonella†	No antibiotic recommended for outpatient treatment. If hospitalization is required: Trimethoprim-sulfamethoxazole (TMP/SMX) or Norfloxacin or Chloramphenicol
Campylobacter	Erythromycin Norfloxacin
Clostridium	Vancomycin or Metronidazole
Yersinia enterocolictica	Generally self-limited and no antibiotic is necessary unless septicemia develops; then IV aminoglycosides or IV moxalactam
Entamoeba	Metronidazole and Iodoquinol
Giardia lamblia	Metronidazole or Quinacrine HCl or Furazolidone (only one that comes as a suspension and thus especially useful in young children)
Cryptosporidium	No effective antibiotic known

*These are not used routinely in the emergency department.
†Because of increasing incidence of resistance, Ampicillin is reserved for culture-sensitive organisms.

Admission

Patients are admitted if one or more of the following criteria apply:

1. Toxic or possibly bacteremic appearance, as indicated by high fever, shaking chills, or a high white blood cell count.
2. Severe dehydration or inability to keep up with fluid loss resulting from persistent vomiting or copious diarrhea.
3. Lack of appropriate response to treatment in the emergency department. Orthostatic vital signs remain abnormal in spite of vigorous intravenous fluid replacement.
4. Underlying medical condition or extremes of age.
5. Severe disease in very old or very young patients.

Outpatient Management

Outpatient management is selected if

1. The patient is hemodynamically stable, and orthostatic vital signs show no abnormality after volume repletion.
2. Vomiting has ceased and the patient is able to tolerate oral fluids.
3. The patient is likely to follow up with care. If stool cultures are taken because of a suspected bacterial or parasitic cause, reevaluation and consideration for antibiotic therapy in 48 hours are essential.

The great majority of patients can be safely managed at home. Most patients do not undergo electrolyte derangements unless they are very ill or have renal insufficiency. Liberal use of intravenous fluids in the emergency department and the availability of glucose-electrolyte oral solutions allow outpatient therapy even in some significantly dehydrated patients. Most patients do not need to drink commercially prepared solutions. They will do well with diluted fruit juices, powdered fruit drinks such as lemonade or Kool-Aid, and the noncola, nondiet soft drinks. Table 7–5 provides a sample discharge instruction sheet for the patient.

PROBLEM After 3 liters of fluid given over 4½ hours, the patient began to feel much better. He was able to take liquids by mouth and no longer had any abnormalities in orthostatic vital signs. His repeat temperature was 100.4°F (38°C).

This patient qualifies for outpatient management. A stool specimen is taken for culture because the patient's diarrhea appears "infectious" owing to the positive test for blood. The results are returned to the emergency physician and the patient's primary physician. Both are responsible for ensuring that the patient is improving or, if not, that a treatable cause of the diarrhea is covered with an appropriate antibiotic. The patient and family are given verbal and written instructions about diet, continued rehydration, and reasons for a return visit.

DOCUMENTATION

1. Frequency and duration of the diarrhea.
2. Character of the stools—especially blood, pus or mucus.
3. Exogenous factors—medications, food, travel, sexual practice, and exposure to known infections.
4. Associated symptoms—fever, vomiting, abdominal pain, weight loss.
5. Pertinent past medical history.
6. General appearance and state of hydration.
7. Vital signs and orthostatic changes.
8. Results of abdominal examination and rectal examination.
9. Stool guaiac and fecal leukocyte results.
10. Response to therapy.
11. Diagnosis—at least the major category, e.g., invasive versus noninvasive diarrhea.
12. Discharge plan for follow-up.

TABLE 7–5. Sample Discharge Instruction Sheet for Patients with Infectious Diarrheas

Impression	The doctor believes your problem is an infection of your intestines. You should get better over the next 2 to 5 days.
Home Care Instructions	Rest.
	Drink plenty of fluids that contain *sugar*, such as fruit juices, Kool-Aid, lemonade, and soda pop.
	Avoid all colas (Pepsi, Coke, etc.), diet beverages, milk, and alcohol.
	Take acetaminophen (Tylenol) for pain.
	Do not take any other medications unless approved by the doctor.
	Do not allow others to come in contact with your stools.
	Call back in 3 days (phone) for your results if any cultures were done.
Warning signs	Contact your doctor or return to emergency at once if you are:
	1. Unable to keep fluids down for 24 hours (8 to 16 hours in young children).
	2. Having increased vomiting, diarrhea, or pain.
	3. Having red or black vomitus or stools.
	4. Not better in 2 days.
	5. Worse in any way.

SUMMARY AND FINAL POINTS

- Differentiation of acute invasive diarrhea from noninvasive diarrhea can often be accomplished by the history and physical examination alone.
- Invasive bacterial diarrhea is recognized by the presence of fever, marked abdominal cramping, volume depletion, and fecal leukocytes and blood.
- Because the specific cause of diarrhea cannot be identified during the emergency department visit, emergency management is directed at the common result of any diarrheal disorder, volume depletion.
- The fecal leukocyte smear test is used when the clinical evaluation does not clearly point to either an invasive or noninvasive cause.
- Acute invasive as well as toxin-induced diarrheas are generally self-limited diseases.
- Stool cultures are obtained only in patients in whom invasive organisms are suspected.
- Liberal use of intravenous fluids, antiemetics, and pain medications in the emergency department can provide significant comfort to patients prior to discharge.
- Management decisions regarding the use of antibiotics, repeat cultures, and job, work, or public health concerns depend on the specific organism isolated and the patient's current clinical status.
- Most patients with acute diarrhea can be managed at home with symptomatic therapy and oral fluids containing sugar.

BIBLIOGRAPHY

Texts

1. Fine K, Krejs G, Fordtran J: Diarrhea. In Sleisenger M, Fordtran J. Gastrointestinal Disease (4th ed). Philadelphia, Saunders, 1989, pp. 290–316.
2. Hoeprich P, Jordan M: Infectious Diseases (4th ed). Philadelphia, Lippincott, 1989, pp. 685–756.

Journal Articles

1. DuBois D, Binder L: Usefulness of stool Wright's stain in the emergency department. J Emerg Med 6:483–486, 1988.
2. DuPont AL: Nonfluid therapy and selected chemoprophylaxis of acute diarrhea. Am J Med 78(Suppl 6B):81–89, 1985.
3. Guerrant RK, Sluetds DS, Thorson SM: Evaluation and diagnosis of acute infectious diarrhea. Am J Med 78 (Suppl 6B):91–97, 1985.
4. Kimmey M: Infectious diarrhea. Emerg Med Clin North Am 3(1):127–142, 1985.
5. National Institutes of Health: Consensus Conference on Traveler's Diarrhea JAMA 253(18):2700–2704, 1985.
6. Oral fluids for dehydration. Med Lett 29(743):63–64, 1987.
7. Pichler HE, Diridl G, Strickler K, et al: Clinical efficacy of ciprofloxacin compared with placebo in bacterial diarrhea. Am J Med 82(Suppl 4A):329–332, 1987.
8. Rolston KV, et al: Diarrhea in patients infected with human immunodeficiency virus. Am J Med 86(1):137–138, 1989.
9. Siegel D, et al: A predictive value of stool examination in acute diarrhea. Arch Pathol Lab Med 11:715–718, 1987.

CHAPTER 8

NAUSEA AND VOMITING

GREGG A. PANE, M.D.

PROBLEM A 47 year old man presented to the emergency department complaining of nausea and epigastric discomfort for the past 3 hours. He did not want to come to the hospital but became concerned after experiencing slight light-headedness and diaphoresis.

QUESTIONS TO CONSIDER

1. What are the major life-threatening illnesses in patients presenting with nausea and vomiting?
2. What are serious sequelae of vomiting?
3. Which findings from the history and physical examination are most helpful in evaluating the patient with vomiting?
4. What are the therapeutic goals for stabilizing these patients?
5. Which patients with nausea and vomiting are candidates for hospital admission?
6. If a patient is discharged from the emergency department, what diet instructions are given, and when is follow-up arranged?

INTRODUCTION

Nausea and vomiting are common symptoms of a variety of organic and functional disorders. Nausea is a vague unpleasant sensation that often precedes vomiting. Vomiting is the forceful expulsion of gastric contents through the mouth.

Three related actions are retching, regurgitation, and rumination. *Retching* is spasmodic respiratory activity against a closed glottis that precedes vomiting. *Regurgitation* is the retrograde movement of esophageal or gastroduodenal material into the oropharynx. It is not preceded by nausea or accompanied by abdominal muscular activity characteristic of vomiting. *Rumination* denotes the asymptomatic regurgitation of food, followed by rechewing and reswallowing.

The act of vomiting involves forceful contraction of the abdominal wall musculature, contraction of the pylorus and antrum, relaxation of the cardiac sphincter, esophageal dilation, and glottic closure (Fig. 8–1).

This complicated mechanism is controlled by the vomiting center, located in the lateral reticular formation deep within the medulla. The vomiting center is influenced by the chemoreceptor trigger zone (CTZ), which is located in the floor of the fourth ventricle, and by vagal and sympathetic afferent pathways from the pharynx, gastrointestinal tract, heart, and genitalia. The CTZ pathway mediates the nausea and vomiting characteristic of uremia, motion sickness, diabetic ketoacidosis, drugs, and general anesthetics. Central dopamine receptors probably play a role in mediating vomiting; thus dopamine agonists (L-dopa, apomorphine) cause emesis, whereas dopamine antagonists (phenothiazines, metoclopramide) are antiemetics (Fig. 8–2).

Vagal and sympathetic afferent pathways bypass the CTZ to stimulate the vomiting

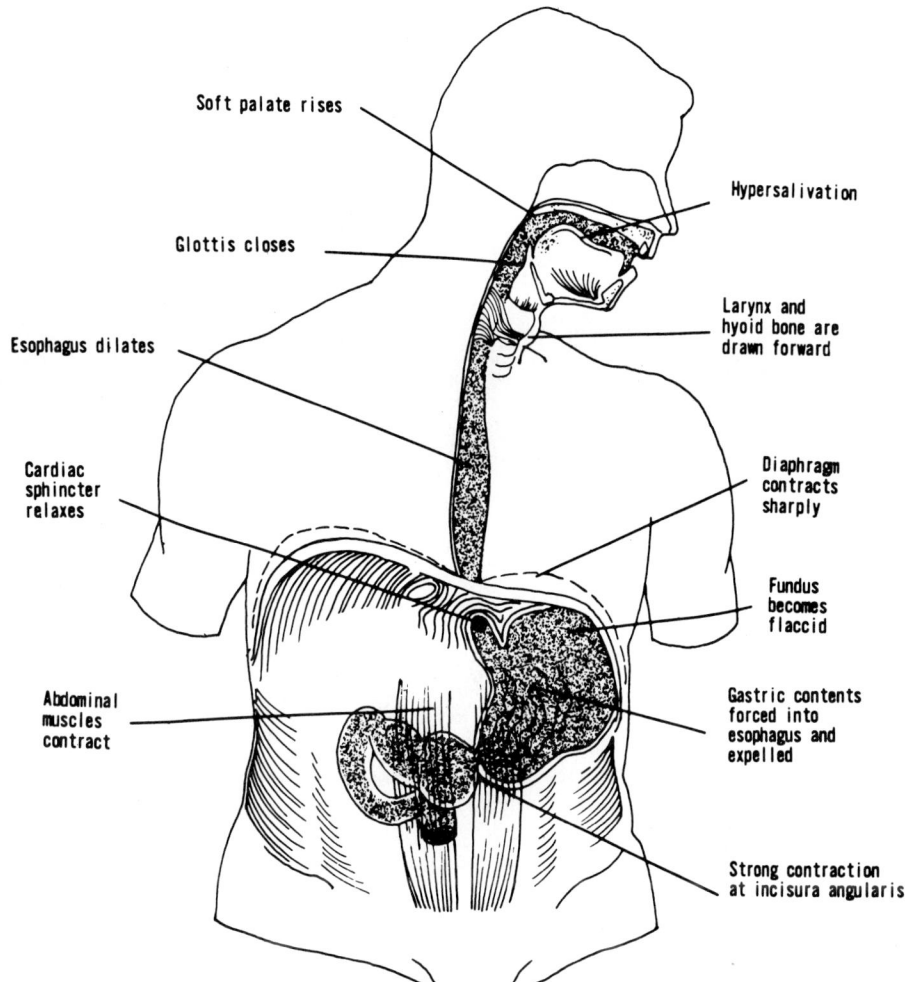

FIGURE 8–1. Muscles involved in the act of vomiting. (Reproduced from Searle AT: Research in the Service of Medicine 44:2, 1956.)

center directly in a number of instances, e.g., in patients with myocardial infarction or renal and biliary colic and in those who have ingested substances noxious to the stomach mucosa. Hypersalivation usually accompanies vomiting owing to the close proximity of the vomiting and salivation centers in the medulla.

The most common causes of nausea and vomiting are acute gastroenteritis, febrile systemic illnesses, drug effects, other gastrointestinal diseases, and central nervous system disorders.

Serious consequences of vomiting include aspiration, esophageal mucosal tears (Mallory-Weiss syndrome), esophageal rupture (Boerhaave's syndrome), and volume depletion. Protracted vomiting can cause several metabolic derangements. These include hypokalemia, due primarily to urinary loss in exchange for sodium, and hypochloremic metabolic alkalosis, secondary to hydrochloric acid loss in emesis. Both are perpetuated by urinary bicarbonate reabsorption associated with intravascular volume depletion.

PREHOSPITAL CARE

The patient with severe nausea and vomiting occasionally uses the prehospital care system. Assessing the patient's hemodynamic status and identifying serious causes or

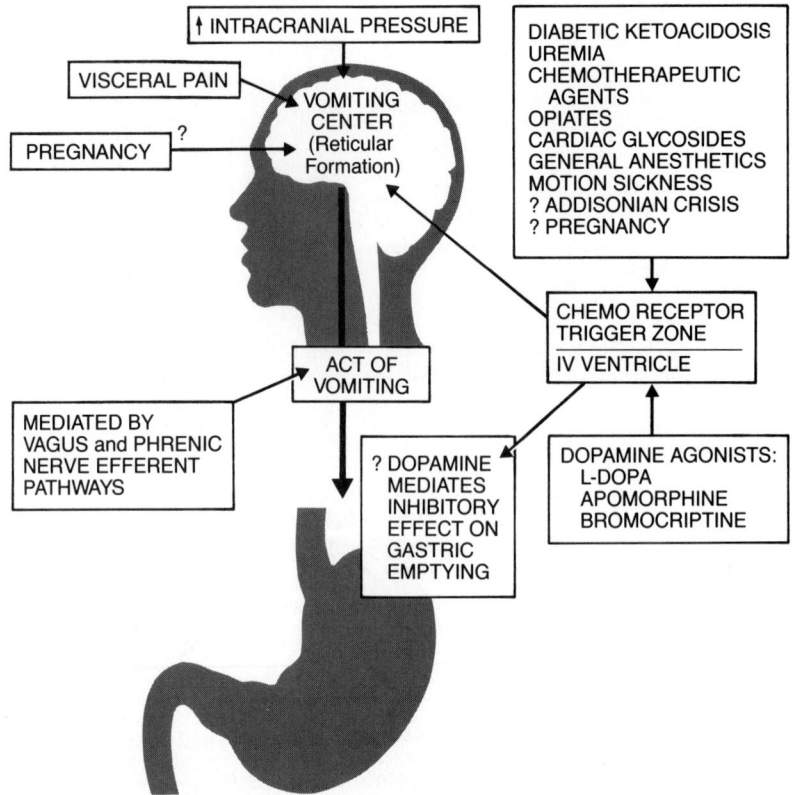

FIGURE 8–2. Central nervous system control of vomiting. (Reproduced with permission from Hanson JS, McCallum RW: The diagnosis and management of nausea and vomiting. Am J Gastroenterol 80(3):210–219, 1985, © by American College of Gastroenterology.)

sequelae of vomiting are the important foci of care in the field. Information gathered by prehospital care personnel includes the following:

History

1. How long has the patient been vomiting?
2. Is there any blood in the vomitus?
3. Are there symptoms of hypovolemia, e.g., postural dizziness?
4. Are there associated symptoms pointing to serious underlying disease?
   a. Headache suggests central nervous system (CNS) pathology, e.g., meningitis, hemorrhage, mass lesions.
   b. Altered mental status raises concerns about CNS pathology, hypoxia, metabolic disorders, or drug ingestion.
   c. Abdominal pain is a sign of an acute abdominal event such as a ruptured viscus or pancreatitis.
   d. Chest pain may indicate ischemic heart disease (IHD).
5. Is there a significant medical history, for example, known IHD, diabetes mellitus, hypertension, or depression?

Physical Examination

1. Vital signs are taken, specifically to check for hypovolemia.
2. The remainder of the examination is directed by the associated symptoms.

Intervention

1. Supplemental oxygen is given, as necessary.
2. Cardiac monitoring is performed if there are symptoms of IHD or signs suggesting volume depletion.
3. Intravenous access is obtained and volume resuscitation given with isotonic crystalloid at a rate and volume guided by the estimated amount of fluid loss.

INITIAL APPROACH IN THE EMERGENCY DEPARTMENT

The initial approach to the patient with nausea and vomiting in the emergency department is very similar to the sequence described under Prehospital Care. Its purpose is to assess the hemodynamic status of the patient, search for potentially catastrophic underlying disease, identify the sequelae of vomiting, and begin stabilization as necessary.

History

1. The prehospital information is repeated and verified.
2. Are there any known allergies?
3. When did the patient eat his last meal? What was eaten? The possibility of "food poisoning" is important to consider. It is usually corroborated by the knowledge that someone else was ill after eating similar food.

Physical Examination

1. The patient's level of consciousness and adequacy of the airway are assessed.
2. The abdomen is examined specifically for signs of an "acute" abdomen—abdominal pain with rebound tenderness, guarding, or distention.
3. A rapid neurologic assessment is performed, primarily evaluating the level and content of consciousness.
4. Vital signs are repeated and findings supporting volume depletion are sought. If the patient is not hypotensive, the orthostatic vital signs are checked. These are obtained by first determining the pulse and blood pressure when the patient has been supine for 3 minutes and then repeating them after the patient has been standing for 1 minute. A positive result is a rise of 20 beats or more in the pulse rate or a drop of 20 mm Hg or more in systolic blood pressure or the presence of significant symptoms, e.g., syncope or dizziness.

Intervention

1. Intravenous (IV) access is established if there are signs and symptoms of volume depletion or systemic diseases.
2. Fluid resuscitation is begun or continued, using an isotonic crystalloid solution. If treatment was started by the rescue squad, the patient's response to this treatment is checked, and infusion rates are adjusted accordingly.
3. Cardiac monitoring is initiated.
4. In volume-depleted patients or patients with persistent vomiting, early diagnostic tests include a complete blood count, serum electrolytes, blood urea nitrogen (BUN), and creatinine. The vomitus is routinely tested for hemoglobin (Gastro-occult test).
5. If the patient has problems that are related to a specific underlying disease, they are treated appropriately, e.g., hypertension (see Chap. 13), myocardial infarction (see Chap. 10), cerebrovascular hemorrhage (see Chap. 49). These measures are often instituted simultaneously with initial data gathering in unstable patients.

PROBLEM The patient's history of nausea, epigastric discomfort, and lightheadedness aroused the suspicion of the triage nurse. The initial vital signs taken in triage were blood pressure 150/90 mm Hg, heart rate 90 beats/min, respiratory rate 14/min, temperature 37°C (98.7°F). The patient stated that he was feeling better. His wife commented that he was "not a complainer" and had never had symptoms like this previously. The patient was triaged immediately to a monitored bed in the emergency department. He was placed on oxygen, and a cardiac monitor and IV access were established. The doctor was asked to see the patient ahead of less potentially ill patients.

Although the patient was apparently stable and was feeling somewhat better, the triage nurse knew that this patient's symptoms and stoicism could combine to mask a potentially catastrophic problem, ischemic heart disease. A high index of suspicion for serious disease is essential at the triage desk. An experienced nurse in this setting is invaluable. The importance of a complete evaluation had to be clearly conveyed to the patient and his wife. The personality profile obtained from his wife was an important and skilled use of triage time.

DATA GATHERING

Because the differential diagnosis of nausea and vomiting is large, the goal of data gathering is to narrow the differential to the likely organ system. This process is often aided by assessing the associated symptoms and their relation to the vomiting.

History

1. *When did the vomiting begin and how long has it lasted? Was it preceded by nausea? Is it a single episode or has it occurred in the past?*
   Acute episodes are far more common and also can represent catastrophic disease. Persistent vomiting is more likely to have serious sequelae. The rare finding of vomiting without nausea is highly suggestive of CNS disease, usually a mass lesion.
2. *How severe is the vomiting? How many times has it occurred? Has there been significant retching on an empty stomach—"dry heaves"?*
   Although not useful in differentiating the cause, the severity of vomiting does direct the emergency physician to the need for symptomatic relief and makes him aware of possible complications.
3. *Does the vomiting occur at a certain time of day?*
   Early morning vomiting can indicate pregnancy.
4. *Is the vomiting related to a particular stimulus, such as meals or motion?*
   Gastrointestinal abnormalities may be stimulated by food. Vestibular system abnormalities are usually very sensitive to motion.
5. *What is the character of the emesis? Does it contain undigested food, bile, or blood?*
   Undigested food may represent suddenness of onset, gastrointestinal mucosal irritation, or high gastrointestinal obstruction. Bilious vomiting points to an obstruction below the opening of the common bile duct. If there is blood in the emesis, the timing of its appearance (before or after vomiting began) is important. If before, bleeding from the upper airway, pharynx, or upper gastrointestinal tract may have induced the vomiting. If after, a Mallory-Weiss tear or gastric irritation may be a complicating factor.
6. *Has the patient attempted to treat the problem? If so, how?*
   Dietary changes or the lack thereof are explored. The use of aspirin may increase the potential for bleeding.

TABLE 8–1. Associated Symptoms with Nausea and Vomiting
and Organ Systems That Can Cause Them

Organ System	Symptom
Central nervous system	Headache, altered mental status, dizziness, paresis, altered vision
Peripheral nervous system—sensory	Severe pain of any origin
Vestibular	Vertigo, dizziness
Eye	Altered vision, headache
Cardiovascular	Chest pain, dizziness, syncope, fleeting changes in vision
Gastrointestinal, including gallbladder and pancreas	Abdominal pain, back pain
Genitourinary	Back pain, abdominal pain, vaginal bleeding

7. *How is the patient feeling at present?*
   This question is often overlooked. Since most illnesses are dynamic, its course from onset to the decision to come to the emergency department to arrival in the department and the interview is very important. If nausea and vomiting are persisting, symptomatic care is often best for the patient.
8. *Can the degree of fluid loss and dehydration be estimated? Is there a history of syncope or dizziness? Can blood loss be estimated?*
9. *Are there associated symptoms? Did they precede the vomiting or result from it?*
   The symptoms of abdominal pain, chest pain, headache, and altered mental status are reviewed in detail (Table 8–1) (see also Chaps. 5, 10, 45, and 46, respectively).
10. *Could the patient have ingested something as a suicide gesture or attempt?*
11. *The patient's past medical history is reviewed. Has the patient had prior gastrointestinal disease, diabetes mellitus, renal failure, hypertension, or alcohol or substance abuse? Is there a past history of abdominal surgery? What medications is the patient taking? When was the last dose taken?*
12. *Are old medical records available?*

Physical Examination

Vital Signs. The findings of hypovolemia were discussed earlier under Initial Approach in the Emergency Department. Fever with vomiting is suggestive of a viral infection or a genitourinary infection.

General Examination. After the initial survey, the condition of the patient is reassessed. Specific areas consistent with symptoms are checked carefully.

Skin

Skin Turgor. Poor skin turgor and dry mucous membranes indicate the presence of 15% to 20% dehydration of some duration.

Clammy Skin. Cool, clammy skin is found in the presence of increased sympathetic nervous system activity. It is considered a useful clue to significant disease.

Head, Eyes, Ears, Nose, and Throat. Since CNS problems may play a major role in nausea and vomiting, a careful examination of this area is necessary.

Head. The head is palpated for signs of tenderness from headache or head trauma.

Eyes. Visual acuity is assessed, and a funduscopic examination for papilledema and retinal hemorrhage is performed. Extraocular movement (EOM) is assessed. Nystagmus may indicate the presence of central or peripheral nervous system disorders. Horizontal nystagmus is seen in some CNS, vestibular, and drug-induced diseases. Vertical nystagmus originates primarily from CNS disorders.

Ears. The status of hearing is checked, and intact tympanic membranes are examined. Signs of middle ear infection and impacted wax in the external ear canal are sought.

Mouth and Throat. The status of mucosal hydration may reflect the volume status of the entire body. An intact gag reflex is important. Occasionally, signs of systemic disease may be seen, e.g., petechiae in meningococcemia.

Neck. The neck is evaluated for the presence of meningismus.

Chest. Rales may indicate congestive heart failure or myocardial infarction. Pulmonary disorders rarely present as nausea and vomiting.

Abdomen. A careful examination of the abdomen can help to localize the source of nausea and vomiting. Tenderness with rebound or guarding is consistent with a diagnosis of appendicitis, cholecystitis, or a perforated viscus. Since pancreatitis originates in a retroperitoneal organ, peritoneal signs are uncommon. Distention with tympany is present in patients with gastric outlet obstruction, gastric retention, and bowel obstruction. Peristaltic waves may be associated with gastric outlet obstruction and hypertrophic pyloric stenosis but are absent in the presence of gastric retention. If pain exists without other signs, it is localized to an abdominal quadrant; such pain must be differentiated from muscle wall pain.

Back. Localized back pain, particularly CVA tenderness, is a useful finding in patients with genitourinary abnormalities.

Pelvic Region. A bimanual examination is done, searching for lower abdominal tenderness and uterine or adnexal masses.

Rectal Examination. The rectum is examined for localized tenderness and the presence of hemoglobin in the stool.

Neurologic Examination. The patient is observed to detect signs of an altered level of consciousness, cranial nerve palsies, signs of autonomic or peripheral neuropathy, focal paresis, or sensory abnormalities.

PROBLEM After the data were gathered, the patient stated that the nausea and epigastric discomfort were much improved. He no longer felt lightheaded. His symptoms had begun suddenly while he was cheering and jumping up while watching a basketball game on television. These symptoms (lightheadedness and a slight headache) evolved to nausea and vomiting (twice) during 2 hours. There was no blood or bile in the emesis. He denied head trauma, chest pain, abdominal pain, or recent use of medication.

The patient was afebrile, had a blood pressure of 160/90 mm Hg, and a regular heart rhythm of 86 beats/min. He did not appear dehydrated. While standing during the taking of orthostatic vital signs, the patient said that he was becoming lightheaded again and vomited once. Chest and abdominal examinations revealed slight epigastric tenderness on deep palpation and slight chest wall tenderness over the left chest. Results of the neurologic examination were normal except for the "soft" finding of slight meningismus.

Improvement in such a patient's condition in the hospital is relatively common. The return of symptoms while standing is not. This finding, plus the slightly elevated blood pressure, pointed to possible cardiovascular problems. The "slight meningismus" raised the suspicion of CNS disease. The patient's high tolerance of discomfort may contribute toward the lack of progressive localizing systemic signs.

DECISION PRIORITIES AND PRELIMINARY DIFFERENTIAL DIAGNOSIS

At this point, three priorities assist in establishing the preliminary differential diagnosis:

1. *What is the hemodynamic status of the patient?*
   If the patient has unstable vital signs on admission, volume loss is estimated and fluid replacement started immediately. The patient's response to treatment is assessed serially. If the patient is less ill but continues to vomit, a potentially deteriorating condition is suspected. The first goal is stabilization. The method

used to estimate the volume loss based on the vital signs is detailed in Chapters 4 and 39.

2. *Is the patient's nausea and vomiting persisting?*
Patients come to the emergency department for relief of symptoms. Early in the course of care, often before a definitive diagnosis has been made, the emergency physician may need to treat the primary complaint. Symptomatic relief is very appropriate for the patient with the very unpleasant sensation of persistent nausea and vomiting. Reducing the intensity or frequency of symptoms will increase the patient's comfort and cooperation. As opposed to treating a symptom such as abdominal pain, relieving nausea and vomiting does nothing to undermine the process of observing the patient's course or developing a preliminary differential diagnosis.

Early treatment with an antiemetic such as hydroxazine (Vistaril) 25 to 50 mg intramuscularly (IM), prochlorperazine (Compazine) 5 to 10 mg IM, or promethazine (Phenergan) 25 to 50 mg IM is usually appropriate. If the patient does not respond to initial treatment with one of these drugs, some insight is gained into the severity of the illness, and the probability of a serious underlying disorder is heightened.

Isotonic fluid replacement (500 to 1000 ml in adults) can be beneficial, even in the hemodynamically stable patient. Replacing intracellular volume losses that occurred before intravenous volume changes may simply make the patient feel better. There is empiric evidence to support this action. The antiemetic may allow the patient to take the fluid orally rather than intravenously.

3. *Is a potentially catastrophic disease causing the nausea and vomiting?*
There are five major clinically "catastrophic" types of disorders in which nausea and vomiting may play a prominent role.

1. CNS lesions—meningitis, intracerebral hemorrhage, mass lesions.
2. Drug intoxication—therapeutic (e.g., digitalis), illicit (e.g., heroin), or poisoning (e.g., methanol).
3. Ischemic heart disease—unstable angina, myocardial infarction.
4. Acute intra-abdominal events—ischemic bowel disease, intestinal obstruction, pancreatitis, ectopic pregnancy.
5. Metabolic disorder—ketoacidosis (occurs primarily in diabetics), hyperkalemia (occurs primarily in renal failure patients).

These five types of disorders and the diseases occurring within them are the basis for the preliminary differential diagnosis of nausea and vomiting in the emergency department. The patient's history, especially the associated symptoms, and the results of the physical examination are gauged against these possibilities. If the findings support a suspicion about one or more of these sources, laboratory tests are directed toward a specific diagnosis. The goal of management is to prevent complications of the potential problem.

One might question the need to expend this effort when gastroenteritis is certainly the most common cause of nausea and vomiting seen in the emergency department. The principles of emergency medicine emphasize concern about potentially catastrophic disorders compared with common disorders. Gastroenteritis is a diagnosis of exclusion and can be a serious diagnostic trap if it is evoked before more serious illnesses are considered. Each of the above disorders has been mislabelled "gastroenteritis." The diagnosis provided no benefit to either the patient or the physician.

PROBLEM The patient remained hemodynamically stable and had no further vomiting. The presence of nausea, mild meningismus, mild headache, and mild hypertension could be a "viral syndrome" but at this point pointed to the possibility of a CNS lesion or meningitis. Because the patient was a male, had no medical problems, was not taking medications, and denied any illicit drug usage, hyperkalemia and drug intoxication appeared much less likely. Because of the slight epigastric discomfort and the history of abdominal surgery, neither an occult myocardial ischemia nor an acute intra-abdominal problem could be ruled out.

At this point, after the history and physical examination, the diagnosis was not clear. There were vague findings suggestive of a CNS lesion, occult myocardial ischemia, or an abdominal event. Because these were not ruled out, selected diagnostic adjuncts were needed. Close monitoring was continued. The preliminary differential diagnosis was discussed with the patient and his wife.

DIAGNOSTIC ADJUNCTS

The broad differential diagnosis for nausea and vomiting makes it impossible to recommend any standard series of tests. Tests are selected according to the etiologies implied by the history and the results of the physical examination. The following lists are guidelines only.

Laboratory Studies

Complete Blood Count. Although acute recent hemorrhage due to hematemesis does not always result in anemia, a low hematocrit can be an indicator of significant blood loss or chronic anemia. An increased hemoglobin and hematocrit are consistent with a diagnosis of dehydration. A complete blood count (CBC) is usually ordered in patients with hematemesis or unstable vital signs. Hemoglobin and hematocrit measurements may suffice because the white blood cell count is seldom useful. Evaluation of platelets has a role primarily in patients with active bleeding.

Serum Electrolytes. Measurement of serum electrolytes is ordered in patients with protracted vomiting and significant volume depletion. The classic electrolyte abnormality seen in patients with protracted vomiting is hypochloremic hypokalemic metabolic alkalosis.

Blood Urea Nitrogen and Creatinine. The blood urea nitrogen (BUN) and creatinine measurements are ordered for reasons similar to those governing measurement of electrolytes. An elevated BUN-creatinine ratio (normal, 20:1) may signify severe dehydration.

Pregnancy Test. A urine pregnancy test is ordered for all females of childbearing age who present with nausea and a history of menstrual abnormalities.

Amylase Level. Determination of amylase level is ordered in patients suspected of having pancreatitis.

Radiologic Imaging

Abdominal Radiographs. An abdominal series, including anteroposterior, supine, and upright views, is requested too often in patients with nausea and vomiting. Such films are ordered to *confirm suspicion* of a *specific disorder*. Upright films are ordered in patients suspected of bowel obstruction or perforation. They are particularly useful in patients with a history of prior surgery. Plain films may be diagnostic in patients with suspected renal tract calculi.

Head CT Scan. CT scans are considered in all patients in whom cerebral disease is suspected or when there is a history of significant head trauma.

Contrast Studies and Endoscopy. These studies may be necessary to diagnose and occasionally treat mechanical obstruction of the bowel, e.g., intussusception, sigmoid volvulus.

Electrocardiogram

A 12-lead electrocardiogram (ECG) is ordered for patients with persistent vomiting and associated symptoms consistent with a diagnosis of ischemic heart disease. Chest pain, diaphoresis, and acute onset of fatigue (particularly in the elderly) are all reasons justifying this study.

Other Tests

Stool Examination. If diarrhea accompanies the nausea and vomiting, the stool is examined for white blood cells using a Wright stain. The presence of white cells is a positive indicator of bacterial gastroenteritis. A recent history of travel in a patient with vomiting and diarrhea may be an indication to examine the stool for ova and parasites. Blood in the stool is useful for detecting occult gastrointestinal bleeding from below the duodenum. Ischemic bowel or inflammatory bowel disease may manifest as vomiting and lower gastrointestinal bleeding.

PROBLEM The emergency physician ordered an ECG, a CBC, and an abdominal radiograph series. They were all normal. A CT scan of the head was then ordered. Electrolyte levels, CBC, and an abdominal series are often overordered, especially in young, healthy patients with a relatively short duration of vomiting. In contrast, one need not hesitate to order pertinent tests. In this case, the suspicion of ischemic heart disease might have been supported by the ECG. The head CT is more difficult to justify fully, but the history and physical examination results were supportive of a possible subarachnoid hemorrhage.

REFINED DIFFERENTIAL DIAGNOSIS

Once catastrophic causes are ruled out, the emergency physician attempts to match the data gathered with the organ system or cause most commonly associated with nausea and vomiting. These systems are the central nervous system, alimentary system, cardiovascular system, drug-related and metabolic causes, psychological causes, and miscellaneous causes. Commonly seen disorders in each system are listed in Table 8–2. A few observations about each system are given below.

Central Nervous System

Increased intracranial pressure caused by an intracerebral disease may be manifest as projectile vomiting without nausea. Vascular events such as subarachnoid hemorrhage or acute intracerebral bleeding are often associated with an acute and sudden onset of severe symptoms. A history of recent head trauma with associated nausea suggests subdural epidural hematoma as a diagnosis. Headache, vomiting, visual complaints, and a history of recurrent episodes are common findings in patients with migraine headache. Labyrinthine disease typically manifests with vertigo, nausea, and vomiting.

Alimentary System

The most common alimentary cause of vomiting is gastroenteritis. Association of nausea and vomiting with diarrhea, abdominal cramps, and myalgias of more than 24 to 48 hours' duration is virtually diagnostic of acute viral gastroenteritis. An acute onset in a previously well patient can also suggest an infectious or toxic agent such as food poisoning.

Delayed (more than 1 hour after a meal) and recurrent vomiting is characteristic of gastric outlet obstruction (usually secondary to peptic ulcer disease) or gastric retention

TABLE 8–2. Specific Disorders in Each of Six Major Areas Associated with Nausea and Vomiting

Central nervous system
  Cerebral lesions, e.g., infection, mass lesions with increased intracranial pressure, hemorrhage
  Migraine
  Labyrinthine disorders (Ménière's disease, motion sickness)

Cardiovascular
  Ischemic heart disease
  Congestive heart failure
  Dysrhythmia, usually tachycardia

Alimentary
  Gastrointestinal
    Gastroenteritis*
    Viral food poisoning, particularly that due to *Staphylococcus*
    Appendicitis
    Intestinal obstruction
    Paralytic ileus
  Gastroduodenal
    Peptic ulcer disease, e.g., gastritis*
    Gastric outlet obstruction
    Gastric atony
    Postgastric surgery
  Hepatobiliary
    Cholecystitis and cholelithiasis*
    Acute hepatitis
    Cirrhosis of the liver
  Pancreatitis

Drug-related and metabolic origin
  Drugs and chemicals—theophylline, digitalis, erythromycin*
  Metabolic acidosis
  Renal failure, with or without hyperkalemia
  Electrolyte abnormalities (hyponatremia, hypercalcemia, hyperkalemia)
  Endocrine disorders: hyperthyroidism, adrenal insufficiency, diabetes mellitus

Psychologic origin
  Emotional and environmental stress*
  Surreptitious vomiting
  Cyclic vomiting (infants and children)
  Bulimia

Miscellaneous
  Acute febrile illness
  Deep visceral pain, e.g., renal, colic, salpingitis
  Radiation sickness
  Glaucoma
  Pregnancy

*Most common causes.

(commonly seen with diabetes mellitus due to vagal neuropathy). Chronic nausea and vomiting is often caused by mechanical obstruction, such as gastric outlet obstruction from peptic ulcer disease, gastric carcinoma, or motility disorders, e.g., diabetic gastroparesis.

Inflammatory processes in both the hepatobiliary and pancreatic systems can present as nausea and vomiting. The retroperitoneal position of the pancreas may make localization more difficult. A history of ethanol abuse is suggestive of pancreatic involvement.

Cardiovascular System

Though ischemic heart disease (IHD) is a serious cause of nausea and vomiting, the symptoms are also found in some patients with dysrhythmia or congestive heart failure.

Drug-Related and Metabolic Causes

Drug overdose, intoxication, and drug side effects are common causes of nausea and vomiting. A medication history is elicited from the patient, and the use of drugs such as theophylline and digitalis is specifically questioned. Metabolic acidosis, particularly diabetic ketoacidosis, may present only as nausea and vomiting. The past medical history and laboratory results can help to identify patients with renal failure and endocrine disorders such as adrenal insufficiency, hyperthyroidism, and diabetes mellitus.

Psychological System

Any acute or chronic emotional or environmental stress can precipitate nausea or vomiting. Psychogenic vomiting is suspected if there is a long history of vomiting, maintenance of adequate nutrition, vomiting during or shortly after meals, vomiting that is of little concern to the patient, evidence of psychological disturbance, and normal appetite. There is a higher incidence of this type of vomiting in females.

Miscellaneous Causes

Acute febrile illness, e.g., otitis media, pneumonia, or meningitis, particularly in pediatric patients, is a common cause of acute nausea and vomiting. Deep visceral pain from any source is an important cause of nausea and vomiting. It is often seen in patients with renal colic or salpingitis. Early morning vomiting and a history of menstrual irregularities in females of childbearing age is caused by pregnancy until proved otherwise.

In refining any differential diagnosis, particularly when the range of choice is wide, serial examinations of the patient are essential. By weighing all the available data and information, despite an unclear history and supporting data, the emergency physician can often reach a correct "ball park" diagnosis leading to management and disposition of the patient.

PROBLEM When he was reevaluated 30 to 40 minutes later, the patient had developed increasing headache and had vomited a second time. There were physical findings of meningismus. The result of the head CT scan showed an acute subarachnoid hemorrhage.

It is fortunate that the triage nurse's suspicions caused her to move the patient into the treatment area immediately. This person could easily have been triaged as a nonacute case and asked to wait in the lounge area until a bed was available. This case typifies a problem characteristic of emergency medicine, that of sorting out seriously ill patients who present with minor problems. Emergency physicians and nurses often develop a "sixth sense" about patients at risk based on the principles of the specialty and on experience.

PRINCIPLES OF MANAGEMENT

The major objectives of therapy for the vomiting patient are to restore volume losses, control emesis, and treat the underlying disease. Many patients who do not have severe underlying disease often respond to the first two modes of therapy. Cases that are refractory to therapy or that have a potentially serious underlying cause need aggressive management tailored to the specific problem.

Volume Restoration

Fluid resuscitation in significantly dehydrated patients is accomplished with intravenous administration of isotonic crystalloid solution. Adult patients without cardiovascular disease usually tolerate 500 to 1000 ml initially. Additional fluid is given according to the clinical response. Older patients and those with cardiovascular disease receive smaller aliquots of fluid, e.g., repeated 200-ml boluses. These are accompanied by frequent checks of vital signs and pulmonary condition.

Significant volume depletion due to vomiting can occur in the absence of physical findings or orthostatic changes, especially in younger patients. These patients often experience subjective improvement after receiving fluids given by the oral or intravenous route. Patients who appear to respond to fluids given intravenously are tested with oral fluids while still in the emergency department. They need to be able to take fluids by mouth to continue fluid management at home.

Emesis Control

The patient with severe nausea or vomiting in the emergency department can be given an antiemetic either through an intramuscular injection or by rectal suppository. This will help to prevent ongoing fluid losses and will aid the patient's symptoms.

Most antiemetics are either antidopaminergic or antihistamine drugs. The antidopaminergic drugs are the most effective for suppressing nausea and vomiting in most cases. They have a greater incidence of extrapyramidal reactions. Though slightly less effective, the antihistamine drugs are relatively free of extrapyramidal reactions. Each antiemetic class acts through different mechanisms. The antihistamine agents dampen the neuropathways originating in the labyrinth and reduce the nerve impulse. The antidopaminergic drugs depress the chemoreceptor trigger zone and act directly on the vomiting center itself. Anticholinergic agents, e.g., scopolamine, are used less commonly. They act by reducing the excitability of the labyrinth receptors. These receptors depress conduction in vestibular cerebellar pathways or prevent recruitment of impulses at the chemoreceptor trigger zone.

Among antihistamine agents, the most commonly used drug is hydroxyzine (Vistaril). Promethazine hydrochloride (Phenergan) and prochlorperazine (Compazine) are the most commonly used antidopaminergic drugs.

Treatment of Underlying Disease

Most of the diseases listed in Table 8–2 are treated according to accepted standards. One newer treatment is metoclopramide (Reglan), a dopamine antagonist that stimulates gastric motility. It is used in people with disorders that cause delayed gastric emptying without mechanical obstruction such as diabetic gastroparesis and postgastrectomy states.

SPECIAL CONSIDERATIONS

Pediatric Patients

Infant regurgitation is often due to gastroesophageal reflux and faulty feeding technique. It often needs to be distinguished from true vomiting. Vomiting in newborns may be secondary to hypertrophic pyloric stenosis, sepsis, intracranial hemorrhage, volvulus, congenital bowel obstruction or stenosis, tracheoesophageal fistula, narcotic addiction, or endocrine-metabolic disorders (adrenal insufficiency, inborn errors of metabolism).

Vomiting in infants and children may be the earliest and only sign of infection (otitis media, pneumonia, gastroenteritis, meningitis), mechanical obstruction of the gastrointestinal tract (volvulus, intussusception), or increased intracranial pressure (tumor, hydrocephalus, hemorrhage, edema). Encephalitis and Reye's syndrome are considered if vomiting is accompanied by a sudden and marked change in mental status.

Cyclic vomiting is a syndrome of recurrent prolonged vomiting attacks without apparent cause. The onset occurs suddenly, usually before age 6, and patients are asymptomatic between attacks. Organic disease must be ruled out to establish this diagnosis. Additional information on the effects of nausea and vomiting in children is given in Chapter 39.

Geriatric Patients

Isolated complaints of nausea and vomiting in elderly patients are often warnings of a serious underlying disease. Elderly patients are often difficult to evaluate because they are unable to cooperate in data gathering; complaints may be nonspecific and multiple; classic signs and symptoms are often delayed, altered, or absent; and the interactions of many prescribed drugs may modify the typical presentations of disease. In the elderly, heightened suspicion is needed, and attention is directed toward searching for intracerebral events, drug intoxication, dehydration, bowel obstruction, causes of an "acute" abdomen, sepsis, hyperthyroidism, and myocardial infarction.

One should avoid attempting to "explain away" apparently inconsistent or vague findings. Recurrent examinations are extremely important, and the physician should not hesitate to order necessary laboratory and special diagnostic studies. Decisions are made in a conservative manner.

DISPOSITION AND FOLLOW-UP

Admission

Admitting the patient to the hospital is appropriate when:
1. The patient has a significant underlying disease. This includes both potentially catastrophic problems and most of the diseases listed in Table 8–2.
2. Patients have an unclear diagnosis and respond poorly to fluid and antiemetic therapy.
3. There is uncontrolled emesis refractory to medication.
4. Patients are at the extremes of age and have no diagnosis or respond poorly to treatment.
5. The diagnosis is unclear and there are poor prospects for timely follow-up, e.g., the patient has no family, no transportation, is indigent, is a drug abuser or an alcoholic, has a language barrier, etc. This category is subject to broad interpretation.

Discharge

Patients are considered for discharge if the following conditions are met:
1. No serious underlying illness is present.
2. There is a good response to fluid and antiemetic therapy.
3. The patient is able to take clear liquids prior to discharge.
4. There are good prospects for follow-up and observation at home. No orthostatic changes are present.

The patient's family and primary physician can help in deciding the disposition. Close follow-up is arranged for all discharged undiagnosed patients, preferably with their primary physician, in 24 to 48 hours. At discharge the gradual return to a normal diet is explained, as are doses of any medications prescribed (Table 8–3). A clear message is given to return to the emergency department if recurrence of symptoms or deterioration in condition occurs.

PROBLEM The patient was admitted to the hospital with a diagnosis of subarachnoid hemorrhage. The emergency physician consulted with the neurosurgeon on call and discussed the diagnosis with the patient and family members.

Not all cases turn out this well. Patients complaining of nausea and vomiting may have a variety of underlying disorders. Although it is usually easy to differentiate the sickest patients from those with the most benign conditions, between these extremes there is great uncertainty in predicting outcome.

TABLE 8–3. Example of Patient Discharge Sheet for Nausea and Vomiting

1. For 12–24 hours: Clear liquid diet (frequent small amounts of liquid).
    a. Plain flavored gelatin—Jello water (prepare with twice the normal amount of water). Drink at room temperature.
    b. Gatorade, Kool-Aid, or noncaffeine-containing soft drinks such as 7-Up or ginger ale.
    c. Clear broth or bouillon.
    d. Decaffeinated tea, sugar.
2. Obtain extra rest, both physical and mental.
3. Take medications as prescribed by the emergency physician.
4. Watch for signs of dehydration—excessive dryness of the tongue, no tears when crying, sunken eyes. If your symptoms have not improved or become worse within 24 hours, contact your family doctor or clinic.
5. Soft diet. Gradually begin with three small meals and two to three small snacks.
6. After 24 hours with improvement on clear liquids, the following foods can be included in a soft diet:
    a. Milk and milk-based drinks, soft drinks without caffeine, decaffeinated tea
    b. Plain meats—baked, broiled, roasted, or boiled
    c. Mild cheese such as American or mild Colby
    d. Cooked or canned vegetables such as green beans, peas, carrots, or squash
    e. Canned or cooked fruits
    f. Plainly prepared potatoes, rice, or noodles
    g. Mild cream or broth soups (no chili)
    h. Fruit juices (if juices cause distress, they may be taken in the middle of a meal instead of on an empty stomach).
    i. For children: bananas or applesauce
    j. Foods to avoid: highly seasoned foods, fatty or fried foods, raw vegetables, and fresh fruit (bananas are all right), popcorn, regular and decaffeinated coffee, regular tea, soft drinks with caffeine (most colas).
7. Gradually resume regular diet and activity.

DOCUMENTATION

1. Onset and duration of vomiting.
2. Description of emesis.
3. Presence of symptoms suggesting underlying etiology, e.g., trauma, headache, fever, or diarrhea, and their timing relative to onset.
4. Pertinent past medical history, especially gastrointestinal, cardiac, and CNS disorders.
5. Menstrual history.
6. Medications taken.
7. Vital signs including orthostatic changes.
8. Signs of dehydration.
9. Complete abdominal examination results.
10. Complete neurologic examination results.
11. Therapeutic intervention and response.
12. Diagnosis, including a brief sentence of the rationale for discharge if the diagnosis is unclear.

SUMMARY AND FINAL POINTS

- True vomiting is differentiated from retching, regurgitation, or rumination.
- The timing of associated symptoms relative to the onset of nausea and vomiting is important in separating underlying disease from complications.
- A careful physical examination is performed to seek evidence of dehydration and possible causes. High-yield areas are the abdominal and neurologic examinations.
- The most common causes of nausea and vomiting are gastroenteritis, febrile illnesses, and drug effects.
- Patients who have been recently discharged from the emergency department with "acute gastroenteritis" and return with persistent symptoms are considered at high risk for underlying disease.

- Vomiting can be caused by serious illness, e.g., myocardial infarction, cerebral hemorrhage, volvulus, Reye's syndrome.
- The complications of vomiting can be serious. These include aspiration, Mallory-Weiss syndrome, electrolyte disorders, and dehydration.
- A urine pregnancy test is ordered for females of childbearing age who are vomiting. This includes those taking birth control pills and those who are post-tubal ligation.
- Patients with gastroenteritis often respond very well to fluid and antiemetic therapy in the emergency department. They may require no formal laboratory testing.
- Patients with chronic nausea and vomiting may have a mechanical cause of intestinal obstruction. If plain radiographs are normal, barium studies or endoscopy can be scheduled after the emergency department visit.
- Elderly patients in whom the underlying cause of vomiting is unclear or who have a marginal response to therapy are usually admitted to the hospital.
- Discharge instructions are clearly written, giving guidelines about following a graduated diet, use of medication, conditions prompting return to the emergency department, and follow-up plans.

BIBLIOGRAPHY

Texts

1. Feldman M: Nausea and vomiting. In Sleisenger MH, Fordtran JS (eds): Gastrointestinal Diseases. Philadelphia, Saunders, 1983.
2. Westell C: Vomiting. In Hart FD (ed): French's Index of Differential Diagnosis. Bristol, John Wright and Sons, 1979.

Journal Articles

1. Book LS: Vomiting and diarrhea. Pediatrics 74:950–954, 1984.
2. Clarke RSJ: Nausea and vomiting. Br J Anaesthesiol 56:19–27, 1984.
3. Hanson JS, McCallum RW: The diagnosis and management of nausea and vomiting. Am J Gastroenterol 80(3):210–218, 1985.
4. Malagelada JR, Camilleri M: Unexplained vomiting: A diagnostic challenge. Ann Intern Med 101:211–218, 1984.
5. Stonham J, Ross S: Antiemetics. Br J Hosp Med 31(5):354–359, 1989.
6. Wruble LD, Rosenthal RH, Webb WL: Psychogenic vomiting: A review. Am J Gastroenterol 77(5):318–321, 1982.

CHAPTER 9

ABDOMINAL TRAUMA

WILLIAM C. DALSEY, M.D.

PROBLEM A rescue squad was called to the scene of a motor vehicle accident involving a 23 year old male driver who collided head-on with a truck.

QUESTIONS TO CONSIDER

1. What potential catastrophic injuries are considered in all patients with abdominal trauma?
2. What points of the history and physical examination can help to differentiate serious from benign injury?
3. When does the patient need rapid surgical intervention?
4. Which laboratory, radiographic, and specialized tests are necessary to evaluate the extent of injury?
5. What are the roles of diagnostic peritoneal lavage and computed tomography?
6. How does the approach differ in managing blunt as opposed to penetrating abdominal trauma?
7. Are there important age-related differences in assessing patients with abdominal trauma?

INTRODUCTION

Abdominal trauma is defined anatomically as trauma to the anterior thoracoabdominal area, which extends from the nipple line to the inguinal creases and posteriorly from the tips of the scapula to the gluteal creases of the buttocks (Fig. 9–1). The abdominal cavity and its contents vary in location based on the position of the diaphragm when the injury occurs. Trauma may damage any of the contents of either the intraperitoneal cavity or the retroperitoneal space. The severity or location of the injury may not be easily determined by physical examination because many of the anatomic structures are difficult to palpate, and the source of pain is often difficult to localize. Patients can have referred pain to the shoulders, scapula, chest, flanks, and back or diffuse abdominal pain relayed by both parietal and visceral pain receptors. Retroperitoneal injury is even more difficult to determine by physical examination. As in all patients with traumatic injuries, alcohol intoxication or head injury may make data-gathering unreliable. A high index of suspicion is necessary to prevent misdiagnosis or delayed diagnosis of significant abdominal injuries.

Abdominal trauma may be either an isolated injury, or it may be one of multiple injuries. It is seen in 20% to 40% of patients with multiple trauma and contributes significantly to morbidity and mortality. It is the fourth most common isolated injury following extremity, head, and neck injuries. In any case, males are affected more often than females by a 2:1 ratio.

Blunt abdominal trauma is five times more common than penetrating injury. It has an overall mortality of 10% to 30%. The relative incidence of individual organ injury in the blunt trauma victim is listed in the left column of Table 9–1.

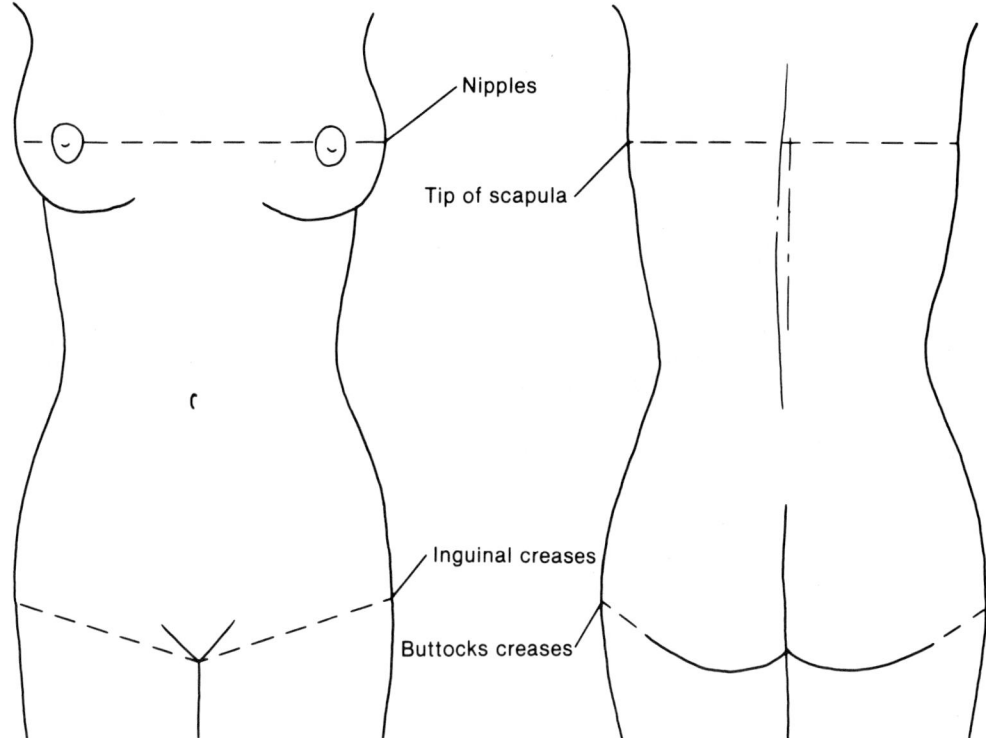

FIGURE 9–1. *The anatomic surface boundaries of the abdomen. Anteriorly, the abdomen extends from the nipple line to the inguinal creases; posteriorly, it extends from the tips of the scapula to the gluteal creases of the buttocks.*

Penetrating trauma results from high- or low-velocity projectiles, stabbing, or foreign bodies. The relative incidence of individual organ injury in penetrating abdominal trauma is listed in the right column of Table 9–1. Gunshot wounds produce a high incidence (70% to 80%) of significant intra-abdominal organ injury (Table 9–2). Stab wounds

TABLE 9–1. Relative Incidence of Organ Injury in Blunt vs Penetrating Abdominal Trauma

Blunt		Penetrating	
Organ	*Percentage*	*Organ*	*Percentage*
Spleen	25	Liver	37
Intestine	15	Small bowel	26
Liver	15	Stomach	19
Retroperitoneal hematoma	13	Colon	16.5
Kidney	12	Major vascular and retroperitoneal	11
Mesentery	5		
Pancreas	3	Mesentery and omentum	9.5
Diaphragm	2	Spleen	7
Urinary bladder	6	Diaphragm	5.5
Urethra	2	Kidney	5
Vascular	2	Pancreas	3.5
		Duodenum	2.5
		Biliary system	1
		Other (uterus, sciatic plexus, bladder, muscle, ovary, vagina, adrenal)	1

From Zuidema GD, Rutherford RB, Ballinger WF: The Management of Trauma (4th ed). Philadelphia, Saunders, 1985.

TABLE 9–2. Visceral Injury with Penetrating Abdominal Wounds

	Stab Wounds	Gunshot Wounds
Peritoneal violation and visceral injury	26%	77%
Peritoneal violation without significant injury	42%	3%
No peritoneal penetration	32%	20%

penetrating the intraperitoneal cavity injure the abdominal organs in 25% of patients. The mortality of gunshot wounds varies from 10% to 20%, whereas stab wounds have a mortality of less than 5%.

In the case of gunshot wounds or "ballistic" injuries, the energy delivered to the body is determined approximately by the mass of the object times its velocity squared ($E = mv^2$). The impact velocity of the bullet is an important determinant of damage potential. Most "assault-type" weapons have muzzle velocities of more than 2000 feet/sec (high), whereas most handguns have muzzle velocities of less than 1000 feet/sec (low). Therefore, wounds due to high-velocity bullets are much more devastating because they have much greater energy. The mortality from high-velocity injuries is over 50%. Solid organs may be shattered directly by the concussive effect of such a missile or indirectly by the dissipation of its kinetic energy. This damage may occur even when the organ has not actually been hit by the bullet or projectile, so the path of the wound is not a reliable indicator of what organs might be injured. Projectiles also take irregular paths or may hit bone, thereby causing secondary projectiles, both of which result in injury outside the direct path of the wound.

Early death in patients with abdominal trauma results from uncontrolled hemorrhage after vascular or solid organ injury. Rarely, diaphragmatic rupture with herniation of abdominal contents into the thorax may cause death due to respiratory compromise. Late deaths result from sepsis, unrecognized delayed bleeding, an occult injury, or disruption of the hollow organs (bowel, gallbladder, and urinary bladder), pancreas, or kidneys.

PREHOSPITAL CARE

Since limiting time in the field is essential, only basic data are quickly obtained by the rescue squad. Optimal resuscitation and definitive management are best accomplished in the hospital.

History

1. What is the mechanism of injury (blunt or penetrating)?
2. Are more immediately life-threatening injuries present, particularly injuries of the chest, head, or neck?
3. A detailed description of the location, severity, and character of any pain is *unnecessary*.
4. If the patient is a victim of a motor vehicle accident, what is the status of the steering wheel? Was a seat belt used?

Physical Examination

1. What are the vital signs?
2. Does the patient have any airway injury or respiratory distress?
3. What is the patient's color and peripheral perfusion?
4. Any other potentially life-threatening injuries are described.

Intervention

Field stabilization for trauma patients includes the following actions:
1. Airway intervention and ventilatory support as necessary.

2. Supplemental oxygen, usually at 4 to 6 liters/min by nasal cannula or face mask in the spontaneously breathing patient.

3. Spinal immobilization and extrication of the patient from the vehicle if necessary.

4. Cardiac monitoring and serial taking of vital signs. Hemodynamic changes are observed during transport.

5. If it does not result in a significant transport delay, one or two 14- to 16-gauge intravenous (IV) lines are placed, and isotonic crystalloid solution is administered.

6. Pneumatic antishock garments (PASG) may be used, although their efficacy has not been proved. Many authorities advocate that their use be limited to specialized indications, e.g., the splinting of pelvic fractures.

PROBLEM On arrival at the scene and after initial assessment, the rescue squad radioed the base station and reported that the patient was awake and alert but intoxicated. He was the driver of a medium-sized car that had collided head-on with a tractor trailer 15 minutes earlier. Each was travelling at about 35 miles per hour. The windshield and steering wheel were intact, and he was wearing a seatbelt. He had no other symptoms other than moderately severe abdominal pain. There was no other evidence of injury. Vital signs were pulse 130 beats/min, respirations 18/min, and blood pressure 100/50 mm Hg. The squad placed the patient on nasal oxygen at 6 liters/min and started a 16-gauge IV line with Ringer's lactate at a wide-open rate. The electrocardiographic (ECG) monitor showed sinus tachycardia. The driver of the tractor trailer was anxious but unhurt.

Although the patient appeared stable, the severity of the accident, the complaint of abdominal pain associated with an increased pulse rate, and the presence of intoxication raised the suspicion of a potentially severe intra-abdominal injury with significant hemorrhage. Rapid transport was appropriate. Close observation and monitoring for changes in the patient's condition can be expected of the rescue personnel. It is useful to make a brief inquiry about the status of other people involved in the accident.

INITIAL APPROACH IN THE EMERGENCY DEPARTMENT

The important goals of the initial approach are stabilizing the patient's condition and determining the need for operative intervention. The following sequence is often completed in a simultaneous manner. Assessment of airway and breathing always initiates the approach.

History

1. A brief description of the event itself and the events that have occurred during transport is obtained from prehospital care personnel.

2. If possible, the history taken from the patient includes current symptoms such as shortness of breath or abdominal pain.

3. The mechanism of injury from the patient's perspective is briefly reviewed and corroborated with the description given by the rescue squad.

Physical Examination

1. Vital signs are obtained, and the circulatory and ventilatory status is assessed. Early recognition of hemorrhagic shock indicates the need for aggressive fluid resuscitation and early surgical management. Patients with significant hemorrhage appear restless, pale, and clammy and have poor capillary refill. Repeated monitoring of vital signs may give the first clues of a deteriorating condition due to intra-abdominal bleeding.

2. Only after the ventilatory and circulation needs of the patient are addressed can an adequate secondary examination be accomplished, which includes examining the chest and abdomen and a brief assessment of neurologic function.

Examination of the abdomen focuses on whether a "surgical abdomen" is present, i.e., whether there is rigidity, rebound tenderness, or gross distention. The back and flanks are visualized as part of the abdominal examination because they are common sites of unsuspected wounds or injuries.

3. Associated findings of rib fractures or neurologic deficit increase the risk that significant intra-abdominal injury exists.

Intervention

1. Oxygen at 4 to 6 liters/min and airway stabilization with intubation and ventilatory assistance are given as necessary.
2. Depending on the patient's condition and the field care given previously, one to two large-bore (14- to 16-gauge) peripheral IV lines are inserted, and isotonic crystalloid is infused. Blood administration sets are used in all patients with potentially significant injury.
3. Cardiac monitoring is continued. Vital signs are repeated frequently, every 5 to 10 minutes, to track the patient's course.
4. In patients with significant trauma, initial laboratory tests are ordered. These include a type and screen or cross-match for 6 units of blood. A complete blood count, amylase, and urinalysis are ordered. Ethanol level, glucose, electrolytes, and coagulation studies are ordered if appropriate.
5. An anteroposterior portable chest radiograph is obtained to screen rapidly for life-threatening thoracic disorders, e.g., pneumothorax, transected aorta, herniated diaphragm.
6. Other bedside tests and procedures complement the physical examination.
    a. A *spun hematocrit* is obtained. A low hematocrit is presumed to represent significant bleeding. However, a normal hematocrit does not exclude bleeding because it may take several hours for a decrease due to hemodilution to occur. Serial hematocrits of decreasing values represent ongoing hemorrhage.
    b. Urine dipstick analysis for blood may give an early clue to a potentially significant urologic injury.
    c. The patient is examined for urethral injury, and in males the position of the prostate on rectal examination is noted. If the patient is unstable or if diagnostic peritoneal lavage or surgery is planned, a urinary catheter is placed. The catheter decompresses the bladder, provides urine for examination, and allows urinary output to be monitored. A catheter is not placed if urethral disruption is suspected because of blood at the urethral meatus, pelvic instability, or an abnormally positioned prostate.
    d. Placement of a large nasogastric tube with suction allows emptying and decompression of the stomach. The presence of blood, bile, or feces in the aspirate may indicate a significant intra-abdominal injury.

PROBLEM In the emergency department, the patient was alert and admitted to having consumed "two beers" shortly before the accident. He had no shortness of breath or neurologic symptoms. He complained of abdominal pain in the epigastric area. The squad reported that there had been no change in his condition enroute. The patient was undressed and placed on a cardiac monitor. His repeat vital signs were: blood pressure 100/60 mm Hg, pulse 130 beats/min, and respiratory rate 20/min. The chest was not obviously injured, and breath sounds were equal. The abdomen was diffusely tender with rebound tenderness, but bowel sounds were present. He moved all four extremities and had no neck tenderness. A second intravenous line was started, and an initial bolus of 1000 ml of isotonic crystalloid was given. A blood sample was sent for CBC, electrolyte panel, coagulation studies, and a type and cross-match for 6 units of blood. A portable anteroposterior chest radiograph was unremarkable. A nasogastric tube was inserted, and a small quantity of nonbloody gastric fluid returned through it. An indwelling urinary catheter was placed, and the urine dipstick test for blood showed negative results. The emergency physician called the trauma surgeon to consult on the patient.

The need to evaluate a trauma victim rapidly and thoroughly requires an organized and systematic approach. Initial assessment and treatment often are completed simultaneously. Assigning tasks to individuals prior to the patient's arrival can improve the overall management of these cases. The protocols and skills derived from repetition are two reasons for the success of the "trauma center" concept.

DATA GATHERING

As in all patients with traumatic injury, the goal of data gathering is to establish the patient's "clinical" status before the injury, the nature and degree of the forces involved, the patient's physiologic response to the injury, and evolving signs and symptoms. Changing clinical status points to undiscovered problems and complications of the injury. An extended history and physical examination are possible only if the patient remains hemodynamically stable.

History

Key historical points include the following:

1. *When did the accident occur?*
   The time from the initial trauma incident is a critical factor in managing the abdominally injured patient. The primary reason is that blood loss can occur rapidly, leading to irreversible shock.
2. *What are the specific details about the mechanism of injury?*
   Questions are often specific to the nature of injury:
   a. *Motor vehicle accident.* Speed, size of vehicles, position of patient, damage to vehicles, use of seatbelt, ejection from car?
   b. *Motorcycle.* Speed, distance thrown, protective clothing and helmet?
   c. *Fall.* Distance, surface of landing, secondary impacts while falling?
   d. *Gunshot wound.* High- versus low-velocity weapon, distance from gun, multiple shots?
   e. *Knife wound.* Length of blade, direction of blade, multiple stabbing?
3. *Why did the injury occur?*
   The "why" addresses the possibility of another disease process, including intoxication, that caused or contributed to the event. The use of ethanol prior to injury is unfortunately so common that it warrants specific inquiry.
4. *What are the patient's symptoms?*
   The symptoms, such as the character, location, and severity of abdominal pain, or symptoms related to other organ systems, e.g., shortness of breath, provide clues to the extent and severity of injury.
5. *Is there a history of allergy?*
   Allergies, particularly allergies to antibiotics, contrast material, or anesthetics, can severely complicate treatment and are routinely recorded.
6. *Is the patient currently taking medications?*
   Medication use provides insight into current illness and information about the potential risk of interactions from pharmaceuticals given during treatment.
7. *Are there current illnesses or a significant past medical history?*
   Prior abdominal surgery can influence interpretation of diagnostic tests and

treatment decisions. The presence of preexisting heart disease or diabetes may provide clues about the original cause of trauma.
8. *What is the tetanus immunization history?*
9. *When did the patient last eat or drink?*
This is necessary to plan for anesthesia if surgery is necessary. If intake was recent, the potential for vomiting and risk of aspiration are increased.

Physical Examination

The physical examination is an insensitive indicator of the presence or severity of the underlying injury. After the initial assessment, a secondary head to toe examination of the patient is carried out as described in Chapter 4, Multiple Trauma. Listed below are the aspects of an examination relevant to abdominal injury.

General Appearance. Skin color, temperature, presence of diaphoresis, and capillary refill help to assess the adequacy of the patient's perfusion and oxygenation. Hypoperfusion is presumed to be hemorrhagic in origin. Intra-abdominal bleeding is a common source, but retroperitoneal, pelvic, and chest cavity bleeding are all possibilities.

Neck. Evaluation for tenderness or deformity may support a diagnosis of spinal injury. Spinal cord injuries may render the examination of the abdomen useless by interrupting the normal visceral and peritoneal pain pathways.

Chest. In patients with abdominal trauma, associated thoracic injuries are common and need to be identified early. The reverse is true as well. For example, lower rib fractures may indicate the possibility of splenic or liver injury. Penetrating injury of the thorax can easily extend into the abdomen. Rupture of the diaphragm and herniation of the abdominal contents into the chest may compromise the patient's ventilation. Anterior and posterior evaluation for signs of penetrating injury, adequacy of bilateral excursion, bilateral breath sounds, bowel sounds in the chest, heart sounds, palpable fractures, subcutaneous emphysema, and tympany may aid in the diagnosis of life-threatening injuries.

Abdomen

1. Visualizing the abdomen also includes visualizing the flanks and back. Injury and intra-abdominal bleeding are suggested by signs of abrasion, penetrating injury, abdominal wall swelling or hematoma, and abdominal distention; distention is more indicative of a ruptured viscus and free air. In the adult, the peritoneal cavity can accommodate most of the patient's blood volume with only moderate distention.

2. On auscultation, the presence or absence of bowel sounds is a poor indicator of acute injury. The ileus associated with a silent abdomen has not usually appeared. Bruits may indicate vascular injury, but they are insensitive findings and are seldom heard in a noisy emergency department.

3. Palpation and percussion may identify abdominal distention, local and rebound tenderness, guarding, hepatic or splenic masses, flank tenderness or masses, palpable spinal injury, and bladder distention. Signs of peritoneal irritation such as guarding and rebound tenderness are useful indications of underlying injury, but they are insensitive predictors of pathology—e.g., up to one-third of patients with intra-abdominal hemorrhage may show no evidence of peritoneal irritation. Such signs may be masked by intoxication, spinal injuries, and analgesics. Unequal femoral pulses may suggest abdominal aortic injury but are not reliable in this regard.

4. All patients require pelvic and rectal examinations and visual inspection and palpation of their external genitalia. During the latter examination one looks for blood at the external urethra, representing urethral injury, and distant signs of abdominal injury, e.g., blood in the scrotum. A high-riding prostate on rectal examination or palpable pelvic fracture also suggests possible urologic injury. Patients in whom urethral injury is suspected should not have an indwelling urinary catheter inserted until their injuries are better evaluated. Unless there is active vaginal bleeding, the initial pelvic examination is usually confined to a gentle bimanual examination.

Bony Pelvis. It is important to check the stability of the bony pelvis in this assessment. It is a complex anatomic area with a large potential space for blood loss.

Extremities. Penetrating injuries may extend great distances to involve the intra-abdominal organs. The presence of femoral fractures indicates that significant forces caused the injury; thus the possibility of intra-abdominal injury is increased.

Neurologic. The patient's mental status and ability to respond to stimuli may point to an intracranial injury or may reflect the adequacy of cerebral perfusion. The peripheral loss of sensation, muscular activity, muscular tone, peripheral reflexes, cerebral and autonomic reflexes, rectal tone, and the presence of priapism all may indicate a spinal injury. A change in neuroreceptiveness has a major influence on the accuracy of examination findings in abdominal trauma.

PROBLEM On secondary examination, the patient showed no evidence of other injury. The main finding was diffuse upper abdominal tenderness with mild rebound and guarding. Rectal and genital examinations showed no abnormalities. After the infusion of 1000 ml of isotonic crystalloid, the patient's pulse rate dropped to 110 beats/min and the systolic pressure rose to 110 mm Hg. Because the patient was showing some hemodynamic improvement, the emergency physician decided, after discussion with the surgeon, that further testing rather than immediate surgical intervention was appropriate.

The patient has been rapidly and systematically evaluated and appropriately treated. Localized signs and symptoms that appear on the secondary examination allow an isolated area of injury to be considered for the first time. Early surgical consultation is important in providing prompt definitive care. Patients waiting for the surgeon may undergo further diagnostic assessment. Any patient whose condition deteriorates hemodynamically needs aggressive treatment and early laparotomy.

DECISION PRIORITIES AND PRELIMINARY DIFFERENTIAL DIAGNOSIS

The primary differential diagnoses and decisions involve the patient's hemodynamic stability, the need for surgical intervention, and the role of the abdominal injury in terms of the patient's total body trauma. Before further evaluation and diagnostic efforts are made, patients are placed in one of three categories of potential life-threatening injury.

Immediate Operation. Some patients require *immediate operative intervention* because of the potential for immediate threat to life. The conditions include the following:

1. Hemodynamically unstable trauma patients require stabilization simultaneously with data gathering. Isolated abdominal trauma may be immediately life-threatening if there is severe uncontrolled hemorrhage. These patients remain in shock despite vigorous isotonic replacement with crystalloid and blood.

2. Patients with an evisceration or visible peritoneal contents require immediate operation. The eviscerated bowel is kept moist with saline and a sterile dressing and is not returned into the abdomen. Occasionally, the omentum, looking like a piece of fat, will protrude from a wound. It must not be mistaken as subcutaneous fat in the abdominal wall. It is kept moist with saline and a sterile dressing.

3. Diaphragmatic rupture with impairment of adequate ventilation from bowel contents also requires immediate action.

4. Most authorities recommend exploratory laparotomy if the peritoneum is violated. The question is timing. Any patient with a penetrating injury requires prompt surgical consultation to assist in evaluating the extent of damage. Unstable patients who do not respond to resuscitative effort are candidates for early surgery. A penetrating knife or object retained in place is not removed in the emergency department. The patient is stabilized while movement of the object is prevented. Removal is completed in the operating suite under controlled conditions.

5. Sudden deterioration or hemodynamic collapse of the patient may require an emergency department thoracotomy to gain proximal vascular control. This is accomplished by cross-clamping the descending aorta manually or by using an appropriate vascular clamp.

Hemodynamic Stability with Signs of Blunt Abdominal Trauma. Hemodynamically stable patients who have sustained blunt abdominal trauma are a more difficult diagnostic challenge. Patients who progress to abdominal distention, localized tenderness with significant guarding, peritoneal findings, or evidence of intra-abdominal bleeding require surgical exploration. If the physical examination is unreliable, e.g., if the patient is intoxicated or has an altered mental status, the diagnostic adjuncts discussed below can be helpful. They should never delay definitive intervention if the patient's condition continues to deteriorate. Serial measurements of vital signs and repeated abdominal examinations are essential during the "observation" period while more definitive diagnoses are being formulated.

Stable Vital Signs with Minimal Findings. As with many traumatic events, a number of patients will have stable vital signs and minimal physical findings. The deciding factor for further testing or observation in these patients is the mechanism of injury and the severity of the forces involved. If both are minimal, the patient in considered for disposition. If either or both are significant, e.g., in patients with a tangential gunshot wound or a fall of more than 15 feet, more time and information are necessary before a decision is made.

Site of Injury. A question, unrelated to severity, is useful to ask at this stage: *Is the patient's injury intra-abdominal, retroperitoneal, or both?*

The retroperitoneal space can contain 1500 to 2500 ml of blood. It is poorly localized by the neurosensory system, and serious injuries in this location may manifest few localizing signs. Injury to the retroperitoneal organs, such as part of the duodenum, pancreas, and kidneys, are a continual concern in evaluating the patient with abdominal trauma. Unexplained hemodynamic instability must include retroperitoneal hemorrhage in the list of possible causes.

PROBLEM This patient now fits under the category of hemodynamic stability with signs of blunt trauma. There had been an episode of hemodynamic instability, which improved with therapy. The symptoms suggested serious underlying problems but were not so serious as to require immediate surgical intervention. The possibility of retroperitoneal injury existed. Further observation and diagnostic testing were necessary.

DIAGNOSTIC ADJUNCTS

The benefits of diagnostic testing in patients with abdominal trauma have steadily increased. More tests are becoming definitive, such as computed tomography, but they are always placed in the context of the patient's injury and condition. In most cases, at least a CBC and urinalysis are ordered. In patients with severe injury, all of the tests listed are requested.

Laboratory Studies

Complete Blood Count. A complete blood count (CBC) is obtained in all patients with abdominal injuries. In unstable patients, a spun hematocrit is done in the emergency department. This simply establishes a baseline to follow. A normal level tells nothing, and a low level may represent the patient's status prior to the injury. Hemoglobin and hematocrit results are interpreted to estimate the blood's available oxygen-carrying capacity. White blood cell counts may be elevated in patients with splenic injury, or elevation may occur as a result of the sympathetic discharge accompanying trauma. This is very common and renders the white count nondiagnostic. Platelet estimates may vary greatly and are useful only if they are under 100,000/cm^3. All such measurements represent "baseline values" and can be repeated during the continuing care of the patient.

Urinalysis. Injury to the urinary tract is frequently associated with abdominal trauma. Any blood (2 to 3 red blood cells/high-power field) found in the urine is considered significant but is not necessarily indicative of serious genitourinary trauma. Recent improvements in the sensitivity of urine dipstick testing have made it a suitable screening test for urinary hemoglobin. If blood is present, an intravenous pyelogram is indicated; it may be combined with a urethrogram and cystogram depending on the injury and findings.

Amylase. Although uncommon, pancreatic injury occurs in patients with either penetrating or blunt trauma. An abnormal amylase value is often the only indicator of injury to the pancreas, but it is nonspecific.

Other Laboratory Tests. Other laboratory tests are indicated as necessary: glucose, blood urea nitrogen (BUN), and creatinine determinations, platelet count, coagulation studies, electrolytes, ethanol level, and toxicology screening. Blood type and screen or cross-matching is ordered if hemorrhage is suspected, the number of blood units depending on the estimated severity of injury; 4 to 6 units are a reasonable first estimate.

Radiologic Imaging

Plain Radiographs. Plain radiographs ordered include supine and upright abdominal films and upright posteroanterior and lateral or anteroposterior portable views of the chest. If the patient cannot sit, an anteroposterior supine chest and a decubitus abdominal view are performed. The presence of free air suggests a bowel perforation and warrants surgical consultation for exploratory laparotomy. Bullets and other foreign bodies may be localized by plain radiographs. Films taken in two different planes are needed to determine foreign body position in the abdomen. Plain radiographs of the abdomen are not sensitive. If abnormalities are seen, they may be diagnostic, but normal or nondiagnostic plain films do not rule out the possibility of significant injury. If localized ileus, mass effect, or radiographic evidence of intra-abdominal or retroperitoneal blood is present, additional testing or exploration is necessary.

Intravenous Pyelogram. The double-dose single-shot intravenous pyelogram (IVP) is the technique most commonly used in patients with abdominal trauma to establish the presence and function of both kidneys. It helps to delineate the renal vasculature and renal injury. It may also demonstrate ureteral injury. The standard IVP provides a more complete view of the entire urinary system, but it requires significantly more time.

Urethrogram and Cystogram. This is the best diagnostic test if there is a suspected urethral or bladder injury. Ninety percent of bladder disruptions caused by blunt injury are retroperitoneal and are usually identified by extravasation of dye. Urethral or bladder injury is suspected if there is gross blood at the urethral meatus, gross hematuria, a palpable urethral disruption, or a high-riding, free-floating prostate on rectal examination. Penetrating injury in a lower abdominal location or the presence of a pelvic fracture significantly increases the risk of this injury. Injury to the urethra or bladder requires urologic consultation. A suprapubic cystostomy may be required to provide urinary bladder drainage.

Contrast Duodenography. Contrast radiographs may improve the sensitivity of plain radiographs in diagnosing perforations and injury of the upper gastrointestinal tract, particularly of the small bowel, which are not well seen by other imaging methods. Pancreatic injury may also be suspected, but this diagnosis frequently requires more specific testing.

Ultrasound. Commonly used by surgeons as a diagnostic adjunct in the rapid evaluation of abdominal trauma in Europe, ultrasound is under investigation in the United States. It can be used in the emergency department to identify intra-abdominal bleeding and injury to solid organs, kidney, spleen, or liver.

Angiography. Angiography is the gold standard for evaluating vascular injury. It is not commonly used for initial assessment of abdominal trauma because most patients with major vascular injury are unstable and need rapid surgical exploration. It may be used to evaluate inguinal vessels or renal vasculature. It is the method of choice for assessment of patients with uncontrolled retroperitoneal bleeding from pelvic fractures.

Other Tests

Diagnostic Peritoneal Lavage and Computed Tomography. Diagnostic peritoneal lavage (DPL) or computed tomography (CT) is considered whenever there is a suspected intra-abdominal injury in a hemodynamically stable patient. The choice depends on the clinical circumstances and currently varies between institutions. The criteria for selecting these diagnostic procedures include (1) presence of abdominal tenderness, (2) obtunded mental state (due to head injury, drugs or alcohol), (3) a need for anesthesia for treatment of other surgical injuries, and (4) significant mechanism of injury (high-speed collision, motorcycle accident, fall from a height). Any one of these criteria is considered sufficient for performing one of these tests. They are not indicated if the patient is hemodynamically unstable and requires immediate surgical intervention or if the decision to perform an exploratory laparotomy has already been made. Relative contraindications, specifically for DPL, include pediatric patients, pregnancy, patients with multiple prior abdominal surgical procedures, or those in whom the bladder and stomach cannot be decompressed.

As the established standard for the determination of intra-abdominal bleeding, DPL is both sensitive (indicating bleeding in 97% of cases) and accurate. Criteria for interpreting DPL include evaluation of red blood cells, white blood cells, and amylase (Table 9–3). The major advantages of this test are its quickness, cost effectiveness, reliability, and low complication rate. It does not, however, delineate the location or severity of injury. DPL may miss significant retroperitoneal injuries, diaphragmatic injury, and bowel or bladder injuries that do not result in significant bleeding. A false negative result may occur if prior surgery or infection has resulted in significant abdominal adhesions, preventing blood from freely entering the peritoneal cavity.

The indications for a CT scan are similar to those for DPL. A CT scan will identify the presence of blood and assess the location of bleeding and the severity of organ injury. It is contraindicated in hemodynamically unstable patients and those needing emergent laparotomy. It is the diagnostic modality of choice in pediatric patients or whenever a DPL is relatively contraindicated. Its sensitivity for detecting significant intraperitoneal injury under ideal circumstances and with optimal technique is greater than 95%. CT scans can detect most cases of intraperitoneal (when there is more than 250 ml of blood) and significant retroperitoneal bleeding. Another advantage is its ability to identify the extent of specific injury to solid organs (spleen, liver, kidneys), and it may reduce the need for exploratory laparotomy. To optimize the results of this test, both oral and intravenous contrast media are used. CT scanning is less capable of identifying diaphrag-

TABLE 9–3. Interpretive Criteria for Diagnostic Peritoneal Lavage

Test results are considered positive if:	Test results are considered indeterminate if:
More than 10 ml of gross blood are aspirated	RBCs total >50,000/ml and < 100,000/ml
Lavage fluid exits via Foley catheter or chest tube	WBCs total > 100/ml and < 500/ml
There is a grossly bloody lavage return	Amylase totals > 75 and < 175 IU
RBCs total > 100,000/ml*	**Test results are considered negative if:**
WBCs total > 500/ml	RBCs total < 50,000/ml
Amylase totals > 175 IU	WBCs total < 100/ml
Urine, feces, bile, or particulate matter are found in the lavage fluid	Amylase totals < 75 IU

RBCs = red blood cells, WBCs = white blood cells, DPL = diagnostic peritoneal lavage.
*If gunshot wounds of the abdomen are assessed using DPL, the RBC count considered positive falls to 5000/ml.

matic, pancreatic, and hollow viscous injury, and it may miss early findings of these injuries in a large percentage of cases. CT scans are relatively expensive, time-consuming, and dependent on the technical quality of the equipment and the experience of the operator and interpreter.

Local Exploration of Stab Wounds. Surgical exposure and direct observation may be warranted to determine the presence of violation of the peritoneum in the evaluation of stab wounds. If a wound penetrates the peritoneum, most authorities recommend diagnostic peritoneal lavage or exploratory laparotomy. Wounds are not probed to determine the violation of the peritoneum because the technique is inaccurate and risks causing increased bleeding. Surgical consultation is important whenever there is significant concern of peritoneal violation by the emergency physician.

PROBLEM A contrast CT scan of the abdomen showed a laceration of the left lobe of the liver with free blood in the peritoneum. The first hematocrit taken in the emergency department was 28%. Urinalysis and amylase values were unremarkable. Infusion of 2 units of packed red cells was started prior to transferring the patient to the operating room. Other test results, including coagulation studies and platelet count, were normal. The patient's vital signs at the time of transfer were blood pressure 110/70 mm Hg and pulse rate 100 beats/min.

Whenever trauma patients leave the emergency department, they should be accompanied by trained personnel to monitor their clinical status. If unmonitored patients are delayed in the radiology department and left unattended, catastrophic changes in their condition may occur.

REFINED DIFFERENTIAL DIAGNOSIS

The differential diagnosis of abdominal injury relies on an understanding of the anatomy of the abdomen and a high degree of suspicion. Solid organ structures may be significantly injured by both direct and indirect trauma. Hollow structures may rupture or perforate without causing localizing findings. Penetrating injuries with unsuspected paths of injury may be caused by secondary missile formation and concussive effects. The mechanism and location of trauma may help to formulate the initial differential diagnosis, but the true extent of organ involvement can be known only after a definitive CT scan or laparotomy is performed. Table 9–4 lists the signs and symptoms of various injuries of the intra-abdominal organs and guidelines for their diagnosis and management.

PRINCIPLES OF MANAGEMENT

The basic principles of management of the patient with abdominal trauma are the same as those for any trauma patient: airway and ventilatory control, volume resuscitation, and recognition of the need for surgical intervention. The goal is to balance the risk of unnecessary laparotomy with the increased morbidity and mortality associated with delayed surgery. The need for immediate surgical intervention was discussed earlier in Decision Priorities. The following guidelines are useful for patients in whom the decision is not so clear-cut.

Blunt Abdominal Trauma

Figure 9–2 presents the management of blunt abdominal trauma in the form of an algorithm. If the patient is hemodynamically stable, a decision as to whether to perform a DPL or CT scan is made. As mentioned, a CT scan is often preferred in children and in patients with previous abdominal incisions. If the DPL or scan shows positive results,

TABLE 9-4. Differential Diagnosis of Abdominal Injury by Major Organs

Injury	Clinical Signs and Symptoms	Possible Associated Injuries	Diagnosis and Management
Liver injury	Pain or tenderness in right upper quadrant Signs of hypovolemic shock Referred pain to right shoulder from diaphragmatic irritation	Lacerated bowel Right lower rib fractures Hepatic vascular injury Renal injury	Liver injury can range from minor parenchymal injury with confined subcapsular bleeding to massive organ injury with uncontrolled hemorrhage Significant injury or hemorrhage may be determined in hemodynamically stable patients by peritoneal lavage or CT scanning CT scanning may delineate extent of injury, but the management of minor injuries with minimal bleeding remains controversial Significant injury or bleeding requires surgery; in children, conservative expectant management is favored whenever possible Surgical consultation is indicated for all suspected liver injuries Patients with subcapsular hematomas are protected from further trauma that might result in rupture of the capsule
Splenic injury	Tenderness and pain in left upper quadrant Kehr's sign: referred pain to left shoulder from diaphragmatic irritation Muscle spasm, guarding, rigidity Signs of hypoperfusion	Stomach, bowel and pancreatic injury Renal injury Diaphragmatic injury Left lower rib fractures 20% of fractures of 9th to 10th ribs have associated splenic injury	Splenic injury may range from relatively minor parenchymal injury with confined bleeding within a subcapsular hematoma to complete parenchymal or vascular disruption with uncontrolled hemorrhage Splenic injuries are the most common cause of intraperitoneal bleeding from blunt abdominal trauma Enlarged spleen with medial displacement of the gastric bubble on plain film CT scan can delineate the extent of injury and bleeding. It is a useful adjunct in hemodynamically stable patients A splenectomy is required for unstable patients or those with massive injury A splenorrhaphy may be attempted in less damaged spleens, and minor injuries (particularly in children) may be treated conservatively by close observation and expectant management
Pancreatic injury	Mild epigastric pain and tenderness that may decrease initially and then worsen after several hours Guarding and muscle spasm (relatively rare) Signs of hypovolemic shock (may be delayed) Ileus Severe back pain	Seatbelt-associated injuries Duodenal injury	Lack of significant acute physical findings from this retroperitoneal structure often make initial diagnosis difficult A high amylase level in lavage fluid or evidence on CT scan coupled with a high degree of suspicion may result in early diagnosis Undiagnosed injury may result in necrosis with subsequent pancreatitis, delayed bleeding, peritonitis, or cyst formation No definitive diagnostic test exists for early and accurate diagnoses of these injuries following injury Requires surgical intervention when suspected
Ruptured or perforated gastrointestinal tract (hollow viscus)	Epigastric pain, tenderness, gastrointestinal pain, or guarding; blood in nasogastric fluid or bowels Ileus and distention Free air in peritoneum	Mesenteric vascular injury Solid organ injury (liver and spleen) Most often due to penetrating injury	High mortality rate (15%–20%) due to other injuries Free intraperitoneal rupture or air on plain film is presumed to be a perforation of the gastrointestinal tract. These patients require exploratory laparotomy Immediate symptoms and physical findings may be unremarkable, but over 48–72 hours gradually increasing pain and tenderness may indicate peritonitis from occult injury Significant injury from blunt trauma may be difficult to diagnose initially when the injury involves the retroperitoneal portion of the duodenum. Contrast duodenography, CT scan, or exploratory laparotomy may aid in the diagnosis. Perforation in blunt trauma occurs at the points of fixed attachment, particularly the duodenum Patients with suspected bowel perforation are given antibiotics in anticipation of surgery and a nasogastric tube to remove gastrointestinal contents Bile or urine in peritoneal lavage fluid suggests biliary perforation or genitourinary disruption; both require surgical consultation and management
Inferior vena cava	More often due to penetrating trauma Signs of hypoperfusion Signs of retroperitoneal hematoma Abdominal distention, tenderness, and rigidity	Bowel perforation Spinal cord injury Retroperitoneal hematoma	In suspected inferior vena cava injury, intravenous access for fluid resuscitation is placed above the diaphragm Vascular injury may cause significant hemorrhage and needs both aggressive resuscitation and immediate surgery This injury is frequently catastrophic; DPL and CT scans may show hemorrhage while angiography and exploratory laparotomy define the extent of injury. Aggressive fluid resuscitation with acute surgical repair is necessary

Injury	Signs/Symptoms	Associated Injuries	Management
Perforation of aorta or vascular rupture	Abdominal distention, tenderness, and rigidity; Bruits and lost or decreased distal pulses; Signs of hypoperfusion	Bowel perforation; Spinal fractures	Emergency department thoracotomy to access the aorta and control bleeding may be required in catastrophic bleeding; The use of PASG to minimize bleeding is controversial
Genitourinary (kidneys, ureters, urethra, and bladder)	Signs of retroperitoneal hematoma; Flank or abdominal pain and tenderness; Flank swelling or ecchymosis; Blood at urethral orifice; Hematuria (95%); Suprapubic tenderness or ecchymosis; Displaced prostate; Retroperitoneal hemorrhage; Distended bladder; Suprapubic mass from blood or urine	Pelvic fracture, e.g., 90% of bladder injuries are associated with a pelvic fracture; Vascular injuries; Spinal fractures; Liver and spleen injuries	Gross hematuria, anuria, and intraperitoneal injury; Suspected renal injury can be evaluated by IVP, angiography, and contrast CT scan; Suspected urethral injury should be evaluated by urethrogram prior to placement of an indwelling urinary catheter; Suspected bladder injury or disruption can be evaluated by cystogram, cystoscopy, and CT scanning; In renal injury due to blunt trauma the bleeding is usually confined by Gerota's fascia and the capsule. Therefore, if bleeding is limited, patients may be managed conservatively with supportive care and observation; Penetrating renal injury with uncontrolled bleeding or renal vascular injury usually requires surgical management; Transected or damaged ureters require surgical repair or external drainage; intraperitoneal bladder disruption will require surgical repair; retroperitoneal rupture needs urinary diversion with suprapubic cystostomy; Urethral injury is frequently managed conservatively; however, urinary diversion must be provided by a carefully placed indwelling urinary catheter or suprapubic cystostomy. Urologic consultation is obtained prior to any procedure
Fractured pelvis	Pain and tenderness in pelvis; Referred pain to abdomen or back; Palpable fractures, crepitus or instability; Signs of hypoperfusion or retroperitoneal bleeding	Urethral, bladder, and rectal injury; Vascular injury and retroperitoneal bleeding; Spinal fractures; Uterine and vaginal injury	Patients with significant blunt abdominal injury and the possibility of a pelvic fracture require pelvic radiographs. The pelvis is a ring structure and usually fractures in more than one place; Pelvic fractures may result in uncontrolled life-threatening retroperitoneal hemorrhage and may require aggressive fluid resuscitation and early consultation; Pelvic stabilization with PASG or external fixation may minimize pain and bleeding; Uncontrolled bleeding may require angiography and selective embolization
Diaphragmatic injury	Ventilation compromise from herniation of intra-abdominal contents; Bowel sounds in thorax; Hypovolemic shock; Stomach, bowel, or nasogastric tube in thorax on chest x-ray; Thoracic aspiration of bile, gastric contents, or feces or drainage from chest tube. 95% of lesions are on left side	Liver and spleen injury; Renal injury; Lung and thoracic injury; Stomach and bowel injury	No single diagnostic test will identify all diaphragmatic injuries; Plain chest radiographs with stomach, bowel, or nasogastric tube in the thorax, or CT scans with thoracic windows, and contrast upper gastrointestinal radiographs may help diagnose these injuries; Thoracic aspiration of bowel contents or drainage from a chest tube indicates diaphragmatic or esophageal rupture; Surgical exploration may be required to diagnose these injuries, and when identified, these injuries need surgical repair; Stabilization focuses on maintaining adequate ventilation
Abdominal wall injury	Pain or tenderness localized to traumatized area; Hematoma or localized swelling; Increased pain with stress of rectus muscles	Any intra-abdominal injury; Liver or spleen injury	Abdominal wall injury is often difficult to differentiate from underlying or concomitant intra-abdominal injury and, therefore, is regarded as a diagnosis of exclusion; Conservative management is appropriate; Significant hematomas of the abdominal wall and along the rectus sheath can complicate DPL or lead to false-positive results; CT scan can determine the presence of a significant soft tissue hematoma, which may result from direct injury or dissection from retroperitoneal bleeding
Uterine and ovarian injury	Vaginal bleeding or lacerations; Lower abdominal pain, tenderness, and guarding; Tender or enlarged uterus or ovaries on bimanual examination; Hypovolemic shock, particularly from uterine trauma when pregnant (abruptio placentae or uterine rupture)	Other intra-abdominal injury; Pelvic fractures; Pelvic vascular injuries; Bladder and urethral injury	Uterine disruption or injury may result in significant bleeding and may require hysterectomy; During pregnancy, blunt abdominal trauma may cause a placental abruption, and patients with abdominal pain or vaginal bleeding require obstetric consultation and fetal monitoring; Vaginal lacerations are identified by direct examination with a speculum. They frequently require surgical repair

DPL = diagnostic peritoneal lavage; PASG = pneumatic antishock garment.

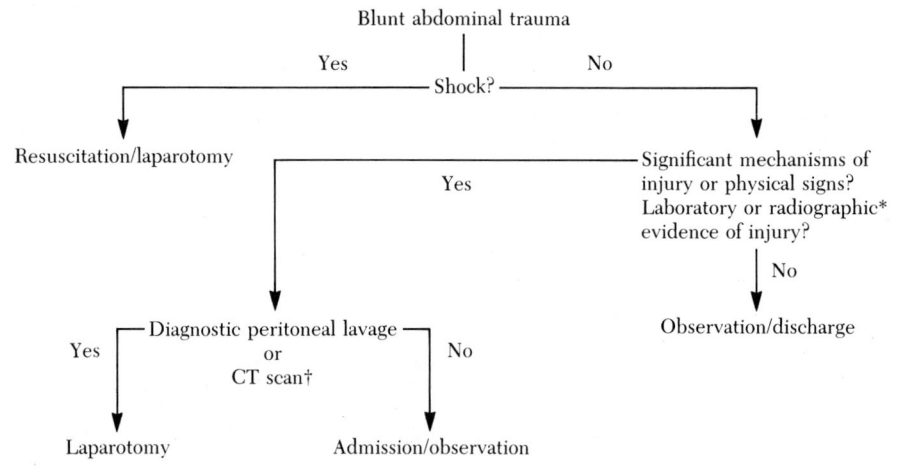

*Free air on plain radiography indicates a need for laparotomy
†Obtained only if patient's hemodynamic condition is stable

FIGURE 9–2. *Algorithm for recommended management of blunt abdominal trauma.*

surgery is usually performed. In recent years, however, patients with known liver or spleen lacerations have been managed successfully with in-hospital observation and without surgery.

Penetrating Abdominal Trauma

Almost all gunshot wounds to the abdomen require surgical exploration. This includes any wounds within the bounds of the abdomen as illustrated in Figure 9–1. Occasionally, a gunshot wound will penetrate the chest, and there will be uncertainty as to whether the abdominal cavity has been violated. After management of the chest wound, a DPL can be performed to detect any intraperitoneal injury. As noted in Table 9–3, the red blood cell count defining a positive result is lowered in such a case to 5000/ml. If the lavage shows negative results but doubt remains, a laparotomy is performed.

Stab wounds are managed according to the algorithm shown in Figure 9–3. If the patient is hemodynamically stable, local wound exploration is done. It is essential to determine whether the peritoneum has been violated. This is done by determining that the posterior fascia of the abdominal musculature has been penetrated. In some centers, a laparotomy is performed if the peritoneum has been entered. Another strategy, supported by the finding that up to 30% of penetrating stab wounds do not injure the vital organs, is to perform a DPL and then explore the abdomen based on those results. If laparotomy is not done, all patients with suspected peritoneal violation are observed for 24 hours for signs of visceral injury.

Other Measures in Management

Abdominal traumatic injuries with skin abrasions or penetrating injury are treated with tetanus prophylaxis. Patients with penetrating injuries and those requiring emergent surgery are also treated with appropriate antibiotics. Prophylactic antibiotics, e.g., clindamicin plus gentamicin, with the capability of combatting bowel organisms have been shown to reduce the morbidity of penetrating wounds. These measures are important because they may be overlooked after the patient leaves the emergency department. The actual skin wounds themselves can be closed primarily with sutures if they are clean, sharp, and not devitalized. Otherwise, they can be left to heal by secondary intention or

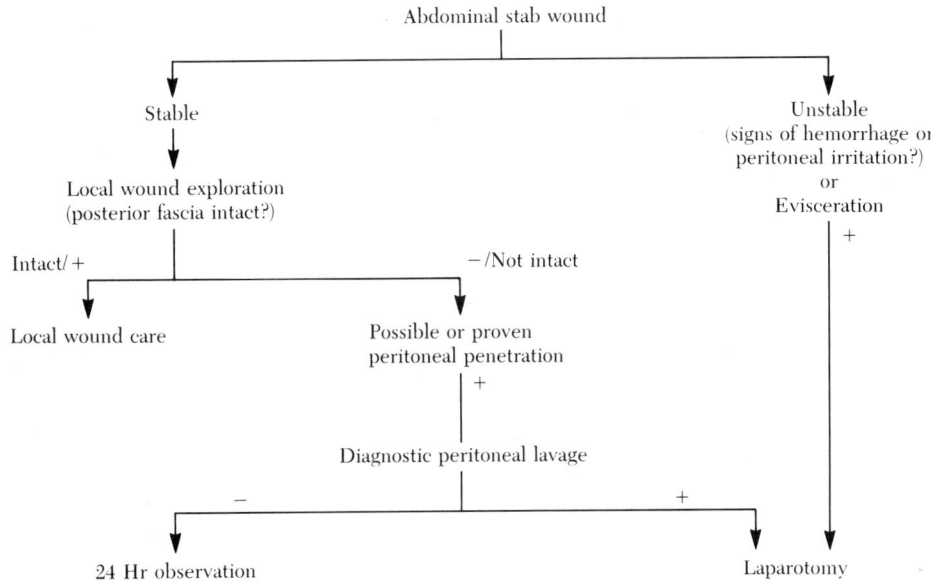

FIGURE 9–3. *Algorithm for recommended management of abdominal stab wounds.*

closed over drains. Occasionally the skin wound due to a gunshot can be completely excised and closed primarily.

Specific management recommendations for individual injuries of different organs are listed in Table 9–4.

PROBLEM After rapid induction of anesthesia, a laparotomy revealed an 8-cm laceration of the left lobe of the liver that had violated the liver capsule. Approximately 1500 ml of blood were found to be in the peritoneum. Further careful exploration of the abdomen was unremarkable except for a small tear of the mesentery of the small bowel. All bleeding was controlled. A total of 6 units of packed red cells and 6 liters of lactated Ringer's solution were necessary to restore hemodynamic stability. The patient was transferred to the postoperative recovery unit.

SPECIAL CONSIDERATIONS

Pediatric Patients

Pediatric patients with abdominal trauma provide unique challenges. Treating injured infants or children can be extremely stressful to health care providers. Intravenous access is often difficult and may require venous cutdowns or intraosseous infusion. Fluid administration is carefully followed to provide adequate volume resuscitation without causing fluid overload or electrolyte complications. The soft, less muscular abdominal wall may provide less protection, and there is a greater possibility of significant organ injury from blunt abdominal trauma. Pediatric abdominal injuries are more frequently managed by close in-hospital serial evaluations than by aggressive surgical operative management. In most pediatric patients, CT scans have replaced DPL in the evaluation of abdominal trauma. Surgical consultation is initiated early in patient management.

Pregnant Patients

Abdominal trauma in pregnancy is a difficult management problem. The emergency physician must attend to both the mother and the fetus. Generally, what is best for the mother is best for the fetus. If radiographs are needed, they are obtained with awareness of the radiation exposure involved. If the mother needs resuscitation or surgery, aggressive treatment will benefit both the fetus and the mother.

Vaginal bleeding, abdominal pain, cramping, decreased fetal movements, or changes in fetal heart rate are clues to potentially significant injury. Unlike the situation in nonpregnant patients, even relatively minor trauma may result in significant complications. The most common problem is separation of the placenta or abruptio placentae. Premature labor or spontaneous abortion also frequently occurs. Most authorities advocate ultrasonography and a period of at least 6 hours of fetal monitoring following abdominal trauma. Therefore, most pregnant patients sustaining abdominal trauma will require obstetric consultation. Penetrating trauma may cause injury to the fetus as well as the mother, but treatment of the mother takes precedence. Blunt trauma, particularly that resulting from motor vehicle accidents, is the most common cause of abdominal trauma in pregnancy. Even when the mother is seriously injured in the first trimester, uterine and fetal trauma are uncommon. Complete uterine rupture is more likely to occur in patients who are nearer term and in such situations is usually catastrophic, with sudden fetal demise and maternal hemorrhagic shock. An injury to the fetus is more likely to occur in the third trimester for obvious reasons. If the mother dies or is mortally injured, the emergency physician may be faced with the necessity of performing an emergent Caesarean section.

Geriatric Patients

As in a variety of other circumstances, the geriatric patient with abdominal trauma is more difficult to diagnose, requires more diagnostic adjuncts, and has more complications and a higher mortality. An awareness of these problems directs the emergency physician to take a very conservative approach and frequently to admit these patients for observation.

DISPOSITION AND FOLLOW-UP

Disposition plans begin on entry to the emergency department and are reformulated throughout the patient's course of care. The majority of patients with abdominal trauma require admission to the hospital at least for observation. There are some patients who, after appropriate evaluation in the emergency department accompanied by a several-hour period of observation with repeated examinations, can be safely sent home. The following are general guidelines for disposition of patients with abdominal trauma.

Admission

Patients who are admitted include:
1. All patients requiring surgery or peritoneal lavage.
2. Patients with unexplained pain, tenderness, or vomiting that does not resolve during observation.
3. All patients with gunshot wounds.
4. Abdominal trauma patients with other systemic injuries.
5. Patients with significant alcohol or drug intoxication that does not clear rapidly.
6. Patients with significant head injury and impaired mentation.

Discharge

Patients who can be safely discharged include:
1. Blunt trauma patients with pain or tenderness that resolves under observation. These patients have not shown any sign of hemodynamic instability or chemical impairment. A negative CT scan of the abdomen is part of the discharge criteria if the

mechanism and forces of injury involved usually cause a high incidence of intra-abdominal injury.

2. Patients with superficial stab wounds in whom the peritoneum has been shown to be clearly intact after local wound exploration.

DOCUMENTATION

1. Time, mechanism, and severity of trauma.
2. Vital signs and condition of patient at initial prehospital evaluation.
3. Prehospital stabilization measures and changes occurring in patient's condition en route.
4. Patient's symptoms on arrival in the emergency department; e.g., abdominal pain, shortness of breath.
5. Vital signs on arrival, including level of consciousness.
6. Results of initial physical assessment with attention paid to abdominal findings.
7. Interventions attempted and patient's response to them.
8. Findings on each repeated examination.
9. Laboratory study results and radiographic findings.
10. Results of DPL or CT scans.
11. Diagnosis, disposition, and patient's condition on leaving the emergency department.

SUMMARY AND FINAL POINTS

- In patients with abdominal trauma there is often little correlation between the physical findings and the extent of injury.
- Trauma to the abdomen is anatomically defined as any injury to the anterior thoracoabdominal area extending from the nipples to the inguinal creases and posteriorly from the tips of the scapula to the gluteal creases of the buttocks.
- Abdominal trauma is separated into blunt versus penetrating injury. Penetrating trauma (gunshot and stab wounds) is more likely to cause damage to the vascular and bowel structures than blunt trauma.
- Early death in patients with abdominal trauma occurs secondary to uncontrolled hemorrhage due to vascular or solid organ injury (liver, spleen, kidneys).
- The cornerstone of successful management of abdominal trauma patients is aggressive resuscitation for hemorrhagic shock, ventilatory support, and early surgical intervention.
- Visualizing and examining the backs and flanks of a patient with abdominal trauma are part of the complete examination.
- Hemodynamically stable patients who have sustained blunt trauma are more difficult to diagnose than patients with penetrating trauma. In general, there are four types of patients with acute abdominal trauma that require immediate surgery: (1) patients who are hemodynamically unstable and who do not respond to volume resuscitation; (2) patients with gunshot wounds; (3) patients with gross evisceration; and (4) patients with significant diaphragmatic herniation of bowel contents into the chest.
- Diagnostic peritoneal lavage is the preferred method for determining whether there is free blood in the abdomen of an adult. This procedure has been replaced by abdominal computed tomography in children.
- Violation of the peritoneum is an indication for exploration of any stab wound of the abdomen.

BIBLIOGRAPHY

Texts
1. Weiner SL, Barrett J: Trauma Management. Philadelphia, Saunders, 1986.
2. Zuidema GD, Rutherford RB, Ballinger WF: The Management of Trauma (4th ed). Philadelphia, Saunders, 1985.

Journal Articles
1. Davis JJ, Cohn I, Jr, Naver FC: Diagnosis and management of blunt abdominal trauma. Ann Surg 183:672–678, 1976.
2. Netterville RE, Hardy JD: Penetrating wounds of the abdomen. Analysis of 55 cases with problems in management. Ann Surg 166:232, 1967.
3. Feliciano DV: Abdominal vascular injuries. Surg Clin North Am 6(4):741–755, 1988.
4. Frame SB, Browder IW, Lang EK, et al: Computed tomography versus diagnostic peritoneal lavage: Usefulness in immediate diagnosis of blunt abdominal trauma. Ann Emerg Med 18(5):513–516, 1989.
5. Kurtzman RS: Radiology of blunt abdominal trauma. Surg Clin North Am 57(1):211–226, 1977.
6. Madden MR: Occult diaphragmatic injury from stab wounds to the lower chest and abdomen. J Trauma 29(3):292–298, 1989.
7. Moore EE, Marx JA: Penetrating abdominal wounds: Rationale for exploratory laparotomy. JAMA 253:2705–2708, 1985.
8. Philippart A: Blunt abdominal trauma in childhood. Surg Clin North Am 57(1):151–163, 1977.
9. Snyder HS: Blunt pelvic trauma. Am J Emerg Med 6(6):618–627, 1988.
10. Thompson JS, Moore EE, VonDuyer-Moore S: The evolution of abdominal stab wound management. J Trauma 20:478–484, 1980.

SECTION THREE

CARDIOVASCULAR DISORDERS

CHAPTER 10

ACUTE CHEST PAIN

GLENN C. HAMILTON, M.D.

PROBLEM 1 The rescue squad brought a 73 year old female to the emergency department. She complained of lower chest and epigastric discomfort persisting for 12 hours. The discomfort was described as "indigestion." She noted slight nausea and increased belching since it began.

QUESTIONS TO CONSIDER

1. What are the six potentially catastrophic illnesses to consider immediately in all patients presenting with acute chest pain?
2. What points of the history and physical examination can help differentiate serious from benign disease?
3. How can chest pain be categorized to facilitate the diagnostic approach?
4. What ancillary tests or maneuvers are available to assist in the chest pain evaluation? How useful are they?
5. How is the disposition decided between intensive care admission, intermediate care admission, and discharge?
6. What are the age-related differences important in evaluating the patient with acute chest pain?
7. What is myocardial salvage therapy and when is it recommended?

INTRODUCTION

Discomfort in the chest is derived from many separate anatomic structures. It is described not only as pain but also "pressure," "burning," "ache," or "choking." Many thoracic structures are innervated by sensory fibers from the spinal cord segments C2 to T5 and the tenth (X) cranial nerve. All may be involved in the sensation of "pain in the chest." This broad innervation accounts for the referral of pain from intrathoracic structures to the jaw, arm, shoulder, or back. Superficial pain is easier to localize than visceral pain. The origin of visceral pain correlates poorly with the place where it is perceived.

American men have a 20% chance of manifesting coronary artery disease (CAD) in their lifetime. Although its incidence is declining, CAD accounts for over 500,000 deaths per year in the United States. Cardiovascular disease has the dual hazard of being both common and potentially catastrophic. It accounts for 10% to 30% of all undifferentiated chest pain cases presenting to the emergency department. Therefore, despite other diagnostic concerns, determining the potential for the cardiovascular origin of acute chest pain is a primary goal.

Evaluating acute chest pain is a challenging pursuit for the emergency physician. It is the presenting complaint in 5% to 7% of emergency department visits. Although 97% of emergency department patients with the eventual diagnosis of myocardial infarction (MI) or unstable angina are admitted, errors due to misdiagnosis of cardiovascular disease are the second most common source of medicolegal problems in emergency medicine. Defining the cause of acute chest pain is difficult because:

- The patient's ability to describe the symptoms can greatly influence the outcome of the evaluation.
- The severity of the pain correlates poorly with its life-threatening potential.
- There is little correlation between the location of the pain and its source.
- More than one disease process may cause the pain.
- Because of the broad innervation, a number of different pathologic processes in a variety of organs may present in a similar manner.
- The situation is dynamic. *At any time in the evaluative process, the patient may require rapid therapeutic intervention for shock, increased pain, dysrhythmia, or cardiac arrest.*

In many cases an extensive inpatient evaluation is the only means of making a correct diagnosis. Yet in caring for a patient with chest pain, the emergency physician must differentiate rapidly between potentially catastrophic disease and benign illness, determine the probability of ischemic heart disease, anticipate management, and proceed to disposition. The data-gathering and observation skills necessary to diagnose chest pain correctly are developed by serial exposure and close follow-up of these patients.

PREHOSPITAL CARE

PROBLEM 1 The 73 year old female was at home when the lower chest discomfort and nausea began 12 hours earlier. The rescue squad was called by her family, and they have contacted the emergency department by radio.

The information from the rescue squad should be given and acknowledged quickly and professionally. Only the most pertinent data are necessary.

History
1. What is the location, severity, character, and duration of the pain?
2. Are there associated symptoms, e.g., diaphoresis, shortness of breath?
3. What is the medical history? Is there a known history of coronary artery disease, hypertension, or diabetes mellitus?

Physical examination
1. What is the patient's color? Degree of discomfort?
2. What are the patient's vital signs, including level of consciousness?
3. Any prominent, pertinent physical findings are described.

Interventions
1. By patient? Result?
2. By the rescue squad? Result?
3. What is the transport time?

From this information, one can often gauge "how ill" the patient seems. Radio orders are given as necessary, and the nursing staff is notified of the patient's status and arrival time.

Each rescue squad has a different level of ability depending on their training and medical control. Familiarity with the capability of the unit is essential for the emergency physician. Field stabilization for the patient with chest pain includes:

Cardiac Monitor. The rhythm is observed initially and in transit. Verbally describing it is usually sufficient. Sending the rhythm strip by radio telemetry is seldom necessary unless the patient has a complex rhythm or decisions about lidocaine prophylaxis must be made. Lidocaine is considered if there are multiple premature ventricular contractions (PVCs), multifocal PVCs, or ventricular tachycardia.

Oxygen. Oxygen is given at 2 to 4 liters/minute by nasal cannula, since masks are poorly tolerated. Lower flows (1 to 2 liters/minute) are recommended if severe obstructive pulmonary disease is present because of the potential for carbon dioxide retention.

Intravenous (IV) Line. A heparin lock is established if the patient's vital signs are stable. An alternative is IV access maintained with 5% dextrose in water at a keep-open rate. An isotonic crystalloid may be the fluid of choice if significant hypotension is present. Intravenous line placement is essential unless serial attempts result in significant time delay.

Analgesia. Pain is often relieved with oxygen and reassurance. Sublingual nitroglycerin (NTG, tablet or aerosol, 0.3 or 0.4 mg q 5 minutes × 3) may give relief if ischemic heart disease (IHD) is seriously considered. Optimally, before NTG administration, an IV line is established and the blood pressure (BP) is measured. Caution is exercised and problems anticipated if the systolic BP is less than 110 mm Hg. Repeat BP readings are taken 2 to 3 minutes after the NTG dose. Nalbuphine (Nubain), morphine sulfate, or a nitrous oxide–oxygen (Nitronox) mixture may be available in certain areas.

Patient Comfort. The rescue squad should explain the situation and reassure the patient and family before transport. Depending on state laws, lights with no siren is the preferred mode to transport alert patients with chest pain.

PROBLEM 1 The rescue squad reported that the patient's pain was in the lower chest. It was described as a "burning indigestion," moderate in intensity, and lasting about 12 hours. The patient complained of nausea, belching, and increasing pain during the past 4 hours. Vital signs were BP 180/90 mm Hg, pulse 100 beats/min, respirations 18/min. Patient was approximately 5 feet tall and weighed 200 pounds. She was sweating slightly and was slightly pale. She seemed in distress but was tolerating the pain. The patient had taken Alka-Seltzer without experiencing relief. The squad had placed oxygen via a nasal cannula at 2 liters/min and had started an IV line with D/W 5% at a keep-open rate. A monitored rhythm showed sinus tachycardia. Transport time was 15 minutes. The patient has known hypertension, treated with a daily "water pill."

Although nothing "catastrophic" is apparent, the patient's age, weight, pain pattern, associated symptoms, and slightly increased blood pressure and pulse should raise suspicions about serious illness. Because the history is atypical for ischemic heart disease, administration of nitroglycerin is not indicated in the field. Lidocaine prophylaxis is not necessary either. Ambulance transport and observation with cardiac monitoring are appropriate. At the close of radio contact it is useful to request the rescue squad to bring in the patient's medication. The rescue personnel are expected to allay the initial fears of the patient and family about coming to the hospital.

INITIAL APPROACH IN THE EMERGENCY DEPARTMENT

With few exceptions, such as superficial chest wall pain due to injury, *all* patients with chest pain are brought immediately into the acute care area of the emergency department and are seen by a physician. The physician must anticipate the need to manage the airway, correct dysrhythmias, stabilize hypotension, and provide pain relief at any time. The following activities are part of the initial assessment and stabilization:

1. History. Confirmation of the rescue squad history is obtained.
2. Physical examination
    a. Repeat vital signs are taken and compared with values from the prehospital setting.
    b. The patient is undressed. A rapid physical assessment is done. Attention is directed to the level of consciousness, pain tolerance, skin color, and auscultation of heart and lungs. Any cardiac murmurs or pulmonary rales are noted. The latter finding may suggest left ventricular insufficiency and a cardiac inability to tolerate aggressive volume repletion.

3. Intervention
   a. Cardiac monitoring is reestablished and a rhythm strip recorded. Supplemental oxygen is given, and an IV line is placed or the established access is checked.
   b. Requesting a 12-lead ECG is often appropriate at this point. With the advent of myocardial salvage therapies, the appearance of "classic" MI changes on the ECG can significantly expand the management plan in the emergency department.

The clinical appearance of the patient may require treatment to supersede or proceed concomitantly with the preliminary assessment. The "sixth sense" of the experienced emergency nurse and physician is very helpful in assessing the severity of illness of each patient.

PROBLEM 1 The patient was brought into the acute care area, and the physician was asked to see her. Her family was referred to registration. All points of the assessment and stabilization routine were accomplished and her status remained unchanged. Repeat vital signs were BP 200/100 mm Hg, pulse 100 beats/min, respirations 18/min, temperature afebrile. Her color was slightly pale. The monitor showed a sinus tachycardia with an occasional premature ventricular beat.

Even when busy, it is useful to observe quickly the arrival of a chest pain patient. This is the best opportunity to meet the patient and further question the rescue personnel, who otherwise may leave quickly. One must shift from the "audio" impression given by prior radio contact to the "video" reality of the patient's presence. It is surprising how many patients change abruptly, seldom for the better, upon arrival at the hospital. In this patient there was little change from the vital signs taken in the field. Further intervention, e.g., nitroglycerin, could wait until more data were gathered.

DATA GATHERING

History

A careful history is the most important factor in the assessment of the patient with acute chest pain. It is of particular value in identifying patients who are at high risk for potentially catastrophic illness.

The physician must appreciate the psychologic impact the pain, emergency setting, and interview have on the patient. When confronted by a complex or confusing history, early reassurance and a chronologic sequencing of the event will provide a structure for the patient's recollection. The physician should derive an organized framework of the evolving illness. The history is guided but not led. Key historical points include the following:

Characteristics of the Pain

Character or Quality of Pain. The patient is asked to describe the "discomfort" rather than the "pain." The words "heaviness," "pressure," or "crushing" may describe the sensation. "Burning" pain is problematic because it has the same frequency of association with myocardial infarction as with upper gastrointestinal disorders. The symptoms are first assumed to be cardiac in origin. Other descriptive terms less typical of cardiac pain are "stabbing," "shooting," and "aching." These words are often used to describe the severity of pain rather than the character. Make sure the meaning of each word is mutually understood.

Onset. Circumstance and pattern of onset are important. Were there any episodes of discomfort prior to this episode? Was it related to exercise, stress, or after a meal?

Site and Radiation. The patient is asked whether the pain is centrally or laterally located in the thorax. Whether it "goes anywhere else" is important to ascertain. Wait before prompting with a list of possible referral sites.

Severity. Severity may be measured against the "worst pain" the patient has previously experienced. A 1 to 10 pain severity scale may help the patient be more precise.

Duration and Pattern of Pain. The total time of the episode, the length of individual episodes of discomfort, and the varying degree of symptoms are details of importance. Has there been a recent change in any?

Factors that Relieve or Worsen the Pain. The influence of time of day, meals, exercise, cold exposure, reaching or stretching, deep inspiration, and cough on increasing or decreasing the pain can help to differentiate superficial from visceral pain and ischemic cardiac pain from pain of other origins. Response to therapy can give useful information about the source of pain, the patient's perception of pain, and the patient's medical sophistication.

Previous History of Pain. How does this pain compare to previous episodes or a prior documented myocardial infarction or angina?

Associated Symptoms. Other symptoms may suggest a visceral origin for the pain.

1. *Diaphoresis.* "Sweating" is an important symptom that is often associated with serious pathology. It must be separated from the sensation of being "warm" or "flushed."

2. *Dyspnea.* "Shortness of breath" is the subjective sensation of working harder to breathe associated with decreased lung compliance. It is differentiated from hyperventilation and anxiety.

3. *Dizziness* or *syncope.* Dizziness is the term used for symptoms ranging from "lightheadedness" to true vertigo. Syncope, a true loss of consciousness with or without chest pain, requires patient admission for evaluation.

4. *Nausea, vomiting, belching.* All these symptoms can be nonspecific responses to deep pain. Belching is further explored in context of the pain episode and response to therapy.

Risk Factors

Identifying risk factors has not been found to increase the diagnostic accuracy of chest pain assessment. They do influence the physician's judgment of the probability of ischemic heart disease (IHD). Factors that correlate well with IHD are:

1. Age. The incidence of coronary artery disease in the general population increases with each decade, e.g., 30 to 39 years (8%), 40 to 49 years (24%), 50 to 59 years (44%), 60 to 69 years (56%)

2. Male sex. Risk is increased in men, particularly in the younger age groups

3. Hypertension. Hypertension is also a risk factor for dissecting aneurysm

4. Diabetes mellitus

5. Cigarette smoking. Only 2 pack-years or more are required to be a risk factor

6. Known history of arteriosclerotic vascular disease

Other factors less well correlated with IHD but supportive of suspicion:

1. Sedentary versus active lifestyle
2. Stress level
3. Obesity
4. Type A personality
5. Gout
6. Family history of high-risk factors including IHD. Although difficult to correlate, there are patterns not to be ignored, e.g., sudden death in the patient's immediate family at a young age.

Past Medical History

1. Surgical history. The physician should ask about chest or neck trauma and the details of any surgery.

2. Medications. Information about medications—what, why, how faithfully taken, and perceived side effects—offers insight into the patient's understanding of illness and compliance with treatment.

3. Allergies, especially to medications, are always important to determine.

Two actions are automatic to maximize efficiency early during care. First, the patient's old chart is ordered. The chart can clarify a confusing history, supply a comparison ECG, list a complex and poorly recalled medical regimen, and reveal a supporting or an unconsidered prior diagnosis, e.g., drug-seeking behavior. Second, supplemental corroborating information is sought by talking with family, friends, and the patient's private physician. These data also help to assess the patient's living circumstances and support systems.

PROBLEM 1 *Note to the reader: From this point on the case is written to demonstrate errors leading to an unfortunate outcome. Evaluating patients with chest pain has a number of pitfalls. Many are included here.*

The physician's history from the patient was not amplified in the chart. There was a brief nursing note repeating the history given by the paramedic. The physician wrote, "History as above" and went on to the physical examination. Information available from the daughter in the waiting room was not obtained.

This is pseudoefficiency. Time demands of emergency medicine may compromise one's assessment, but the basic principles of care, such as "A detailed history is the most important diagnostic tool in chest pain assessment" and "If it isn't recorded on the chart, it wasn't done," cannot be ignored. This may not be the situation literally, but in this case the history the physician actually obtained is lost forever. Shortcuts of this type tend to reflect shortcuts in the interview. Additional history the physician may have learned was instead of 12 hours' lower chest and epigastric pain only, during the last 4 hours the patient's pain had changed from epigastric to substernal in location and was more a "fullness" and "burning" sensation than pain. There was no radiation of pain. She came to the hospital after trying Alka-Seltzer but experiencing no relief. She noted a little "sweatiness" earlier in the day and was mildly nauseated at the time. A lesser sensation of pressure was noted on two occasions during the last 2 days, each lasting 10 to 15 minutes before disappearing. The patient denied any previous pain history. She gave a family history of hypertension and stated that two brothers and one uncle had died of "heart attacks." The daughter in the waiting room would have added that her mother was rather stoic and distrustful of doctors and that 2 days earlier she had called her and complained of "pressure between her breasts" when going out into the cold air.

Physical Examination

The physical examination may complement the history but is not often a deciding factor in the diagnosis of acute chest pain. It can supply important information when guided by a few principles:

1. The history directs the emphasis of the examination.
2. The vital signs and general appearance are the most important determinants in separating deep visceral from superficial pain.
3. The examination should seek evidence supporting the presence of atherosclerotic vascular disease.
4. Evidence of myocardial ischemia is most often found when the pain is present.
5. Specific evidence of catastrophic illness is sought first, e.g., unequal pulses (aortic dissection) or hyperresonance on chest percussion (pneumothorax); then the examiner moves on to more subtle findings or less serious diagnoses.

The important components of the physical examination are listed in Table 10–1.

TABLE 10–1. Important Components of the Physical Examination in Acute Chest Pain

Area of Examination	Important Components	Comments
Vital signs	Heart rate/pulse	Tachycardia (>95 beats/min) is common. Vagal response to visceral pain may result in bradycardia (<60 beats/min). Assess symmetry and quality of pulses
	Blood pressure	Often elevated owing to increased sympathetic tone. Hypotension is always a serious sign
	Respiratory rate	Tachypnea is one of the earliest signs of shock. A common response to pain
	Fever	Suggests infectious or inflammatory process
General appearance	Position, movement, color, diaphoresis	Rough gauge of "distress," though interpretation is complicated by patient pain tolerance or denial
Eyes	External—xanthelasma Iris—arcus senilis Fundus—arteriovenous nicking and thickening of capillary wall (i.e., "copper wiring")	All indications of atherosclerotic status
Neck	Inspection, palpation, auscultation	Check position of trachea and jugular venous distention. Palpate the carotid pulse for rate and quality. Crepitant subcutaneous emphysema may be noted. Auscultate for bruits and for referred aortic stenosis murmur
Chest wall	Palpation	Superficial, reproducible and localized pain is one of the few findings helpful in ruling out visceral disease. Still, 5% of documented MI patients have this finding. Subcutaneous emphysema may be noted
Lungs	Percussion	Particularly useful in pulmonary effusion and pneumothorax
	Auscultation	Listen for signs of consolidation, rales, wheezes
Cardiac	Palpation	Feel for size and lateral shift of apex, also rocking motion due to akinetic myocardium
	Auscultation	Examination while pain is present yields a higher return. Listen for S_3 and S_4 heart sounds and mitral insufficiency murmur due to papillary muscle dysfunction. Pericardial rubs heard best with the patient sitting up and leaning forward
Abdomen	Inspection, auscultation, percussion, palpation	Rectal and pelvic examinations are not deferred if history suggests origin of pain related to these areas
Extremities	Upper extremity	Ask patient to reach or stretch and observe pain response to motion
	Lower extremity	Note edema, signs of circulatory insufficiency, or thrombophlebitis
Neurologic	Altered sensation, motor function	Assess the cervical spine and dermatomes that radiate to the chest (C_2 to T_5)

Bedside Tests

A few bedside tests may aid in differentiating the site of chest pain. None is diagnostic, but each can assist in directing attention toward an organ system.

1. Pulmonary system. Intentional hyperventilation for 1 to 3 minutes may reproduce psychogenic central pain or consistently aggravate pleuritic pain.

2. Gastrointestinal system. A "GI cocktail" composed of 10 to 15 ml 1% viscous Xylocaine and 15 to 30 ml of antacid may relieve esophageal pain in 2 to 3 minutes. A positive result on this test increases the probability that the esophagus is the cause of the pain. The test is not standardized and does not "rule out" ischemic heart disease. Taken too quickly, the mixture may induce vomiting.

3. Cardiac system. When the history is suggestive but not convincing for angina pectoris, a trial of NTG resulting in the complete relief of pain in less than 3 minutes

increases the probability of ischemic heart disease. This test is not diagnostic of any disease. It produces false-positive results in 20% of patients, presumably owing to placebo effect or esophageal relaxation.

PROBLEM 1 The patient looked her stated age of 73 years. She was obese and in mild distress from the discomfort. Vital signs were BP 170/100 mm Hg, pulse 90 beats/min, respirations 18/min, temperature afebrile. The results of the physical examination were recorded as follows:

    Thorax—WNL, some xiphoid tenderness
    Lungs—Clear
    Heart—Distant heart tones (pendulous breasts), no murmur
    Abdomen—Mild epigastric discomfort and tenderness
    Extremities—Pulses symmetric, no edema, no cyanosis

This record provides adequate information, although data on the head, cervical spine status, eye, and patient's response to bedside tests or maneuvers were not recorded. The xiphoid area almost always has some tenderness. From the chart it is difficult to tell the patient's pain tolerance.

DECISION PRIORITIES AND PRELIMINARY DIFFERENTIAL DIAGNOSIS

Simultaneously with the initial stabilization of the patient and data gathering, the physician develops decision priorities and forms a preliminary differential diagnosis by answering these four questions:

1. *Which pattern (location/character) does the patient's complaint best fit: central, lateral pleuritic, lateral nonpleuritic?*

   Categorizing the patient complaint in this way quickly divides the diagnostic pursuit into high probability (central) and lower probability (lateral) locations for acute visceral pathology. This scheme is not without potential sources of error, e.g., both pneumothorax and pulmonary embolism may present as lateral or lateral pleuritic pain. It is useful as a *beginning* and can be modified as experience with the patient and in the practice of emergency medicine grows.

2. *If the pattern is central, is there a potentially catastrophic disease requiring immediate intervention?*

   Unless the pain is obviously superficial and totally reproducible by palpation, the historical features of the pain or discomfort and the physical examination must be compared with the typical and atypical presentations of six immediately life-threatening diseases (Table 10–2): *myocardial infarction, unstable angina, aortic dissection, pulmonary embolism, tension pneumothorax, and esophageal rupture.* Any patient presenting in *shock* with central chest pain has one of these six emergent problems until proved otherwise.

   After these six diseases are considered, the physician decides on either immediate intervention or further evaluation. The first goal remains establishing the presence of an immediately life-threatening disease. If it is not present, the second goal is to evaluate the potential for other serious conditions that may require intervention. Uppermost in the differential diagnosis is the potential for occult ischemic heart disease (IHD).

3. *If catastrophic disease is not present, is there a continued risk of ischemic heart disease?*

   Ischemic heart disease is common, often subtle, dynamic, possibly lethal, and generally treatable. To determine its presence, the physician reviews the history. The Chest Pain Decision Rule adds a weighted value to the elements of the history (Table 10–3).

   The rule was developed from an office setting but can apply to patients seen

TABLE 10–2. Causes and Differentiation of Potentially Catastrophic Illness Presenting with Central Chest Pain or Discomfort

	Pain History	Associated Symptoms	Supporting History	Prevalence in Emergency Department	Physical Examination	Useful Tests	Atypical or Additional Aspects
1. Ischemic heart disease							
a. Myocardial infarction	Discomfort is usually moderately severe to severe and rapid in onset. May be more "pressure" than pain. Usually retrosternal, may radiate to neck, jaw, both arms and sides of chest (left more than right). Lasts more than 15–30 min and is unrelieved by NTG	Diaphoresis, nausea, vomiting, dyspnea	May be precipitated by emotional stress or exertion. Prodromal pain pattern often elicited. Previous history of MI or angina. Over 40 years old, positive risk factors, and male sex increase possibility	Common	Patients are anxious, restless, uncomfortable, and may be confused. Blood pressure is usually elevated but normo- and hypotension can be seen. The heart rate is usually increased, but bradycardia can be seen. Patients may be diaphoretic, and show peripheral poor perfusion. There are no diagnostic examination findings for MI, although S_3 and S_4 heart sounds and mitral regurgitant murmur are supportive	ECG changes (new Q waves or ST segment–T-wave changes) occur in 80% of patients. At present, there is limited use of cardiac enzymes (CPK-MB) in selected populations (e.g., elderly, patients presenting late in course)	Pain may present as "indigestion," "burning," or "unable to describe." Other atypical presentations include altered mental status, cerebrovascular accident, angina pattern without extended pain, severe fatigue. Elderly may present with weakness, congestive heart failure, or chest tightness. Twenty-five percent of nonfatal MIs are unrecognized by patient. The pain may have resolved by the time of evaluation
b. Unstable angina	Changes in pattern of preexisting angina with more severe, prolonged, or frequent pain. Angina at rest or new-onset angina (duration less than 1 month) with minimal exertion. Unpredictable response to NTG and rest	Often minimal. May have mild diaphoresis, nausea, dyspnea with pain	Not clearly related to precipitating factors. May be a decrease in amount of physical activity that initiates pain. Previous history of MI or angina. Over 40 years old, presence of risk factors, and male sex increase probability	Common	Nonspecific findings of a transient nature, e.g., S_3, S_4, or mitral regurgitant murmur	Often no ECG or enzyme changes	May be pain free at presentation. Full history is essential. Fewer than 15% of patients hospitalized for unstable angina go on to acute MI

Table continued on following page

TABLE 10–2. Causes and Differentiation of Potentially Catastrophic Illness Presenting with Central Chest Pain or Discomfort
Continued

	Pain History	Associated Symptoms	Supporting History	Prevalence in Emergency Department	Physical Examination	Useful Tests	Atypical or Additional Aspects
2. Aortic dissection	Ninety percent of patients have rapid-onset severe chest pain that is maximal at beginning. Radiates anteriorly or to the back interscapular area. Pain often migrates with a "tearing" sensation	Neurologic complications of stroke, peripheral neuropathy, paresis or paraplegia. Extremity ischemia possible	History of hypertension in 70–90% of patients. 3:1 ratio males to females; Marfan's syndrome and congenital bicuspid aortic valves have increased incidence	Rare	Often poorly perfused peripherally but with elevated BP. In 50–60% of cases there is asymmetric decrease or absence of peripheral pulses. Fifty percent of proximal dissections cause aortic insufficiency. Occasional vascular occlusions: coronary (1–2%), mesentery, renal, spinal cord. New-onset pericardial friction rub or aortic insufficiency murmur supportive of diagnosis	ECG usually shows left ventricular hypertrophy, nonspecific changes. Chest film shows abnormal aortic silhouette (90%). Aortic angiography has diagnostic accuracy of 95–99%. Ultrasound, CT, MRI most useful in screening more stable cases	It is rare for patient to present pain free. May present with neurologic complications. Physical examination findings may be minimal. May present with congestive heart failure secondary to insufficiency or MI from coronary insufficiency
3. Pulmonary embolism	Pain is more often lateral-pleuritic. Central pain is more consistent with massive embolus. Abrupt in onset and maximal at beginning	Dyspnea and apprehension play a prominent role. Cough accompanies about half the cases. Hemoptysis occurs in less than 20%	Usually some period of immobilization has occurred, e.g., postoperative. Pregnancy, oral contraceptives, heart disease thrombophlebitis, previous embolus are all risk factors	Rare in ambulatory patients	Patients are anxious and have a respiratory rate over 16/min. Tachycardia, inspiratory rales, and an increased pulmonic second sound are common. Fever, phlebitis, and diaphoresis are seen in 30–40% of patients. Wheezes and peripheral cyanosis less common	Arterial blood gases show $P_{O_2} < 80$ mm Hg in 90%. Widened A–a gradient is a useful screen. Chest film is usually normal, though up to 40% show some volume loss, oligemia, or signs of consolidation due to pulmonary infarction. Lung perfusion scan rules out this diagnosis if negative	Patients may present with dyspnea with or without bronchospasm. Severe abdominal pain can be the primary complaint

4. Pneumothorax	Pain is usually acute and maximal at onset. It is more often lateral-pleuritic, but central pain does occur	Dyspnea has a prominent role. Hypotension and altered mental states occur in tension pneumothorax	Chest trauma, previous episode, or asthenic body type	Infrequent	Decreased breath sounds, increased tympany on percussion. Elevated pressure in neck veins and tracheal deviation occur in tension pneumothorax	Chest film definitive. Inspiratory and expiratory films may enhance contrast between air and lung parenchyma. Tension pneumothorax should be diagnosed on physical examination	May be subtle in COPD, asthma, cystic fibrosis. Can be complicated by pneumomediastinum
5. Esophageal rupture	Pain is usually preceded by vomiting and is abrupt in onset. Pain is persistent and unrelieved, localized along the esophagus, and increased by swallowing and neck flexion	Diaphoresis, dyspnea (late), shock	Older individual with known gastrointestinal problems. History of violent emesis, foreign body, caustic ingestion, or blunt trauma	Rare	Signs of lung consolidation, subcutaneous emphysema may be present	Chest film usually has mediastinal air, a left-sided pleural effusion, pneumothorax, or a widened mediastinum. pH of pleural effusion is < 6.0. Diagnosis supported by water-soluble contrast esophagram or esophagoscopy	Patient may present in shock state. This entity often considered late in differential diagnostic process

NTG = nitroglycerin; CT = computed tomography; MRI = magnetic resonance imaging; COPD = chronic obstructive pulmonary disease.

TABLE 10–3. Chest Pain Decision Rule

Weight	Pain Characteristics
+3	Substernal location
+3	Pain radiates to left arm
+2	Pain described as "pressure"
+3	Pain elicited by exertion
+2	Patient must stop all activities when pain occurs
+7	Pain relieved promptly by nitroglycerin
+6	History of MI
−2	Pain is "sharp"
−3	Pain is "pleuritic"
−3	Pain is positional (by moving arms or torso)

Note: To calculate score, add weighting for each characteristic. According to Sox et al., if score is ≤ 1, pain is nonischemic. If score is > 1, pain is considered ischemic. In outpatients in their study, sensitivity was 100% and specificity was 65% for ischemic versus nonischemic pain.

Adapted from Sox HC, Margulies I, Sox CH: Psychologically mediated effects of diagnostic tests. Ann Intern Med 95(6):681, 1981. With permission.

in the emergency department. Before testing, the patient over 40 years old with acute chest pain has a 15% to 30% chance of having an acute MI. If a patient meets the historical criteria for ischemia, further testing may help in stratifying him or her into high- versus low-probability groups. If the criteria are not met, and the patient has sharp or stabbing pleuritic pain that is positional or is reproduced on palpation, there is an almost 0% chance that the pain is due to myocardial ischemia. A 35% probability of a false-positive diagnosis remains.

4. *If the risk of ischemic heart disease is low, what other possibilities for the symptoms are logical?*

If the discomfort is central but does not appear to be catastrophic or ischemic in nature, the organ system approach outlined in the section on Refined Differential Diagnosis is followed. The possibility of serious illness is continually reviewed in the patient with acute central chest pain or discomfort.

If the pain is of the lateral pleuritic pattern, it usually originates from the pleura or the chest wall. The most important concerns at this time are whether pulmonary embolism or pneumothorax is present and whether the patient data are correlated with the information given in Table 10–2. If the risk of embolism is high, e.g., in pregnant patients or those with recent surgery or distal thrombophlebitis, or if the physical examination raises suspicion, the work-up proceeds with arterial blood gas analysis, chest radiography, and a ventilation-perfusion lung scan. Pneumothorax is considered next. It is confirmed by radiograph unless circumstances warrant immediate intervention. Other diagnoses such as infection, rib fracture, muscle injury, or muscle spasm are considered after embolism and pneumothorax are ruled out.

Lateral nonpleuritic pain as an isolated symptom is usually not life-threatening. It commonly represents pain of musculoskeletal, neurologic, or psychogenic origin. Its evaluation becomes part of the organ system approach described in the section on Refined Differential Diagnosis.

PROBLEM 1 The patient's condition was preliminarily categorized as central chest pain of nonischemic origin. An ECG and chest radiograph were ordered.

The major reason for not emphasizing cardiac ischemia as the cause of the patient's symptoms was an inadequate history, at least as recorded on the chart. In patients with acute chest pain, a cardiac etiology is the first diagnosis to rule out. A serious error in emergency medicine is forming an early diagnosis and not reconsidering it throughout the examination. An early diagnosis can give the physician a false sense of security and limit the search for more information.

DIAGNOSTIC ADJUNCTS

Electrocardiogram

A 12-lead ECG is performed on most adult patients presenting with acute chest pain. Patients with lateral pleuritic or lateral nonpleuritic pain often do not need an ECG. The test remains popular among physicians and patients, although it seldom changes the outcome of care. If the results are positive, the probability of ischemia in patients with equivocal histories is increased, and the test allows more precise diagnosis of monitored dysrhythmias. The ECG changes in three types of IHD are listed in Table 10–4. About 60% of patients with an acute MI will have new ST-segment changes on ECG.

The ECG is best for "ruling in" myocardial infarction. A single emergency department ECG in a patient with "classic" changes of MI shows false-positive results in only 2.3% of patients. Therefore, classic changes are highly specific, and finding them nearly establishes the diagnosis, even in a patient with a weak history for MI. Myocardial salvage therapy is considered when these changes are found. Classic changes of MI on ECG are rare in cases of nonischemic chest pain.

Problems occur when a single ECG tracing is used to rule out MI. Twenty percent of ECGs in patients diagnosed as having myocardial infarctions are read as normal in the emergency department. The ECG is often "over-read," looking for subtle changes that may or may not represent ischemic heart disease. Comparison with previous ECGs may improve the yield of positive results and increases the physician's propensity to admit the patient. The absence of classic ECG findings alone does not significantly alter the probability of myocardial infarction if the history is highly suggestive. For example, in a patient with a history that is 90% probable for myocardial infarction, the probability would be increased to 99.5% if the ECG showed the classic changes of MI, but if the ECG did not show such changes, the probability of infarction would decrease only to 80%. Negative ECG results in patients with histories showing a low probability for MI may lower the chances but do not remove myocardial infarction as a possible cause.

Radiologic Imaging

The results of the history and physical examination direct the radiographic assessment. Posteroanterior (PA) and lateral chest radiographs are most useful for diagnosing cardiac- and pulmonary-related pain and for assessing congestive heart failure. Patients with undiagnosed central chest pain are not sent to the radiology department. An anteroposterior (AP) upright portable film is an adequate screening view for serious pathology. Inspiratory-expiratory films may be beneficial in patients with suspected pneumothorax. Tables 10–2 and 10–5 list the findings characteristic of specific problems. In patients with IHD, most of the radiographic findings are interpreted as normal.

Cervical or thoracic spine films may be taken if nerve compression is suspected. Abdominal films usually yield few results but may be considered if abdominal pathology is suspected. Most organs in the upper abdominal quadrants can produce pain that is referred to the chest. Gallbladder disease and peptic ulcer disease are particularly common sources of such pain.

TABLE 10–4. ECG Findings in Ischemic Chest Pain

Classic MI	Q waves ≥ 0.04 sec duration. ST-segment depression (greater than 1 mm) or ST-segment elevation (greater than 1 mm) is seen, depending on the degree and location of ischemia
Subendocardial infarction	Persistent T-wave inversion and ST-segment depression occur in several limb or precordial leads
Unstable anginal pain	Most often has no ECG changes. Elevation or depression ST segments may be seen. Symmetric inversion of T waves

Note: Conduction abnormalities and blocks also may be seen in infarct and ischemia.

Other imaging or contrast techniques have not played a major role in emergency department diagnosis. Two exceptions are the use of computer tomography in patients with suspected dissecting aneurysm and technetium-99m lung scans in patients with suspected pulmonary embolism. Technetium-99m pyrophosphate myocardial scanning is both sensitive and specific for myocardial damage but is not clinically useful for 24 to 36 hours after the onset of pain. Emergency coronary arteriography is becoming more readily available as myocardial salvage techniques become more established.

Laboratory Studies

Creatine Kinase (CK). The combination of the history, ECG findings, and serial cardiac enzyme determinations, particularly creatine kinase with or without fractionation, is the basis for the diagnosis of myocardial infarction. Therefore, CK measurements would logically serve as a useful tool in evaluating acute chest pain. Unfractionated CK levels have not proved useful because CK comes from a variety of sources. In contrast, 98% of the MB isoenzyme of fractionated CK arises from within myocardial muscle. Though studies continue, CK-MB levels have demonstrated variable diagnostic capability in identifying myocardial ischemia as the source of acute chest pain. At present, CK-MB levels may be drawn in patients at high risk, e.g., elderly or diabetic patients, who have equivocal histories and ECG results. The duration of pain should be greater than 3 hours. The measurements have a potential but undefined role in emergency observation units, where a second level may be determined after 12 to 24 hours.

Other Cardiac Enzymes. Lactate dehydrogenase (LDH) with or without isoenzymes and aspartate aminotransferase (AST) may be diagnostic in the patient arriving 24 hours after a chest pain episode.

Serum Myoglobin. Serum myoglobin levels may rise 60 minutes after cardiac ischemia begins, reaching peak levels 4 to 6 hours later. At 3 hours, the test result shows a high correlation with MI. More studies of the value of this test in the emergency department are necessary. It is not routinely available.

Other Studies. In preparing for hospital admission, these laboratory studies are commonly ordered: complete blood count (CBC), arterial blood gases (ABG), electrolytes, blood urea nitrogen (BUN), creatinine, and hemostasis studies. Most are baseline assessments rather than specific assessments for chest pain.

PROBLEM 1 An ECG was performed and interpreted as having only nonspecific ST–T-wave changes in the chest leads. An old ECG was available to the physician, but it was "in another building." Therefore no comparison of new and old ECGs was done. No other laboratory tests were performed.

Comparison of old and new ECG results does not greatly improve the predictive capability of the test for ischemic heart disease. Interestingly, "new" ECG changes based on comparison of ECG test results lead to increased frequency of admission to the hospital. The impact of ECG comparison on critical care versus monitored bed selection is unknown.

This patient's ECG results showed subtle changes of an ischemic nature compared to the ECG taken 1 year earlier. Although not definitive, the opportunity for a raised level of suspicion was missed by not pushing for more responsiveness from the hospital record retrieval system.

REFINED DIFFERENTIAL DIAGNOSIS

Once the clinical examination, laboratory test results, response to therapy, and observation data are available, the physician can reassess the preliminary differential diagnosis based on the presence of central or lateral pain. One must confirm or resolve any persistent concerns about the presence of the six catastrophic diseases or the potential for ischemic heart disease.

Beyond this point, the physician may approach the problem by matching the patient data with patterns typical of organ systems and with common diseases within those systems (Table 10–5). In order of frequency, central pain may arise from chest wall structures, psychogenic factors, esophagus, nonischemic myocardium, pericardium, or lung. Lateral pain usually originates in the chest wall, psychogenic factors, or lung.

It is serial experience and follow-up of patients that allow the trained emergency physician to weigh the multiple bits of data and, despite a vague atypical history or lack of supporting data, reach a correct disposition, if not diagnosis. There is no reason to order multiple laboratory tests and produce a "shotgun" diagnosis. The level of uncertainty is not reduced in most cases.

PROBLEM 1 With the history, physical examination, and laboratory test results assembled by the physician, the most likely origin of the pain was thought to be gastrointestinal. The highest probability in this category was esophagitis. Although the patient did not improve with one dose of antacid in the emergency department, she was readied for discharge.

No additional history or repeat physical examination was recorded. It must be assumed that the patient was relatively pain free or at least not actively complaining about it. Because of failure to gather complete data from all sources, the physician chose the wrong diagnosis. A careful history would have pointed to new-onset angina with a recent change in pattern. Even at this late point in care the outcome can still be influenced in both the patient's and the physician's favor. Please continue reading to see how.

PRINCIPLES OF MANAGEMENT

General Principles

The underlying principle of management is the same as that for the initial diagnosis—always anticipate the worst possible diagnosis. In patients with acute chest pain, management is guided by anticipating four major complications. The majority of patients with pain, discomfort, or associated signs and symptoms of a suspicious nature should receive:

1. Oxygen to prevent *hypoxia*, commonly from ventilation-perfusion mismatch.
2. Electrocardiographic monitoring to seek *dysrhythmias*. Most are ventricular in origin. They are treated with antidysrhythmic medication or electrical conversion, or both.
3. An intravenous line or heparin lock for possible *hypotension* and drug administration. The origin of hypotension is usually cardiac pump failure or hypovolemia, or a combination. They are first treated with volume repletion, then inotropic or chronotropic agents once adequate volume is restored.
4. Analgesia to relieve suffering and stress. The drug is selected after assessing the nature of the pain, patient tolerance, and the suspicion or probability of catastrophic disease.

Specific Principles

The six potentially catastrophic diseases have specific therapies.
Ischemic Heart Disease (Myocardial Infarction or Unstable Angina)
1. Patients with unstable angina or new-onset angina are treated with nitroglycerin and beta-adrenergic blocking drugs.

TABLE 10–5. Other Chest Pain Syndromes and Common Causes by Organ System

	Typical Pain Pattern of Organ System	Diagnosis	Supporting History	Physical Examination	Tests (Diagnostic and Exclusionary)	Comments
Cardiac nonischemic	Dull, aching recurrent pain unrelated to exercises or meals. Or it may be a sharp, stabbing pleuritic-type pain that does not change with chest wall motion. May be severe	a. Pericarditis	Pain is often worse when supine, but improves sitting up. Often preceded by viral illness or underlying disease (SLE or uremia)	Friction rub may be heard, often fleeting. Patient may need to be on hands and knees for rub to be heard	ECG pattern typical for ST-segment elevation across the precordial leads. Erythrocyte sedimentation rate may be elevated	More common in 20 to 50 year olds. A common sequela of myocardial infarction or cardiac surgery
		b. Mitral valve prolapse	Women often with long history of undiagnosed chest pain. May have associated symptoms such as palpitations, sharp chest pain	Often mid to late systolic mitral regurgitant murmur with or without click	Echocardiogram diagnostic; ECG may show extra systoles, ST-T-wave changes	Approximately 5% of young women in United States
Pulmonary	Peripheral pleuritic pain pattern, sharp, stabbing with respiratory variations. Dyspnea often more prominent complaint	a. Upper airway–tracheobronchitis	Associated viral illness and cough, usually minimally productive. Low-grade fever	Ear, nose and throat may be involved; lungs—upper airway. Rhonchi, possible wheezes	Examination and history usually are sufficient, unless sputum examination is desired	Very common
		b. Lower airway–pneumonia	Fever, cough often productive; general malaise	Patient is ill-looking, lung sounds consistent with early pneumonitis or consolidation. Fever	Sputum examination and chest film diagnostic. Cultures necessary to be specific	Atypical causes on the rise
		c. Pleurisy	May follow viral infection. Localized laterally	Rarely rub is heard on auscultation. Chest wall usually not tender	No other tests, chest film usually not helpful unless effusion is noted	Coxsackie B virus causes unique severe spasmatic pain—pleurodynia
Gastrointestinal	Dull, deep aching with occasional severe increases in degree. Long history of recurrence. May be "burning" or "pressure." Occasionally associated with bad taste or burning in hypopharynx, particularly after ingesting alcohol or spicy foods	a. Esophagitis	"Heartburn," worse bending over or supine. Improves with antacids	No typical findings except epigastric discomfort	Definitive tests: esophagoscopy, biopsy, or acid stimulation test—not available in the emergency department	Very common differential diagnostic concern in emergency department. One needs to become facile in discriminating

		Description	Findings	Comments
	b. Esophageal spasm	Constricting chest pain often occurring at time of swallowing. Long recurrent history. May be associated with hot or cold foods or drink or pills	No typical findings except epigastric discomfort	Responds to "GI cocktail" and nitroglycerin. Usually short-lived. Often, responds in emergency department
	c. Peptic ulcer disease, gastritis	Persistent, recurrent aching pain or burning. May relate to meals. Often some improvement after antacids	No typical findings except epigastric discomfort	Barium swallow may assist. Definitive tests: manometry with stimulation (not readily available)
Musculoskeletal	a. Costochondritis	Younger patient, previous history	Often chest wall tenderness, seldom swelling or redness	May see response to antacid trial. Esophagoscopy and contrast not readily available
	b. Xiphoiditis	Similar to costochondritis, located at xiphoid		ECG negative, may not be required. Pain may decrease with local anesthetic
Neurogenic	a. Cervical/thoracic spine	Dull, persistent aching or stabbing pain. Recurrent, long history		Very common differential consideration. Requires analgesia and reassurance. Do not settle on this diagnosis too quickly
		Long history, older patient or patient with known neck trauma	Increased pain with neck, torso motion. Dermatomal pattern. Pain may increase with Valsalva maneuver	Cervical spine films often negative. May see degeneration or osteophytes
Psychogenic	a. Hyperventilation	Usually substernal pressure or lateral "cardiac apex" discomfort associated with considerable concern or anxiety	Difficult to determine on physical examination	Unless obvious, usually considered part of exclusion process. Myelography or MRI occasionally necessary
		Associated breathlessness, occasional cirumoral and distal extremity tingling	May ask patient to hyperventilate to recreate pain. Confirmation with ABGs. ECG may show T-wave inversion that reverses after pain episode	Usually occurs in younger population. They respond well to reassurance and short-term anxiolytics. Do not settle on this diagnosis too quickly
	b. Situational stress			

SLE = systemic lupus erythematosus; ABG = arterial blood gases; MRI = magnetic resonance imaging.

2. Stabilizing acute myocardial infarction includes the following:
    a. Supplemental oxygen, to improve the oxygen supply–demand imbalance
    b. Intravenous narcotic analgesia, as necessary. The dose is adjusted in the context of patient tolerance, cardiac hemodynamics, and side effects of the medication, i.e., nausea, atrioventricular (AV) block.
    c. Antidysrhythmia treatment or prophylaxis is initially accomplished with lidocaine. The dose is adjusted for age, the presence of liver disease or congestive heart failure, and patient symptoms related to administering it.
    d. Anticipation of major complications, as noted under General Treatment Principles.
    e. In selected patients with infarctions less than 6 hours old who meet a number of other screening criteria (e.g., age under 75 years old, no active or previous ulcer history), myocardial salvage therapy is begun in the emergency department. This is a protocol-based intervention performed by a team of emergency physicians, cardiologists, nurses, and the cardiac catheterization laboratory personnel. It includes one or more of the following agents or procedures:
        (1) Intravenous nitroglycerin
        (2) Intravenous beta-blockade or calcium channel blockers
        (3) Thrombolytic agents, such as streptokinase or tissue plasminogen activator (tPA)
        (4) Platelet inhibiting agents, e.g., aspirin
        (5) Coronary angioplasty
        (6) Acute coronary revascularization surgery
    This is a rapidly evolving and expanding area of major importance to both patient and the emergency physician.

Aortic Dissection

Therapy is directed toward decreasing the "pulse" of the pressure wave to impede progression of the dissection. This goal is accomplished initially by achieving controlled hypotension and suppressed myocardial contractility using sodium nitroprusside and beta-adrenergic blockade.

Pulmonary Embolism

Because the majority of pulmonary emboli are thrombotic in origin, initial therapy is intravenous heparin. Therapy is started immediately if there is a strong suspicion of embolism based on clinical data, arterial blood gas measurements, or chest radiograph or lung scan interpretation. The goals of therapy are to inhibit the growth of thromboemboli, promote clot resolution, and prevent recurrence. Thrombolytic therapy may be considered in circumstances of massive embolism and hypotension.

Tension Pneumothorax

Rapid decompression with needle thoracostomy can be lifesaving. The goal is to decrease the intrapleural pressure below that of the right ventricular filling pressure, allowing blood to return to the heart. A thoracostomy tube is inserted after the initial needle decompression.

Esophageal Rupture

Early diagnosis and treatment of accompanying hypotension are important stabilizing efforts while waiting for the surgeon. Antibiotics are given only after discussion with the consultant.

SPECIAL CONSIDERATIONS

Pediatric Patients

Previously healthy children less than 14 years old who present with acute chest pain without a history of trauma and without significant physical findings generally do not have serious disease. A precise history can be obtained from the child if effort is directed toward achieving maximum information. The parents often incorporate their own concerns into the story but may not share their main concern about "heart problems." Musculoskeletal syndromes, hyperventilation, and functional problems are common causes. They present as either short-lived localized stabbing pain or a dull persistent "chest ache" in a child who is otherwise normal. Lateral pleuritic pain is associated with viral illnesses, e.g., pleurodynia, pneumonitis. ECG and additional laboratory studies are usually not indicated.

Organic diseases causing acute chest pain in the pediatric population may include the following:

1. Pain of cardiac origin: pericarditis, mitral valve prolapse, aortic stenosis, pulmonary stenosis, anomalous coronary vessels
2. Pain of esophageal origin: strictures, esophagitis
3. Pain of toxic origin: alcohol, cocaine
4. Pain of hematologic or oncologic origin: leukemia, sickle cell anemia, neuroblastoma
5. Pain of metabolic origin: diabetes mellitus, hyperlipoproteinemia syndromes

Geriatric Patients

The sources of acute chest pain in geriatric patients do not differ significantly from those in the general adult population. Unfortunately, the presentation of serious ischemic heart disease is often atypical. "Classic" chest pain may be elicited in only 30% of elderly patients with myocardial infarction, and ischemic heart disease may present without chest discomfort at all. Instead of pain, the presenting complaint may be sudden progressive dyspnea, abdominal or epigastric fullness, extreme fatigue, confusion, or syncope. The associated symptoms of diaphoresis are significantly less common in the elderly. Because the history may be misleading or difficult to obtain, ancillary testing takes on more significance in this population. ECG changes may be more difficult to interpret owing to a longer history of ischemic problems. Enzyme changes do not help make the diagnosis in the emergency department, although CPK-MB levels are being investigated.

The emergency physician must be aware of the increased risk of silent atypical MI in the elderly. Suspicion of MI should always be raised when elderly patients are in a medically stressful situation, such as occurs with general anesthesia, hypotensive states, hypoxia, systemic infection, or anemia. Even after timely diagnosis, geriatric patients with MI have a mortality (30% to 40%) that is double that of their younger counterparts. They also have more post-MI complications including heart block, cardiogenic shock, myocardial rupture, and pulmonary edema.

Diabetic Patients

Patients with diabetes mellitus, type I or II, are at high risk for ischemic heart disease. They have the dual problem of early atherosclerosis and the atypical pattern of chest pain similar to that seen in the geriatric population.

DISPOSITION AND FOLLOW-UP

Disposition plans usually progress in concert with patient evaluation. Most plans are formulated at the time of the initial stabilization and preliminary differential diagnosis. The same deciding factors are used:

1. *Is there a high probability of catastrophic disease?*
   Disposition is admission with appropriate treatment as necessary.
2. *Is there a high probability of ischemic heart disease?*
   This diagnosis is based on the *history*. It may be supported by the physical examination, laboratory test results, response to therapy, and observation. The

disposition is admission unless there are unique reasons to decide otherwise (e.g., stable angina patient in for a prescription refill or another problem).

The disposition process may be facilitated in the future by computer-based predictive instruments. Presently, these probability generators are most useful for training. One system increased the physician's diagnostic accuracy from 83% to 91%, decreased the cardiac care unit admissions from 23% to 14%, and did not increase the 3% inappropriate discharge rate. Another computer protocol reduced the admission of patients without infarction to intensive care by 11.5% without jeopardizing the patients who required intensive care. These programs are an adjunct, not a replacement, for a careful history and a physician's experience.

The possibility of ischemic heart disease, concerns about its progression and sequelae, and the lack of definitive tests for identifying its presence are sources of tremendous stress on the decision-making capabilities of the emergency physician. About 90% of all patients evaluated in an emergency department and found to have a myocardial infarction are appropriately admitted to the intensive care unit. Another 7% are brought into the hospital, and 3% or less are discharged. Only 20% to 30% of all patients admitted to the intensive care unit with acute chest pain prove to have a myocardial infarction. Therefore, another disposition issue must be resolved.

3. *If a patient is admitted, are there guidelines for choosing between intensive care and intermediate care?*
   The few studies examining this decision have focused on the use of the ECG. An ECG interpreted as "normal" during the initial evaluation in the emergency department correlates with a 0.6% chance of a serious hospital complication. An "abnormal" ECG result correlates with a 14% chance. Therefore, patients with a normal ECG who are admitted as "rule-out" myocardial infarction are considered for admission to an intermediate care area with telemetry and trained nursing staff. Patients diagnosed as having unstable angina rather than myocardial infarction may also fall into a low-risk group for complications. Admission to an intermediate care unit may be appropriate for them as well.

4. *What is done with the patient in whom the diagnosis remains elusive?*
   This point is often reached, so an approach to this clinical dilemma is essential. A great deal of information has been assembled, a number of diagnoses have been considered, and the patient has survived to the present. The following steps will help resolve the disposition:
   a. Reassess the information. Has the patient's history been fully explored? Have all sources of information been used? Would other tests supply useful data?
   b. Reassess the patient and support system. Is there a reason the patient may not be telling the truth or giving only part of the story? Does the patient have significant stoicism or denial? How medically sophisticated are the patient and supporting individuals? Will they be compliant with medication regimens and plans for follow-up?
   c. Have the diagnostic possibilities been reviewed and a decision made on at least an organ system as the most likely site of pain?
   d. Importantly, the case is discussed with the patient's primary physician, if available. The diagnostic process and concerns are thus shared with a colleague. *Decisions of importance are not made in a vacuum.*

   After this review, if doubt remains or if the primary organ system causing pain is suspected as cardiac, the patient is admitted to a monitored bed for observation. An emergency department observation unit is also an appropriate disposition.

   If potentially catastrophic illness, including ischemic heart disease, is ruled out as well as possible, the assessment is repeated quickly. "Are you sure there is nothing else? How is your pain today?" If the patient is without disabling pain and is clinically stable, plans are made for discharge. The care given is documented and a sentence is included about serious disorders believed to be ruled out and the organ system considered as the site of pain. An analgesic or other useful medications, e.g., antacids, are prescribed. The findings are discussed with the patient and family, and mention is made of the "serious problems" that are considered unlikely. Given sufficient information to decrease their anxiety, most people understand that all the answers cannot be supplied in a limited time frame.

It is critical to arrange close follow-up for patients being discharged with the complaint of acute chest pain, whether the diagnosis has been made or not. Optimally, both the emergency physician and the primary physician or consultant participate in follow-up activities. Any patient in the diagnostic "gray zone" in regard to acute chest pain who is discharged from the emergency department is contacted within 24 hours. Any patient who voluntarily recontacts or revisits the emergency department because of persistent or recurrent chest pain is strongly considered a candidate for admission. Such a patient is evaluated as if he had a "new" chief complaint to avoid being lulled into believing the diagnosis made on the first visit.

PROBLEM 1 The patient was discharged home on antacid therapy. The following morning, just before the treating physician was leaving his night shift, she called the emergency department to speak to the physician. She described a slightly stronger pain in the epigastric area and a slight amount of sweating after going home. A second similar episode lasting 10 to 20 minutes awakened her just before her call. The physician stated that the antacids take some time to work and that she should avoid hot foods. The patient called back about 2 hours later, but the physician had left. She was found dead at her home approximately 4 hours later. An autopsy found a new inferior myocardial infarction.

The most worrisome patients in emergency medicine are often the ones that are discharged home. This physician neglected a cardinal rule of emergency medical practice: "Listen to, rather than explain away, a patient who has returned. Do not form a rigid mindset about any diagnosis." Better patient education, a follow-up system in the emergency department, more responsiveness on the part of the treating physician, and arranged referral to the primary physician might have favorably influenced the outcome of this case. "Come on back, we'd like to see you again. Particularly if things are not working out," must be the continual parting message in the emergency department. It is always smarter to rule out serious disease in the hospital than to have it ruled in at home.

DOCUMENTATION

1. Onset, duration, location, radiation, exacerbating or relieving factors, and associated symptoms of the pain
2. Risk factors for cardiac disease
3. Other illnesses and past pertinent history
4. Medications taken
5. Physical appearance, vital signs, and findings of the physical examination
6. Response to therapy
7. Laboratory findings, including ECG and ECG findings compared to those on previous ECG, if available
8. Reasons for reaching final diagnosis and disposition (only one to two sentences are needed)
9. Follow-up arrangements, if patient is not admitted

PROBLEM 1 The total documentation in this case read as follows:

> History as above
> Obese WF
> Thorax—WNL, some xiphoid tenderness
> Lungs—clear
> Heart—distant heart tones (pendulous breasts), no murmur
> Abdomen—mild epigastric tenderness
> Extremities—no edema
> Diagnosis: Esophagitis
> Treatment: Antacids, D/C (discharge) to PMD (primary medical doctor)
> ECG—WNL

The physician is vulnerable medicolegally because of poor documentation. Compare this information to that described in the nine areas listed in the Documentation section. Each has a purpose in communication and collectively creates a high-quality record from the emergency department. The importance of a few sentences in documenting one's thoughts on a complex or confusing patient with acute chest pain who is being discharged from the emergency department is not to be underestimated.

Despite the untimely death of this patient, the hospital generated and forwarded a bill. The physician did not notify the risk management department of the hospital nor know that the bill had been sent. This is a not-uncommon progenitor of legal action on the part of the individuals or family members receiving the bill!

> Total time in the emergency department—2 hours, 45 minutes
> Charges:

Ambulance fee:	$100.00
Hospital fee:	50.00
Physician fee—medium level care:	55.00
ECG and interpretation:	60.00
Monitor:	20.00
IV:	15.00
Mylanta—first dose:	2.00
TOTAL:	$302.00

SUMMARY AND FINAL POINTS

- Acute chest pain is a complex complaint that requires a careful, detailed history.
- The physical examination focuses on signs of catastrophic illness, arteriosclerosis, and duplicating the chest discomfort.
- The initial differential diagnosis of acute chest pain may be based on the location and character of the pain.
- The six potentially catastrophic illnesses to be considered first are myocardial infarction, unstable angina, pneumothorax, dissection of the aorta, pulmonary embolism, and esophageal rupture.
- A single ECG is helpful for ruling in ischemic heart disease if it shows positive results. "Normal" results do not rule it out.
- Cardiac enzyme concentrations as presently available are not useful for ruling out ischemic heart disease in most patients with acute chest pain evaluated in the emergency department.
- Patients without a clear diagnosis are best reevaluated and the case discussed with another physician. If a clear decision cannot be reached, it is preferable to admit the patient for observation and further evaluation.
- Elderly patients with IHD may present without chest pain. A high index of suspicion is necessary in this age group.

BIBLIOGRAPHY

Texts

1. Braunwald E (ed): Heart Disease (3rd ed). Philadelphia, W.B. Saunders, 1984.
2. Griner PF, Panzer RJ, Greenland P: Clinical Diagnosis and the Laboratory: Logical Strategies for Common Medical Problems. Chicago, Year Book, 1986.
3. Levene DL, Billings RF, Davies GM, et al: Chest Pain: An Integrated Diagnostic Approach. Philadelphia, Lea & Febiger, 1977.
4. Pepine CJ (ed): Acute Myocardial Infarction. Cardiovascular Clinics, Vol. 20, No. 1. Philadelphia, F.A. Davis, 1989.
5. American College of Emergency Physicians: Clinical Policy for Management of Adult Patients Presenting with a Chief Complaint of Chest Pain, with No History of Trauma. Dallas, American College of Emergency Physicians, 1990.

Journal Articles

1. Behar S, Schor S, Kariv I, et al: Evaluation of the electrocardiogram in emergency room as a decision-making tool. Chest 71:486, 1977.
2. Brush JE, Brand DA, Acampora et al: The use of the initial electrocardiogram to predict in-hospital complications of acute myocardial infarction. N Engl J Med 312:1137–1141, 1985.
3. Cohen PE: Silent myocardial ischemia: Classification, prevalence and prognosis. Am J Med 79(Suppl 3A):2–6, 1985.
4. DeSanctis RW: Aortic dissection. N Engl J Med 317:1060–1067, 1987.
5. Gibler WB, Gibler DC, Weinshenker E, et al: Myoglobin as an early indicator of acute myocardial infarction. Ann Emerg Med 16:851–856, 1987.
6. Goldman L, Cook EF, Brand DA, et al: A computer protocol to predict myocardial infarction in emergency department patients with chest pain. N Engl J Med 318:797–803, 1988.
7. Lee TH, Cook EF, Weisberg M, et al: Acute chest pain in the emergency room. Arch Intern Med 145:65–69, 1985.
8. Richter JE, Bradley LA, Castell DO: Esophageal chest pain: Current controversies in pathogenesis, diagnosis, and therapy. Ann Intern Med 110:66–78, 1989.
9. Start ME, Vacek JL: The initial electrocardiogram during admission for myocardial infarction. Arch Intern Med 147:843–846, 1987.
10. Nowakowski JF: Use of cardiac enzymes in the evaluation of acute chest pain. Ann Emerg Med 15:354–360, 1986.
11. Ornato JP: Computer-assisted diagnosis of chest pain. In Ornato JP: Cardiovascular Emergencies, Vol. 9. Clinics in Emergency Medicine. New York, Churchill Livingstone, 1986, pp 1–22.
12. Posen MW, D'Agostino RB, Selker HP, et al: A predictive instrument to improve coronary care unit admission practices in acute ischemic heart disease. N Engl J Med 310:1273–1278, 1984.
13. Schneider RR, Seckler SG: Evaluation of acute chest pain. Med Clin North Am 65(1):53–66, 1981.
14. Selbst SM: Evaluation of chest pain in children. Pediatr Rev 8:56–62, 1986.
15. Shoemaker WC, Kram HB, Appel PL: Therapy of shock based on pathophysiology, monitoring, and outcome prediction. Crit Care Med 18:519–525, 1990.

CHAPTER 11

PALPITATIONS

M. ANDREW LEVITT, D.O.

PROBLEM 1 A 29 year old male presents for medical attention because he feels weak and his "heart is beating funny."

PROBLEM 2 A 63 year old female calls the rescue squad because she feels that her heart "is doing flip flops in her chest."

QUESTIONS TO CONSIDER

1. What are palpitations?
2. What cardiac dysrhythmias can cause a patient to complain of palpitations?
3. What are the causes of palpitations? What conditions require immediate attention?
4. What specific data are obtained in a patient presenting with palpitations?
5. What ancillary tests are helpful in evaluating and treating a patient with palpitations?
6. In the patient presenting with a wide complex tachycardia, how can the origin of the tachydysrhythmia be determined?
7. Are there patients with palpitations who can be discharged with follow-up care?

INTRODUCTION

Palpitations is a term commonly used by physicians but infrequently by patients. Most patients use terms such as *pounding, fluttering, skipping, jumping, racing, quivering,* or *flip-flopping* to describe the abnormal feeling produced by an irregular or fast heart beat.

Palpitations can be defined as the perception of an abnormal beating of the heart. The sensation is generally anxiety producing and is most often due to cardiac rhythm disturbances. The patient feels the changes in the cardiac output caused by the dysrhythmia. Cardiac output depends on stroke volume and heart rate. Extrasystoles produce an increase in the stroke volume in the beat following the premature beat. This results from increased filling time during the compensatory pause. Tachydysrhythmias are associated with increased heart rates and decreased stroke volume. Variations in cardiac output may be minimal and intermittent, such as those produced by occasional extrasystoles. These are usually felt as a discomfort in the chest. A decreased cardiac output may be sustained, producing significant compromise in systemic perfusion. These patients may complain of persistent dizziness, weakness, confusion, chest pain, or syncope.

Palpitation is a relatively common presenting complaint in the emergency department. Though its prevalence is unknown, the "abnormal" cardiac rhythms are the cause of symptoms in about 90% of cases. They are the focus of this chapter. Psychogenic conditions are next in frequency.

PREHOSPITAL CARE

Prehospital management of these patients is directed to determine hemodynamic stability, monitor the patient for cardiac deterioration and end-organ hypoperfusion, and give emergent treatment for patients who are unstable. The following information is important to the staff in the emergency department.

History

1. Is there a previous history of palpitations; if so, how were they treated?
2. Are there associated symptoms of chest pain, dyspnea, diaphoresis, light-headedness, or confusion?
3. What has patient done for the palpitations? What was the result?
4. Is there a personal or family history of cardiovascular disease or history of drug ingestion?

Physical Examination

1. Vital signs are most important.
2. General appearance, including tolerance of symptoms, presence of cyanosis, diaphoresis.
3. Presence of jugular venous distention, peripheral edema.
4. Symmetry and quality of breath sounds.
5. Level of consciousness.

Intervention

The patient's condition is unstable if there is hypotension, decreasing level of consciousness, chest pain, or congestive heart failure. The appropriate treatment is as follows:

1. Transportation to the hospital *as rapidly as possible*.
2. Oxygen supplement by nasal cannula beginning at 2 liters/min and adjusted as tolerated.
3. Frequent blood pressure monitoring.
4. Electrocardiographic (ECG) monitoring to interpret and monitor changes in rhythm.
5. Intravenous (IV) access with 5% dextrose in water (D/W 5%) at a keep-open rate (TKO) in case drugs or fluids need to be given.
6. If the findings are the result of a tachydysrhythmia and the hemodynamic parameters deteriorate, electrical cardioversion at 50 to 100 joules is attempted. This order usually comes from an emergency physician at the base hospital.

PROBLEM 1 The patient related no previous history of palpitations, and his only associated symptom was a vague complaint of weakness. He was reported as awake and alert with a blood pressure of 118/80 mm Hg and a heart rate of 250 beats/min. Results of his physical examination were benign. An IV line of D/W 5% at TKO and nasal oxygen at 2 liters/min were started. ECG monitoring showed a wide-complex tachycardia.

PROBLEM 2 The patient related a history of congestive heart failure and was taking digoxin and hydrochlorthiazide. Her only other complaint was that of mild nausea. Her blood pressure was reported as 152/92 mm Hg and her heart rate as 72 beats/min and irregular. The ECG monitor showed wide premature contractions and a sinus rhythm. An IV line of D/W 5% given at TKO and oxygen 2 liters/min by nasal cannula were ordered.

Both patients may have serious diseases, but their conditions are stable. Definitive treatment will be started in the emergency department.

INITIAL APPROACH IN THE EMERGENCY DEPARTMENT

On arrival in the emergency department, the patient is placed in a cardiac room with continuous ECG monitoring. Hemodynamic status is quickly assessed to detect deterioration. These patients are often very apprehensive about their symptoms. This anxiety may be out of proportion to their actual risk of dying. The physician's demeanor and appropriate reassurance will go far to lessen their fears.

1. An assessment is made to determine whether the patient is alert, has good skin color and temperature, or complains of chest pain, dyspnea, or dizziness. If at any time the patient's condition deteriorates, cardioversion may be indicated.
2. Blood pressure and pulse rate are rechecked.
3. The patient is placed on the emergency department ECG monitor.
4. Oxygen by nasal cannula is administered.
5. The IV line is confirmed or established.
6. A 12-lead ECG is obtained. It is extremely important to obtain an ECG recording while the symptoms are present. The type of dysrhythmia can be determined early in the patient's care, and reassurance given as appropriate.

Table 11–1 lists the immediate life-threatening dysrhythmias that are to be anticipated and treated as necessary.

DATA GATHERING

The history and physical examination will help to determine whether cardiovascular disease is present and assess end-organ perfusion.

History

1. What is the *sensation* being *felt?* Are the *palpitations regular* or *irregular?* Are they present while the patient is on the ECG monitor? There is a great deal of variability in patients' perceptions of abnormal heart beats. The palpitations may be more noticeable at rest than with activity. Transient and episodic dysrhythmias may be more symptomatic than persistent rhythm disturbances.
2. Have there been *similar events* in the past? Does the patient have a *history* of *preexcitation syndrome?* The patient's response to key words such as Wolff-Parkinson-White syndrome, atrial fibrillation, atrial flutter, and ventricular tachycardia is sought. Does the patient have a history of experiencing palpitations with anxiety-producing events? It is important to remember that patients with a past history of specific dysrhythmias may have another disorder this time.
3. Are there *associated symptoms?* Does the patient have chest pain, lightheadedness, dizziness, or loss of consciousness? These symptoms may indicate a decreased cardiac output and poor cerebral or myocardial perfusion.
4. *Past medical history.* Is there a history of cardiovascular, pulmonary, or thyroid disease? The patient's age and cardiovascular history can help differentiate between wide-complex tachycardias. If the patient is older than 35 years and has a history of congestive

TABLE 11–1. Palpitations from Serious Dysrhythmias

Dysrhythmia	Immediate Intervention
Ventricular tachycardia	Stable—lidocaine
	Unstable—synchronized cardioversion
Myocardial infarction with PVCs	Prophylactic lidocaine
Supraventricular tachycardia with hypotension or poor end-organ perfusion	Synchronized cardioversion
Sinus tachycardia due to systemic disease (hypoxia, shock)	Treat underlying condition (oxygen, fluids, pressors)

heart failure, myocardial infarction, or angina pectoris, there is an 85% to 100% probability that a wide-complex tachycardia is ventricular in origin. No historical information is highly predictive of paroxysmal supraventricular tachycardia (PSVT) with aberrancy.

5. Is the patient on cardiac *medications* or diuretics? Some cardiac medications such as digoxin may cause extrasystoles. Diuretics may cause hypokalemia, which can cause dysrhythmias and exacerbate digoxin toxicity. Other medications such as quinidine or procainamide indicate that the patient has had problems with dysrhythmias in the past.

6. *Predisposing drugs.* Has the patient taken cocaine, alcohol, or caffeine? Cocaine can cause cardiac dysrhythmias as well as acute myocardial infarction. Alcohol is associated with atrial fibrillation in what has been termed the "holiday heart" syndrome. Caffeine can cause premature contractions.

Physical Examination

General Appearance. Is the patient cold, clammy, or ashen? These may be symptoms of decreased skin perfusion and early shock.

Vital Signs. Hypotension may indicate decreased cardiac output from the dysrhythmia or shock due to a systemic illness with a compensatory sinus tachycardia. An irregularly irregular pulse usually indicates atrial fibrillation or multifocal atrial tachycardia. A regularly irregular rhythm is usually caused by premature atrial or ventricular contractions.

Cardiovascular System. The cardiac examination includes auscultation for heart sounds, murmurs, clicks, rubs, and gallops as well as careful attention to neck veins. The finding of cannon waves in the neck, changing loudness of the first heart sound, and changes in systolic blood pressure on successive beats are all suggestive of independent contractions of the atria and ventricles. These findings are characteristic of ventricular tachycardia; however, their absence does not exclude ventricular tachycardia. Ventricular tachycardia may occur in the presence of atrial fibrillation or in conjunction with ventriculoatrial conduction. Murmurs or clicks may be indicative of valvular heart disease. The mitral valve prolapse syndrome is associated with both atrial and ventricular dysrhythmias.

Pulmonary System. Wheezing, rales, or rhonchi on lung examination may indicate a pulmonary cause for the palpitations. Acute pulmonary edema secondary to dysrhythmias indicates cardiac decompensation and the need for electrical cardioversion.

Abdominal Signs. Tenderness, guarding, or rigidity on abdominal examination may indicate a systemic cause for dysrhythmias or shock.

Extremities. Lower extremity swelling, tenderness, warmth, or erythema may indicate deep venous thrombosis and possible pulmonary embolus as a cause for the palpitations.

Neurologic Signs. Is the patient alert, oriented, and responding appropriately to questions? Decreased mentation may indicate the need for immediate electrical cardioversion.

DECISION PRIORITIES AND PRELIMINARY DIFFERENTIAL DIAGNOSIS

Following the directed history and physical examination, the physician attempts to answer several key questions.

1. *Is there a cardiogenic problem associated with the subjective complaint of palpitations?*

    If the patient has a history of dysrhythmias or cardiac disease, an irregular rhythm, tachycardia, or abnormalities on cardiac examination, cardiac dysrhythmias must be suspected. It is not unusual, however, for the symptoms and dysrhythmia to be resolved prior to the patient's arrival in the emergency department. Patients with palpitations are placed on a continuous ECG monitor to be observed for dysrhythmias in the emergency department. If the patient is having symptoms but no dysrhythmia appears on ECG, it is unlikely that the palpitations are associated with a cardiogenic problem.

2. *Does the patient have a life-threatening dysrhythmia?*
Specific attention is directed toward diagnosing serious cardiac or systemic disease that may cause palpitations. These diseases were listed in Table 11–1.

3. *What is the etiology of the cardiogenic palpitations?*
Multiple systemic diseases may cause palpitations. Primary cardiovascular disease is the cause of dysrhythmias in some patients. In other patients metabolic, endocrine, infectious, psychogenic, and toxic etiologies exist. Table 11–2 reviews the common causes of atrial and ventricular dysrhythmias causing palpitations.

PROBLEM 1 The patient was awake and alert and was still complaining of weakness. Heart rate was 250 beats/min, BP was 188/80 mm Hg. Results of the cardiac examination were unremarkable. He was placed on a continuous ECG monitor, which showed a wide-complex tachycardia. Results of examination otherwise were benign.

This patient had a cardiac dysrhythmia that was causing palpitations. He did not show significant problems, maintaining end-organ perfusion despite the rapid heart rate. The most likely cause of the dysrhythmia, based on the patient's age and rapid rate, is paroxysmal supraventricular tachycardia with aberrant conduction. Ventricular tachycardia (VT) is a possibility.

PROBLEM 2 The patient's condition, described previously, remained unchanged. She

TABLE 11–2. Etiologies for Dysrhythmias Causing Palpitations

System	Disease	Comment
Cardiovascular	Sick sinus (tachy-brady) syndrome	History of rapid and slow heart rhythms, near syncope or syncope
	Preexcitation syndrome	12-lead ECG shows short interval or delta wave and documented episodes of tachydysrhythmia
	Coronary artery disease	Documented by stress test or angiography or history suggestive of angina
	Myocardial infarction	History may be suggestive, i.e., substernal crushing chest pain
	Valvular heart disease	Patient may relate history of murmurs or cardiac auscultation may reveal murmurs
	Mitral valve	Patient may relate known history or family history or have click or midsystolic murmur on cardiac examination
Metabolic	Hypokalemia	Suggested by diuretic use and confirmed by serum measurement
	Hypoxia	Suggested by respiratory complaints, presence of cyanosis, and tachypnea; and confirmed by ABG
Endocrine	Thyrotoxicosis	Tachycardia, fever, dehydration, history of thyroid disease. Confirmation by thyroid function testing
	Pheochromocytoma	Hypertension, tachycardia, elevated catecholamine levels
Infections	Septicemia	An infection may be present and will need to be diagnosed and treated
Psychogenic	Anxiety	Diagnosis of exclusion
Toxins	Tobacco, caffeine, epinephrine, alcohol, cocaine, amphetamines, atropine, digoxin, thyroid replacement	History of ingestion or confirmation of ingestion by urine or serum testing

still complained of some nausea and her heart "flip-flopping in her chest." On the ECG monitor the heart appeared to be in a sinus rhythm with frequent unifocal premature ventricular contractions (PVCs). Results of examination were otherwise benign.

The palpitations are of cardiac origin. There are several possible causes for the dysrhythmia. The PVCs do not seem to be associated with the history of an acute myocardial infarction. In light of the complaint of nausea, history of taking digoxin, and presence of frequent PVCs, digoxin toxicity is a possibility. Additionally, she was taking diuretics. Therefore, hypokalemia in combination with the digoxin could potentiate the PVCs.

DIAGNOSTIC ADJUNCTS

Electrocardiography, laboratory studies, and radiographs can be valuable in defining the etiology of cardiac palpitations.

Electrocardiogram

A 12-lead ECG with rhythm strip is mandatory in all patients to determine the presence of an underlying rhythm disturbance or evidence of myocardial infarction. Even if the symptoms have resolved, a 12-lead ECG may demonstrate an underlying preexcitation syndrome. Preexcitation syndromes, such as Wolff-Parkinson-White (WPW), Mahaim, or Lown-Ganong-Levine (LGL) syndromes, are characterized by a short PR interval. They may have a widened QRS pattern and a delta wave.

Laboratory Studies

Serum Electrolytes. Measuring serum electrolyte levels, particularly potassium, is indicated if the patient is taking a diuretic or digoxin or is suspected of having renal failure. Potassium imbalance can cause dysrhythmias and potentiate digoxin toxicity.

Arterial Blood Gases. Determination of arterial blood gases (ABGs) is indicated if the patient has dyspnea, pleuritic chest pain, cyanosis, hypotension, or abnormalities on pulmonary examination. Hypoxia or acidosis can cause dysrhythmias. Hyperventilation syndromes may be perceived as palpitations without dysrhythmias.

Thyroid Function Tests. These tests are indicated when the patient has signs or symptoms of hyperthyroidism such as heat intolerance, weight loss, ophthalmic signs, or goiter. The results will not be available during the emergency department evaluation and treatment.

Drug Levels. In patients taking digoxin, quinidine or aminophylline, blood levels are checked to determine the toxicity or adequacy of the medication. A toxicology screen that includes cocaine may help diagnose an unknown sinus tachycardia.

Radiologic Imaging

Plain Films. A *chest radiograph* may be helpful if the patient has dyspnea, shortness of breath, rales, distended neck veins, or decreased breath sounds. Radiographic evidence of pulmonary edema indicates cardiac decompensation and the need for prompt intervention.

Other Tests

Holter monitoring is indicated for patients who do not have symptoms in the emergency department but where palpitations may have been caused by dysrhythmias. The ECG monitor is attached to the patient and worn for 24 hours while the patient keeps a record

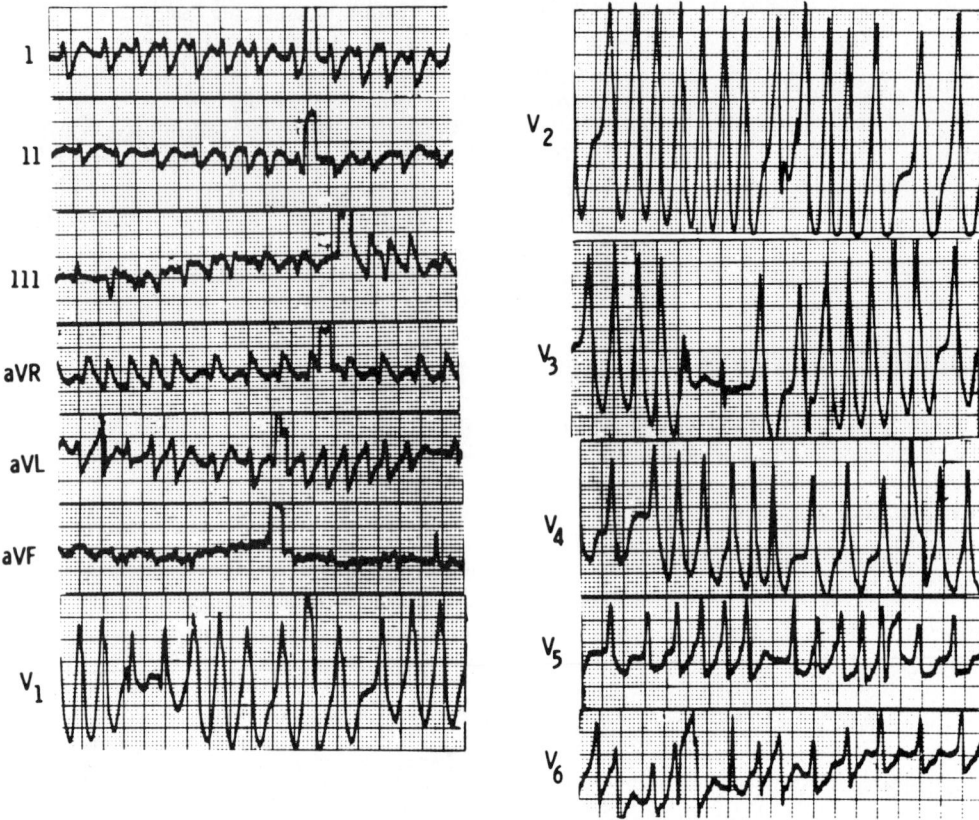

FIGURE 11-1. This is the 12-lead electrocardiogram of the patient in Problem 1. This is wide-complex tachycardia. (Used with permission from Chung EK: Principles of Cardiac Arrhythmias (4th ed). © 1989, the Williams & Wilkins Co., Baltimore.)

of all symptoms and activities. The ECG is subsequently analyzed for dysrhythmias and correlated with symptoms.

PROBLEM 1 The 12-lead ECG for this patient is shown in Figure 11-1. The next step is to determine if this wide-complex tachycardia is ventricular or supraventricular in origin.

PROBLEM 2 The digoxin level was found to be 3.2 mg/ml (normal range 0.8 to 2.0 mg/ml). Additionally, the serum potassium was 3.0 mEq/liter (normal range, 3.5 to 5.0 mEq/liter). The emergency physician concluded that this patient's PVCs and nausea resulted from digoxin toxicity and hypokalemia. The 12-lead ECG results and additional blood tests including serum electrolytes and blood gases were all within normal limits.

REFINED DIFFERENTIAL DIAGNOSIS

The recognition of cardiac dysrhythmias is usually straightforward based on results of the 12-lead ECG and rhythm strip.

Common Cardiac Rhythms Causing Palpitations

Atrial Fibrillation. Atrial fibrillation is represented by rapid chaotic atrial foci stimulating the atrioventricular (AV) node (Fig. 11-2). The ventricular response is limited

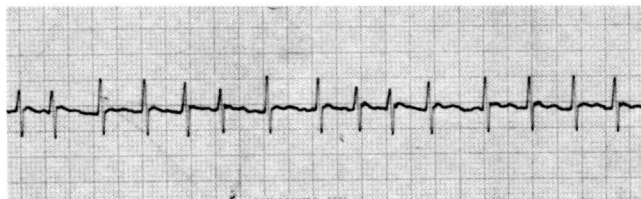

Rapid atrial fibrillation

FIGURE 11-2. *Atrial fibrillation. (From Eisenberg MS, Cummins RO, Ho MT (eds): Code Blue: Cardiac Arrest and Resuscitation. Philadelphia, W.B. Saunders, 1987.)*

by the refractoriness of the AV node. Patients with a normal AV node will have a rapid ventricular response. Myocardial contractions are irregularly irregular. Cardiac output is compromised because of the rate and lack of atrial kick. Causes of atrial fibrillation include coronary artery disease, congestive heart failure, mitral stenosis, hypertensive heart disease, pericarditis, and alcohol abuse.

Atrial Flutter. Atrial flutter is characterized by regular rapid atrial contractions of about 300/min with a variable ventricular response (Fig. 11-3). A characteristic sawtooth pattern of atrial contractions is often seen. Causes include coronary artery disease, mitral stenosis, atrial septal defect, chronic lung disease, pulmonary embolus, and thyrotoxicosis.

Paroxysmal Supraventricular Tachycardia (PSVT). PSVT arises from a reentry circuit involving the AV node (Fig. 11-4). The rapid rate may result in decreased cardiac output. The patient may feel faint or may develop syncope. More frequently, he experiences a rapid forceful heartbeat accompanied by anxiety. Patients with preexcitation syndromes have accessory conduction pathways that predispose them to supraventricular tachycardias. Wolff-Parkinson-White syndrome (WPW) is present in less than 0.2% of the population. Tachycardias are reported in up to 85% of patients with WPW. Preexcitation syndromes through other accessory pathways are not as prevalent as WPW. Supraventricular tachycardias with heart block are commonly associated with digitalis toxicity. Recently, with a better understanding of digitalis dosage and the use of serum level measurements, digitalis toxic tachycardias are less commonly seen.

Multifocal Atrial Tachycardias (MAT). These tachycardias result from multiple atrial foci conducted through the AV node, resulting in an irregular supraventricular tachycardia with multiform P waves. It occurs most commonly in elderly people and is usually associated with serious disease such as hypoxia due to chronic lung disease, theophylline toxicity, and diabetes mellitus. Heart block is usually not part of this dysrhythmia.

Premature Atrial Contraction (PAC). PAC originates from an ectopic atrial focus outside of the sinoatrial (SA) node. It is usually conducted through the AV node, resulting in a narrow QRS complex. PACs are frequently seen in patients without organic heart disease. They may precede more serious dysrhythmias such as atrial fibrillation. Their causes include pericarditis, electrolyte abnormalities, hypoxia, and drug toxicities from theophylline, caffeine, or sympathomimetics.

Ventricular Premature Beats (VPBs). This abnormality arises from an ectopic

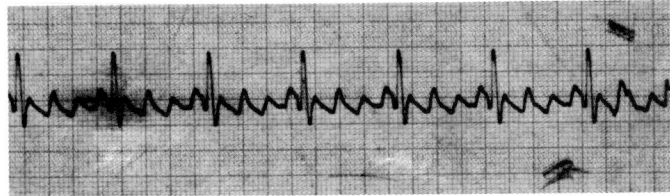

Atrial flutter

FIGURE 11-3. *Atrial flutter. (From Eisenberg MS, Cummins RO, Ho MT (eds): Code Blue: Cardiac Arrest and Resuscitation. Philadelphia, W.B. Saunders, 1987.)*

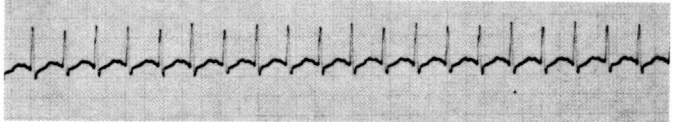

Paroxysmal supraventricular tachycardia (PSVT)

FIGURE 11–4. *Paroxysmal supraventricular tachycardia (PSVT). (From Eisenberg MS, Cummins RO, Ho MT (eds): Code Blue: Cardiac Arrest and Resuscitation. Philadelphia, W.B. Saunders, 1987.)*

ventricular focus and may represent a benign or serious dysrhythmia. A VPB occurring near the vulnerable period, the middle third of the T wave, may result in ventricular tachycardia or fibrillation. Studies have demonstrated that approximately 20% of men without known organic heart disease have VPBs over a 24-hour period. The incidence increases with age to such an extent that VPBs are detected in 80% of men over age 60. The key distinction between benign and malignant VPBs is whether the patient has underlying organic heart disease. Organic heart disease may be evident from other aspects of the patient's history, physical examination, or ECG. The causes of VPBs include ischemia, hypokalemia, hypoxia, valvular heart disease such as mitral valve prolapse, digitalis toxicity, and congenital heart diseases.

Ventricular Tachycardia (VT). Ventricular tachycardia is characterized by three or more VPBs in succession (Fig. 11–5). Sustained VT lasts longer than 30 seconds, usually producing hemodynamic decompensation and symptoms of dizziness, chest pain, palpitations, and lethargy. Occasionally, patients in VT will have minimal symptoms. Causes of VT are similar to those listed for VPB.

Wide-Complex Tachycardia. A confusing diagnostic dilemma is the differentiation of wide-complex tachycardias. The confusion is in determining whether the origin is ventricular or supraventricular (see Fig. 11–1). Clinical studies have shown that physicians misinterpret VT as PSVT approximately 40% of the time and therefore potentially treat the dysrhythmia inappropriately.

Clinical investigations have attempted to differentiate between these rhythms by means of electrocardiographic criteria (see Table 11–3). If AV dissociation is seen during the tachycardia, the dysrhythmia is more likely to be ventricular in origin. Approximately 50% of patients with ventricular tachycardia have AV dissociation. Irregular R–R intervals suggest atrial fibrillation with aberrancy and rapid ventricular response. However, ventricular tachycardia may present with irregular R–R intervals. A QRS width of less than 0.14 second was found in all patients with supraventricular tachycardia (SVT) and aberrant conduction in one study. In contrast, 60% of patients with ventricular tachycardia had a QRS width of greater than 0.14 second. None of the patients in these studies had a preexisting bundle branch block; thus, if a bundle branch block is present during sinus rhythm or if the patient is taking antidysrhythmic drugs, the QRS width may be less helpful. A left-axis deviation of greater than 30 degrees in the frontal plane is suggestive of a ventricular origin.

The QRS configuration in the precordial lead V_1 may help sort out the wide-complex

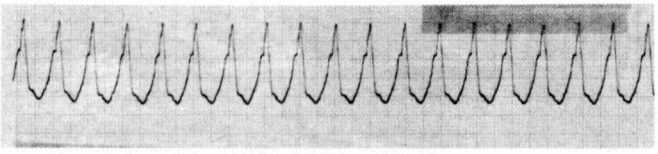

Ventricular tachycardia

FIGURE 11–5. *Ventricular tachycardia. (From Eisenberg MS, Cummins RO, Ho MT (eds): Code Blue: Cardiac Arrest and Resuscitation. Philadelphia, W.B. Saunders, 1987.)*

TABLE 11–3. Criteria for Diagnosing Origin of Wide-Complex Tachycardia on Electrocardiogram

1. AV dissociation during tachycardia favors a ventricular origin, although cases have been reported with aberrant conduction.
2. Irregular R–R intervals may suggest atrial fibrillation with aberrant and rapid ventricular response, but ventricular tachycardia may present with irregular R–R intervals.
3. QRS width of more than 0.14 second suggests ventricular tachycardia. If a bundle branch block is present during sinus rhythm or if the patient is taking antiarrhythmic drugs, this sign is less definite.
4. Left axis deviation in the frontal plane suggests a ventricular origin.
5. Monophasic or biphasic right bundle branch block in lead V_1 is highly suggestive of a ventricular origin.
6. Triphasic right bundle branch block in lead V_1 were found in ventricular and supraventricular tachycardia. A left-axis deviation and a R/S ratio of less than 1 in lead V_6 is suggestive of ventricular origin.
7. In the presence of left bundle branch block, only lead V_6 was found to be helpful. Q–R and Q–S complexes in this lead point to a ventricular origin of tachycardia.

tachycardias (Fig. 11–6). A monophasic or biphasic QRS configuration is more suggestive of a ventricular origin. A triphasic QRS configuration is more suggestive of SVT with aberrant conduction. A left-axis deviation that is present along with an R/S ratio of less than 1 in lead V_6 suggests a ventricular origin (Fig. 11–7). In the presence of a left bundle branch block configuration, QRS findings are of little help. Only the presence of a Q–R or Q–S complex in lead V_6 suggests a ventricular origin (Fig. 11–8).

In conclusion, no one criterion is able to predict with 100% accuracy whether the rhythm is ventricular or supraventricular in origin. Several criteria are suggestive of the rhythm's origin.

PROBLEM 1 The patient's ECG (see Fig. 11–1) showed a wide-complex tachycardia.

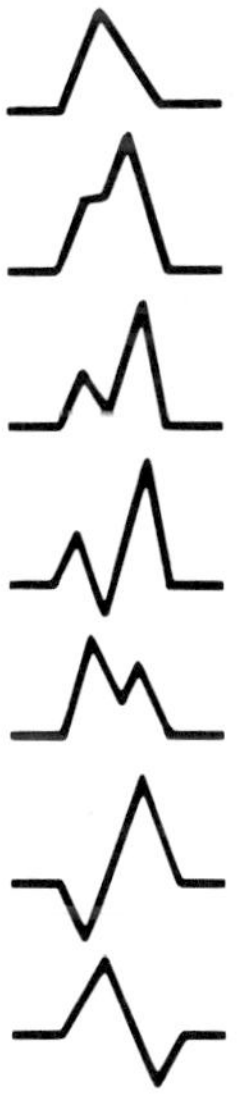

Type Complex	Aberrant*	Ventricular Tachycardia*
1	–	15
2	11	17
3	19	3
4	38	3
5	–	7
6	1	16
7	–	4
	69	65

FIGURE 11–6. *Types of right bundle branch block patterns of the QRS complex in lead V_1 in patients with supraventricular tachycardia and aberrant conduction and patients with ventricular tachycardia. Note that triphasic QRS complexes are not found exclusively in aberrant conduction. Asterisk indicates number of patients in each group for a QRS configuration.*

Type Complex	Aberrant*	Ventricular Tachycardia*
1	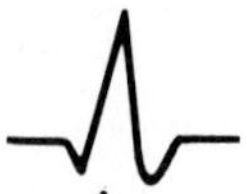 44	3
2	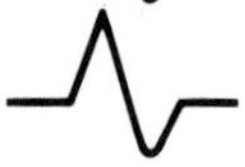 21	15
3	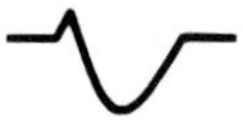 4	27
4	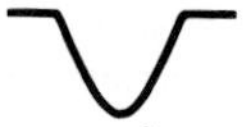 –	16
5	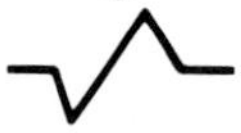 –	3
6	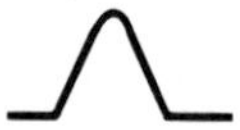 –	1
	69	65

FIGURE 11–7. Types of right bundle branch block patterns of the QRS complex in lead V_6. Note that small or absent R waves in lead V_6 suggest a ventricular origin of the tachycardia. Asterisk indicates number of patients in each group for a QRS configuration.

Applying the aforementioned criteria may help to determine the origin of this tachycardia. The irregular R–R intervals suggest atrial fibrillation with aberrant conduction and rapid ventricular response. The QRS width varies but for the most part is less than 0.14 second, suggesting a supraventricular origin. There are occasional normally conducted atrial fibrillation beats. There does not appear to be left-axis deviation. A biphasic

Type Complex	Aberrant*	Ventricular Tachycardia*
1	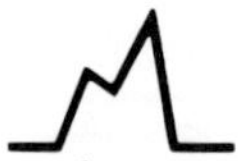 14	15
2	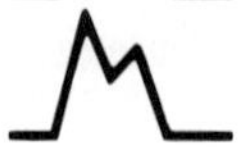 17	14
3	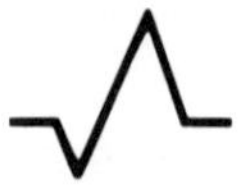	5
4	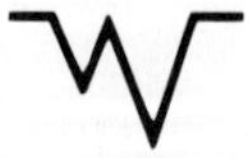	1
	31	35

FIGURE 11–8. Types of left bundle branch block patterns of the QRS complex in lead V_6. Only rarely can the site of origin of the tachycardia be accurately predicted from QRS configuration alone. Asterisk indicates number of patients in each group for a QRS configuration.

pattern of the QRS in V_1 suggests a ventricular origin. These criteria suggest a supraventricular origin for the patient's rhythm.

PRINCIPLES OF MANAGEMENT

The management of patients with palpitations is directed by the following principles.

Immediate Interventions

It is assumed that the patient has a life-threatening dysrhythmia until proved otherwise. Vital signs and end-organ perfusion are frequently reassessed. Supplemental oxygen is provided. IV access is established, anticipating the need for pharmacologic intervention. The ECG rhythm is continuously monitored.

Cardioversion

Prompt electrical cardioversion is indicated if the patient's condition deteriorates or if there is poor end-organ perfusion as manifested by cardiac chest pain, decreased mental status, or acute pulmonary edema. Studies have shown that physicians often spend too much time attempting to make a definitive diagnosis while they allow serious dysrhythmias such as ventricular tachycardia to remain. These dysrhythmias may deteriorate into ventricular fibrillation and cardiac arrest.

Treatment of Specific Dysrhythmias

Atrial Fibrillation. The treatment of patients in atrial fibrillation depends on the ventricular rate and its influence on the hemodynamic state and end-organ perfusion. Patients whose condition is unstable are given electrical cardioversion using synchronized sequential countershocks of 100, 200, 300, and 400 joules. Patients in stable condition are treated initially with intravenous digoxin, verapamil, or propranolol to slow the ventricular rate.

Atrial Flutter. Atrial flutter is very sensitive to electrical cardioversion. Synchronized cardioversion at 25 to 50 joules will often convert this dysrhythmia to a sinus rhythm. Alternatively, intravenous digitalis, propranolol, or verapamil may be used to slow the ventricular response and convert the dysrhythmia to a sinus rhythm. Correction of the underlying etiology such as hypoxia should be addressed at the same time.

Multifocal Atrial Tachycardia. Multifocal atrial tachycardias are treated by addressing the underlying medical problems. Improvement of the pulmonary problem or withdrawal of theophylline will generally correct the dysrhythmia.

Premature Atrial Contractions. Premature atrial contractions have no specific treatment. Underlying etiologies such as use of caffeine or theophylline are addressed through patient education.

Ventricular Premature Beats. Ventricular premature beats are addressed by determining their cause and their potential for deteriorating into ventricular tachycardia or ventricular fibrillation. In patients with suspected acute ischemia, VPBs are treated if they (1) are frequent (more than 5/min); (2) show the R wave of the VPB close to the T wave of the underlying rhythm; (3) occur in runs of couplets or triplets; or (4) are multifocal. Treatment with intravenous lidocaine is started with a loading dose of 1 mg/kg and a maintenance dose of 2 mg/min. An underlying cause such as hypoxia or hypokalemia is treated specifically. In patients with VPBs without suspected organic heart disease, further tests to define the nature of the VPBs are indicated. Cardiology consultation and Holter monitoring are appropriate, depending on the clinical setting.

Ventricular Tachycardia. If ventricular dysrhythmias are found, lidocaine is the treatment of choice in the stable patient. DC cardioversion is the treatment of choice for the unstable patient. Figure 11–9 is the specific algorithm recommended by the American Heart Association for the treatment of ventricular tachycardia.

Paroxysmal Supraventricular Tachycardia. If PSVT is present, vagal maneuvers such as carotid sinus massage and the Valsalva maneuver may be employed. If unsuccessful, verapamil or adenosine will usually terminate the dysrhythmia. Adenosine is given as a rapid IV bolus, 6 mg over 2 seconds. If unsuccessful, it may be followed within a few minutes by a 12-mg bolus. Verapamil is given as 5 mg IV and may be repeated in 10 to 15 minutes if there is no response. Verapamil *is avoided* in patients with *wide-complex tachycardias*. Additionally, it is usually avoided in patients who are hypotensive or in congestive heart failure. Alternatively, digoxin may be used if a more gradual slowing of the heart rate is appropriate. Other drugs such as quinidine, procainamide, and propranolol may be employed in selected patients. DC cardioversion with 50 to 100 joules is the treatment of choice in a patient in an unstable or rapidly deteriorating condition.

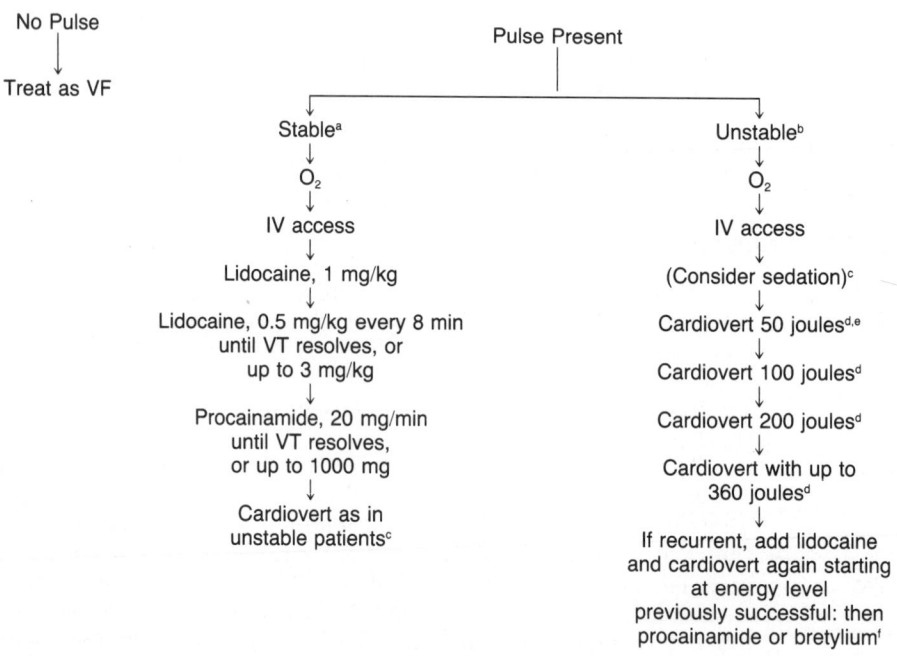

FIGURE 11–9. *This sequence was developed to assist in teaching how to treat a broad range of patients with sustained ventricular tachycardia (VT). Some patients may require care not specified herein. This algorithm should not be construed as prohibiting such flexibility. The flow of the algorithm presumes that VT is continuing. VF indicates ventricular fibrillation; IV, intravenous.*

[a]*If the patient becomes unstable (see footnote b for definition) at any time, move to the "Unstable" arm of the algorithm.*

[b]*Unstable = symptoms (e.g., chest pain, dyspnea), hypotension (systolic blood pressure <90 mm Hg), congestive heart failure, ischemia, or infarction.*

[c]*Sedation should be considered for all patients, including those defined in footnote b as unstable, except those who are hemodynamically unstable (e.g., hypotensive, in pulmonary edema, or unconscious).*

[d]*If hypotension, pulmonary edema, or unconsciousness is present, unsynchronized cardioversion should be done to avoid the delay associated with synchronization.*

[e]*In the absence of hypotension, pulmonary edema, or unconsciousness, a precordial thump may be employed prior to cardioversion.*

[f]*Once VT has resolved, begin an IV infusion of the antiarrhythmic agent that has aided the resolution of the VT. If hypotensive, in pulmonary edema, or unconscious, use lidocaine if cardioversion alone is unsuccessful, followed by bretylium. In all other patients, the recommended order of therapy is lidocaine, procainamide, and then bretylium. (Reproduced with permission. © Textbook of Advanced Life Support, 1987. Copyright American Heart Association.)*

Wide-Complex Tachycardias. Because it is difficult to determine the origin of a dysrhythmia by the ECG, it is important to determine a therapeutic approach that is appropriate for both VT and SVT with aberrant conduction (Fig. 11-10). Lidocaine, procainamide, and bretylium have all been shown to be effective in treating ventricular tachycardia. Choosing a drug for treatment of SVT with aberrant conduction is more difficult if an accessory pathway exists.

Verapamil, digoxin, and lidocaine have been reported to induce hemodynamic deterioration in WPW patients presenting in atrial fibrillation with wide-complex tachycardia. This deterioration has been secondary to the development of ventricular fibrillation or an accelerated ventricular response. That is why this subset of WPW patients with atrial fibrillation presenting as a wide-complex tachycardia is of greatest concern in designing a treatment protocol. Additionally, if verapamil is administered to a patient in ventricular tachycardia that is mistaken for PSVT with aberrant conduction, deterioration may occur.

The drug of choice for patients with stable wide-complex tachycardia is procainamide. If the rhythm is ventricular in origin, procainamide should abolish the rhythm. If the rhythm is SVT with aberrant conduction through an accessory pathway, procainamide will block the accessory pathway, terminating the tachycardia. The efficacy of procainamide in decreasing antegrade and, to a lesser extent, retrograde conduction through the accessory tract has been demonstrated. Additionally, procainamide has not been reported to cause deterioration in a WPW patient who presents in atrial fibrillation with a wide-complex rapid ventricular response.

If the patient's condition is stable, vagal maneuvers such as carotid massage and the Valsalva maneuver might be attempted first. These maneuvers, however, may not be beneficial because they have minimal effect on the accessory pathway. If unsuccessful, pharmacologic intervention can be considered.

If the patient's condition is unstable, as represented by hypotension, angina, decreased mental status, or heart failure, DC cardioversion is indicated. Intravenous diazepam is titrated to sedate the patient before cardioversion is attempted. One regimen is to give 2 mg every 2 minutes until the patient can no longer count backwards by two's. Close monitoring of the patient's hemodynamic and respiratory status is essential.

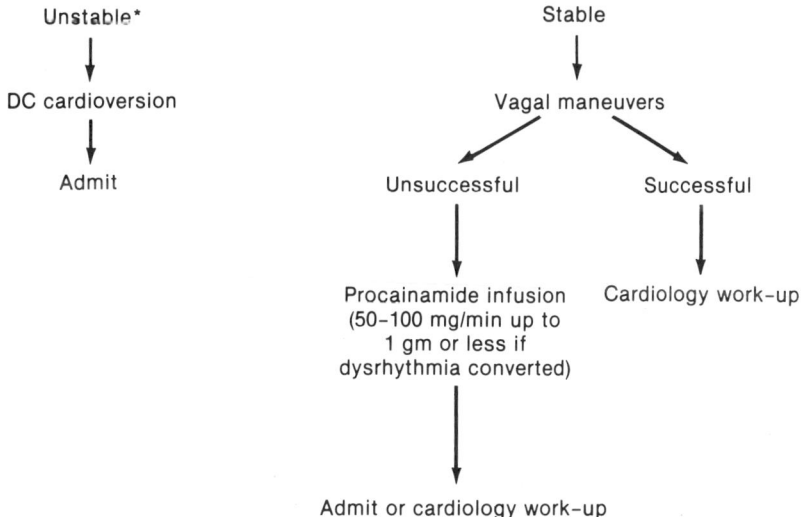

FIGURE 11-10. Therapeutic approach to the patient with a wide-complex tachycardia (unstable or stable). (Unstable is defined by hemodynamic parameters or clinical finding, e.g., chest pain, decreased mentation.)

Treatment of Noncardiac Causes of Dysrhythmias

Management of specific noncardiac causes of dysrhythmias is based on the specific abnormality detected. Drugs or toxins such as caffeine, alcohol, or cocaine are identified and the patient educated about their use. Medications are reevaluated based on their indications and toxicity.

Metabolic problems are specifically addressed. Potassium is slowly replaced while the patient is on an ECG monitor. Oxygen supplementation may be needed to correct hypoxia. Propranolol can control the effects of thyrotoxicosis.

Treatment of Palpitations Without Dysrhythmias

If there is no evidence of dysrhythmia as the cause of palpitations the patient is reassured and referred to his or her primary physician for further work-up. It is possible that the dysrhythmia was not present during the ECG monitoring in the emergency department. If the patient had no symptoms of palpitations while being monitored, it is uncertain whether dysrhythmias were responsible for his previous perception of palpitations. A Holter monitor worn for 24 hours while the patient keeps a diary of symptoms may eliminate the uncertainty.

PROBLEM 1 (To the reader: This portion of the problem points out an error in therapy for teaching purposes.) The 29 year old male was treated with verapamil based on the rhythm strip being interpreted as PSVT. He promptly developed ventricular fibrillation but was successfully defibrillated, and normal sinus rhythm returned.

The 12-lead ECG offers a clue that this rhythm probably is atrial fibrillation in a patient with WPW (irregular R–R intervals with 1:1 conduction, giving a ventricular rate of up to 300) with antegrade conduction down an accessory pathway (a wide QRS complex). This rhythm has been reported to deteriorate with verapamil use. There are two options for treating this rhythm—cardioversion or IV procainamide. Following defibrillation, the patient returned to a sinus rhythm (Fig. 11–11). Note the classic findings for WPW, a wide initial upstroke of the QRS complex (delta wave) and a short P–R interval.

PROBLEM 2 Two treatment modalities are appropriate for this patient. The first is to stop the digoxin. The degree of digoxin toxicity is not severe and requires no additional therapy. The second is to replace the potassium orally.

SPECIAL CONSIDERATIONS

Pediatric Patients

Paroxysmal supraventricular tachycardia is the most common dysrhythmia seen in children. Infants with PSVT may have associated systemic illness, drug toxicity, congenital heart disease, or preexcitation syndromes; however, up to 50% of infants with PSVT have no obvious cause for their dysrhythmias. Older children and teenagers are more likely to have dysrhythmias and palpitations that are due to preexcitation syndromes such as WPW.

The treatment of children with dysrhythmias depends on the adequacy of end-organ perfusion. Patients in unstable condition are immediately given cardioversion with 1 to 2 joules/kg of energy. Patients in stable condition are often treated with digoxin. Verapamil is used less frequently in children because it can cause severe hypotension. Early consultation with a pediatric cardiologist is prudent.

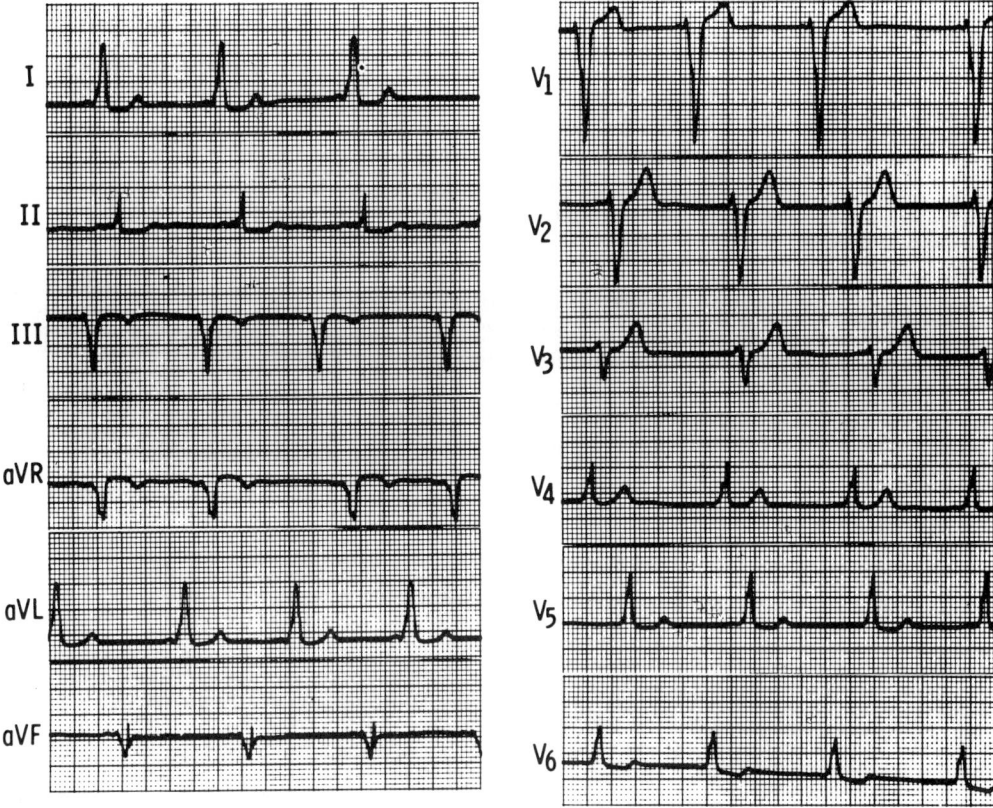

FIGURE 11-11. Wolff-Parkinson-White syndrome (type B). The P-R interval is 0.09 second, whereas the QRS interval is 0.14 second. (Used with permission from Chung EK: Principles of Cardiac Arrhythmias, 4th ed. © 1989, the Williams & Wilkins Co., Baltimore.)

It is important to remember that normal heart rates vary at different ages. Tachycardias are significant according to the following scheme:

- Newborn to 3 months, over 205 beats/min
- 3 months to 2 years, over 190 beats/min
- 2 years to 10 years, over 140 beats/min

Geriatric Patients

Elderly patients are more likely than other patients to have dysrhythmias that are due to serious heart disease. The emergency physician should readily admit elderly patients to a monitored bed in the hospital to investigate coronary artery disease and ventricular dysrhythmias. Cardiac medications such as verapamil are used with caution in the elderly because of their potent effects on hemodynamics as well as the cardiac conduction system.

DISPOSITION AND FOLLOW-UP

Once the patient's condition has been stabilized and the dysrhythmia diagnosed, the question is whether to admit the patient to the hospital. The best way to make this decision is to ask oneself a series of questions illustrating the underlying principles.

1. *Is there severe underlying disease that warrants admission?*

   If the palpitations are due to serious disease or a malignant dysrhythmia, the patient is admitted. Serious diseases include acute myocardial infarction, pulmonary embolus, and significant digoxin toxicity. Malignant dysrhythmias include ventricular tachycardia and frequent or multifocal PVCs that have the potential to deteriorate into ventricular fibrillation. If no serious disease is suspected or demonstrated, the next question is asked.

2. *Was any deterioration of vital signs evident during the evaluation and treatment?*
If the patient had a significant drop in blood pressure, change in mental status, deterioration of rhythm (PSVT to VT), or respiratory arrest, admission is warranted. If the patient remained stable, the next question is asked.

3. *Was the episode of dysrhythmia (if present) sustained or intermittent? Is the patient old or young?*
If the patient is young, admission is rarely needed even if the dysrhythmia was sustained (unless the criteria in questions 1 and 2 are met). In older patients, the tendency is to be conservative and admit the patient. Older patients are often less able to tolerate dysrhythmias and are more likely to have severe underlying disease. Admission is more appropriate for a patient with a sustained dysrhythmia than for a patient with an intermittent one.

4. *Does the patient have a previous history of this presentation, and if so, what was the outcome?*
If the patient previously had severe complications from the dysrhythmia (i.e., MI, cardiac arrest), admission is strongly considered.

If after reviewing these questions it seems that the patient may be sent home, telephone consultation with a cardiologist is prudent. This measure will ensure appropriate follow-up for the patient, and a joint decision can be reached in regard to chronic therapy.

PROBLEM 1 This patient was admitted because of the deterioration in vital signs caused by the verapamil. This particular rhythm (WPW with atrial fibrillation) is associated with a higher incidence of morbidity and mortality than other PSVTs.

PROBLEM 2 In consideration of the patient's age and two ongoing problems (hypokalemia and digoxin toxicity), it is best to admit this patient.

DOCUMENTATION

1. Any previous history of the complaint and what happened previously (complications, treatment, diagnosis)
2. Associated symptoms
3. Cardiopulmonary examination
4. Any deterioration of the patient's condition during the course of evaluation and treatment
5. Medications
6. Laboratory findings, including the ECG and its interpretation
7. Any treatment initiated and the response to that treatment
8. If the patient was not admitted, the kind of follow-up that has been arranged and whether this has been discussed with the follow-up physician

SUMMARY AND FINAL POINTS

- The sensation that physicians term palpitations may be described by a variety of terms by the patient.
- A wide range of underlying causes, from anxiety to acute myocardial infarction, may precipitate palpitations.

- A 12-lead ECG and blood tests may be helpful in determining both the rhythm disturbance if it is present and the cause of the palpitations.
- The patient presenting with a wide-complex tachycardia needs special evaluation and treatment.
- The patient presenting with a wide-complex tachycardia and underlying atrial fibrillation *should not* be treated with *verapamil, digoxin, or lidocaine*.
- Procainamide is the drug of choice for treating wide-complex tachycardia.
- Disposition of patients presenting with palpitations can be based on a series of questions as discussed in the text.

BIBLIOGRAPHY

Texts

1. Goldberger E: Treatment of Cardiac Emergencies (4th ed). St. Louis, C.V. Mosby, 1985.
2. Chou T: Electrocardiography in Clinical Practice (2nd ed). Orlando, Grune & Stratton, 1986.

Journal Articles

1. Levitt MA: Supraventricular tachycardia with aberrant conduction versus ventricular tachycardia: Differentiation and diagnosis. Am J Emerg Med 6:273, 1988.
2. Stewart RB, Brady GH, Green HL: Wide-complex tachycardia: Misdiagnosis and outcome after emergent therapy. Ann Emerg Med 104:766–771, 1986.
3. Wellens HJJ, Bar F, Lie KL: The value of the electrocardiogram in the differential diagnosis of tachycardia with a widened QRS complex. Am J Med 64:27–33, 1978.
4. Wellens HJJ, Bar F, Vanagt E, et al: Medical treatment of ventricular tachycardia: Considerations in the selection of patients for surgical treatment. Am J Cardiol 49:186–193, 1982.
5. Baerman JM, Morady F, DiCarlo LA, et al: Differentiation of ventricular tachycardia from supraventricular tachycardia with aberration: Value of the clinical history. Ann Emerg Med 16:40, 1987.
6. Jacob AS, Nielson DH, Gianelly RE: Fatal ventricular fibrillation following verapamil in Wolff, Parkinson, White syndrome with atrial fibrillation. Ann Emerg Med 14:159–160, 1985.
7. Akhtar M, Gilbert CJ, Shenasa M: Effect of lidocaine on atrioventricular response via the accessory pathway in patients with Wolff, Parkinson, White syndrome. Circulation 63:435, 1981.
8. Wellens HJ: The wide QRS tachycardia (editorial). Ann Intern Med 104:879, 1986.
9. Steinman RT, Herrera C, Schuger CD, et al: Wide QRS tachycardia in the conscious adult. JAMA 261:1013–1016, 1989.
10. Ornato JP, Hallagan LF, Reese WA, et al: Treatment of paroxysmal supraventricular tachycardia in the emergency department by clinical decision analysis. Am J Emerg Med 6:555–560, 1988.
11. DiMarco JP, Miles W, Akhtar M, et al: Adenosine for paroxysmal supraventricular tachycardia. Ann Intern Med 113:104–110, 1990.

CHAPTER 12

SYNCOPE

KYM A. SALNESS, M.D.
ARTHUR B. SANDERS, M.D.

PROBLEM 1 A 17 year old high school athlete who "can't stand the sight of blood" had a "fainting spell" during routine blood drawing. He lost consciousness and had some involuntary muscle contractions of his arms and legs.

PROBLEM 2 An 80 year old man with history of atherosclerotic coronary artery disease collapsed suddenly and lost consciousness while watering his garden.

PROBLEM 3 A 25 year old female medical student collapsed suddenly at home. She had been ill for several days with left lower quadrant abdominal pain.

QUESTIONS TO CONSIDER

1. What is syncope?
2. What potentially life-threatening illnesses are considered in patients presenting with syncope?
3. What immediate diagnostic and therapeutic measures have priority during evaluation of the postsyncope patient?
4. What information is most valuable for establishing the differential diagnosis of syncope?
5. What ancillary tests are useful for evaluating patients with syncope?
6. What are the most common causes of syncope in patients presenting to the emergency department?
7. What are the appropriate management strategies and disposition options for patients with syncope?

INTRODUCTION

Syncope is defined as a brief loss of consciousness characterized by unresponsiveness, loss of postural tone and collapse, with or without minor muscle twitching, with spontaneous recovery. After a brief period of unconsciousness, the patient has a complete recovery of function without a postictal phase. Unfortunately, neither patients nor health care providers consistently adhere to this strict definition. The variability of presentation and imprecise descriptions leave considerable room for confusion and misunderstanding in the diagnosis and discussion of "syncopal episodes." The term *syncope* is only to be used if the description of events is consistent with the above definition.

Consciousness is maintained through activity of the reticular activating system (RAS) in the brain stem. Loss of consciousness is due to injury or disease in the RAS or bilateral cerebral hemispheric dysfunction. The problem may be either a primary neurologic disease or secondary to toxins, inadequate nutrients, or inadequate cerebral blood flow. The primary nutrients for the brain are oxygen and glucose. Cerebral perfusion pressure is determined by the mean arterial pressure minus the intracranial pressure. Neurologic disease or injury can raise the intracranial pressure and compromise cerebral perfusion. More commonly, however, patients with syncope experience a temporary decrease in mean arterial pressure. Arterial pressure is dependent on multiple factors as outlined in Figure 12-1, including cardiac output (CO), peripheral vascular resistance (PVR), heart rate (HR), stroke volume (SV), myocardial contractility, preload, and afterload.

Circumstances that affect any of these hemodynamic parameters can decrease the arterial pressure and cerebral blood flow, causing syncope. If the heart rate is slowed owing to increased vagal tone or heart block, the CO decreases, and arterial pressure falls. Normally, the peripheral vascular resistance increases in an attempt to compensate for the bradycardia and raise the arterial pressure. Hypovolemia decreases the preload, stroke volume, and cardiac output. When a patient who is hypovolemic stands up, he may experience syncope because the CO is not adequate to support a cerebral perfusion pressure necessary to maintain consciousness. In attempting to compensate for hypovolemia the HR and PVR will generally increase.

Syncope is seen relatively frequently in the emergency department. It may be caused by serious illness, e.g., cardiac dysrhythmias, or benign conditions, e.g., a simple faint. In approximately 37% of patients seen in emergency departments following a syncopal episode a vasovagal or psychogenic cause is found. These patients have a benign clinical course even after several years of follow-up. Cardiac syncope occurs in approximately 13% of patients with transient loss of consciousness and heralds a poor long-term prognosis. Approximately 21% to 30% of patients with cardiac syncope will die within 1 year despite medical treatment. In other patients, almost one-fifth have orthostatic hypotension, and up to 42% of patients have no clear cause for the syncope. Patients who have cerebrovascular disease or drug or metabolic causes of syncope have poorer long-term prognoses than the general population.

PREHOSPITAL CARE

Prehospital care providers responding to a syncopal patient may find a range of clinical presentations; the patient may be unresponsive to all stimuli or awake and alert and embarrassed by all the attention. The rescue squad must be prepared to treat the serious, life-threatening conditions that can cause syncope and should obtain the following information.

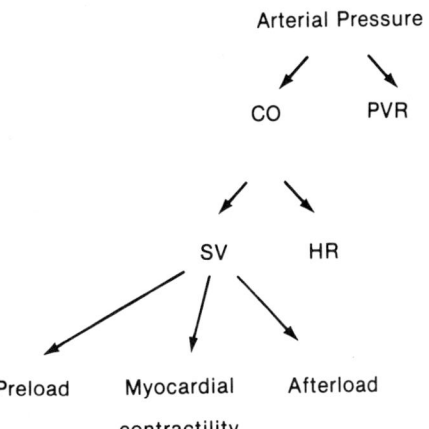

FIGURE 12-1. Components of arterial pressure. CO = cardiac output; PVR = peripheral vascular resistance; SV = stroke volume; HR = heart rate.

History

1. Can the patient or witnesses describe what happened?
2. Was there an inciting event?
3. Has this situation occurred previously?
4. Is the patient now alert and oriented?
5. Is the patient taking medications?
6. Does the patient have specific complaints or injuries related to the syncope?

Physical Examination

1. General appearance—skin color and warmth, mentation, and response to questions
2. Vital signs
3. Airway, breath sounds
4. Gross neurologic function
5. Any sites of injury resulting from syncope

Intervention

1. Oxygen supplement is usually given at 2 to 4 liters/min by nasal cannula.
2. An intravenous catheter is placed for the administration of medications and volume replacement. If dehydration or blood loss is suspected by the history or vital signs, 200 to 300 ml of isotonic crystalloid is rapidly administered and the hydration status reassessed.
3. A cardiac monitor is attached and continuously monitored for dysrhythmias. Symptomatic bradycardias may be treated with atropine. The treatment of tachycardias is discussed in Chapter 11.
4. If there is a decreased level of consciousness, the rescue squad is ordered to draw a clotted tube of blood and administer intravenously the following medications: (a) 100 mg thiamine to treat Wernicke's encephalopathy, which may be provoked by a glucose load; (b) 25 to 50 gm of 50% dextrose to treat hypoglycemia; (c) 2 mg of naloxone to reverse the effects of having taken opiates or some of their derivatives.

PROBLEM 2 The 80 year old man had a blood pressure (BP) of 130/90 mm Hg, pulse 60 beats/min, respirations 16/min. He was alert and responded appropriately to questions. He moved all four extremities. He had no secondary injury.

Because of this patient's age and history of cardiac disease the base station physician was concerned about serious diseases. The patient was placed on oxygen and a cardiac monitor. An IV line with D/W 5% was started in case medications were needed.

PROBLEM 3 The 25 year old female was confused; her skin was cool and gray. Her vital signs were blood pressure of 80/50 mm Hg, pulse 120 beats/min, respirations 20/min. Her boyfriend said that she was a marathon runner and normally had low blood pressure.

Despite the history from the boyfriend, a systolic pressure of 80 mm Hg by palpation and a pulse of 120 beats/min are disturbing. The patient's cool skin and confusion are indications of a shock state. A large-bore IV line with normal saline was started, and the patient was given thiamine, glucose, and naloxone. The rescue squad was ordered to transport this patient as quickly as possible (lights and siren). A rapid crystalloid infusion was ordered while en route.

INITIAL APPROACH IN THE EMERGENCY DEPARTMENT

The initial concern in the emergency department is to stabilize abnormal vital signs and anticipate a recurrence of the syncope.

1. The patency and protection of the airway and breathing are assessed.
2. Measurement of vital signs is repeated and compared with those of the rescue squad.
3. The intravenous line, supplemental oxygen, and cardiac monitor are confirmed or started as necessary.
4. The cardiac monitor is observed for any evidence of dysrhythmias.
5. The rescue squad is asked if thiamine, glucose, and naloxone were given and what was the response. The clotted blood drawn by the rescue squad is secured for later laboratory studies, primarily glucose determination.
6. The physical examination is focused on whether the patient is alert, oriented, and aware of what happened. If the patient remains unresponsive, it is more appropriate to classify the problem as *altered mental status* (see Chap. 45) rather than *syncope*.
7. The patient is asked to move all extremities; signs of asymmetric motor strength that may represent a gross neurologic deficit are sought.
8. The patient is questioned about any injury that may have occurred during the syncopal episode, and a brief physical examination is made of the affected area.

PROBLEM 3 The young woman's mental status did not respond to the thiamine, glucose, and naloxone. She received 300 ml of normal saline during transport, but her vital signs remained BP 80/50 mm Hg, pulse 130 beats/min, respirations 20/min. A second IV line was not started by the rescue squad because of lack of time.

This patient is more likely to be in shock. A second IV line is best started immediately while the emergency physician begins the data-gathering process. Her persistent unresponsive mental status is moving her out of the "pure" syncope category.

This patient must receive an urgent fluid resuscitation while the history and physical examination are being completed. Normal saline at a wide open rate is ordered in each line. Early laboratory studies include hemoglobin/hematocrit and blood type and screen.

DATA GATHERING

History

An accurate history of the event is crucial for determining the appropriate diagnosis. It is often useful to talk to family, friends, or bystanders as well as to the rescue personnel on the scene. It is important to remember that syncope is a dynamic event in which the patient's status is changing frequently.

Precipitating Event. What events immediately preceded the syncopal episode? Did the patient say anything?

1. Was there an *inciting event?* Physical or emotional stress such as a fight or extreme anger are common preceding syncope.
2. Was a *prodrome* experienced by the patient such as pallor, chest or abdominal pain, weakness, confusion, diaphoresis, nausea, or anxiety? Each of these may point to a serious cause of the event.

Position. Was the event preceded by the patient suddenly *assuming* the *upright position?* Was there any *head turning* or *neck pressure?* The first question explores the possible role of postural hypotension, the second the possibility of a hypersensitive carotid sinus or vascular obstruction of one or more vessels supplying the brain.

Situation. Did any activity like urination, defecation, Valsalva maneuver, or hyperventilation occur prior to the syncopal episode? Were there any noxious stimuli?

Review of Systems

1. Is there any reason to suspect *dehydration* or *volume loss?* Dehydration could be caused by strenuous activity, diuretics, gastrointestinal losses, or poor fluid intake.
2. Is there any history suggesting *chronic anemia* or *recent blood loss* (gastrointestinal tract bleeding or excessive menstrual loss)? Is there any possible occult blood loss from obscure but critical sites such as a leaking abdominal aneurysm or ruptured ectopic pregnancy?
3. Was there any *chest pain* or *palpitations?*
4. Did the patient have any *seizure* activity, weakness, or other neurologic symptoms?
5. Could the patient be *pregnant?*
6. Was the fall the *cause* or the *result* of the loss of consciousness? Was there any trauma to the head, chest, abdomen, or extremities?

Past Medical History

1. Has the patient ever *sustained* a *syncopal episode before?*
2. Is there any history of *cardiac disease?* Any history of paroxysmal supraventricular tachycardia (PSVT), heart blocks, ventricular arrhythmias, valvular heart disease, cardiac medications, or prior placement of an external pacemaker?
3. Does the patient have a history of seizures, carotid artery disease, transient cerebral ischemia, or stroke? Is there a history of an abdominal aneurysm?
4. Is there a history of bleeding problems or peptic ulcer disease?
5. Is the patient a diabetic? Insulin dependent? If so, what is the usual dose, when was it last given, and when was the last meal?
6. Since pulmonary embolus can be a cause of syncope, careful inquiries should be made about past pulmonary embolus, venous thrombosis, and leg pain or swelling.

Medications. A review of pertinent medications may be helpful. Quinidine causes syncope in 0.5% of patients taking it. In addition, digoxin, lithium, diuretics, nitroglycerin, propranolol, and other beta blockers can contribute to orthostatic hypotension or syncope. Other intoxicants such as cocaine can cause cardiac dysrhythmias, and alcohol and narcotics produce an altered mental status.

Physical Examination

The goal of the physical examination is to determine whether there are findings that confirm the origin of the patient's syncope and whether injuries resulted from the episode. Specific elements of this examination are listed in Table 12–1.

PROBLEM 1 The 17 year old passed out after having his blood drawn at a student health center. He felt nauseated while the blood was being drawn but did not remember passing out. He had never passed out before and had no medical problems. Findings on physical examination were unremarkable.

In this patient a precipitating event and some nausea occurred prior to syncope. It is important to get an exact description of what happened when he passed out. A call to the phlebotomist at the student health center confirmed some muscle twitching but no tonic-clonic movements. The patient recovered and knew where he was within a minute of falling to the ground.

PROBLEM 2 The 80 year old man was watering his garden. No prodrome or precipitating event occurred. He was unconscious for "a few minutes," according to his wife, and had no muscle movement. He had never fainted before but had had a heart attack 5 years previously. The patient was not orthostatic.

Physical examination revealed a systolic murmur in the aortic and pulmonary area, which radiated to the carotids.

Because there was no prodrome or precipitating event, cardiac etiologies are highly probable in this elderly gentleman. The "heart attack" history and systolic murmur (aortic stenosis?) are supporting evidence.

DECISION PRIORITIES AND PRELIMINARY DIFFERENTIAL DIAGNOSIS

Following the history and physical examination, the emergency physician formulates a preliminary differential diagnosis based on the following questions.

1. *Does the patient have true syncope?*
   Syncope is often confused with other conditions like dizziness, weakness, vertigo, "faintness" or "lightheadedness," transient confusion, or inability to stand. Occasionally stroke, coma, transient cerebral ischemia, or seizures are labeled syncope. Furthermore, some patients with incomplete loss of consciousness, altered mental status, or loss of postural tone are described as having "presyncope." The history of a transient loss of consciousness with sudden collapse and spontaneous recovery is important for a diagnosis of true syncope.

TABLE 12–1. Directed Physical Examination in Patients with Syncope

Area of Examination	Important Findings	Significance
Vital signs	Pulse—rate and regularity	Atrial or ventricular tachycardias (pulse > 100/min). Heart blocks can cause bradycardias and syncope. Irregular pulse may indicate premature contraction or heart blocks
	Blood pressure, orthostatic pressure, and pulse	Shock from any cause can decrease cerebral blood flow and cause syncope. Orthostatic pressure and pulse may indicate hypovolemic cause
	Respiratory rate	Tachypnea may indicate hypoxia or pulmonary embolus
	Temperature	Fever may indicate sepsis
General appearance	Responsiveness, skin color, diaphoresis	Signs of decreased organ perfusion
Head, eyes, ears, nose, throat	Point tenderness or ecchymosis	May indicate trauma from fall
	Funduscopic examination, papilledema	Increased intracranial pressure, diabetic retinopathy, retinal hemorrhages from CNS bleeding
	Breath, oral mucosa	Ketones from ingestion, ketoacidosis, or dehydration
Neck	Tenderness, carotid bruits	Cervical spine trauma, source of cerebral emboli
Lungs	Percussion, auscultation: consolidation, decreased breath sounds, rales, wheezing	Hypoxia due to pulmonary embolus, infection, bronchospasm, or congestive heart failure
Cardiac system	Systolic ejection murmur, particularly changing with the Valsalva maneuver; gallop, rub, prosthetic valves	Aortic stenosis murmur decreases and IHSS murmur increases with Valsalva maneuver; new murmur
Abdomen and rectum	Pulsatile masses, peritoneal signs, stool hemotest	Abdominal aneurysm, intra-abdominal catastrophe, gastrointestinal bleeding
Pelvis	Uterine bleeding, tenderness, adnexal mass	Ectopic pregnancy, pelvic infection
Extremities	Cyanosis, pallor, capillary refill, leg pain, swelling	Evidence of peripheral perfusion and deep vein thrombophlebitis
Neurologic	Cranial nerves, motor, sensation, reflexes, mental status	Focal neurologic signs may indicate intracranial process or primary neurologic disease

2. *Did a life-threatening event cause the syncope? Is it ongoing?*
   The patient's vital signs and the cardiac monitor will generally indicate any immediate threats. Specific diseases to be considered first include:
   a. Cardiac dysrhythmia with hypotension. Vital signs, chest pain, level of mentation, and the cardiac monitor may indicate a dysrhythmia that must be immediately treated.
   b. Acute blood loss. The patient will often exhibit orthostatic hypotension and be pale and cold ("shocky"). The physical examination usually indicates the source of blood loss, such as abdominal pain or vaginal bleeding.
   c. Hypoxia. An acute pulmonary event such as a pulmonary embolus may cause syncope. Stress or exercise may also cause syncope if the patient has a limited physiologic ability to respond, e.g., if the patient has idiopathic hypertrophic subaortic stenosis (IHSS).
   d. Hypoglycemia. The patient usually has a history of diabetes mellitus and responds to an infusion of 50% dextrose.
3. *If there is no immediate life-threatening process, what organ systems are likely to be involved?*
   The major systems to be assessed are the cardiovascular, neurologic, metabolic, and psychologic systems (Table 12–2). Most of these patients have cardiovascular problems that cause decreased blood flow to the reticular activating system. Primary neurologic diseases are the next most common cause. Metabolic abnormalities or psychological problems are also significant causes of syncope. A specific cause of syncope is not determined even after a full hospital or outpatient evaluation in about 20% of patients.

DIAGNOSTIC ADJUNCTS

Routine screening laboratory tests, radiographs, and electrocardiograms performed on *all* patients with temporary loss of consciousness or syncope yield few results and are *not cost-effective*. A young person with a simple faint precipitated by a plausible situation who is now fully recovered may not benefit from any additional tests. Diagnostic adjuncts are considered in all older patients and in those younger patients in whom the cause is unclear.

TABLE 12–2. Etiology of Syncope and Temporary Loss of Consciousness

Cardiovascular System	**Situational Syncope**
Vasovagal faint	Micturition, defecation, cough, Valsalva maneuver
Cardiopulmonary	**Pregnancy**
Aortic stenosis	Anemia, hemodynamic predisposition to faint
Myocardial infarction	Ruptured ectopic pregnancy (blood loss)
Dysrhythmias	**Neurologic System**
(rapid: PSVT or ventricular tachycardia)	Transient ischemic attack
(slow: sick sinus syndrome, AV blocks)	Stroke (completed or stroke in evolution)
Pericardial tamponade, pericarditis	Seizures
Faulty prosthetic valve	Occult head trauma
Pacemaker failure	**Metabolic**
Pulmonary embolus	Intoxication
Carotid sinus hypersensitivity	Alcohol, sedative hypnotics, opiates
Orthostatic hypotension	Medications
Medications	Cardiac, hypertensive drugs
Chronic illness	**Psychological**
Autonomic neuropathy	Hysterical
Volume loss	**Uncertain Etiology**
Sudden massive occult blood loss	
Leaking abdominal aneurysm	
Ruptured ectopic pregnancy	

PSVT = paroxysmal supraventricular tachycardia.

Laboratory Studies

1. Hematocrit–hemoglobin is ordered for patients in whom anemia or active blood loss is suspected by the history and physical examination. Measurements may be repeated if blood loss continues.
2. Blood type and cross-match are obtained for patients who are orthostatic, hypotensive, or if massive blood loss is suspected, as in patients with ectopic pregnancy or leaking abdominal aneurysm.
3. Electrolytes are obtained in patients taking diuretics or when severe dehydration is suspected based on orthostatic measurements and clinical history.
4. Glucose concentration is checked in all patients with persistently altered mental status prior to administration of glucose.
5. Arterial blood gases are obtained in patients who have unexplained pleuritic chest pain, shortness of breath, or tachypnea associated with syncope.
6. A pregnancy test may be needed, since ectopic pregnancy must be considered in all women of childbearing age with syncope.

Electrocardiogram (ECG)

All patients with unexplained syncope and possible cardiovascular disease receive a 12-lead ECG and cardiac monitoring.

Radiologic Imaging

Computer tomography (CT) of the head is indicated for patients with focal neurologic signs, unexplained seizures, suspected stroke, or persistently altered mental status postsyncope.

Special Tests

Holter Monitor. A Holter monitor may provide useful information in patients who are discharged from the hospital but need to have additional ECG recordings made during their normal activity at home. The ECG monitor is attached to the patient and worn for 24 hours while the patient keeps a diary of all symptoms and activities. Subsequently the ECG record is analyzed for dysrhythmias and correlated with symptoms.

Electroencephalogram (EEG). Routine EEG testing for all syncopal patients is unnecessary. It is performed in patients in whom seizure is the most likely cause of syncope, and in those difficult patients with no other likely cause of syncope in whom an occult seizure disorder is being ruled out. It is a test seldom performed in the emergency department.

PROBLEM 1 No ancillary tests were ordered on the 17 year old. He was observed in the emergency department. His history was consistent with true syncope. There did not seem to be any life-threatening causes, and a reasonable explanation for his "spell" was apparent.

PROBLEM 2 The ECG on the 80 year old man showed nonspecific ST–T-wave changes. The cardiac monitor picked up occasional evidence of premature ventricular contractions (PVCs). A complete blood count (CBC), electrolytes, and glucose concentration were normal.

The etiology of syncope remains elusive in this patient. The knowledge that he is a patient with cardiovascular risk factors is very worrisome.

PROBLEM 3 The 25 year old medical student felt much better after receiving 2 liters of isotonic crystalloid. Her BP was 110/70 mm Hg, pulse 100 beats/min, respirations 16/min. She said she had not been eating well but would improve her diet after this episode. She was eager to return home so she could study for an exam.

This patient was resuscitated with isotonic crystalloid, but the cause of her hypovolemia remained unclear. Attributing it to her poor appetite is a diagnosis of exclusion. The emergency physician insisted on performing laboratory tests. A CBC, electrolytes, glucose, and urine pregnancy test are ordered. A blood type and cross-match are requested on this patient with unexplained shock presenting as syncope.

REFINED DIFFERENTIAL DIAGNOSIS

The history, physical examination, and ancillary tests support a definitive diagnosis in most patients presenting with syncope. Table 12–3 reviews the common causes of syncope. These include vasovagal faint, cardiac dysrhythmias, orthostatic hypotension, seizures, situational syncope, primary neurologic diseases, and metabolic abnormalities.

Vasovagal Faint

The *vasovagal faint* is the most common cause of syncope in patients under age 40. Less frequently, fainting may occur in older patients and pregnant women. It is caused by sudden vagal stimulation accompanied by a failure of sympathetic nerve response. Accordingly, when such a patient has collapsed and is unconscious on the ground, the pulse rate is usually slow at 40 to 60 beats/min, and blood pressure is low at approximately 60 to 80 mm Hg systolic.

Given the right set of circumstances, almost anyone can experience a fainting episode. Predisposing conditions associated with a vasovagal faint are hunger, exhaustion, alcohol, a stuffy, closed warm room, strong smells, or noxious sensory input. Noxious stimulation includes any unpleasant physical or psychological event. Additionally, medical

TABLE 12–3. Common Causes of Syncope

Disease Entity	History	Physical	Ancillary Tests	Comments
Vasovagal faint	Past fainting history; predictable stimulus; sudden collapse with complete recovery	Young, healthy. Immediate recovery after event: low BP, slow pulse, then normal examination results	Unremarkable	Young, healthy, rapid return to normal
Orthostatic hypotension	Past illness, prolonged bed rest, dehydration, medications. Sudden upright position associated with collapse	May be unremarkable except for postural changes in vital signs.	Orthostatic changes in BP and heart rate	Check for dehydration or sudden blood loss; review medications
Cardiac dysrhythmias	Past medical history: Cardiac history, sudden collapse, older patient, may be associated with chest pain	May be within normal limits or may have irregular heart rate	Monitor rhythm, ECG, rule out MI. Outpatient Holter monitor helpful	Older patients with cardiac history have serious 1-yr mortality with syncope. Admit patient with pacemaker and syncope
Situational syncope	May have had similar prior experience. Sudden collapse. History of Valsalva or micturition, or cough	May be within normal limits	Not generally helpful. Results of carotid sinus massage may be dramatic	Be careful with carotid massage
Seizure	Usually positive past history; loss of bladder control, tongue biting, generalized convulsion	Postictal state is common postevent; otherwise may be within normal limits	EEG may be helpful	In simple syncope, motor activity is usually not generalized and is not accompanied by tongue biting or loss of bladder control
Metabolic abnormality	Usually *not* sudden collapse with complete recovery as in true syncope	Generalized weakness, associated confusion	Serum glucose, hematocrit	Most often related to glucose abnormality or exogenous toxins
Primary neurologic disease	Older patients, atherosclerosis or hypertensive vascular disease	Fixed or transient neurological deficit. BP elevated	CT scan of head may be positive	Rarely is simple true syncope associated with a neurologic deficit

conditions such as anemia, dehydration, certain medications (vasodilators), and electrolyte abnormalities may predispose patients to a vasovagal faint.

Many patients who faint experience a prodrome lasting a few moments before actually collapsing. The patient is aware of feeling very uncomfortable and often complains of being warm and diaphoretic, lightheaded, or nauseated. The patient may be confused just prior to collapsing and may try to sit or lie down. This frequently results in an unprotected fall and possible injury. While lying on the ground unconscious, the patient may exhibit eye rolling, lip smacking, a few generalized muscle spasms, or tonic movement. Very rarely urinary incontinence, tongue biting, or true tonic-clonic movements occur. The faint is rapidly resolved within 1 or 2 minutes as the cardiac output increases while the patient is lying in a horizontal position. There is no postictal state, and the patient becomes alert and responsive. The rate of the resolution may vary because of age, the continued presence of noxious stimuli, and possible injury from the fall.

Cardiac Syncope

Cardiac causes of syncope frequently have a serious predisposing cause and a worse prognosis than vasovagal faint. Valvular heart disease such as aortic stenosis or idiopathic hypertrophic subaortic stenosis (IHSS) can be associated with syncope. Exertional syncope in a patient with undiagnosed aortic stenosis or IHSS is a serious herald of critical outflow obstruction and perhaps coronary artery hypoperfusion. The classic systolic murmur heard at the base of a hypertrophic dynamic heart may be the only finding.

As many as 10% of patients with *acute myocardial infarction* will have syncope. In some patients syncope is related to ventricular dysrhythmias and in others to sudden uncompensated changes in cardiac output. A careful history and the ECG record is necessary in making the diagnosis.

A number of cardiac conduction disorders can cause an abrupt fall in cardiac output and subsequent syncope. Many of these are associated with atherosclerotic coronary artery disease (ASCAD) and acute ischemia or chronic degeneration of the conduction system. Conduction disorders are manifest as heart blocks at the sinoatrial (SA) node (sick sinus syndrome), atrioventricular (AV) node (second- or third-degree block), or bundle of His (fascicular block). Tachycardias such as ventricular tachycardia or supraventricular tachycardia can also decrease cardiac output and lead to syncope (see Chap. 11).

The sick sinus (bradytachy) syndrome is characterized by abnormal sinoatrial function causing episodes of bradycardia as well as tachycardia. The bradycardias can consist of sinus rhythm, usually less than 50 beats/min, or sinus arrest with junctional escape beats. Syncopal episodes occur most frequently during bradycardia. Sick sinus syndrome can be caused by degeneration of the sinus node, atherosclerotic heart disease, rheumatic heart disease, cardiomyopathy, or congenital abnormalities of the conduction system. It has also been associated with a previous diphtheria infection. Electrophysiologic studies can help to define the sick sinus syndrome if the diagnosis is uncertain.

Atrioventricular blocks are seen in approximately 11% of patients with cardiac syncope. First-degree heart block, a prolongation of the P–R interval, indicates disease in the AV conduction system but by itself should not be associated with syncope (Fig. 12–2).

In second-degree heart block some supraventricular impulses are conducted to the ventricles while others are not. In Mobitz type I block, the P–R interval increases until a P wave is not conducted (Fig. 12–3). It is associated with myocardial infarction, digitalis toxicity, and increased vagal tone. Type I block generally has a benign prognosis and is not usually the cause of syncope. Mobitz type II block is characterized by a fixed P–R interval with dropped beats in a regular or irregular pattern (Fig. 12–4). Type II block can cause significant hemodynamic compromise and syncope. Causes include myocardial infarction, myocarditis, and degenerative disease of the conduction system.

Third-degree heart block is marked by complete AV dissociation (Fig. 12–5). Causes

FIRST-DEGREE ATRIOVENTRICULAR BLOCK

Diagnostic Criteria	Causes
Rate: 60–100/min *Rhythm:* regular *P wave:* normal *P:QRS:* 1:1; PR interval is >0.20 sec	Coronary artery disease, digoxin, rheumatic fever, congenital conditions

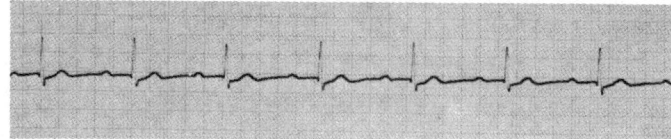

First-degree atrioventricular block

FIGURE 12–2. First-degree atrioventricular block. (From Eisenberg MS, Cummins RO, Ho MT (eds): Code Blue: Cardiac Arrest and Resuscitation. Philadelphia, W.B. Saunders, 1987.)

include acute myocardial infarction, digitalis toxicity, congenital anomalies, and degenerative disease of the conduction system. Third-degree heart block can lead to significant hemodynamic compromise and syncope.

Fascicular blocks are another important consideration in cardiac causes of syncope. The bundle of His bifurcates into right and left bundle branches. The left bundle is thought to further divide into anterior and posterior fascicles. Thus three fascicles transmit impulses to the ventricles. There is concern that patients with syncope who demonstrate bifascicular disease on ECG may be predisposed to complete heart block. Patients with left bundle branch block or right bundle branch block with left anterior hemiblock have bifascicular blocks. These patients need continued cardiac monitoring and electrophysiologic studies to define their conduction disease and subsequent treatment.

A number of cardiac medications can lead to serious toxicity and may cause conduction

SECOND-DEGREE ATRIOVENTRICULAR BLOCK, MOBITZ TYPE I (WENCKEBACH)

Diagnostic Criteria	Causes
Rate: atrial rate is greater than ventricular rate *Rhythm:* atrial rhythm is regular; ventricular rhythm is irregular *P wave:* normal *P:QRS:* PR interval becomes progressively lengthened until a QRS is dropped; PP interval remains constant	Myocardial infarction, rheumatic fever, digitalis toxicity

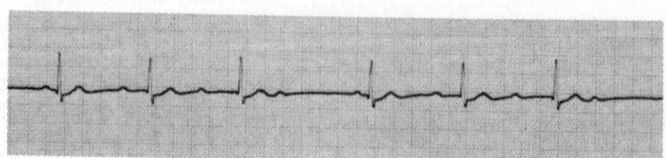

Second-degree atrioventricular block, Mobitz Type I (Wenckebach)

FIGURE 12–3. Second-degree atrioventricular block, Mobitz type I (Wenckebach). (From Eisenberg MS, Cummins RO, Ho MT (eds): Code Blue: Cardiac Arrest and Resuscitation. Philadelphia, W.B. Saunders, 1987.)

SECOND-DEGREE ATRIOVENTRICULAR BLOCK, MOBITZ TYPE II

Diagnostic Criteria	Causes
Rate: atrial rate is greater than ventricular rate *Rhythm:* atrial rate is regular; ventricular rate may be regular or irregular *P wave:* normal; PR interval is normal, and QRS usually shows bundle branch block *P:QRS:* ratio may be 2:1, 3:1, 4:1, or 3:2; ratio may vary over time; ratios of 2:1 are difficult to distinguish from Mobitz Type I; if in doubt, treat as Mobitz Type II	Myocardial infarction, digitalis toxicity

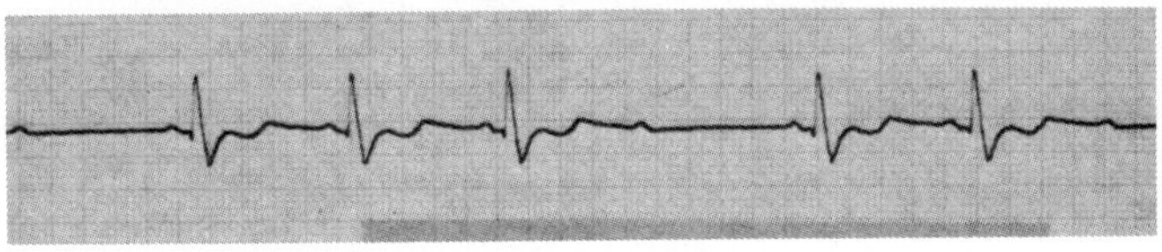

Second-degree atrioventricular block, Mobitz Type II

FIGURE 12–4. *Second-degree atrioventricular block, Mobitz type II. (From Eisenberg MS, Cummins RO, Ho MT (eds): Code Blue: Cardiac Arrest and Resuscitation. Philadelphia, W.B. Saunders, 1987.)*

disturbances and syncope. Digoxin toxicity can result in sinus node stimulation with the AV node conduction delay resulting in paroxysmal supraventricular tachycardia (PSVT) with block. Quinidine can cause conduction delays marked by Q–T prolongation and eventually bizarre ventricular dysrhythmias. Calcium channel blockers and beta blockers can cause conduction delays and bradydysrhythmias.

THIRD-DEGREE ATRIOVENTRICULAR BLOCK, COMPLETE HEART BLOCK

Diagnostic Criteria	Causes
Rate: atrial rate is greater than ventricular rate *Rhythm:* atrial rate is 60–100/min; ventricular rate is 40–60/min if junctional escape beats occur; ventricular rate is 20–40/min if ventricular rate escape beats occur *P wave:* normal *P:QRS:* no relationship; atria and ventricles are independently contracting *QRS:* normal if junction escape beats occur; >0.11 sec if ventricular escape beats occur	Coronary heart disease, myocardial infarction, myocarditis, drug toxicity (digitalis, procainamide, quinidine, verapamil)

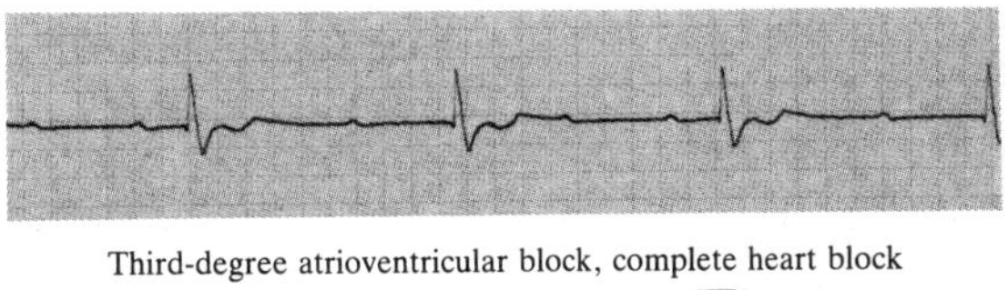

Third-degree atrioventricular block, complete heart block

FIGURE 12–5. *Third-degree atrioventricular block, complete heart block. (From Eisenberg MS, Cummins RO, Ho MT (eds): Code Blue: Cardiac Arrest and Resuscitation. Philadelphia, W.B. Saunders, 1987.)*

Orthostatic Hypotension

A fall in blood pressure after a quick change in position from lying to standing is a frequent cause of syncope or near syncope. The causes of orthostatic hypotension include prolonged inactivity and bed rest, medications (vasodilators, antihypertensive drugs), central nervous system disorders (Parkinson's disease), and autonomic neuropathies (chronic alcoholism and diabetes). Other causes of orthostatic hypotension include acute blood loss and dehydration due to diuretics, poor oral intake, excess sweating, or gastrointestinal loss.

Situational Syncope

Situational syncope may occur under specific circumstances. It has been described following micturition, defecation, cough, and the Valsalva maneuver. The inciting event produces vagal stimulation and bradycardia without immediate sympathetic stimulation, resulting in transient loss of consciousness.

Seizures can cause a temporary loss of consciousness. The patient is frequently seen in a postictal state, which gradually resolves. The work-up and management of seizures in the emergency department are discussed in Chapter 48.

Metabolic Abnormalities

Metabolic abnormalities such as hypoxia, hypoglycemia, and hyponatremia can be associated with syncope. Generalized weakness and confusion often accompany these conditions.

Neurologic Diseases

Primary neurologic diseases such as stroke can produce syncope. These are often accompanied by focal neurologic deficits and are discussed further in Chapter 49.

PROBLEM 2 The patient's history was highly suspicious for syncope of cardiac origin, vasovagal faint, or situational syncope. His past cardiac history, abnormal ECG results, and the aortic murmur heard on the physical examination indicate significant valvular and coronary artery disease.

PROBLEM 3 The medical student's response to volume replacement is indicative of volume loss. The question remains as to the site and source of loss.

PRINCIPLES OF MANAGEMENT

Management of the patient with syncope is based on the following general principles:
1. Reversible causes of syncope are immediately addressed.
2. Recurrences or complications are anticipated.
3. Specific etiologies of syncope are addressed.

As discussed previously, airway and breathing are assessed, and supplemental oxygen is provided. Circulation is maintained with IV isotonic crystalloid. An ECG monitor is placed, and dysrhythmias are promptly treated. Thiamine, glucose, and naloxone are given if the patient does not have a normal level of consciousness when initially seen.

Vasovagal Faint

Patients who clearly have had a simple vasovagal faint are observed for 1 to 2 hours, rechecking the vital signs including orthostatic measurements and observing the cardiac rhythm. No specific treatment is required other than reassurance and patient education.

Cardiac Dysrhythmias

Tachycardias. Patients with ventricular tachycardia or ventricular fibrillation require defibrillation, intravenous lidocaine, and additional medication as necessary to control their dysrhythmias (see Chap. 11). These patients may have an irritable cardiac focus due to acute ischemia, ventricular aneurysm, electrolyte imbalance, or digoxin toxicity.

Bradycardia. Patients with a bradycardic dysrhythmia usually have serious disease in the conduction system or acute or cardiac medication toxicity. If they are symptomatic these patients may be treated with intravenous atropine. If atropine is unsuccessful in decreasing the symptoms, a transcutaneous or transvenous pacemaker is indicated. Isoproterenol has been used temporarily if a pacemaker cannot be promptly inserted.

Orthostatic Hypotension

Patients presenting with syncope due to orthostatic hypotension are rehydrated with normal saline until the symptoms and orthostasis improve. A search for the source of volume depletion is mandatory. If blood loss is the cause of orthostasis, blood transfusion and surgical consultation must be considered depending on the cause of the bleeding. Some patients with chronic illness and multiple medications will have orthostatic hypotension and syncope after rapidly rising from the horizontal position. These patients may only need reassurance and education.

Other Causes

Situational syncope requires no specific emergency department treatment. Patients are educated about the inciting events. Metabolic abnormalities are treated according to the laboratory test results. Patients with seizures and primary neurologic diseases are treated for specific entities in conjunction with neurologic consultants (see Chaps. 48 and 49).

PROBLEM 3 While waiting for the laboratory test results to come back, the 25 year old female became lethargic. Repeat BP was 70/40 mm Hg, pulse 140 beats/min, respirations 24/min. Her extremities were cold and clammy, and the left lower quadrant pain had returned.

Fluid resuscitation was begun a second time. Blood was drawn for type and cross-match. Because of her age and abdominal pain, the emergency physician suspected ectopic pregnancy. The laboratory was called and asked to complete the pregnancy tests urgently. The obstetric consultant was called to see the patient for immediate operative intervention. The patient was taken to the operating room, where an ectopic pregnancy was found and removed. Eight hundred milliliters of blood was in her peritoneal cavity.

This patient's course could have been disastrous. Her initial hemodynamic response to fluids was misleading. A pregnancy test and type and cross-match should have been ordered as part of the initial evaluation.

SPECIAL CONSIDERATIONS

Pediatric Patients

The most common causes of syncope in children are vasovagal episodes, orthostatic hypotension, and breath-holding spells. Cardiovascular disease is much less common than in adults; when present, it is frequently associated with congenital heart disease such as aortic or pulmonic stenosis, tetralogy of Fallot, or pulmonary hypertension. It is sometimes difficult to distinguish true syncope from seizures. The clinical history, postictal state, and associated signs and symptoms such as incontinence and tongue biting may help the clinician to make the appropriate diagnosis. Children with syncope should be scheduled for follow-up visits to a pediatrician.

Geriatric Patients

A substantial percentage of patients with true syncope in the geriatric age group will be found to have a serious and potentially fatal cause for the disorder. These causes include acute myocardial infarction, bradydysrhythmias or tachyarrhythmias, cerebrovascular accident, or serious blood loss.

Geriatric patients presenting with apparent orthostatic syncope often require an extensive evaluation. This finding is noted in up to 20% of patients over 65 years of age. These patients may be taking a number of medications capable of causing syncope, e.g., beta blockers, calcium channel blockers, or diuretics. Assessment of these patients may be complicated by poor history, mild dehydration, autonomic nervous system dysfunction, and recent prolonged bed rest. Hypertension is a known risk factor.

Testing for orthostatic hypotension is done carefully. In this age group, a reduction of 20 mm Hg or more in the systolic blood pressure within 3 minutes of standing up is a significant risk for falls and syncope. Also, minimal cardioacceleration (< 10 beats/min) with hypotension suggests an impaired baroreceptor reflex or cardiac response.

Geriatric patients need to be carefully evaluated for serious causes and sequelae of syncope. They need to be observed, educated, and protected so that they do not sustain a secondary injury related to orthostatic hypotension and syncope.

DISPOSITION AND FOLLOW-UP

Admission

The disposition of patients with syncope depends on the presumed etiology. Patients with the following etiologies are admitted to the hospital.

Cardiac Disorders. Patients with syncope due to cardiac causes have a 21% to 30% 1-year mortality. Therefore, admission to a cardiac-monitored bed is mandatory. These patients include those with ventricular tachycardia, second- or third-degree heart block, bifascicular conduction defects, or PSVT with hypotension. Some of these patients require sophisticated diagnostic testing procedures in the coronary catheterization or electrophysiology laboratory to precisely determine the dysrhythmia.

Patients with a pacemaker who present with syncope are admitted to the hospital even if their pacemaker appears to be functioning adequately. In many of these patients a malfunction of the pacemaker, the battery, or at the electrode-cardiac muscle implant site may be beginning. Although they now appear stable, their syncopal episode may herald pacemaker malfunction.

Patients with newly diagnosed aortic stenosis causing syncope are admitted for monitoring, catheterization, and valvular intervention. Other patients with a known prosthetic valve who have a new or changed murmur or any evidence suggesting valvular malfunction require admission to the hospital with cardiothoracic consultation to consider prosthetic valve replacement.

Orthostatic Hypotension. Patients with syncope due to acute blood loss need urgent volume and blood resuscitation, surgical consultation, and admission to the hospital.

Situational Syncope. The unusual patient who is found to have *new* onset of situational syncope, such as micturition, defecation, or cough syncope, may benefit from admission to rule out other serious diseases.

Drugs. Patients with syncope that is attributed to medications need a review of their medication dose and indications by their primary care physician. Most patients with medication-induced syncope are admitted and observed in the hospital.

Discharge

Patients may be discharged from the emergency department under the following circumstances:

Vasovagal Faint. The young person with a simple, clear, vasovagal faint can be discharged after a brief period of observation. The patient is educated to avoid inciting stimuli and to take appropriate precautions when the prodrome occurs.

Cardiac Etiology. An exception to the rule to admit all syncopal patients with cardiac causes is the young patient with previously known, predictable, and controllable PSVT. If the dysrhythmia is easily converted and the patient has not been hypotensive or experienced chest pain, discharge with close follow-up by a primary physician is appropriate (see Chap. 11).

Orthostatic Hypotension. Dehydrated patients are rehydrated and sent home. Specific treatment is given for the cause of the dehydration such as diarrhea and vomiting. On discharge, the patient should be able to tolerate oral fluids.

Situational Syncope. If situational syncope has been previously diagnosed and other causes of syncope have been ruled out, the patient is discharged with suggestions for altering behavior to minimize future risk; follow-up arrangements are made with the primary care physician.

Drugs. Patients found to be intoxicated by alcohol are observed until their mental status is normal. They are examined and, if no serious problems are found, discharged. Care is taken to ensure that no other drugs have been ingested. Other, more serious intoxications (i.e., tricyclic antidepressants or opiates) will require specific and supportive therapy (see Chap. 19).

Uncertain Etiology

In a substantial number of patients the precise diagnosis or etiology is not clear in the emergency department. For this group of patients, hospitalization is considered under the following circumstances:

1. Elderly patients. Mortality for syncope increases for patients over 70 years of age.
2. Patients with demonstrated or suspected heart disease.
3. Patients who have an abrupt onset of syncope without prodrome (consistent with a dysrhythmia).
4. Patients who fall and sustain a significant injury.

In approximately 40% of patients presenting with syncope a clear etiology is not identified even after extensive inpatient evaluation. If the patient is under 70 years of age, the long-term prognosis for these patients is no different from that in the general population.

PROBLEM 1 The patient was observed for 1 hour, during which repeated examinations and vital signs were normal. He was discharged and advised about precautions to be taken when inciting events occur.

PROBLEM 2 The patient was admitted to a monitored bed to be observed for dysrhythmias. Work-up during hospitalization revealed the presence of hemodynamically significant aortic stenosis and coronary artery disease.

DOCUMENTATION

1. Precise description of the event including prodrome, precipitating situation, and recovery period.
2. Past cardiac or neurologic problems. Prior syncope?
3. Medications, drugs, intoxicants taken.

4. Examination: (a) General examination results: stable or unstable condition; (b) obvious blood loss if present; (c) vital signs; (d) results of a careful cardiac and neurologic examination.
5. Interpretation of ECG and cardiac monitor.
6. Laboratory studies.
7. Results of repeated cardiac, neurologic.
8. Any response to interventions (glucose, naloxone).
9. Assessment—likely diagnosis; how were serious diseases ruled out?
10. Follow-up arranged and, if patient is not admitted, document who patient is leaving with.

SUMMARY AND FINAL POINTS

- Syncope is defined as a transient loss of consciousness characterized by unresponsiveness and loss of postural tone with spontaneous recovery.
- The most common cause of true syncope in young people is a simple vasovagal faint. An appropriate predisposition, inciting event, and stressful environment are usually present.
- In as many as 40% of patients a precise diagnosis of the etiology of the syncopal episode will never be made.
- In approximately 13% of patients with syncope there is a cardiac cause. The 12 year mortality for this group is 21% to 30%.
- Older patients with syncope are assumed to have serious dysrhythmias until proved otherwise.
- Syncope may present as an injury. Patients are questioned closely about the cause of falls, and secondary problems are actively sought in patients after a syncopal episode.

BIBLIOGRAPHY

Texts

1. Eagle KA, Haber E, DeSanctis RW, et al (eds): The Practice of Cardiology (2nd ed). Boston, Little, Brown, 1989.

Journal Articles

1. Lee RT, Cook EF, Day SC, et al: Long-term survival after transient loss of consciousness. J Ger Intern Med 3:337–343, 1988.
2. Kapoor WN, Karpf M, Maher Y, et al: Syncope of unknown origin. The far more cost-effective approach to the diagnostic evaluation. JAMA 247:2687–2691, 1982.
3. Day SC, Cook EF, Funkenstein H, et al: Evaluation and outcome of emergency room patients with transient loss of consciousness. Am J Med 72:15–23, 1982.
4. DiCarlo LA, Jr, Morady F: Evaluation of the patient with syncope. Cardiol Clin 3(4):499–514, 1985.
5. Dohrmann ML, Cheitlin MD. Cardiogenic syncope. Seizure versus syncope. Neurolog Clin 4(3):549–562, 1986.
6. Eagle KA, Black HSR, Cook EF, et al: Evaluation of prognostic classification for patients with syncope. Am J Med 79:455–460, 1985.
7. Kapoor WN, Karpf M, Wieand S, et al: A prospective evaluation and follow-up of patients with syncope. N Engl J Med 309:197–204, 1983.
8. Linzer M: Syncope. South Med J 80(5):545–553, 1987.
9. Lipsitz LA: Orthostatic hypotension in the elderly. N Engl J Med 321:952–956, 1989.
10. Martin GJ, Adams SL, Martin HG, et al: Prospective evaluation of syncope. Ann Emerg Med 13:21–26, 1984.
11. Morady F: The evaluation of syncope with electrophysiologic studies. Cardiol Clin 4(3):515–526, 1986.

CHAPTER 13

HYPERTENSION

RONALD B. LOW, M.D.

PROBLEM 1 A 55 year old obese woman complained of dyspnea, malaise, and vague chest and back pain. Her symptoms began 20 minutes earlier and became progressively worse. Vital signs were blood pressure 230/150 mm Hg, pulse 128 beats/min, and respiratory rate 32/min.

PROBLEM 2 A 76 year old male tripped over a grandchild's toy and presented with pain in his right knee and ankle. Vital signs were blood pressure 200/120 mm Hg, pulse 98 beats/min, and respiratory rate 20/min.

QUESTIONS TO CONSIDER

1. What blood pressure levels define mild, moderate, and severe hypertension?
2. What organs are common sites of damage by hypertension?
3. What is a hypertensive emergency? What is a hypertensive urgency?
4. In a hypertensive emergency, what symptoms and signs might one see with ongoing organ damage?
5. How are hypertensive emergencies managed? Hypertensive urgencies?
6. When is sodium nitroprusside indicated for control of hypertension?
7. Which patients with hypertension can be discharged, and what follow-up arrangements are necessary?
8. What are the unique aspects of hypertension in pregnancy?

INTRODUCTION

Hypertension affects more than 20% of the adult population and about 3% of the pediatric population. Chronic hypertension is a major cause of morbidity and mortality in the United States. Over the course of years, untreated hypertension causes substantial long-term morbidity and mortality due to stroke, congestive heart failure, peripheral vascular disease, sudden death, and, to a lesser extent, myocardial infarction.

Hypertension is a physical finding that is usually not accompanied by symptoms. Thus, detection of patients with hypertension is problematic, and elevated pressures deserve appropriate follow-up. In the emergency department an elevated blood pressure reading is often unrelated to the patient's chief complaint. Approximately one-third of patients with elevated blood pressure measured in the emergency department have significant hypertension; another third have borderline hypertension, and the remainder are normotensive on follow-up visits.

Hypertension is classified according to the degree of elevated blood pressure into mild, moderate, and severe categories. Table 13–1 lists the values that define mild, moderate, and severe hypertension. Hypertension is most common in a mild or moderate form. Diagnosis of mild and moderate hypertension in asymptomatic cases requires two blood pressure measurements taken days apart. Severe hypertension is diagnosed and

TABLE 13–1. Classification of Blood Pressure (in Patients over 18 Years Old)

Blood Pressure (mm Hg)	Category
Diastolic	
<85	Normal blood pressure
85–90	High normal blood pressure
90–104	Mild hypertension
105–114	Moderate hypertension
≥115	Severe hypertension
Systolic (when diastolic BP < 90 mm Hg)	
<140	Normal blood pressure
140–159	Borderline isolated systolic hypertension
≥160	Isolated systolic hypertension

Adapted from the 1988 Joint National Committee of the National High Blood Pressure Education Program of the National Heart, Lung and Blood Institute, Bethesda, MD. These committee definitions are for averages of two or more blood pressure measurements. Measurements in the severe range need to be controlled before the patient leaves the emergency department.

managed from a single blood pressure reading with or without symptoms indicative of organ damage.

Rarely, elevated blood pressure causes rapidly progressive end-organ damage. This is a *hypertensive emergency* and usually does not occur until the diastolic blood pressure is at least 115 mm Hg. A blood pressure in this range without rapidly progressive end-organ damage is considered a *hypertensive urgency*. Prompt diagnosis and treatment of hypertensive emergencies may save organ function and the patient's life. Preeclampsia and eclampsia, both hypertensive emergencies of pregnancy, can occur at lower blood pressures (see Special Considerations). In emergency medicine most clinical management efforts are devoted to the diagnosis and management of hypertensive urgencies and emergencies.

Hypertension results from any disorder affecting the circulation that increases cardiac output or total peripheral resistance. These changes can result from normal and pathologic processes in the autonomic, cardiovascular, renal, and endocrine systems. Each of these systems is eventually evaluated in the assessment of the hypertensive patient.

The organ systems primarily involved in hypertensive emergencies are also insidiously damaged by mild and moderate hypertension. These are the central nervous, cardiovascular, and renal systems. In the central nervous system excessive elevation of blood pressure produces cerebral hyperfusion, dilation of arterioles, and loss of the integrity of the blood-brain barrier. These effects in turn result in increased intracranial pressure, cerebral edema, and, eventually, decreased blood flow. Patients with chronic uncontrolled mild to moderate hypertension have reset their cerebral autoregulation mechanism. In these patients, adequate cerebral blood flow is not maintained when the arterial pressure is low. Therefore, overzealous treatment of the hypertensive patient may result in significant compromise of cerebral blood flow. In the cardiovascular system, acute significant elevations in the diastolic pressure cause increases in the cardiac afterload. This increase results in increased myocardial work and oxygen demand to maintain cardiac output. This cardiovascular stress can lead to angina, myocardial infarction, or heart failure. The kidney is subject to arteriolar vasoconstriction, arteriolitis, parenchymal damage, and hormonal changes that can result in decreased renal function.

PREHOSPITAL CARE

The ability to diagnose and treat hypertensive emergencies before the patient arrives in the emergency department is limited. Prehospital management is directed toward the presenting symptom, e.g., chest pain, shortness of breath, or headache.

History

1. Is there chest or abdominal pain? When did it start? Was the onset sudden or insidious? What is the character of the pain? Does anything make the pain better or worse?
2. For females of childbearing age, is the woman pregnant? If she is, is there an antecedent history of obstetric problems?
3. Is there a severe headache, weakness, visual problems, or change in mentation?
4. Is there any trouble breathing?
5. Is the patient known to be hypertensive? Has he or she ever been given medications for high blood pressure?
6. What medications does the patient take? Is there any circumstantial evidence of drug abuse such as needle tracks or drug paraphernalia at the scene?

Physical Examination

1. *Vital signs.* The blood pressure is taken from both arms. Reassessments are repeated every few minutes during transport. It can be difficult to obtain accurate blood pressure measurements in a moving ambulance.
2. *Cardiovascular system.* Does the patient have rales, distended neck veins, or peripheral edema?
3. *Neurologic system.* Does the patient's mental status appear to be appropriate? Are there any gross neurologic deficits?

Intervention

1. Oxygen supplement by nasal cannula at 2 to 4 liters/min is given if there are any respiratory signs or symptoms.
2. An intravenous (IV) catheter is placed. The initial fluid is dextrose in water 5% (D/W 5%) at a keep-open rate.
3. A cardiac monitor is placed and observed for dysrhythmias.
4. Patients with central chest pain may be given sublingual nitroglycerin. If administered, the blood pressure response is monitored closely after dosing.
5. Patients with suspected pulmonary edema and a long transport time may be given morphine sulfate and furosemide. This treatment depends on the rescue squad's capabilities.

PROBLEM 1 The rescue squad stated that the patient was in moderate respiratory distress. Rales were heard halfway up the lung fields. Her neck veins (external jugular) were distended, and she had 2+ pitting edema in the lower extremities. Medications found in the patient's home included furosemide (Lasix), clonidine (Catapres), glyburide (Diabeta), and alprazolam (Xanax).

This patient has serious disease. Her potential diagnoses include myocardial infarction, pulmonary edema, dissecting aortic aneurysm, and clonidine or alprazolam withdrawal. Oxygen, nitroglycerin, furosemide, and morphine are ordered for treatment of hypertension, chest pain, and probable pulmonary edema. Because a dissecting aneurysm is a possibility, the squad is instructed to proceed to the nearest center capable of performing cardiopulmonary bypass. This equipment is not available in every setting.

PROBLEM 2 This patient had pain and tenderness in the lower extremity but no other complaints or obvious problems. His medication history was significant in that "a couple of blood pressure pills" of unknown type had been prescribed previously. The patient was noncompliant and did not refill the rather expensive prescription.

This patient may have serious orthopedic injuries, but the medics have not discovered any evidence of a hypertensive emergency. He was treated as a patient with a hypertensive urgency and was given oxygen by nasal cannula and intravenous access established. D/W 5% was infused at a keep-open rate.

INITIAL APPROACH IN THE EMERGENCY DEPARTMENT

Patients classed as hypertensive emergencies are seen immediately and are placed in the resuscitation area. These emergencies are suspected in patients with diastolic pressures greater than 115 mm Hg who have evidence of end-organ damage. The accompanying finding may be altered mental status, severe headache, new focal neurologic deficits (including visual problems), seizures, chest or back pain, dyspnea, tachypnea, or hematuria. These patients undergo diagnostic and therapeutic maneuvers simultaneously.

1. Vital signs including blood pressure are repeated in both arms. Pulses are compared in all extremities.
2. An oxygen supplement is maintained at 2 to 4 liters/min by nasal cannula. Higher flow rates may be necessary.
3. Intravenous access is established or confirmed. D/W 5% is given at a keep-open rate.
4. A cardiac monitor is placed followed by a 12-lead electrocardiogram (ECG).
5. The prehospital history is confirmed. The questions are the same if the patient arrives in the emergency department by private car.
6. What is the patient's response and blood pressure response to any treatment given by the rescue squad?
7. The physical examination is repeated with the important addition of a funduscopic examination for papilledema or retinal hemorrhage.
8. Immediate laboratory studies including urinalysis, complete blood count, serum electrolytes, blood urea nitrogen (BUN), creatinine, and glucose are ordered.
9. Emergency management consists in administering parenteral antihypertensive medications in hypertensive emergencies. The medications are selected depending on the end-organ affected (Table 13–2). They are reviewed in detail under Principles of Management.

Patients with hypertensive urgencies are seen promptly, although intervention is significantly less aggressive. In patients with uncomplicated mild or moderate hypertension, the primary presenting complaint is addressed first.

DATA GATHERING

The history and physical examination allow the physician to assess the end-organ effects and search for primary causes of hypertension.

History

Symptoms. What is the *time course* and *character* of the symptoms? Hypertensive emergencies usually have a rapid onset and fast (minutes to hours) progression.

Neurologic Signs. Does the patient have *headache, seizures,* and *visual disturbances* or other *focal neurologic findings* that are found with hypertensive encephalopathy, intracranial hemorrhage, eclampsia or preeclampsia, or pheochromocytoma?

Chest Pain. Is *chest pain present?* Ischemic cardiac pain is typically dull and boring and is often described as a feeling that something heavy is sitting on the patient's chest.

TABLE 13–2. Drugs Used to Control Hypertensive Emergencies and Urgencies

Drug	Class	Dose and Route	Onset	Duration	Comments
Parenteral					
Nitroprusside	Direct-acting vasodilator	0.025–10.0 μg/kg/min infusion	<1 min	3.5 min	Very potent, easily titratable. Dilates arteries and veins. May cause nausea, vomiting, diaphoresis
Diazoxide	Vasodilator	50–100 mg IV at 5- to 10-min intervals	3–5 min	12–24 hr	Used less often recently. Combined with furosemide because of urinary retention. Can cause flushing, tachypnea, headache, vomiting, and hyperglycemia
Trimethaphan	Ganglionic blocker	1–20[a] mg/min infusion	1–5 min	10 min	Anticholinergic side effects, e.g., urinary retention, pupillary dilatation, dry mouth
Labetalol	Alpha and beta blocker	2 mg/min IV to 300 mg total dose; 100–600 ≈ 1 hr mg PO b.i.d.	≤5 min	3–6 hr	Contraindicated in patients with asthma, CHF. May cause nausea, vomiting, burning in throat. Postural dizziness reported
Propranolol	Beta blocker	1–10 mg loading dose at 2–4 mg/hr; 40–240 mg PO b.i.d.	1 min <1 hr	2 hr 12 hr	Used in conjunction with other drugs in patients with severe hypertension. May need concomitant alpha blockade. Contraindications: CHF, asthma, diabetes
Esmolol	Beta blocker	50–200 μg/min IV	<1 min	10 min	Short-acting. See entry under propranolol
Hydralazine	Arteriolar dilator	10–20 mg IV	10–30 min	2–4 hr	May precipitate angina; main use is in patients with eclampsia and preeclampsia
Furosemide	Diuresis, venodilation	40–80 mg IV over 2 min	5 min	2 hr	Used in conjunction with other drugs; rare ototoxicity
Nitroglycerin	Direct-acting vasodilator	5–200 μg/min infusion, 0.15–0.6 μg sublingually	<1 min	5 min	Titratable. Dilates veins and coronaries, has some effect on peripheral arteries
Magnesium sulfate	Vasodilator, nerve stabilizer	2–4 gm IV load over 5 min, then 1–2 gm/hr	Minutes	Hours[b]	Main benefit is stabilization of nerves; used for patients with eclampsia and preeclampsia
Oral					
Clonidine	Sympatholytic	0.2 mg PO load, then 0.1 mg/hr	30–60 min	6–8 hr	Sedating; rebound hypertension
Nifedipine	Calcium channel blocker	10–20 mg PO	15–30 min	3–5 hr	Rare overshoot hypotension. May precipitate angina, MI
Captopril	ACE inhibitor	6.5–50.0 mg PO	15 min	4–6 hr	Variable response; overshoot hypotension
Labetalol and nitroglycerin		Available in oral or IV preparation			

Abbreviations: CHF = congestive heart failure; ACE = angiotensin converting enzyme.
[a]The upper limit of the dose of trimethaphan varies considerably in the literature from 5–20 mg/min; some authorities give no upper limit for the dose.
[b]The excretion rate varies with renal function, which is often abnormal in these patients. Serum levels should be monitored and are usually kept in the 7–10 mEq/liter range. If deep tendon reflexes disappear, the dose is probably too high; pathologically brisk reflexes suggest that a higher dose is needed.

Pain from a dissecting aortic aneurysm often radiates to the back and is described as a "tearing" sensation.

Congestive Heart Failure. Is there *shortness of breath, dyspnea* on exertion, *orthopnea,* or *peripheral edema* that may be suggestive of congestive heart failure?

Hematuria. Is *hematuria* present? A history of hematuria is highly suggestive of accelerated renal hypertension; this condition may have few other signs or symptoms until other organ systems start to fail.

Pregnancy. Is the patient *pregnant?* If so, the diastolic blood pressure at which the patient may have a hypertensive emergency or urgency is lowered to 100 mm Hg.

Similar Episodes. Have *similar episodes* occurred in the *past?* Are there precipitating factors? Are there treatments that have been effective? Episodes of congestive heart failure (CHF), pulmonary edema, aortic aneurysm, coronary artery ischemia, and eclampsia or preeclampsia tend to recur.

Past Medical History. Is there a history of hypertension, cardiovascular disease, or renal disease? Does the patient have a history of endocrinopathy, especially diabetes, medullary carcinoma of the thyroid, or pheochromocytoma? Diabetics are at increased risk of underlying renal disease, ischemic heart disease, and peripheral arterial disease. Patients with medullary carcinoma of the thyroid are at increased risk of developing pheochromocytoma.

Drug History. The *medication* history, including illicit drugs, alcohol, and compliance with prescribed medications, is important. The use of "uppers," including cocaine, amphetamines, and phenylpropanolamine (the main component of over-the-counter diet pills), can increase blood pressure, sometimes dramatically. Young, healthy patients can develop myocardial infarction and stroke as a side effect of these medications. Similar problems occur when patients on a monoamine oxidase (MAO) inhibitor (e.g., phenelzine [Nardil]), prescribed for depression ingest food with tyramine or certain drugs, e.g., pseudoephedrine. Sudden cessation of antihypertensive medication, especially clonidine, may lead to rebound hypertension, a condition in which the blood pressure rises above the level it was before treatment was begun.

Physical Examination

Appearance. Level of consciousness, evidence of distress, diaphoresis, and skin color are assessed.

Blood Pressure. Blood pressure in these patients can be very labile. The evolving underlying disease and the drugs used for treatment can cause wide swings that require close monitoring. Blood pressure measurements are taken in both arms and repeated every 3 to 5 minutes at a minimum.

Noninvasive blood pressure measurements can be significantly inaccurate. The blood pressure cuff must be of the appropriate size. The bladder of the cuff should encircle at least two-thirds of the arm, and the width of the cuff should be 40% of the circumference of the arm at the midpoint (or 20% wider than the diameter). Most cuffs are labeled so that the appropriate size can be verified for each patient. Palpation of an artery while the blood pressure cuff is being inflated or released is one of the least accurate ways of determining blood pressure. Auscultating for Korotkov sounds is the standard means of measurement. After the pressure is increased 20 to 30 mm Hg above the point where a palpable medial pulse is lost, the systolic pressure is recorded when the heart beat is heard clearly and at every beat as the cuff pressure is lowered. The diastolic level is recorded when the heart beat sounds begin to muffle and when they disappear. Which of the two points is more accurate is still controversial. The point at which sound becomes absent is more commonly recorded. Listening with a Doppler device for the onset of arterial pulsations while the cuff is slowly released is as accurate as any other noninvasive method of detecting systolic pressure, although this method gives comparatively little information about the mean and diastolic pressures.

Oscillometric devices, also called automatic noninvasive blood pressure monitors (such as Accutorr or Lifestat monitors), are useful when repeated measurements are necessary. They most accurately measure mean pressure; systolic and diastolic readings are subject to greater error. These devices can be set to measure automatically every few minutes.

Compared to noninvasive methods, invasive blood pressure measurement with an arterial line is considerably more accurate and gives continual information. This monitoring method is feasible in some emergency departments and is the ideal method for monitoring unstable hypertensive patients. When this method cannot be used, the best alternative is to use an oscillometric device that automatically repeats measurements.

Eye. Papilledema, fundal hemorrhage, and vasospasm occur as acute, ongoing hypertensive damage. The term *malignant hypertension* is applied to a diastolic blood pressure of more than 130 to 140 mm Hg with papilledema. Although the term is used less now than formerly, it appropriately describes the high potential for morbidity and mortality that is associated with these two findings. Chronic changes of hypertension (arteriovenous nicking, silver wiring) or diabetes (arteriolar aneurysms, cotton-wool exudates) may suggest an undiagnosed or long-standing underlying problem.

Cardiovascular Examination. The heart is auscultated for murmurs, gallops, and extra sounds; the neck is inspected for jugular venous distention; pulmonary rales and peripheral edema are sought. Patients with congestive heart failure may have S_3 gallops, rales, jugular venous distention, and peripheral edema. Aortic dissections involving the aortic root may cause a diastolic murmur of aortic regurgitation. Continuous (lasting through systole and diastole) murmurs may be heard in patients with coarctation of the aorta. Peripheral edema is often seen in pregnant patients with preeclampsia.

Pulmonary Findings. The major findings are those of pulmonary edema secondary to CHF. Increased respiratory rate and effort combined with diffuse fine rales are highly suggestive.

Abdomen. The gravid uterus is a sine qua non of eclampsia/preeclampsia; if the uterus is gravid, what are the fetal heart tones? The abdomen and flanks are carefully auscultated for bruits. The presence of a bruit suggests the presence of an arterial aneurysm or stenosis; the absence of a bruit does not rule them out. A pulsatile abdominal mass is palpated in up to 60% to 70% of cases of aortic aneurysm. If found, an aneurysm is assumed to be present until proved otherwise.

Peripheral Pulses. If a dissecting aneurysm is suspected, peripheral pulses are compared and rechecked often. Other conditions can cause different blood pressures in arteries of different extremities, such as peripheral arteriosclerosis or coarctation of the aorta.

Neurologic Findings. The neurologic examination includes an estimate of the mental status and cranial nerve, motor, sensation, deep tendon reflex, and plantar (Babinski) responses. Altered mental status and focal deficits may be seen with hypertensive encephalopathy, intracranial hemorrhage, and eclampsia or preeclampsia.

PROBLEM 1 On presentation to the emergency department, the patient was markedly dyspneic; she gave only brief answers to questions. She was not accompanied by her family. She had developed dyspnea during the past 2 hours that had worsened in the past 30 minutes. Her vague, nonlocalized chest and back pain came on at the same time and persisted. She described previous hospitalizations for "heart trouble" but could not give any details. She denied a history of renal disease, hematuria, or flank pain. She confirmed taking furosemide (Lasix), clonidine (Catapres), glyburide (Diabeta), and alprazolam (Xanax). She denied taking any other prescribed, over-the-counter, or recreational drugs. She stated that she complied with the prescribed medications.

The patient was sitting forward, using accessory muscles of respiration, and breathing at a rate of 36 breaths/min. She had rales extending throughout both lung fields. Seven centimeters of jugular venous distention were present. Heart sounds were difficult to hear over the rales. Results of the neurologic and abdominal examinations were unremarkable. Blood pressure was about 220/130 mm Hg in all extremities. The pulse rate was 130 beats/min.

PROBLEM 2 The patient was awake and alert, complaining that the pain in the right knee and ankle prevented him from ambulating. He stated he had had no symptoms of hypertension for "a good long time" and was supposed to be taking three different medications to control his blood pressure. He had not taken the medication for "several days because he had been feeling well." He had a past medical history of diabetes mellitus controlled with diet.

The patient was sitting with his right lower extremity splinted. Results of the neurologic examination were unremarkable except that funduscopic examination revealed arteriovenous nicking. Lungs were clear, and no extra sounds were noted. Abdominal examination was normal. Distal pulses were intact, and blood pressure was 200/120 mm Hg in both arms and in the left lower extremity. The pulse rate was 90 beats/min, and the respiratory rate was 18/min.

DECISION PRIORITIES AND PRELIMINARY DIFFERENTIAL DIAGNOSIS

After gathering the data, the emergency physician must first ask: *Is the hypertension producing any organ damage?*

The physiologic systems at risk are the central nervous system (including the eye), the cardiovascular system, and the renal system.

Central Nervous System. Hypertensive encephalopathy and cerebral vascular accidents due to severe hypertension may cause significant neurologic dysfunction and damage. Hypertensive encephalopathy involves the entire brain, although the damage is not uniform. At autopsy petechial hemorrhages and multiple small infarctions are found, often accompanied by edema. Some areas are relatively spared, and other areas are more heavily damaged. Thus, neurologic manifestations vary from patient to patient. Typically, hypertensive encephalopathy evolves over hours to days. Patients complain of headache, nausea, and vomiting. They may have an altered mental status or focal neurologic findings including blindness, cranial nerve dysfunction, aphasia, and hemiparesis. In addition to or separate from encephalopathy, patients with severe hypertension often develop intracerebral hemorrhage. Differentiation between hypertensive encephalopathy and intracranial hemorrhage is important because treatment for hypertensive encephalopathy is more aggressive than for hypertension associated with intracranial hemorrhage. Intracranial hemorrhages are usually seen on CT, and a hemorrhage too small to be seen on CT is unlikely to result in an elevated blood pressure.

Cardiovascular System. Patients with cardiovascular damage secondary to hypertensive crisis may manifest hypertensive pulmonary edema, aortic dissection, myocardial infarction, or unstable angina. Myocardial oxygen consumption is increased because of the greater afterload in patients who are hypertensive. This increase can lead to ischemia in patients with underlying cardiovascular disease. One-third of patients with a myocardial infarction have diastolic pressures of over 100 mm Hg. This elevation usually lasts for only a few hours.

Pulmonary edema is often the initial manifestation of a hypertensive emergency. An acute ischemic cardiac event or other factors such as salt overload are diagnosed as precipitants. More often, there is no clear precipitating event. Pulmonary edema may be present in a subtle or dramatic manner. The patient may complain of orthopnea and dyspnea on exertion or may demonstrate fine rales, mild tachypnea, and anxiety. Severe pulmonary edema manifests as extreme dyspnea, cough, frothy sputum, profound diaphoresis, cyanosis, pallor, and a frantic appearance.

Aortic dissection classically presents (in 75% to 85% of cases) with a sudden onset of severe tearing chest pain. The pain radiates to the epigastrium, extremities, or, more typically, the back. These patients may have diminished blood pressure distal to the site of the dissection. This finding varies from patient to patient. The findings for a given patient often change as the dissection progresses. If the aneurysm involves a carotid artery or the coronary arteries, the illness may present as a cerebrovascular accident (CVA) or myocardial infarction (MI). Proximal aortic dissection may lead to acute aortic insufficiency or dissection into the pericardium, which can cause acute cardiac tamponade. Up to 20% of patients have some degree of congestive heart failure. Though hypertension is the rule, patients may be normotensive or hypotensive. The finding of unequal blood pressures or pulses or ischemia in two sites is consistent with a dissecting aneurysm.

Renal System. Acute renal failure may present as a hypertensive emergency. The patient may complain of hematuria or peripheral edema. Laboratory testing is usually necessary to confirm this diagnosis.

PROBLEM 1 The woman was in acute distress. The blood pressure, rales, jugular venous distention, respiration distress, and history identified her as a patient with a hypertensive emergency, probably with hypertensive pulmonary edema, although an aortic dissection was a possibility.

PROBLEM 2 The patient did not exhibit neurologic, cardiovascular, or renal end-organ damage. He had a hypertensive urgency and an unrelated orthopedic injury.

DIAGNOSTIC ADJUNCTS

Diagnostic tests help to confirm the presence of end-organ damage caused by severe hypertension and can help to differentiate primary from secondary causes of hypertension.

Laboratory Studies

Blood Urea Nitrogen, Creatinine, Electrolytes, Glucose, and Complete Blood Count. These tests are indicated in all patients with significant hypertension. Blood urea nitrogen (BUN) and creatinine values may rise steeply, indicating a significant loss of renal function. An elevated glucose concentration may disclose the existence of diabetes mellitus. Hypokalemia may indicate the presence of hyperaldosteronism or high-renin forms of hypertension. Microangiopathic hemolytic anemia is suspected if broken red cells are noted in the peripheral smear, and the red cell count is decreased.

Urinalysis. Urinalysis is indicated in all patients with significant hypertension. In patients with ongoing renal damage, blood and protein leak into the urine and are usually discovered by testing with a urine dipstick. These tests are quite sensitive, although other causes besides hypertensive renal damage may result in protein or blood being found in the specimen. Test strips can also detect glucosuria, which may be due to diabetes mellitus. On microscopic examination, red cell casts imply glomerulonephritis; white cell casts suggest pyelonephritis. Proteinuria with red cells or red cell casts often indicates the presence of acute renal dysfunction secondary to hypertension.

Drug Screen. Urine or serum drug analysis is indicated in any hypertensive patient in whom drug abuse is suspected. Drug screening can clarify whether or not the patient suffers from the toxic effects of cocaine or other "uppers." Screening tests detect the presence of cocaine and most amphetamines; they do not give quantitative information about the amount of substance ingested by the patient.

Electrocardiogram

A 12-lead ECG is indicated for all patients with severe hypertension. Patients with ischemic heart disease may have ECG evidence of ischemia. Most patients with an evolving myocardial infarction will develop ECG changes within hours after the onset of the infarction. Left ventricular hypertrophy is very suggestive of chronic hypertension. The ECG is abnormal in 80% of 90% of patients with aortic dissection.

Radiologic Imaging

Radiographs. Posteroanterior (PA) and lateral chest radiographs are ordered in all patients with hypertensive emergency or urgency. They are highly sensitive for findings of pulmonary edema. Early in the process of pulmonary edema, vascular markings become blurred, and interstitial edema may be seen. These changes are subtle and are often missed. Normally, the dependent vessels are larger than the upper ones. As pulmonary edema progresses beyond the early stages, the upper vessels enlarge. This is called *cephalization* of flow. In the latter stages of pulmonary edema the lungs become diffusely hazy. Frequently cardiomegaly or left ventricular hypertrophy is noted. When the disease has progressed to this advanced stage, the changes are easy to see and are universally present.

Chest radiographs of patients with aortic aneurysms typically show widening of the superior mediastinum with "blurring of the aortic knob." If the vascular intima is calcified, the aortic wall will appear abnormally thick. These diagnostic findings are present in 80% of cases. Coarctation of the aorta can appear on the chest radiograph as disproportionate widening on the arteries proximal to the site of the coarctation; there may also be a narrowing "three sign" of the aorta at the site of the coarctation. In asymptomatic patients the left ventricle is often enlarged, suggesting a chronic problem.

Computed Tomography. CT of the head is needed for the patient with neurologic findings. CT will detect an intracranial bleed with a high degree of accuracy (see Chaps. 45 and 49).

Aortography, CT Scan of Chest. Aortography or chest CT scan is indicated for the patient in whom a dissecting aortic aneurysm is suspected. Both tests reveal the dissection with a very high degree of accuracy, although a few false-negative tests have been reported. CT is usually performed more quickly than aortography, but aortography usually provides more accurate information about the location of intimal tears. This information is important for surgical management. Performance of both tests improves the diagnostic accuracy.

PROBLEM 1 The cardiac monitor showed a sinus rhythm with a heart rate of 130 beats/min. Twelve-lead ECG was interpreted as a sinus tachycardia with borderline left ventricular hypertrophy. There were no ischemic changes. A chest radiograph was read as marked cardiomegaly and distended pulmonary vasculature with cephalization of flow. The aorta appeared normal. A Foley catheter was placed and drained 100 ml of clear yellow urine, which on dipstick testing proved negative for glucose, protein, and blood.

PROBLEM 2 Twelve-lead ECG showed a normal sinus rhythm with borderline left ventricular hypertrophy. Chest radiograph was unremarkable. Urine dipstick testing results showed no protein, glucose, or blood.

REFINED DIFFERENTIAL DIAGNOSIS

Following the history, physical examination, and ancillary tests, the physician should be able to determine definitely the answers to the following three questions:

1. *Is a hypertensive emergency present?*
   The answer to this question depends on the demonstration of ongoing end-organ damage of hypertension as manifested by progressive neurologic, cardiovascular, or renal dysfunction.
2. *Is a hypertensive urgency present?*

The patient with a sustained diastolic pressure greater than 115 mm Hg without signs or symptoms of end-organ damage has a hypertensive urgency. Such patients are at risk for end-organ damage if the blood pressure is not brought under control.

3. *Is the hypertension essential or secondary to another disease process?*

The last question may not be pertinent to most management decisions in the emergency department. It is important to maintain a broad differential outlook and consider definitive care beyond the emergency department. The great majority (90% to 95%) of patients have essential hypertension with no underlying cause. Of those 5% to 10% of patients with secondary hypertension, approximately half have diseases in which the hypertension is potentially curable. The most common causes of secondary hypertension are chronic renal disease, renal artery stenosis, primary aldosteronism, coarctation of the aorta, Cushing's syndrome, pheochromocytomas, and drug-induced hypertension.

Renal Artery Stenosis

Renal artery stenosis is the most common potentially curable cause of hypertension. It is seen in approximately 1% to 5% of hypertensive patients. Compromised renal perfusion caused by the stenosis promotes the secretion of renin. Renin produces an increase in angiotensin II, a potent vasoconstrictor, which also increases sympathetic vasomotor activity. Renal artery stenosis occurs most commonly in two groups of patients, elderly males with atherosclerotic disease and young women with fibrous dysplasia of the renal artery. An abdominal bruit is present in 40% to 80% of patients with renal artery stenosis. Other clinical findings that have been associated with renovascular hypertension include severe hypertensive retinopathy (papilledema, flame hemorrhages, cotton-wool exudates), acute onset of severe hypertension, hypertension resistant to treatment, thin body habitus, and hypokalemia. Diagnostic studies include renal arteriography and renal vein renin sampling.

Aldosteronism

Mineralocorticoid excess or aldosteronism is an uncommon but potentially curable cause of hypertension. Patients with mineralocorticoid excess experience sodium retention, volume expansion, and increased cardiac output. The degree of hypertension is usually mild to moderate. Patients typically demonstrate hypokalemia and increased potassium excretion on laboratory evaluation. Aldosteronism may be due primarily to an adrenal adenoma or hyperplasia or secondary to other diseases such as Cushing's syndrome, congenital adrenal hyperplasia, or exogenous mineralocorticoids such as heavy licorice ingestion containing glycyrrhizic acid. Patients have elevated levels of aldosterone that do not suppress normally with volume expansion.

Renal Disease

Chronic renal disease is the most common form of secondary hypertension. It occurs in more than 80% of patients with end-stage renal disease.

Pheochromocytoma

Pheochromocytoma is an uncommon cause of reversible hypertension. It represents a tumor of chromaffin cells, usually in the adrenal medulla, producing excess catecholamines, epinephrine, and norepinephrine that cause paroxysmal hypertension. Ten percent of pheochromocytomas are extra-adrenal. Patients usually complain of a pounding, severe headache, palpitations, and excessive perspiration. Episodes of hypertension may be paroxysmal with normotensive, symptom-free intervals in 50% of patients. Laboratory tests may show hyperglycemia. Pheochromocytomas are associated with specific diseases, including medullary thyroid carcinoma, hyperparathyroidism, neurofibromatosis, cerebellar hemangioblastoma, mucosal neuromas, and intestinal ganglioneuromatosis. About 10% of patients have a family history of pheochromocytoma. Biochemical tests such as those determining fasting levels of plasma catecholamines and urinary vanillylmandelic acid can help to make the diagnosis.

Drugs

Medications are an important cause of secondary hypertension. Drugs such as cocaine and amphetamines may produce severe hypertensive crisis. In addition, withdrawal from drugs such as alcohol or clonidine may precipitate severe hypertension. Finally, some drugs such as monoamine oxidase (MAO) inhibitors may react with tyramine-containing foods such as red wine, aged cheese, beer, and pickled herring to produce a hypertensive emergency.

PROBLEM 1 The laboratory findings reinforced the working diagnosis of hypertensive congestive heart failure with pulmonary edema. In this patient, as in others, more than one cause may be producing the situation—for instance, both clonidine withdrawal and hypertensive pulmonary edema could be operative. The chest radiograph findings and the normal peripheral pulses made an aortic aneurysm unlikely. The normal results of urine analysis made renovascular disease improbable. The normal neurologic findings decreased the possibility of an intracranial event. The patient was not of childbearing age. The relatively normal ECG findings suggested that ischemic heart disease was unlikely, but this could not be ruled out. The patient continued to require cardiac monitoring and serial ECGs during treatment and recovery.

PRINCIPLES OF MANAGEMENT
General Management

The management of patients with hypertensive emergency or urgency depends on the following principles:
  1. Blood pressure is gradually lowered as appropriate for the degree of crisis.
  2. Complications of hypertensive crisis including myocardial infarction, CNS hemorrhage, pulmonary edema, and renal failure are treated.
  3. The possibility of underlying secondary hypertension is addressed.

As with other conditions seen by emergency physicians, it is prudent to search for the most catastrophic illnesses first. Hypertensive emergencies, as the name would imply, are treated aggressively. The goal of therapy is to reduce blood pressure within minutes. Since a too rapid reduction can cause cerebral and myocardial ischemia, the level to which the pressure is reduced depends on which underlying pathologic processes are involved. Fifteen to twenty percent reduction from the initial blood pressure is a reasonable first goal; the patient is then reassessed. There is no need to correct the blood pressure to "normal" levels, and it is often dangerous to do so.

Pharmacologic agents are necessary for the treatment of patients with hypertensive emergencies and urgencies. Patients with hypertensive emergencies are treated with intravenous medications under close hemodynamic supervision and with cardiac monitoring. Optimally, an arterial catheter continuously measures the systolic, diastolic, and mean blood pressures. Serial external measurements by blood pressure cuff usually suffices. The intravenous medication is titrated to the desired blood pressure and the clinical response. The most common drugs used to control hypertensive emergencies are listed in Table 13–2 and briefly discussed below.

Drugs for Hypertensive Emergencies

1. *Nitroprusside* is widely used for hypertensive emergencies. It is an arterial and venous dilator that acts rapidly, thus decreasing both preload and afterload. It has minimal effect on cardiac output and myocardial blood flow. When nitroprusside is administered over a prolonged period of time, thiocyanate intoxication may occur.

2. *Diazoxide* is a direct arteriolar dilator that has little effect on preload. Patients often have a reflex tachycardia with increased myocardial oxygen consumption. Blood flow to the brain and kidneys is maintained. There are problems maintaining a controlled, smooth reduction in blood pressure with diazoxide. It should not be used in patients with cardiovascular diseases.

3. *Labetalol* is an alpha-1 and beta blocker that has a direct vasodilatory effect. It reduces systolic arterial pressure and total peripheral vascular resistance without producing reflex tachycardia. Cerebral and renal blood flows are maintained despite reductions in blood pressure. It is safe for patients with severe renal insufficiency.

4. *Nitroglycerin* is an arterial and venous dilator that also dilates the large coronary arteries. It has a greater effect on the capacitance (venous) vessels. Administered intravenously, it is effective in lowering the preload and afterload immediately. It is particularly useful for hypertensive emergencies with coronary insufficiency.

Drugs for Hypertensive Urgencies

Oral or sublingual medications are commonly used for the treatment of hypertensive urgencies (see Table 13–2).

1. *Nifedipine* is a calcium channel blocker that dilates the peripheral and coronary arteries. It causes a slight increase in heart rate. Following oral or sublingual administration of nifedipine, blood pressure effects are seen in 15 to 60 minutes.

2. *Clonidine* is a central alpha-2 agonist that decreases sympathetic activity and blocks catecholamine release. It may cause sedative and anticholinergic effects such as dry mouth.

Specific Management
Hypertensive Emergencies

Hypertensive Encephalopathy. Ongoing neurologic damage necessitates prompt control of blood pressure, ideally within 1 hour. Normally, sodium nitroprusside is the drug of choice for these patients because it produces no inherent CNS side effects. Intravenous labetalol can also be used.

Other Intracranial Hypertensive Emergencies. Subdural and epidural hematomas are best treated with prompt surgery. Treatment of intraparenchymal and subarachnoid hemorrhages is problematic. Unfortunately, most cerebrovascular hemorrhages due to hypertension belong in these categories. In many patients, the CNS "barostat" is reset, and some elevation in the mean arterial pressure is necessary to maintain cerebral perfusion. Therefore, it is dangerous to lower the pressure too quickly. The blood pressure is initially reduced by only 15% to 20%. The patient is then reassessed, and if stable, another 15% to 20% decrease is attempted. The goal is to lower the diastolic pressure into the 100- to 110-mm Hg range. Nitroprusside and labetalol are the drugs of choice. These patients may benefit from treatment that reduces intracranial pressure with mannitol and hyperventilation (see Chaps. 49 and 50).

Hypertensive Pulmonary Edema. Nitrates are excellent drugs in this situation. They dilate both arteries and veins, reducing preload and afterload. Nitroglycerin also dilates the coronary arteries and is especially useful when patients have concomitant angina. Nitroprusside is relatively more effective in dilating the peripheral arteries and reducing afterload. Furosemide (Lasix) and bumetanide (Bumex) are also used to increase venous capacitance and diurese excess water. Morphine sulfate is given intravenously to reduce sympathetic overflow, dilate the veins, and reduce anxiety. Some authors report success using nifedipine. The goal of blood pressure reduction is to maximize perfusion and minimize cardiac work. This is attained most precisely by titrating the antihypertensive drugs while following arterial pressure, pulmonary artery wedge pressure, and cardiac output.

Acute Aortic Dissection. The therapeutic goal is to quickly reduce the mean arterial blood pressure and the rate of rise of aortic pulse pressure during the cardiac cycle (dP/dt). Nitroprusside is administered with a beta blocker such as propranolol or esmolol to decrease mean arterial pressure while reducing dP/dt. The beta blocker is titrated to avoid sudden heart failure or bronchial spasm. Invasive arterial line monitoring is especially useful in these patients because it allows one to see the pressure wave and monitor dP/dt. Labetalol may be used by itself or in combination with nitroprusside. Trimethaphan was once the standard agent but is now rarely used because of the unpleasant side effects of ganglionic blockade. Type A aneurysms, which involve the ascending aorta, require surgical intervention. Uncomplicated type B (DeBakey type III) aneurysms, which involve only the descending aorta, may be treated medically. Early mortality occurs in up to 50% of these patients if they are not treated properly.

Hypertensive Renal Failure. Symptoms of this emergency may not become evident until the patient suffers severe renal failure. Prompt treatment may salvage some damaged but still viable renal tissue. Because almost all of these patients have elevated renin levels, angiotensin converting enzyme (ACE) inhibitors, captopril, and enalapril are useful. Unfortunately, it takes a few hours for these drugs to produce an antihypertensive effect. Treatment is usually begun with nitroprusside, nifedipine, or labetalol.

Pharmacologically Induced Hypertension. In hypertension induced by circulating catecholamines (e.g., by MAO inhibitors and sympathomimetic agents or by pheochromocytoma) labetalol may block the excessive adrenergic stimulation. Phentolamine (Regitine) may be needed as a more potent alpha blocker. If the initial response to these drugs is inadequate, nitroprusside is often effective.

Withdrawal from Antihypertensives. Relatively sudden withdrawal from antihypertensive agents may lead to "rebound" hypertension above baseline hypertensive states. This rebound is not a problem with diuretics, but it is with agents that block sympathetic tone, especially clonidine (Catapres). It occurs in 1% to 5% of patients who abruptly stop taking the drug. The time course varies with the agent involved. With clonidine, the onset of rebound hypertension typically begins 18 to 20 hours following the last dose. Hypertensive urgency due to clonidine withdrawal responds well to reinstitution of the drug. Patients with specific end-organ damage may be treated like other hypertensive emergencies described above.

Withdrawal from CNS Depressants. As patients withdraw from CNS depressants they enter a relatively sustained hyperadrenergic state characterized by tachycardia, tachypnea, hypertension, and fever. The time course of the withdrawal process varies with the involved drug. In general, the longer the half-life of the drug, the longer the withdrawal process. Ethanol withdrawal evolves over a period of about 4 days, diazepam (Valium) withdrawal over about 9 days. If untreated, withdrawal sometimes progresses to profound vasomotor instability, characterized by alternating hyperadrenergic and hypoadrenergic states such as delirium tremens. Delirium tremens has a significant mortality, so it is important to diagnose and treat these patients early. A wide variety of CNS depressants have been used successfully to treat withdrawal. Chlordiazepoxide (Librium) and diazepam are both relatively inexpensive, have desirable pharmacokinetic properties, and cause minimal respiratory depression. These agents can be used to treat most patients with depressant withdrawal. Narcotic withdrawal usually does not require any treatment; if treatment is necessary, clonidine or methadone is often used.

Hypertensive Urgencies

Patients with hypertensive urgency need to have their blood pressure reduced in the emergency department. The goal is to lower the blood pressure within hours to a safe level. Rapidly progressive organ damage is not a feature of hypertensive urgency, so there is little reason to lower blood pressure rapidly over a span of minutes. As in patients with a hypertensive emergency, it is risky to lower the blood pressure to "normal" levels. A mean arterial pressure of 120 torr (about 150–180/100–110 mm Hg) is a good target. Oral nifedipine, labetalol, clonidine, and captopril are all relatively safe and effective drugs for treatment of these patients. It is usually safe to treat patients in the "gray zone" between hypertensive urgency and hypertensive emergency with nifedipine, monitoring them carefully for blood pressure control and evidence of progressive end-organ damage.

Moderate and Mild Hypertension

Patients with relatively mild high blood pressure and no ongoing end-organ damage need no emergency department intervention. They are referred for follow-up.

PROBLEM 1 The patient was given 15 mg of morphine over 40 to 60 minutes in 2- to 3-mg increments. Furosemide 80 mg was given intravenously, and 10 mg of nifedipine was given sublingually. The patient's blood pressure decreased to 180/90 mm Hg, and her anxiety diminished in concert with her ability to breathe.

This patient was appropriately treated for hypertensive pulmonary edema. Lowering the blood pressure decreased the afterload and myocardial oxygen consumption. She needs continued intensive care monitoring of her arterial and pulmonary artery wedge pressures. If the blood pressure had not responded to these measures, more aggressive therapy would include nitroprusside.

PROBLEM 2 This patient's blood pressure decreased to 170/85 mm Hg after he was given 10 mg of nifedipine by mouth. He was given another 10 mg capsule to take before bedtime (in 5 hours, 7 hours after his last dose).

Although blood pressure control may not always be this easy, it is important to decrease the pressure to some degree. Since a significant "afterdrop" in pressure can occur up to 24 hours after initiating therapy, it is important not to seek too tight control initially.

SPECIAL CONSIDERATIONS

Pregnancy

Pregnant patients are more sensitive to the effects of hypertension than are other adults. The American College of Obstetrics and Gynecology defines *hypertension of pregnancy* as (1) a diastolic pressure of greater than 90 mm Hg or greater than 15 mm Hg above baseline or (2) a systolic pressure of greater than 140 mm Hg or 30 mm Hg above baseline. These patients are at increased risk for complications, including fetal mortality, eclampsia, and preeclampsia. Preeclampsia may involve hypertension, edema, proteinuria, microangiopathic hemolytic anemia, thrombocytopenia, and abnormal results of liver enzyme tests. Eclampsia is preeclampsia accompanied by new-onset seizures. Eclampsia and preeclampsia occur only in the latter part of gestation, so in most cases the diagnosis of pregnancy is not in doubt. Pregnant patients are at increased risk for preeclampsia if:
1. Previous episodes of preeclampsia have occurred.
2. Multiple gestations exist.
3. A hydatidiform mole is present.
4. There is a family history of preeclampsia.

5. The patient belongs to the lower socioeconomic classes.
6. The patient is a child or an older primigravid woman.

Patients with eclampsia or preeclampsia typically have hyperactive deep tendon reflexes. The visual and optic funduscopic changes described in the earlier section on hypertensive encephalopathy place them at risk for cerebral hemorrhage. Magnesium sulfate is the drug of choice for treatment of the neurologic symptoms, and it may also help to lower the blood pressure. Hydralazine is the drug of choice for blood pressure control, especially antepartum because it preserves uterine blood flow. Although these agents help to control the disease, delivery is the only cure for preeclampsia and eclampsia.

Pediatric Patients

The issue of asymptomatic hypertension in children has been the source of much discussion. There is evidence that many of these children, if left untreated for an extended period of time, will develop the complications of hypertension as adults. It is prudent to refer children with high blood pressure to specialists for further evaluation. To determine which children are hypertensive one must refer to tables or graphs of normal values for children. Children are considered hypertensive if they consistently have blood pressures above the ninety-fifth percentile for age.

DISPOSITION AND FOLLOW-UP

Disposition of the patient depends on accurate classification of the hypertension, assessment of end-organ damage, and response to treatment.

Admission

All patients with hypertensive emergencies are admitted. Essentially all require close monitoring in the intensive care unit. Rarely patients are sent to a "monitored bed" if the blood pressure has been controlled in the emergency department and there is no longer a need for intravenous agents. Repeated blood pressure measurements are still necessary.

Discharge

Patients with uncomplicated hypertensive urgencies are discharged from the emergency department if they respond appropriately to initial therapy. Generally, an appropriate response means that the blood pressure was lowered below the severe level, the patient tolerated the treatment without significant side effects, and no evidence of end-organ damage was apparent on initial assessment. Often the drug used to bring the blood pressure under control is continued on an outpatient basis. These patients need prompt follow-up, usually within a day. It is appropriate to consult with the physician who will follow the patient by telephone. An agreement is necessary on outpatient medication and a follow-up appointment. If follow-up cannot be arranged, the patient should return to the emergency department in 24 hours. If there is doubt about how well the blood pressure has been controlled, the patient is admitted.

Patients with moderate hypertension, mild hypertension, or isolated systolic hypertension are referred for follow-up to their primary physician. Many patients with isolated elevated blood pressure measurements are found to have chronic hypertension, and their long-term prognosis is greatly improved if they are correctly diagnosed and treated.

PROBLEM 1 The patient's condition continued to stabilize in the emergency department. She was transferred to an intensive care unit, where she spent 2 days. She was discharged from the hospital after 5 days with a diagnosis of hypertensive congestive heart failure. She was well at 4-month follow-up.

PROBLEM 2 Follow-up with the patient's personal physician was arranged for the next morning. His blood pressure was controlled with outpatient therapy.

DOCUMENTATION

1. History
   Chief complaint
   Past history of hypertension
   Cardiac or renal problems
   Drug history
2. Physical examination
   Serial blood pressure measurements taken at multiple extremities
   Neurologic examination including examination of the optic fundus
   Cardiovascular examination including peripheral pulses
   Presence or absence of vascular bruits
3. Laboratory tests
   ECG, urinalysis, chest radiograph, renal function, and electrolyte measurements
4. Assessment
   Presence or absence of neurologic, cardiovascular, or renal end-organ damage
   Underlying etiology of hypertension
5. Treatment
   Specific treatment given and its effect
   Flow sheet often very useful
   All procedures such as arterial lines are carefully documented
6. Diagnosis
7. Plans for discharge and follow-up

SUMMARY AND FINAL POINTS

- Most of the patients seen in the emergency department with elevated blood pressure have mild or moderate hypertension. They do not need immediate treatment and are referred for further care.
- Patients with severe hypertension have either a hypertensive urgency or a hypertensive emergency. The end-organ systems at special risk are the neurologic system (including the eyes), the cardiovascular system, and the renal system.
- The blood pressure cuff must be of the appropriate size and must be correctly applied. The blood pressure is measured in at least two extremities, and the pulses are palpated in all extremities.
- A careful physical examination is important to search for end-organ effects of severe hypertension.
- Drugs, especially cocaine, are in wide use. Abrupt cessation of antihypertensive medications can produce severe rebound hypertension.
- Pregnant women become hypertensive at relatively low blood pressures. Their blood pressure readings must be compared to baseline values for the same patient.
- Patients sent home after treatment of hypertensive urgency are given prompt (usually next day) follow-up.

BIBLIOGRAPHY

Texts

1. Wollam GL, Hall WD: Hypertension Management—Clinical Practice and Therapeutic Dilemmas. Chicago, Year Book, 1988.

Journal Articles

1. Bennett NM, Shea S: Hypertensive emergency: Case criteria, sociodemographic profile and previous care of 100 cases. Am J Public Health 78:636–640, 1987.
2. Bertel O, Marx BE: Hypertensive emergencies. Nephron 47 (Suppl 1): 51–56, 1987.
3. Chernow SM, Iserson KV, Criss E: Use of the emergency department for hypertension screening: A prospective study. Ann Emerg Med 16:180–182, 1987.
4. Drugs for hypertensive emergencies. Medical Letter on Drugs and Therapeutics 29(733):18–20, 1987.
5. Gonzalez DC, Venkata SR: New approaches for the treatment of hypertensive urgencies and emergencies. Chest 93(1):193–195, 1988.
6. Houston MC: The comparative effects of clonidine hydrochloride and nifedipine in the treatment of hypertensive crises. Am Heart J 115(1):152–159, 1988.
7. Jackson RE: Hypertension in the emergency department. Emerg Clin North Am 6:173–196, 1988.

005# SECTION FOUR

CUTANEOUS DISORDERS

CHAPTER 14

RASH

EVE NORTON, M.D.

PROBLEM 1 A 50 year old ill-appearing male was brought to the emergency department with fever and altered mental status. Several 0.5-cm solid, red, nonscaling, flat-topped lesions were visible on his ankles. They did not blanch on pressure and were palpable.

PROBLEM 2 A 24 year old male presented with a painless, solid, red, slightly scaling rash on the trunk and neck. He also had pink-red, annular lesions surrounded by a collarette of scale on his palms and soles.

PROBLEM 3 A 30 year old female presented with pruritic, linear, clear, fluid-filled bullous lesions on her arms. The lesions involved only the forearms.

QUESTIONS TO CONSIDER

1. Which rashes are manifestations of potentially life-threatening cutaneous diseases or serious systemic disease?
2. Why is the initial appearance of the skin lesion important?
3. What is the significance of the initial site and distribution of the skin lesion?
4. What history and physical data are necessary for a dermatologic work-up in the emergency department?
5. What ancillary tests may be performed to give additional diagnostic information?
6. Once the lesion or rash has been defined, what specific management strategy is indicated?
7. Which patients with a cutaneous disorder need to be admitted? Which patients require referral to a dermatologist?

INTRODUCTION

The emergency physician is confronted with a wide variety of skin disorders. In some settings complaints related to the skin make up 5% to 8% of all visits. Though rarely life-threatening, skin lesions and rashes are a source of considerable discomfort and anxiety.

The skin is composed of three layers: the epidermis, the dermis, and the subcutaneous layer. In addition to these layers, the skin contains various adnexal structures such as hair follicles, nails, sebaceous glands, eccrine sweat glands and apocrine sweat glands, and cutaneous blood vessels and nerves (Fig. 14–1).

The epidermis is the outermost layer of skin. In this layer reside the melanocytes, which produce the skin pigment melanin. Melanin serves as the protective filter against ultraviolet radiation. The outermost layer of the epidermis, the stratum corneum, with its interlocking sheets of keratin and lipid is responsible for the barrier function of the skin. The dermal-epidermal junction is a complex region. It is the site of immunoglobulin and complement depositions and the site of blister formation in many vesiculobullous

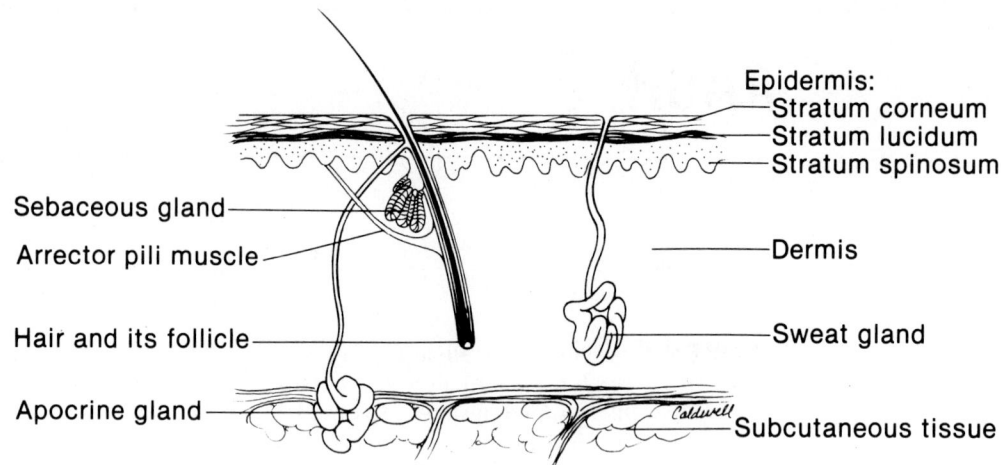

FIGURE 14–1. Cross-sectional anatomy of the skin.

diseases. The dermis makes up the bulk of the skin. Major components of the dermis are the collagen and elastin fibers and the ground substance, which is responsible for the strength and elasticity of the skin. The subcutaneous layer consists mostly of fat cells intermingled with connective tissue. It provides a protective cushion against trauma.

The cutaneous blood supply consists of arterioles connected to capillary loops, which are associated with venules to form the vascular network in the dermis. These blood vessels regulate temperature by vasodilation and vasoconstriction. Cutaneous sensation is mediated by both myelinated and nonmyelinated sensory nerves terminating in the dermis. Itching is a unique cutaneous sensation that probably represents a type of weak pain. Scratching converts the intolerable sensation of itching to the more familiar sensation of pain and can relieve the pruritus.

The skin serves as a strategic interface between the body and the external environment. It functions as a physical barrier, maintains temperature control, offers protection from ultraviolet light, and operates as a source of sensory input to the body.

TERMINOLOGY

To describe a cutaneous disorder appropriately, a common language must be used and understood by all clinicians. These descriptive terms are crucial in the development of a differential diagnosis.

- Lesion: General term for any single, small area of skin disease.
- Rash: A more extensive process that is generally made up of many lesions. See Tables 14–1 and 14–2 for further terms and definitions.

INITIAL APPROACH IN THE EMERGENCY DEPARTMENT

Most cutaneous disorders presenting in the emergency department are not life-threatening, and the patient is not systemically ill. In these cases it is appropriate to begin with a detailed dermatologic history and a physical examination. However, the clinician must be able to recognize the patient with a serious cutaneous disorder or a cutaneous manifestation of a serious systemic illness.

TABLE 14–1. Basic Terminology

Primary Skin Lesions: Initial, Basic Lesion
- Macule: An area of color change <2 cm in diameter. Is not palpable. Visible margins only. May be red, brown, yellow, or white.
- Patch: Macules >2 cm in diameter.
- Papule: A palpable mass <1.5 cm in diameter. May be red, brown, yellow, white, or skin-colored. May be flat-topped, dome-shaped, or pointed. May have a smooth surface or have surface changes, such as scale, crust, erosion, or ulceration.
- Plaque: A flat-topped, palpable lesion >1.5 cm in diameter. Papule that has enlarged in length and width but not depth.
- Nodule: A papule that has enlarged in length, width, and depth. More than 1.5 cm in diameter. May be solid, edematous, or cystic and may be dome-shaped or have sloped shoulders.
- Wheal: An edematous papule containing nonloculated fluid.
- Vesicle: A fluid-filled papule <1 cm in diameter in which the fluid is loculated. Usually skin-colored because they contain clear fluid.
- Bulla: A vesicle >1 cm in diameter.
- Petechiae: A circumscribed deposit of blood <0.5 cm in diameter.
- Purpura: A circumscribed deposit of blood >0.5 cm in diameter.

Secondary Skin Lesions:
Develop during the evolutionary process of the cutaneous disorder or are created by scratching or infection
- Scales: Shedding of excess keratin from surface epithelial cells. Reflects abnormal keratinization. Loose flakes of scale are white or gray and rough on palpation. Compacted scale is translucent and shiny and smooth on palpation.
- Crust: A collection of dried serum and cellular debris. Usually yellow or yellow-brown in color unless red blood cells are involved—then the crust is black.
- Excoriation: Linear or angular erosions due to scratching.
- Lichenification: An area of thickened epidermis that results from habitual rubbing. The normal skin markings are accentuated and may be accompanied by a mild amount of scaling.

History

Are there any other symptoms not related to the lesions or rash? Key symptoms to be covered briefly include:
1. Shortness of breath, chest pain
2. Hoarseness or voice change, trouble swallowing
3. Malaise, headache, visual disturbances
4. Neck stiffness, mental status changes
5. Abdominal pain, nausea, vomiting
6. Arthralgias
7. Easy bruisability, mucosal bleeding

Physical Examination

1. General appearance: Most patients who are systemically ill look ill.
2. Are there any airway problems? A patient with urticaria may have laryngeal edema or wheezing leading to airway compromise.

TABLE 14–2. Other Descriptive Terms

- Margination: The shape of a lesion as viewed in cross section, representing the transition from normal to diseased skin. If that transition occurs abruptly (dome-shaped, square shoulders), the lesion is sharply marginated. If the transition zone is gradual (slope shoulders), it is poorly marginated. This term is helpful in distinguishing the papulosquamous diseases with their sharp margins from the eczematous diseases, which have poor margination.
- Configuration: The shape of a lesion as viewed from above.
- Linear or angular: Suggests that external factors are causative agents, as in contact dermatitis.
- Annular: A ring-shaped lesion. This shape implies outward extension with central clearing.
- Discoid: A lesion with outward extension without central clearing.
- Nummular: A coin-shaped lesion without central clearing.
- Iris or target: A ring-shaped lesion with a central bull's-eye.

254 — CUTANEOUS DISORDERS

3. The vital signs are obtained.
4. A brief survey of the lesions or rash is performed. Is the rash extensive? Bigger is not necessarily worse, but it can imply a serious problem. Is there mucosal involvement?
5. Is there generalized lymphadenopathy?

Interventions

As with any potential life-threatening process, the following basic measures are carried out to ensure the safety of the patient:

1. The patient is transferred to a higher level care area within the emergency department. Patients with rash of whatever cause are often triaged to a basic exam room.
2. Oxygen per nasal cannula can be beneficial, particularly in a patient with compromised respiration. Occasionally, more definitive airway management may be necessary.
3. Intravenous access is established. An isotonic crystalloid solution is the fluid of choice.

PROBLEM 1 This 50 year old man looked ill and was lying quietly on the stretcher. His temperature was 102°F (38.9°C), blood pressure 100/70 mm Hg, and pulse was 120 beats/min. His respiratory rate was 20/min. He complained of malaise and chills. He had a headache, felt sleepy, and said that the light bothered his eyes.

Even without recognizing the skin lesions, it is apparent that a serious process is ongoing. The patient is systemically ill. The patient may not volunteer information about "insignificant skin lesions"; therefore it is imperative that the patient be fully undressed and the entire body examined.

DATA GATHERING

In dermatology it is often useful to perform a brief initial overview examination of the rash or lesion to guide the data-gathering process. An appropriate dermatologic history and physical examination includes all of the following points.

History

1. *What was the date of onset?*
   This will help determine if the patient has an acute process such as contact dermatitis or a chronic problem like psoriasis.
2. *Where was the site of onset?*
   If the lesions are confined to a particular anatomic site, the scope of the differential diagnosis is automatically limited. Has it spread? If so, to what areas? What areas are spared? A patient with a rash in the clothing distribution which spares the axilla has a dermatitis due to some constituent of clothing. But if the axilla is involved, the rash is usually a dermatitis due to a component of an antiperspirant or deodorant.
3. *Does the lesion or rash exhibit periodicity?*
   Hand lesions that improve on weekends are probably due to a work-related irritant dermatitis.
4. *What makes the lesion better and what makes it worse?*
   Pruritus associated with urticarial lesions will improve with cool compresses and worsen with a hot shower.
5. *Does anyone else at home or at work have a similar rash? Are there any known exposures to contagious diseases?*
   Scabies and flea bites can affect the entire household.

6. *What are the patient's occupation, hobbies, and recreational activities?*
7. *Are there any associated local symptoms such as pain or itching?*
   A painless penile lesion may be the chancre of primary syphilis, whereas painful penile lesions may represent chancroid. Patients with lesions of scabies or urticaria almost always describe intense pruritus.
8. *What treatment, if any, has been given for the lesion or rash?*
   Many patients attempt to treat their condition prior to seeking medical advice. The treatment may alter the appearance of the rash.
9. *Is the patient taking any medication or has he recently finished taking medication? Has the patient used any illicit intravenous drugs?*
   In the case of a possible drug eruption rash, this information is crucial. One should not forget to ask about over-the-counter medications and contraceptives.
10. *Does the patient have any allergies?*
    This question includes allergies to external agents, food allergies, and drug allergies.
11. *What is the patient's past medical history?*
    The past medical history should include any previous cutaneous disorders.

Physical Examination

The physical examination is crucial in making the correct diagnosis, since dermatology is a visual specialty. Although the focus in dermatology is on the skin and its related structures, it must always be kept in mind that the patient may have a potentially life-threatening dermatosis.

1. Adequate exposure and lighting are needed. The entire skin needs to be examined to avoid missing important information.
2. Are any of the initial lesions still present? A lesion can change over time or with scratching or rubbing and can confuse the examiner. A fresh lesion, if present, is most helpful in pinpointing the diagnosis.
3. The lesion or rash is palpated wearing gloves. Is the lesion or rash palpable? Is the skin texture rough or smooth? Is the lesion or rash wet? Is the skin surrounding the lesion cool or warm to the touch?
4. The size and configuration of the lesion or rash are noted.
5. It is also noted whether the lesion or rash has sharp margins or is poorly marginated.
6. The distribution of the lesions or rash is described accurately.
7. A general physical examination is completed to look for other associated findings that may contribute to the diagnosis.

PROBLEM 2 The lesions on the 24 year old black male were distributed on the trunk and neck with involvement of the palms and soles.

There are a limited number of rashes that involve the palms and soles. This unique distribution helps to limit the scope of the differential diagnosis.

PROBLEM 3 The 30 year old white female with the arm lesions stated that they began 3 days ago on her wrists. They spread to her forearms, but no other areas were involved. She had had similar lesions last spring, but they weren't as bad and resolved spontaneously after several weeks. Calamine lotion made the rash slightly better. No one else at home or at work had any similar lesions. The patient was an accountant and a weekend gardener. Five days ago, she was gardening while wearing gloves and a short sleeved shirt. The lesions were not painful but were very itchy.

From the historical data gathered, the importance of the patient's gardening hobby and the connection between the forearm distribution of the lesions and her exposed forearms during this activity became apparent.

DECISION PRIORITIES AND PRELIMINARY DIFFERENTIAL DIAGNOSIS

The descriptive approach to dermatology based on the Lynch algorithm allows placement of an unknown lesion or rash into a major diagnostic group. To begin the process of developing a differential diagnosis, the questions listed in Figure 14–2 are asked in order to describe the lesion or rash. This information is then used to make an accurate diagnosis based on the choices in the major diagnostic groups (Table 14–3). How well this approach works can be illustrated by referring to the problem cases.

PROBLEM 1 This patient had several solid, red, nonscaling, flat-topped lesions. Following

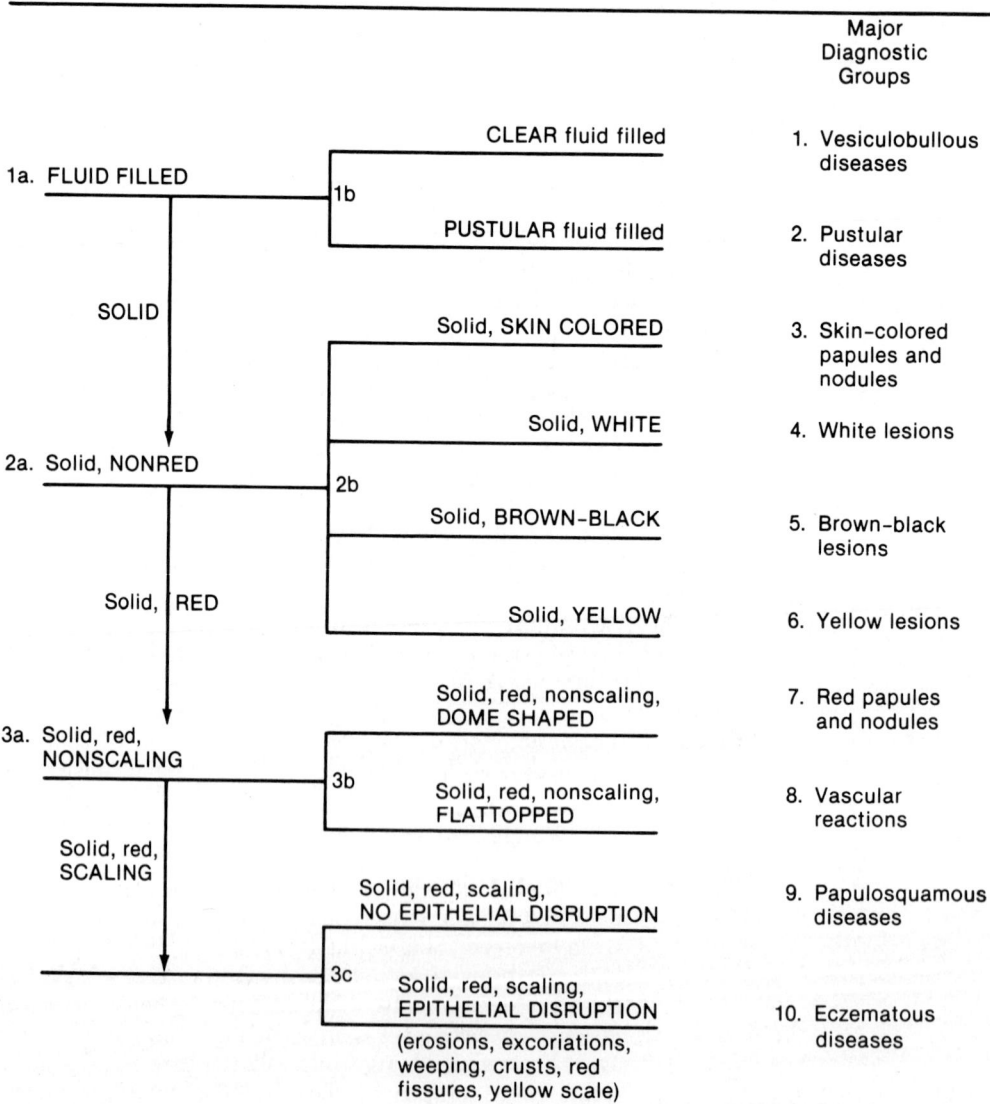

FIGURE 14–2. A rapid method to place rashes into major diagnostic groups is illustrated by this algorithm. Basic descriptors for the consistency, color, and appearance of the rash allow for the initial group selection. (Modified from Lynch PJ, Edminster SC: Dermatology for the nondermatologist. Ann Emerg Med 13(8):603–606, 1984.)

TABLE 14–3. The Lynch Algorithm*

I. Vesiculobullous diseases
   A. Vesicular disease
      1. Herpes simplex
      2. Varicella-zoster
      3. Vesicular tinea pedis
      4. Dyshidrosis (pompholyx)
      5. Scabies
      6. Dermatitis herpetiformis
   B. Bullous disease
      1. Poison-ivy-type contact dermatitis
      2. Bullous impetigo
      3. Erythema multiforme bullosum (Stevens Johnson syndrome)
      4. Pemphigoid
      5. Pemphigus
II. Pustular diseases
   A. True (soft pustules)
      1. Acne vulgaris
      2. Rosacea (acne rosacea)
      3. Bacterial folliculitis
      4. Fungal folliculitis
      5. Candidiasis
      6. Systemic bacterial infection (e.g., gonorrhea)
   B. Pseudopustules
      (See white papules, group IV)
III. Skin-colored lesions
   A. Keratotic (rough-surfaced lesions)
      1. Warts: verruca vulgaris, paronychial, and plantar warts
      2. Actinic keratoses
      3. Seborrheic keratoses
      4. Corns and calluses
   B. Nonkeratotic (smooth lesions)
      1. Warts: genital warts, flat warts
      2. Basal and squamous cell carcinoma (with or without ulceration)
      3. Epidermoid ("sebaceous") cysts
      4. Lipomas
      5. Molluscum contagiosum
      6. Nevi: intradermal
IV. White lesions
   A. White patches and plaques
      1. Pityriasis alba
      2. Pityriasis (tinea) versicolor
      3. Vitiligo
      4. Postinflammatory hypopigmentation
   B. White papules
      1. Milia
      2. Keratosis pilaris
      3. Molluscum contagiosum
      4. Sebaceous gland hyperplasia
V. Brown lesions
   A. Brown macules
      1. Freckles
      2. Lentigenes
      3. Nevi: junctional
   B. Brown papules and nodules
      1. Nevi: compound and intradermal
      2. Seborrheic keratoses
      3. Melanoma
   C. Brown patches and plaques
      1. Café au lait patches
      2. Postinflammatory hyperpigmentation
      3. Giant congenital nevi
   D. Generalized hyperpigmentation
      1. Secondary to systemic disease
      2. Secondary to medication
      3. Postinflammatory hyperpigmentation

VI. Yellow lesions
   A. Smooth yellow lesions
      1. Xanthelasma
      2. Necrobiosis lipoidica diabeticorum
      3. Sebaceous gland hyperplasia
   B. Rough yellow lesions
      1. Actinic keratoses
      2. Any crusted lesion (see vesiculobullous diseases, eczematous and insect bites)
VII. Inflammatory papules and nodules
   A. Nonscaling red papules
      1. Insect bites
      2. Cherry angiomas
      3. Spider angiomas
      4. Granuloma annulare
      5. See nonconfluent papules, group IX
   B. Nonscaling red nodules
      1. Furuncles
      2. Inflamed epidermoid cysts
      3. Hidradenitis suppurativa
      4. Erythema nodosum
VIII. Vascular reactions
   A. Nonpurpuric (blanchable) leasions
      1. Toxic erythema: exanthems, medications, photosensitivity
      2. Urticaria: infection, medications
      3. Erythema multiforme
      4. Cellulitis (erysipelas)
   B. Purpuric lesions
      1. Neutrophilic vasculitis
         a. Meningococcemia
         b. RMSF
         c. Palpable purpura
      2. Actinic ("senile") purpura
      3. Petechia and ecchymoses secondary to medications
IX. Papulosquamous diseases
   A. Prominent plaque formation
      1. Psoriasis vulgaris
      2. Tinea: corporis, capitis, pedis, cruris
      3. Lupus erythematosus: discoid type
      4. Parapsoriasis-mycosis fungoides
   B. Nonconfluent papules
      1. Pityriasis rosea
      2. Lichen planus
      3. Syphilis: secondary
      4. Psoriasis: guttate type
X. Eczematous diseases
   A. Excoriations prominent
      1. Atopic dermatitis (neurodermatitis, lichen simplex chronicus, infantile eczema)
      2. Dyshidrotic eczema
      3. Stasis dermatitis
      4. Tinea: cruris, capitis, pedis
      5. Psoriasis in atopic individuals
      6. Candidiasis
   B. Little or no excoriation
      1. Seborrheic dermatitis
      2. Contact dermatitis
      3. Xerotic (asteatotic) eczema
      4. Impetigo
   C. Eczematous reaction patterns (seen with more than one of the above eczematous diseases)
      1. Hand and foot eczema
      2. Diaper dermatitis
      3. Nummular eczema
      4. Exfoliative erythrodermatitis
      5. Autoeczematization (autosensitization, "Id" reaction)

*Once a major diagnostic group has been selected, the individual diagnostic possibilities are explored by using the list under each heading as an aid to further patient questioning and examination.
Modified from Lynch PJ, Edminster SC: Dermatology for the nondermatologist. Ann Emerg Med 13(8):603–606, 1984, Fig. 2.

the algorithm, it is apparent that these lesions belonged in the vascular reaction group. Since they did not blanch on pressure, the differential lay with the purpuric lesions. The patient stated that he was taking no medications; therefore, petechiae and ecchymoses due to medication were ruled out. Actinic or senile purpura occurs on sun-damaged skin. Since this patient was a businessman with little outdoor activity, it is unlikely that this is the diagnosis. That leaves the diagnosis of neutrophilic vasculitis. This type of vasculitis is caused by medications, infection, autoimmune disease, and certain malignancies. The lesions of neutrophilic or leukocytoclastic vasculitis consist entirely of petechiae and are associated with perivascular inflammation resulting in palpable lesions (palpable purpura). This description corresponds to the lesions found on this patient. From the initial assessment of this patient, it was apparent that he had symptoms consistent with meningitis. Therefore, a major diagnostic concern would be meningococcemia.

PROBLEM 2 This patient had a solid red, scaling rash. There were no signs of excoriation, fissures, or crusts, so there was no epithelial disruption. The major diagnostic group for this rash is papulosquamous diseases. On physical examination, the lesions appeared as discrete palpable masses less than 1.5 cm in diameter. By definition, these are nonconfluent papules. Table 14–3 delineates four possible diagnoses in this group. The distribution of pityriasis rosea in the typical Christmas tree pattern without involvement of the palms and soles did not fit this patient. A lichen planus rash occurs on the trunk but rarely involves the palms and soles. The papules of lichen planus are more violet than red in color, distinguishing them from other lesions. Because the color and distribution were wrong, lichen planus could be ruled out. Guttate psoriasis is often triggered by a streptococcal infection and consists of a widespread papular rash. The papules may be arranged in a linear manner along a scratch. This provocation of lesions by trauma is called Koebner's reaction and is distinctive for psoriasis and lichen planus. This patient gave no history of a recent sore throat and had no evidence of Koebner's reaction. It appeared, therefore, that secondary syphilis was the most likely diagnosis.

PROBLEM 3 In this case, the clear fluid-filled lesions fulfilled the criteria for vesiculobullous diseases. The lesions were greater than 1 cm in diameter and therefore belonged in the bullous disease category. From the complete physical examination, it was clear that this patient had discrete localized lesions. Erythema multiforme bullosum, pemphigoid, and pemphigus can automatically be ruled out because all these are disorders with extensive cutaneous and mucous membrane involvement. Bullous impetigo usually occurs on the face, hands, elbows, and knees but can occur on the arms and legs. The blisters rupture, leaving a crust, and pus may accumulate under the crusts. Poison ivy-type contact dermatitis occurs in exposed areas and may have a unilateral or asymmetric distribution. Vesicles and bullae occur on top of inflammatory plaques. Weeping and crusting can occur, but no pus is seen unless there is secondary infection. A linear and angular configuration resulting from antigen deposition in scratch marks is distinctive of this disorder. Because of the linear configuration and the strong history of exposure, poison ivy dermatitis was the most likely diagnosis in this patient.

DIAGNOSTIC ADJUNCTS

A few simple tests done in the emergency department can give immediate information that can aid in making the diagnosis of a cutaneous disorder.

Diascopy

A glass slide is firmly placed against a solid, red, nonscaling lesion. It is used to determine whether the lesion blanches with pressure as do the wheals of urticaria. A nonblanchable lesion implies extravasated blood such as occurs in the petechiae of meningococcemia.

Potassium Hydroxide Preparation

This test is helpful in confirming or ruling out the presence of a fungal infection and in identifying the causative mite in suspected cases of scabies. To determine the presence of fungal disease, the lesions are scraped vigorously with the edge of a microscope slide or a No. 15 scalpel blade after moistening the skin slightly with tap water. The best areas to use for obtaining a specimen include the underside of the roof of a blister, moist macerated areas, the rim of a lesion, under the nail or paronychial fold, and the base of a plucked hair. The scrapings are placed on a glass slide, one to two drops of 10% potassium hydroxide (KOH) solution are added, and the slide is covered with a glass cover slip. The specimen is gently heated over an alcohol flame. Right after heating the specimen is examined under the microscope at $10\times$ and $40\times$ objective power with low illumination. The presence or absence of hyphae or spores is determined. They may resemble grapes on a branch or spaghetti and meatballs, or long thin hyphae may be present with few spores. For the diagnosis of scabies, a fresh lesion at the end of a burrow should be selected. The best areas are the wrist, between the fingers, and the shaft of the penis. With a No. 15 scalpel blade, the top of the lesion is removed. The base of the lesion is scraped and the specimen is placed on a glass slide. Two drops of 10% KOH solution are added and a cover slip is put in place. The specimen is viewed under $10\times$ magnification, searching for the mite, egg, or fecal deposits. No heating is necessary.

Tzanck Smear

The presence of multinucleated giant cells with intranuclear inclusions on a specially prepared smear is diagnostic of herpes simplex, herpes zoster, and varicella. To make a Tzanck smear, the top of the vesicle or bulla is removed with a scalpel blade. The base of the lesion is gently scraped and the material smeared on a microscope slide. After letting it air dry, the specimen is stained with Giemsa or routine Wright's stain. A drop of immersion oil and a cover slip are added, and the specimen is examined under $10\times$ and $40\times$ objective power for the multinucleated giant cells.

Gram's Stain

Gram's stain is rarely helpful in making the diagnosis of a cutaneous lesion. Pustules, crusts, or exudates may have overlying skin colonization with bacteria, making interpretation of the Gram's stained specimen confusing. In the case of gonorrhea, a Gram's stained specimen of the cervical or penile discharge that exhibits gram-negative intracellular diplococci is diagnostic for the disease. The organisms are not recoverable from the skin lesions in patients with disseminated gonococcemia.

Wood's Lamp Examination

A Wood's lamp is a low-output ultraviolet lamp. Examination of certain skin lesions with a Wood's lamp will show a characteristic fluorescent pattern. In patients with tinea capitis due to *Microsporum* sharply marginated, bright blue-green patches are visible on the scalp when it is examined with the Wood's lamp. In patients with erythrasma, which is an erythematous patch affecting the intertriginous areas and caused by a bacterium, a red fluorescence of the skin is seen on examination with a Wood's lamp. This sign is extremely helpful because erythrasma looks very similar to the lesions of tinea cruris, which do not fluoresce. Hypopigmented lesions do not fluoresce but are more visible when examined under a Wood's lamp in a darkened room. This procedure may also lead to better identification of the skin lesions of tinea versicolor and vitiligo and the ash leaf spots of tuberous sclerosis.

VDRL/RPR

A serologic test (Venereal Disease Research Laboratories [VDRL]/rapid protein reagin [RPR]) is performed in any case of suspected syphilis or in patients who have a rash, usually in a generalized, maculopapular distribution, that cannot be explained. Syphilis can masquerade as other, more benign dermatoses such as pityriasis rosea.

REFINED DIFFERENTIAL DIAGNOSIS

Using the major diagnostic groups as a guideline, several dermatologic manifestations of serious systemic illness and common dermatologic disorders can be described in more detail.

Potential Life-Threatening Dermatoses
Vesiculobullous Diseases

Erythema Multiforme Bullosum. Erythema multiforme bullosum is a variant of erythema multiforme characterized by bullous lesions. *Stevens-Johnson syndrome* (SJS) is erythema multiforme with extensive mucosal lesions as well as bullous-cutaneous lesions. *Toxic epidermal necrolysis* (TEN) is a variant of erythema multiforme characterized by extensive cutaneous bullae associated with epidermal sloughing. Causes of erythema multiforme and its variants include medications, especially sulfa drugs, bacterial, viral, and fungal infections, and autoimmune diseases.

Patients with SJS present with vesicles and ulcerations of the mucous membranes of the lips, buccal cavity, eyes, nostrils, and genitalia. Bullous lesions appear on the hands and feet and the trunk. These patients appear extremely toxic and have a high fever and malaise. They have difficulty with oral intake, and urinary retention may result from the painful mucosal lesions. Eye involvement can be severe, and blindness can result. Mortality is 5%. The rash of TEN begins on the face and is followed by widespread erythema and extensive formation of bullae. The bullae and large sheets of epidermis can be lifted off the dermis. Because of the subepidermal cleavage plane, extensive fluid loss can occur. The mucous membranes are usually involved as in SJS. These patients are extremely toxic with fever and malaise. They have signs of dehydration and vascular collapse due to fluid losses. Mortality is 10% to 30%.

Pustular Diseases

Gonococcemia. Disseminated gonococcemia occurs in 1% to 3% of patients with gonorrhea. It usually occurs 3 to 21 days after the initial infecting contact. The skin lesions are often few in number and tend to occur on the palms, fingers, and soles. The lesions are umbilicated pustules with a red halo. Occasionally erythematous macules, tender hemorrhagic papules, or hemorrhagic necrotic bullae may be seen. A flulike illness precedes the migratory polyarthralgias and the pustules by 1 to 3 weeks. Although gonococcemia is relatively benign, life-threatening complications of meningitis, endocarditis, myocarditis, pericarditis, or hepatitis can develop if the disease is left untreated.

Vascular Reactions

Meningococcemia. Meningococcemia is a rapidly progressive and potentially lethal infection due to *Neisseria meningitis*. It often follows a mild upper respiratory infection. The patient looks toxic and has a fever. He may complain of headache, nausea, and vomiting. Meningeal signs may or may not be present. Mental status changes, such as aggressive behavior, confusion, or stupor may occur. Five to ten percent of patients have a fulminant onset characterized by vasomotor collapse and shock. Seventy-five percent of patients have skin lesions that consist of palpable petechiae with pale gray centers. They usually occur on the wrists, ankles, and flanks and in the axillae. The lesions may progress to purpura fulminans.

Rocky Mountain Spotted Fever. This tick-borne rickettsial disease occurs mostly in the spring and summer. The incubation period from tick bite to illness is about 7 days. The classic triad of symptoms of Rocky Mountain spotted fever (RMSF) is fever, rash, and a history of tick exposure; this triad occurs in only 67% of patients with the disease. RMSF begins with a prodrome of fever, chills, severe frontal headache, arthralgias, and myalgias. The rash begins on day 2 to 4 of the illness as erythematous macules, which become palpable petechiae and finally hemorrhagic vesicles. The rash begins on the palms, wrists, soles, and ankles and spreads to involve the entire body. Abdominal pain, hepatomegaly, splenomegaly, conjunctivitis, lymphadenopathy, and meningismus are frequently seen. Mortality in untreated cases ranges from 20% in children to 80% in adults.

Urticaria with Anaphylaxis. Urticaria represents the skin manifestations of an allergic reaction. Urticarial lesions are transient edematous papules or wheals that extend to form large flat plaques. Urticaria can involve any part of the body. Itching is usually a prominent feature. Urticaria is triggered by a wide variety of agents. Possible causes include medications, infections, insect venom, autoimmune diseases, dysproteinemias, malignancies, and foods, dyes, and preservatives. IgE-mediated systemic involvement in addition to skin lesions represents anaphylaxis and is a true emergency. The hallmarks of anaphylaxis include hoarseness, trouble in swallowing, stridor, wheezing, and respiratory arrest. Hypotension and vascular collapse may occur owing to vasodilation and capillary permeability. Other findings include apprehension, a sense of impending doom, headache, increased lacrimation, rhinorrhea, abdominal pain, and pelvic pain from uterine contractions. Angioneurotic edema is a variant of urticaria with painless subcutaneous swelling of the face involving the eyelids, lips, and tongue. It may be hereditary or sporadic and may result in laryngeal edema and airway compromise.

Cellulitis. Cellulitis is a localized deep infection involving both the dermis and the subcutaneous tissue. It is usually caused by *Streptococcus pyogenes* or *Staphylococcus aureus* and is often precipitated by minor trauma or preexisting lymphatic stasis. Cellulitis occurs most frequently on the extremities and the face. The lesion is deeply indurated, erythematous, warm, edematous, tender, and poorly marginated. Regional adenopathy may be prominent. There may be systemic spread of the infection manifested by fever and malaise.

Common Dermatoses
Vesiculobullous Diseases

Herpes Simplex. Herpes simplex is caused by *Herpesvirus hominis* types I and II. They result in herpes labialis or herpes genitalis eruptions. Recurrent infections are quite common and are triggered by sunburn, coryza, fever, and stress for type I, and trauma during intercourse, vaginitis, menses, and stress for type II. There is a preeruptive syndrome that consists of burning and tingling of the skin prior to the appearance of lesions. Herpes labialis lesions present as a tight cluster of small vesicles on an erythematous base or arising from normal skin in the perioral area. The vesicles are fragile and rupture easily, leaving an irregularly shaped erosion. Herpes genitalis is similar to herpes labialis in appearance except that more vesicles are present, and they are less tightly clustered. Primary and recurrent lesions are painful. The diagnosis can be confirmed by Tzanck smear or viral culture.

Scabies. This infestation is due to the mite *Sarcoptes scabiei*. The female mite burrows within the stratum corneum and deposits eggs within the epidermis. Transmission of the disease usually depends on direct person-to-person contact but can occur through contaminated clothing or bed linens. Once contracted, it is spread by scratching. The lesions of scabies are quite pruritic, especially after several weeks of infestation, when allergic sensitization occurs. Although scabies is a vesicular disease, few intact vesicles are seen because of the intense scratching, which leaves excoriated inflammatory papules. If present, the vesicles are oval or elongated, reflecting their development as a burrow for the mite. The lesions are distributed in the web spaces of the hands, around the elbows, on the anterior axillary folds, and over the buttocks. The breasts in women and the penis in men are often involved. Long-standing cases involve the trunk and extremities, but the face is spared (except in infants). The diagnosis is confirmed by demonstration of the mite, eggs, or feces in material obtained from unroofing the lesion.

Papulosquamous Diseases

Tinea. Tinea is a superficial fungal infection affecting the feet, the groin area, the body, or the scalp. The diagnosis can be made from KOH preparations and fungal cultures. Tinea pedis involves the feet and usually begins with fissures in the web space between the fourth and fifth toes that appear white and macerated. The infection can spread to involve the toenails, but it does not extend to the dorsal surface of the foot. It is worsened by occlusive footwear, which promotes a warm, moist environment that encourages growth of the dermatophyte.

Tinea cruris involves the groin area and begins as a sharply marginated red plaque in the inguinoscrotal crease. It advances to the inner thighs and may extend to the gluteal cleft and buttocks but tends to spare the penis and scrotum. It is more common in men and does not occur prior to puberty. Tinea corporis involves the neck, arms, legs, or trunk. Annular tinea corporis is the classic "ringworm" infection, which begins as an erythematous, sharply marginated, scaling plaque that enlarges and becomes clear in the center. The annular form rarely consists of more than one or two lesions. Other forms of tinea corporis present as multiple annular lesions with gyrate or serpiginous borders.

Tinea capitis involves the scalp and occurs in two forms. The noninflammatory form presents with patchy, scaling areas containing short stubby hairs. If the hairs are broken off at the surface of the scalp, a characteristic black dot appearance results. This type of infestation is extremely common in black children. The inflammatory type consists of exudative, crusted patches, draining nodules, or massive swellings with multiple pustules and draining sinuses; it can easily be confused with a bacterial infection. To make the diagnosis in either type, use a plucked broken-off hair rather than scalp scrapings for the KOH preparation or culture.

Tinea can be complicated by an "id" reaction, an idiopathic vesicular eruption of the palms and lateral borders of the fingers distant from the fungal infection site.

Pityriasis Rosea. This disorder most often affects healthy young people between the ages of 10 and 30 years. The cause is unknown. Most patients are asymptomatic, but some may complain of extreme pruritus. Because secondary syphilis can mimic the rash of pityriasis rosea, it is advisable to perform a VDRL test in most instances. In 50% of patients a large erythematous scaling plaque may be present that may be oval or annular and precedes the rash. This is known as the herald patch. This patch is followed by an eruption of 50 to 100 isolated, oval erythematous, nonconfluent papules 1 cm in diameter. These oval lesions run parallel to the rib lines in the typical Christmas tree distribution. The lesions are found on the trunk, neck, and inner aspects of the arms and thighs. The face is always spared.

Eczematous Diseases

Contact Dermatitis. Contact dermatitis is an inflammatory response of the skin to an external agent. There are two major types: irritant contact dermatitis and allergic contact dermatitis.

Irritant contact dermatitis is more common than allergic contact dermatitis. Strong irritants will produce skin changes almost immediately after a single exposure. Examples of these are thermal burns and chemical burns due to strong acid or alkaline solutions. These are painful lesions. Weak irritants cause skin changes after repeated exposures to the irritant; these are due to changes in the moisture content of the skin. The changes result in skin that is too dry or too wet. Examples of weak irritants are detergents, hot water, and solvents. Irritant dermatitis can involve any area of the skin, but the hands are most frequently affected. Exposure to strong irritants produces erythema, swelling, blister formation, ulceration, or skin necrosis. Low-grade irritants causing drying of the skin result in minimal redness with cracks and fissure and scale formation. When exposure to low-grade irritants results in maceration, the area is bright red with small amounts of weeping, and scale formation is not prominent.

Allergic contact dermatitis is the result of inflammatory changes that are due to sensitization to chemical antigens. The inflammatory response does not occur on the first exposure to the antigen, and sensitization may not occur for months or years. The most common antigens responsible for allergic contact dermatitis are pentadecacatechols of poison ivy, nickel, formaldehyde, neomycin, benzocaine, parabens, ethylenediamine, chromates in cements and cutting oils, and uncured epoxy resins in fiberglass. Proof of causation can be made by patch testing. The affected area exhibits prominent erythema and edema. Weeping and crusting will be present in acute cases, whereas in chronic cases scale formation is more prominent. Vesicles are seen only in poison ivy dermatitis. Asymmetric or unilateral lesions may suggest an external causation. Linear configuration of lesions is a clue to causation by external agents. Pruritus is usually a prominent feature.

Drug Eruptions

Drug eruptions transcend classification because they can present in many different forms. No drug is "safe," and drugs vary in their ability to produce a reaction. The same drug can produce a variety of reactions. Drug reactions often occur after a course of therapy has been completed. The most likely culprit is the drug most recently prescribed. However, a reaction can develop after a drug has been taken continuously for months or years.

Exanthems. A morbilliform rash is the most common expression of a drug rash and accounts for 50% of all cases. This rash appears as discrete or confluent erythematous macules and papules distributed on the trunk, face, and extremities. Palms, soles, and mucous membranes are not usually involved. The penicillins, sulfonamides, phenytoin, and barbiturates are the most frequent causes of this type of drug eruption.

Urticaria. Typical urticarial lesions consist of edematous papules or wheals, and anaphylaxis accounts for 25% of drug rashes. Penicillin and its derivatives are the most common drugs associated with urticaria and anaphylaxis. Aspirin and nonsteroidal anti-inflammatory agents also cause this type of rash. Codeine causes urticaria by triggering the release of histamine by nonimmunologic mechanisms. Serum sickness is characterized by urticaria, fever, myalgias, arthritis, and lymphadenopathy. It usually begins 7 to 10 days after administration of the drug and is due to circulating immune complexes. Penicillin, sulfonamides, phenytoin, and thiazides can produce this type of reaction.

Erythema Multiforme and Erythema Multiforme Bullosum. The penicillins, phenytoin, sulfonamides, thiazide diuretics, phenothiazines, chloropropamide, pyrazolone, and allopurinol have been implicated in erythema multiforme. The rash may present as the typical minor form of erythema multiforme or may progress to the life-threatening bullous forms (TEN, SJS).

Exfoliative Dermatitis. The generalized eczematous reaction characteristic of exfoliative dermatitis is most likely to be triggered by gold therapy or phenytoin.

Acneiform Dermatitis. Acneiform dermatitis has the appearance of acne vulgaris but without the formation of comedones and cysts. It has a sudden onset and is commonly caused by steroids, phenytoin, or lithium.

Vasculitis or Palpable Purpura. Vasculitis results in a petechial rash or widespread palpable purpura that affects the legs most severely. Sulfonamides, thiazide diuretics, pyrazolone, triouracils, phenytoin, penicillin, indomethacin, cimetidine, and quinidine are the most likely culprits.

Localized Reaction. Drug eruptions may also manifest as localized reactions. A fixed drug reaction presents as a recurrent erythematous, oral plaque in the same site with each exposure to the drug. It is associated with tetracycline, chlordiazepoxide, sulfonamides, and phenobarbital. The tender erythematous plaques or nodules of erythema nodosum may occur in response to oral contraceptive use or sulfonamide, penicillin, or salicylate therapy. These lesions are extremely painful and are most always located on the anterior legs.

Photosensitivity. Certain drugs may be responsible for photoeruptions. A phototoxic eruption resembles an exaggerated sunburn in light-exposed areas. Compounds that absorb ultraviolet energy, such as tetracycline and its derivatives, can cause this condition. A photoallergic reaction is the result of a cell-mediated immune response that is elicited by light exposure. It resembles an allergic contact dermatitis and is usually due to topical drugs.

PRINCIPLES OF MANAGEMENT

Management of a cutaneous lesion or rash includes general therapeutic techniques of skin care as well as specific therapy for the particular disease state.

General Therapy

Wet Dressing. Wet dressings are indicated for any scaly eruption of an acute nature such as eczema as well as for crusted, exudative lesions. They provide an antipruritic effect, cause evaporative heat loss, which reduces inflammation, and effectively debride crusts to prevent secondary infection and maceration from fluid entrapment. There are three types of wet dressings: compresses (wet cloths soaked in solution), soaks (immersion of the involved part in solution), and baths. Soaking solutions include normal saline, Burrow's solution (1 tablet of Domeboro [aluminum sulfate and calcium acetate] diluted in a pint or quart of cold water), acetic acid (¼ cup vinegar in 1 quart of cool water), and Aveeno (colloidal oatmeal added to a cool bath).

Topical Medications and Lubricants. Topical medications and lubricants are commonly used in treatment of cutaneous disorders. They come in a variety of different vehicles, including powders, lotions, gels, creams, ointments, and pastes. Powders work best for intertriginous areas because of their ability to absorb moisture and alleviate maceration. Lotions are mild lubricants. Calamine lotion also absorbs moisture and dries out exudative lesions. Gels spread easily and work well in hair-bearing areas. Creams are good lubricants for acute exudative processes and are associated with the best patient compliance. Ointments are the best lubricants and should be the first choice for a dry chronic disorder. They should not be used on acutely oozing lesions because they are nearly occlusive.

Antipruritics and Anesthetics

Topical. Anesthetics such as lidocaine (5% ointment) may be helpful in relieving pain and itching. Benzocaine (Americaine) preparations can cause allergic contact sensitization. Antihistamines, such as diphenhydramine cream and diphenhydramine mixed with calamine lotion (Caladryl), are very popular over-the-counter remedies. They are prescribed cautiously because of the risk of allergic sensitization. Mixtures that contain menthol, phenol, and camphor can be mixed together and added to a standard lotion or cream. They produce a cooling sensation and are helpful in relieving itching.

For painful oral ulcerations and erosions it is useful to know how to prescribe "magic mouthwash." It consists of 4 oz of diphenhydramine elixir, 4 oz of Kaopectate, and 100 ml of viscous lidocaine. The patient is instructed to swish and swallow 1 teaspoon 30 minutes before each meal.

Systemic. Antihistamines are most helpful in cases of itching due to urticaria. There are approximately 30 histamine H_1 antagonists, and there is little difference between their antipruritic capabilities. Diphenhydramine (Benadryl) is probably the most sedating and should be used only at night. The histamine H_2 blockers (cimetidine and ranitidine) may be helpful in patients with chronic urticaria used in conjunction with an H_1 antihistamine. Although not a true antihistamine, hydroxyzine (Atarax) has both antihistaminic and tranquilizing properties. It is often the drug of choice for the relief of itching.

Specific Therapy
Steroids

Topical. Corticosteroids of various potency have been incorporated into lotions, gels, creams, and ointments. They are extremely useful for treatment of the eczematous disease group, moderately useful for the papulosquamous disease group, and somewhat useful for the vesiculobullous disease group. The topical steroids are divided into groups based on potency (Table 14–4). It is only necessary to learn one or two products from each group. The low-potency steroids will work for almost all acute and subacute eczematous diseases. The intermediate-potency group is used for resistant eczematous diseases and for most papulosquamous diseases. The high-potency group is necessary for eczematous diseases of the palms and soles and for resistant papulosquamous diseases. Only low-potency, nonfluorinated preparations are used for the face and groin; otherwise the patient will develop steroid acne and cutaneous atrophy or groin striae. Steroids are applied twice a day. A good time is right after bathing.

Systemic. Systemic corticosteroids are necessary when the severity or extensiveness of the cutaneous disorder precludes topical use. For example, an allergic contact dermatitis that involves the face or the trunk as well as the extremities is treated with systemic steroids. Other dermatoses treated with systemic steroids include erythema multiforme bullosum, urticaria, and several other disease states affecting a large total body surface area. Chronic eczema and psoriasis are not treated with systemic steroids in spite of their effectiveness. Their effect on a chronic illness is only transient, and there is an increased

TABLE 14–4. Topical Steroids

Potency	Use
Low Potency	
Hydrocortisone 1%, 2.5%	Acute and subacute eczematous disorders
Hydrocortisone valerate 0.2% (Westcort)	
Betamethasone valerate 0.01% (Valisone)	
Triamcinolone acetonide 0.025% (Kenalog, Aristocort)	
Intermediate Potency	
Betamethasone valerate 0.1% (Valisone)	Resistant eczematous discomforts, papulosquamous disorders
Desonide 0.05% (Tridesilon)	
Triamcinolone acetonide 0.1% (Kenalog, Aristocort)	
High Potency	
Dexamethasone 0.25% (Topicort)	Eczematous disorders of palms and soles; resistant papulosquamous disorders
Triamcinolone acetonide 0.5% (Kenalog, Aristocort)	
Fluocinonide 0.05% (Lidex, Topsyn)	

risk of adverse effects with long-term use of steroids. The most effective way to give systemic steroids is by the short-burst method. Forty to sixty milligrams of prednisone is given daily for 7 to 10 days, then discontinued without tapering. There do not appear to be any problems with pituitary-adrenal suppression using this approach. A longer treatment period usually involves a 7- to 10-day taper.

Antifungal Agents

Topical. Both clotrimazole (Lotrimin) and miconazole (Monistat) are effective against yeasts and dermatophytes. They are effective for all candidal infections as well as in tinea corporis, tinea cruris, and tinea versicolor. They are applied twice a day for 2 to 4 weeks.

Systemic. Systemic antifungal agents, such as griseofulvin (GrisPEG) and ketaconazole (Nizoral) are necessary for chronic fungal infections of the nails (onychomycosis), palms, soles (tinea pedis), and tinea capitis. They may be used for cases of extensive tinea corporis. Griseofulvin is not effective for candidal infections; however, ketaconazole is effective for both dermatophyte and candidal infections and appears to have less toxicity than griseofulvin. Often the patient must be treated for 1 month to 1 year depending on the type of infection.

Antibacterials

Topical. Topical antibiotics are helpful in the treatment of mild impetigo. Mupirocin ointment (Bactroban) is effective against both staphylococcal and streptococcal organisms. Studies have shown it to be as efficacious as oral erythromycin in the treatment of impetigo. It is applied to the affected area three times a day for 5 days.

Systemic. Ninety percent of all skin infections are caused by *Staphylococcus aureus* or group A *Streptococcus*. Penicillin is the drug of choice for streptococcal infections. An antistaphylococcal agent such as dicloxacillin is effective for staphylococcal infections. Erythromycin is effective against both organisms. Tetracycline and cephalosporins are second-line antibiotics for skin infections. Tetracycline is the drug of choice in acne, but erythromycin can be used as well, although it is not as effective. Systemic infections with cutaneous manifestations are treated with the antibiotic that is specifically effective against the causative organism.

Scabicides

Lindane (Kwell cream, lotion, or shampoo) is the treatment of choice for scabies. It is also effective against head and pubic lice. It is safe in infants and children if used properly. Crotamiton (Eurax) 10% cream or lotion is somewhat less effective than lindane, but it is also less toxic and an antipruritic.

SPECIAL CONSIDERATIONS

Pediatric Patients

Emergency dermatologic treatment transcends all age groups. However, the age of the patient can help to key in to the appropriate diagnosis. The pediatric age group deserves special mention because there are several cutaneous disorders that are more likely to occur in this group as well as some that are not likely to occur. For example, allergic contact dermatitis is unusual in this age group because it takes several months or even years to become sensitized to most common allergens. The typical cutaneous disorders in children are often infectious in origin. Some pediatric age-specific cutaneous disorders are listed in Table 14–5.

TABLE 14–5. Pediatric Cutaneous Disorders

Disease	Cause	Skin Presentation	Associated Signs and Symptoms	Therapy
Scarlet fever	Group A beta-hemolytic *Streptococcus*	Nearly confluent punctate papules, sandpaper texture. Begins on neck and chest and spreads to abdomen and extremities. Petechiae may be found in creases. Desquamation occurs	Fever, exudative pharyngitis and tonsillitis, strawberry tongue, cervical lymphadenopathy	Penicillin, erythromycin
Roseola (measles)	Paramyxovirus	Erythematous maculopapular rash begins on face and spreads to body and extremities. Desquamation occurs except on palms and soles. Koplik spots: white papules on red base on buccal mucosa opposite second molar	Fever, coryza, cough, conjunctivitis. Pneumonia, encephalitis, hemorrhagic measles can occur	Supportive/symptomatic
Rubella (German measles)	Togavirus	Erythematous maculopapular rash begins on face and spreads to trunk and extremities	Upper respiratory symptoms, fever, malaise, lymphadenopathy. Arthritis, encephalitis, hemorrhagic German measles are complications	Supportive/symptomatic
Varicella (chicken pox)	Varicella virus	Vesicles (2–4 mm) on an erythematous base progress to pustules and crusts. Rash begins on trunk and face and spreads to extremities. Lesions are present in all stages simultaneously. Pruritus is present. Patient may have mucous membrane lesions and almost always has scalp lesions. Tzanck smear is positive	Fever, malaise. Varicella bullosum, pneumonia, encephalitis, DIC, and secondary infection of lesions are complications	Cool compresses, calamine lotion. Antibiotics for secondary infection
Erythema infectiosum (fifth disease)	Probably caused by parvovirus	Erythematous plaques on cheeks; "slapped-cheeks" appearance 2–4 days later, a reticulated erythema appears on extensor surfaces of extremities and buttocks. No mucous membrane involvement	Headache, malaise, nausea, myalgias	Supportive/symptomatic

Table continued on following page

TABLE 14–5. Pediatric Cutaneous Disorders *Continued*

Disease	Cause	Skin Presentation	Associated Signs and Symptoms	Therapy
Roseola infantum	Response to several different viruses: echovirus, coxsackie virus, adenovirus	Discrete pink macules begin on trunk and may spread to extremities. Face is usually spared	High fever, rash coincides with defervescence	Supportive/symptomatic
Hand, foot, mouth disease	Coxsackie virus A-16, B-5	Maculopapular and vesicular lesions on palms and soles. Vesicles and ulcerations on tongue, buccal mucosa, soft palate, and gums	Pharyngitis, fever	Supportive/symptomatic
Exanthem	Coxsackie virus A-9, B-5	Pinkish-red maculopapular rash. Occasionally petechiae are present. A-9 virus causes generalized face and trunk lesions. B-5 virus causes generalized lesions. No mucous membrane involvement	Fever, adenopathy. Aseptic meningitis can occur	Supportive/symptomatic
Impetigo	Nonbullous: streptococcus Bullous: staphylococcus	Nonbullous: erythematous papule or vesicle that spreads to form an erosion covered with honey-colored crust. Usually involves the face. Bullous: erythematous macules that vesiculate and enlarge to produce bullae that contain purulent exudate. Rupture easily, usually involve face, trunk, or buttocks	None	Nonbullous: penicillin, erythromycin Bullous: oxacillin, dicloxacillin, erythromycin. Both: gentle washing with soap and water three times a day
Kawasaki's syndrome (mucocutaneous lymph node syndrome)	Unknown	Erythematous rash; resembles urticaria involving trunk and extremities. Can be maculopapular as in measles. Vesiculopapular eruption may occur on knees and elbows. Oral cavity: edema and erythema of lips, strawberry tongue; no mouth ulcers	Major criteria: Fever, conjunctivitis, firm indurated edema of hands and feet which later desquamates. Lymphadenopathy present. Associated signs: urethritis, arthritis, aseptic meningitis, diarrhea, hepatitis, jaundice. Twenty per cent of patients will have cardiac involvement: CHF, pericardial effusion, dysrhythmias, coronary artery aneurysms, valvular dysfunction	Hospitalize. High-dose aspirin therapy: 80 mg/kg/day until fever subsides, then 10 mg/kg/day

DIC = disseminated intravascular coagulation; CHF = congestive heart failure.

DISPOSITION AND FOLLOW-UP

Several general principles are recommended to arrange appropriate follow-up for the patient.

Admission

Patients with cutaneous disorders who have lost the generalized protective barrier function of the skin are admitted. Examples of disorders in this category include toxic epidermal necrolysis and Stevens-Johnson syndrome. Also, patients with evidence of extensive systemic involvement, airway compromise, suspected sepsis, or an immunocompromised state require inpatient therapy. These criteria include such disorders as gonococcemia, meningococcemia, Kawasaki's disease, and anaphylaxis.

Emergency Department Observation

Emergency department observation with discharge within 12 to 24 hours or less is appropriate for disorders that resolve rapidly after emergency department therapy. These disorders include anaphylaxis not requiring intubation and responding promptly to therapy, angioneurotic edema, and urticaria.

Discharge to Home

Most cutaneous disorders take at least a week or longer to resolve. It is important to schedule follow-up appropriately to allow time for improvement or resolution. It is also important to let the patient know how long the condition will last to prevent unrealistic expectations and frustration if the condition is not cured immediately.

Close Follow-Up. Close follow-up implies physician contact in 2 to 3 days by phone, a repeat emergency department visit, or an appointment with the referral physician. This is appropriate for cutaneous disorders with minimal systemic involvement. The patient must be able to tolerate the prescribed outpatient therapy. Examples of disorders in this group include cellulitis and the childhood exanthems.

Expedient Follow-Up with a Dermatologist. In certain situations the patient is referred to a dermatologist within a week or less. Examples include unknown or unclear cutaneous disorders, suspected melanoma, and known treatment failures.

Routine Dermatology Follow-Up. Certain cutaneous disorders are always referred to a dermatologist for follow-up. These include chronic dermatologic disorders such as psoriasis, acne, tinea pedis, tinea capitis, onychomycosis, chronic urticaria, and atopic dermatitis, and disorders requiring specific dermatologic work-ups.

Appropriately Timed Follow-Up with a Primary Care Physician. Minor cutaneous disorders that do not meet the criteria for the preceding categories are referred after a course of therapy to the patient's primary physician.

DOCUMENTATION

1. Thorough dermatologic history
2. Complete description of the lesion or rash
3. Indication that serious or life-threatening dermatoses have been considered and ruled out if the patient is to be sent home
4. Emergency department diagnostic efforts
5. Presumed diagnosis
6. Emergency department interventions and recommended home treatment
7. Disposition

SUMMARY AND FINAL POINTS

- Although the majority of patients who present to the emergency department with rashes do not have serious complications of that rash or an underlying systemic disorder, the possibility has to be kept in mind.
- All patients require a systemic overview before focusing on the cutaneous complaint.
- By learning the appropriate terminology and descriptors and then performing a thorough dermatologic history and physical examination, the algorithm outlined in this chapter will lead the clinician to workable differential diagnosis.
- The emergency physician has a finite number of dermatologic therapies available. The benefits and risks of each are to be well understood before prescribing them to the patient.

BIBLIOGRAPHY

Texts

1. Dobson RL, Abele DC: The Practice of Dermatology. Philadelphia, Harper & Row, 1985.
2. Habif TP: Clinical Dermatology. St. Louis, C.V. Mosby, 1985.
3. Lynch PJ: Dermatology for the House Officer. Baltimore, Williams & Wilkins, 1982.

Journal Articles

1. Buxton PK: ABC of dermatology: Fungal and yeast infections. Br Med J 296: 420–422, 1988.
2. Elgart M: Differentiation of childhood exanthems. Hosp Med 21–35, Aug. 1988.
3. Lynch PJ, Edminster SC: Dermatology for the nondermatologist. Ann Emerg Med 13(8):603–606, 1984.
4. Pariser RJ, Pariser DM: Primary care physicians' errors in handling cutaneous disorders. J Am Acad Dermatol 17(2): 239–245, 1987.
5. Rosen T: The alarming dermatoses. Emerg Med 23–60, Sept. 15, 1986.

CHAPTER 15

WOUND CARE

BRIAN ZINK, M.D.

PROBLEM 1 A 28 year old man was caught breaking into a store by police and was attacked by a police dog. The dog bit him on the head, the left shoulder, and the back. He was escorted to the emergency department.

PROBLEM 2 A 54 year old woman stumbled and fell while raking leaves. Her right lower leg was impaled on a broken stick. She pulled the stick out and came to the hospital 6 hours later.

QUESTIONS TO CONSIDER

1. What types of wounds are commonly seen in the emergency department?
2. What are the elements of a complete yet efficient wound evaluation?
3. What techniques and equipment are needed for emergency wound cleansing, exploration, and closure?
4. How is anesthesia best achieved in emergency wound care?
5. What factors determine whether a wound can be treated in the emergency department or whether surgical consultation is needed?
6. What factors affect wound healing?
7. Which subsets of patients are more likely to experience complications with wounds?
8. When are antibiotics necessary in wound care?
9. Which patients require tetanus, hepatitis, or rabies prophylaxis?
10. What types of dressings, follow-up instructions, and referral are needed for outpatient wound care?

INTRODUCTION

Wounds of all types rival upper respiratory infections as the most common reason for seeking medical care. In emergency departments minor wounds may comprise from 5% to 40% of all diagnoses. Minor wounds are more common in children, during warmer months, in laborers, and in those who work and play outdoors. The most common wounds are hand lacerations, minor burns, and puncture wounds.

Skin Anatomy

The major components of the skin are the epidermis, dermis, and fascia.
Epidermis. The epidermis is the thick, totally cellular outer segment that does not contain blood, lymphatic vessels, or connective tissue. Wounds that violate only the epidermis, such as first-degree burns or superficial scratches, are usually minor.
Dermis. The dermis is the deeper layer of the skin that contains vascular, nervous, and structural connective tissues. It also houses the four skin appendages derived from the epidermis—hair follicles, eccrine and apocrine sweat glands, and sebaceous glands. The dermis is readily visible in wounds that require closure, and its proper approximation is essential to good wound healing and final cosmetic appearance.

Fascia. Beneath the dermis is the subcutaneous tissue. This tissue is divided into two layers of fascia. The superficial fascia is a web of connective tissue interspersed with fat. It is readily identifiable in wounds. The deep fascia is a dense, thin fibrous layer that supports and protects the underlying muscle and bony tissue. Any violation of the deep fascia signifies a more complicated wound. The subcutaneous tissue contains spaces in which blood or pus may accumulate. It must be cleansed and debrided properly to prevent unwanted bleeding or infection.

There are regional differences to consider when repairing the skin. The scalp is special because of its extremely rich blood supply and the presence of a fibrous layer, the galea aponeurotica. The palms and soles are notable for their thick epidermis. The eyelids have a very thin dermis, whereas the back has a thick dermis.

Mechanisms of Injury

Lacerations are often described as resulting from shearing, tension, or compression forces. A shearing-type laceration is the simple dissection of the skin by a sharp object. An example is a cut from a razor blade or knife. Little physical force is imparted to the tissue adjacent to the laceration. For this reason there is less necrosis, inflammation, and edema in simple shear lacerations. They usually heal without complications or severe scarring. Tension lacerations result when the skin is ripped apart by the application of blunt force at an angle to the skin. The force is transmitted to adjacent tissue, and considerable injury is typical. The wound tends to be irregular and jagged. Often a triangular flap of skin is created. Compression lacerations occur when an opposing force presses the skin against bone, causing the skin to burst. An example of a compression laceration is a cut over the supraorbital ridge in a boxer who is struck with great force by his opponent's glove. These lacerations are irregular, often stellate, and are associated with a great deal of damage in the adjoining skin and soft tissues. This type of injury requires far less bacterial contamination to become infected. Many lacerations have components from each of these types of forces.

Abrasions are wounds produced by the forcible avulsion of skin layers to a certain depth. The forces causing abrasions are usually applied horizontally to the skin. For example, "road rash" is a type of abrasion seen in motorcycle accident victims who have slid along asphalt. Such abrasions may be extensive and are usually contaminated with soil, gravel, or tar. Depending on their thickness, abrasions may require the same treatment as burns.

Puncture wounds are frequently seen in the emergency department. Because these wounds are much deeper than they are wide, they are difficult to explore and decontaminate. There is a greater risk of inoculation of bacteria or foreign material into the wound. In some cases, penetration to bone may occur, with a resulting risk of osteomyelitis.

Burns result from thermal injury to the skin and are classified on the basis of penetration. Superficial (first-degree) burns involve only the epidermis and do not cause blistering. An example of a first-degree burn is a mild sunburn. A second-degree burn, or partial-thickness burn, penetrates into the dermis but spares the nerves and vascular tissue. This type of burn usually blisters and is painful. A third-degree, or full-thickness, burn extends to the depths of the dermis and causes coagulation of blood and lymphatic vessels and destroys nervous tissue. It usually appears pale and is not painful.

Another type of injury to the skin is a local hypothermic injury, or frostbite. After prolonged exposure to cold temperatures, the skin cells may freeze. Intense vasoconstriction causes hypoperfusion and occlusion of small blood vessels. Like burns, frostbite can be graded as first-, second-, or third-degree, depending on the depth of injury.

Wound Healing

Wound healing is a dynamic process initiated at the time of the insult to the skin. It is not complete for many months. It is a natural, predictable process, but can be affected by a number of outside factors. The stages of wound healing are summarized below.

Inflammatory Stage (0 to 3 Days). In this stage there is tissue reaction to trauma. Disruption of soft tissue and blood vessels activates the clotting system and aggregation of platelets. Leukocytes and mast cells release histamine and other enzymes and factors. Release of these substances produces local capillary vasodilatation. Leukocytes are chemotactically drawn to the site. An exudate of serum and white cells develops. The clinical result is redness, warmth, and edema at the wound site.

Destructive Stage (2 to 5 Days). Polymorphonuclear leukocytes are active in the wound and are later joined by macrophages. The wound is cleared of devitalized tissue and blood products. Macrophages are thought to recruit fibroblasts into the wound. Epithelialization begins in the epidermal part of the wound.

Proliferative Stage (3 to 24 Days). Fibroblasts organize and synthesize collagen, and new blood vessels are formed. This combination of fresh fibrous tissue and new blood vessels is called *granulation tissue*.

Maturation Stage (24 Days to 1 Year). Special modified fibroblasts, called myofibroblasts, appear at the edges of the wound. When these cells contract, the wound also undergoes contraction as fibrous tissue matures and reorganizes.

The outer appearance of the scar passes through several stages. In the first month, the scar is weak, soft, and undeveloped. In the next 2 months it becomes redder, firmer, and stronger. After 3 months the scar gradually softens, becomes more pliable, elastic, and paler in color. The scar continues to contract over time.

Despite rapid recellularization, a wound does not regain its original strength quickly. At 2 weeks, the wound has only 5% of its tensile strength. At 1 month, it has about 35%. It takes 6 to 12 months for maximum strength to develop. For this reason, a wound may need protection even after it appears well healed.

Wounds in areas with a poor blood supply are more prone to infection and take longer to heal. Patients with chronic diseases such as diabetes or lung, liver, or kidney disease, vascular impairment, or alcoholism have poorer wound healing and a higher rate of infection. Malnutrition also impairs wound healing. Steroids are the most widely implicated drugs that impair wound healing, but cytotoxic agents, antibiotics, nonsteroidal anti-inflammatory agents, and topical ointments and creams may also have an effect.

The most important negative influence on wound healing is wound infection. It occurs in about 5% of wounds treated in the emergency department. It is sometimes difficult to tell merely by observation whether a wound is infected, since the normal inflammatory response in wounded tissues may simulate infection. A pure definition of *wound infection* is the presence of greater than 100,000 colony-forming units of bacteria per gram of tissue. By far the most common organism implicated in wound infections is *Staphylococcus aureus*. Certain wounds are prone to infections with particular organisms. For example, puncture wounds of the feet are associated with a high incidence of *Pseudomonas* infections, and cat bites often become infected with *Pasteurella multocida*. Table 15–1 lists those factors that predispose to impaired wound healing and increase the risk of infection.

Wound healing is sometimes classified clinically according to the timing of treatment. *Primary union*, or healing by first intention, refers to closure of the wound by sutures or staples, usually within the first 6 hours after the injury. This "golden period" is often extended up to 12 hours or longer if the wound is not contaminated and is located in a part of the body with good vascular supply, such as the face. In *secondary union* the wound is allowed to granulate in from bottom to top. It is used in wounds more than 12 hours old, those having tissue loss or avulsion, or contaminated to the degree that primary union is not deemed feasible. *Tertiary union*, or delayed closure, is used in contaminated wounds that are initially cleansed and then are observed for 4 to 6 days for development of infection (with or without concomitant antibiotic use). If no infection develops, the wound is closed with sutures. This usually means granulation tissue is incorporated in the closure.

Some people have problems with excessive scar formation. Hypertrophic scars are common in children, in dark-skinned races, and in people with burns. A hypertrophic

TABLE 15-1. Factors Associated with Impaired Wound Healing and Increased Infection

Wound characteristics	Patient characteristics
Age of wound greater than 6 hr when treated	Advanced age
Wound location in an area with poor blood supply	Malnourished
Crushing, macerating mechanism of injury	Poor hygiene
Contamination with soil, foreign material	Alcoholism
Wound care, technical elements	Diabetes mellitus
Use of detergent scrub solutions	Peripheral vascular disease
Inadequate cleansing and irrigation	Uremia
Anesthetics containing epinephrine	Liver disease
Inadequate hemostasis, wound hematoma	Connective tissue diseases
Reactive suture material	Hypoxia
Excessive suture tension	Severe anemia
Tincture of benzoin	**Drug use**
	Corticosteroids
	Nonsteroidal anti-inflammatory agents
	Colchicine
	Anticoagulants
	Antineoplastic agents
	Penicillamine

Modified from Trott A: Principles and Techniques of Minor Wound Care. New Hyde Park, NY, Medical Examination Publishing Co, 1985, pp. 24 and 31.

scar is raised and may be more sensitive than a normal scar but does not extend past the original wound margins. A keloid scar represents the extreme of excessive scar formation; in this case, a disorder in collagen deposition produces a large, fibrous growth that extends beyond the limits of the original scar. Keloid scars are most common in blacks and are more common if a foreign body is retained in the wound.

PREHOSPITAL CARE

The role of prehospital care providers in the assessment and initial management of wounds is an important one. The primary functions of the rescue squad are to control hemorrhage, reduce contamination of the wound, and splint injured extremities safely. The following items are the responsibilities of the rescue squad.

History

1. How much time has elapsed since injury?
2. What is the mechanism of injury?

Physical Examination

1. The patient's vital signs are assessed for evidence of hemodynamic instability.
2. Any associated conditions or injuries are noted.
3. Extremities are assessed for evidence of obvious neurovascular or bone injury.

Intervention

1. Patency of the airway is ensured.
2. Intravenous access is established in patients with large wounds or those in whom hemodynamic compromise is possible.
3. Hemorrhage is controlled in the prehospital setting either by direct manual pressure or by bandages that exert pressure, and by elevation of the extremity. The use of tourniquets or clamping of bleeding vessels is not necessary and may lead to further tissue injury.

4. To reduce contamination, soiled clothing is cut away and a sterile dressing, either dry or moistened with saline, is applied.

5. Fractures are splinted as they are found. Fractures are not manipulated in the prehospital setting. In open fractures, this may draw debris into the wound.

6. A special situation exists in the prehospital care of patients with amputated digits or extremities. Hemorrhage may be severe in these cases, but it is again controlled with direct pressure. The prehospital care provider must assume that an amputated part can be surgically reimplanted. The final decision is made at the hospital, not in the field. The amputated part is wrapped in dry, sterile sheets or plastic and then placed in a cold container or bag of ice.

INITIAL APPROACH IN THE EMERGENCY DEPARTMENT

Patients with wounds are usually anxious, frightened about impending treatment, and in some degree of pain. They perceive their wounds as very real emergencies, no matter how minor the injury, and dislike waiting for treatment. They often are greatly concerned about the cosmetic appearance of the wound. Many wounds result from assaults, fights, robberies, animal bites, or careless mistakes or accidents. Patients bring the stresses from these events with them to the emergency department. The initial emergency department management of wounded patients is aimed at reducing anxiety, relieving pain, and moving the patient quickly through the emergency system. The exception to this goal is the intoxicated patient, who initially may be impossible to assess. In such a case, it is best to wait until the effect of alcohol or drugs is reduced to the point where the patient can be evaluated and treated properly.

1. The time from injury and the mechanism of injury are carefully determined because this information will have a significant impact on the timing and direction of care of the wound.

2. Because there are many drugs that potentially could be administered, it is important to establish an allergy history.

3. Full vital signs must be recorded in all wounded patients.

4. Clothing is removed to permit a complete examination depending on the location of the wound.

5. Rings, watches, jewelry, and other objects or apparel are also removed if they will interfere with the examination and treatment. Rings or watches must be removed early from an injured extremity before edema makes removal impossible.

6. Depending on the nature of the wound or wounds, a primary survey of the patient is carried out; priority is given to the patency of the airway and adequacy of the respiratory effort.

7. The circulatory system is evaluated, paying particular attention to blood pressure, heart rate, and capillary refill. Hypotension can occur from seemingly minor wounds. Scalp lacerations are notorious for bleeding vigorously. Early hemorrhagic shock may present only as an elevation of the heart rate or narrowing of the pulse pressure. If active hemorrhage is seen during the initial assessment, it should be controlled with elevation and direct pressure.

8. In extremities, a careful neurovascular examination is performed distal to the wound to ensure proper function before anesthetics or other treatments are administered.

9. Early surgical consultation is obtained in any case of life- or limb-threatening injury.

10. Once initially assessed, the wound is covered and protected with a temporary dressing such as a moistened saline gauze pad.

11. Unless significant pain is present, e.g., a burn or wound with fracture, analgesia is usually not given until after a more complete examination has been done.

PROBLEM 1 In this patient, multiple dog bite wounds were noted about the head, back, and left shoulder. The injuries had occurred 1 hour prior to admission. The patient was alert and talking. Vital signs were unremarkable. He had a recent tetanus immunization. A brief examination revealed that the airway was intact and there was no evident neurovascular injury to the left arm. Moistened saline gauze pads were applied to the wounds, and preparations were made to evaluate and repair the wounds further.

In spite of the dramatic appearance of the patient's lacerations, attention is paid first to potential life- or limb-threatening injuries. An appropriate evaluation of the areas of most concern is carried out. Once the basic evaluation is completed and serious problems have been addressed, the individual wounds are managed.

DATA GATHERING

Obtaining a history from a patient with a wound is not usually a time-consuming task. The standard format for taking a wound history and examining a wound is outlined below.

History

1. *When* did the wound occur? The longer the lapse of time between the injury and the repair, the greater the chance for infection.
2. *How* did it occur, i.e., what was the *mechanism of injury?* As discussed previously, the mechanisms of injury have a significant impact on outcome.
3. Is there *pain* or *numbness?* Both can be indicative of neurovascular compromise in injuries of an extremity.
4. Was there significant *bleeding?* Note both the amount and intensity.
5. Is there a sensation of a *foreign body?* Is there the possibility of one being present? A reported sensation of a foreign body by the patient is very accurate.
6. In *older* or *infected* wounds, is there *warmth* or *exudate?* These are indicators of infection.
7. Was any *prior treatment* given, e.g., cleansing or application of agents to the wound?
8. Depending on the region of the wound, specific questions are directed to *functional status*. For example, evaluation of head wounds includes questioning about loss of consciousness, headache, vomiting, visual changes, and gait abnormalities. With hand wounds, the patient's occupation, handedness, and present impairment are assessed.
9. Past *medical* history
    a. The patient's history of *tetanus immunization* is most important. In some cases, vaccination against hepatitis B virus may also be important.
    b. Are there *underlying medical diseases?* Specifically, diabetes mellitus, peripheral vascular disease, or a bleeding disorder is most important.
    c. *Habits* such as smoking, alcohol abuse, and drug use history are ascertained.
    d. What are the patient's *current medications?* Compliance?
    e. Patients with *acquired immune deficiency syndrome* (AIDS) or positive *human immunodeficiency virus* (HIV) blood tests must be identified. This knowledge is important for predicting wound infection and for the safety of staff working with the patient.

Physical Examination

Physical examination of the patient with a wound begins with a survey of the vital signs and an assessment of the patient's general appearance and state of health. A young, previously healthy woman who hit her thumbnail with a hammer does not need a general examination as part of her emergency department treatment. An elderly alcoholic who fell down some stairs and has a scalp laceration does need a full, systematic examination.

The examination of a wound includes the following observations:
1. Measurement or estimation of wound length, width, and depth.
2. Identification of dermis and subcutaneous tissue.
3. Degree of contamination and presence of foreign bodies.
4. Assessment of vascularity and amount and type of bleeding.
5. Maceration and necrosis of tissues.
6. If the wound is a facial wound, its anatomic position in relation to skin tension lines is important in predicting whether the scar will widen as it matures. This is valuable to discuss with the patient.
7. Anatomic position of the wound in reference to joints and skin creases.
8. A functional examination of the neuromuscular and vascular system distal to the injured area is performed. This examination is extremely important in forearm and hand injuries, in which tendon, nerve, and vascular damage is common. Sensation, motor function, tendon integrity, and capillary refill are tested in all extremity injuries. In children, this part of the assessment is best done before examining the wound. Better cooperation is obtained.

PROBLEM 2 The patient stated that the wound had occurred 6 hours before, when she fell against a broken stick that was part of her compost pile. The stick impaled her lower leg, but she pulled it out. Since she experienced minimal pain and bleeding, she continued with her yard work. Before coming to the hospital, she applied a warm tea bag to the wound. Further questioning about her past history revealed that she was a heavy cigarette smoker, had adult-onset diabetes mellitus, and was taking a pill for high blood pressure. She complained of having "poor circulation." She could not remember the time of her last tetanus immunization. On examination, a jagged, macerated 6-cm flap laceration containing dirt and bark fragments was found over the lateral midtibial surface.

There are several elements of the history that will influence the decision about the care of this wound. The wound is "old," tetanus-prone, and may contain foreign material. It occurred in a dirty environment. The lower leg is not a highly vascular area, and the blood supply of this patient may be more limited than normal, since the wound did not bleed. Other factors that may impair the blood supply and wound healing are heavy smoking, diabetes, high blood pressure, and a possible history of peripheral vascular disease. Clearly, this woman is not the average patient with a leg wound.

DECISION PRIORITIES AND PRELIMINARY DIFFERENTIAL DIAGNOSIS

Once the history has been taken and the wound explored, it is useful to ask a series of questions that may influence decisions about management.

1. *Are the anatomic boundaries of the wound understood?*
   This question directs the physician to two areas. First, the physician should understand the normal anatomy in the area of the wound and anticipate the structures that might be injured. Second, knowledge of the full extent of the wound is necessary to decide whether the wound should be closed and how many layers it will take.
2. *Is there a potential for a foreign body in the wound?*
   A foreign body increases the risk of infection, may impede healing, and can cause pain and internal damage after wound closure. Penetrating injuries, falls onto gravel or glass, and injuries due to explosions are all notorious for involving hidden foreign bodies. Every effort is made to find and remove them.
3. *Are the distal neurovascular, muscle, and tendon functions consistent with the anatomic location of the wound and the findings on exploration?*

Any discrepancy between function and wound location needs an explanation. This usually requires a reexamination of both the distal functions and the anatomic structures involved in the wound.

4. *Are there factors that may promote infection or impair wound healing?*
   These factors (Table 15–1) are reviewed while care of the wound is planned. Decisions about closure, type of suture, number of layers, necessity of drainage, use of antibiotics, types of dressing, need for hospitalization, and timing of follow-up are influenced by these factors.

5. *Does the emergency physician have the skill and the time to care for this wound properly?*
   Although it is expected that a trained emergency physician will be able to care for a wide variety of wounds, it is wise to know when an injury repair is beyond one's skill or, more often, beyond the time available to do it right. A wound closure that might require 30 minutes is appropriate and satisfying on a quiet Sunday morning but may need to be referred on a busy Saturday night. Both the emergency physician and the surgical consultant must be aware of the balance between skills and the available time in deciding which cases are cared for by whom.

DIAGNOSTIC ADJUNCTS

Laboratory tests and diagnostic imaging procedures, other than plain radiographs, are only occasionally helpful in the management of wounds.

Laboratory Studies

Blood tests are of minimal use in treating wounds. The hemoglobin and hematocrit may help in assessing blood loss. Serologic tests for hepatitis are obtained in patients injured by a potentially contaminated source (e.g., needle or scalpel). (See Chap. 18.)

Radiologic Imaging

Plain radiographs are useful in detecting bony abnormalities and joint involvement in wounds. They are commonly used in high-risk situations to identify and localize foreign bodies and to show soft tissue changes, such as edema or gas in the tissues. Glass foreign bodies will show up on radiographs about 90% of the time, even if the glass does not contain lead. Metal foreign bodies are almost always visible on radiographs. Less dense substances such as plastic and wood usually are not visible on plain radiographs but may be visualized by computed tomography. They may show as a "filling defect" on plain films. If there are questions about the best imaging technique to use to identify a foreign body, a discussion with the radiologist is usually very helpful.

PRINCIPLES OF MANAGEMENT

Once the wound and its impact on the patient have been assessed, management includes wound preparation, closure techniques, and wound aftercare.

Wound Preparation

Wound preparation is divided into five areas of concern: anesthesia delivery, cleansing and debridement, hemostasis, suture materials, and assessment.

Wound Anesthesia. Adequate pain relief prior to closure is foremost in the minds of most wounded patients. A number of local anesthetic agents are used. The properties, onset and duration of action, and maximum doses of three agents are summarized in Table 15–2. Lidocaine and mepivacaine are the most commonly used. For a longer duration of anesthesia, bupivacaine is favored. The addition of epinephrine to an anesthetic agent causes vasoconstriction in the wound field and prolongs the action of the anesthetic. Its use is limited to well-vascularized tissues. Fingers, toes, the ears, the nose, and the distal parts of flap lacerations may suffer ischemic necrosis if epinephrine is used with the anesthetic agent. If a patient has a number of lacerations or very large lacerations, care must be taken to keep track of the amount of local anesthetic agent administered. As a benchmark, no more than 30 ml of 1% lidocaine (300 mg since 1% = 10 mg/ml) in a 60-kg person (5 mg/kg) may be used. Seizures or even cardiac arrest may result from acute overdose of lidocaine and related agents. Diphenhydramine (Benadryl) in a 1% solution is an effective local anesthetic. It may be used in the rare patient who is allergic to the commonly used agents.

An alternate type of anesthesia, that which is applied topically rather than infiltrated, is used primarily in children. If effective, it can be used for total anesthesia. Because it does not always fully take effect, it is also used to decrease the pain of infiltrative anesthesia. The preparation most commonly used is called TAC and is a mixture of tetracaine 0.5%, epinephrine 1%, and cocaine 4%. A cotton ball or gauze soaked in the solution is applied directly to the wound. Vasoconstriction and anesthesia result after 5 to 10 minutes of contact. Some clinicians feel that wound infections are more common with this preparation. The solution can cause systemic toxicity if it is absorbed through mucosal surfaces, and the ratios and percentages of the components in the mixture must be known.

Techniques of wound anesthesia are closely related to the type of wound repair used. Local anesthesia is obtained by local infiltration into and around the wound or by a regional block. Local infiltration into the dermis and subcutaneous tissues is used for most simple, common wounds and when distortion of the wound by an anesthetic agent is not a problem. The anesthetic is injected either adjacent and parallel to the wound edge in a sequential fashion or directly into the dermis or subcutaneous tissue through the open wound edge. It is important to aspirate for blood before the injection to avoid injecting the anesthetic into a vein or artery. Enough anesthetic agent is infiltrated to cause a wheal or elevation in the dermal tissues. Usually a 25- or 27-gauge needle provides a big enough lumen for infiltration yet is narrow enough to reduce pain during the injection. Slow infiltration is tolerated better than rapid injection because the pain is caused more by the rate and degree of tissue distortion than by the presence of the needle. Talking with the patient is helpful to provide distraction and a modicum of "vocal anesthesia."

Regional anesthesia (nerve block) is provided by injecting the agent at a site distant from the wound that blocks sensation in the area. It is imperative to know the anatomy of the nerves and the area they supply for regional anesthesia to be effective. Regional anesthesia usually requires less anesthetic agent, does not distort the appearance of the wound, and may be less painful than local anesthesia. However, the techniques may be

TABLE 15–2. Anesthetic Agents in Wound Care

Agent	Concentration	Onset of Action (Infiltration/Block)	Maximum Dosage
Lidocaine (Xylocaine)	1% or 2%	Immediate/4–10 min Duration: 1–2 hr	4.5 mg/kg = 30 ml of 1% solution (for average adult)
Mepivacaine (Carbocaine)	1% or 2%	Immediate/6–10 min Duration: 1.5–2.5 hr	5 mg/kg = 35 ml of 1% solution
Bupivacaine (Marcaine)	0.25%	Slower/8–12 min Duration: 6–8 hr	3 mg/kg = 80 ml of 0.25% solution

Modified from Trott A: Principles and Techniques of Minor Wound Care. New Hyde Park, NY, Medical Examination Publishing Co, 1985, p. 48.

difficult to master, the anesthesia may take a longer time to work, and the area anesthetized is usually larger than the wound.

Many techniques have been described for blocking various nerves, including digital, supraorbital, infraorbital, mental, median, ulnar, radial, sural, and posterior tibial nerve blocks. The basic technique used in all these blocks is locating the nerve first by identifying reliable local landmarks. A needle is inserted to the approximate level of the nerve. If paresthesias are produced, the needle is withdrawn slightly, then 1 to 3 ml of anesthetic agent is infiltrated on either side of the nerve. The amount depends on the size of the nerve to be blocked. A digital nerve block is shown in Figure 15–1.

Wound Cleansing and Preparation. Cleaning a wound is an unglamorous task but is extremely important in preventing wound infection. Sterile water or normal saline is poured over the wound to remove gross contamination. The skin surface is further cleaned by applying an antibacterial solution. The physician can then anesthetize the wound to reduce pain during the remaining cleansing procedure. Once the skin surface is clean, particulate matter in the wound is best removed by using medium-pressure irrigation. A large syringe and an 18-gauge needle produce a jet of saline that can dislodge particles and reduce the number of bacteria in the wound. After the wound has been generously irrigated with saline (more than 150 ml is recommended in wounds >3 to 4 cm), an antibacterial solution is commonly used. Preparations containing isopropyl alcohol and those with detergents are not used in wounds because of the tissue toxic properties of these solutions. Povidone iodine solution (not the surgical scrub) does not cause tissue damage when used in open wounds and has good antibacterial activity. After the wound has been cleansed and irrigated, povidone iodine solution can be applied to the wound and allowed to stand for 2 or 3 minutes and then rinsed. Povidone iodine must be used cautiously in wounds on the face because it is irritating to the eyes. Direct mechanical scrubbing has a role in wound cleaning. Optimally, it is done with a fine-pore sponge and a surfactant solution (e.g., Shur Clens).

Removing or shaving hair around a wound is necessary only if this makes it significantly easier to repair the wound. Hair can be cleansed the same way as skin. The perception that shaving hair around wounds prevents wound infections is not documented. Shaving may violate skin integrity and increase the likelihood of infection. Scalp wounds are easier to close if a small area of hair around the wound is clipped with scissors. This may also be true in extremity or trunk wounds in individuals with thick body hair. Another method of keeping the hair out of the wound is to apply a water-soluble lubricant to the hair and mat it down away from the wound. The eyebrows are not shaved because of the alteration in appearance that results with new hair growth.

Hemostasis. Once a wound has been cleansed and prepared for treatment, the amount of bleeding is assessed. In many cases, manipulation of the wound during cleansing and anesthesia opens up previously coagulated blood vessels, and fresh bleeding occurs. Bleeding is usually controlled by elevation of the part, direct pressure, and patience. If bleeding is not controlled by these measures, the next alternatives depend on the location of the wound. In head, scalp, and truncal wounds, the placement of deep sutures and fascial closure can help to occlude bleeding vessels. It is very important to have as bloodless a field as possible when evaluating extremity injuries for nerve, artery, and tendon damage. One way to accomplish this is to elevate the extremity to promote venous drainage and then apply a blood pressure cuff proximally, and inflate it to 20 to 40 mm Hg above systolic pressure. This measure will prevent bleeding at the wound site and can be tolerated by most patients for up to 20 minutes.

Suture Materials and Equipment. One can practice good wound care with a limited amount of materials and equipment. A standard suture tray containing a needle holder, toothed forceps, skin hooks, iris scissors and bandage scissors, hemostats, and a scalpel handle can be prepared and sterilized. Sterile accessory materials placed on the opened tray include gauze sponges, a basin or cups, and towels for draping.

The most practical needle holder for emergency use is the 4½-inch variety with serrated carbide-tipped jaws. This has the strength to hold large needles in larger

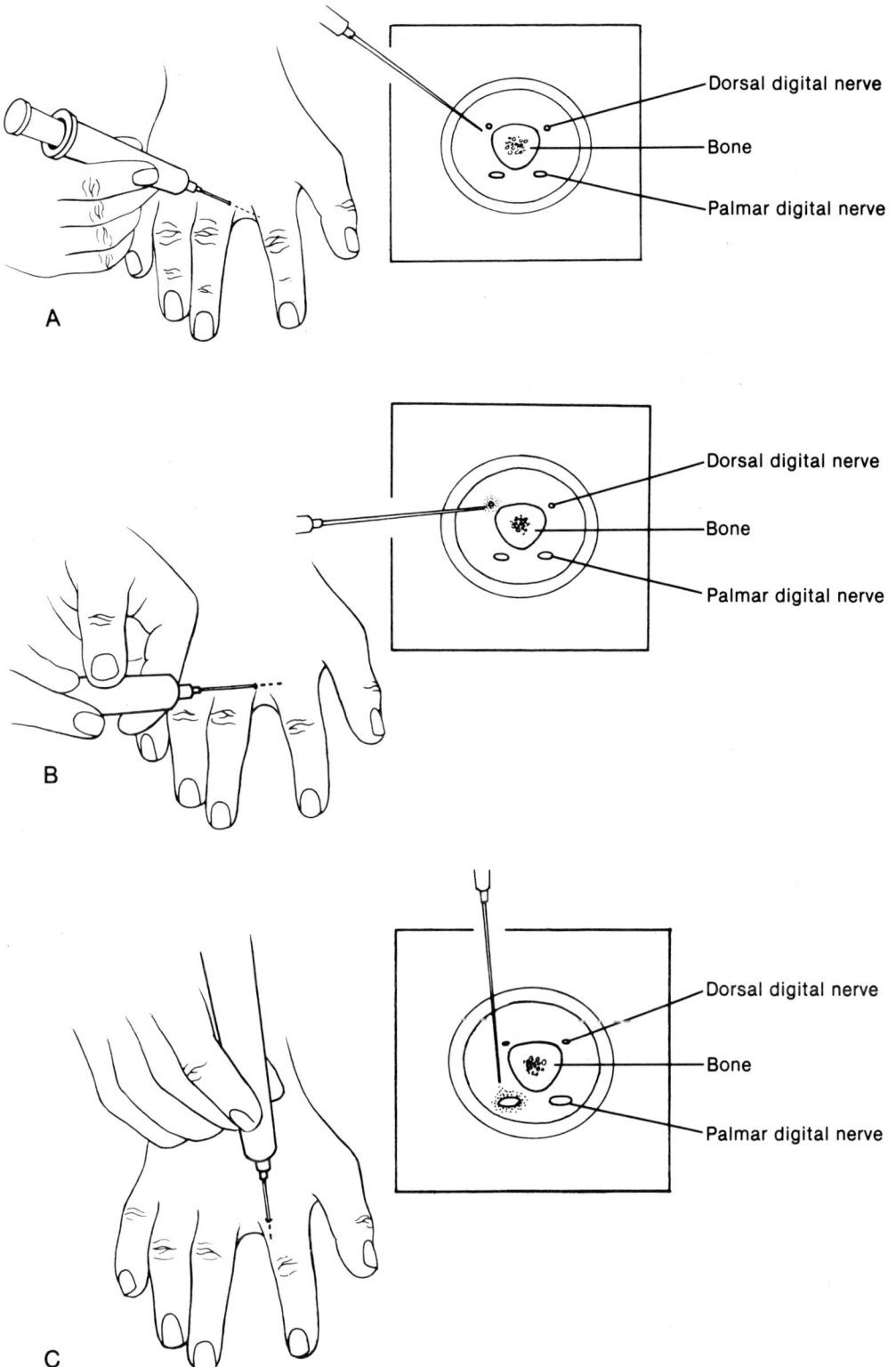

FIGURE 15–1. A, *Technique for digital nerve block. The needle is introduced at the proximal portion of the proximal phalanx well back into the web space. It is advanced until it touches bone.* B, *The needle is slightly withdrawn and 1 ml of anesthetic solution is delivered to the dorsal digital nerve.* C, *Without exiting the skin, the needle is then passed along the shaft of the proximal phalanx to the palmar surface of the digit and 1 ml of anesthetic solution is delivered to the palmar digital nerve.*

lacerations but is small enough to be used with more delicate closures. Forceps with teeth aid in manipulating and exposing underlying tissue. They should not be clamped on the external skin surface. Skin hooks, or a substitute, are used to provide better exposure in deep wounds. Iris scissors are both curved and straight and are used only for debriding tissue. Hemostats are used more to expose and explore the wound. Rarely, in large or deep wounds, they are used to clamp tissues or an exposed bleeding small vessel.

The choice of suture material for emergency department purposes can be limited to two types for external sutures and two absorbable types for buried or deep sutures. Nylon and polypropylene are synthetic materials used for external skin sutures. Compared with traditional silk sutures, they have low tissue reactivity and pass easily through tissues. An undesirable feature is their poor knot-holding ability, which necessitates the tying of extra "security" knots when placing the sutures. The two main absorbable suture materials are polyglactin (PG 910) and polyglycolic acid (PGA). PG 910 has greater tensile strength, but PGA is easier to manipulate and tie, especially in small wounds. Another absorbable material, chromic catgut, is used primarily in intraoral lacerations.

Suture size and the type of suture needle used depend on the type of laceration. Table 15–3 provides guidelines for selecting suture materials in different areas of the body. Needles are either of the tapered or cutting variety. A tapered needle is round in cross section. A cutting needle has an edge and is triangular in cross section. Most suturing in the emergency department is done with a cutting needle. The smallest size appropriate for the job is chosen.

Not all wounds require sutures. Small, nongaping lacerations often can be closed with wound tapes (e.g., Steri-Strips). These are also used as adjuncts to suturing. For example, they can be placed between widely spaced sutures to help keep the skin edges together. Some emergency physicians routinely use a stapling device to close straight, uncomplicated wounds of the arms, legs, trunk, and scalp. The metal staples can be placed more quickly than sutures and provide good wound edge eversion. They are not effective in jagged, irregular lacerations or with thin, delicate skin.

Wound Assessment and Debridement. Before a wound is repaired or closed, it must be assessed and explored, as described earlier in the section on physical examination. Once it is thoroughly explored, a need for debridement may be apparent.

Wound debridement is the resection of tissue for the purpose of reducing wound infection or changing the appearance of the wound. Nonviable tissue can act as a nidus for infection and inflammation. It is cut away from the surrounding tissue with a scalpel or iris scissors. Foreign material ground into the wound and not washed away by irrigation is removed in the same manner.

Excision of viable tissue from a wound is sometimes necessary to improve the closure and cosmetic appearance of the wound. The irregular edges of some lacerations can be

TABLE 15–3. Suggested Guidelines for Suture Materials and Size for Body Area

Body Area	Deep Closure	Superficial Closure
Scalp	4–0 PGA[a]	4–0, 3–0 nylon[d]
Facial structures	5–0 PGA	6–0 nylon
Trunk	4–0 PGA	5–0, 4–0 nylon
Hand	5–0 PGA	5–0 nylon
Extremities	4–0 PGA	5–0, 4–0 nylon
Oral mucosa	—	5–0 chromic gut
Deep fascia	4–0 PG910[b]	—
"Pull out" dermal or subcuticular	6–0, 4–0, 5–0 polypropylene[c]	—

[a] PGA, polyglycolic acid (Dexon).
[b] PG 910, polyglactin 910 (Vicryl).
[c] Polypropylene (Prolene).
[d] Nylon (Ethilon, Dermalon).
Prolene can be readily substituted. Polyglycolic acid (PGA) will meet most needs for deep dermal and superficial fascia closure, but polyglactin 910 is an acceptable alternative.

sharply excised to make the wound edges smooth and straight. In circular or gaping, jagged wounds, skin may be excised to convert the shape of the wound to an ellipse, which is more easily closed.

PROBLEM 1 The patient weighed 75 kg. He had two 3-cm dog bites in the scalp, a 5-cm bite or laceration of the left shoulder, and six puncture wounds, each less than 1 to 2 cm, on the upper left back. There was minimal devitalization of the wound margins.

Before an anesthetic was administered, the maximum total dosage was calculated. For plain 1% lidocaine, the maximum dose is 5 mg/kg (375 mg for this patient) or 37.5 ml of a 1% solution. Care is taken to properly anesthetize the wounds while not exceeding this limit. Cleansing with povidone iodine and thorough irrigation were carried out, and debridement of devitalized wound margins was performed. Nylon nonabsorbable external sutures were chosen for repair. Deep, absorbable sutures were not needed and in this situation could increase the likelihood of wound infection.

Basic Closure Techniques

Percutaneous Closure. Placing a simple suture starts with the proper loading of the suture needle into the needle holder. The needle is clamped in the tips of the needle holder at a right angle to the needle holder about one-third of the way between its connection to the suture (swedge) and its point. The needle point is then placed at a 90-degree angle to the skin. The skin is punctured, and with a smooth rolling motion of the wrist, the needle is advanced (Fig. 15–2). In a straight, nonbeveled laceration, the needle should emerge from the skin equidistant to the wound edge. The path of the needle should be as wide (or wider) at its base as it is near the surface (Fig. 15–3). This will evert the wound edges and result in a flatter, less noticeable scar. In a beveled laceration, a larger "bite" of tissue is taken on the beveled side of the laceration.

The number of skin sutures placed in a laceration and the distance between sutures depend on the location of the laceration and the skin tension in the area. In general, the fewest number of sutures that will close the laceration with minimal wound edge tension and no gaping between sutures is the appropriate number.

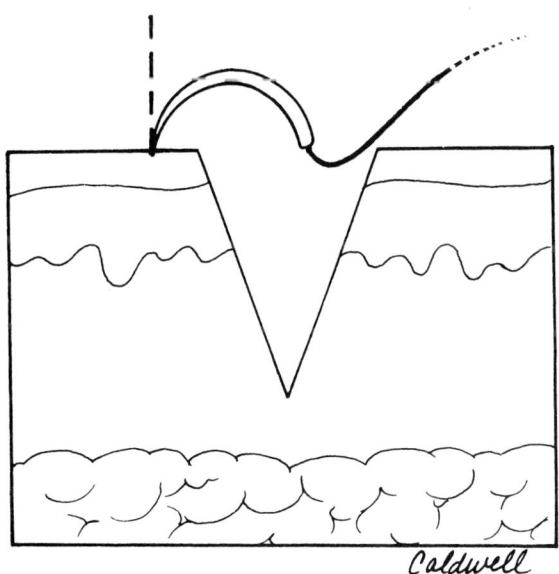

FIGURE 15–2. Technique for wound edge eversion. The needle is introduced at a 90-degree angle to the skin.

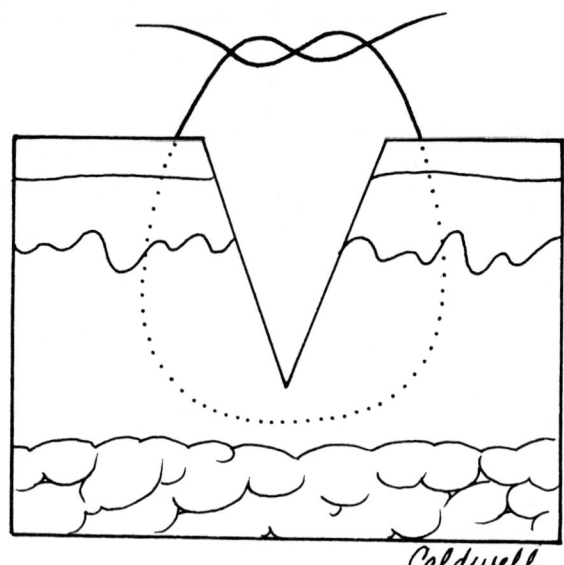

FIGURE 15–3. *By using proper needle placement technique, as illustrated in Figure 5–2, the correct suture configuration will be achieved.*

Deep Closure. A simple deep suture is used to approximate the subcutaneous tissues and dermis. By readjoining tissue, pockets of "dead space" are eliminated. This technique is thought to help reduce hematoma collection and the threat of infection. Also, the tension on skin sutures is reduced, and fewer skin sutures are necessary. The most important element in this type of suture is identifying and matching the layers of tissue to avoid buckling or an uneven closure. A skin hook is helpful to lift the dermis and better observe the juxtaposition of the opposite sides. The deep suture knot is buried in the wound as shown in Figure 15–4. The need for deep sutures depends on the location of the wound and is currently a controversial topic. The risk of promoting infection by introducing foreign material into the wound must be weighed against any benefits in wound approximation and cosmetic appearance. In hand wounds, deep sutures are almost never needed. In the face, trunk, and extremities, deep sutures are more commonly used in larger lacerations. The rich vascularity of the face and head makes infection less likely, even when deep sutures are used. In general, a wound is closed with as few deep sutures as possible.

Mattress Technique. The simple interrupted skin suture and deep suture described above can be used to close most lacerations. In some cases special techniques or suture methods are needed. For widely gaping wounds, vertical and horizontal mattress sutures provide extra strength and good wound edge eversion (Fig. 15–5A, B). Another technique used to reduce the tension on the skin edges in gaping wounds is undermining of the dermis and superficial fascia, separating these layers from their underlying attachments. Iris scissors work best for this technique.

Running Technique. In straight, long lacerations, such as those made by a knife or razor blade, a running suture, placed either through the skin or subcuticularly, may give a better cosmetic result and is faster to place than interrupted sutures. The disadvantages are that if the suture breaks the entire wound is disrupted, and if infection develops it is not possible to open part of the wound selectively for drainage as it is with interrupted sutures (Fig. 15–6).

Corner or Flap Suture. With irregular, jagged lacerations, flaps of tissue are often produced. The tips of these flaps are often contused and partially necrotic and may have a compromised blood supply. Securing a suture in this friable tissue is difficult and may further impair blood flow. A flap or corner suture is used in these situations (Fig. 15–7).

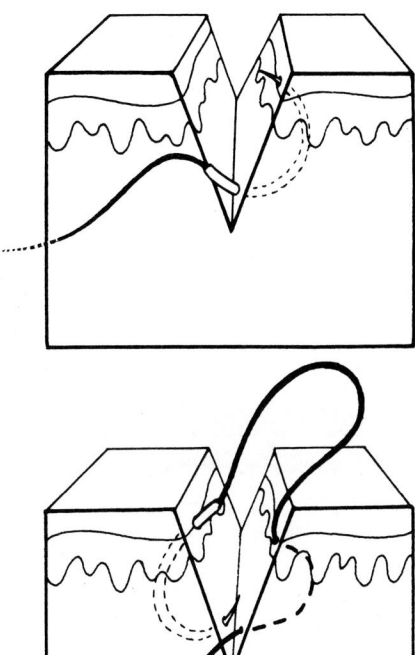

FIGURE 15–4. Technique for placement of a deep suture closure. The needle is introduced in the subcutaneous tissue and brought vertically through the dermis. The needle is rearmed with the needle holder and introduced into the dermis on the direct opposite wound surface. The needle is exited from the subcutaneous tissue close to the original entry point. The knot is tied. Care is taken to avoid tying the knot over the dermal portion of the suture loop.

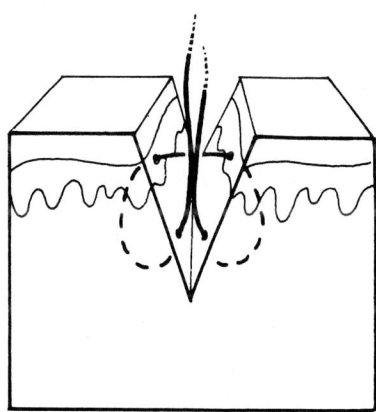

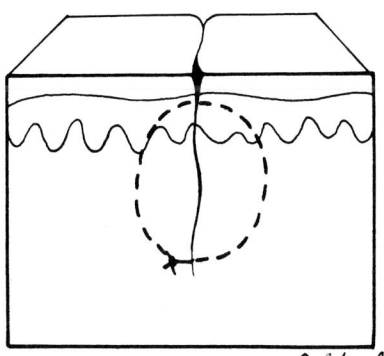

286 — CUTANEOUS DISORDERS

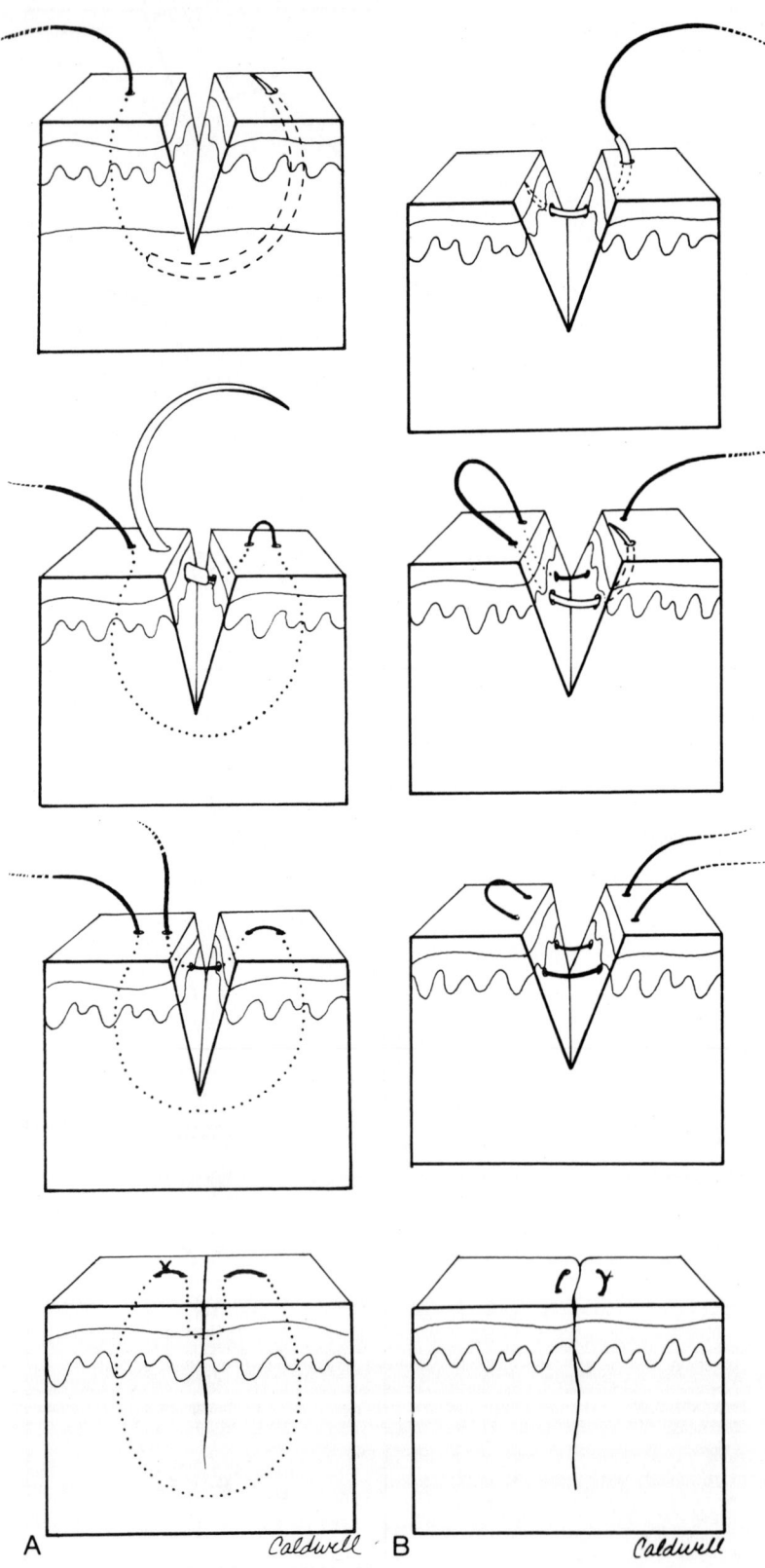

FIGURE 15–5. Technique for mattress sutures. A, Vertical mattress. A deep bite, followed by a superficial bite to the dermis, completes the vertical mattress suture. B, Horizontal mattress. Two bites through the dermis, placed at the same level, form a horizontal mattress suture.

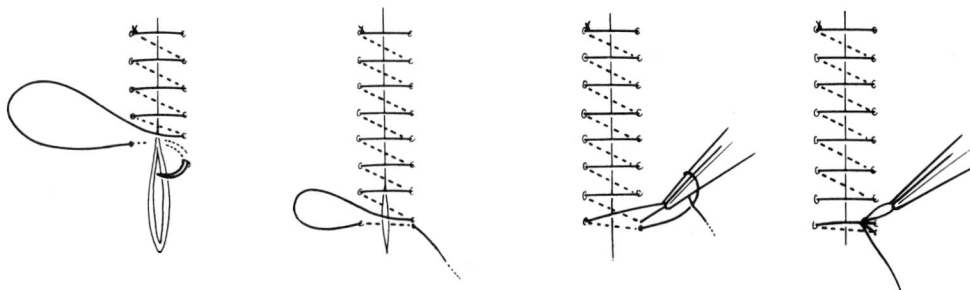

FIGURE 15-6. Technique for running suture closure. This suture is started by placing a standard tie at the extreme right-hand portion of the laceration (left side for left-handed operators). The suture material is not cut and tissue bites are taken at a 45-degree angle to the wound direction. The superficial portions lay at a 90-degree angle. The securing knot is fashioned, as illustrated, by using the final loop as the anchor for the needle holder. Several throws are made in the standard manner.

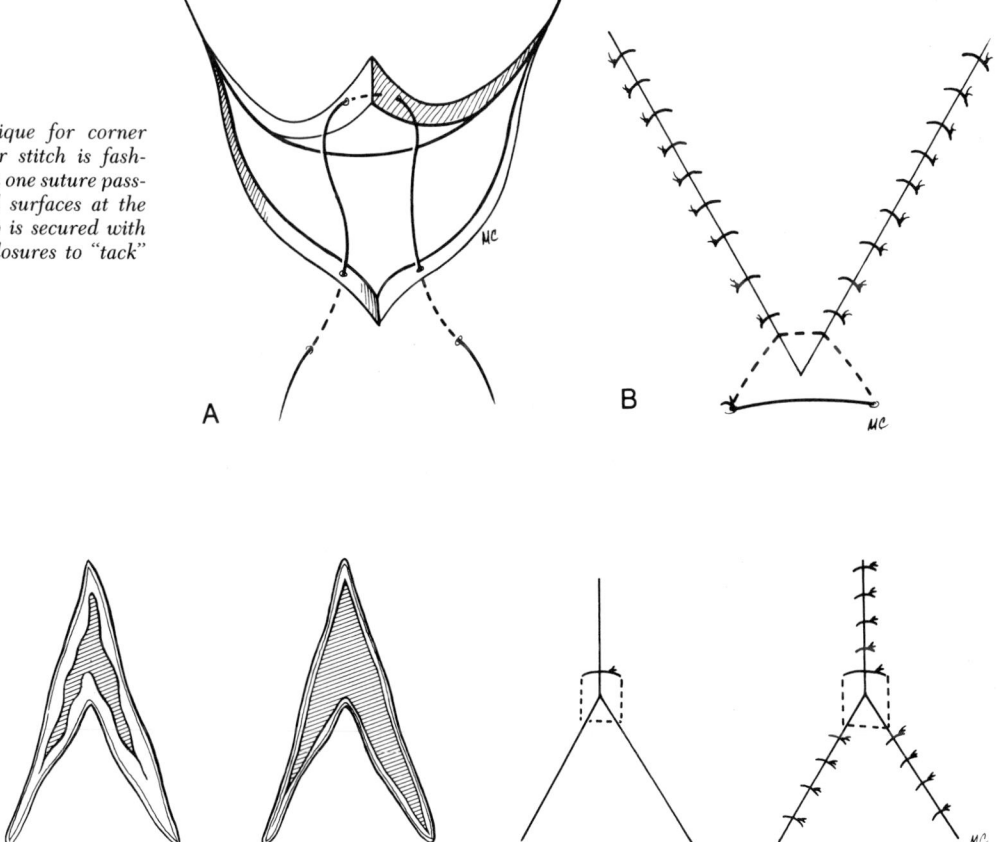

FIGURE 15-7. Technique for corner closure. A, The corner stitch is fashioned as illustrated with one suture passing through all wound surfaces at the same level. B, The flap is secured with small bite superficial closures to "tack" down the flap.

FIGURE 15-8. Technique for V-Y closure of a flap with irregular edges. All devitalized edges of the flap are trimmed back with tissue scissors. This debridement often leaves a flap that is inadequate to close the resulting defect. A modified corner suture is placed as illustrated to convert the wound to a Y. The remainder of the wound is closed with superficial sutures.

If the edges of a flap laceration are necrotic and require debridement, a simple flap suture will not suffice. In this case, the V shape of the flap is converted into a Y shape by using a flap (corner) suture and simple interrupted sutures (Fig. 15–8).

PROBLEM 2 The wound was a 6-cm jagged flap laceration at the midtibial level of the lateral aspect of the right leg. The edges of the wound and the flap were macerated and necrotic. There was contamination of the wound by dirt particles and bark fragments. On exploration there was no evident damage to muscle tissue or bone. The wound was anesthetized, prepared with povidone iodine solution, and irrigated using a 30-ml syringe and a 20-gauge needle to produce a medium-pressure jet. A total of 500 ml of normal saline was combined with a thorough exploration to remove all of the foreign material.

Because of the poor vascularity of this patient's leg, deep sutures were not considered for closing the wound. The irregular flap presented a problem, which was addressed first by debriding the necrotic wound edges. Next, a flap suture was placed using 4–0 nylon, which converted the wound to a Y shape. Seven simple interrupted sutures of 4–0 nylon were used to close the remainder of the Y.

SPECIAL CONSIDERATIONS

Scalp Wounds

The scalp is anatomically different from other areas of skin. Hair usually obscures a wound, making it difficult to evaluate. The dermis of the scalp is quite thick, and it sits on a very dense layer of connective tissue (superficial fascia), which contains a rich network of arterial and venous vessels. This abundant vascular supply leads to brisk bleeding when the scalp is lacerated, which can produce hemorrhagic shock even in seemingly minor wounds. This bleeding is made worse by the stiffness of the connective tissue, which prevents the normal constriction of injured blood vessels. Beneath the thick connective tissue layer is the galea aponeurotica, composed of dense, fibrous tissue that attaches to the frontalis muscle anteriorly and the occipitalis muscle posteriorly. Under the galea aponeurotica is a thin layer of loose connective tissue, which overlies the periosteum. Most wound care authorities believe it is essential to identify and close lacerations in the galea aponeurotica because a large defect in this layer may lead to abnormal contraction of the frontalis muscle. Also, there is great potential for extension of hematoma and infection in the loose connective tissue layer deep to the galea, and its closure can prevent hematoma formation and reduce the chance of infection.

Facial Wounds

Facial injuries are of special concern to the physician as well as the patient. The challenge is to maintain the cosmetic appearance of the face. In general, deep buried sutures are placed in the dermis to close the wound and keep the tension off the skin sutures. Skin sutures are placed to align the superficial tissues. Debridement may be used to delineate the wound edges, but the amount of tissue removed is kept small. Smaller suture material is used, and greater attention is paid to skin tension lines. In some cases definitive repair cannot be done in the emergency department. After surgical consultation the wound is closed to align the tissues, and the patient is referred for further care.

1. Eyelid lacerations are explored for involvement of the orbicularis oculi muscle or the tarsal plate. A simple 6–0 suture closure is usually used. If there is involvement of the medial canthus or internal margin of the lid (gray line), an ophthalmologist or plastic surgeon is consulted.

2. Nasal injuries require internal as well as external exploration. Trauma to the nose may produce a septal hematoma, which is a collection of blood under pressure in the mucosa covering the septal cartilage. If left unevacuated, a septal hematoma can lead to necrosis of part of the septum.

3. Intraoral lacerations often appear gaping and ragged but as a rule heal quickly with minimal repair. For large intraoral lacerations a few chromic, absorbable or nonabsorbable silk sutures are placed to approximate the irregular mucosal edges. Lacerations of less than 2 cm in the mouth do not usually need sutures unless they are actively bleeding.

4. Lip lacerations are challenging to repair because of the importance of exactly readjoining the disrupted tissue. If it is lacerated, the vermilion border, which is the thin line of transition between the lip and the facial skin, must be properly realigned. Failure to do this results in a very noticeable scar on the lip. Anesthetic blocks for the lip are ideal in this situation because they do not distort the anatomy in the area. Some physicians find it helpful to realign the vermilion border with the initial suture when closing lip lacerations.

5. The ear has a thin layer of skin over its cartilage foundation. When traumatized, a collection of blood in and adjacent to the cartilage (perichondrial hematoma) may exert pressure on the cartilage, causing impaired healing and necrosis. A grossly disfigured ear can result. Perichondrial hematomas should be incised and drained and then covered with a special pressure dressing. If extensive underlying damage to the cartilage is found, an ear, nose, and throat (ENT) surgeon should be consulted. For uncomplicated ear lacerations, closure with 6–0 nylon simple interrupted sutures is sufficient.

Foreign Bodies

In almost all wounds a foreign body must be suspected. Common foreign bodies are glass and metal fragments, wood chips, gravel, and dirt particles. Radiographs may be helpful, as noted in the Diagnostic Adjuncts section. Some foreign bodies are superficial and easy to remove, but deeper ones, particularly those penetrating the sole of the foot, are often very difficult to find. When normal wound cleansing and exploration do not reveal a foreign body that is suspected by the history or identified on radiographs, a decision must be made about removal. In some cases the removal attempt may cause more damage than leaving the foreign body in the tissues. If composed of an inert substance such as glass, metal, or plastic, a foreign body is less likely to cause tissue reaction and infection. Removal of inert foreign bodies is advisable but not at the expense of major tissue damage. Noninert foreign bodies are composed of organic material such as wood or vegetable matter, which may decay in the body and cause marked tissue reaction and infection. All noninert foreign bodies are removed from a wound. Foreign bodies requiring removal are best approached by extending the original wound. Splinter forceps may make it easier to pull thin, sharp foreign bodies out of the wound. If exploration involves dissection along nerves, tendons, large blood vessels, or into joints, it is carried out in the operating room.

Burns

Many burns seen in the emergency setting can be handled on an outpatient basis. Those burns usually requiring admission to the hospital are summarized in Table 15–4. Emergency department treatment of superficial- and partial-thickness burns involves providing pain relief with cool water immersion and parenteral medications if needed, followed by gentle cleansing of the burned area with a mild soap solution. In first-degree burns the application of an antibiotic cream is not necessary, and the patient can be treated with a systemic anti-inflammatory agent such as ibuprofen. Some people report a soothing effect with aloe vera preparations. If the first-degree burn blisters, it should be rechecked. Partial-thickness burns are debrided of broken blisters, but intact blisters

TABLE 15–4. Guidelines for Hospital Admission of Burn Victims

Partial-thickness burns >15% surface area (>10% body surface area of child)
Full-thickness burns >3% surface area
Suspected inhalation injury
Age <2 or >65 years
Partial- or full-thickness burns of hands, face, perineum, or feet
Electrical burns
Severe underlying systemic disease
Acute alcohol or drug abuse
Suspected child abuse

are not disturbed. A topical antibiotic cream or ointment, such as silver sulfadiazine, is applied. A nonadherent dressing base is placed next, followed by fluffed gauze bandages and a gauze wrap. The dressing is changed once daily by the patient. In 24 to 48 hours the patient is rechecked for further debridement, if necessary, and for signs of infection.

Bites

Animal and human bites usually occur on the extremities, where a less generous vascular supply predisposes to infection. Cat bites are most likely (40% to 50% incidence) to become infected. The bacteria primarily responsible for infection from a cat bite is *Pasteurella multocida*. It usually causes redness, warmth, and pain in and around the bite within 24 hours. Dog bites have about a 4% to 6% incidence of infection. Human bites have a significant rate of infection—about 25% to 30%. Extensive irrigation and debridement of devitalized tissue can reduce the chances of infection in animal bites. Dog bites, if seen within 6 to 8 hours, can be closed with sutures. Because of the low incidence of infection, dog bites to the face may be sutured even up to 24 hours after the injury. In the hands and feet, dog bites are usually left to heal by secondary union. Cat bites are often puncture wounds and are not closed unless the cosmetic concerns of scarring outweigh the risk of infection. Prophylactic antibiotics are used in animal bites for older wounds (over 8 hours), hand wounds, deep puncture wounds that cannot be adequately cleaned, and in high-risk patients. The penicillinase-resistant penicillins have good activity against *P. multocida* and *Staphylococcus* and *Streptococcus* species. All are common in bite infections.

The risk of rabies in animal bites is very low, but, given the lethality of the disease, all bites are considered for possible rabies prophylaxis. Guidelines are available for rabies prophylaxis. They are summarized in Table 15–5.

PROBLEM 1 Because the wounds were not too old, were in well-vascularized areas, and could be cleansed well, the head and shoulder wounds were judged to be acceptable for primary closure. The back wounds were small puncture wounds that were not in a cosmetically significant area. They were left open to heal by secondary intention. Rabies is always a consideration in dog bites, but in the setting of a provoked attack, and with documentation of the dog's rabies vaccination, there was no need to provide rabies prophylaxis.

Wound Aftercare

Tetanus Prophylaxis. Before a wounded patient leaves the emergency department, the matter of tetanus prophylaxis is addressed. The patient's immunization history is obtained. The risk of tetanus is highest in people who have never been fully immunized. The elderly and people not native to the United States are at highest risk. The decision to provide tetanus prophylaxis is based on the patient's immunization history and the

TABLE 15–5. A Guide to Rabies Postexposure Prophylaxis

Animal Species	Condition of Animal at Time of Attack	Treatment of Exposed Person[a]
Domestic: dog or cat	Healthy and available for 10 days of observation	None, unless animal develops rabies[b]
	Rabid or suspected rabid	RIG[c] and HDCV
	Unknown (escaped)	Consult public health officials if treatment is indicated, give RIG[c] and HDCV
Wild: skunk, bat, fox, coyote, raccoon, bobcat, and other carnivores	Regard as rabid unless proven negative by laboratory tests[d]	RIG[c] and HDCV
Other: livestock, rodents, and lagomorphs (rabbits and hares)	Consider individually. Local and state public health officials should be consulted on questions about the need for rabies prophylaxis. Bites of squirrels, hamsters, guinea pigs, gerbils, chipmunks, rats, mice, other rodents, rabbits, and hares almost never call for *antirabies* prophylaxis.	

From Advisory Committee on Immunization Practices: Rabies Prevention—U.S., 1984. MMWR 33:393–402, 407–408, 1984.

[a]All bites and wounds should immediately be cleansed thoroughly with soap and water. If antirabies treatment is indicated, both rabies immune globulin (RIG) and human diploid cell rabies vaccine (HDCV) should be given as soon as possible, regardless of the interval from exposure. Local reactions to vaccines are common but do not contraindicate continuing treatment. Discontinue vaccine treatment if fluorescent-antibody tests of the animal are negative for rabies.

[b]During the usual holding period of 10 days, begin treatment with RIG and vaccine (preferably with HDCV) at the first sign of rabies in a dog or cat that has bitten someone. The symptomatic animal should be killed immediately and tested.

[c]If RIG is not available, use antirabies serum, equine; do not use more than the recommended dosage.

[d]The animal should be killed and tested as soon as possible. Holding for observation is not recommended.

assessment of the wound. Table 15–6 lists current tetanus immunization recommendations.

Bandaging. Dressings or bandages are used on wounds to provide protection, prevent contamination, and absorb wound drainage. The standard dressing consists of an occlusive, nonadherent pad placed next to the skin, covered by thicker layers of gauze that can absorb wound drainage. Tape is used to secure the bandage to the skin. An occlusive layer is used over the wound because it provides more rapid epithelialization and decreased formation of fibrous tissue at the wound surface. It is also easier and less painful to change because it does not adhere to the wound. There are a variety of materials for bandaging wounds and many ways of applying bandages. Occlusive dressings are divided into film dressings (Telfa, Tegaderm) and hydrocolloid dressings (Duoderm).

TABLE 15–6. Summary Guide to Tetanus Prophylaxis in Routine Wound Management—United States, 1985

History of Adsorbed Tetanus Toxoid (Doses)	Clean, Minor Wounds		All Other Wounds[a]	
	Td[b]	TIG	Td[b]	TIG
Unknown or < three	Yes	No	Yes	Yes
≥ Three[c]	No[d]	No	No[e]	No

From Advisory Committee on Immunization Practices: Diphtheria, tetanus, and pertussis: Guidelines for vaccine prophylaxis and other preventive measures—U.S., 1985. MMWR 34:405–414, 419–426, 1985.

[a]Such as, but not limited to, wounds contaminated with dirt, feces, soil, saliva, etc., puncture wounds, avulsions, and wounds resulting from missiles, crushing, burns, and frostbite.

[b]For children under 7 years old: DTP (DT, if pertussis vaccine is contraindicated) is preferred to tetanus toxoid alone. For persons 7 years old and older, Td is preferred to tetanus toxoid alone.

[c]If only three doses of *fluid* toxoid have been received, a fourth dose of toxoid, preferably an adsorbed toxoid, should be given.

[d]Yes, if more than 10 years since last dose.

[e]Yes, if more than 5 years since last dose. (More frequent boosters are not needed and can accentuate side effects.)

Even occlusion from regular petroleum-based antibiotic ointment (polysporin, bacitracin) has demonstrated benefit. For many minor wounds a simple Band-Aid type dressing will suffice. For larger wounds or for wounds that are likely to have significant exudate, a more substantial bandage is needed. Many physicians do not bandage small face or scalp lacerations, preferring to apply an antibiotic ointment and leave the wound uncovered. If a bandage is applied circumferentially, as on an extremity, care must be taken to make it loose enough so that blood flow is not impaired. The timing of bandage changes depends on the nature of the wound and patient activity. If the wound has little drainage and little chance of infection and if the patient can keep it clean and dry, the bandage can be left on for several days. If there is significant drainage or if the bandage becomes soiled or wet, it is changed daily or more frequently.

Antibiotics

For simple, uncomplicated minor wounds and lacerations, there is no good clinical evidence that systemic antibiotics provide protection against the development of wound infection. Several randomized controlled studies support this conclusion. On the other hand, clinical and empiric experience suggests that there are certain wounds and clinical circumstances that warrant antibiotic intervention. If the decision is made to initiate antibiotic therapy, evidence indicates the initial dose has to be administered as soon as possible. Antibiotics may lose their protective effect when given more than 3 hours after injury and bacterial contamination. The following guidelines indicate wounds for which oral antibiotics on an outpatient basis are considered. The initial dose, either oral or parenteral, is administered prior to the discharge of the patient.

- Wounds more than 8 to 12 hours old, especially of the hands and lower extremities.
- Wounds due to a crushing (compression) mechanism with the potential for devitalization or requiring extensive revision.
- Significantly contaminated wounds requiring extensive cleansing and debridement.
- Wounds involving violation of the ear cartilage.
- Wounds involving the joint spaces, tendon, or bone.
- Mammalian bites, particularly human and cat bites.
- Extensive or contaminated wounds in patients with preexisting valvular heart disease.
- Wounds in persons with conditions of immunosuppression or impaired host defenses (e.g., diabetes mellitus).

The choice of systemic prophylactic antibiotic should take into account the fact that the most common infecting agent is *Staphylococcus aureus*. However, gram-negative organisms occur with significant frequency and need to be covered as well. Because of their broad activity against gram-positive and gram-negative organisms, including penicillinase-producing *S. aureus*, first-generation cephalosporins are a reasonable choice when prophylaxis is advisable. Examples include cephalexin (Keflex) and cefadroxil (Duricef). Some authorities feel that coverage for gram-positive organisms alone is sufficient and recommend using the less expensive dicloxacillin. For penicillin-allergic patients, erythromycin or ciprofloxacin can be used. In most situations requiring prophylaxis, 3 to 5 days of therapy should suffice.

DISPOSITION AND FOLLOW-UP

Outpatient Management

A large component of the eventual outcome of a wound is the care and treatment given after the patient leaves the emergency department. It is essential to educate patients about their wounds and to give them specific instructions about aftercare.

The timing and number of follow-up visits depend on patient compliance and reliability as well as the perceived risk of wound complications. Some wounds need minimal follow-up. Examples of these are first-degree burns and clean lacerations or abrasions. Some wounds, such as hand injuries, need to be checked every 24 to 48 hours for infection and to be rebandaged. Second-degree burns and extensive animal bites also belong in this category. Suture removal is also done according to the individual needs of each wound. Guidelines are given in Table 15–7. Generally, sutures are removed from facial wounds in 3 to 5 days, from the scalp in 7 to 10 days, from the trunk and upper extremities in 7 to 12 days, and from the lower extremity in 10 to 14 days. The person responsible for follow-up care varies with the community. The key element in follow-up is making clear to the patient, in writing, the time and place of the follow-up appointment.

Pain relief once the patient leaves the emergency department is accomplished in a number of ways. For many wounds, immobilization, elevation, and ice application can minimize pain. Some people will require systemic analgesic medications. For musculoskeletal injuries a nonsteroidal anti-inflammatory agent such as aspirin or ibuprofen provides good analgesia. Some wounds are extremely painful, and some patients have a lower tolerance for pain. In these cases an oral narcotic medication (e.g., acetaminophen with codeine) may be necessary. Examples of injuries that might need narcotics are extensive burns or abrasions and crush injuries of the digits.

Inpatient Management

Certain wounds are considered for inpatient management. The general principles behind inpatient management include the possible need for surgical intervention, the need for intravenous antibiotic prophylaxis, complicating secondary illnesses, the need for extensive nursing care, and an inability to care for oneself. Specific indications include:

- Complex, contaminated lacerations, particularly of the face or distal extremities.
- Suspected penetration of bone, tendon, or joint space.
- Extensive animal or human bite wounds, particularly of the hand or foot.
- Second-degree burns covering more than 10% of the body surface area.
- Serious underlying illness such as diabetes mellitus.

PROBLEM 1 The patient had wounds that required close follow-up. The chance of an infection in the first 24 hours after a dog bite is great enough to warrant a follow-up check at this time. If the wound looks good at 24 hours, further follow-up can be scheduled at 72 hours or later. The patient was given written instructions to return for follow-up the next day. He was instructed to watch for signs of infection and to keep the bandages in place and the wound clean and dry.

PROBLEM 2 The patient was given tetanus toxoid, 0.5 ml IM, after it was determined that she had received tetanus immunization 15 years earlier. Several factors, noted earlier, increased the risk for infection of the patient's wound. Given

TABLE 15–7. Suture Removal Intervals (Days)

Face	3–5
Eyelid	4
Ear	4–5
Nose	3–5
Scalp	7–10
Neck	5–7
Trunk	7–10
Arm	8–10
Hand	8–12
Leg	12–14
Foot	10–12
Extensor surface of joints	10–14

the patient's diabetes, poor vasculature, and the degree of contamination of the wound, the emergency physician elected to give the patient prophylactic antibiotics. Cephalexin, 500 mg every 6 hours for 5 days, was prescribed. Because antibiotics do not obviate the need for close follow-up, the physician arranged a follow-up appointment in 24 hours with her primary physician for a wound check. The patient also received written instructions on recognizing signs of infection and keeping the wound bandaged, clean, and dry.

DOCUMENTATION

1. Mechanism of injury
2. Time of injury
3. Prehospital treatment
4. Tetanus history and any immunization given
5. Physical examination record
   a. Vital signs
   b. Anatomic description or drawing of the wound
   c. Wound dimensions
   d. Functional examination results
   e. Neuromuscular and vascular examination results
6. Concise description of treatment. The findings of wound exploration are described. The anesthesia used, type and amount of irrigation solution, and number and type of sutures are included.
7. The most important documentation consists of the follow-up and referral plan. The advice given to the patient on how to care for the wound is recorded. The plan for wound rechecks and suture removal is recorded, and a copy is given to the patient. If a specialist is consulted, the phone conversation is summarized on the record, and specific mention of the follow-up appointment becomes part of the record.

SUMMARY AND FINAL POINTS

- The mechanism of injury is an important clinical factor because it can have a significant impact on wound healing.
- After 2 weeks, repaired wounds have recovered only 5% of the original tensile strength of the skin. They are susceptible to re-opening for a short period of time after suture removal.
- Wound infections are uncommon but occur in 5% of patients, *Staphylococcus aureus* is the most common infecting organism.
- Determining the elapsed time since injury is important because the chance of wound infection increases with each passing hour prior to repair.
- In evaluating patients with wounds and lacerations, it is important to determine whether a serious underlying condition caused the wound (e.g., syncope, seizures) or whether the actual surface injury is accompanied by a functional deficit, e.g., neurovascular or tendon interruption.
- Inert foreign bodies, such as glass, metal, or gravel, are almost always visible on radiographs. Noninert objects, such as wood, thorns, and dirt, are not radiopaque and need to be identified visually.
- Wound cleansing and irrigation are the cornerstones of wound care. Neither good wound closure techniques nor antibiotics can overcome superficial or inadequate wound preparation.
- Although deep closures with absorbable suture material are important to reduce wound

- tension and close deep spaces, they act like foreign bodies. As few as possible are used to accomplish the task intended for them.
- Tetanus remains an important worldwide disease. Proper tetanus prophylaxis must be ensured for every patient, particularly those over the age of 50 who might not have been properly immunized as children.
- All wounds heal better with properly applied occlusive dressings or frequent application of a petroleum-based antibiotic ointment.
- During the early follow-up period, pain that results from most wounds is successfully managed with non-narcotic analgesic, appropriate dressings, immobilization, and elevation of the area.

BIBLIOGRAPHY

Texts

1. Trott AT: Wounds and Lacerations: Emergency Care and Closure. St. Louis, C.V. Mosby, 1990.
2. Zukin DD, Simon RR: Emergency Wound Care: Principles and Practice. Rockville, MD, Aspen Publications, 1987.

Journal Articles

1. Edlich RF, Rodeheaver GT, Morgan RF, et al: Principles of emergency wound management. Ann Emerg Med 17:1284–1302, 1988.
2. Fariss BL, Foresman PA, Rodeheaver GT, et al: Anesthetic properties of bupivacaine and lidocaine for infiltration anesthesia. J Emerg Med 5:275–262, 1987.
3. Haury B, Rodeheaver GT, Venski J, et al: Debridement: An essential component of wound care. Am J Surg 135:238–242, 1978.
4. Hotter A: Physiologic aspects and clinical implications of wound healing. Heart Lung 11:522–530, 1982.
5. Rodeheaver G, Bellamy W, Kody M, et al: Bactericidal activity and toxicity of iodine-containing solutions in wounds. Arch Surg 117:181–185, 1982.
6. Stevenson T, Thacker J, Rodeheaver G, et al: Cleansing the traumatic wound by high-pressure syringe irrigation. J Am Coll Emerg Phys 5:17–21, 1976.
7. Swanson N, Tromovitch T: Suture materials: Properties, uses and abuses. Int J Dermatol 21:373–378, 1982.
8. Tandberg D: Glass in the hand and foot. JAMA 248:1872–1874, 1982.
9. Thirlby R, Blair A: The value of prophylactic antibiotics for simple lacerations. Surg Gynecol Obstet 156:212–216, 1983.
10. Trott AT: Mechanisms of surface soft tissue trauma. Ann Emerg Med 17:1279–1283, 1988.

SECTION FIVE

IMMUNOLOGIC DISORDERS

CHAPTER 16

ANAPHYLAXIS

DAVID N. ZULL, M.D.

PROBLEM 1 A 23 year old female came to the emergency department after she developed diffuse pruritus, lip swelling, dizziness, shortness of breath, and a lump in her throat while jogging. One hour earlier she had eaten a crab salad.

PROBLEM 2 A 45 year old female developed acute massive swelling of her lips, mouth, and tongue after taking the first dose of amoxicillin prescribed for bronchitis. She was in marked respiratory distress with audible stridor and hoarse, garbled speech. Her husband called the rescue squad.

PROBLEM 3 A 28 year old male was brought to the emergency department after a syncopal episode at home. Shortly before passing out he had taken ibuprofen for a backache. In the field, his blood pressure was unobtainable, but a thready pulse of 140 was noted. His skin was diffusely flushed, and the lungs were clear.

QUESTIONS TO CONSIDER

1. What is the pathophysiologic basis for anaphylactic and anaphylactoid reactions?
2. What are the various causes of anaphylaxis in the outpatient setting? Which of these most commonly lead to death?
3. What are the various clinical presentations of patients with anaphylactic reactions?
4. What are the differential diagnostic considerations in patients with apparent anaphylaxis?
5. What is the basic treatment approach for a patient with anaphylaxis?
6. What are the therapeutic alternatives in a patient with imminent airway obstruction or refractory shock?

INTRODUCTION

Anaphylaxis is an acute, life-threatening allergic reaction characterized by urticaria, angioedema, hypotension, bronchospasm, laryngeal edema, or abdominal colic. The clinical presentation may vary from localized angioedema to generalized organ system involvement to sudden respiratory or cardiovascular collapse. No age is exempt; however, the elderly and infants are rarely affected. Episodes of anaphylaxis tend to be more severe if they occur after age 40. There is no male-female predominance.

The constellation of symptoms that comprise an anaphylactic reaction results from the massive release of chemical mediators from mast cells and basophils throughout the body on exposure to a foreign substance (Fig. 16–1). For anaphylaxis to occur, previous exposure to the substance and synthesis of antigen-specific IgE by B lymphocytes is necessary. This IgE then binds to the surface of mast cells and basophils throughout the body. On reexposure, the antigen binds to the IgE on mast cells. This antigen-IgE

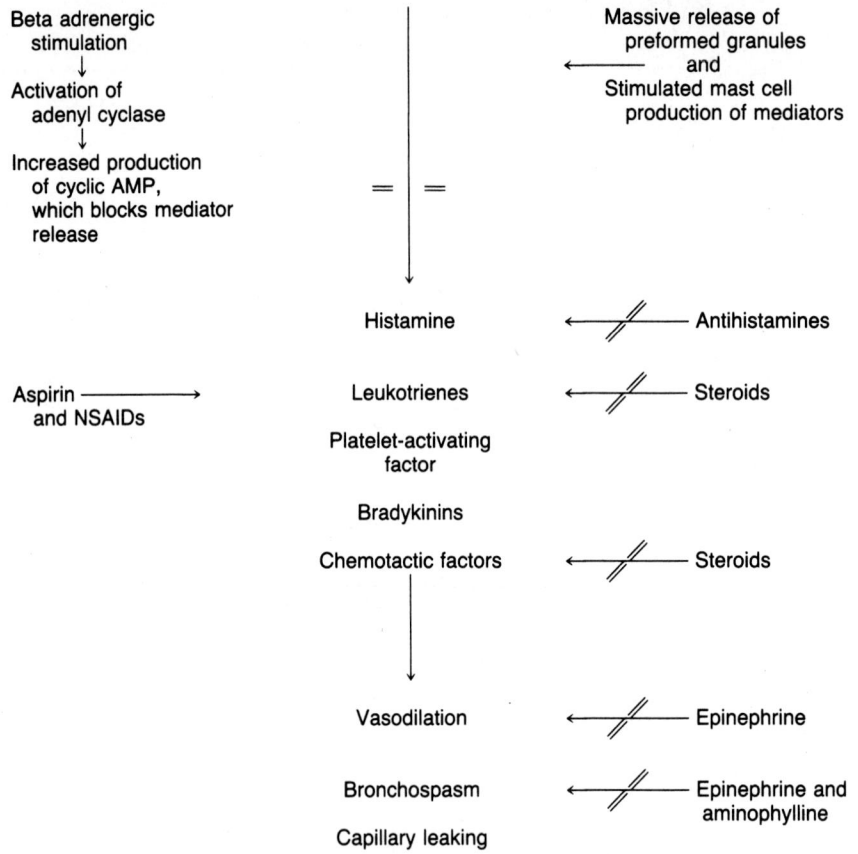

FIGURE 16–1. *Mechanism of anaphylactic reactions.*

interaction on the mast cell surface leads to release of preformed granules containing histamine, prostaglandins, and kallikrein and to the synthesis of leukotrienes. The term *anaphylactoid reaction* is often used to denote a syndrome clinically identical to anaphylaxis in which the release of mediators from mast cells is a direct degranulating response independent of antigen-IgE interaction.

Most of the chemical mediators released in anaphylaxis lead to vasodilation and capillary leaks, resulting in hypotension, urticaria, and angioedema of the skin, upper airway mucosa, and gastrointestinal tract. Leukotrienes are also released. They are byproducts of arachidonic acid and prostaglandin metabolism that are very potent bronchoconstrictors.

The following medications can modulate mediator release from mast cells or alter the end-organ response to these mediators (Fig. 16–1).

1. Beta-adrenergic drugs promote the synthesis of cyclic AMP inside mast cells. Increases in the concentration of intracellular cyclic AMP inhibit degranulation of mast cells, thereby stopping the ongoing reaction as well as dilating bronchial smooth muscle.

2. Antihistamines competitively block histamine at its tissue receptor sites.

3. The anti-inflammatory effect of steroids appears to have a delayed benefit in decreasing angioedema and relieving bronchospasm. Steroids may also interfere with leukotriene production.

4. Aspirin and the nonsteroidal anti-inflammatory drugs (NSAIDs) block the cyclo-oxygenase enzyme, thereby shunting prostaglandin synthesis to leukotriene production.

It is estimated that 15% of the population will develop urticaria sometime during their lifetime; however, the prevalence of anaphylaxis is less than 1%. The ratio of mild to severe to fatal anaphylaxis is roughly 200:20:1.

PREHOSPITAL CARE

Self-Treatment

Some patients will have initiated treatment on their own by means of self-treatment kits such as the Ana-Kit (Miles Pharmaceuticals) or Epi-Pen (Center Labs). These kits are generally reserved for patients with idiopathic anaphylaxis, bee sting allergy, and sometimes food allergy. The Ana-Kit contains a preloaded syringe with two doses of 0.3 ml of epinephrine and two 25-mg diphenhydramine tablets. The Epi-Pen is a self-contained autoinjector device that looks like a pen and delivers 0.3 ml of epinephrine by pushing the pen against the thigh. Epi-Pen Jr. delivers 0.15 ml.

Rescue Squad

Recognition of the manifestations of acute anaphylaxis in the field is usually straightforward, especially when all features of the syndrome are present (Problem 1). Confusion may arise, however, when one clinical feature predominates, such as airway obstruction (Problem 2) or syncope or hypotension (Problem 3). The rescue squad and the base hospital personnel should maintain a high index of suspicion for anaphylaxis in such situations. Delay in proper treatment for even a few minutes may lead to the patient's demise.

History

1. Did the patient complain of itching, localized or generalized edema, difficulty in breathing, lightheadedness, or fainting?
2. Did symptoms begin after exposure to medications or other possible allergens such as bites or stings?
3. Does the patient have a history of previous allergic reactions?

Physical Examination

1. Is there evidence of a rash, wheals, or urticaria?
2. Is there facial, lip, or tongue swelling?
3. Does the patient exhibit stridor or wheezing?
4. Is there tachycardia or hypotension?

Intervention

1. If the diagnosis of anaphylaxis is clear or strongly suspected in a patient with respiratory or hemodynamic compromise, epinephrine is given without delay, 0.3 ml (1/1000 dilution) for an adult or 0.01 ml/kg for a child, subcutaneously or intramuscularly.
2. Field stabilization also includes establishment of a large-bore intravenous (IV) line with an isotonic crystalloid infusate. If the patient is clinically in shock, fluids are given with the line wide open, and a second line is established.
3. If refractory shock or imminent airway obstruction results, epinephrine is prepared for IV use (see later section, Initial Approach in the Emergency Department).
4. Although of secondary importance, the rescue personnel should consider administering steroids and antihistamines, if these medications are available.

INITIAL APPROACH IN THE EMERGENCY DEPARTMENT

Urticaria is often an isolated phenomenon, but it is also the most common early manifestation of anaphylaxis. The severity of the reaction is proportionate to the rapidity of onset; hence, an eruption occurring over a few minutes tends to be more severe and has greater systemic involvement than a reaction that develops over several hours or days.

History

Since the major threats to life in patients with anaphylaxis are airway obstruction and shock, immediate questioning focuses on the following:

1. Laryngeal edema. Do you feel a lump in your throat? Is it difficult to swallow? Does your voice seem hoarse to you? Do you feel short of breath or is it difficult getting air in? Do you feel swelling or tingling of your lips, tongue, or throat? This last question is important because any angioedema about the mouth may be a harbinger of laryngeal edema.

2. Hypotension. Do you feel dizzy, lightheaded, or confused? Did you pass out at any time?

Physical Examination

Initial physical examination also focuses on potential life-threatening issues:

1. Vital signs: Is there hypotension, tachycardia, or tachypnea?
2. General appearance: Does the patient look sick, apprehensive, pale, cyanotic? Does the voice sound hoarse? Are there supraclavicular retractions?
3. HEENT: Is there edema of the lips, uvula, tongue, or posterior pharynx?
4. Lungs: Is there inspiratory stridor? Is there wheezing or poor air movement?
5. Skin: Are there urticarial wheals, a diffuse flush, or angioedema of the face or hands?

Intervention

If the answer to any of these questions is affirmative, or if there are positive physical findings as described above, treatment must be administered immediately.

Oxygen. Supplemental oxygen by nonrebreathing mask at a flow rate of 10 to 12 liters/min will maximize oxygenation during the episode of decreased ventilation.

Intravenous Access. If not established in the prehospital setting, an intravenous line is placed to allow administration of fluids as well as medications.

Cardiac Monitoring. Cardiac monitoring is essential for detecting dysrhythmias, which may be secondary to hypoxia, hypoperfusion, or therapeutic drugs.

Epinephrine. Epinephrine is "the cornerstone of anaphylaxis therapy." The beta-adrenergic effect stops the ongoing release of mediators from mast cells and dilates the bronchial smooth muscle. The alpha-adrenergic effect causes vasoconstriction, thereby raising the blood pressure and decreasing swelling of edematous tissues. Dosage is 0.3 ml (1/1000) subcutaneously or intramuscularly (IM) in an adult and 0.01 ml/kg in a child. This dose may be repeated at 10- to 20-minute intervals. The IM route is preferred if the patient is hypotensive.

Intravenous epinephrine is reserved for patients in shock or with imminent upper airway obstruction. Intravenous dosage consists of 0.1 mg (1 ml of cardiac epinephrine, 1/10,000) diluted in 10 ml of normal saline and given by slow IV push over 5 to 10 minutes while carefully monitoring the patient's cardiac rhythm. This dose may be repeated at 10-minute intervals, or the patient may be put on an epinephrine drip made by adding 1 mg of epinephrine to 250 ml of D/W 5%, to run at 1 to 4 µg/min (15 to 60 microdrops/min). The drip is safer and easier to titrate but also contains a much smaller dose of epinephrine. If frequent premature ventricular contractions (PVCs) or chest pain develop, therapy is held for a few minutes and then resumed at a lower infusion rate.

Airway Management. Laryngeal edema and upper airway obstruction may progress rapidly to an acute stage, resulting in sudden death. In most instances, airway obstruction is heralded by angioedema of the lips, uvula, tongue, and oropharynx. When these signs are observed, a cricothroidotomy kit is placed at the bedside, and the emergency physician must be prepared to perform a cricothyroidotomy.

The patient with marked upper airway angioedema is best kept in the upright position so that the edematous tissues do not fall back and obstruct the airway. The patient is reassured and asked to breathe slowly, and secretions are gently suctioned as necessary. The physician should be at the bedside constantly until a trend of improvement is established.

Crystalloid Administration. Hypotension in anaphylaxis is secondary to marked vasodilation and capillary leaking. As a result, volume loading is a rational therapeutic approach in conjunction with epinephrine therapy. Most adults are given 1 liter of isotonic crystalloid as fast as it will run in, and a second liter can be titrated to response, usually over the next hour. Similarly, children should receive a bolus of 20 ml/kg up to 1 liter. Elderly adults and those with heart disease are not excluded from aggressive fluid resuscitation, but frequent checks are made for the development of rales or neck vein distention. Invasive hemodynamic monitoring should be considered.

Adjuncts to Hypotension Management. The Trendelenburg position is routine unless airway management contraindicates it. A MAST suit may be very effective and is considered in any patient with refractory hypotension. Dopamine infusion has an advantage over epinephrine infusion in that most physicians and nurses are more familiar with it.

PROBLEM 1 The complaint of a "lump in the throat" may be related to uvular edema, but concomitant, life-threatening laryngeal edema must also be considered. Subcutaneous epinephrine was given immediately. The patient's vital signs were not significantly altered: blood pressure, 90/55 mm Hg, pulse 110 beats/min, respirations 28/min. Faint wheezing, which was present prior to therapy, quickly resolved, but the lip and uvular edema remained unchanged. Oxygen, an intravenous line, and a cardiac monitor were placed, and the patient felt more comfortable.

Intravenous epinephrine is not needed in this case unless there is deterioration. Additional doses of subcutaneous epinephrine are likely to result in complete resolution of the remaining symptoms.

PROBLEM 2 This patient's complaints were similar to those of the patient described in Problem 1 at the onset but rapidly progressed to severe respiratory distress. Subcutaneous epinephrine administered early in the course might have been effective, but by the time the paramedics arrived to administer it, it had no effect. On arrival in the emergency department the patient was agitated, sitting bolt upright, struggling with secretions, and barely able to speak or swallow. Blood pressure was 110/70 mm Hg, pulse was 120 beats/min, respirations were 20/min. There was massive edema of the oropharynx, stridor, and suprasternal retractions. Intravenous epinephrine was administered by slow push, but the patient's condition continued to deteriorate. Attempts at intubation were futile owing to the angioedema of the palate and supraglottic area. As preparations for cricothyroidotomy were made, complete obstruction developed, and the patient could not be ventilated by bag-mask. Immediate cricothyroidotomy was performed, and the patient was ventilated with 50% oxygen.

PROBLEM 3 On arrival of the rescue squad, this patient was in shock. Intravenous saline and subcutaneous epinephrine were started. On arrival in the emergency department, intramuscular epinephrine was administered, and after two doses as well as 1 liter of normal saline, the blood pressure was 65 mm Hg and the pulse was 140 beats/min. A second large-bore IV line was started to allow more fluid to be administered. After 2 liters of saline had been given, the blood pressure had risen to only 75 mm Hg. Intravenous epinephrine was started by slow push (0.1 mg or 1 ml of cardiac epinephrine in 10 ml of saline given over 5 minutes). The blood pressure promptly rose to 122/75 mm Hg, and the pulse fell to 120. After 20 minutes, however, the blood pressure fell to 85/50 mm Hg. An epinephrine drip at 4 µg/min was started with good blood pressure response. This patient also received 4 liters of normal saline in the first 90 minutes in the emergency department, and the fluid was continued at 500 ml/hr as the epinephrine drip was tapered.

DATA GATHERING

Patients may present in extremis and be unable to provide any historical information. More often, information about the events that took place and possible precipitating agents is obtainable.

History

Onset. What were the *initial symptoms*, and how did they *progress*? Symptoms may develop immediately after exposure and are usually present within 30 minutes. Exposure to antigens by the oral route may result in a delay of symptoms for 2 to 3 hours, however.

Route. Was there *exposure* to possible *antigens* by an invasive route? The more direct the access to the systemic circulation, the greater the likelihood of a severe reaction. Therefore, intravenous exposures are the most dangerous, followed in order by intramuscular, subcutaneous, intradermal, mucous membrane, and skin exposures.

Timing and Dosage. Have there been frequent *recurrent exposures* to the possible antigen? Recurrent exposures increase the risk of sensitization.

Antigen Potency. What are the *possible offending agents*? A review of the patient's step-by-step actions during the previous 4 hours will usually identify potential offending agents. Antibiotics are a common etiologic factor, penicillin being the most common cause of life-threatening anaphylaxis. Stings of insects of the order Hymenoptera are the second most common cause. Iodinated radiographic contrast media are also potent antigens. Foods, especially shellfish, and common analgesics such as aspirin and the nonsteroidal anti-inflammatory agents are also common offenders and are specifically inquired about.

Duration. *How long* have the *symptoms* persisted? There is wide clinical variability, but symptoms generally do not last for more than 3 to 4 hours. Angioedema, however, is very slow to resolve and may last for 6 hours or more.

PROBLEM 3 This weekend athlete had taken ibuprofen for a backache about 30 minutes before passing out. Further history obtained after treatment revealed that he had been taking this medication before exercising for some time. He estimated that he had taken one to two tablets weekly for many months.

This is a pattern that is consistent with development of sensitization. Onset in this case is quite rapid for an oral exposure but is consistent with the severe reaction that later developed in this patient.

Physical Examination

The physical examination may be deceptively normal. Most findings relate to the skin or respiratory tract (Table 16–1). With the onset of premonitory symptoms such as pruritus

TABLE 16–1. Symptoms and Signs of Anaphylaxis

Reaction	Symptoms	Signs
Urticaria	Itching	Raised wheals diffusely wandering, evanescent
Angioedema	Nonpruritic tingling	Swelling of lips, eyes, hands; without heat or erythema
Laryngeal edema	Hoarseness Dysphagia Lump in throat Airway obstruction, sudden death	Inspiratory stridor, intercostal and supraclavicular retractions, cyanosis
Bronchospasm	Cough, dyspnea, chest tightness	Wheezing, tachypnea, retractions
Vasodilation	Dizziness Syncope Confusion	Hypotension (mild to severe), tachycardia, oliguria
Rhinitis	Nasal congestion, itching, and rhinorrhea	Mucosal edema
Conjunctivitis	Tearing Itching	Lid edema and injection
Gastroenteritis	Cramping Diarrhea Vomiting	Normal examination or increased bowel sound activity

of the palms or a lump in the throat, there are often no objective findings. Acute hypotension resulting in syncope or coma may not be accompanied by other manifestations of anaphylaxis. The onset of angioedema of the skin and mucous membranes is often very subtle. In all these circumstances the symptoms should be recognized as signs of possible anaphylaxis, and the patient's word not doubted despite normal findings on physical examination.

Vital Signs. Hypotension, tachypnea, and tachycardia are common. Fever is not part of the picture of anaphylaxis and suggests an infectious etiology or a delayed drug reaction such as serum sickness.

Skin. Over 90% of patients have some combination of urticaria or angioedema. Urticaria is edema of the upper dermis and appears as raised erythematous wheals covering most of the body surface in evanescent, pruritic patches. Angioedema is edema of the deep dermis and appears as puffy, nonpitting, uninflamed areas of the skin or mucous membranes. Angioedema is generally painless and nonpruritic, and patients note only tingling and swelling in the affected areas. Angioedema tends to be most prominent about the face, lips, and hands. Edema of the mucous membranes often appears gelatinous and translucent in nature; the uvula is often likened to a pealed white grape.

Lungs. Evidence of intercostal and supraclavicular retractions is sought, and auscultation for inspiratory stridor, wheezing, and air movement is performed. Generally, bronchospasm is mild in patients with anaphylaxis unless the patient has a previous history of asthma. Rales and pulmonary edema are not part of anaphylaxis except as rare terminal events.

Heart. Cardiac rate and rhythm are noted, since ventricular dysrhythmias and myocardial infarction may occur in anaphylaxis. Cardiac involvement is thought to be secondary to hypotension, hypoxia, epinephrine therapy, or combined factors.

Abdomen. Although mild cramping is common, results of the examination are generally normal. Rarely, diarrhea and hematochezia may occur, and a rectal examination may be indicated.

DECISION PRIORITIES AND PRELIMINARY DIFFERENTIAL DIAGNOSIS

After data gathering and observing the initial response to any treatment, two important questions can usually be answered.

1. *When confronted by a patient in shock or with acute upper respiratory distress, the first question to answer is: Is this anaphylaxis? If not, what other problem is present?*

    The diagnosis of anaphylaxis is obvious when antigen exposure is rapidly followed by urticaria, angioedema, bronchospasm, upper airway edema, and hypotension. When there is a delay in the development of symptoms so that cause and effect are not clear or expression of the syndrome is only partial, other entities are considered (Table 16–2).

    Whether a patient has an anaphylactic reaction, an anaphylactoid reaction, severe bronchospasm, or severe urticaria is of no immediate importance because the treatment is the same. All these conditions are potentially life-threatening, and all require immediate treatment as outlined above.

    Hereditary angioedema is a rare autosomal dominant disorder characterized by repeated episodes of angioedema of the skin, upper airway, and gut. Episodes generally date from adolescence and are frequently provoked by minor trauma. The gastrointestinal involvement is very prominent, often mimicking an acute condition of the abdomen. Urticaria is not seen in this disorder, and patients do not respond to epinephrine.

    Viral or bacterial infections of the upper airway such as croup, epiglottitis, and peritonsillar abscess may have a similar respiratory presentation, but the association of fever, cough, sore throat, and dysphagia will usually provide adequate differentiation of these problems.

    Scombroid fish poisoning may present as severe urticaria, nausea, vomiting, headache, and dysphagia. This syndrome occurs shortly after ingestion of fish with a high histidine content (tuna or mahi mahi) that is spoiled slightly so that histidine is broken down to histamine.

    Chinese restaurant syndrome is secondary to monosodium glutamate ingestion and may resemble anaphylaxis; however, the prominence of headache and burning chest discomfort is unique.

    Systemic *mastocytosis* and the *carcinoid syndrome* are extremely rare disorders associated with neoplastic processes that can mimic allergy by their episodes of flushing and hypotension.

    Munchausen's syndrome, in which patients may feign symptoms of stridor and obstruction as part of hysteria, is very rare.

2. *If the problem is anaphylaxis, what is the precipitating agent?*

    The agents most likely to be responsible for anaphylaxis are identified in Table 16–3.

PROBLEMS 1, 2, and 3 The acute development of angioedema, airway compromise, or shock after exposure to common inciting agents leaves little doubt about the cause of the patient's symptoms in each case. Frequently, the inciting agent is not this obvious. The physician and patient must reconstruct the events preceding the episode to detect possible offending agents. Every effort is made to identify the cause, since a recurrence may result in even more severe symptoms.

TABLE 16–2. Differential Diagnosis of Anaphylaxis

Anaphylactoid reactions	Scombroid fish poisoning
Acute, severe urticaria	Chinese restaurant syndrome
Acute, severe bronchospasm	Systemic mastocytosis
Hereditary angioedema	Carcinoid syndrome
Upper airway infections	Munchausen's syndrome

TABLE 16–3. Etiologic Factors

1. *Antibiotics.* Penicillin is the most common cause of life-threatening anaphylaxis, with 100 to 200 deaths per year reported in the United States. Approximately 1% of the population is sensitive to penicillin, most manifesting urticaria alone; however, of 100,000 patients treated with penicillin, 25 will develop severe anaphylaxis, and one patient will die. Penicillins include ampicillin, dicloxacillin, and related drugs. Cephalosporins will cross-react at a rate of 5% to 16%, but the likelihood is much greater if the penicillin anaphylaxis is life-threatening. Other antibiotics are unusual causes of anaphylaxis. However, sulfonamides are commonly implicated in drug rash, serum sickness, and Stevens-Johnson syndrome.
2. *Bee Stings.* Stings from insects of the order Hymenoptera constitute the second most common cause of life-threatening anaphylaxis in the United States, resulting in 50 to 80 deaths per year. This is not surprising because 0.4% to 1.0% of the population reports a history of bee sting allergy. Yellow jackets, honey bees, wasps, hornets, bumble bees, and fire ants comprise this group. Most stings occur in July and August and although 90% of victims are less than 20 years old, more than 90% of fatalities occur in those over 20.
3. *Iodinated Contrast Media.* These compounds can result in anaphylactoid reactions in 1% to 2% of patients undergoing intravenous infusion for intravenous pyelography or CT scanning. One to ten of 100,000 administrations may result in death, with 40 to 50 deaths per year reported in the United States.
4. *Foods and Food Additives.* Foods are probably the most common cause of mild anaphylaxis seen in the outpatient setting, but life-threatening reactions do occur. Shellfish, nuts, legumes, seeds, and eggs are most often implicated. Food additives such as sulfites may be occasionally responsible.
5. *Aspirin and Nonsteroidal Anti-inflammatory Drugs.* These compounds are also a common cause of anaphylaxis in the emergency department setting. Aspirin and NSAIDs are so frequently used by the general public that they are often overlooked as a potential cause of an acute allergic reaction.
6. *Complete Proteins.* These include streptokinase, chymopapaine, insulin, vaccines, toxoids, antisera and other blood products, allergy extracts, and seminal fluid.
7. *Physical Factors.* Exercise is being increasingly recognized as a cause of anaphylaxis. These reactions are not predictable or reproducible, and food or drug ingestion before exercise may be related to the result in some patients (Problem 1). Cold may induce urticaria or mild anaphylaxis in some patients.
8. *Anesthetic Agents.* Induction agents and muscle relaxants used in facilitating intubation are increasingly recognized as a cause of anaphylactic shock.
9. *Miscellaneous Drugs.* Included in this category are morphine, thiamine, enalapril, local anesthetics, and vitamin K.
10. *Idiopathic Causes.* Twenty-five to thirty per cent of anaphylactic reactions fall into this category, even after thorough evaluation by an allergist.

DIAGNOSTIC ADJUNCTS

Although there are no tests that are specifically helpful in the diagnosis of anaphylaxis, some laboratory, radiologic, and electrocardiographic tests may assist in ruling out other diagnoses or in detecting complications resulting from the anaphylactic syndrome.

Laboratory Studies

1. A *complete blood count* may be helpful in supporting the diagnosis of an upper airway infection and may be abnormal in patients with a neoplastic syndrome.
2. *Serum electrolytes and renal function tests* are useful for patients who have been in shock or who are receiving large volumes of fluids.
3. *Arterial blood gases* are very helpful in evaluating the patient's oxygenation and ventilatory status.

Radiologic Imaging

1. *Chest radiography* plays no role in the acute management of the patient with anaphylaxis unless the patient requires intubation and the film is obtained to check tube placement.
2. A *plain film soft tissue lateral view of the neck* may be used in diagnosing epiglottitis.

Electrocardiography

The stress of airway compromise or shock can precipitate myocardial ischemia or dysrhythmias, especially in older patients and in those with preexisting cardiac disease.

PRINCIPLES OF MANAGEMENT

The therapeutic approach to the patient with anaphylaxis includes general supportive care, cessation of exposure to the antigen, and blocking of the anaphylactic or anaphylactoid process on a cellular or biochemical level. As outlined in Figure 16–1, these processes can be blocked at multiple sites using catecholamines, antihistamines, steroids, and aminophylline.

General Supportive Care. All patients with suspected anaphylaxis are placed on a cardiac monitor, and oxygen and an intravenous line are initiated.

Cessation of Antigen Exposure. As long as exposure to the antigen continues, the anaphylactic reaction will continue. Medications, especially intravenous infusions, that may be causative are of course stopped, and stingers from honey bees are removed.

Catecholamines. Beta-adrenergic stimulation leads to activation of adenyl cyclase and the production of cyclic AMP, which in turn blocks the release of vasoactive substances from the mast cell granules and also produces bronchodilation. Alpha-adrenergic stimulation produces vasoconstriction. With its combined alpha- and beta-adrenergic activity, epinephrine is an excellent agent to use in countering this syndrome. (See earlier section on initial approach for dosage guidelines.)

Antihistamines. Antihistamines block the effect of histamine after it is released. The H_1 and H_2 antagonists are used together in patients with severe reactions because they act synergistically. The H_1 antagonists, diphenhydramine and hydroxyzine, can be given intramuscularly or intravenously in the acute situation (1 mg/kg up to a total dose of 75 mg) and may be given orally after discharge. The H_2 antagonists, cimetidine and ranitidine, are used intravenously in doses of 300 mg and 50 mg, respectively, and may also be used orally when the acute episode is resolving. The H_1 antagonists are respiratory depressants and are used with caution in patients with marginal respiratory status. Cimetidine inhibits theophylline metabolism and may lead to toxic blood levels.

Steroids. Steroids stabilize membranes and deter the release of preformed granules in mast cells. Additionally, they block the effects of leukotrienes and chemotactic factors and reduce capillary leaking.

They are administered to all patients with systemic anaphylaxis, excluding perhaps those whose symptoms are very mild and resolve with a single subcutaneous dose of epinephrine. Steroids are thought to prevent reexacerbation of symptoms that may occur several hours later in some patients. Extrapolating from clinical studies done in patients with status asthmaticus, large doses of steroids given immediately when the patient presents appear to have clinical benefit in the emergency setting.

Recommended doses are:

Methylprednisolone	50 to 125 mg IV push (adult)
	1 to 2 mg/kg (child)
Hydrocortisone	250 to 500 mg IV push (adult)
	4 to 7 mg/kg (child)

This dose may be repeated at 4-hour intervals if symptoms persist; otherwise rapid tapering of oral steroids is suggested. Prednisone, 40 to 50 mg given in 6 to 12 hours and then tapered daily over 3 days, is suggested.

Beta-Adrenergic Agents—Inhaled. Bronchospasm may also be treated by inhaled beta-adrenergic agonists, such as metaproterenol or salbutamol. These drugs potentiate the beta-stimulating effects of epinephrine. Cardiac dysrhythmias are possible complications.

Aminophylline. Bronchospasm in patients with anaphylaxis is usually very responsive to epinephrine. However, patients with a history of asthma may require aminophylline loading in a dose of 5.6 mg/kg given over 30 minutes. If the patient is currently taking theophylline, the present blood level of the drug is determined and then 1 mg/kg will increase the theophylline level every 2 mg/100 ml until the desired level is reached.

Repeated Examination. Throughout the course of therapy, the vital signs are assessed frequently, the airway is checked for angioedema of the uvula or oropharynx, the lungs are auscultated for wheezes or stridor, and the patient is questioned for symptoms of hoarseness, dysphagia, lump in the throat, or dyspnea. Most anaphylactic episodes clear within 2 to 4 hours, but, especially with oral exposures, the duration of symptoms may be much longer. Observation should continue until symptoms are minimal or absent for a number of hours.

PROBLEM 1 The rapid resolution of this patient's angioedema and bronchospasm with subcutaneous epinephrine made further aggressive intervention unnecessary. Oral antihistamines are helpful in treating subsequent symptoms. The patient is cautioned to avoid shellfish in the future.

PROBLEM 2 Severe, persistent upper airway compromise necessitating cricothyroidotomy required continued aggressive therapy and monitoring. Intravenous steroids were used to reduce further development of angioedema, and aminophylline or a beta-adrenergic agent would be used if bronchospasm developed.

PROBLEM 3 Again, this patient who presented in shock had a good response to epinephrine but also benefited from early intravenous steroid administration. Continued intensive care monitoring is essential.

SPECIAL CONSIDERATIONS

The Geriatric or Cardiac Patient

There is great concern among physicians about the use of epinephrine in this patient group. Certainly, if the episode is mild, steroids and antihistamines alone may suffice. Cautious fluid resuscitation with saline is the initial treatment of choice for hypotension. Epinephrine should not be withheld in patients with potential upper airway obstruction or those with hypotension that is unresponsive to volume loading.

Although full doses of subcutaneous epinephrine have been shown to be safe in the treatment of elderly asthmatics, an initial test dose of 0.15 ml (1/1000) subcutaneously is prudent in cardiac patients. They are monitored carefully for 15 minutes after the dose is given. If no chest pain or dysrhythmias develop, another test dose or a full dose may be administered. Intravenous epinephrine is avoided in this patient group unless death appears imminent without its use.

Beta-Adrenergic Blocker–Aggravated Anaphylaxis

Patients taking beta blockers may have an accentuated allergic reaction that is resistant to epinephrine therapy. Epinephrine may produce only a net alpha-adrenergic effect characterized by paradoxical bradycardia. In this setting a pure beta agonist such as isoproterenol may be preferred. In addition, the MAST suit may be a helpful adjunct for treating hypotension, and atropine is effective for treating bradyarrhythmias. The drug of choice, however, is glucagon, which increases intracellular cyclic AMP by a mechanism separate from beta-receptor stimulation. It is given in a dose of 1 mg by IV push over 2 minutes and repeated once. Nausea and vomiting are common side affects of the drug.

DISPOSITION AND FOLLOW-UP

Disposition will depend on the severity of the reaction and the degree of resolution that occurs with emergency department treatment.

Admission

- Any patient who has had life-threatening manifestations such as shock or upper airway obstruction, even if these were resolved with acute therapy.
- Patients with a slow or incomplete response to therapy (unless urticaria or very minimal angioedema of the skin or uvula remains).
- Patients who have experienced any worsening of symptoms during emergency department evaluation and treatment.
- Elderly, debilitated, or cardiac patients.

Admission to Critical Care Unit

- Patients with hypotension not responding to fluid resuscitation and epinephrine subcutaneously or intramuscularly.
- Patients with any potential upper airway obstruction with persistent symptoms or signs of upper airway angioedema.
- Any patient who required intravenous epinephrine.
- Patients with beta-blocker–accentuated anaphylaxis.

Discharge

- Patients who have experienced complete and rapid resolution of symptoms after minimal therapy (e.g., one or two doses of subcutaneous epinephrine) and who have been observed in the emergency department for 3 to 4 hours. Also, such patients should have a companion to observe them at home.
- What is the plan for the patient who goes home?
  1. Prednisone 40 mg given initially and then tapered over 3 days. In a small percentage of patients, a secondary exacerbation of symptoms occurs within 12 hours of the initial onset despite earlier complete resolution. Steroids appear to be effective in preventing this late recrudescence.
  2. Diphenhydramine 25 mg every 4 to 6 hours for rash or itching.
  3. Avoidance of any potential inciting causes.
  4. Physician follow-up arranged in 24 hours.

PROBLEM 1 The symptoms cleared completely after two doses of epinephrine were given subcutaneously. After 4 hours of observation there was no recurrence. The patient was released to go home and was given a prescription for oral antihistamines; her family agreed to continue observation at home and to return to the emergency department if symptoms recurred.

PROBLEMS 2 AND 3 These two patients, both having experienced severe, persistent reactions, required admission to an intensive care unit for continued monitoring and treatment.

DOCUMENTATION

1. Time of onset, prodromal symptoms, and progression of symptoms.
2. All events preceding the onset by 4 to 6 hours (medications, activity, exposures, food).

3. Allergic history (similar reactions are noted).
4. Medications (including over-the-counter preparations and recreational drugs).
5. Angioedema of the uvula and other mucous membranes, if present.
6. Response to therapy.
7. Step-by-step progress notes on symptoms, signs, and therapy at frequent intervals.
8. Diagnosis and suspected etiologies.
9. If patient is not admitted: disposition, follow-up plan, and outpatient treatment regimen.

SUMMARY AND FINAL POINTS

- Anaphylaxis is an acute, life-threatening clinical syndrome in which airway compromise and hypotension are the most common causes of death and severe morbidity.
- There are numerous potential etiologic factors that can be elucidated by some detective work.
- Symptoms and signs of airway angioedema are always sought and are considered warning signs of airway obstruction.
- Epinephrine is the cornerstone of therapy and in extreme instances is given by the intravenous route.
- Fluid resuscitation is of critical importance in the treatment of patients with hypotension.
- In-house observation is indicated for all but the most mild and transient anaphylactic reactions.

BIBLIOGRAPHY

Texts

1. Weiszer I: Allergic emergencies. In Patterson R (ed): Allergic Diseases: Diagnosis and Management (3rd ed). Philadelphia, J.B. Lippincott, 1985.
2. Kniker WT: Anaphylaxis in children and adults. In Bierman CW, Pearlman DS (eds): Allergic Diseases from Infancy to Adulthood. Philadelphia, W.B. Saunders, 1988.

Journal Articles

1. Barach EM, Nowack RM: Epinephrine for treatment of anaphylactic shock. JAMA 25:2118–2122, 1984.
2. Bickell WH, Dice WH: Military anti-shock trousers in a patient with adrenergic-resistant anaphylaxis. Ann Emerg Med 13:189–190, 1984.
3. Fisher M: Anaphylaxis. DM 33(8):433–479, 1987.
4. Greenberger PA: Contrast media reactions. J Allerg Clin Immunol 74:600–605, 1984.
5. Lucke WC, Thomas TH: Anaphylaxis: Pathophysiology, clinical presentations, and treatment. J Emerg Med 1:83–95, 1983.
6. O'Leary MR, Smith MS: Penicillin anaphylaxis. Am J Emerg Med 4:241–247, 1986.
7. Muelleman RL, Gatz M, Salomone JA, et al: Hemodynamic and respiratory effects of thyrotropin-releasing hormone and epinephrine in anaphylactic shock. Ann Emerg Med 18(5):534–541, 1989.
8. Patterson R, Valentine M: Anaphylaxis and related allergic emergencies including reactions due to insect stings. JAMA 248:2632–2636, 1982.
9. Perkin RM, Anas NG: Mechanisms and management of anaphylactic shock, not responding to traditional therapy. Ann Allergy 54:202–208, 1985.
10. Silverman HJ, Van Hook C, Haponik EF: Hemodynamic changes in human anaphylaxis. Am J Med 77:341–344, 1984.
11. Stark BJ, Sullivan TJ: Biphasic and protracted anaphylaxis. J Allerg Clin Immunol 78:76–82, 1986.
12. Sue MA, Noritake DT, Klaustermeyer WB, et al: Penicillin anaphylaxis: Fatality in elderly patients without a history of penicillin allergy. Am J Emerg Med 6(5):456–458, 1988.
13. Yunginger JW, Sweeney KG, Sturner WQ, et al: Fatal food-induced anaphylaxis. JAMA 260(10):1450–1452, 1988.

SECTION SIX

INFECTIOUS DISORDERS

CHAPTER 17

SUSPECTED SEPSIS

CLOYD GATRELL, M.D.

PROBLEM A 73 year old man arrived at the emergency department by private car. The accompanying family members said he "hadn't been acting right." The man stated vigorously that he "felt fine" and did not wish to be evaluated.

QUESTIONS TO CONSIDER

1. What signs and symptoms are diagnostic of a septic emergency?
2. How can the emergency physician identify the patient with subtle signs of early sepsis?
3. What underlying conditions predispose a person to sepsis?
4. What are the most likely anatomic sources and etiologic agents of sepsis? How are they identified?
5. How does the underlying pathophysiologic source and infectious agent dictate therapy?
6. Which antibiotics provide optimal antimicrobial coverage?

INTRODUCTION

Bacteremia, viremia, and fungemia denote pathogens in the bloodstream. *Sepsis* and *septicemia* are broad terms describing systemic signs and symptoms resulting from any of these microorganisms or their toxins. Sepsis may progress to septic shock, a severe systemic response manifested by hypotension, hypoperfusion, disordered temperature regulation, and derangements of organ function. Mediators of these effects include a variety of endotoxins and exotoxins. Endotoxins are elements of bacterial cell walls, whereas exotoxins are agents released by the functioning cell. An exotoxin may produce a specific disease such as diphtheria, tetanus, or toxic shock syndrome. In contrast, endotoxin from a variety of gram-negative organisms may cause clinically identical septic shock states. The host response to sepsis is variable and complex.

The overall incidence of sepsis due to various organisms is not known. Virtually any class of microorganism can cause sepsis and septic shock, but gram-negative aerobic bacteria are the most common offenders. The term *septic shock* is often used as if it were synonymous with *gram-negative bacteremic shock*. Gram-negative sepsis occurs in approximately 1% of hospitalized patients. The primary pathogen is *Escherichia coli*, followed by *Klebsiella* and *Pseudomonas* species. The most common sources are the pulmonary, genitourinary, and digestive tracts. *Staphylococcus* and *Streptococcus* species account for most cases of gram-positive sepsis. The skin and wounds are the most common sources. If not complicated by septic shock, gram-negative sepsis has a mortality of 10% or less. Septic shock develops in 25% to 50% of patients with gram-negative bacteremia and increases the mortality to 40% to 60% of cases.

Sepsis has been exhaustively studied but is still incompletely understood. Gram-

---

These are the personal opinions of the author and are not to be construed as official views of Madigan Army Medical Center or the Department of Defense.

negative endotoxin, also called lipopolysaccharide, consists of an O antigen side chain specific for each bacterial serotype, a common R core antigen, and a lipid A moiety. Endotoxin stimulates macrophage production of cachectin, also called tumor necrosis factor. It activates complement, the coagulation and fibrinolytic cascades, and such mediators as prostaglandins, leukotrienes, thromboxane, and bradykinin. The peptidoglycan-teichoic acid complex in gram-positive cell walls appears to play a similar role.

Early sepsis is a hyperdynamic metabolic state that is often termed *warm shock*. Physiologically, there is vasodilatation, increased cardiac output, and good peripheral perfusion. These are clinically reflected by warm, dry skin, bounding pulses and widened pulse pressure, and normal capillary refill. Despite these outward signs, there is impairment of both oxygen extraction and cellular metabolism. Continued sepsis rapidly leads to *cold shock*. Vasodilatation and vascular permeability result in decreased circulating blood volume. Systemic vascular resistance rises in an attempt to maintain core perfusion. Dilatation of arterioles and constriction of venules cause pooling and stasis in the capillaries. The extremities become cool and clammy, and thready pulses, poor capillary refill, or actual cyanosis ensues. The poor tissue perfusion and impaired cellular metabolism exhaust energy reserves and lead to profound acidosis. The final stage is multiorgan failure with circulatory collapse and death. This continuum is illustrated in Figure 17–1.

PREHOSPITAL CARE

Common presentations for ambulance patients with possible sepsis include coma and other alterations of mental status, or fever and increased debilitation in the elderly.

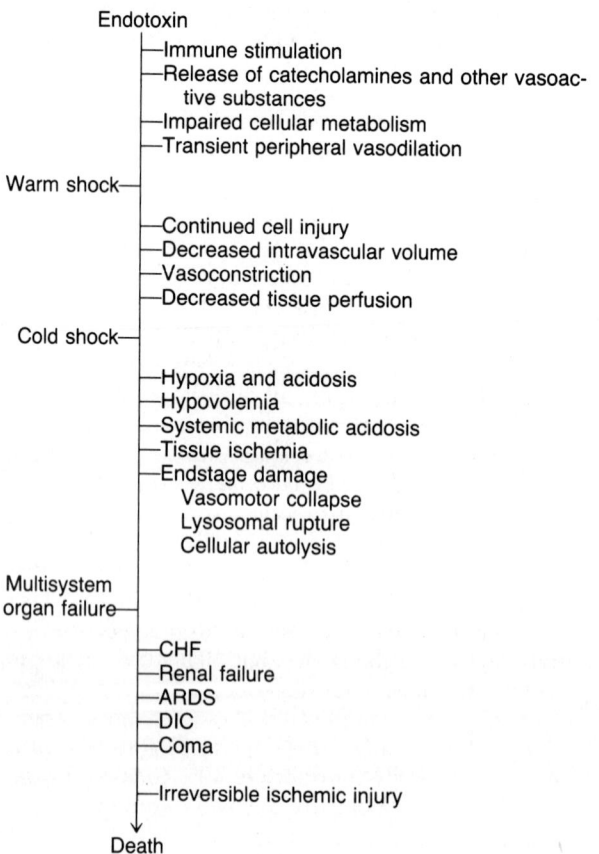

FIGURE 17–1. *The sepsis continuum. (From Zimmerman JJ, Dietrich KA: Current perspectives on septic shock. Pediatr Clin North Am 34:131–163, 1987. Reproduced with permission.)*

Various structural, metabolic, and infectious causes can mimic the presentation of sepsis. Therefore, the rescue squad must quickly gather information relevant to the cause of the patient's condition and provide initial treatment for any complications of sepsis such as airway difficulty, hypotension, altered mental status, or seizures. Assessment and intervention usually take place concurrently.

History

1. *What were the circumstances of the patient's illness? Is there shortness of breath, chest pain, or confusion?*
2. *Does the patient have a condition predisposing to sepsis, such as diabetes or cancer?*

Physical Examination

1. Vital signs, including accurate measurement of respiratory rate and blood pressure, guide decisions about the level of hemodynamic and ventilatory support the patient will need.
2. The chest and abdomen are examined briefly. Is there an increase in secretions or difficulty breathing? Is there evidence of emesis or bleeding?
3. A brief neurologic assessment is carried out looking for alterations in consciousness or obvious focal findings. The Glasgow Coma Scale is useful for prehospital measurement of altered mental status (see Chap. 45).
4. Are there clues in the surroundings such as medications (to be brought to the emergency department), liquor bottles, or drug paraphernalia? Any of these may or may not be relevant, but all resources are gathered at this stage.

Interventions

Oxygen. Oxygen at 4 to 6 liters/min is given by face mask. Patients with sepsis are at high risk for hypoxemia.

Cardiac Monitor. Any potentially critically ill patient requires monitoring during transport.

Large-Bore Intravenous Access. One or two 14- or 16-gauge peripheral IV lines are started. If local protocols permit, pretherapy blood samples are extremely helpful. Blood in a red-top (clot) tube is collected for determining glucose and electrolyte abnormalities that could cause altered mental status. The intravenous solution of choice is an isotonic crystalloid, either lactated Ringer's or normal saline. Fluid infusion rates are dictated by the vital signs and the circumstances. A pneumatic antishock garment (PASG) may help raise blood pressure in hypotensive patients.

Intravenous Medications. If mental status is altered, immediate benefit may be gained by giving 2 mg of naloxone, 50 to 100 ml of 50% dextrose (25 to 50 gm), and 100 mg of thiamine. A normal or high reading on a glucose test-strip may preclude the 50% dextrose infusion. Thiamine is recommended to avoid precipitating Wernicke's encephalopathy with dextrose infusion but is not a standard order on all rescue squads.

INITIAL APPROACH IN THE EMERGENCY DEPARTMENT

The emergency physician continues and expands the care initiated by the rescue squad. For patients not arriving by ambulance, the physician must start from the beginning. The initial goal of the emergency team is to determine the hemodynamic status and decide what resuscitation the patient needs.

History

1. *What are the events surrounding the change in this patient's condition? Are these sudden changes, or are they associated with recent or prolonged illness?*
Progressive change following a recent illness suggests sepsis or a metabolic derangement.
2. *Does the patient have an obvious serious underlying illness susceptible to septic complications, such as an immunosuppressive disorder?*
3. *Are there subtle signs of early sepsis, such as an unexplained alteration in mental status (seen especially in the elderly and infants), environmentally unrelated hypothermia, poor feeding (infants), or tachypnea without pneumonia?*
4. *Are there allergies that limit antibiotic choices?*

Physical Examination

Vital Signs. Fever is much more common in septic patients, but hypothermia is seen in 5% of cases and occurs more often at the extremes of age. A normal or high systolic blood pressure and a widened pulse pressure can be caused by sepsis. Hypotension and a narrow pulse pressure are seen in late sepsis and in other types of shock. Tachypnea with full respirations is consistent with early sepsis. Rapid, shallow respirations are consistent with late sepsis.

Skin. Skin temperature and appearance are noted. Warm skin in the presence of hypotension is seen in only a few conditions, sepsis being the most common. Cool, clammy skin may be present but is much less specific. Petechiae, purpura, and diffuse erythema are occasionally seen in the septic patient.

Heart and Lungs. Cardiopulmonary assessment is performed rapidly to detect potentially diagnostic findings and to assess hemodynamic function. Rales, especially if unilateral, may indicate a pulmonary source of sepsis.

Interventions

Oxygen Supplementation. Although any patient with altered mental status deserves oxygen, the impaired ability to extract and use oxygen in patients with sepsis makes it especially important. A rapid respiratory rate also indicates the need for supplemental oxygen. As in the prehospital care setting, oxygen can be initiated at 4 to 6 liters/min by nasal cannula. If the patient shows a significant degree of respiratory distress or is in shock, definitive airway management is necessary.

Fluid Therapy. Fluid resuscitation is critical in patients who are already hypotensive; however, it should not be neglected in those with evidence of sepsis and "normal vital signs." These patients are vasodilated and relatively hypovolemic. Fever and probable poor oral intake during the early stages of the illness also place them at risk for relative hypovolemia. In any case, these patients will require a substantial amount of intravenous fluids to restore volume. In an adult, a fluid bolus of 250 to 500 ml of isotonic crystalloid is a reasonable starting point regardless of the patient's blood pressure.

PASG. The pneumatic antishock garment is controversial but makes therapeutic sense in some septic patients. In early septic shock, vasodilatation is often present. Since the PASG increases systemic vascular resistance, it may augment peripheral tone, improve central and peripheral tone, and improve central perfusion. In patients with cold shock and peripheral vasoconstriction, the PASG is not useful.

Laboratory Studies. Laboratory tests are often ordered early in the care of these patients. The diagnosis is made clinically and is supported by the results of laboratory tests. A complete blood count, urinalysis, arterial blood gas determination, and chest radiograph may be all that are necessary initially.

PROBLEM The patient continued to deny any complaint. The nurse noted that he was disoriented about date and place. He gave coherent but inappropriate responses. The patient was transferred by the nurse to a monitored bed, disrobed, and gowned. Vital signs were blood pressure 160/60 mm Hg, pulse 110 beats/min, respiratory rate 24/min, and oral temperature 97.6°F (36.4°C). An intravenous line of normal saline was begun, the cardiac monitor attached, and the doctor notified.

Up to this point, the patient had been managed correctly. The nurse appropriately recognized the potential seriousness of the problem, moved the patient to a monitored area, and provided appropriate monitoring and IV access. This patient was given priority by the physician.

DATA GATHERING

The critical information needed is the presentation of the current problem and the presence of underlying conditions that would make the patient more vulnerable to sepsis.

History

1. *Present illness*
   a. Is *fever* present? Although most febrile illnesses are not associated with sepsis, antecedent fever and chills raise the possibility.
   b. Are there *symptoms* or *signs* related to *infection*? Cough, shortness of breath, productive sputum, purulent sinus drainage, or dysuria and frequency are symptoms referable to the common foci for sepsis. New skin lesions or joint inflammation may indicate infection.
   c. Are there *changes in behavior*, *appetite*, or *mentation*? These are nonspecific responses to a variety of diseases. Infection is a common finding in patients with these changes, particularly at the extremes of age.
2. *Predisposing conditions*
   a. What is the *age* of the patient? The very young and the very old are more vulnerable to sepsis and tend to have nonspecific presentations.
   b. Has there been *recent medical intervention*? Iatrogenic conditions include urologic or gynecologic instrumentation (including delivery), indwelling urinary or vascular catheters, surgery, cancer chemotherapy, post-transplant immune therapy, and steroid use.
   c. Is there a *synthetic* or *prosthetic device* in place? The presence of a prosthetic heart valve, vascular graft, or ventriculoperitoneal shunt increases the risk of sepsis.
   d. Is there *evidence* of *drug abuse*? Parenteral drug abuse introduces nonsterile matter into the bloodstream.
   e. What *underlying diseases* are *present*? Chronic conditions predisposing to sepsis include congenital and acquired immune deficiencies, malignancies (especially hematologic), surgical or functional hyposplenism (including sickle cell disease), decubitus ulcers and other skin problems, alcoholism and cirrhosis, chronic renal failure, diabetes, connective tissue diseases (such as systemic lupus erythematosus), and malnutrition.

Physical Examination

A complete physical examination is essential for any patient at risk for sepsis. Complete disrobing is essential. The only findings may be subtle skin lesions covered by the patient's clothing.

Vital Signs

Blood Pressure. Common blood pressure and pulse pressure findings have already been discussed.

Pulse. Tachycardia may be either a compensatory response to the vasodilatation of early sepsis or the result of fever.

Temperature. Fever is an obvious indicator that sepsis may be present. In the very young, very old, or hyperventilating patient, determination of a rectal temperature is advised because oral readings may be unreliable. Hypothermia is common in patients with sepsis, especially in neonates or the elderly. Sepsis is found in about one-third of adults admitted to an urban hospital for hypothermia. Hypothermia in septic shock has an ominous prognosis.

Respiratory Rate. A careful respiratory count by both nurse and physician is essential. Tachypnea is a nonspecific but sensitive finding in early sepsis. It may also indicate a pulmonary focus for the underlying infection.

Skin

A careful skin examination may supply one or more clues of septicemia. Sepsis causes skin lesions through five major mechanisms: disseminated intravascular coagulation (DIC), vascular invasion and occlusion by microorganisms, immune complexes and vasculitis, endocarditic emboli, and vascular effects of toxins.

DIC may be manifest by bleeding from venipuncture sites or by nonblanching acrocyanosis that may progress to large ecchymoses, which blister and necrose to cause symmetric peripheral gangrene (SPG). In SPG the distal portions of two or more extremities are involved, but there is no large-vessel obstruction. The responsible organism is most often *Neisseria meningitidis*, but the lesions are sterile.

Vascular invasion by bacteria causes the petechiae of Rocky Mountain spotted fever, the purpuric lesions of meningococcemia, and ecthyma gangrenosum, which is usually linked to *Pseudomonas*. Smears from the lesions often demonstrate the organism. Ecthyma gangrenosum begins as a central vesicle that ruptures, leaving a necrotic base surrounded by a halo of normal skin and a pink outer rim.

Neisseria can cause immune vasculitis with delayed maculopapular lesions. These are far more common with *N. gonorrheae* than with *N. meningitidis*. In blacks they start as an area of darkened skin with a blistered edge. In whites there is an erythematous macule that progresses through papular, vesicular, and hemorrhagic stages.

Classically, endocarditis due to *Streptococcus viridans* causes embolic lesions. Other organisms can cause them as well. The classic Janeway lesions are raised pustular or purpuric lesions that measure up to several centimeters in diameter. Osler's nodes are painful erythematous nodules that range from a few millimeters to a centimeter in size and have a pale center. Both are found mostly on the palms and soles. Smears from both show large numbers of organisms.

Toxic shock syndrome exemplifies skin lesions caused by a toxin. The characteristic rash is a diffuse, macular erythema that blanches with pressure. It clears in 3 to 4 days and is followed by peeling, particularly of the hands and feet. Associated signs include pharyngitis, acute synovitis, and conjunctivitis.

General Physical Examination

This part of the examination should address possible infectious foci, including:
1. The neck for meningismus or lymphadenopathy.
2. The ENT area (which is often overlooked) for sinus tenderness and unilateral nasal drainage; thrush, oral ulcers, gingivitis, and dental abscesses; and otitis and pharyngitis. The thyroid gland is assessed for size and tenderness.
3. The chest for localized or diffuse rales, or dullness and decreased fremitus indicating possible pneumonia.

4. The heart for pathologic murmurs or rubs. Bacterial endocarditis may be present if there is a newly diagnosed murmur.

5. The abdomen for ascites, localized tenderness, masses, or evidence of an acute surgical condition, particularly peritonitis.

6. The back for costovertebral tenderness and evidence of urinary tract infection.

7. The genitorectal area for pelvic or prostate infection.

8. The extremities for needle marks and swollen lymph nodes. Lymphadenopathy may be a clue to underlying malignancy or acquired immunodeficiency syndrome (AIDS).

PROBLEM Because the patient denied any complaint, the history was taken largely from the accompanying family members. They reported that he had been doing well until the evening before admission. He did not eat his supper and occasionally spoke in an incoherent manner. They were worried that this might be the first sign of senility and planned to call his doctor in the morning. By morning he was increasingly confused and his physician recommended that he be brought to the emergency department. The past medical history indicated that he was a heavy smoker and had had episodes of acute bronchitis. Significant findings on physical examination included disorientation to time and place, rales in the left chest, and moderate cyanosis of the lips and fingers. Repeated vital signs remained the same except for a rectal temperature of 102.6°F (39.2°C).

In spite of the "stable" blood pressure, this patient has early but clear evidence of a septic process. The widened pulse pressure, tachycardia, and elevated temperature suggest serious infection, possibly pneumonia. However, the peripheral skin findings suggest a more insidious and dangerous derangement.

DECISION PRIORITIES AND PRELIMINARY DIFFERENTIAL DIAGNOSIS

Initial management and the preliminary diagnosis are based on two questions:

First, what is the hemodynamic and mental status of the patient? Whatever the etiology, the status of the circulatory system and the central nervous system direct any life-saving interventions needed. Though mentioned elsewhere in this and other chapters, it bears repeating that the critical priorities are airway management, volume resuscitation, oxygenation, and replacement of CNS metabolic substrates (e.g., glucose).

Second, what are the potential sites of infection? Often there is no readily appreciable site in the patient who appears to be septic. The physician must decide whether there is an occult focus or a nonseptic condition.

Several conditions associated with hemodynamic instability and abnormal temperature may be confused with sepsis:

1. Purulent pericarditis or pancreatitis may be associated with fever and hypotension. The characteristic pain patterns of these two conditions usually help to distinguish them from sepsis.

2. Patients with gastrointestinal bleeding, myxedema coma, or diabetic ketoacidosis may be hypothermic and hypotensive. Blood can usually be found on rectal examination or nasogastric aspirate in the first group; bradycardia, hypoventilation, and myxedema help set the second apart; and acetone odor on the breath and diabetic history may identify the third.

3. Patients who are chronically malnourished may also be hypotensive and hypothermic. Although body habitus identifies them, they are also at increased risk for sepsis.

4. Patients with environmental hypothermia are often hypotensive, but the history is usually clear in these cases.

5. Substantial drug ingestions are often associated with hypothermia. Patients with salicylate intoxication may present with fever, confusion, increased respiratory rate and

depth, and later, hypotension. Anticholinergic overdose can cause fever, altered mental status, and hypotension or hypertension.

6. With septic pulmonary emboli, evidence of intravenous drug abuse usually can be found.

7. Certain endocrine disorders masquerade as or can be precipitated by infection. Adrenal insufficiency and crisis can be very subtle, although skin pigment changes may be present. If fever is also present, there is probably superimposed infection. Thyroid storm can produce findings typical of sepsis and may be difficult to differentiate from it.

DIAGNOSTIC ADJUNCTS

The basic laboratory tests available to the emergency physician are helpful in identifying the anatomic source and severity of sepsis. They also assist in differentiating other disorders from sepsis. The following tests are regularly obtained in the emergency department.

Laboratory

Urinalysis. The most frequently identifiable source of sepsis is the urinary tract.

Complete Blood Count and Differential Cell Count. Leukocytosis is a common but nonspecific finding. Leukopenia is more significant and suggests a poor prognosis. The differential cell count interprets the number of new cells being produced. A shift toward more immature forms (bands) denotes significant infection or inflammation. The presence of toxic granulation in neutrophils suggests serious infection. The results of this test rarely affect management unless they show severe granulocytopenia, anemia, or thrombocytopenia that requires correction.

Serum Electrolytes. Serum electrolyte values confirm the low bicarbonate concentration associated with metabolic acidosis. They also help to identify other conditions such as adrenal insufficiency (marked by decreased sodium and elevated potassium levels).

Renal and Liver Function Tests. Blood urea nitrogen (BUN) and creatinine rise in patients in early septic shock. A similar pattern is seen with liver enzymes, such as aspartate aminotransferase (AST) and alanine aminotransferase (ALT).

Hemostasis Studies. Since sepsis brings the risk of disseminated intravascular coagulation, a peripheral smear (looking for low numbers of platelets and broken red cells), a platelet count, and a prothrombin time are usually ordered. More testing is done if DIC is suggested by these "screening" tests or if there are physical findings of unusual bleeding, petechiae, or purpura. Tests for fibrinogen levels, fibrin split products, and partial thromboplastin time belong in this category.

Arterial Blood Gases. When there is a question about the presence of sepsis, an arterial blood gas (ABG) analysis is often helpful. Classically, its values evolve from respiratory alkalosis in early sepsis to relative hypoxemia and mild metabolic acidosis, and then to profound hypoxemia and acidosis.

Microbiologic Studies

Gram's Stain. Smears are examined from any sputum that can be obtained, suspicious skin lesions, ascites fluid, or pleural effusions.

Lumbar Puncture. A lumbar puncture (LP) is essential if altered mental status or meningeal signs accompany suspected sepsis. If there are lateralizing neurologic signs, papilledema, or a potential brain mass lesion, the LP is deferred until after a CT scan has been done. In these cases, the first dose of antibiotics is given while the arrangements are being made. Early treatment may be lifesaving, and a single dose of antibiotic will not appreciably interfere with cerebrospinal fluid (CSF) cell count, protein, Gram's stain, or rapid antigen testing.

Rapid antigen testing is more sensitive than Gram's stains and can direct specific antibiotic therapy before cultures give results. Commercial latex agglutination assays can detect antigens from *Streptococcus pneumoniae, Neisseria meningitidis, Hemophilus influenzae,* and other pathogens in serum, urine, or CSF. The kits are simple and give results within minutes. Counterimmunoelectrophoresis (CIE) takes about an hour and is less sensitive. Enzyme-linked immunoassay (ELISA) offers greater sensitivity and specificity but is slower and is not generally available.

Blood and Body Fluid Cultures. Cultures do not provide results in time to help emergency management but they are essential to guide inpatient therapy. Cultures are done on any body fluids obtained: urine, blood, CSF, ascites, pleural effusions, and sputum. An induced specimen of sputum should be taken to minimize contamination by oral flora. More than 91% of documented cases of bacteremia in adults can be detected with a single blood culture. A second culture increases the yield to 99%.

Radiologic Imaging

Chest Radiograph. Posteroanterior and lateral chest films are required in all suspected septic patients for possible diagnostic as well as management purposes.

Sinus Radiographs. Sinus films are ordered if headache or facial or dental pain is a prominent feature.

Special Studies. If intra-abdominal or retroperitoneal abscesses are suspected, ultrasonography, computed tomography (CT), magnetic resonance imaging, or radionuclide scanning is indicated. These studies are usually performed after admission.

PROBLEM Laboratory values were significantly abnormal. The patient had a P_{O_2} of 60, P_{CO_1} of 30, and a pH of 7.31 on room air. The hemostasis profile revealed an elevated prothrombin time (16 seconds) and a platelet count of 80,000/mm^3. A lobar infiltrate of the left lower lobe was found on the chest radiograph. A lumbar puncture was performed after careful fundoscopy and neurologic assessment revealed no abnormalities. The CSF was clear and no white cells or bacteria were seen.

The laboratory values have defined the extent of the disease process more clearly. The patient is hypoxemic and in the early stages of metabolic acidosis. Of particular concern is the abnormal coagulation profile, which suggests disseminated intravascular coagulation. The lumbar puncture is appropriate in this patient because of his abnormal mental status. In spite of a clear source of infection in the lungs, he could have a concomitant meningitis.

REFINED DIFFERENTIAL DIAGNOSIS

After the diagnostic adjunct data are available, a specific site of infection is usually located. The most common sources of sepsis are the urinary tract, lungs, central nervous system, abdomen, and skin. In a number of cases the source cannot be identified.

Sepsis Due to Urinary Tract Infections

The genitourinary tract is the most common focus of sepsis. It is unclear how or why a given individual progresses from normal colonization, asymptomatic bacteriuria, and uncomplicated lower urinary tract infection to upper tract involvement, systemic infection, and sepsis. In most cases, the organisms are gram-negative aerobes that gain retrograde access to the urinary tract. About 90% of cases are caused by *Escherichia coli*, 5% by *Klebsiella-Enterobacter*, and most of the remainder by *Proteus, Enterococci, Staphylococcus aureas,* and *S. epidermidis*.

In infancy and childhood, such infections are often related to congenital anomalies, particularly in males. In infants under 2 years of age, nonspecific vomiting, failure to thrive, and fever may be the only symptoms. Urinary tract infections are extremely common in adolescent and young adult females but systemic infections and sepsis are rare. One exception is pregnancy, during which the combined effects of progesterone and the gravid uterus tend to cause urinary stasis and obstruction. In middle age, renal stones, diabetes, and other underlying conditions begin to play a greater predisposing role. By far the majority of cases of urinary sepsis occur in old age. There is general deterioration of physiologic responsiveness, including the immune system. Debilitation may compromise local hygiene. Patients unable to care for themselves may have indwelling or external urinary catheters. Male prostatic hyperplasia and female perineal relaxation set the stage for urinary stasis and infection. The increasing incidence of diabetes, malignancy, and other immune-compromising diseases contributes to the number of cases in this age group.

Sepsis Due to Pulmonary Infections

The pulmonary system is the second leading site of sepsis. In neonates, it may start with an intrauterine infection caused by such organisms as *Toxoplasma* or *Listeria*. Aspiration of amniotic fluid or birth canal secretions can lead to pneumonia and sepsis within days of birth; group B streptococcus and gram-negative bacilli are the dominant organisms, while *Hemophilus influenzae* and *S. aureus* are less frequent. During the first 2 to 3 months of life *Chlamydia* may cause a diffuse, slowly progressive pneumonia with little fever but marked respiratory distress.

Beyond the neonatal period, the emergency physician most often sees community-acquired pulmonary infections. *Streptococcus pneumoniae*, *H. influenzae*, *S. aureus*, and *Legionella pneumophila* are the organisms most likely to cause sepsis. The evaluation must consider the clinical setting and address such factors as occupational history, exposure to animals, recent travel, and sexual history. Underlying conditions such as congestive heart failure, diabetes, alcoholism, and chronic lung disease are present in about 80% of adults with serious pulmonary infections and sepsis. Patients with chronic obstructive pulmonary disease (COPD) tend to be colonized with *S. pneumoniae* and *H. influenzae*, whereas cystic fibrosis causes increased risk of infection with *S. aureus* and *Pseudomonas*. The risk of *Pneumocystis* infection in AIDS patients is well known. Necrotizing lesions, cavities, or empyema raise concern about infection with *S. aureus*; aspiration may be complicated by *E. coli*, *Klebsiella pneumoniae*, or *Pseudomonas*.

Sepsis Due to Central Nervous System Infections

Sepsis related to CNS infections is devastating but fortunately less common than other sources of infection (see Chap. 47). Most meningitis is caused by extension of organisms normally colonizing the nasopharynx. However, it can arise by hematogenous spread from infections elsewhere. Predisposing conditions include traumatic or congenital defects ranging from skull fractures to apparently minor sacral dimpling associated with dermal sinuses, and underlying diseases that compromise immunity. In the newborn period, *E. coli* and group B streptococci account for 50% to 75% of cases. *Pneumococcus*, *Meningococcus*, and *H. influenzae* cause 40% of cases of meningitis seen in adults. Considering all ages, *Pneumococcus* is the single most common organism. *Neisseria meningitidis* occurs primarily among young adults and *H. influenzae* among children. *Listeria* infects primarily neonates and elderly patients. Less common pathogens can be acquired by swimming in contaminated water or by exposure to pigeons, rodents, or domestic animals.

The diagnostic triad of meningitis is fever, headache, and meningismis. The latter two signs are not helpful in neonates or infants. Patients with CNS sepsis often also have vomiting, altered mental status, or seizures. Subdural empyema, brain abscess, or epidural abscess in the head or spine may be misdiagnosed as meningitis. Focal signs of these lesions may be subtle, and require an alert clinician. Such patients have a high mortality unless the focus is surgically drained. Apparent meningitis following sinusitis, mastoiditis, or more distal septic foci warrants a CT scan to rule out a CNS abscess.

Sepsis Due to Abdominal Infections

Intra-abdominal sepsis is usually heralded by fever, abdominal pain, and peritoneal signs; anorexia, nausea, vomiting, and diarrhea may also be present. Primary peritonitis is infection of the abdominal cavity without an evident source. The organisms may seed the peritoneum after hematogenous or transmural spread from the intestine. The incidence of this disease in children has decreased markedly, presumably because of the increased use of oral antibiotics in respiratory illness. Among adults, primary peritonitis occurs most often in patients with alcoholic cirrhosis and ascites. Pelvic pathogens can migrate through the fallopian tubes into the abdomen without necessarily causing clinical pelvic infection. The main organisms in children are *Streptococcus pneumoniae* and group A streptococci. In adults, *E. coli* is more common than these two, and anaerobic gram-negative or polymicrobial pathogens are less common still. In young women, *Neisseria gonorrheae*, *Chlamydia*, and anaerobic organisms associated with pelvic inflammatory disease are usual. By definition, primary peritonitis means that conditions affecting specific abdominal organs are not present. This is often difficult to determine without laparotomy unless there is a known predisposing condition and a history of prior occurrences.

The causes of secondary peritonitis are as many as there are conditions affecting the abdominal or retroperitoneal organs. Secondary peritonitis may be precipitated by obstruction, perforation, vascular compromise, or surgical procedures. The pathogens released vary by location and organ. Endotoxins produced by anaerobic gram-negative organisms tend to be weaker than those of the aerobes. The bacterial count rises with organs located further distally in the gut. The stomach and proximal small intestine contain low numbers of gram-positive organisms native to the oral cavity. The ileum contains both aerobic *E. coli* and enterococcal anaerobes such as *Bacteroides*. In the colon, anaerobes outnumber aerobic gram-negative organisms by three or four orders of magnitude. Achlorhydria or blood in the proximal gut increases the bacterial count; in the colon, antibiotic therapy affects the mix but does not decrease the number of organisms. Vaginal and cervical secretions contain a polymicrobial population, with anaerobes about 10 times more common than aerobes.

Sepsis Due to Skin Infections

The majority of skin infections are caused by staphylococci or streptococci and are not associated with systemic signs of sepsis. The risk of serious skin infection and sepsis increases in patients with surgical or traumatic wounds, burns, eczema, proliferative disorders, microvascular disease, or other underlying problems.

Sacral decubiti or diabetic lower extremity ulcers have a polymicrobial population that includes gram-negative and anaerobic organisms. The ulcers provide a route of entry of pathogens into an already compromised patient. Sepsis prevention or treatment requires broad antibiotic coverage and prolonged, scrupulous wound care.

A variety of gangrenous conditions may follow skin infections. Streptococcal gangrene is a rare complication of group A streptococcal infection after a minor extremity injury. Necrotizing fasciitis is a combined aerobic and anaerobic infection that extends down to the deep fascia on the legs, abdominal wall, or perineum. Fournier's gangrene is a fulminant mixed anaerobic and facultative infection of the scrotum that spreads throughout the perineum and abdominal wall, initially sparing the testis and epididymis. Clostridial wound infections cause anaerobic cellulitis or, less often, gas gangrene. *Staphylococcus aureus*, by itself or mixed with anaerobic and aerobic streptococci, can cause purulent myositis after minor puncture wounds. Any of these patients may be acutely ill and show signs of sepsis. Prompt, aggressive surgical debridement is lifesaving. Appropriate antibiotics are essential adjuncts.

Sepsis Due to Unknown Sources

In many septic patients a source of infection is not identified in the emergency department. Cardiopulmonary support and empiric antibiotic therapy are instituted as necessary. A scrupulous search is made for retained foreign bodies or surgical prostheses. Although uncommon in most U.S. populations, mycobacteria, malaria, rickettsia, and fungi are also occasionally identified in the emergency department. Abdominal abscesses frequently cause sepsis without an evident source. Questions about previous abdominal surgery, endoscopy, laparoscopy, chronic bowel disease, or ovarian cysts may yield clues. Osteomyelitis, sinusitis, dental abscesses, and brain abscesses are less common and are difficult to diagnose in the obtunded patient. CT, gallium scans, and other efforts to localize infection must continue after the patient has been admitted.

Adults in frank septic shock without an evident source have almost 100% mortality. In part, that figure reflects a number of elderly or immunocompromised patients who are too unstable or not candidates for advanced studies.

PROBLEM With the completion of the clinical, laboratory, and radiographic evaluation, it was clear that this patient had sepsis of pulmonary origin. Although his blood pressure was still within the normal range, it was obvious that inadequate oxygen and nutrients were being delivered to the microcirculation. He was managed in the anticipation that full-blown life-threatening signs of sepsis might develop.

PRINCIPLES OF MANAGEMENT

Emergency management of the septic patient is directed toward airway support and oxygenation, maintenance of tissue perfusion and organ function through fluid therapy and vasoactive drugs, and initiation of antimicrobial therapy to eliminate the pathogen or pathogens.

Standard Therapies

Airway and Ventilatory Support. Many septic patients require airway protection because their level of consciousness is depressed. Early endotracheal intubation and mechanical ventilation may also help prevent the adult respiratory distress syndrome (ARDS), the most common cause of death in patients in septic shock. Mechanical ventilation and positive end-expiratory pressure (PEEP) maximize oxygenation in patients with ARDS, but this benefit must be balanced against the adverse effects of these interventions on venous return and cardiac output. Even before chest film abnormalities or hypoxemia is evident, interstitial accumulation of water and neutrophils decreases pulmonary compliance and increases the work of breathing. Blood and oxygen are diverted from other organs, aggravating metabolic acidosis. Mechanical ventilation reduces the work of breathing and its contribution to metabolic acidosis. It also facilitates compensatory hyperventilation.

Hemodynamic Support

Fluid Therapy. Sepsis is a hypermetabolic state associated with increased oxygen demands, but vasodilatation and hypotension impair oxygen delivery. Cellular mechanisms remain largely intact early on, with oxygen utilization responding to increased oxygen delivery. The goal of fluid therapy is to maximize perfusion and oxygen delivery to the tissue. Early therapy emphasizes crystalloid, whereas colloids may have a role later in the course of care. Colloids are usually part of inpatient management.

Invasive Monitoring. Right and left heart filling pressures do not correlate during sepsis, so central venous pressure is an inadequate monitor of cardiovascular status. In any septic patient who is hypotensive or has a widened pulse pressure suggestive of "warm shock" a Swan-Ganz pulmonary artery catheter should be placed as soon as feasible. Measurements from this catheter allow correlation of fluid therapy with left heart filling pressures, as reflected in the pulmonary artery wedge pressure (PAWP) and cardiac output (CO). Repeated fluid boluses are given until they no longer increase CO, and the PAWP does not exceed a high normal level. Data obtained by means of the Swan-Ganz catheter can also help to confirm the presence of suspected sepsis. Low systemic vascular resistance in the presence of high cardiac output is very suggestive. A small difference in Po_2 between the central mixed venous and arterial samples suggests impaired tissue oxygen extraction, as seen in shock.

Invasive hemodynamic monitoring may not be available in all emergency departments. Pulse oximetry for measuring oxygen saturation and continuous automatic blood pressure cuffs are useful alternatives during stabilization in the emergency department.

Vasoactive Drugs. Maintenance of a mean arterial pressure (MAP) of at least 60 mm Hg in adults is generally desirable to maintain tissue perfusion. Vasoactive drugs may help if MAP does not rise with fluid therapy. Higher than normal doses may be needed because sepsis can dampen cardiovascular responsiveness. Dopamine and dobutamine are the usual choices because they maximize cardiac output and MAP without markedly worsening vasoconstriction. Dopamine has a more potent pressor effect because it has alpha- as well as beta-adrenergic properties. At low doses, its dopaminergic effect stimulates preferential blood flow to the kidneys and other vital sites. Dobutamine has mainly an inotropic effect and is preferable in patients with fluid overload. Both drugs are usually begun at a low level and titrated to the desired response. Vasodilators such as nitroprusside and phentolamine, an alpha-adrenergic blocker, may be used with dopamine and dobutamine to reduce afterload and enhance CO. This goal is accomplished after invasive hemodynamic monitoring has been established and the values analyzed.

Antibiotics. Traditional therapy for sepsis consists of synergistic combination of an aminoglycoside with a beta-lactam antibiotic (a penicillin or cephalosporin). A third agent is added if gram-negative anaerobes are a major concern. New cephalosporins, other beta lactams, and combinations of semisynthetic penicillins with beta-lactamase inhibitors (ticarcillin and clavulanate, or ampicillin and sulbactam) are altering this approach.

All cephalosporins cover a relatively broad spectrum of gram-positive and gram-negative organisms. In general, first-generation agents such as cefazolin and cephradine have better activity against gram-positive pathogens. Among second-generation agents, cefaclor and cefuroxime add coverage of *H. influenzae, Branhamella catarrhalis, Bacterioides fragilis*, and other anaerobes. Third-generation agents are exceptionally useful in serious gram-negative infections. They have minimal inhibitory concentrations that are much lower than those of the aminoglycosides, and their low toxicity allows higher doses. Single agent therapy with ceftazidime is highly effective against *Pseudomonas*, perhaps even in neutropenic patients. Ceftriaxone has the longest half-life and the widest use among the other third-generation cephalosporins.

Other beta lactams include aztreonam and imipenem. Aztreonam is more active against gram-negative bacteria but not against gram-positive pathogens or anaerobes. Its penetration into the CSF has not been established. It has a monocyclic nucleus and therefore little cross-sensitivity with the bicyclic penicillins and cephalosporins. Imipenem, with cilastatin, is highly resistant to beta lactamases. It has wide activity against aerobic gram-positive, gram-negative, and anaerobic organisms and is an effective single drug treatment for *Pseudomonas* infections. Combination with cilastatin inhibits renal antibiotic breakdown, yielding higher and more prolonged serum levels.

The fluoroquinolone class includes norfloxacin, which has been approved only for urinary infections, and ciprofloxacin, which has broad gram-negative activity. It covers virtually all bacterial causes of enteritis and has moderate activity against gram-positives but less against anaerobes.

The use of erythromycin has increased since the recognition of *Legionella* and *Chlamydia* species as major pathogens. Trimethoprim/sulfamethoxazole is the drug of choice in patients with *Pneumocystis carinii* infections.

Appropriate antibiotics can halve the mortality from sepsis. Since the specific organism and its sensitivity are often not known initially, empiric decisions are based on the anatomic source of the infection, where it was acquired (locally or traveling, hospital or community), and historic bacterial sensitivity patterns. Patient factors to be considered include age, the existence of allergies, underlying status, and the presence of renal or hepatic disease that would affect drug metabolism. Table 17–1 includes recommendations for selected conditions.

Adjunctive Therapies

Steroids. The question of whether to give exogenous glucocorticoids to patients in septic shock has been debated for many years. Potential benefits include stabilization of lysosomal membranes, prevention of cachectin release, inhibition of complement-mediated leukocyte aggregation, and blocking of beta-endorphin release. A typical regimen is methyl prednisolone 30 mg/kg, repeated once or twice at 4-hour intervals if shock persists. Animal studies have shown that improved survival results if steroids precede septic shock. A few human studies have shown improved survival when steroids are given within 1 to 4 hours of the diagnosis or onset of shock. Others have shown increased mortality, particularly with repeated doses of steroids. A number of studies have shown hemodynamic improvement and higher short-term survival but no change in overall mortality. The most recent consensus is that steroids are not beneficial.

Narcotic Antagonists. Endogenous opioids released during sepsis may depress cardiovascular function. Naloxone has improved blood pressure in some septic patients, but other patients became worse. Naltrexone, a longer-acting opiate antagonist, and thyrotropin-releasing hormone, which blocks many of the nonanalgesic properties of opiates, are also being evaluated. None are standard therapy for sepsis at present.

Nonsteroidal Anti-inflammatory Drugs. Because of the role of prostaglandins, thromboxanes, and leukotrienes as mediators in sepsis, a variety of nonsteroidal anti-inflammatory drugs (NSAIDs) have been studied in animal septic shock models with promising results. However, it is too early to tell if they will produce clinical benefits.

Immune Therapy. Bactericidal antibiotics liberate toxic cell wall components as bacteria are killed. The cascade of harmful endotoxin effects continues despite the reduction in bacteremia. Elevated levels of complement activation products appear to correlate with fatal outcome in sepsis. Specific antibody therapy may reduce end-organ damage and mortality. Anti-C5a and other antisera have shown promise in animal studies. Human monoclonal antibody against endotoxin core lipopolysaccharide is currently undergoing multicenter clinical trials.

PROBLEM The patient was given 500 ml of normal saline because of the presumed relative hypovolemia. Supplemental oxygen was maintained at 6 liters/min. Vital signs were monitored every 10 minutes, and any changes were reported to the physician. Because the organisms could include *S. pneumoniae, H. influenzae, K. pneumoniae,* or other pathogens, immediate antibiotic therapy was begun with a third-generation cephalosporin and erythromycin.

SPECIAL CONSIDERATIONS

Toxic Shock Syndrome

Coagulase-positive *S. aureus* may produce toxic shock syndrome toxin-1 (TSST-1), formerly called pyrogenic exotoxin C or enterotoxin F. The toxin causes a syndrome with

TABLE 17–1. Empiric Antibiotics for Community-Acquired Adult Sepsis

Setting	Common Organisms	Antibiotics of Choice Primary	Alternate
Urinary tract			
Normal anatomy	Enterobacteriaceae	A third-geration cephalosporin	Ampicillin + aminoglycoside
Abnormal anatomy	Pseudomonas	Ceftazidime	Ciprofloxacin
Biliary tract	Enterobacteriaceae Enterococci Bacteroides	Third-generation cephalosporin + metronidazole or clindamycin; or ticarcillin/clavulanate	Mezlocillin, aztreonam, or aminoglycoside + metronidazole
Peritonitis, secondary	Enterobacteriaceae Enterococci Bacteroides	Third-generation cephalosporin + metronidazole	Cefoxitin or ticarcillin/clavulanate
Pneumonia			
Previously healthy	Pneumococcus Group A Streptococcus Mycoplasma Legionella Chlamydia	Erythromycin + cefazolin	Erythromycin + aminoglycoside
DM, COPD, EtOH	Same as above, plus Hemophilus influenzae, Branhamella catarrhalis, Klebsiella	Erythromycin + third-generation cephalosporin	Erythromycin + TMP/SMX
Neutropenic	Same as above, plus cytomegalovirus, Aspergillus	Ceftazidime + aminoglycoside + erythromycin +/− vancomycin	Aztreonam + aminoglycoside + erythromycin +/− vancomycin
HIV+	Same as above, plus Pneumocystis, cytomegalovirus, herpesvirus	TMP/SMX +/− erythromycin	Pentamidine +/− erythromycin
Cystic fibrosis	Pseudomonas Staphylococcus aureus	Aminoglycoside + nafcillin or vancomycin	Ceftazidime + nafcillin or vancomycin
Post-influenza	Staphylococcus aureus	Nafcillin	Vancomycin
Meningitis			
Previously healthy	Meningococcus Pneumococcus Group A Streptococcus	Penicillin G (high dose)	Ceftriaxone, ampicillin, or chloramphenicol
Elderly, DM, EtOH	Same as above, plus Enterobacteriaceae, Listeria, Hemophilus influenzae	Penicillin G or ampicillin + third-generation cephalosporin	Chloramphenicol
Decubitus ulcer	Staphylococcus aureus Group A Streptococcus Anaerobic Streptococcus Enterobacteriaceae Pseudomonas	Clindamycin + aminoglycoside, ticarcillin/clavulanate, or ceftazidime	Ciprofloxacin + metronidazole of clindamycin
Unknown source	Enterobacteriaceae Staphylococcus aureus Group A or D Streptococcus Pneumococcus Bacteroides	Third-generation cephalosporin or ticarcillin/clavulanate	Cefoxitin + aminoglycoside; or nafcillin + aminoglycoside + clindamycin
Neutropenic	Enterobacteriaceae Staphylococcus aureus Staphylococcus epidermidis Pseudomonas	Vancomycin + mezlocillin + aminoglycoside; or vancomycin + ceftazidime + aminoglycoside	Nafcillin + aztreonam + aminoglycoside

DM = diabetes mellitus; COPD = chronic obstructive pulmonary disease; EtOH = alcoholism; TMP/SMX = trimethoprim/sulfamethoxazole.

high fever, myalgias, vomiting, watery diarrhea, and hypotension. There are prominent cutaneous symptoms, as described above. Most cases originate with a vaginal infection and are associated with tampon use. Nonmenstrual TSS is often related to surgical procedures. The wounds usually appear noninfected, but S. aureus (most commonly phage group 1, type 29) appears on culture. Patients are not usually bacteremic, but the exotoxin has direct harmful effects. TSST-1 also activates some of the mediators prominent in gram-negative shock and may result in multiple organ failure. Intensive care unit (ICU) monitoring, supportive care, and antistaphylococcal antibiotics are essential, and the prognosis is good. Any offending foreign body must be removed. Menstruating TSS patients must avoid tampon use for at least 6 months after recovery.

Acquired Immune Deficiency Syndrome

Acquired immune deficiency syndrome (AIDS) is caused by the human immunodeficiency virus (HIV). The incidence of HIV infection is highest among homosexual and bisexual men, prostitutes, parenteral drug abusers, blood product recipients, and residents of certain developing countries. HIV lowers the T_4 helper-inducer lymphocyte population, reducing cellular immunity. This reduction makes the patient susceptible to opportunistic infections, such as those with cytomegalovirus, *Pneumocystis*, *Myobacteria*, *Toxoplasma*, and *Candida*.

More recently, HIV infection has also been shown to reduce the humoral immunity mediated by B lymphocytes. There is diffuse elevation of immune globulin levels but poor antibody response to specific antigens. Community-acquired bacterial infections in AIDS patients most often involve encapsulated organisms, such as *S. pneumoniae*, *H. influenzae*, *E. coli*, *Klebsiella*, and group B streptococci. AIDS patients hospitalized because of opportunistic infections are at particular risk for gram-negative sepsis.

The initial presentation of HIV infection may be an emergency department visit for a flulike illness, malaise and weight loss, diarrhea, pneumonia, or mucocutaneous lesions. Persistent generalized lymphadenopathy often predates any opportunistic or bacterial infection. *Pneumocystis carinii* pneumonia is the most common serious infection associated with AIDS. It may present with weeks of a relatively nonproductive cough and progressive shortness of breath. Chest radiograph most often shows a diffuse, interstitial infiltrate. Kaposi's sarcoma prompts the diagnosis of many AIDS patients. It is an angioproliferative condition causing violaceous or erythematous macular-nodular lesions on mucosa or skin. Oral thrush in an adult not taking antibiotics or otherwise compromised suggests AIDS. Oral or genital herpes may also be the presenting problem, but these are obviously seen in many patients without HIV infection.

HIV-infected patients may not be identified to the emergency department. Laboratory clues are common but nonspecific, such as anemia, leukopenia, and thrombocytopenia. Although a rapid latex agglutination test for HIV-antibody was licensed in the United States in 1989, HIV testing is limited by law in many areas. The emergency department potential for such tests is yet to be determined. Health care personnel must scrupulously avoid exposure to body fluids during all patient evaluations and resuscitations. (See Chap. 18.)

Neonatal Sepsis

Sepsis during the first 4 days of life is usually acquired in the birth canal. Such "early onset" neonatal sepsis is most frequently caused by group B streptococci, *E. coli*, *N. gonorrheae*, and herpes simplex. Less often, enterococci, *Listeria monocytogenes*, and gram-negative bacilli are responsible. Early onset neonatal sepsis among babies delivered at home may be seen as an emergency department problem. The trend toward discharging newborns on day 2 or 3 of life may bring more cases of early onset neonatal sepsis to the emergency department.

"Late onset" neonatal sepsis (between days 5 and 30) reflects nosocomial infection or community exposure. It involves the same organisms plus staphylococci, *Pseudomonas*, enteric bacilli, and *Candida*.

Low birth weight, prematurity, prolonged rupture of membranes, resuscitation (especially procedures requiring endotracheal intubation or umbilical catheterization), and meconium staining indicate an increased risk of sepsis. Clinical signs are nonspecific.

Parents may bring the baby to the emergency department because of poor feeding, lethargy, or irritability. Jaundice and hepatomegaly may be clues. Cardiorespiratory symptoms may include irregular or rapid respirations; flaring, grunting, or retractions; and pallor, cyanosis, or mottling. Either fever or hypothermia may be present. Any neonate who "doesn't look right" in the emergency department needs to be considered for admission. Any neonate with fever or temperature instability must be treated for presumed sepsis. Intravenous access is often difficult; umbilical catheterization and intraosseous infusion are useful alternatives. If diagnostic tests do not suggest a specific pathogen, empiric therapy must be started. The pattern of nosocomial infections in the nursery must be considered when choosing antibiotics.

The fetus receives immunoglobulin G (IgG) transplacentally during the last few weeks of pregnancy but only those antibodies that are present in the maternal circulation. Babies born prematurely miss some of the antibody transfer. Neonates may thus have both qualitative and quantitative deficiencies of immune globulin. Intravenous IgG enhances opsonic activity against encapsulated organisms and may become standard therapy in neonates with sepsis.

DISPOSITION AND FOLLOW-UP

Any patient with suspected sepsis is admitted to the hospital. Sepsis does not usually progress to shock in patients younger than 40 except during the neonatal period, in pregnant women, or in the presence of underlying disease. Young, generally healthy patients with signs and symptoms of sepsis who are hemodynamically stable may be managed in an intermediate care unit with close monitoring capability. Older patients with suspected sepsis and those with hemodynamic instability or complicating underlying disease are admitted to an intensive care unit.

PROBLEM The patient was stabilized and admitted to the intensive care unit. His age, abnormal vital signs, altered mentation, and potential for deterioration warranted close hemodynamic monitoring.

DOCUMENTATION

1. Succinct history of the present problem and notation of underlying conditions predisposing to sepsis.
2. Full vital signs (including rectal temperature, when indicated), with serial determinations as indicated.
3. General appearance of illness or well-being as well as the specific findings on physical examination.
4. Laboratory results.
5. Final note outlining the course of the illness and the response to treatment in the emergency department.

SUMMARY AND FINAL POINTS

- Although all classes of microorganisms can cause sepsis, the great majority of cases are due to gram-negative aerobic bacilli. The most common pathogen is *Escherichia coli*.
- Early sepsis can be very subtle in its clinical presentation. The only clues may be altered mental status, tachypnea, or unexplained hypothermia.
- The most common sources of sepsis are the urinary tract and lungs.
- Skin lesions can provide clues to the etiology of sepsis. Dermatologic manifestations

include nonblanching acrocyanosis, purpura, maculopapular rashes, endocarditic lesions, and diffuse macular erythema.
- Differentiating between sepsis and other conditions is not always possible in the emergency department. The clinical findings characteristic of sepsis, particularly the hemodynamic changes, are found in acute myocardial infarction, thyrotoxicosis, hemorrhagic shock, environmental hypothermia, and some drug overdoses.
- Although diagnostic adjuncts can be useful in revealing the etiology of sepsis, they are more often helpful in determining the degree of hemodynamic and metabolic derangement of the patient.
- Sepsis without an identifiable source is not uncommon and carries a high mortality rate.
- A normal blood pressure in a patient with sepsis does not reflect adequate tissue perfusion and delivery of oxygen. Patients with normal blood pressure readings are candidates for invasive monitoring and vigorous fluid resuscitation.
- The choice between isotonic crystalloid and colloid fluid resuscitation remains controversial. However, in the emergency department setting, volume repletion begins with a crystalloid.
- The goal of initial, empiric antibiotic therapy in septic patients is to provide coverage of a broad range of gram-positive and gram-negative organisms. Traditional choices have been a penicillin and an aminoglycoside. Recent therapeutic trials suggest that a single broad-spectrum cephalosporin (third-generation) is as efficacious as combination therapy.

BIBLIOGRAPHY

Texts

1. Mandell GL, Douglas RG Jr, Bennett JE (eds): Principles and Practice of Infectious Diseases (3rd ed). New York, Churchill Livingstone, 1990.
2. Sanford JP: Guide to Antimicrobial Therapy. West Bethesda, MD, Antimicrobial Therapy, 1989.

Journal Articles

1. Chaisson RE: Medical management of AIDS. Infections due to encapsulated bacteria, Salmonella, Shigella, and Campylobacter. Infec Dis Clin North Am 2:475–484, 1988.
2. Dunn DL: Immunotherapeutic advances in the treatment of gram-negative bacterial sepsis. World J Surg 11:233–240, 1987.
3. Ellrodt AG: Sepsis and septic shock. Emerg Med Clin North Am 4:809–840, 1986.
4. Jacobs ER, Bone RC: Clinical indicators in sepsis and septic adult respiratory distress syndrome. Med Clin North Am 70:921–933, 1986.
5. Kingston ME, Mackey D: Skin clues in the diagnosis of life-threatening infections. Rev Infect Dis 8:1–11, 1986.
6. Long WM, Sprung CL: Corticosteroids, nonsteroidal anti-inflammatory drugs, and naloxone in the sepsis syndrome. World J Surg 1:218–225, 1987.
7. Luce JM: Pathogenesis and management of septic shock. Chest 91:883–888, 1987.
8. Lyman JL: Use of blood cultures in the emergency department. Ann Emerg Med 15:308–311, 1986.
9. Molloy M, Vukelja SJ, Yelland G, et al: Postoperative toxic shock syndrome. Milit Med 154:74–76, 1989.
10. Rackow EC, Astiz ME, Weil MH: Cellular oxygen metabolism during sepsis and shock. The relationship of oxygen consumption to oxygen delivery. JAMA 259:1989–1993, 1988.
11. Shenep JH, Flynn PM, Barrett FF, et al: Serial quantitation of endotoxemia and bacteremia during therapy for gram-negative bacterial sepsis. J Infect Dis 157:565–568, 1988.
12. Whimbey E, Gold JWM, Plsky B, et al: Bacteremia and fungemia in patients with the acquired immunodeficiency syndrome. Ann Intern Med 104:511–514, 1986.
13. Zimmerman JJ, Dietrich KA: Current perspectives on septic shock. Pediatr Clin North Am 34:131–163, 1987.

CHAPTER 18

ACCIDENTAL EXPOSURE TO BIOLOGIC AGENTS

RAYMOND P. TEN EYCK, M.D.

PROBLEM A 32 year old female nurse presented with a history of just having accidentally stuck her right index finger on a discarded hypodermic needle from an unknown source while disposing of an intravenous catheter needle. She reported that her last tetanus immunization had been received less than 1 year ago.

QUESTIONS TO CONSIDER

1. Which infectious diseases present the main occupational threat to health care workers?
2. What is the risk of a health care worker becoming seropositive for human immunodeficiency virus (HIV) after a percutaneous or mucosal exposure to a patient who either has clinical acquired immunodeficiency syndrome (AIDS) or is HIV positive without symptoms?
3. What steps should be taken in the emergency department to evaluate a health care worker who has had a percutaneous or mucosal exposure to an HIV-positive patient?
4. What precautions should all health care workers take to prevent possible infection from contact with HIV, hepatitis, and other biologic hazards?
5. What are the appropriate steps involved in the evaluation of a health care worker who has been exposed to hepatitis B?
6. What are the indications for using immune globulin, hepatitis B immune globulin, and hepatitis B vaccine in the postexposure prophylaxis of hepatitis?
7. For which etiologic agents of bacterial meningitis is prophylaxis recommended for contacts and under what circumstances should health care workers receive prophylaxis?
8. What are the risks to a health care worker from exposure to patients with herpes simplex or varicella zoster infections and what prophylactic measures should be considered?

INTRODUCTION

Emergency physicians and nurses have traditionally been at high risk from exposure to biologic agents owing to the unscreened nature of the patient population cared for in the emergency department and to the frequent need for immediate interventions that are commonly invasive in nature. These biologic risks can compromise the ability of emergency department personnel to practice as well as posing a significant risk to their physical well-being. Today, this awareness is intensified by concerns about the risk of contracting AIDS in addition to the traditional hazards of hepatitis, bacterial meningitis, herpes simplex, and varicella zoster.

The Centers for Disease Control (CDC) recommends that all patients be considered potentially infected with HIV. The prevalence of HIV infections in the United States has been estimated to be 0.04% based on data from blood donor screening. However, in a recent study performed at a high volume inner-city emergency department, the point prevalence was found to be 3% and was as high as 19% in some study subgroups. Although epidemiologic evidence points only toward transmission by blood, vaginal secretions, semen, and possibly breast milk, HIV has also been isolated from samples of human urine, saliva, tears, amniotic fluid, and cerebrospinal fluid.

Infection from exposure to hepatitis is a more frequent occurrence. Approximately 38% of hepatitis cases in the United States are attributable to hepatitis A. However, hepatitis A represents a minimal risk to health care workers unless they have not utilized appropriate barrier precautions when they are exposed to the feces of an infected patient.

Hepatitis B virus (HBV) infections account for about 43% of hepatitis cases in the United States. Only 0.1% to 0.5% of the population are carriers of HBV. However, certain groups are considered high risk including immigrants or refugees from countries with a high endemic rate of HBV infection, patients from institutions for the mentally retarded, illicit parenteral drug abusers, homosexual men, hemodialysis patients, and household contacts of HBV carriers. Nonimmunized health care workers have a low prevalence of serologic markers to HBV. Thus, those exposed to infected body fluids by the percutaneous or mucosal routes are at risk for infection.

Patients with bacterial meningitis represent a minimal risk to health care providers. *Neisseria meningiditis* (meningococcal) meningitis and *Hemophilus influenzae* meningitis pose a threat only to people who have established intimate contact with an infected patient.

Another group of potential biologic hazards in the emergency department is herpes simplex and varicella zoster virus particles that are shed from patients with these diseases. Herpes simplex virus type 1 (HSV-1) has been isolated from the salivary secretions of 2% to 9% of asymptomatic adults, 11% of a group of college students with pharyngitis, and 78% of salivary samples from patients with acute oral lesions. In a population attending a clinic for sexually transmitted diseases, herpes simplex virus type 2 (HSV-2) was isolated from the genital tract of 0.3% to 5.4% of males and 1.6% to 8% of females. The major risk to immunocompetent health care workers exposed to HSV through patient contact is herpetic whitlow, although infection of the eye or perianal area is theoretically possible secondary to finger contamination.

Health care providers may be exposed to varicella zoster virus (VZ) from patients presenting with varicella (chicken pox) or herpes zoster (shingles). Immunocompetent health care providers with prior VZ infection are at no significant risk from exposure to these patients. Although most workers can be expected to have circulating antibodies, there is still a small but significant number who do not.

INITIAL APPROACH IN THE EMERGENCY DEPARTMENT

In the emergency department, the potentially infected patient (with HIV or HBV) presents personnel with several risks, particularly if the patient requires invasive procedures. Although HIV is the most deadly risk, the chances of a health care provider contracting hepatitis B are statistically greater. However, the recommendations given for protecting health care providers from HIV transmission will also help to protect them from exposure to other biologic agents. The CDC recommends that "universal blood and body fluid precautions" should be used for all patients (Table 18–1). Emphasis should be placed on the immediate disposal of used needles without recapping as well as other sharp instruments used on the patient.

DATA GATHERING

The evaluation needed for any health care provider with a potential infectious exposure depends primarily on the history. Because health care workers are seen shortly after

TABLE 18–1. Universal Precautions

Threat	Prevention
Skin or mucous membrane exposure to blood or other body fluids	Gloves: All exposures Masks, eyewear, face shields: Procedures likely to generate droplets Gowns, aprons: Procedures generating splashes Washing: All contaminated skin surfaces Bag-mask ventilation devices in all resuscitation areas
Penetrating injuries with contaminated needles or instruments	Place all sharp items in a puncture-proof container immediately after use without manipulation (e.g., recapping needles)
Exudative lesions	Refrain from direct patient contact

exposure in most cases, little information is available from the physical examination other than establishment of a normal baseline or documentation of preexisting abnormalities.

History

Several key historical points should be noted during the examination of the exposed victim both in the case cited and with other types of exposures.

1. *Significant exposures* include needle sticks, mucous membrane exposures, and contamination of the care provider's skin with a patient's blood or other body fluids in areas where the barrier function of the skin has been compromised by disease or injury.

2. Every attempt should be made to identify the *infectious status* of the *source patient* (the patient from whom the blood or body fluid came). The source could be unknown (as in this case), it could be known but the infectious status unknown, or the source could be known along with a documented infectious status.

3. The provider's history of *immunizations* and *relevant* history of *previous infections* should be recorded. These data include the date of the last tetanus immunization. If the nurse had been immunized against hepatitis B, such information as the dates of the injections and the results of postvaccination antibody testing would be noted. Patients who were vaccinated during the early years of the program were often injected in the buttocks area, and consequently the immunogenicity of the vaccine approached only 80%. Currently, it is recommended that the vaccine be given in the deltoid muscle, where its immunogenicity exceeds 90%.

4. Any history of *clinical hepatitis* or positive results of a test for *serologic markers* of hepatitis should be noted.

5. Any history of being *seropositive* for *HIV* is recorded.

6. If the provider was exposed to varicella zoster and denies a prior *history* of having had a *clinical* case of *chickenpox*, results of previous testing for antibody titers to varicella zoster virus are obtained if available.

7. Any treatment or medical problems that would lead to an *immunocompromised state* are noted.

8. The *menstrual history* and the *possibility* of *pregnancy* in a female are important because exposure to these biologic agents could have a direct bearing on management of such patients.

Physical Examination

Physical examination should focus on the signs relevant to the disease process of concern based on the patient's history. Signs of the following problems are carefully sought:
1. Fever
2. Rashes or mucous membrane sores
3. Jaundice

4. Lymphadenopathy or splenomegaly
5. Hepatic tenderness or hepatomegaly
6. Potential wound sites from a needle stick injury

PROBLEM The nurse was agitated and upset when the physician talked with her. She expressed a great deal of concern about her risk of contracting AIDS or hepatitis from the needle stick. She wanted to know how great her risk of infection was and what signs and symptoms she should anticipate.

DIFFERENTIAL DIAGNOSIS: EXPOSURE RISK OF THE HEALTH CARE WORKER

Human Immunodeficiency Virus

As of March 1988, 55,315 adult cases of AIDS had been reported to the CDC. More than 90% of the population of AIDS patients is composed of males between 20 and 49 years of age. The high-risk groups for AIDS include homosexual or bisexual males whether or not they are intravenous drug abusers, heterosexual IV drug abusers, recipients of blood transfusions, hemophiliacs, and heterosexual sex partners of people with AIDS. Between 3% and 6% of people with AIDS have not been shown to belong to any high-risk group.

Parenteral exposure is one of the three demonstrated modes of transmission along with sexual and perinatal exposure. However, very few health care workers with documented parenteral or mucous membrane exposures to HIV patients have become seropositive. The Cooperative Needlestick Surveillance Group has followed 1201 health care workers with documented mucous membrane or parenteral exposure to blood of patients infected with human immunodeficiency virus as of July 1988. Of this group, 963 were tested for HIV antibody at least 180 days after exposure, and positive results were found in only four. Based on surveillance studies, the best estimate of seroconversion after exposure is about 0.4%.

Following transmission of the virus, an acute infection appears in 3 to 6 weeks. The signs and symptoms include fever, arthralgias, sweats, myalgias, sore throat, headaches, nausea, vomiting, diarrhea, lymphadenopathy, splenomegaly, and a transient macular, erythematous rash. This syndrome lasts 3 to 4 days and is followed by a latent period, after which the patient may develop AIDS. Seroconversion generally occurs 6 to 12 weeks after transmission. The clinical manifestations of AIDS, which often do not develop for 4 to 6 years following exposure, are divided into respiratory syndromes, gastrointestinal syndromes, neurologic syndromes, and mucocutaneous syndromes. As mentioned earlier, all patients should be considered to be potentially infected with HIV.

Hepatitis B Virus

Although the mode of transmission of AIDS is similar to that of hepatitis, the demonstrated acquisition of infection is quite different in the health care setting. Compared to the low rate of transmission of HIV mentioned above, the incidence of seroconversion following accidental exposure to hepatitis B virus is 19% to 27% among health care personnel. The prevalence of hepatitis B serologic markers in emergency department personnel and other selected health care personnel is outlined in Table 18–2. Following such an exposure, hepatitis B surface antigen (HBsAg) can be identified in the serum 30 to 60 days later in those who become infected and lasts for variable periods.

Antibodies against the surface antigen develop after the infection has resolved and provide long-term immunity. Antibodies to the HBV core antigen (anti-HBc) develop in all HBV infections and persist indefinitely. IgM anti-HBc is detectable early in an infection and lasts for about 6 months. It is therefore a useful indicator of an acute or

TABLE 18–2. Prevalence of Hepatitis B Serologic Markers in Selected Health Care Personnel

Group	Prevalence Rate
Healthy adults	4–5%
Laboratory technicians	18.8–25%
Surgeons	28%
Internists	18%
Pathologists	9.1–27%
Emergency nurses	30%
Emergency medical technicians	18–25%
Emergency physicians	11.7%

From Trott A: Hepatitis B exposure and the emergency physician. Am J Emerg Med 5:54, 1987.

recent infection. The third hepatitis antigen is hepatitis B e antigen (HBeAg). The presence of this antigen correlates with high levels of infectivity, whereas the presence of the corresponding antibody (anti-HBe) correlates with lower infectivity.

The incubation period of hepatitis B virus infections is 45 to 160 days, and the symptoms are generally insidious in onset. The clinical signs and symptoms include anorexia, malaise, nausea, vomiting, jaundice, abdominal pain, rashes, arthritis, and arthralgias.

Bacterial Meningitis

In patients with an acute meningitis syndrome the signs and symptoms of both systemic and central nervous system compromise usually have a rapid onset. These signs include fever, headache, nausea, altered sensorium, and neck stiffness. The reported incidence of bacterial meningitis in the United States is 2.9 cases per 100,000 population annually. About 70% of cases occur in children under 5 years of age. *Hemophilus influenzae* has become the leading cause of meningitis in the United States. When *H. influenzae* or *Neisseria meningitidis* is the infectious agent of meningitis, prophylaxis is recommended for persons having intimate contact with the patient. In the case of health care workers, prophylaxis is recommended only when intimate contact with the body fluids of a patient with meningococcal meningitis occurs.

Herpes

As mentioned in the introduction to this chapter, herpetic whitlow is the major risk to health care workers exposed to herpes simplex virus (HSV). Most cases of whitlow are caused by HSV-1, but cases have been reported in which HSV-2 was the infectious agent. Herpetic whitlow does represent a diagnostic challenge. Infection occurs when breaks in the skin are exposed to vesicular fluid, oropharyngeal secretions, or tracheal secretions. The lesions appear after 3 to 7 days along with edema, erythema, and tenderness of the infected finger. Painful, deep-seated vesicles then develop on the paronychial or volar surface of the distal phalanx. These lack the tense pulp characteristic of bacterial infections. Systemic symptoms including fever, chills, lymphadenopathy, and lymphangitis can occur. The vesicular fluid can become turbid, mistakenly suggesting a pyogenic infection. The vesicles coalesce or ulcerate, and after 10 to 14 days the pain rapidly subsides, and the lesions dry and heal without scarring.

Varicella zoster virus represents a smaller risk to health care providers. Many health care workers who do not recall having chickenpox as a child have serologic evidence of prior exposure. By age 10, 60% to 70% of children have antibodies indicating prior infection. About 96% of adults in the United States are immune to VZ. However, for those without a history of exposure, serologic testing may be indicated, particularly in pregnant health care workers. If they actually have negative results on tests for serologic markers to VZ, they are at risk if exposed to patients with chickenpox and, to a lesser extent, to patients with shingles.

PROBLEM The nurse appeared to be reassured after the physician's explanation of her risk of infection. She stated that she had been in good health and took no medication except birth control pills. She denied any past history of hepatitis or of immunization against hepatitis B.

DIAGNOSTIC ADJUNCTS: SEROLOGIC TESTING—MANAGEMENT PRINCIPLES FOR THE EXPOSURE VICTIM

Human Immunodeficiency Virus

Because the source patient cannot be identified in the case cited, the decisions about HIV testing and follow-up for the nurse need to be made on an individual basis guided by the prevalence of HIV in the institution's patient population and the nurse's concern about possible infection. If there is a high prevalence of HIV infection, or if the nurse is extremely concerned, the physician should proceed as if the source were HIV positive. Under any circumstances, the nurse should be offered serologic evaluation for HIV infection as outlined in Table 18–3. Although seroconversion in an exposed health care worker ordinarily does not occur until 6 to 12 weeks after infection, the initial test result serves as a baseline for the detection of a preexisting HIV infection. If the result is seronegative on the initial test, the patient should be retested at 6 weeks, 12 weeks, and 6 months after exposure to determine whether infection from the incident occurred. If the result remains negative at 6 months, the physician can assume that HIV transmission has not occurred. During this 6-month period, particularly during the first 12 weeks, the patient should consider himself or herself potentially infective and follow the Public Health Service recommendations for prevention of HIV transmission. These recommendations include refraining from breastfeeding and from blood, semen, or organ donation. In addition, the patient should either abstain from sexual intercourse or use measures to prevent HIV transmission during intercourse. The patient should also be advised to report any febrile illnesses during the 12-week period following exposure because such illness may represent an acute HIV infection, which is different from AIDS (which may develop later). The patient also requires referral for initial follow-up with his or her private physician to discuss fully the chances of infection, the patient's concerns, and the recommended alterations in lifestyle pending the results of serologic tests. These topics should be addressed in the emergency department but usually cannot be fully explored in the emergency department environment. In the case described here, unless the nurse were shown to be HIV positive, there would be no reason to restrict her from further patient contact while she underwent follow-up testing. The same precautions recommended to protect the nurse should provide appropriate protection for her patients should she be found to be one of the few health care providers who become HIV seropositive after exposure. If this were to occur, decisions about her future patient care

TABLE 18–3. Evaluation of Health Care Workers with Parenteral, Mucous Membrane, or Cutaneous Exposure to Blood or Other Body Fluids

Source Patient Status	Initial Clinical and Serologic Evaluation	Serologic Retest		
		At 6 Weeks[a]	At 12 Weeks	At 6 Months
Has AIDS, is HIV positive, or refuses test	Yes	Yes	Yes	Yes
HIV-negative, low risk of HIV infection	Yes	No	No	No
HIV-negative, high risk[b] of HIV infection	Yes	No	Yes	No

[a] Retesting is needed only if the patient was seronegative on a previous testing.
[b] Groups comprising the majority of AIDS patients including homosexual or bisexual males, IV drug abusers, patients with hemophilia or coagulation disorders, heterosexual sex partners of persons with AIDS.

activities should be made by the nurse in conjunction with her personal physician and the medical director and personnel health service staff of the employing institution.

If the source patient in this case were known, HIV testing would be performed on a blood sample taken from the source patient. If the sample were found to be positive for HIV antibody or if the patient refused to have a blood sample drawn, the nurse would need to be counselled and followed as indicated above. If the source patient proved to be HIV negative and was not from a high-risk group, the nurse would not need testing beyond the initial evaluation. If the patient was HIV negative but belonged to a high-risk group, the nurse would need an additional serologic test at 12 weeks to confirm that transmission had not occurred.

One additional consideration of note in this evaluation is that informed consent is needed to draw a blood sample for HIV testing from the source patient. The results of the study must be handled confidentially and the test results revealed only to the patient and others as required by law. The laws limiting who can be notified of the test results without the patient's consent vary from area to area. In some instances, even those at risk of infection from the patient are not entitled to notification by medical personnel. Consequently, it is important that patients who are found to be seropositive are properly counselled by an appropriately trained individual. It is also important to ensure that the patient will not be denied needed care once he or she is found to be seropositive.

Testing is done by a series of steps starting with repeated enzyme-linked immunoassays (ELISA) and followed by a more specific assay such as the Western blot if repeated ELISAs show positive results. The ELISA has a specificity of approximately 99% when it is performed under optimal conditions and repeated assays are done in a patient infected for 12 weeks or more. The sensitivity of repeated ELISAs is also approximately 99%. Further specificity is gained by using the Western blot assay to validate samples that are repeatedly found to be positive by ELISA. This assay has a specificity of 99.9% when used in this manner. The sensitivity of the Western blot test is comparable to that of the ELISA.

One additional concern in the management of patients with exposure to HIV is that of prophylaxis. Currently, no prophylactic measures are available. The CDC does not recommend the use of immune globulin in these patients. Although this product has been shown to be free of the AIDS virus, it also has not been shown to be of any benefit in this setting. Some institutions have offered the antiviral agent zidovudine for post-exposure prophylaxis.

Hepatitis B Virus

The CDC recommendations for hepatitis B prophylaxis for various situations following percutaneous exposure are outlined in Table 18–4. Some of these scenarios are amplified below to describe instances in which ancillary testing would be indicated for the nurse in the problem case if the circumstances of exposure had been different.

If the nurse had stuck herself with a needle from an HBsAg-positive source and had received one or more doses of hepatitis B vaccine, she would need to be tested for an adequate antibody response if such a response had not been demonstrated within the past 12 months. If an adequate level of antibody were demonstrated (10 sample ratio units or more by radioimmunoassay or positive ELISA), either in the past 12 months or following the exposure, no further testing or treatment would be required. However, if antibody levels were found to be inadequate, the recommended treatment would be based on the patient's prior history of vaccination as outlined below:

1. If the patient never completed the original series of three shots, hepatitis B immune globulin (HBIG [0.06 ml/kg IM]) would be administered immediately and the vaccination series completed as scheduled.

2. If the original vaccination series was completed and the antibody level was shown

TABLE 18-4. Recommendations for Hepatitis B Prophylaxis Following Percutaneous Exposure

Source	Exposed Person	
	Unvaccinated	*Vaccinated*
HBsAg-positive	1. HBIG given once immediately[a] 2. Initiate HB vaccine[b] series	1. Test exposed person for anti-HBs[c] 2. If inadequate antibody,[d] give HBIG (once) immediately plus HB vaccine booster dose
Known source High-risk HBsAg-positive	1. Initiate HB vaccine series 2. Test source for HbsAg; if positive, give HBIG once	Test source for HBsAg only if exposed person is a vaccine nonresponder; if source is HBsAg-positive, give HBIG once immediately plus HB vaccine booster dose
Low-risk HBsAg-positive	Initiate HB vaccine series	Nothing required
Unknown source	Initiate HB vaccine series	Nothing required

[a] HBIG dose 0.06 ml/kg IM.
[b] HB vaccine dose 20 μg IM for adults; 10 μg IM for infants or children under 10 years of age. First dose within 1 week; second and third doses, 1 and 6 months later.
[c] See text for details.
[d] Less than 10 sample ratio units by radioimmunoassay, negative by enzyme immunoassay.
From Advisory Committee for Immunization Practices: Recommendations for protection against viral hepatitis. Morbid Mortal Weekly Rep 34:331, 1985.

to be adequate at one time, a booster dose of 20 μg (1 ml) of hepatitis B vaccine should be administered.

3. If the patient had completed the series but had never demonstrated adequate levels of antibodies, a dose of HBIG should be given immediately along with a booster of hepatitis B vaccine. As always, the vaccine should be given in the deltoid with the HBIG administered at a different site.

The patient should be cautioned to obtain immediate follow-up if the signs and symptoms of an acute hepatitis infection appear. Unless the patient was late in presenting and the signs and symptoms of an acute infection had already developed, the nurse in this case could return to work without restrictions.

Screening of health care workers with significant exposure to hepatitis A virus is not recommended because prophylaxis with immune globulin (IG) is less expensive than the screening test. These health care providers should be given IG (0.02 ml/kg) as a single IM injection. IG should also be considered if the source patient has a high risk for non-A, non-B hepatitis (e.g., the source patient has a recent history of multiple blood transfusions).

Tetanus

A more common concern for the nurse who sustained a needle stick injury is the need for tetanus prophylaxis. Because her last tetanus immunization had been given within the previous year, she did not require any additional prophylaxis with tetanus toxoid. Table 18-5 shows the CDCs summary guide to tetanus prophylaxis in routine wound care. Of particular interest is the definition of wounds that are not considered clean (see footnote a). This definition encompasses the majority of wounds seen in the emergency department including puncture wounds. Therefore, when evaluating a patient with a needle stick injury, a booster of diphtheria-tetanus toxoid (0.5 ml IM) is needed if more than 5 years have passed since the last booster and the patient had the original three-shot series. If the patient has not completed the initial series, a booster of diphtheria-tetanus toxoid should be given (with provisions made to complete the series as needed), and 250 to 500 units of tetanus immune globulin should be given IM at another site.

Bacterial Meningitis

In dealing with exposure to *H. influenzae* or meningococcal meningitis, the prophylactic agent of choice is rifampin. Prophylaxis is not routinely recommended for health care

TABLE 18–5. Summary Guide to Tetanus Prophylaxis in Routine Wound Management, 1985

History of Absorbed Tetanus Toxoid	Clean Minor Wounds		All Other Wounds[a]	
	Td[b]	TIG	Td[b]	TIG
Unknown or <3 doses	Yes	No	Yes	Yes
>3 doses[c]	No[d]	No	No[e]	No

[a]Such as, but not limited to, wounds contaminated with dirt, feces, soil, saliva, etc., puncture wounds, avulsions, and wounds resulting from missiles, crushing injuries, burns, and frostbite.
[b]For children <7 years of age; diphtheria, pertussis, and tetanus (DTP) (diphtheria and tetanus [DT], if pertussis vaccine is contraindicated) is preferred to tetanus toxoid alone. For persons >7 years of age, Td is preferred to tetanus toxoid alone.
[c]If only three doses of fluid toxoid have been received, then a fourth dose of toxoid, preferably an absorbed toxoid, should be given.
[d]Yes, if more than 10 years have elapsed since last dose.
[e]Yes, if more than 5 years have elapsed since last dose.
From Centers for Disease Control: Tetanus—United States, 1985–1986. Morbid Mortal Weekly Rep 36:479, 1987.

workers who have delivered care to a patient infected with one of these agents. However, personnel exposed to the saliva of a patient with meningococcal meningitis during mouth-to-mouth resuscitation warrant consideration for prophylaxis with rifampin. Therefore, a provider who delivered mouth-to-mouth resuscitation to such a patient would require treatment. However, other providers involved in a resuscitation would not require prophylaxis if they did not have intimate contact with the patient's body fluids. Although prophylaxis is recommended for household contacts as well as for some day care contacts of patients with *H. influenzae* meningitis, it is not currently recommended for health care workers. Rifampin should be prescribed for the exposed provider in the dose of 600 mg (20 mg/kg in children) orally once daily for 4 days. This prophylaxis should be administered as soon as possible (within 14 days). Rifampin prophylaxis is contraindicated in pregnant patients because it has been shown to be teratogenic in laboratory animals.

Patients taking this regimen should be warned that it causes an orange discoloration of the urine, discoloration of soft contact lenses, and decreased effectiveness of oral contraceptives. No further follow-up is indicated unless the patient develops signs of an acute systemic infection. Providers need not be restricted from work if they follow normal precautions against infection that protect them as well as their patients.

Herpes

The varicella zoster exposure should not generally be a problem because of the high incidence of protective antibodies in the adult population. However, health care workers with a history of exposure who deny having had a clinical case of chickenpox should probably have a screening test for antibodies to VZ if they are either pregnant, immunosuppressed, or working with immunosuppressed patients. If the test shows positive results, the worker can be reassured. If results are negative, or if testing cannot be done, VZ immune globulin (VZIG) should be given (125 mg/10 kg IM) to the immunosuppressed health care worker and considered for the pregnant patient.

All exposed seronegative health care workers should be restricted from working around immunocompromised patients. This small percentage of the population without immunity is at risk of developing overt disease, which is contagious before it is apparent. They should be seen in follow-up by the personnel health services staff of the employing institution or by their private physician before returning to work with these patients. If the health care worker is pregnant or immunocompromised, follow-up is indicated if he or she develops symptoms of chickenpox (which occasionally occurs even if VZIG is administered).

No prophylactic agents are available for herpes simplex. The prevention of whitlow depends on the use of gloves on both hands whenever the oral cavity, the genital region, or obvious herpetic lesions are examined. The key to managing health care workers presenting with whitlow is recognizing the lesion and avoiding surgical intervention or antibiotics unless secondary infection is present. Treatment should be conservative and should consist of analgesia, elevation, and immobilization as indicated for comfort.

An equally important concern is the health care worker who presents to the emergency department as the source patient. For example, a patient with an active case of herpes labialis should not return to an environment where he or she will expose immunocompromised, pregnant, or neonatal patients to the infection. Although they may still shed the virus after the lesions have healed, as many other people may shed HSV, the titers of HSV in cultures from patients with active lesions are 100 to 1000 times higher than in asymptomatic workers.

Similarly, if a health care worker has active whitlow lesions, he or she should wear gloves when dealing with patients to avoid infecting them.

PROBLEM The nurse asks the physician how much emergency department evaluation is needed because her ward is short of nurses and she would like to get back to work. She also wants to know what, if any, follow-up is required.

A patient with a needle stick injury from an unknown source can be contaminated with several agents, many of which would not alter the general approach to wound care, i.e., local cleansing and provision of a tetanus booster if indicated. The agents that required further consideration in this scenario are HIV, HBV, and tetanus. Under current guidelines, this patient should be offered serologic testing for HIV and does not require a tetanus shot. Because she has never been immunized for hepatitis B, she should begin the hepatitis B vaccine series as recommended in Table 18–4.

DOCUMENTATION

Key points that require documentation in the chart of a health care worker with exposure to a transmissible infection include:
1. The type of exposure sustained.
2. The infectious status of the source patient.
3. The health care worker's history of immunizations and relevant history of previous infections.
4. The possibility of pregnancy in female patients.
5. Current illnesses.
6. Vital signs and examination findings suggesting current infections or an immunocompromised state.
7. Screening laboratory tests ordered from the emergency department.
8. Instructions given for follow-up.
9. Counselling that was given concerning risks of the incident to the patient and to others both in and out of the health care environment.

SUMMARY AND FINAL POINTS

- Health care workers are at ever increasing risk of exposure to biologic agents in their daily practice. The main defense against these risks is adherence to well-defined preventive measures in which all patients are considered to be infectious. The proper steps needed for evaluation and treatment are determined by defining the nature of the exposure, the patient's immune status relative to the particular agent, and the actual infectious status of the source patient if known.
- In some instances it is more cost-effective to treat the patient than it is to define all of the parameters.

- In other instances, no treatment is available. Nonetheless, the evaluation can provide peace of mind or may be of significant medicolegal importance in the future.

BIBLIOGRAPHY

Text
1. Nelson WE: Textbook of Pediatrics (13th ed). Philadelphia, Saunders, 1987.

Journal Articles
1. Advisory Council for Immunization Practices: Meningococcal vaccines. Morbid Mortal Weekly Rep 34:255–259, 1985.
2. Advisory Council for Immunization Practices: Recommendations for protection against viral hepatitis. Morbid Mortal Weekly Rep 34:313–335, 1985.
3. Advisory Council for Immunization Practices: Update on hepatitis B prevention. Morbid Mortal Weekly Rep 36:353–366, 1987.
4. Advisory Council on Immunization Practices: Update: Prevention of *Haemophilus influenzae* type b disease. Morbid Mortal Weekly Rep 35:170–180, 1986.
5. Advisory Council on Immunization Practices: Update: Prevention of *Haemophilus influenzae* type b disease. Morbid Mortal Weekly Rep 37:13–16, 1988.
6. Centers for Disease Control: Recommendations for prevention of HIV transmission in health-care settings. Morbid Mortal Weekly Rep 36:3S–18S, 1987.
7. Centers for Disease Control: Tetanus United States, 1985–1986. Morbid Mortal Weekly Rep 36:4477–4481, 1987.
8. Centers for Disease Control: Update: Acquired immunodeficiency syndrome and human immunodeficiency virus infection among health-care workers. Morbid Mortal Weekly Rep 37:229–234, 1988.
9. Corey L, Spear PG: Infection with herpes simplex viruses, Part 1. N Engl J Med 314:686–691, 1986.
10. Corey L, Spear PG: Infection with herpes simplex viruses, Part 2. N Engl J Med 314:749–756, 1986.
11. Kelen GD: Human immunodeficiency virus and the emergency department: Risks and risk protection for health care providers. Ann Emerg Med 19:242–248, 1990.
12. Marcus R: Surveillance of health care workers exposed to blood from patients infected with the human immunodeficiency virus. N Engl J Med 319:1118–1123, 1988.
13. Trott A: Hepatitis B exposure and the emergency physician. Am J Emerg Med 5:54–59, 1987.

SECTION SEVEN

TOXICOLOGIC/ENVIRONMENTAL DISORDERS

CHAPTER 19

THE POISONED PATIENT

TIMOTHY L. TURNBULL, M.D.
MARTIN J. SMILKSTEIN, M.D.

PROBLEM 1 A 45 year old male was found unresponsive by his son at home.

PROBLEM 2 A 15 year old female was brought to the emergency department by her parents after she took 10 "sleeping tablets" in response to an argument with her parents. She was alert and asymptomatic.

PROBLEM 3 A 35 year old auto mechanic presented with severe headache, nausea, and vomiting.

PROBLEM 4 A 65 year old patient with chronic obstructive pulmonary disease (COPD) and congestive heart failure (CHF) presented with nausea, palpitations, and the "jitters."

PROBLEM 5 A 2½ year old boy was brought to the emergency department by his mother, who found him playing with an opened bottle of furniture polish. He coughed a few times at home but in the emergency department was asymptomatic.

PROBLEM 6 A 21 year old student took "a bunch of Tylenol No. 3 tablets" according to her family. In the emergency department she was short of breath and wouldn't talk.

QUESTIONS TO CONSIDER

1. What are the different ways in which a poisoned patient can present to the emergency department?
2. How are historical information and physical findings used to identify an unknown intoxicant?
3. What is the role of the laboratory in the evaluation of the poisoned patient?
4. What general principles of management are applicable to most poisonings?
5. Which poisonings are treated with a specific antidote?
6. Which poisoned patients require intensive care monitoring and which can be safely discharged from the emergency department?
7. Which patients require psychiatric evaluation?

INTRODUCTION

Poisoning is a problem of enormous magnitude. In 1987, members of the American Association of Poison Control Centers (AAPCC) cataloged nearly 1.2 million toxic exposures. Owing to lack of information from many regions of the country, this figure greatly underestimates the actual incidence of poisoning. Toxic ingestions may account for 10% to 20% of all hospital admissions and about 10% of all ambulance runs. These statistics are of particular interest to emergency physicians because initial care for the great majority of poisoned patients is provided in the emergency department.

As the problem cases illustrate, the poisoned patient can present for emergency care in a variety of ways. Most poisonings are accidental. However, almost 10% are intentional and are often associated with suicidal ideation. Most occur at home, though the number of recognized toxic exposures occurring in the workplace is increasing.

A history of ingestion is often unavailable, and the diagnosis must be inferred from the clinical circumstances. At other times it is obvious that a toxic ingestion has occurred, but the actual offending agent is unknown. Patients who ingest potentially poisonous substances in quantities sufficient to cause toxicity usually manifest signs or symptoms on presentation. Occasionally, if presentation is very early or if the pathophysiologic process is slow, indicators of toxicity may not be seen initially but develop later, after the initial evaluation is completed.

Poisoning tends to be more commonly associated with certain groups of patients. According to AAPCC data, children less than 6 years of age are involved in two-thirds of all exposures. Because children can rarely give good histories, a potentially toxic ingestion can easily go unrecognized in this age group, and any unusual symptoms should prompt suspicion. Similarly, drug abusers and depressed and potentially suicidal patients are viewed as being at high risk for poisoning.

Although not directly suggestive of poisoning, other settings or clinical circumstances that may be associated with toxic exposures include fires, in which victims are often exposed to toxic gases; farm work, during which victims may be exposed to pesticides; trauma, which frequently occurs in the company of substance abuse; serious cardiac arrhythmias in young patients who have no history of cardiac disease; and any unexplained alteration in mental status in any patient.

PREHOSPITAL CARE

Management of the poisoned patient frequently begins before the patient reaches the emergency department. Prehospital personnel can play a pivotal role in both the diagnosis and treatment of a person with a toxic ingestion.

History

Since a reliable history may or may not be obtainable from the patient, the rescue squad can be invaluable in obtaining information from family members, friends, or other witnesses at the scene. Whenever possible, the scene is surveyed for prescription bottles, syringes, open containers of chemicals, and other potentially valuable diagnostic clues. When possible, the following information is obtained:
1. Type, amount, and timing of ingestion or exposure.
2. Symptoms (variable depending on the type of substance involved).
3. Circumstances leading to the exposure (accidental or intentional).
4. Home remedies used (e.g., syrup of ipecac).
5. Past medical or psychiatric history.

Physical Examination

A brief physical examination is also conducted to establish the need for in-field management. The examination includes assessment of (1) the patency and protection of the airway and ventilation; (2) vital signs; (3) mental status; and (4) pupillary size and reactivity.

Intervention

Airway. When ventilation is compromised or airway protective mechanisms are impaired, as evidenced by loss of the gag reflex, the paramedics begin airway management at the scene (Chap. 2). Assisted ventilation is instituted whenever ventilation is of insufficient rate or depth.

Oxygen. Supplemental oxygen is administered at an initial rate of 2 to 4 liters/min. If there is exposure to a toxic gas such as carbon monoxide or secondary toxic pulmonary effects such as pulmonary edema, high flow oxygen (10 to 12 liters/min) is given by means of a nonrebreathing mask.

Intravenous Access. If a significant ingestion of a toxic substance is suspected, intravenous (IV) access is established. If it is started primarily to administer medications, 5% dextrose in water is an appropriate infusate. If hypotension is present or is likely to be a problem, an isotonic crystalloid solution is preferred.

Cardiac Monitor. Cardiac monitoring is useful to observe the effects of a cardiotoxic drug or any hemodynamically unstable patient.

Treatment for Altered Mental Status

Hypoglycemia Screening. A 50% dextrose solution (25 to 50 gm) is administered intravenously to reverse the effects of an occult hypoglycemic reaction. In some systems, a rapid quantitative or semiquantitative glucose determination using a glucose oxidase reagent strip is used as an alternative to empiric treatment. Thiamine 100 mg IV or IM is given first, if available.

Empiric Treatment for Narcotic Overdose. Naloxone (Narcan) is given to reverse the effects of a possible opioid overdose. It may also have an effect in patients suffering from an overdose of ethanol, barbiturates, phenothiazines, or benzodiazepines. Large doses (2 mg) are generally preferred except when opioid dependence is suspected. In this situation, smaller doses (0.4 mg) are used and are titrated to the clinical response, since large doses can precipitate violent withdrawal reactions and greatly complicate patient management during transport.

Decontamination. Prompt decontamination of the skin or eyes with copious irrigation may significantly reduce exposure to pesticides or the damage incurred from caustics.

Dilution. Dilution by ingestion of 4 to 6 oz of milk or water may be appropriate early in the management of patients with some caustic ingestions. This treatment is not routinely indicated.

Elimination. Syrup of ipecac–induced emesis and activated charcoal, although advocated for prehospital use by some, are generally reserved for use with ingestions of highly toxic substances when transport times are prolonged. Syrup of ipecac is recommended by some authors as a home remedy in cases of pediatric ingestion. Prehospital personnel are usually aware of this possibility.

INITIAL APPROACH IN THE EMERGENCY DEPARTMENT

Although many poisoned patients are transported by ambulance and may have been stabilized to some degree before they reach the emergency department, many more present directly to the emergency department. Their medical condition will vary greatly. Because the time course and the ultimate outcome of a toxic ingestion are unpredictable, all patients are evaluated without delay.

Primary Survey

The initial priorities for the emergency physician are the same as those for paramedics. The patency and security of the airway, the rate and depth of breathing, and the adequacy of arterial perfusion (circulation) are assessed (the ABCs of emergency care). Simultaneously, a brief preliminary history is elicited to determine the nature of the problem.

Often this information can be provided only by accompanying family or friends. Whenever possible, the type, amount, and time of ingestion are ascertained and any symptoms are noted. Various treatments administered at home or in the field are explored because these may affect emergency department management. Past medical or psychiatric history is also discussed because it can significantly influence both diagnostic and treatment efforts. If no source of a history is available, an emergency department staff member is assigned to go through the patient's clothing and belongings to search for an address or telephone number of a contact.

Emergency Stabilization

Steps to correct abnormalities in vital functions must be taken without delay. Necessary interventions may include
1. Early intubation (Chap. 2)
2. Oxygen administration (Chap. 2)
3. Intravenous access
4. Electrocardiographic monitoring
5. Dysrhythmia control (Chaps. 3 and 11)
6. Seizure control (Chap. 48)
7. Emergency body cooling measures (Chap. 21)

All of these are necessary skills of the emergency physician and are discussed in other chapters.

Therapeutic Measures

The rapidity and extent of further treatment depend on the clinical circumstances as defined by the history and physical examination. Most early treatment measures are similar to prehospital care activity and are usually instituted as part of the initial evaluation.

Decontamination. Voluminous irrigation of the eyes and skin is instituted rapidly when these body surfaces have been exposed to dangerous chemicals such as caustic agents, certain hydrocarbons, and organophosphate pesticides.

Dilution. Dilution of an ingested substance may be performed in cases of caustic ingestion.

Treatment for Altered Mental Status. A 50% dextrose solution (25 to 50 gm of D/W 50%), thiamine 100 mg, and naloxone 2 mg are administered to patients with altered, usually depressed, mental status.

PROBLEM 1 This patient was found unresponsive at home. The patient was spontaneously breathing and had a weak gag reflex. The presence of several empty pill bottles strongly suggested drug overdose. The rescue squad responding to the call established an intravenous line and initiated cardiac monitoring and oxygen therapy. There was no response to 50% dextrose, thiamine, and naloxone. On arrival in the emergency department, the airway was reassessed because its security was in doubt.

Even if a patient does appear to be ventilating properly, lack of a gag reflex in an unresponsive patient represents an unprotected airway and requires endotracheal intubation. Manual ventilation may be necessary immediately in an apneic or bradypneic patient, as well as later if the ventilatory pattern deteriorates. Blood pressure, pulse, and cardiac rhythm are also reassessed. If there is a partial response or if the dose given is obviously inadequate, the medications for altered mental status may be readministered.

PROBLEM 2 This patient had normal vital signs and no symptoms and did not appear ill. The initial management of this case will differ significantly from that of the patient in Problem 1. The aggressiveness of management is guided by the history as well as by the physical presentation. In this particular case, it was subsequently found that the "sleeping pills" were 75-mg tablets of amitriptyline, a tricyclic antidepressant. Overdoses of this medication can result in rapid and profound alterations in mental status, seizures, and cardiovascular collapse even though the results of the initial examination are normal. Therefore, in anticipation of these problems, this patient was managed aggressively with an intravenous line and cardiac monitoring. An artificial airway was not necessary at this time but was readied for use should the patient deteriorate.

DATA GATHERING

History

The history is of paramount importance in the evaluation of poisoned patients. However, the nature of these patients or their condition often precludes their providing any helpful information. They are often young children or people whose thought processes are impaired by mental illness or the agent to which they have been exposed. Even alert and cooperative patients often provide inaccurate historical information.

The physician needs to gather information routinely from other sources, as outlined in the Initial Approach section above. Although this process is valuable in many situations in emergency medicine, it is essential in the case of the poisoned patient. Old medical records are ordered routinely because they may be the only reliable source of information. If necessary, the police are requested to go to the patient's residence in an effort to obtain information. The desired information depends on the clinical circumstances. Its primary purpose is to confirm the poisoning and identify the substance involved.

1. If the situation is that of a possible but still unverified toxic ingestion and the patient is unable to provide a history (as in Problem 1), the following information is usually necessary:
   a. *Situational history*. *Where* was the patient *found* and *what* were the *circumstances*? Were there pills or drug paraphernalia in the area?
   b. *Occupational history*. Is the patient *exposed* to *potentially toxic substances*?
   c. *Past medical history*. Preexisting medical problems may influence therapeutic options, and chronic or terminal illnesses may predispose patients to depression and suicidal ideation.
   d. Is there a previous *history* of *mental illness*?
   e. Is there a history of *substance abuse*?
2. When the exposure is known and the patient is alert and able to provide a reasonable history (as in Problem 2), the following questions may elicit useful information:
   a. What *medications* or *compounds* were *ingested*? The ingestion of multiple drugs is common, although specific questioning is often necessary to obtain the details.
   b. *How much* of each agent was *ingested*? This information is confirmed whenever possible by checking the prescription bottle for the remaining number of pills relative to the initial number. The pharmacist may be called to confirm the number of pills and contents in a prescription.
   c. *When* and *how* did the *exposure take place*? Exposures of more than 2 hours without causing symptoms must be assessed against the expected toxicity of an ingestant. For example, no clinical findings with acetaminophen are to be expected, but similar findings after ingestion of diazepam and ethanol will cause the physician to requestion the patient completely.
   d. Were there any *symptoms following* the *exposure*?
   e. Was the exposure *accidental* or *intentional*?
   f. Was any *treatment* given *at the scene*? Dilution with water or milk, home remedies, and attempts to induce vomiting are common.

3. Occasionally an alert patient will present with symptoms of an unsuspected toxic exposure (Problems 3 and 4). The following information may shed light on the diagnosis:
   a. The *chronology* of the presenting complaint(s).
   b. *Medications*, including any recent dose changes.
   c. Detailed *situational* and *occupational history*.
4. Certain patients may clearly have experienced a toxic exposure but, for whatever reason, are unable to provide any further history (Problems 5 and 6). Aside from the previously mentioned information that can be obtained from other sources, the following information should be sought:
   a. A detailed *psychiatric history* from the chart or from other individuals.
   b. Were any empty *pill bottles* found at home or on the person?
   c. Was there a *suicide note*?

PROBLEM 1 This patient was brought, unresponsive, to the emergency department by paramedics, who stated that he took an overdose of an unknown substance. The patient could provide no history.

In many cases in which paramedics are involved, evidence in the form of pills or prescription bottles is brought to the hospital with the patient. If this has not been done, a relative or police may be sent to the home to retrieve such evidence. A commitment to an aggressive and extensive search for information while the patient is being stabilized will usually yield results.

PROBLEM 4 This 65 year old patient with a past history of COPD and CHF presented with symptoms of nausea, palpitations, and tremor.

Any chronically medicated patient, especially an elderly patient, who presents with nonspecific symptoms should be suspected of drug toxicity. In many cases the patient will be able to list the medications he or she is taking. In other cases, however, the names of the medications are unknown to the patient and must be inferred from the nature of the illness. Corroborating information is then obtained either by reviewing the patient's medical record or, once again, by having someone retrieve pill bottles from the home.

Physical Examination

The physical examination usually reveals no abnormalities immediately after a toxic ingestion. However, once clinical toxicity begins to develop, the patient may manifest physical signs that can serve as clues to the nature of the intoxication. A thorough examination is completed in an effort to identify sometimes subtle findings. Such findings may be useful in evaluating ingestions of both known and unidentified intoxicants. In the former, the clinical picture can either corroborate or contradict the frequently erroneous preliminary history. In the latter setting, the examination may uncover clues implicating a previously unsuspected intoxicant. Then a more vigorous, directed history can be pursued.

Abnormal physical signs are routinely sought in the following general areas:

Vital Signs. Abnormalities of the pulse, respirations, blood pressure, and temperature can be helpful in indicating the need for therapeutic intervention and in suggesting the class of compound causing the abnormality (Table 19–1).

Cardiopulmonary System. The lungs are auscultated to assess the adequacy of air flow. Findings of wheezes, rhonchi, or rales may indicate the presence of bronchitis or pneumonitis due to inhalation of toxic gases or aspiration of gastric contents or pulmonary toxins such as hydrocarbons. Pulmonary edema may result from ingestion of cardiotoxic drugs or agents such as heroin that produce noncardiogenic pulmonary edema.

TABLE 19-1. Vital Sign Abnormalities Associated with Intoxication

Abnormality	Mechanism	Class of Compound
Hypoventilation	CNS depression	Opioids, sedative-hypnotics, alcohols
Hyperventilation	CNS stimulation	Sympathomimetics, theophylline, salicylates Drug withdrawal
	Tissue hypoxia	Carbon monoxide, cyanide, methemoglobinemia, methane (asphyxia), opioids (noncardiogenic pulmonary edema)
	Metabolic acidosis	See Table 19-4
Bradycardia	Parasympathetic	Organophosphates, carbonates
	CNS depression	Opioids, clonidine
	Cardiotoxicity	Digoxin, calcium channel blockers, beta-blockers
Tachycardia	CNS stimulation	Sympathomimetics, theophylline, drug withdrawal
	Cholinergic blockade	Cyclic antidepressants, antihistamines, belladonna alkaloids
Hypotension	Cardiotoxicity	Cyclic antidepressants, beta-blockers, calcium channel blockers
	Loss of vasomotor tone	Cyclic antidepressants, antihypertensive agents, calcium channel blockers, theophylline
	CNS depression	Opioids
	Volume depletion	Iron, other heavy metals, diuretics, lithium (diabetes insipidus), organophosphates (diarrhea)
Hypertension	Alpha-adrenergic stimulation	Sympathomimetics, drug withdrawal
Hypothermia	CNS depression	Barbiturates, opioids
	Loss of thermoregulation	Phenothiazines, ethanol
Hyperthermia	CNS stimulation	Sympathomimetics, phencyclidine, salicylates, drug withdrawal (ethanol, others)
	Cholinergic inhibition	Cyclic antidepressants
	Loss of thermoregulation	Phenothiazines
	Vasodilatation	Belladonna alkaloids, antihistamines, cyclic antidepressants

Neurologic System. Many toxic agents produce alterations in mental status, and some produce pupillary changes that may be helpful in differentiating a specific type of intoxication. Focal findings on the motor, sensory, or reflex examination suggest etiologies other than intoxication.

Mental status. Specific alterations of mental status are suggestive of particular intoxicants. Delirium, often accompanied by severe agitation, is suggestive of sympathomimetic or phencyclidine (PCP) overdose, anticholinergic toxicity, or withdrawal from opioids, alcohol, or sedative-hypnotics. Depression of mental status is typically seen with narcotic or sedative-hypnotic agents.

Pupillary changes. Abnormalities can be very specific for certain classes of intoxicants (Table 19-2). Though careful inspection is often necessary, the pupillary changes associated with poisons or intoxicants typically do not include altered reactivity to light. This is a differentiating point between metabolic and structural causes of altered mental status.

Skin. Skin color, moisture, and the presence of lesions or needle tracks are noted. An unusually red color of the skin is sometimes present with anticholinergic, boric acid,

TABLE 19-2. Toxic Pupillary Abnormalities

Abnormality	Mechanism	Compound
Miosis	CNS depression	Opioids Chloral hydrate
	Cholinergic stimulation	Organophosphates, carbamates Pilocarpine
	Alpha-adrenergic block	Clonidine Phenothiazines
Mydriasis	Cholinergic inhibition	Cyclic antidepressants, antihistamines, belladonna alkaloids
	Alpha-adrenergic stimulation	Sympathomimetics, drug withdrawal

cyanide, or carbon monoxide intoxication. Cyanosis refractory to oxygen therapy suggests methemoglobinemia. Extremely moist skin suggests cholinergic or sympathomimetic overdose, whereas dry skin is more consistent with anticholinergic toxicity.

Large blisters or bullae may be present in areas subjected to pressure, such as the heels, in intoxications with carbon monoxide, barbiturates, or glutethimide. Needle tracks from intravenous drug abuse are typically associated with heroin, but other agents such as cocaine are commonly abused by the intravenous route as well.

ENT Examination. The oral mucosa is evaluated for evidence of burns due to caustic ingestions, and any specific odor of the breath is noted (Table 19–3). Ulcerated lesions of the nasal mucosa may be seen in persons who have snorted cocaine.

DECISION PRIORITIES AND PRELIMINARY DIFFERENTIAL DIAGNOSIS

The first question to be answered is: Has this patient experienced a toxic ingestion?

Most commonly, this question is asked after a patient presents with an altered level of consciousness. Other causes of mental status change are outlined in Chapter 45. The variability of presentations of toxic ingestions makes it prudent to consider poisoning in any patient who presents with any mental status abnormality of unclear origin. An obvious ingestion involving an identified intoxicant represents no diagnostic dilemma. In most such cases, the physician needs only to establish whether toxicity has occurred or the likelihood that it will.

When the intoxicant has not been clearly identified, a second question is asked: *Does this patient's presentation fit a clinical pattern consistent with a class of toxic substances? To rephrase, are clinical toxidromes present?*

Clinical "toxidromes" (toxic syndromes) are combinations of signs and symptoms that together suggest a particular class of intoxicant. The constellation of clinical findings can be very toxin-specific. The following toxic syndromes are most commonly seen in the emergency department:

Opioids

All opioids are central nervous system depressants and are capable of causing global depression of vital functions. The classic triad for opioid intoxication is

- Coma
- Respiratory depression
- Pinpoint pupils

Hypotension and bradycardia may also be present.

TABLE 19–3. Odors Associated with Toxic Agents

Fruity	Ethanol
	Isopropanol
Mothballs	Camphor
	Naphthalene
	Paradichlorobenzene
Bitter almonds	Cyanide
Silver polish	Cyanide
Stove gas	Carbon monoxide[a]
Rotten eggs	Hydrogen sulfide
Garlic	Arsenic
	Parathion
Wintergreen	Methylsalicylate
Peanuts	Vacor
Vinyl upholstery	Ethchlorvynol

[a]Pure carbon monoxide is odorless.

Cholinergics

Intoxication from organophosphate or carbamate insecticides is evidenced by parasympathetic signs and symptoms. This syndrome is described by the acronym SLUDGE:

- *S*alivation
- *L*acrimation
- *U*rination
- *D*efecation
- *G*astric cramping
- *E*mesis

These patients often appear to be "drowning in their own secretions," demonstrating bronchorrhea, bronchospasm, and pulmonary edema. Mental status will vary from confusion and agitation to coma and seizures. Muscle fasciculations leading to weakness and paralysis may be prominent. Profuse sweating and an odor of garlic may also be present.

Anticholinergics

Compounds such as antihistamines, belladonna alkaloids, and cyclic antidepressants cause a combination of signs and symptoms attributable to their central and peripheral anticholinergic effects. This toxidrome may be remembered by means of the following mnemonic:

- "Hot as a hare" (hyperpyrexia)
- "Red as a beet" (cutaneous vasodilatation)
- "Dry as a bone" (decreased salivation)
- "Blind as a bat" (cycloplegia and mydriasis)
- "Mad as a hatter" (delirium and hallucinations)

Tachycardia, urinary retention and decreased gastrointestinal motility are typical as well.

Sympathomimetics

Compounds such as cocaine and amphetamines are not only central nervous system stimulants but also have a significant effect on the sympathetic portion of the autonomic nervous system. Therefore, the toxidrome seen with overdoses of these compounds suggests total body "overdrive." Drug withdrawal from ethanol and other substances of potential abuse can manifest a similar hyperadrenergic state. This syndrome is characterized by

- Hypertension
- Tachycardia
- Hyperpyrexia
- Mydriasis
- Anxiety or delirium

Toxicity due to phencyclidine (PCP), although not a sympathomimetic agent, may present in a similar manner.

Sedative-Hypnotics

Compounds such as barbiturates and benzodiazepines cause both depressed mental status and respiratory depression. Unlike with the opioids, pupillary changes with these drugs are unpredictable, although a slowing in reaction to light is common. The barbiturates may cause vesicles or bullae to develop at pressure points. Characteristic signs are

- Confusion or coma

- Respiratory depression
- Hypotension
- Hypothermia
- Variable pupillary changes
- Vesicles or bullae ("barb burns")

Salicylates

Salicylates are common components of both prescription and nonprescription preparations. Toxicity may result from intentional or accidental overdose and is extremely common in all age groups. Characteristic signs are

- Fever
- Tachypnea
- Vomiting
- Lethargy (rarely coma)
- Tinnitus

Phenothiazines and Butyrophenones

These antipsychotic tranquilizers are frequently available to patients who are at high risk for intentional overdose. Toxicity is evident by

- Postural hypotension
- Hypothermia
- Lethargy, coma, convulsions
- Miosis
- Extrapyramidal reactions, composed of buccal dystonias, opisthotonus, oculogyric crisis, torticollis

Not all patients will demonstrate a specific toxidrome. The effects of individual agents vary somewhat, and polydrug overdose is common. Diagnostic tests are used to confirm ingestion of suspected toxic agents or to identify toxic agents when the presenting signs and symptoms are not specific enough to indicate the toxin.

PROBLEM 6 This patient was unable to give a history, but a family member stated that she had taken an overdose of Tylenol No. 3. On presentation she was unresponsive, tachypneic, and miotic and had wet clothes. She was tearing from both eyes and salivating. She had vomited at home and was incontinent of bowel and bladder contents in the emergency department.

Findings on the physical evaluation were not consistent with acetaminophen or opioid toxicity. A different toxidrome is present here. The recognition of this discrepancy by an alert emergency physician resulted in further inquiry. Eventually, one of the family remembered that the patient "might have" consumed some liquid from an old pop bottle in the garage. When the bottle was retrieved, the liquid was identified as an organophosphate pesticide.

DIAGNOSTIC ADJUNCTS

Diagnostic testing is performed for several reasons:

- To rule out or identify a nontoxic medical problem.
- To rule out or identify a particular toxic agent.
- To identify certain manifestations of toxicity.

- To provide prognostic information.
- To guide therapy.

To order tests in a rational and judicious manner, the emergency physician must be aware of the indications for and limitations of the diagnostic tests available to the emergency department.

Laboratory Studies

Complete Blood Count and Differential. The presence of leukocytosis with a "left shift" in the differential cell count generally suggests infection, but ingestions of iron, theophylline, and hydrocarbons may produce an absolute leukocytosis.

Serum Electrolytes. These tests facilitate the diagnosis of numerous metabolic disturbances; however, their greatest value in evaluating the poisoned patient is their determination of the "anion gap."

$$\text{Anion gap} = Na^+ - (HCO_3^- + Cl^-)$$

The normal anion gap of 8 to 12 mEq/liter is due to the presence of unmeasured anions such as sulfates, phosphates, and negatively charged proteins. Poisoning due to certain toxic compounds can cause an increase in the anion gap as the compounds form more unmeasured anions. This finding is usually associated with a metabolic acidosis (Table 19–4).

Blood Urea Nitrogen and Creatinine. In the poisoned patient, these tests are useful to identify the presence of a preexisting renal dysfunction that could influence management and for providing a useful baseline when the poison involved is potentially nephrotoxic. Rarely, abnormalities are suggestive of acute nephrotoxicity.

Serum Glucose. Either hypoglycemia or hyperglycemia may be due to the effect of toxic compounds. The "blood sugar" concentration may have prognostic, diagnostic, and therapeutic significance.

Serum Osmolality. Serum osmolality is most useful when an osmotically active intoxicant such as methanol, ethylene glycol, isopropanol, or ethanol is suspected. These compounds increase the "osmolal gap," the difference between the calculated and measured osmolalities. The measured osmolality is determined by the laboratory. The calculated osmolality is determined by the equation:

$$\text{Osmolality} = 2[Na] + \frac{[\text{glucose}]}{18} + \frac{[\text{BUN}]}{3} + \frac{[\text{ethanol}]}{5}$$

A difference greater than 10 mOsm/liter reflects the presence of one or more of the aforementioned compounds.

Toxicology Screens. These "screens" are a diverse group of *qualitative* assays used to identify the presence of any of a predetermined array of toxic compounds in the urine, blood, or gastric fluid. Unfortunately, use of a toxicology screen in the emergency department may be problematic. Results are often unavailable on a stat basis. Further-

TABLE 19–4. Causes of a High Anion-Gap Metabolic Acidosis (AMUDPILE)

Aspirin
Methanol
Uremia
Diabetic ketoacidosis[a]
Paraldehyde, phenformin
Iron,[b] isoniazid[b]
Lactic acid
Ethylene glycol, ethanol[b]

[a]Ethanol and starvation can also lead to ketoacidosis.
[b]These agents also produce lactic acidosis.

TABLE 19–5. Drugs Screened by the Enzyme-Mediated Immunoassay for Toxins (EMIT)

Amphetamines	Marijuana
Barbiturates	Opiates[a]
Benzodiazepines	Phencyclidine
Cocaine	Tricyclic antidepressants[b]
Ethanol	

[a] Specifically identifies methadone and propoxyphene.
[b] Not part of the basic screen but often added.

more, "tox" screens are frequently inaccurate, demonstrating significant limitations in both sensitivity and specificity. They are also relatively expensive. Considering the relative infrequency with which results from these screens influence management or outcome, this cost is usually not justified. A standard toxicology screen may be of use when there are occupational, medicolegal, or forensic concerns.

One type of toxicology screen that has gained acceptance for emergency department use is the enzyme-mediated immunoassay (EMIT). This assay is simple and quick, with turnaround times of 2 to 4 hours, and it has intermediate accuracy and specificity. The EMIT-dau (CIBA) screens for common drugs of abuse (Table 19–5) are performed on a urine sample. When interpreting screen results the physician must bear in mind that when the screen shows negative results certain drugs may be present but in undetectable quantities. Ideally, this screen is selected when the result will make a significant change in the therapy planned for the patient.

Quantitative Toxicology Studies. Quantitative blood levels can be obtained for a variety of potentially toxic compounds (Table 19–6). If ingestion of one of these compounds is known or suspected, a properly interpreted drug blood level can provide both diagnostic and prognostic information. Proper use of the various blood levels depends mostly on the timing of the test with respect to the absorptive course of the involved compound. The most useful information about the toxicity or potential toxicity of a particular compound is obtained when the blood sample is taken when the compound is at or near peak concentration. Unfortunately, individual variations in absorptive capacity and unreliable information about the actual time of ingestion often make it impossible to know when peak concentration occurs. Furthermore, early blood levels may be useful for making prognoses even before peak concentration is reached. Multiple drug levels are frequently required to determine whether drug concentration is rising or falling.

Radiographic Imaging

Chest Radiography. The chest radiograph is important in the evaluation of a patient exposed to pulmonary toxic agents such as hydrocarbons, toxic gases, or paraquat. It may also be useful in the baseline assessment of patients who ingest potentially toxic quantities of drugs that cause noncardiogenic pulmonary edema (e.g., salicylates, methaqualone, heroin).

Abdominal Radiography. Supine and upright view plain films of the abdomen can be useful by revealing the presence of radiopaque agents in the gastrointestinal tract. Compounds commonly visualized radiographically include chloral hydrate, enterically

TABLE 19–6. Clinically Useful Quantitative Blood Levels

Acetaminophen	Lithium
Carbon monoxide (carboxyhemoglobin)	Methanol
Digoxin	Methemoglobin
Ethanol	Phenobarbital
Ethylene glycol	Phenytoin
Iron	Procainamide
Isopropanol	Salicylates
Lidocaine	Theophylline

coated potassium tablets, ferrous sulfate, and other heavy metals. The radiograph is also useful for evaluation of "body packers"—individuals who swallow large amounts of cocaine or heroin encased in balloons or condoms for purposes of smuggling (Chap. 23).

Electrocardiography

The duration of the various measurable intervals of the electrocardiographic complex (P–R, QRS, and Q–T) may provide important clues as to whether or not agents such as cyclic antidepressants are affecting the cardiac conduction system.

PROBLEM 1 This patient was found unresponsive at home with empty pill bottles nearby. One bottle had contained thirty 1-mg tablets of lorazepam, the other fifty 325-mg tablets of acetaminophen. Laboratory results were obtained as follows: Blood glucose, 90 mg/dl; BUN, 14 mg/dl; sodium, 140 mEq/liter; potassium, 4.0 mEq/liter; chloride, 100 mEq/liter; bicarbonate, 10 mEq/liter; pH, 7.26; serum osmolality, 350 mOsm/kg. Acetaminophen level was unavailable.

The patient had an acidosis. Without arterial blood gas measurements, it could not be clearly determined if there was a respiratory component. However, the anion gap ($Na^+ - [Cl^- + HCO_3^-]$) was abnormally elevated at 30 mEq/liter and the serum bicarbonate was low. Therefore, the acidosis had to be at least partly metabolic. Since neither lorazepam nor acetaminophen causes metabolic acidosis, another problem existed. The osmolal gap gave a clue in that it was elevated at 50 mOsm/liter. Two compounds that can cause a high anion-gap metabolic acidosis, as well as increasing the osmolal gap, are methanol and ethylene glycol. Ethanol will also increase the osmolal gap, and its use can result in a mild lactic acidosis or ketoacidosis. It was reasonable to presume that the patient had ingested one of these compounds. Specific blood level measurements were ordered, and treatment was started for presumptive methanol or ethylene glycol intoxication (Chap. 20). The methanol level subsequently proved to be 30 mg/dl.

PRINCIPLES OF MANAGEMENT

Although the gathering of clinical and laboratory data is essential for accurate identification of both the toxic compound and the degree of toxicity, medical management often cannot be delayed until a definitive diagnosis is made. Diagnosis and management are therefore dynamic and interrelated processes. Early medical treatment can often forestall the development of toxicity that might otherwise have occurred had treatment been delayed pending accurate diagnosis. The potential benefit of each intervention is weighed against its posssible adverse effects, particularly when used in a situation of clinical uncertainty.

Because of the vast array of potentially toxic compounds and the diversity with which ingestions of these are managed, assistance in management is routinely sought from standard references. Perhaps the most comprehensive and practically useful of all such references is a compendium of information called Poisindex. This resource is available for use in both a microfiche system and a computer-display system, one of which can be found in most hospital emergency departments. Poisindex provides up-to-date therapeutic information that is specific for each toxic compound or class of compounds.

Certain principles of management have general applicability:
1. Emergency stabilization
2. Decontamination
3. Minimization of absorption
4. Maximization of elimination
5. Use of antagonist agents

Emergency Stabilization

This phase of management is relatively nonspecific but always takes priority over other phases. Emergency stabilization refers to support of the vital functions—airway, breathing, and circulation. It has been covered earlier in this chapter.

Decontamination

Decontamination refers to irrigating the eyes, cleansing the skin, and diluting the stomach contents, as discussed in the sections on prehospital management and initial approach.

Minimization of Absorption

Limiting the absorption of a toxic compound can be accomplished in numerous ways. When the compound is an inhalant or a toxic gas, the best means of limiting pulmonary absorption is to ensure access to fresh air and then administer oxygen. When the intoxicant is dermally absorbed, as with organophosphate pesticides, the best course of action is to scrub the skin, using a series of detergent washings. Gastrointestinal decontamination involves gastric emptying, use of activated charcoal, and chemical catharsis.

Gastric Emptying. Gastric emptying is achieved by one of two methods: *induced emesis* or *gastric lavage*. Historically, emesis has been achieved in a variety of ways, including forced ingestion of salt water, pharyngeal stimulation, and drug induction. The most reliable method is the use of the drug apomorphine or syrup of ipecac. These compounds cause emesis in more than 90% of cases. Although apomorphine is no longer used because of its side effects, syrup of ipecac is still widely employed and is recommended as a first-line treatment for many toxic ingestions. Although syrup of ipecac can be purchased without a prescription, it is to be used judiciously. Contraindications to its use are summarized in Table 19–7. Optimally this compound is administered as early as possible after the ingestion. (Its average time for inducing vomiting is 17 minutes.) Even then, ipecac-induced emesis results in only partial emptying of stomach contents.

The alternative to induced emesis is gastric lavage. This is a procedure referred to by the lay public as "pumping the stomach." The procedure involves passage of a large-bore orogastric tube (36 to 40 Fr in an adult) into the stomach and flushing the stomach of its contents with various kinds of fluids. Multiple 200- to 300-ml aliquots of fluid are sequentially instilled into the tube, allowed to mix with the gastric contents, and then drained by gravity. Recommendations for the volume of fluid that constitutes an optimal lavage vary. The most practical guideline is to continue lavage until the fluid is clear of any debris.

Gastric lavage is associated with some potential adverse effects. Hemorrhage, laryngospasm, esophageal tears, gastric perforation, pyriform sinus trauma, and aspiration are all possible. The most imminent danger is that of aspiration. Prior to using lavage, the physician must assess the ability of the patient to protect his airway by checking the gag reflex. If the gag is absent or weak and gastric lavage is necessary, the patient must first be intubated endotracheally. Even if the patient is able to protect his airway, there

TABLE 19–7. Contraindications to Syrup of Ipecac Usage

1. Infant age <6 months
2. Elderly patient
3. Actual or impending loss of airway reflexes due to coma, seizure, cardiovascular collapse
4. Rapidly acting CNS depressant, e.g., cyclic antidepressants, isoniazid, propoxyphene, propranolol
5. Caustic ingestions
6. Certain hydrocarbon ingestions
7. Hemorrhagic diathesis
8. Digoxin toxicity (increased vagal tone)

is still a small risk of aspiration. This risk can be minimized by placing the patient in the Trendelenburg and left lateral decubitus positions during lavage.

Like syrup of ipecac–induced emesis, gastric lavage cannot be relied on to completely empty the stomach of its contents. It is particularly inefficacious when pill fragments are large or of the slow-release variety. Although no data clearly indicate one approach to be more effective than another, gastric lavage is currently preferred over ipecac-induced emesis for most cases in which gastric emptying is indicated. Ipecac-induced emesis is advantageous for treating children who cannot be effectively treated by lavage owing to the need for small tube sizes, for ingestions of large or sustained-release tablets, or for ingestions of agents such as iron-containing compounds or lithium that are not well adsorbed by activated charcoal.

Currently, there is a declining emphasis on gastric emptying. The trend has been toward a more selective approach to using this intervention. Emptying the stomach is no longer indicated for the management of ingestions of low-toxic or nontoxic potential. It is also unlikely to be beneficial for the removal of rapidly absorbed drugs like ethanol and acetaminophen or if spontaneous emesis has already occurred. Furthermore, gastric emptying is contraindicated when the risks of intervention are outweighed by the potential benefits, e.g., in patients with caustic ingestions.

Activated Charcoal. Activated charcoal has been rapidly gaining favor as the most effective modality for reducing the gastrointestinal absorption of toxic compounds. Until recently, the role of this material has been regarded as secondary to that of gastric emptying. The reasons for this are understandable. Even in suspension, activated charcoal has a gritty texture and is unpalatable in appearance. As such, patients are frequently reluctant to drink it. It can result in vomiting and be quite messy, a characteristic that significantly reduces enthusiasm for its use among emergency department nursing staffs. Despite these shortcomings, activated charcoal has become a highly regarded therapeutic modality.

Activated charcoal prevents absorption of a compound by binding molecules of the dissolved portion of the compound to its surface. Its efficacy depends mostly on the surface area available for adsorption. Most available forms are wood-based, but the newer petroleum-based activated charcoals such as Superchar have significantly greater surface areas and are now the agents of choice. A 10:1 ratio of wood-based activated charcoal to ingested compound is effective for most agents *in vitro*. For example, if 10 gm of a compound is ingested, then 100 gm of activated charcoal is administered. This ratio may serve as a rough guideline for treatment, but in practice the best dose is the maximum amount tolerated. The volume of diluent necessary to facilitate administration of activated charcoal limits the maximal tolerated dose to 1 to 2 gm/kg at one time. Should this dose fall short of that required to achieve a 10:1 treatment ratio, either a petroleum-based activated charcoal or multiple doses of a standard activated charcoal may be useful to achieve optimal results.

Recent studies have demonstrated the superiority of activated charcoal to syrup of ipecac–induced emesis in limiting the absorption of certain compounds. Furthermore, activated charcoal is nontoxic. Although there are no absolute contraindications to its use, activated charcoal is withheld in patients who have ingested caustic substances to avoid obscuring the endoscopic examination and in patients who have ingested pure petroleum distillates to avoid emesis. These observations, along with the knowledge that the great majority of toxic compounds will, at least in part, be adsorbed by activated charcoal, greatly expand the possibilities associated with its use. Although activated charcoal is unpalatable and messy to use, abundant data reinforce its position in the early management of a wide variety of toxic ingestions, often in lieu of gastric emptying. Administration in opaque, covered containers and admixture with pleasant-tasting solutions may improve patient cooperation.

Cathartics. Cathartics can counteract the constipating effect of activated charcoal and lessen the intestinal transit time of the drug-charcoal complex, potentially reducing the amount of drug that desorbs from charcoal during its intestinal passage. Although activated charcoal is given simply as an aqueous slurry, the initial dose is usually given with a cathartic agent.

Numerous cathartic agents are available. Saline cathartics such as magnesium citrate or magnesium sulfate are the most commonly used. Standard doses are 4 ml/kg of a 10% solution (up to 300 ml) of the former and 250 mg/kg (up to 30 gm) of the latter. Both cathartics are given as slurries with activated charcoal either orally or by nasogastric tube. A single dose of either is quite safe except in the presence of renal failure. In this setting, a large magnesium load may not be handled well by the kidneys, and symptomatic hypermagnesemia may develop. Repeat dosing with magnesium-containing cathartics can occasionally result in a similar consequence even in patients with normal renal function.

Recently, the osmotic cathartic sorbitol has become more popular. Administered as a 35% to 70% solution, sorbitol is both sweet and viscous. These features lessen the unpalatable characteristics of activated charcoal and increase the likelihood that it will be ingested voluntarily by the patient. Furthermore, some evidence suggests that sorbitol may act more rapidly to produce diarrhea than either magnesium citrate or sulfate. The vigorous catharsis that often follows the use of sorbitol is associated with stomach cramps and can also result in fluid and electrolyte abnormalities in small children. These problems may be lessened by limiting the sorbitol dose and avoiding repeat doses, particularly in children. Current data suggest that the most appropriate dose range is from 0.5 to 1.5 gm/kg. The smaller 0.5 gm/kg dose in a 35% concentration is preferred for children.

Oil-based cathartic agents such as castor oil deserve mention only to be condemned. Use of these cathartics has been associated with a high incidence of aspiration pneumonia in children and is no longer recommended.

Whole bowel irrigation is accomplished by using large volumes of a polyethylene glycol lavage solution such as *Golytely*. Because these solutions are isotonic, their use does not result in fluid or electrolyte imbalance. They may be particularly beneficial in removing cocaine packets found in "body packers" and large quantities of compounds not well adsorbed by activated charcoal, e.g., iron or lithium.

Maximization of Elimination

Although gastric emptying, activated charcoal, and catharsis are useful for limiting the absorption of orally ingested compounds, by the time these interventions are made, a significant amount of compound may have already been absorbed. Elimination of absorbed toxins is often enhanced by hemodialysis, hemoperfusion, forced diuresis, or multidose activated charcoal therapy. These techniques are considered when the compound involved can result in significant tissue toxicity and is amenable to treatment by one of these modalities.

Hemodialysis. Hemodialysis is a procedure in which blood is circulated extracorporeally past a semipermeable dialysis membrane through which certain molecules diffuse passively, thereby being removed from the blood and body. Certain compounds and electrolytes are readily eliminated from the body by this procedure. Dialysis is more effective for compounds that are small, water-soluble, and poorly protein bound (Table 19–8). These are usually compounds that are largely eliminated by the kidney. Therefore, one indication for hemodialysis is intoxication with one of these compounds in the presence of renal dysfunction. Since this procedure is invasive, associated with some adverse consequences, and somewhat expensive, risk-benefit analyses govern its application in each individual case.

Hemoperfusion. Hemoperfusion is similar to hemodialysis in that blood is also

TABLE 19–8. Intoxicants for Which Dialysis Is Especially Useful

Methanol	Salicylate
Ethylene glycol	Lithium
Ethanol	Procainamide

circulated extracorporeally, but the blood passes through a column filled with adsorbent material rather than past a semipermeable membrane. As blood admixes with the adsorbent material, which is usually some form of activated charcoal, molecules of the toxic compound are bound to it electrostatically, thereby being removed from the circulation. Because hemoperfusion does not involve passive diffusion of molecules, some poorly dialyzable, lipid-soluble, protein-bound compounds can be eliminated in significant quantities by this process. Hemoperfusion is recognized as the most valuable modality for eliminating theophylline at very high blood levels. It has also proved useful for eliminating other drugs such as glutethimide, methaqualone, and barbiturates. Many authorities believe that the associated risks of this procedure (hypotension, hemorrhage, and hypocalcemia) do not warrant its use for agents whose effects can be adequately treated by supportive care alone.

Forced Diuresis. Forced diuresis is a relatively noninvasive technique for drug elimination. Significant quantities of some drugs are reabsorbed from the renal tubule after glomerular filtration has occurred. By increasing urine flow by means of volume loading and a diuretic, tubular reabsorption is significantly reduced and elimination of drug enhanced.

Unfortunately, simple forced osmotic diuresis is rarely effective. Satisfactory results are more commonly achieved only after acidifying or alkalinizing the urine, thereby trapping weak bases and weak acids, respectively, within the renal tubule by creating conditions that favor their ionization.

Forced alkaline diuresis is indicated for the treatment of salicylate, phenobarbital, and chlorpropamide intoxication. Alkalinization of the urine traps these weak acids in the urine in the ionized state, preventing their reabsorption by the renal tubules. The hazards of urinary alkalinization are primarily acid-base disturbances that can be forestalled by appropriate monitoring of blood pH. The associated volume loading, on the other hand, can increase the risk of cerebral or pulmonary edema. Fortunately, current evidence now suggests that diuresis is not as important as urinary alkalinization in enhancing drug elimination. Therefore, the problem of volume overload can be avoided simply by pursuing a more moderate approach to diuresis.

Forced acid diuresis has been suggested on theoretical grounds for the elimination of amphetamines and phencyclidine. However, not only is the clinical usefulness of this intervention unproved, it may actually be dangerous. Rhabdomyolysis may occur during severe amphetamine or PCP intoxication, and an acid urine may increase precipitation of the resultant urinary myoglobin, leading to renal failure.

Multidose Activated Charcoal Therapy. Multidose activated charcoal therapy is perhaps the safest means of increasing the rate of drug elimination. Also known as "pulse therapy" or "gastrointestinal dialysis," this treatment is useful to varying degrees for hastening the elimination of a variety of drugs. Originally thought to be applicable primarily to the elimination of drugs with an enterohepatic recirculation, multidose activated charcoal therapy has proved useful for removing phenobarbital, theophylline, and other compounds that do not have this metabolic pathway.

The technique of treatment involves administration of moderate doses of activated charcoal (10 to 50 gm) at frequent intervals (1 to 4 hours) until clinical resolution of toxicity is seen. The persistent presence of activated charcoal in the intestinal lumen creates a gradient between the intestinal fluid and the capillary blood of the gastrointestinal mucosa that favors passage of drug molecules from blood to intestinal fluid, where they are bound and eliminated.

Physiologic Antagonists

Antagonist agents are a diverse group of compounds that block, reverse, slow, or lessen the adverse effects of various intoxicants through a variety of mechanisms. With some exceptions, the actions of antagonists are generally quite specific against certain classes of toxic compounds. Therefore, the physician must know the type of toxic compound

Specific Therapy

Certain drugs are either so commonly encountered in overdose situations or cause such significant morbidity if an overdose is not identified and properly treated that they will be discussed specifically. The alcohols and cocaine are discussed at greater length in Chapters 20 and 23.

Acetaminophen

Acetaminophen is remarkably safe at therapeutic dosages but can cause fatal hepatic necrosis after an overdose. Understanding the toxicity of acetaminophen and the rationale behind antidotal therapy requires an understanding of acetaminophen metabolism. Hepatic metabolism to nontoxic glucuronide and sulfate conjugates accounts for 90% to 95% of the disposition of acetaminophen. A small fraction (1% to 2%) is excreted unchanged in the urine. The remaining drug is converted to a highly reactive, potentially destructive intermediate through the cytochrome P450 mixed function oxidase system. Normally, this intermediate is quickly conjugated with glutathione to nontoxic metabolites. After acetaminophen overdose, however, the rate of glutathione use exceeds the rate of regeneration, glutathione stores become depleted, and the unconjugated toxic intermediate reacts with and destroys hepatocytes. The same reaction can occur in the kidneys, and abnormal results on renal function tests occur in about 10% of patients with hepatotoxicity and, rarely, in patients without liver injury. The true "toxic" dosage of acetaminophen is variable, but ingestions of 7.5 gm in an adult and 150 mg/kg in a child are considered potentially toxic.

Within a few hours of overdose, nonspecific signs and symptoms such as nausea, vomiting, pallor, and diaphoresis may occur, but even severely poisoned patients may remain asymptomatic. During the initial 18 to 24 hours (stage 1) there is no laboratory evidence of hepatic or renal injury. If hepatotoxicity develops, aminotransferase levels

TABLE 19–9. Toxic Compounds and Their Antagonist Agents

Toxic Compound	Antagonist
Carbon monoxide	Oxygen
Opiates	Naloxone (Narcan)
Anticholinergics	Physostigmine
Organophosphates	Atropine, pralidoxime (2-PAM)
Carbamates	Atropine
Nitrates/nitrites (methemoglobinemia)	Methylene blue
Acetaminophen	N-acetyl cysteine (Mucomyst/oral)[a]
Methanol	Ethanol, folate
Ethylene glycol	Ethanol, pyridoxine, thiamine
Cyanide	Lilly cyanide kit:
	Amyl nitrite
	Sodium nitrite
	Sodium thiosulfate
	Hydroxycobalamin[b]
Digoxin	Digoxin-specific FAB antibody fragments (Digibind)
Beta-blockers	Glucagon
Iron	Deferoxamine
Other heavy metals	Dimercaprol (BAL)
	Calcium EDTA
	D-Penicillamine
Benzodiazepines	Flumazenil[b]

[a] Intravenous use of N-acetyl cysteine is under investigation.
[b] Use under investigation.

begin to rise after 18 to 24 hours (stage 2), and this increase is accompanied by symptoms (nausea, vomiting, right upper quadrant pain), signs (hepatic enlargement and tenderness, jaundice), and laboratory abnormalities (hyperbilirubinemia, increased prothrombin time) in proportion to the degree of injury. Peak hepatotoxicity (stage 3) usually occurs 72 to 96 hours after overdose. Aminotransferase levels above 10,000 IU/liter are common. With major overdoses, massive necrosis of the liver can occur, but recovery is the rule. Serum bilirubin concentrations higher than 4 mg/dl and a prothrombin time of more than twice normal have been suggested as more ominous prognostic signs. Recovery (stage 4) usually occurs over a few days but may be slower in severe cases. If patients survive, recovery is complete, with no evidence of chronic hepatotoxicity.

The most important feature of acetaminophen poisoning is that although the signs and symptoms of hepatotoxicity are delayed for 18 to 36 hours, antidotal therapy is most effective if it is started within 8 hours and is relatively ineffective after 16 hours. Because drug histories are unreliable, the plasma acetaminophen concentration is the only reliable method of predicting potential toxicity. It should be measured in all cases of suspected acetaminophen overdose, polydrug overdose, and overdose of drugs of abuse often combined with acetaminophen (e.g., codeine, propoxyphene). The Matthew-Rumack nomogram (Fig. 19–1) is used to predict the severity of toxicity and the need for antidotal therapy. Proper use requires that the blood sample be drawn at least 4 hours postingestion. Patients with acetaminophen concentrations above the line shown in the treatment nomogram are treated with *N*-acetylcysteine (NAC).

NAC serves primarily as a glutathione precursor, but it also is a glutathione substitute, and it increases the supply of substrate for the nontoxic sulfate conjugation pathway. Oral NAC (intravenous NAC is not yet approved in the United States) is an extremely effective antidote if it is started within 8 hours of overdose, and although its efficacy starts to decline thereafter, the current standard of care is to treat patients as late as 24 hours after overdose. The decision to treat with NAC can await determination of acetaminophen levels if they will be available within 8 hours of ingestion of the overdose. If they are not available during that period, it is best to initiate NAC treatment while awaiting results and then to discontinue or continue it accordingly.

In vitro, NAC is adsorbed by activated charcoal, causing some to question whether the use of activated charcoal might significantly decrease the efficacy of NAC. Although this question is still being studied, the best information to date is that this concern is unfounded. In mixed drug overdose, gastric emptying and charcoal are used as indicated, without regard to the presence of acetaminophen. After pure acetaminophen overdose, absorption is rapid. Therefore, gastric emptying is not done more than 2 hours after an overdose, and treatment with activated charcoal is probably logical only within the first few hours after ingestion.

Aspirin

The therapeutic index (the ratio of the maximally tolerated dose to the minimally therapeutic dose) of aspirin (acetylsalicylic acid) is quite low, and toxicity often occurs after repeated dosing with normal or slightly above normal amounts as well as after single acute overdoses.

Aspirin has primary effects on several organ systems. It stimulates the central respiratory system directly, uncouples oxidative phosphorylation, inhibits the Krebs cycle and amino acid metabolism, and interferes with normal hemostasis. As a result, the possible signs and symptoms of poisoning are varied and numerous. Tinnitus is common even with minimal overdoses in the range of 4 gm taken over 24 hours and blood levels greater than 25 mg/dl. Nausea, vomiting, and hyperpnea (with or without tachypnea) are also common. Although slight lethargy and confusion may occur in moderately severe cases, hyperpyrexia or profound central nervous system abnormalities (seizure, coma) imply life-threatening toxicity. Noncardiogenic and cardiogenic pulmonary edema may also occur in severe cases.

366 — TOXICOLOGIC/ENVIRONMENTAL DISORDERS

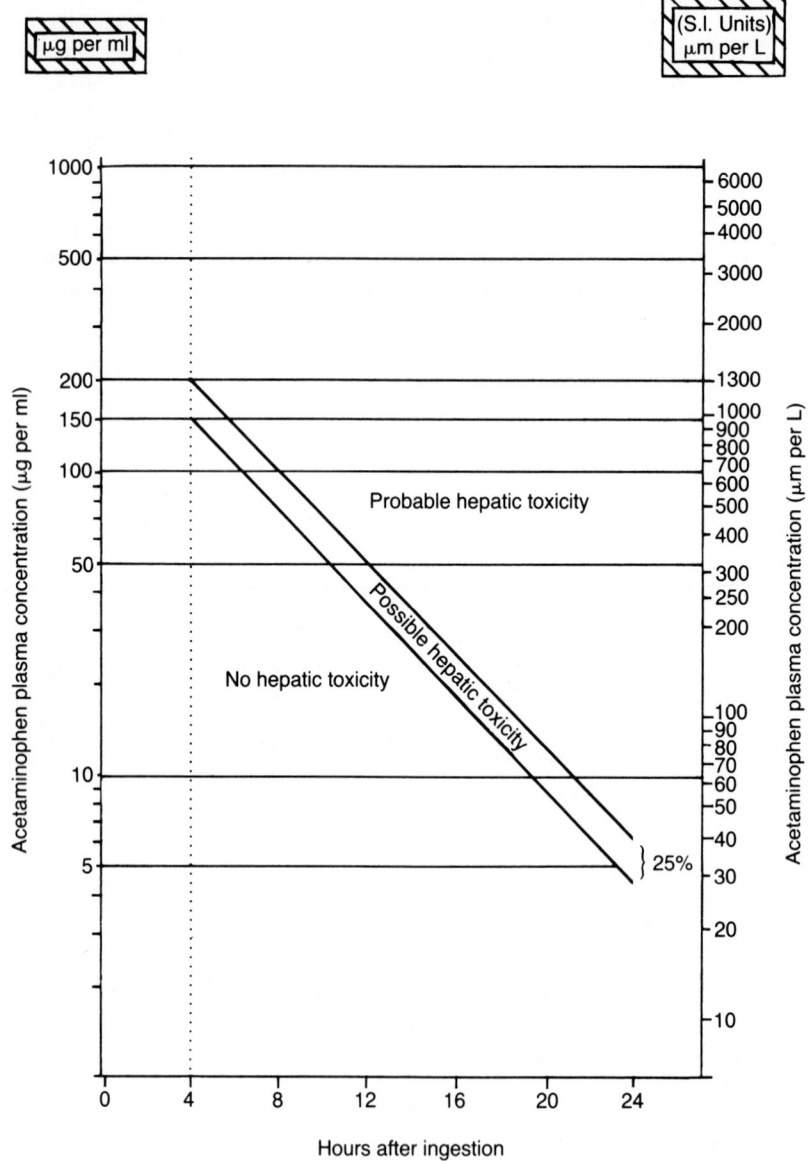

FIGURE 19–1. Rumack-Matthew nomogram for acetaminophen poisoning. (With permission from Micromedex, Inc. Adapted from Pediatrics 55[6], June 1975, with permission from the authors and the publisher. Copyright © Micromedex, Inc. 1974–1985. All rights reserved.)

Of the acid-base disorders caused by salicylates, alkalemia (pH of greater than 7.45) is most common; it is due initially to pure respiratory alkalosis and later to mixed respiratory alkalosis with a lesser metabolic acidosis. In severe cases, especially in children, metabolic acidosis eventually predominates, leading to acidemia (pH of less than 7.35). In addition to primary salicylate-induced acid-base disorders, fever, hyperpnea, and vomiting frequently lead to secondary dehydration and electrolyte abnormalities, which may complicate management. The accumulation of "unmeasured" anions (ketoacids, salicylate, lactate) causes an increase in the anion gap, and salicylate toxicity is considered in any case of an increased anion gap metabolic acidosis. Urine evaluation is also helpful in making the diagnosis. Urine ketones are often present owing to the interference of salicylate with normal glucose and amino acid metabolism. Urine ferric chloride testing provides an extremely sensitive but nonspecific test. This reagent, when mixed with salicylate-containing urine, turns purple. Phenothiazines, alpha-methyldopa, and other agents also produce color changes in ferric chloride–treated urine; however, these colors are clearly distinguishable from that caused by salicylates.

Hepatic salicylate metabolism is limited, and enzyme saturation occurs even at therapeutic dosages. As a result, after an acute overdose or after drug accumulation from repeated doses (chronic toxicity), other routes must be used to enhance elimination. Salicylate exists in both its ionized and unionized forms. Both are readily filtered into the urine, but only the unionized form is reabsorbed. Since the ratio of ionized to unionized drug increases tenfold for each pH unit increase, alkalinization of the urine increases the proportion of ionized salicylate and prevents drug reabsorption (ion trapping). The pK_a (pH at which the concentrations of ionized and unionized drug are equal) of salicylate is 3.5; therefore, increasing urine pH to 7 or higher by administering sodium bicarbonate significantly enhances the urinary elimination of the drug. When alkalinization is not possible or not effective or when more rapid drug removal is indicated, hemodialysis is required. Indications for dialysis include renal failure, pulmonary edema, seizures, any significant alteration in mental status, severe acid-base or electrolyte disturbance, or, in the absence of these, a salicylate level of above 100 mg/dl.

The most common and most serious errors in the management of patients with salicylate poisoning result from a reliance on blood levels rather than on signs and symptoms in assessing patients. In some cases, drug levels accurately reflect actual toxicity. However, in many cases, particularly cases of chronic toxicity, significant increases in tissue levels may occur during a gradual fall in blood levels, resulting in serious symptoms with unimpressive drug levels. This is particularly true in the presence of acidemia. As discussed previously, even small decreases in pH can dramatically increase the proportion of unionized drug. Just as lower pH favors drug reabsorption from the urine, acidemia allows dramatically increased absorption into the tissues from the blood. Since increased toxicity results in further acidosis, the process can accelerate. As a result, acidemia due to salicylate poisoning is always considered an emergency, regardless of the blood level.

Cyclic Antidepressants

Overdose of a cyclic antidepressant is one of the most common toxicologic causes of morbidity and mortality, despite advances in diagnosis and treatment. Several newer agents differ in toxicity from earlier products, but some general principles apply.

Although other non–life-threatening symptoms of toxicity are often evident (anticholinergic syndrome, myoclonic jerks), the major toxic effects of cyclic antidepressants are divided into three areas: dysrhythmias (ectopy, sinus and ventricular tachycardias, QRS and Q–T prolongation), central nervous system abnormalities (delirium, coma, seizures), and hypotension.

Sinus tachycardia due to the anticholinergic effect of cyclic antidepressants is present in more than 80% of cases. Conduction defects and serious rhythm disturbances are due to "quinidine-like" effects. Inhibition of fast inward sodium channels (action potential phase 0) prevents normal rapid depolarization of myocardial cells, slowing conduction and promoting ectopy. On the electrocardiogram, abnormal depolarization may appear only as subtle changes in QRS morphology and vector analysis, or there may be obvious QRS or Q–T prolongation with major axis deviation. Sinus tachycardia with aberrant conduction is common and is often mistaken for ventricular tachycardia.

The onset of toxicity usually occurs early (1 to 3 hours after overdose), and more important, the progression from asymptomatic or minor toxicity to major toxicity is often very abrupt. As a result, syrup of ipecac is not used because loss of the gag reflex and onset of cardiovascular collapse or seizures may occur before emesis is completed. Treatment of conduction defects and tachydysrhythmias starts with alkalinization of the serum to pH 7.45 to 7.55. Unlike the situation in salicylate poisoning, in which alkalinization is undertaken to raise the urine pH and enhance elimination, alkalinization of the serum after cyclic antidepressant overdose is done to diminish the toxic effects of the overdose. The mechanism is still controversial, but serum alkalinization rapidly improves conduction. Both sodium bicarbonate and hyperventilation have been used, but experimentally, the use of bicarbonate appears to be faster and somewhat more effective. Many toxicologists recommend alkalinization whenever the QRS interval is greater than 0.10 second after cyclic antidepressant overdose, and it is certainly indicated whenever hypotension or ventricular dysrhythmias occur. If alkalinization fails, standard antidysrhythmic drugs are used to treat ventricular dysrhythmias, with the exception of class Ia agents (quinidine, diisopyramide, procainamide). Newer class Ic agents (flecainide, ecainide) probably should be excluded as well.

Neurologic manifestations are treated supportively with airway protection, ventilatory support, and rapid control of seizures with diazepam to prevent acidosis and resultant worsening of cardiotoxicity.

Hypotension is caused by both decreased inotropy (quinidine-like effect) and peripheral alpha-adrenergic blockade. Decreased inotropy is best treated with alkalinization, but in most cases of hypotension additional treatment will be needed. A fluid challenge (500 to 2000 ml of isotonic crystalloid solution) will usually correct the hypotension, but vasopressor therapy is required in some patients. Dopamine is often ineffective owing to antidepressant-induced blockade of catecholamine uptake, but direct-acting alpha-adrenergic agents such as norepinephrine or neosynephrine are effective. Despite its ability to reverse anticholinergic signs and symptoms transiently, physostigmine is not recommended to treat cyclic antidepressant toxicity. The limited benefit of this drug is outweighed by occurrences of asystole, seizures, and other complications reported after physostigmine use.

Currently, the QRS duration is the best predictor of subsequent risk for seizures or ventricular dysrhythmias. For older agents, such as amitriptyline, nortriptyline, imipramine, desipramine, doxepin, and protriptyline, only patients who develop a QRS interval of greater than 0.10 second within 6 hours of overdose appear to be at significant risk for subsequent seizures or dysrhythmias. For newer agents, such as amoxapine, loxapine, maprotaline, and trazadone, this relationship may not apply. In fact, refractory seizures and coma have been described without QRS widening after amoxapine overdose.

Carbon Monoxide

Carbon monoxide (CO) poisoning is a major cause of morbidity and mortality that may be easily missed. Combustion of any organic fuel generates CO; thus, in addition to suicidal exposures, accidental home exposures (as from gas water heaters, furnaces, space heaters, fireplaces, barbecues, automobile exhaust) and occupational exposures (as from gasoline-powered tools and machinery) are common. The diagnosis is often difficult because the exposure is not recognized and the symptoms are so nonspecific. Though CO poisoning is a year-round problem, the onset of cold weather is a time these cases are often seen.

CO combines with hemoglobin to form carboxyhemoglobin (COHb) and causes toxicity in three ways: decreased oxygen-carrying capacity (COHb cannot transport oxygen), decreased oxygen delivery (the oxyhemoglobin dissociation curve shifts to the left in the presence of CO), and, possibly, decreased oxygen utilization (cytochrome oxidase is inhibited). The result is cellular asphyxia in proportion to the extent of exposure, with potentially severe multisystem anoxic injury.

There are no methods available to determine the levels of tissue CO; thus, blood COHb levels are used to assess exposure. Smokers, particularly those in urban settings, may have COHb levels as high as 4% to 10%, but they are generally asymptomatic. Levels ranging from 10% to 20% are associated with headache, dyspnea on exertion, and exertional angina in predisposed individuals. These symptoms become worse at COHb levels between 20% and 30%, and dizziness, nausea, vomiting, visual disturbances, and impaired judgment often occur when levels reach 30% to 40%. Levels above 40% are nearly always associated with severe symptoms such as syncope, altered mental status, tachypnea, and tachycardia. At blood COHb levels above 50%, seizures, coma, and marked acidosis are usually evident, and at levels in excess of 60%, fatalities are common. It is critically important to remember that patients often have serious sequelae at levels much lower than the corresponding levels listed. Cases have been reported of clinical toxicity with unmeasurable blood levels. Therefore physician suspicion must remain high.

Treatment consists of supportive care and oxygen. The higher the concentration of oxygen delivered, the more rapidly CO is eliminated from both blood and tissue. Although there is a great variation, COHb levels decrease by 50% (half-life) after about 4 to 6 hours of breathing room air, after 40 to 90 minutes of breathing 100% oxygen, and after 20 minutes in hyperbaric oxygen (HBO) at 3 atm pressure. All symptomatic patients should receive at least 100% oxygen for at least 4 hours or until they are asymptomatic and COHb levels are less than 5% (whichever is longer), and many should receive HBO.

Indications for HBO are controversial but generally include evidence of significant tissue anoxia, as manifested by loss of consciousness, chest pain, ischemic electrocardiographic (ECG) changes, acidosis, hypotension, or any cognitive or neurologic abnormality. In the absence of these signs and symptoms, each HBO center establishes a COHb level above which HBO is offered. These levels vary from 25% to 40%. Because the fetus tolerates CO very poorly, pregnant victims often receive HBO if they have COHb levels as low as 15%. High-risk or difficult to assess groups such as infants, the elderly, and patients with abnormal baseline cardiovascular function also should receive HBO at lower COHb levels.

Supportive care can be complex owing to the multisystemic nature of postanoxic injury. Myocardial infarction, dysrhythmias, shock, pulmonary edema, anoxic encephalopathy, rhabdomyolysis, and renal failure have all been described following CO poisoning. In addition, delayed and permanent neuropsychiatric and neurologic abnormalities occur. The most serious errors in management result from failure to consider the diagnosis, undertreatment because of an unimpressive blood COHb level in patients with ongoing organ dysfunction (i.e., ongoing tissue toxicity), and failure to consider that other victims (family members, neighbors, coworkers) must be assessed and the source of CO established and eliminated.

Caustics

Despite the frequent occurrence and serious morbidity of caustic ingestions, the ideal management method remains highly controversial. Furthermore, management varies among the various types of caustics.

Upper airway edema may occur after ingestion of any caustic substance, and endotracheal intubation is performed if there is any physical evidence of stridor, respiratory distress or cyanosis, or laryngoscopic evidence of impending airway compromise. Intravenous access is established routinely.

Initial care includes attempts to wash the caustic material from the oral mucosa and dilute the ingested agent with 4 to 6 ounces of water or milk. Neutralization of acids or bases is not recommended because of the unproved efficacy of this method and because of concern that the heat of neutralization may add thermal injury to the underlying chemical injury. Spontaneous vomiting is common after caustic ingestions, but induction of emesis is contraindicated because this reexposes the esophagus, hypopharynx, and larynx to the caustic agent, thus increasing the injury. The increased intragastric pressure during emesis also increases the risk of gastric rupture. Similarly, passage of a large-bore orogastric tube is also contraindicated because of the risk of injuring or perforating the hypopharynx, esophagus, or stomach. Whether a small-bore, flexible tube should be used to aspirate the stomach contents after ingestions of large amounts of caustic agents that can lead to systemic toxicity (acids, formaldehyde, and phenols) remains controversial. Activated charcoal does not effectively adsorb most caustics, obscures endoscopic findings, and is contraindicated.

Alkaline corrosives, such as sodium or potassium hydroxide drain cleaners, produce a liquefaction necrosis with deep penetration and marked softening of exposed tissue. Although all portions of the upper alimentary tract are affected, morbidity and mortality are most often due to esophageal injury. Liquefaction of the esophagus may lead to early perforation and mediastinitis, and survivors of this early phase often develop delayed lower esophageal strictures from scar formation. These individuals also have a markedly increased risk of esophageal cancer later in life. Due to the gradual penetration of alkaline corrosives, some authorities recommend that endoscopy be delayed at least 12 hours to allow accurate assessment of the full extent of the injury. In reality, assessment of the extent of involvement and determination of whether tissue injury is superficial, partial-thickness, or full-thickness can be made within a few hours, and allows for earlier planning of therapy.

Surgical management is controversial, but surgical consultation is recommended. Pharmacologic therapy is also highly controversial but includes use of broad spectrum antibiotics in cases of suspected esophageal perforation and high-dose steroids to diminish delayed stricture formation in patients with circumferential partial-thickness esophageal burns.

Acid burns create a coagulation necrosis that often limits the penetration of the acid. Unfortunately, after exposures to large amounts, damage still results in perforation. Acid burns also can affect all exposed areas but, unlike alkalies, more often lead to severe gastric injury (erosive gastritis, hemorrhage, and perforation). Endoscopy is again important in assessment, and management is even more controversial than for injuries due to alkalies. Also unlike alkalies, which have not been shown to cause systemic alkalosis, there is some evidence that acid ingestion can cause systemic acidosis.

Perhaps the most controversial aspect of caustic ingestions concerns the reliability of using signs and symptoms to predict which patients have serious burns requiring endoscopy and further therapy. Previous studies suggested that serious alkaline corrosive esophageal burns could be present without any drooling, vomiting, chest or abdominal pain, stridor, or oropharyngeal burns, but recently this viewpoint has been questioned. Certainly endoscopy is always indicated after ingestion of Clinitest tablets or impacted miniature batteries because they can cause serious local esophageal injury without any initial symptoms or oropharyngeal injury. For other caustics, the controversy continues.

Iron

Iron overdose remains a common toxicologic problem, probably because of both the wide availability of iron-containing preparations and its marketing in colors and shapes that are especially appealing to small children.

Several iron salts containing different amounts of elemental iron are available. Ferrous sulfate (20% iron) is most common, but ferrous gluconate (12%), fumarate (33%), lactate (19%), chloride (28%), and ferrocholinate (13%) are also encountered. Since the most important determinant of toxicity appears to be the amount of elemental iron ingested, these proportions are useful in estimating the iron dose received. Ingestions of less than 20 mg/kg of elemental iron are unlikely to cause toxicity; at between 20 and 60 mg/kg of elemental iron, toxicity is not surprising and is expected after ingestions of over 60 mg/kg of elemental iron.

Toxicity is often categorized into stages. The first stage is due primarily to direct gastrointestinal injury. It occurs from 30 minutes to 6 hours after ingestion and may include nausea, vomiting, hematemesis, abdominal pain, diarrhea, melena, pallor, lethargy, hypotension, and acidosis. The next stage (occurring up to 24 hours after ingestion) is a period of apparent stabilization and improvement that does not always occur. A third stage may occur consisting of cardiovascular collapse and acidosis representing decompensation due to systemic iron toxicity and complications of the initial stage. Hepatotoxicity occasionally occurs 2 to 4 days after ingestion and is sometimes considered a separate stage. The final stage (2 to 4 weeks after ingestion) consists of pyloric or intestinal obstruction due to stricture formation at sites of severe iron-induced injury.

Supportive care, fluid resuscitation, and administration of blood products are provided as needed for volume depletion, hypotension, and gastrointestinal bleeding. Diagnostic assessment of patients with potential iron toxicity includes determination of serum iron and total iron-binding capacity (TIBC), complete blood count, serum chemistries, and abdominal radiographs.

Gastric emptying is attempted if spontaneous vomiting has not occurred or if radiopaque iron is visible in the stomach on plain radiographs. Activated charcoal does not adsorb iron and need not be given. Because diarrhea is common, cathartics are generally not used; they may worsen fluid and electrolyte abnormalities. Whole bowel irrigation using *Golytely* (nonabsorbable isotonic polyethylene glycol solution) to flush iron through the gastrointestinal tract is a new adjunct in management. It does not cause fluid or electrolyte shifts.

Bicarbonate or phosphate solutions have been given orally or enterally to convert iron to a less readily absorbed form. Phosphate solutions can cause dehydration, hypernatremia, hyperphosphatemia, hypocalcemia, and acidosis and have not been shown to be clinically useful. Bicarbonate solution is generally safe, but recent studies cast doubt on its clinical efficacy.

Normally, serum iron is bound to various proteins, and no free iron is present. Serious iron toxicity is due to free iron and therefore does not occur unless the serum iron exceeds the TIBC. As a result, toxicity generally occurs only when serum iron is above 300 μg/dl, and serious toxicity is unusual unless serum iron exceeds 500 μg/dl. Deferoxamine, given intramuscularly or intravenously, chelates free iron to form ferrioxamine, which is then eliminated in the urine, causing the urine to change color to a pink-orange hue ("vin rose" urine). Deferoxamine treatment is indicated when serum iron exceeds TIBC, but often treatment decisions are made without benefit of these values. Any patient with serious symptomatology after iron overdose should receive deferoxamine without waiting for laboratory confirmation. In patients without serious symptoms, hyperglycemia and leukocytosis may indicate elevated serum iron values. A single dose of deferoxamine is often given as a "challenge" to see if the color of the urine changes, indicating the presence of chelatable free iron.

Theophylline

Theophylline toxicity has developed into one of the most important toxicologic problems faced by emergency physicians. Perhaps more than any other kind of poisoning, theophylline toxicity requires the treating physician to understand the principles of pharmacology, general poison management, cardiovascular physiology, and specialized methods of treatment such as hemoperfusion.

Theophylline poisoning generally occurs in one of two settings: acute intentional overdose or accidental gradual (chronic) overdosing. Chronic overdoses may result from dosing calculation errors but probably more common are "appropriate" doses in patients with an impaired ability to metabolize the drug. Any interference with the hepatic metabolism of theophylline can cause toxicity. Alcoholic liver disease, liver congestion due to right-sided heart failure, medications (e.g., erythromycin, propranolol, or cimetidine), and some infections slow metabolism and lead to theophylline toxicity.

Gastrointestinal symptoms (nausea, vomiting, diarrhea) are common regardless of the severity of toxicity. Cardiovascular effects may include sinus tachycardia, premature atrial contractions, supraventricular tachycardias, atrial flutter or fibrillation, ventricular ectopy, ventricular tachycardia, ventricular fibrillation, and refractory hypotension. Central nervous system effects include tremor, anxiety, agitation, and seizures. Laboratory abnormalities are also common and include hypokalemia, lactic acidosis, leukocytosis, hyperglycemia, hypomagnesemia, and hypophosphatemia.

Serum theophylline levels are useful but must be interpreted cautiously. Chronic overdoses result in serious toxicity at much lower drug levels than acute overdoses. In all cases, the degree of symptomatology is the most important factor in determining therapy, but many authors consider a drug level of 60 µg/ml in a patient with a chronic overdose roughly equivalent in significance to a level of 100 µg/ml after an acute overdose. Since morbidity and mortality are significant above these levels, they are used as indications for hemoperfusion. A common, and potentially lethal, mistake is failure to consider the pharmacokinetics of theophylline when interpreting serum levels. Most currently prescribed theophylline preparations are sustained-release formulations, which achieve peak levels as late as 8 to 12 hours after ingestion in therapeutic doses and even later after overdoses. If theophylline levels are obtained earlier, the severity of the overdose may be underestimated unless serial levels are obtained to illustrate the rate of rise and the efficacy of initial attempts to limit absorption. As a result, levels much lower than the commonly used "critical values" may indicate a need for hemoperfusion.

Orogastric lavage is preferable to ipecac to achieve gastric emptying to avoid protracted vomiting, which may interfere with successful administration of activated charcoal. Activated charcoal is a critical part of treatment because it is highly effective in both limiting gastrointestinal absorption and enhancing elimination of theophylline. Large initial doses of activated charcoal (2 gm/kg up to 100 gm) should be used, and frequent repeated doses (0.5 to 1.0 gm/kg every 1 to 2 hours) are given until toxicity has resolved and drug levels have declined. Antiemetics may be needed, and in some cases slow nasogastric instillation facilitates retention of charcoal. Hypokalemia is a common complication and should be corrected. This may reduce the incidence of dysrhythmias. Seizure control is often difficult. Rapid-acting intravenous agents such as benzodiazepines are used initially, followed by phenobarbital loading. Refractory seizures are treated by induction of barbiturate general anesthesia. Fluid challenges may not improve hypotension, and in severe cases vasopressors are also ineffective. In such cases, when hypotension is associated with evidence of shock (increasing acidosis, worsening mental status, or inadequate urine output), beta-blocker therapy is considered. Life-threatening hypotension is probably due more to beta-2 adrenergic-mediated vasodilatation than to decreased cardiac output from beta-1 adrenergic-mediated tachycardia. Propranolol has been useful experimentally and clinically in treating victims of severe theophylline toxicity, but it is considered only in extreme cases.

Extracorporeal theophylline removal using hemodialysis or charcoal hemoperfusion is effective in enhancing drug elimination. Since theophylline is highly protein bound, hemoperfusion is more effective than hemodialysis and is the preferred method of removal when it is available. Indications for extracorporeal removal include seizures, hemodynamically significant dysrhythmias, hypotension, or extremely high theophylline levels. Patients with a rapidly rising drug level or worsening symptoms, despite supportive care and multidose charcoal, are also candidates for hemoperfusion.

Amphetamines and Phencyclidine

Amphetamine toxicity causes nervous system excitation and adrenergic excesses that are similar to the effects of cocaine (Chap. 23), and its complications and treatment are also similar. Phencyclidine toxicity is another important cause of acute agitation. It differs in presentation in several ways from that of cocaine and amphetamine toxicity. PCP is not a sympathomimetic agent, and thus cardiovascular and pupillary findings are much less consistent. Tachycardia and hypertension are common but are not always present. Although pupillary findings vary, miosis is common. Bidirectional nystagmus is the most consistent physical examination finding after PCP intoxication but may be absent. A final distinguishing feature is the waxing and waning mental status of PCP overdosed patients. Unlike cocaine or amphetamine-induced agitation, which occurs early, peaks, and then diminishes progressively, PCP poisoned patients may alternate rapidly and unpredictably between violent agitation and deep coma. As in drug-induced agitation due to other causes, rhabdomyolysis, hyperthermia, and intracranial hemorrhage can result from PCP intoxication.

Sedative-Hypnotics

Sedative-hypnotic abuse is common, and overdose can lead to sedation, respiratory depression, coma, and hypotension. Ethanol, benzodiazepines, barbiturates, and many other medications are included in this broad category, but they may vary in clinical presentation. Benzodiazepines such as diazepam rarely lead to life-threatening toxicity except when used in combination with other agents. Large overdoses of barbiturates commonly cause serious symptoms, including hypotension. Glutethimide (Doriden) overdose is characterized by mydriasis and a prolonged waxing and waning type of mental status depression. The breath or gastric contents of patients with ethchlorvynol (Placidyl) overdose has a characteristic pungent, aromatic, vinyl-like odor. Meprobamate (Miltown) toxicity may also cause prolonged coma, and persistent gastric concretions have been described. Methaqualone (Quaalude) toxicity is now less common; it closely resembles barbiturate overdose. All sedative-hypnotics can produce drug dependence and lead to life-threatening drug withdrawal symptoms.

Opiates

Opiate overdose can result from use of single agents such as intravenous heroin or oral methadone or from combined exposures such as intravenous heroin and cocaine (Speedball), intravenous pentazocine and tripellenimine (Ts and blues), oral glutethimide and codeine (4s and doors). The numerous opioid products available for street use are far exceeded by available prescription formulations (analgesics, cough suppressants). The result is that opioid toxicity is common, comes in many forms, and is always considered in the differential diagnosis of patients with depressed mental status. Opioids characteristically cause sedation, respiratory depression, and miosis. Bradycardia is also common. The opioid antagonist naloxone (Narcan) will rapidly reverse these effects and will precipitate acute withdrawal in opioid dependent patients. Unlike sedative-hypnotic withdrawal, opioid withdrawal is not life-threatening. The safety and efficacy of naloxone and the varied presentations of opioid overdose have led to the routine use of naloxone in the management of patients presenting with altered mental status.

Petroleum Distillates

Petroleum distillates are the breakdown products of crude oil. Examples include kerosene, gasoline, and mineral seal oil. They are a subgroup of the organic compounds called hydrocarbons. Though the figures are thought to represent under-reported values, ingestion of petroleum distillates accounts for an estimated 5% to 25% of all poison deaths in the population younger than 5 years of age. They are commonly ingested because of ease of access, mislabeling of the containers (e.g., kerosene in a pop bottle), and occasionally enticing scenting (e.g., furniture polish). Petroleum distillates can affect the pulmonary, cardiovascular, and central nervous systems. Most toxicity is seen as a chemical pneumonitis secondary to aspiration. This occurs during the ingestion or concomitant with vomiting (resulting from ingestion or therapeutically induced). The aspiration potential of a petroleum distillate is linked to its viscosity and volatility.

Most patients present without symptoms. Other findings include characteristic odor (sometimes so strong it is difficult to localize its origin—skin versus mouth), oral burning, vomiting, belching, abdominal pain, cough or choking, headache, or unusual behavior. Physical findings are consistent with the affected organ system. Most often the examination is normal. There are no specific diagnostic adjuncts, though anteroposterior and lateral views of the chest are usually ordered. Changes can occur quite rapidly, but the process can progress over 72 hours or more. Classically, findings are consistent with a chemical pneumonitis, seen as alveolar infiltrates. If respiratory distress is noted, arterial blood gases are ordered to assess the Po_2.

The serious sequelae of petroleum distillate ingestion are primarily related to pulmonary complications. Since these ingestants are poorly absorbed from the gastrointestinal tract, and vomiting can result in aspiration, induced emesis is not recommended by most authors. Since volatility and viscosity have a role in determining the risk for aspiration, it is important for the emergency physician to categorize the ingestion:

1. Heavy—grease, mineral oil, suntan oil. These are of low toxicity and risk.
2. Medium—kerosene, gasoline. These have a low to moderate risk. Because of their cardiovascular and central nervous system side effects, some authors recommend a large ingestion (more than 1 ml/kg) should be eliminated by induced vomiting. This remains a controversial point, though present evidence points to not inducing vomiting in any of these patients.
3. Light—mineral seal oil. Since the aspiration risk is high, emesis is not recommended.

Other interventions such as gastric lavage, charcoal, steroids, or antibiotics are not recommended. Petroleum distillates may only be the media that contain other toxic substances (e.g., pesticides). It is important to obtain the original container of the substance, if possible.

DISPOSITION AND FOLLOW-UP

Appropriate patient disposition depends on many variables that differ widely from one case of toxic ingestion to the next. Consideration is given to both the medical aspects of the case and the psychosocial circumstances attending it before a final decision is made.

Medical Considerations

Medical considerations are based on the nature of the ingested compound and its manifested or potential toxicity. In the absence of another reason for admission, patients with nontoxic ingestions (Table 19–10) are usually discharged after simple reassurance. Similarly, those who have been exposed to compounds with minimal toxicity can usually be discharged after initial emergency department treatment and a suitable observation period.

Patients who manifest significant clinical evidence of toxicity are usually admitted to the hospital. Those patients who are found to have drug levels in the toxic range may also require admission, even in the absence of symptoms or clinical findings. Although admitted patients tend to require intensive care and monitoring, this is not always necessary. The need for intensive care is generally based on the presence of, or risk for, cardiopulmonary or central nervous system complications that may affect vital functions.

Psychosocial Considerations

The psychosocial elements associated with each case are also taken into account. Toxic ingestions are either intentional or accidental. Intentional ingestions are usually suicide

TABLE 19–10. Substances That Are Nontoxic When Ingested in Small Amounts

Abrasives	Iodophil disinfectant
Adhesives	Laxatives
Antibiotics	Lipstick
Baby-product cosmetics	Lubricants
Ballpoint inks	Lubricating oils
Bath oil	Magic Markers
Bathtub floating toys	Make-up
Bleach (household)	Matches
Body conditioners	Mineral oil
Bubble-bath soaps	Newspaper
Calamine lotion	Paint (indoor, latex)
Candles	Pencil (graphite, coloring)
Caps (toy pistols)	Perfumes
Chalk	Petroleum jelly (Vaseline)
Cigarettes or cigars	Phenolphthalein laxatives
Clay (modeling)	Play-Doh
Colognes	Porous-tip marking pens
Contraceptive pills	Putty (less than 2 oz)
Corticosteroids	Rouge
Cosmetics	Rubber cement
Crayons (marked by AP, CP on label)	Shampoo (liquid)
Dehumidifying packets	Shaving creams, lotions
Detergents (phosphate)	Soap
Deodorants	Spackles
Deodorizers	Suntan cream, lotions
Eye make-up	Sweetening agents (saccharin, cyclamates)
Fabric softeners	
Fertilizer (unless insecticides or herbicides added)	Teething rings
Fishbowl additives	Thermometers (mercury)
Glues and pastes	Toilet water
Grease	Toothpaste (with or without fluoride)
Hair tonics	Vitamins (with or without fluoride)
Hand lotions	Warfarin (most rat poisons)
Hydrogen peroxide (3%)	Water colors
Indelible markers	Zinc oxide
Ink (black, blue)	

Adapted from McPherson MC, Greensheer J: Controversies in the prevention and treatment of poisonings. Pediatr Ann 6:60, 1977.

attempts but may also be gestures. Accidental ingestions or intoxications, on the other hand, are usually caused by either excessive intake of chronically ingested medications, reckless substance abuse, or a child's oral curiosity.

Any *intentional ingestion* that is believed to be the consequence of a suicide attempt requires psychiatric consultation and evaluation. The patient who is a danger to himself may be hospitalized even without his consent, if necessary. Unfortunately, this issue is not "black and white." An intentional ingestion is sometimes the result of a suicide *gesture* rather than a suicide *attempt,* and is the act of a patient who is not self-destructive but wishes to call attention to certain personal problems. The distinction between an actual suicide attempt and a gesture is not always easy to make. When in doubt, the patient is presumed to be suicidal until determined otherwise by a psychiatric evaluation.

Accidental ingestions present other dispositional concerns. For example, the patient who becomes intoxicated after unwittingly ingesting an excessive quantity of a therapeutic drug must be educated about the proper use of the drug prior to discharge. Although such patients are usually admitted for further treatment and observation until sufficient drug metabolism has taken place, some can be safely treated as outpatients. Arrangements are made for timely medical reevaluation and rechecking of blood levels.

The *substance abuser* represents a very special category of patient who frequently requires extensive counselling or rehabilitation to prevent the chronic recurrence of drug toxicity. Although these patients rarely intend to hurt themselves, they are often as self-destructive as suicidal patients. Every effort is made to arrange for some type of rehabilitative care for these patients prior to discharge. An emergency department visit provides an excellent opportunity for treatment of the substance abuser in that the experience may be so terrifying that suggestions about rehabilitation may be heeded even if they had not been before. The emergency physician must avoid cynicism about the future of these patients. The offer for help is repeatedly made, and occasionally the patient accepts.

Children who accidentally ingest toxic compounds are also at risk for recurrence. An effort is routinely made to counsel parents about home safety. At the same time, the family situation is assessed to determine whether or not the ingestion could be a sign of abandonment or some other undesirable family situation that might indicate a need for intervention.

PROBLEM 3 After thorough evaluation, the 35 year old auto mechanic was discovered to have a carboxyhemoglobin level of 15%.

The most serious consequences of carbon monoxide toxicity are cardiac toxicity and neurotoxicity. However, these problems generally occur at levels much greater than 15%. The symptoms experienced by this patient are entirely consistent with the level of 15% and would be expected to resolve with 4 hours of 100% oxygen therapy, at which time discharge may be appropriate. Disposition must, however, include counseling the patient about the potential for recurrent occupational exposure and arranging an investigation into the source of the carbon monoxide in the home or the workplace.

PROBLEM 4 This 65 year old patient was observed to have frequent premature ventricular contractions (PVCs), and a theophylline level of 30 µg/ml was noted. His serum potassium level was normal.

The theophylline level of this patient was in the toxic range. Since theophylline is cardiotoxic, we must assume that the frequent PVCs were a consequence of the excessive serum concentration of this compound. Such a patient is at risk for more serious ventricular dysrhythmias. Since the half-life of theophylline is prolonged in patients with congestive heart failure and with increasing age, we would anticipate metabolism to take place more slowly in this patient and would not expect significant metabolism to take place during a reasonable emergency department observation period. Therefore, this patient was admitted to an intensive care unit for cardiac monitoring.

PROBLEM 5 The child was observed in the emergency department. Repeated examinations were normal. An initial chest radiograph was read as normal. After 4 hours, the child remained asymptomatic. The patient's parents seemed reliable and the hazards of household products were discussed with them. After direct contact and arranging a follow-up visit with their pediatrician for the next day, the child and parents were allowed to leave the emergency department. A list of symptoms that should prompt an immediate return was sent with them. The child did well and remained asymptomatic at home.

DOCUMENTATION

1. The type (including trade name) and amount of all compounds ingested as well as the interval between ingestion and emergency department care.
2. Any symptoms occurring after the ingestion.

3. Any coexistent medical problems that might affect outcome or management.
4. Any potentially interacting medications.
5. Physical findings. Frequent reevaluations may be necessary, particularly in patients with altered mental status.
6. Responses to all therapeutic interventions in the field and in the emergency department, including whether or not pills were recovered with syrup of ipecac–induced emesis or gastric lavage.
7. The time performed and results of all diagnostic tests.
8. The final diagnosis, disposition, and follow-up arrangements. Particular attention is paid to documenting lack of suicidal intent if the patient is to be discharged.

SUMMARY AND FINAL POINTS

Although the incidence of poisoning is high, resultant morbidity and mortality can be kept relatively low by early diagnosis and appropriate treatment. However, the pitfalls associated with the management of toxic ingestions are many. The following caveats can markedly reduce the risk of falling prey to one of them:

- That a poisoning has occurred may not be apparent. *Be suspicious, particularly in high risk groups!*
- Historical information is almost always more important than diagnostic testing for identifying the specific intoxicant(s). Considerable detective work and use of all available individuals and resources are often necessary to get the information needed. These resources *are* available.
- When interpreting physical findings, toxidromes—combinations of symptoms and signs that suggest a particular class of intoxicant—are a useful means of identifying patterns.
- Laboratory studies have value and limitations. Potentially spurious results from poorly chosen tests can cloud the diagnostic picture and may provide a false sense of security.
- Blood levels of the various intoxicants are interpreted in light of the timing of the specimen. Multiple levels may be required to make proper conclusions.
- Preventive and supportive therapy of the poisoned patient should be aggressive. An innocuous clinical presentation can change dramatically over a short period of time.
- When toxicity is in doubt, admission to a setting in which careful monitoring can take place is the indicated course.
- Psychosocial problems and needs may far outweigh the medical concerns. The ingestion or overdose may be a "cry for help."

BIBLIOGRAPHY

Texts

1. Goldfrank LR, Flomenbaum NE, Lewin NA, et al (eds): Toxicologic Emergencies. Norwalk CT, Appleton Century-Crofts, 1986.
2. Rumack BH: Poisindex. Denver CO, Micromedex, 1989.
3. Noji EK, Kelen GD: Manual of Toxicologic Emergencies. Chicago, Year Book Medical Publishers, 1989.
4. Haddad LM, Winchester JF: Clinical Management of Poisoning and Drug Overdose, 2nd ed. Philadelphia, WB Saunders, 1990.

Journal Articles

1. Calleham M, Kassel D: Epidemiology of fatal tricyclic antidepressant ingestion: Implications for management. Ann Emerg Med 14:1–9, 1985.
2. DeBroe ME, Bismuth C, DeGroot G, et al: Haemoperfusion: A useful therapy for a severely poisoned patient. Hum Toxicol 5:11–14, 1986.
3. Kellerman AL: Utilization and yield of drug screening in the emergency department. Am J Emerg Med 6:14, 1988.
4. Krenzelok EP: Role of sorbitol in theophylline elimination. Ann Emerg Med 16:1409–1410, 1987.
5. Kulig K, Bar-Or D, Cantrill SV, et al: Management of acutely poisoned patients without gastric emptying. Ann Emerg Med 14:562–567, 1985.
6. Litovitz TL, Schmitz BF, Matyunas N, et al: 1987 Annual Report of the American Association of Poison Control Centers National Data Collection System. Am J Emerg Med 6:479, 1988.
7. McCarron MM, Wood JD: The cocaine "body packer" syndrome. JAMA 250:1418–1420, 1983.
8. Neuvonen PJ, Olkkola KT: Oral activated charcoal in the treatment of intoxications: Role of single and repeated doses. Med Toxicol 3:33–58, 1988.
9. Olson KR, Benowitz NL, Woo OF, et al: Theophylline overdose: Acute single ingestion versus chronic repeated overmedication. Am J Emerg Med 3:386–394, 1985.
10. Smilkstein MJ, Knapp GL, Kulig KN, et al: Efficacy of oral N-acetylcysteine in the treatment of acetaminophen overdose. N Engl J Med 319(24):1557–1562, 1988.

CHAPTER 20

ALCOHOL INTOXICATION

ROBERT LINDBLAD, M.D.
GARY GELESH, D.O.

PROBLEM A 43 year old male was found lying in the gutter with the heavy odor of ethanol on his breath and clothes. He was arousable only with painful stimulus. His hair was matted, his clothes were torn and wet, and he was without shoes. There was dried blood around his right eyebrow. The police often found him in this condition.

QUESTIONS TO CONSIDER

1. What problems other than ethanol intoxication could be responsible for the patient's condition?
2. What serum ethanol level would account for the patient's mental status?
3. What medications are administered in the initial approach to intoxicated patients with depressed levels of consciousness?
4. How rapidly is ethanol metabolized, and how long will it take for a patient to wake up if the depression is due solely to ethanol ingestion?
5. What common complications of acute and chronic ethanol use may be anticipated during the patient's care?
6. What guidelines can be used to make an appropriate disposition after the patient has been treated in the emergency department?

INTRODUCTION

The use and abuse of ethanol is of enormous social and medical importance. Alcoholism, as defined by the National Council on Alcoholism of the American Medical Association, is "a chronic progressive and potentially fatal disease." It is characterized by tolerance and physical dependency or pathologic organ changes, or both—all the direct or indirect consequence of the alcohol ingested. There are an estimated 18 million alcoholics in the United States and certainly millions more who become intoxicated intermittently. Fifty percent of motor vehicle accidents involve ethanol abuse.

Ethanol consumption ranges from acute intoxication to chronic use with tolerance of its effects. Chronic consumers may be difficult to identify because, contrary to the image of the "derelict," they may be well dressed, successful in business, and avid deniers of their alcoholism.

The evaluation and management of the intoxicated patient are complicated by the effects of the drug. Ethanol is associated with pathologic changes in almost every system of the body (Table 20–1). With chronic abuse, the impairment of judgment and motor coordination that results significantly increases the risk of serious injury, and the depression of the level of consciousness masks many of the usual responses to pain and underlying diseases. The uncooperative, often belligerent patient frequently poses obstacles to even the simplest aspects of evaluation and care.

TABLE 20-1. Systemic Effects of Chronic Alcoholism

Nervous system	**Cardiac effects**
Cerebellar degeneration	Cardiomyopathy
Brain cell degeneration	**Musculoskeletal system**
Peripheral neuropathy	Skeletal myopathies
Seizures	**Hematologic system**
Gastrointestinal tract	Anemia
Esophagitis	Thrombocytopenia
Gastritis	Impaired leukocyte function
Esophageal varices	Hemolytic syndromes
Ulcer disease	**Metabolic effects**
Impaired intestinal absorption	Hypoglycemia
Liver	Hypokalemia
Fatty liver	Hypomagnesemia
Alcoholic hepatitis	Hypocalcemia
Cirrhosis	Hypophosphatemia
Pancreas	Hyperuricemia
Pancreatitis	Hyperlipidemia

The alcohols include ethanol, ethylene glycol, methanol, and isopropyl alcohol. This chapter will emphasize ethanol and briefly address the others in the section on Special Considerations. Alcohols are rapidly absorbed and widely distributed throughout the body. They have properties similar to those of general anesthetics, acting primarily at the cellular membrane level. They are principally metabolized in the liver by the enzyme alcohol dehydrogenase to form a variety of metabolites. Ethanol is converted into acetaldehyde, which in turn is rapidly cleared by acetaldehyde dehydrogenase. Alcohol dehydrogenase is the rate-limiting step of metabolism and has a fixed rate of activity (zero-order kinetics). Therefore, the metabolism of ethanol for any individual will be constant regardless of the initial blood level. The average rate of metabolism is 20 to 30 mg/dl/hr, although there are wide individual variations owing to induction of the liver's microenzyme system with chronic abuse.

The metabolism of ethanol affects many other metabolic pathways. Of prime concern is the inhibition of gluconeogenesis, which results in hypoglycemia, a common finding in intoxicated patients. Hypoglycemia is further exacerbated by the depleted glycogen stores in the liver secondary to chronic malnutrition.

PREHOSPITAL CARE

Providing good medical care for an intoxicated, often belligerent patient is difficult. Patients may place both themselves and the prehospital personnel at risk for injury. Patience, thoroughness, and a clear sense of purpose are essential in evaluating and transporting an intoxicated patient. The patient may be unable to provide any history, and any information obtained from such a patient is potentially unreliable. The most significant historical information is usually obtained from family, friends, or bystanders. If available, the following information is helpful:

History

1. Has the patient been involved in a fight, motor vehicle accident, or other form of trauma?
2. Has there been pain, vomiting, bleeding, or other symptoms of associated medical problems?
3. Are there significant previous medical problems and is the patient currently taking any medication?
4. How much and what type of alcohol has been ingested (gross approximation)?

Physical Examination

1. *Vital signs* may be "unobtainable" owing to poor hygiene, multiple layers of thick dirty clothes, or belligerence. These are not adequate reasons for avoiding these measurements. To the degree possible, vital signs are obtained on all patients, *especially* intoxicated patients.
2. *Evidence of trauma* is sought by examining the patient and the immediate surroundings. Patients found at the bottom of a flight of stairs or down on the sidewalk are treated as if they had incurred trauma even if there is no external evidence of injury on physical examination.
3. *Evidence of medical illness* such as pallor, abdominal tenderness, or abnormal breath sounds is also sought.

Intervention

The initial approach to the intoxicated patient with significant depression of consciousness is based on the presumption that the patient has underlying significant trauma or medical illness. Since active resistance to treatment and transport may occur, negotiating skill is often tested. These discussions are time-limited. Physical intervention and restraint may be necessary.

1. Airway patency and breathing are assessed, and appropriate stabilization is initiated. Cervical spine injury is presumed to have occurred and the neck is immobilized throughout these interventions.
2. In patients with a significantly altered mental status, medications administered in the field include naloxone, thiamine, and glucose. An initial dose of 2 mg of naloxone is adequate for the identification of concomitant narcotic abuse. One to two ampules of 50% dextrose (25 to 50 gm), preceded by 100 mg of thiamine, are usually sufficient to rule out hypoglycemia as a cause of the altered level of consciousness. Values obtained from a rapid glucose test strip may be available but are not to be relied on solely for ruling out hypoglycemia. Normal values in the prehospital setting are rechecked at the hospital. Due to the risk of hypoglycemia with ethanol intoxication, most patients with altered mental status are treated with 1 to 2 ampules of 50% dextrose.
3. Intravenous access is usually established early. A dextrose-containing solution is infused. The flow rate is determined by the hemodynamic status.
4. Any other response is determined by the patient's clinical condition.

PROBLEM The rescue squad reported that the patient was arousable with painful stimuli but then fell back asleep. He had dried blood around his right eyebrow. There were no gross deformities of his extremities, and he moved them all when stimulated. The nearby bar was closed, and there were no other people on the street at the time.

The paramedics followed standing orders for similar cases that included airway inspection, cervical spine immobilization, administration of oxygen, measurement of vital signs, establishment of an intravenous line, and administration of naloxone, thiamine, and dextrose. The patient was transported quickly to the emergency department. His injury potential was high.

INITIAL APPROACH IN THE EMERGENCY DEPARTMENT

The initial approach to the patient first addresses the status of the airway, breathing, and circulation as well as that of the cervical spine. Ethanol consumption is often associated with respiratory depression and a decreased gag reflex. Additionally, significant trauma is frequently an associated finding.

1. Airway patency and protection are established. A nasopharyngeal airway is often helpful if the gag reflex is intact. Suctioning equipment is placed at the bedside.

2. Adequate ventilation is supplied as necessary.

3. The cervical spine is evaluated and immobilized in anticipation of discovery of an injury. Immobilization is maintained and a cross-table lateral plain view of the neck is obtained in any uncooperative patient or those in whom there is a possibility of trauma.

4. If not previously done, IV access is established. An isotonic crystalloid solution is infused at a rate appropriate to the need for volume replacement.

5. Naloxone 2 mg IV will help to identify and reverse concomitant narcotic abuse. Interestingly, it may also improve the depressed mental status that occurs secondary to ethanol ingestion.

6. Thiamine 100 mg IV is administered. Due to malnutrition, thiamine stores are often diminished in alcoholic patients. Thiamine is an important coenzyme in glucose metabolism. If it is absent, the administration of glucose may precipitate a Wernicke's encephalopathy. This encephalopathy is recognizable by the triad of ocular abnormalities (primarily horizontal nystagmus or a bilateral sixth nerve palsy), ataxia, and global confusion. It has a time-dependent reversibility, and a residual deficit can be found in up to 40% of patients. In *any* patient with altered mental status who is suspected to be consuming a poor diet, whether he is an alcoholic or not, thiamine 100 mg is given. This can be administered prior to glucose administration or, if glucose was given in the field, on arrival in the emergency department.

7. Glucose test strips are used to determine initial serum glucose levels. Dextrose 25 to 50 gm is administered to treat hypoglycemia as necessary or if it is suspected.

8. An accurate body temperature is obtained. Rarely will an intoxicated patient cooperate adequately to allow an accurate oral temperature to be recorded. An accurate temperature is crucial in determining both the likelihood of infectious disease and the possibility of hypothermia. Rectal or tympanic membrane measurements are more dependable.

9. The patient is undressed. This important step is often ignored, leading to missed injuries and illnesses.

PROBLEM The intoxicated patient arrived in the emergency department. He was snoring, swore profusely when aroused, spit occasionally, and then fell back to sleep. He was lying on a backboard with a rigid cervical collar in place and had an aroma of alcohol, rotten socks, and urine. His vital signs, taken in the field, were blood pressure 160/90 mm Hg, pulse 96 beats/min, respirations 18/min. Repeat vital signs taken in the emergency department were BP 140/80 mm Hg, pulse 90 beats/min, respirations 16/min, temperature 96.5°F (39.8°C) orally. An intravenous line was established, supplemental oxygen was given by nasal cannula, and naloxone, thiamine, and dextrose were given. A cross-table lateral neck radiograph was read as negative. The cervical collar was left in place until a complete cervical spine series could be done. A repeated temperature taken rectally was 99°F (37.2°C). The patient was completely undressed and placed in a gown. On being asked his name, he replied "None of your business." Asked "Have you ever been to the hospital before?" he replied "Just leave me alone and get out of here!" The staff was not pleased at having the patient in the emergency department.

Initial examination revealed normal vital signs and some hostile responsiveness, which is better than no responsiveness. Close immediate attention is mandatory for accurate assessment of such patients. Many of these patients are *not easy* to manage in a caring manner. Just as in the prehospital setting, a clear sense of purpose and priorities is essential.

DATA GATHERING

History

The acutely intoxicated patient rarely supplies a coherent accurate history. Although it is important to listen to the patient's story, efforts are also directed toward alternative sources to corroborate information. The patient's belongings are searched for phone numbers or addresses, and prior hospital records are requested.

Pertinent questions include:

1. *What is the patient's usual mental status? When was the patient last seen?*
   Acute changes in mental status are usually due to intoxicants, hypoglycemia, head trauma, or a combination of the three. Each is explored if the history supports evidence of an abrupt alteration in thinking.
2. *What are the patient's usual drinking patterns? Preferences? Volumes?*
   Most patients are notoriously inaccurate in describing the volume of ethanol they ingest. The purpose of this questioning is to determine whether variations from the patient's usual drinking habits have occurred. The answers supply some insight into the severity of the patient's alcoholism and the possibility of non-ethanol intoxicants.
3. *Is the patient a potential polydrug abuser?*
   Although most alcoholics stay with ethanol, it often is a "chaser" in polydrug abusers.
4. *Does the patient have known complications of chronic alcoholism?*
   Table 20–1 provides a helpful list of potential sites of organ damage.
5. *Has the patient had withdrawal symptoms from ethanol? If so, what type of symptoms have occurred (see Special Considerations)?*
6. *Could trauma be a causal or contributing factor in the patient's condition?*
7. *What is the past medical history? Have there been any medical, surgical, or psychiatric illnesses? Have there been recent hospitalizations, particularly for detoxification? What medications (e.g., disulfiram [Antabuse]) does the patient take? Does he have any allergies?*

Physical Examination

The physical examination is particularly important in the intoxicated patient. Because the history is often inaccurate, careful examination is critical. Unfortunately, the intoxicated state can hide a variety of findings, particularly those related to pain assessment. Serial examinations are necessary to ensure that the patient "sobers up" and to discover new findings unmasked by the patient's improved mental status. Much of the emphasis is directed toward the areas assessed in the chapters on altered mental status (Chap. 45) and the poisoned patient (Chap. 19). Special attention is paid to findings that support the common complications of alcohol intoxication including head trauma, cervical spine trauma, trauma to the extremities, aspiration pneumonia, pancreatitis, and gastrointestinal bleeding.

General Appearance. The general appearance of the patient is noted, including cautious sampling of the breath odor for ethanol or fruity ketosis. The presence of "alcohol on the breath" is noteworthy, but it does not correlate with blood levels of alcohol, nor does it by itself explain an altered mental status. Signs of chronic alcoholism are sought, including muscle wasting, spider angiomas, palmar erythema, and jaundice. A general inspection for evidence of trauma is also performed at this time, noting lacerations, bruises, or deformities.

Vital Signs. Attention is paid to blood pressure (dehydration, blood loss) and temperature (hypothermia due to exposure, peripheral vasodilatation, and underlying disease; fever due to ingestants or infection).

Head. The skull and facial bones are inspected and palpated.

Eyes, Ears, Nose, and Throat. The tympanic membranes are visualized and pupillary and funduscopic examinations are performed. Evidence of nystagmus is sought when examining the eyes. The oral cavity and nose are examined for signs of trauma, and the neck is palpated for the position of the trachea. The patient is evaluated for neck stiffness (after radiographic clearance).

Thorax. The thorax is inspected for evidence of blunt and penetrating trauma and palpated anteriorly and posteriorly for crepitus or deformity. The lungs and heart are auscultated paying particular attention to the presence of rales or consolidation. These may represent aspiration or underlying infection.

Abdomen. An enlarged abdominal girth may mask or be caused by ascites. Liver and spleen are specifically examined for both size and tenderness. A palpable spleen tip connotes splenomegaly and potential portal hypertension.

Rectum. The rectum is examined for tone, and stool testing is done for gross or occult blood.

Extremities. The extremities are inspected and palpated for bony crepitus, deformity, and pulses.

Neurologic Examination. The level and content of consciousness are evaluated, as are the response to stimulation and the presence of spontaneous movements. An active search for focal neurologic deficiencies is necessary. Cranial nerves are evaluated if the patient is cooperative. Deep tendon reflexes are tested, including plantar responses, and the gait is observed if the patient is able to walk.

PROBLEM The patient fell into a light sleep. He was unable to give any history. Old medical records documented the existence of multiple previous visits for acute intoxication, no allergies, no medications, and a history of withdrawal seizures. On physical examination a 2-cm laceration was found over the right eyebrow, and equal breath sounds were present bilaterally with ecchymosis and crepitus of the right lower ribs in the midaxillary line. The abdomen was soft; there was no guarding, and no grimace was noted on rebound. Bowel sounds were decreased. The spleen was not palpable, and the liver was palpated 2 cm below the right costal margin. Total liver span was 12 cm. No focal deficiencies were found on neurologic testing, including symmetric reflexes and spontaneous movement of all four extremities. The results of rectal examination and stool hemoglobin testing were normal.

The abdominal and neurologic examination results are most difficult to interpret because alcohol intoxication can hide significant pathology. Serial examinations, preferably by the same examiner, are essential for accurate evaluation of the intoxicated patient.

DECISION PRIORITIES AND PRELIMINARY DIFFERENTIAL DIAGNOSIS

Acute intoxication can be associated with many serious conditions. The first decision priorities center around the following questions.

1. *Does the patient have an altered mental status? (See Chap. 45.) If so, what are the possible causes other than ethanol?*
   The major sources of altered mental status associated with alcoholism are listed in Table 20–2. Rapidly reversible conditions are considered and treated first in all intoxicated patients. These include hypoxia, hypotension, hypoglycemia, hypothermia, and substance abuse. If acute trauma has occurred, epidural hematoma, subarachnoid bleed, cerebral contusion or concussion, or subdural hematoma is considered. Subdural hematoma is seen in alcoholics secondary to both repeated trauma and cerebral atrophy leading to spontaneous rupture of the communicating veins. Seizure disorders are commonly associated with alcoholism,

TABLE 20–2. Differential Diagnosis of Impaired Level of Consciousness in the Alcohol-Intoxicated Patient

Metabolic
  Hypoglycemia, diabetic ketoacidosis, uremia, hyponatremia, hypercalcemia, hepatic encephalopathy
Respiratory
  Hypoxia
Environmental
  Hypothermia
Toxicologic
  Narcotics, benzodiazepines, sedative hypnotics, ethanol, methanol, ethylene glycol, isopropyl alcohol, carbon monoxide
Infectious
  Meningitis/encephalitis, sepsis
Trauma
  Hypotension, epidural hematoma, subarachnoid bleed, concussion, or contusion
CNS disorders
  Cerebrovascular accident, tumor, seizure or postictal state, subdural hematoma

and many patients present in a postictal state. Phenytoin toxicity, with signs of ataxia and dysarthria, often mimics acute intoxication but does not usually produce coma. The degree of assessment needed to find these causes may vary from nothing beyond data gathering to the full use of laboratory studies and radiologic imaging. The methods of assessment used depend on the patient's symptoms and their course during treatment. How far to go with an individual patient is based on experience in emergency medical practice. When in doubt, the physician should err on the side of added assessment.

2. *What role does ethanol play in the patient's presentation?*

Although the blood ethanol level does not need to be measured in all cases of alcohol intoxication, it is necessary in patients with depressed mental status, known polydrug ingestion, and in those who are not improving in the emergency department (see Diagnostic Adjuncts). The possibility that other alcohols (methanol, ethylene glycol, and isopropyl alcohol) are contributing to and complicating the patient's condition must be considered (see Special Considerations). It is rare for polyalcohol ingestion to occur, but desperate circumstances can prompt this admixture.

PROBLEM Initial examination of this patient did not reveal any immediate life-threatening conditions. He appeared to be intoxicated with no focal neurologic deficits and perhaps to have a broken rib on the right side and a laceration over his right eye.

It is dangerous to allow this first impression to produce a false sense of security. The apparent intoxicated state is a great masquerader. Many of the items listed in the differential diagnosis have been ruled out by the initial examination. Those remaining include drug ingestion other than narcotics, intracranial processes, and a seizure with a resultant postictal state. Phenytoin toxicity would be unlikely with this patient's depressed level of consciousness and lack of nystagmus. Laboratory assessment is necessary, and an expanded differential diagnosis needs to be developed. The patient is monitored with serial examinations.

DIAGNOSTIC ADJUNCTS

Because the history and the physical findings are often limited, the intoxicated patient with altered mental status requires laboratory and radiologic evaluation.

Laboratory Studies

The laboratory work-up of a patient with an altered mental status and alcohol on the breath has essential and optional elements:

Essential Tests
1. Blood ethanol level
2. Electrolyte measurements
3. Blood urea nitrogen–creatinine concentration
4. Glucose concentration
5. Arterial blood gases
6. Complete blood count
7. Urinalysis

Optional Tests
1. Toxicology screen
2. Liver function tests
3. Amylase concentration
4. Hemostatic studies
5. Serum osmolality

Blood Ethanol Level. Intoxicated patients without significant depression of level of consciousness who come to the emergency department for care of an isolated injury or problem generally do not need to have the ethanol level determined. However, this test is important in evaluating the remainder of intoxicated patients. Although there is considerable individual variation, the value correlates approximately with the expected level of consciousness (Table 20–3). When the level does not correlate as expected (e.g., when it is zero), an intensive search to explain the patient's condition is necessary. A blood ethanol level of less than 250 mg/dl in a chronic alcohol consumer does not adequately explain a significantly depressed mental status, e.g., responsive to deep pain only. Measurements of ethanol levels are available rapidly but have the disadvantage of measuring the serum ethanol concentration only. Methanol, ethylene glycol, and isopropyl alcohol levels have to be specifically requested.

Serum ethanol determinations may be requested by law enforcement agencies or by employers for nonmedical purposes. Care is necessary to guarantee that patients' rights are not violated. Individual emergency departments usually have specific protocols to direct this type of evaluation. Although currently used laboratory techniques for ethanol determination do not measure concentrations of other alcohols, skin preparation is done

TABLE 20–3. Serum Ethanol Levels and Corresponding Clinical Findings

0–100 mg/dl
  Altered judgment
  Decreased inhibitions
  Decreased coordination
100 mg/dl
  Legal limit for driving in most states
100–200 mg/dl
  Slurred speech
  Ataxia
  Poor balance
200–300 mg/dl
  Lethargy
  Altered equilibrium
300–400 mg/dl
  Coma, respiratory depression

Note: Chronic ethanol consumption produces tolerance, which results in much higher ethanol levels producing the same clinical findings.

Common Drinks	Absolute Ethanol Content
1 oz 100 proof whiskey	15 ml
One 6-oz glass wine (12% ethanol)	22 ml
One 12-oz beer (5% ethanol)	18 ml

For a 70-kg person, 15 ml of absolute ethanol will increase the blood alcohol level 25 mg/dl.

with nonalcoholic preparations to avoid any question about contamination of specimens that are drawn for legal or employment purposes.

Serum Electrolytes. Electrolyte disturbances are common in patients suffering from complications of chronic alcohol abuse and electrolytes may be abnormal due to acute dehydration. Hyponatremia alone may be responsible for significant alterations in mental status.

An increased anion-gap acidosis is also a common finding. The anion gap is calculated by subtracting the sum of the chloride and bicarbonate concentrations from the sodium concentration. Potassium concentration is negligible in this calculation. The normal range is 8 to 16 mEq/liter. Values greater than this reflect a positive anion gap. A common cause of an anion-gap metabolic acidosis in an alcoholic patient is alcoholic ketoacidosis. This is a result of chronic ethanol abuse and poor nutritional habits associated with protracted vomiting. Other causes of anion-gap metabolic acidosis are listed in Table 20–4 using the mnemonic MUD PILES. Calculation of the anion gap in an intoxicated patient can be very useful. (See Chap. 30.)

Blood Urea Nitrogen (BUN)–Creatinine Concentrations. These tests are useful in evaluating hydration and renal status. Renal failure is another cause of altered mental status.

Serum Glucose Concentration. Hypoglycemia, although initially assessed by reagent strip determination or by empiric treatment with dextrose, is documented or ruled out more definitively by the laboratory determination. Hyperglycemia may also be responsible for altered mental status.

Arterial Blood Gases. Blood gas determinations are extremely helpful in evaluating adequacy of oxygenation, ventilation, and acid-base status.

Complete Blood Count. A complete blood count (CBC) including a platelet estimate is useful if there are signs of bleeding or infection. Bone marrow suppression by chronic ethanol abuse can lead to anemia and thrombocytopenia as well.

Urinalysis. Urinalysis may provide evidence of dehydration, infection, or bleeding.

Serum Amylase Concentration. Amylase determination is most useful in patients complaining of abdominal pain who may have acute pancreatitis due to alcohol abuse.

Liver Function Tests. Patients who have evidence of hepatic dysfunction on physical examination are screened for adequacy of hepatic function.

Hemostatic Studies. Patients with hepatic dysfunction will have a prolonged prothrombin time. This test result appears early in the course of hepatic dysfunction and can be used as a screening test.

Toxicology Studies. Determinations of specific drug levels are ordered as indicated by the history and results of the physical examination. A general screening test is of limited utility but may be useful when there is suspicion of drug abuse but minimal specific guidance is offered by the history and physical examination.

Serum Osmolality. The serum osmolality is measured by assessing the freezing point depression of a liquid. The measured value (normal = 285 – 295 mOsm/kg) is most useful when it is compared to the calculated value.

$$\text{Serum osmolality} = 2 \times (\text{sodium}) + \frac{\text{BUN}}{3} + \frac{\text{glucose}}{18} + \frac{\text{ethanol}}{5}$$

TABLE 20–4. Anion-Gap Metabolic Acidosis

M–Methanol
U–Uremia
D–Diabetic ketoacidosis
P–Paraldehyde
I–Isoniazid
L–Lactic acidosis
E–Ethylene glycol
S–Salicylates

If the difference between the measured and calculated values is greater than 10 mOsm/kg, unmeasured osmotically active molecules are present in the specimen. The alcohols—ethanol, methanol, isopropanol, and ethylene glycol—are the most commonly encountered osmotically active agents.

PROBLEM This patient's alcohol level was found to be 420 mg/dl; Na^+ was 136, K^+ 4.0, Cl 100, CO_2 24, glucose 66, and the urinalysis showed no evidence of blood.

The anion gap, $Na - (Cl + CO_2)$, was 12 mEq/liter, with a normal range of 8 to 16 mEq/liter. There was no evidence of an anion-gap metabolic acidosis based on this calculation.

Does the alcohol level correspond to this patient's level of responsiveness (Table 20–3)? It is important to note that chronic alcohol abusers become increasingly tolerant of the effects of alcohol. Although this patient is somnolent with an alcohol level of 420 mg/dl, an expected finding based on his previous history of ethanol consumption, a novice drinker may well be somnolent with an ethanol level in the 200 to 300 mg/dl range.

Radiologic Imaging

Radiologic evaluation is often difficult owing to the poor cooperation of the patient. Initial films frequently need to be performed in the emergency department. Only when the patient is stable and cooperative is he allowed to leave the department for complete studies. Important radiologic studies to be considered include studies of the cervical spine, chest, pelvic area, and extremities and computed tomography (CT) of the brain.

1. *Cervical spine* evaluation is frequently necessary in an intoxicated patient. If there is any history of head trauma or evidence of head trauma on examination, the neck should be immobilized and a portable, lateral neck film obtained in the emergency department. A complete cervical spine series is obtained when the patient's condition permits it.

2. A *chest radiograph* may reveal an occult pneumonia or evidence of trauma. If there is any evidence of chest trauma, fever, or abnormal findings on lung examination, a chest radiograph is obtained.

3. *Films of the pelvis* are ordered when there is evidence of significant trauma in the pelvic area.

4. *Extremity films* are ordered based on the history and results of the clinical examination.

5. *CT of the head* is considered when there is evidence of head trauma, focal findings on neurologic examination, new-onset or persistent seizures, inappropriate level of responsiveness when the alcohol level is known, and if there is no improvement in or worsening of the neurologic findings with time.

Electrocardiography

A 12-lead electrocardiogram (ECG) is useful for detecting concomitant cardiac disease. In alcoholic patients this can range from the ischemic heart disease problems to dysrhythmogenic alcoholic cardiomyopathy.

PROBLEM The patient was brought in with a cervical collar in place and had already had a cross-table lateral cervical spine film taken during the initial assessment. A complete cervical spine series was done, which showed no abnormalities. A chest radiograph was performed because of the findings of crepitus and ecchymosis of the right chest wall. An isolated seventh rib fracture with no hemothorax or pneumothorax was noted. On his return from the radiology department to the emergency department, the laceration over his right eye was repaired. A repeat examination revealed no new findings, and there was a slight improvement in his willingness to cooperate and in level of responsiveness.

It is important to remember that a cross-table lateral cervical spine film will rule out significant fractures of the cervical spine in only 85% to 90% of cases. It is imperative that a complete cervical spine series be obtained when the patient's condition permits. The ability to complete other medical care, e.g., suturing, varies greatly with the patient's willingness to cooperate. Some areas, such as wounds, may be cleansed and covered.

REFINED DIFFERENTIAL DIAGNOSIS

By adding the data obtained by ancillary testing to the information previously obtained from the history and physical examination, the cause of the patient's altered mental status can be more accurately determined. Metabolic disturbances will have been identified by abnormalities noted in the arterial blood gas and serum chemistry measurements. These test results may also have suggested the presence of alcohols other than ethanol. Hypoxia will also have been detected and treated by this time. If infection is suggested, specific sites of infection, typically the urine or lungs, will have been evaluated.

At this point another important question is addressed: *Are any potential complications of acute or chronic alcoholism present?*

The patient cannot be considered a chronic alcohol abuser without searching for the pathophysiologic effects of the abuse. Table 20–1 serves as a guide for examination and also offers a checklist of possible problems that could affect a satisfactory outcome. The most common disorders associated with chronic alcohol abuse in patients seen in the emergency department are gastrointestinal hemorrhage, seizures, hepatic dysfunction, pancreatitis, anemia, thrombocytopenia, and hypokalemia. Evidence of each of these problems is actively sought in the alcohol-intoxicated patient.

PROBLEM The patient had normal vital signs, no evidence of respiratory compromise, no focal findings on neurologic examination, normal laboratory values, no acidosis, and an elevated serum ethanol level. Although pure ethanol intoxication was the most likely diagnosis, intracranial lesions are not yet ruled out, and other ingestions could also be involved. Serial examinations made over a period of time should further refine this differential diagnosis. This patient was certainly intoxicated. If his blood alcohol level had been 30 mg/dl, the index of suspicion for a concomitant drug ingestion or a significant intracranial process would be raised. A CT of the head would be needed, and more aggressive monitoring would be indicated. However, because the ethanol level was high and the patient had shown slight improvement on neurologic examination, and because the only other findings were a laceration above the eye and an isolated rib fracture, serial examinations were adequate to follow this patient as his alcohol level fell. Intracranial hemorrhage and drug ingestion were not entirely ruled out at this time, but they are less likely diagnoses than pure ethanol intoxication with minor trauma. Again, care must be taken to continue close monitoring and periodic reassessment. At a metabolic rate of 30 mg/dl/hr, this patient will need an estimated 14 hours to be alcohol free. Because he was a chronic abuser, he should be easily arousable and completely awake several hours before then.

PRINCIPLES OF MANAGEMENT

The goals of management are to protect the patient from hurting himself or others, to treat potentially life-threatening conditions without delay, and to ensure appropriate disposition and follow-up. These goals are realized through several management principles:

1. Observation with frequent measurements of vital signs and neurologic assessment.
2. Aggressive evaluation of nonimproving or deteriorating mental status.
3. Continued observation until the patient is able to function and care for himself.
4. Intravenous hydration and nutrition.
5. Restraint by chemical or physical means when needed (to protect the patient or others).

Close observation with frequent neurologic assessment of the intoxicated patient is essential. Vital signs and mental status checks are initially performed every half hour, and a more complete assessment is made every hour until the patient becomes easily arousable. Examinations can then be made every 2 hours to follow the improvement in neurologic function. The mental status examination is the primary tool in the assessment of the intoxicated patient, not the absolute blood ethanol level.

At any point during the observation, a deterioration of neurologic function should prompt an intensive search for the cause. If the patient has shown progressive improvement, a thorough examination is performed. New symptoms or complaints are acknowledged, and further studies are often needed at this point. The patient, now sober, can more reliably report symptoms and is essentially considered a "new" patient requiring a complete assessment.

Maintenance fluids with multivitamins will allow maintenance of venous access and some nutrition for these chronically malnourished patients. Dextrose is part of the IV fluids given. A repeat serum glucose determination may be obtained if the patient's condition does not improve during the observation period. Nevertheless, neither IV fluids, multivitamins, nor dextrose hastens the metabolism of ethanol.

At times, restraints are needed to protect the patient and the staff. Physical restraints are most commonly used because the patient can be controlled without adding new medications to complicate the assessment of a patient whose consciousness is already depressed. Care is taken to check any patient in physical restraints frequently to ensure distal circulation of the extremities and proper placement of the restraints. Adequate personnel, usually at least four people, is necessary to apply the leather restraints to an agitated patient. They are removed first from two opposite extremities, i.e., left arm and right leg, as the patient improves. When the patient is fully cooperative, they are completely removed. Careful documentation of the reason for the restraints is recorded on the chart. Family members or friends, if present, are also informed about the reason for the restraints. The chemical restraint of choice in the agitated intoxicated patient is haloperidol. The initial dosage is 5 to 10 mg given intramuscularly. Elderly patients are given 1 to 2 mg initially. Haloperidol causes minimal sedation with excellent behavior control. It may be used in conjunction with physical restraints to protect the severely agitated patient.

SPECIAL CONSIDERATIONS

Pediatric Patients

Whether the patient is a toddler who drank mouthwash (up to 20% ethanol, 40 proof) or a child who experimented in the liquor cabinet, hypoglycemia is much more common in this age group owing to the low glycogen reserves in children. In one study of intoxicated pediatric patients, hypoglycemia was found in 24%. Fluids with 5% dextrose are given, and the serum glucose level is monitored frequently.

Because these patients have not been previously exposed to ethanol, much smaller amounts and lower serum levels produce significant and even fatal effects. Respiratory depression is common, and support of respiratory function is often needed until ethanol is metabolized.

Other Alcohols: Methanol, Ethylene Glycol, Isopropanol

Although methanol and ethylene glycol differ in toxicity, there are many conceptual similarities between them, and treatment of patients intoxicated with either is essentially identical. Neither agent is itself dangerous, although ethylene glycol and to lesser extent methanol can cause ethanol-like intoxication. Serious toxicity is caused instead by the metabolites that are formed after metabolism by alcohol dehydrogenase. These byproducts include various organic acids that increase the anion gap; therefore, methanol and ethylene glycol intoxications are always considered in the differential diagnosis of increased anion-gap metabolic acidosis. Because determinations of methanol and ethylene glycol serum levels are not readily available, indirect measures such as the anion and osmolal gaps are useful. Before they are metabolized these agents do not increase the anion gap or cause acidosis, but they do cause an increased osmolal gap. After metabolism is complete, the opposite is true. Methanol metabolites can cause sometimes irreversible visual impairment, complete blindness, and central nervous system damage. Ethylene glycol byproducts can cause coma, cardiopulmonary complications, and renal failure. Oxalic acid production from ethylene glycol leads to formation of calcium oxalate crystals in the urine. (See Chap. 30.)

Treatment of both methanol and ethylene glycol intoxication includes attempts to block metabolism of the parent compounds to their toxic byproducts and often hemodialysis to remove both the parent compound and its metabolite. Alcohol dehydrogenase has a much higher affinity for ethanol than for methanol or ethylene glycol; thus metabolism of these agents can be prevented by administration of ethanol either intravenously or orally. Ethanol therapy does not alter the toxicity of previously formed metabolites, and once alcohol dehydrogenase is blocked, there is no other effective route of elimination of the parent compound. As a result, hemodialysis is almost always required in patients with serious intoxications.

Isopropanol, unlike the other alcohols, is metabolized to acetone. Serum acetone levels in such patients will be very high, but there is little or no acidosis. Isopropanol is a strong gastric irritant, and gastritis with bleeding often develops. Otherwise, the presentation of patients with isopropanol intoxication is similar to that of persons with ethanol intoxication, but the condition resolves much more slowly. By doubling the serum isopropanol level, the emergency physician can approximate the equivalent serum ethanol level.

Ethanol Withdrawal

Alcoholic patients may present to the emergency department with acute intoxication or with onset of symptoms due to the sudden reduction or cessation of ethanol intake. Ethanol withdrawal is traditionally divided into four stages:

- Stage 1: Minor withdrawal
  - Insomnia
  - Irritability
  - Tremor
  - Anorexia, nausea
  - Tachycardia
  - Hypertension
  - Hyperthermia (mild)
- Stage 2: Hallucinosis
  - Visual hallucinations (auditory, tactile, and olfactory hallucinations are less common)
- Stage 3: Seizures
  - Generalized, often multiple
- Stage 4: Major withdrawal
  - Global confusion
  - Sympathetic hyperactivity with agitation and diaphoresis

Ethanol withdrawal is probably best viewed as a continuum of symptoms rather than as a series of distinct stages. The vital signs often give an early clue about impending minor withdrawal syndromes. Tachycardia and mild hypertension are almost always present as early findings and, when not due to other medical or traumatic conditions, are predictors of the development of ethanol withdrawal. The onset of major withdrawal symptoms is signified by disorientation to person, place, and time. Some degree of confusion occurs in 5% to 10% of ethanol withdrawal cases, but the profound global confusion traditionally described as delirium tremens occurs in only 1% to 2% of cases. Hallucinations and seizures may occur after minor or major withdrawal syndromes. They are superimposed on other symptoms, rather than being distinct stages of withdrawal.

The pathophysiology of ethanol withdrawal has been extensively studied. Although many factors are involved in the full expression of these syndromes, the effect of ethanol on the inhibitory neurotransmitter gamma aminobutyric acid (GABA) and the subsequent removal of this effect are believed to be the most important mechanisms. There are chloride-dependent receptor sites for GABA in the central nervous system (CNS), and alcohol has been shown to increase the flow of chloride into these receptor sites, producing depression of the CNS. With chronic ethanol use, this effect is reduced or eliminated, and there is a reduction in the influx of chloride, a decrease in the inhibitory effect of GABA, and a resultant sympathetic hyperactivity mediated by norepinephrine. Other contributing factors to the ethanol withdrawal syndromes are metabolic effects (hypomagnesemia, hypokalemia, zinc deficiency), prostaglandin deficiency, and endocrine effects (cortisol excess).

Management of the ethanol withdrawal syndromes is primarily based on preventing the progression of symptoms to the major withdrawal stage by supplying an alternative CNS depressant that can be gradually withdrawn. Additionally, patients may require treatment for tremor, hallucinations, seizures, hyperthermia, dehydration, and malnutrition.

The benzodiazepines are the drugs of choice as temporary replacements for the withdrawn ethanol. They have similar effects in the CNS. Although their primary clinical usefulness lies in their ability to reduce agitation and tremor, they also have significant anticonvulsant activity. Diazepam and chlordiazepoxide, either orally or intravenously, provide good control and can be titrated to the desired effect.

In major withdrawal reactions, the sympathetic hyperactivity may be so great that the benzodiazepines are not sufficient to control the tremor, tachycardia, and hypertension that occur. Beta-adrenergic blocking agents such as propranolol and alpha-adrenergic blocking agents such as clonidine have been used for further control of sympathetic hyperactivity.

Alcoholic hallucinosis often requires no specific intervention. However, in severe cases or when the patient is significantly upset by the hallucinations, treatment is indicated. Haloperidol, administered intramuscularly, is the drug of choice for control of hallucinations in ethanol withdrawal. Phenothiazines are effective but significantly potentiate seizure activity.

Alcohol withdrawal seizures may occur singly or in multiples (two to four) and do not usually require specific anticonvulsant therapy. Status epilepticus, a rare occurrence, is treated as outlined in Chapter 48. If the patient has not had alcohol withdrawal seizures before, a full laboratory and radiologic evaluation to rule out other causes of seizures is indicated.

Associated hyperpyrexia, a temperature over 104°F (40°C), is treated with a cooling blanket or sponging with tepid water and administering acetaminophen. Aspirin is contraindicated owing to its inhibitory effect on platelet aggregation. Any anticoagulant effect is potentially harmful because the alcoholic patient is already at risk for hemorrhagic complications.

Marked dehydration, associated with electrolyte disturbances and malnutrition, is common in patients with major withdrawal syndromes. Isotonic crystalloid (typically 4 to 10 liters) is used to replace fluid losses. Serum electrolytes are measured and replaced as indicated. Hypokalemia and hypomagnesemia are especially common. Depletion of glycogen stores due to chronic malnutrition makes hypoglycemia a concern. Bedside screening with glucose oxidase reagent strips or empiric treatment with dextrose is indicated. Thiamine is essential to prevent the development of Wernicke's encephalopathy, and administration precedes or is concurrent with the use of dextrose. Multivitamin supplements are also recommended.

The disposition of the patient with ethanol withdrawal will vary depending on the severity of the syndrome. Patients with major withdrawal symptoms and those with status epilepticus require management in an intensive care unit. Ethanol withdrawal patients frequently have significant medical conditions secondary to chronic ethanol abuse that will dictate the type of disposition needed. Common examples are gastrointestinal bleeding, hepatic failure, and cardiomyopathy. If there is no evidence of coexisting medical or traumatic illness and the patient has symptoms consistent with a minor withdrawal syndrome, outpatient management is appropriate, with follow-up scheduled in a detoxification program.

DISPOSITION AND FOLLOW-UP

Admission

Admission to the hospital for alcohol intoxication is usually prompted by concomitant disease processes or trauma. Intoxicated patients with pneumonia, hepatitis, pancreatitis, or trauma often warrant admission because patient reliability is poor, self-care inadequate, and follow-up practically nonexistent. Direct admission to a detoxification unit may be possible, but this requires thorough knowledge of the unit and its capabilities. In general, if medical problems are present, a medical admission is the safest course. Transfer to an appropriate detoxification unit can be made a day or two later once the patient's condition has stabilized.

Intensive Care Unit Admission

Intensive care unit (ICU) admission is usually reserved for patients with major withdrawal symptoms, injuries resulting from major motor vehicle accidents, ingestions of methanol or ethylene glycol, or concomitant medical problems such as sepsis, hemorrhage, and myocardial infarction.

Referral

Alcohol abuse needs to be addressed openly and nonjudgmentally by the examining physician. Referral for counseling through a detoxification program or a primary physician is an extremely important and often ignored part of discharge planning.

Discharge

Most acutely intoxicated patients can be safely discharged after appropriate observation in the emergency department. If supportive family or friends are willing and capable of observing the patient at home, earlier discharge from the emergency department may be possible. If no support system is available, the patient is observed in the emergency department until he (or she) is able to care for himself (or herself). Patients must be capable of eating and walking with a steady gait, and oriented to their surroundings before discharge is considered. This may require extended observation.

PROBLEM The patient was awake and alert 10 hours after his arrival in the emergency department. He ambulated to the bathroom on his own and ate a full meal without difficulty. He stated that he was ready to go home.

It appeared that the patient had returned to his normal level of functioning and could safely look after himself. Discharge was appropriate after counseling and referral for treatment of alcoholism. He may be unlikely to follow through, but good practice requires that he be provided with the opportunity to obtain help.

DOCUMENTATION

1. It is inappropriate to record that a patient was "drunk" or "intoxicated." Recording "alcohol on the breath" and describing the behavior that occurred during the emergency department visit is reasonable. The documentation is descriptive and not judgmental.
2. Other information includes history of the event, known complications of ethanol abuse, and pertinent past medical history.
3. Physical examination findings, including stigmata of chronic abuse.
4. If restraints were used, the indications for the restraints (e.g., protecting the patient or the staff) need to be recorded.
5. Serial observation is the key to successful management of these patients, and a record of the results of these examinations must be maintained.
6. Laboratory findings, especially the ethanol level.
7. Of utmost importance is the discharge examination. The patient's mental status, response to his or her environment, ability to walk, and ability to care for himself or herself should be documented.
8. Plans for disposition and referral.

SUMMARY AND FINAL POINTS

- Intoxicated patients are commonly seen in the emergency department; they often have little insight into their own illness or injury and may be openly hostile and belligerent.
- The patient is completely undressed and fully examined.
- Injury to the cervical spine must be ruled out if trauma was possible.
- Reversible conditions are identified and treated: hypotension, hypothermia, hypoglycemia, hypoxia, other substance abuse.
- Deterioration or lack of improvement on serial examination needs aggressive evaluation.
- Observation, serial examinations, and a complete discharge examination are performed.
- Appropriate referral for treatment of alcoholism is an important part of care.

BIBLIOGRAPHY

Texts

1. Ellenhorn M, Darceloux D: Alcohols and glycols. In Ellenhorn M, Darceloux D: Medical Toxicology. New York, Elsevier, 1988, pp. 782–812.
2. Goldfrank L, et al: Metabolic acidosis in the alcoholic: Methanol and ethylene glycol. In Goldfrank L, Starke C: Toxicologic Emergencies. Norwalk, CT, Appleton-Century-Crofts, 1986, pp. 435–444, 452–465.

Journal Articles

1. Adinoff B, Bone GHA, Linnoila M: Acute ethanol poisoning and the ethanol withdrawal syndrome. Med Toxicol 3:172–196, 1988.
2. Airaksinen MM, Peura P: Mechanisms of alcoholic withdrawal syndrome. Med Biol 65:105–112, 1987.
3. Becker C: The alcoholic patient as a toxic emergency. Emerg Med Clin North Am 2:47–62, 1984.
4. George JE: The alcoholic patient in the E.D. Emerg Phys Legal Bull 6:1, 1980.
5. Hoffman RS, Goldfrank LR: Ethanol-associated metabolic disorders. Emerg Med Clin North Am 7(4):943–961, 1989.
6. Isselbacker KJ: Metabolic and hepatic effects of alcohol. N Engl J Med 296:612–616, 1977.
7. Leung AKC: Ethyl alcohol ingestion in children. Clin Pediatr 25:617–619, 1986.
8. Morris JC, Victor M: Alcohol withdrawal seizures. Emerg Med Clin North Am 5(4):827–839, 1987.
9. Reuler JB, et al: Wernicke's encephalopathy. N Engl J Med 312:1035–1039, 1985.
10. Reyna TM, et al: Alcohol related trauma. Ann Surg 201:194–197, 1985.
11. Schuckit M: Genetic aspects of alcoholism. Ann Emerg Med 15:991–996, 1986.
12. Smithline N, Gardner KD: Gaps anionized osmolal. JAMA 236:1599, 1976.
13. Tabkoff B, et al: Alcohol tolerance. Ann Emerg Med 15:1005–1012, 1986.

CHAPTER 21

HEAT ILLNESS

RONALD S. BARRECA, M.D.

PROBLEM 1 A 30 year old male was brought into the emergency department by a friend. According to the patient, he had been playing basketball for approximately two hours when he suddenly experienced muscle cramps in his legs and abdomen. The outside temperature was 94°F (34.4°C), humidity 78%.

PROBLEM 2 A 17 year old male was exercising during the first football practice of the year on a hot August afternoon when he became weak and dizzy and passed out.

PROBLEM 3 A 21 year old military recruit collapsed during training exercises. When the paramedics arrived, they noted that the patient was sweating, unconscious, and very warm to the touch.

QUESTIONS TO CONSIDER

1. What are the major compensatory mechanisms the body uses to combat heat stress?
2. What factors predispose to heat illness?
3. In what ways are the adverse effects of heat on the body manifested?
4. What are the major forms of heat illness and what are the different pathophysiologic characteristics of each?
5. What are the complications of heat stroke?
6. What methods are most effective in lowering body temperature?
7. Which patients with heat-related illness require admission to the hospital?
8. What measures are effective in preventing heat illness?

INTRODUCTION

References to heat illness date as far back as 24 BC, when it was reported that an entire Roman army succumbed to heat illness. Summer heat kills 4000 or more people per year in the United States. The population at risk includes not only the elderly and debilitated but also the young and otherwise healthy who exercise strenuously in adverse conditions. Heat illness is the second leading cause of death in athletes (head and spine injuries are number one). One percent of marathon runners suffer heat illness.

Heat illness is not a single entity but a *spectrum* of disorders that result from the body's attempts to maintain a normal temperature in the face of an environmental or internal heat load. Internal heat production from basal metabolism generates about 70 kilocalories (kcal)/hr. A 70-kg man would experience a 1°C rise in temperature per hour if there were no mechanism to dissipate this heat. Exercise can produce tremendous amounts of heat, ranging from 300 to 1000 kcal/hr. Without heat dissipation the temperature of a vigorously exercising man would increase 5 to 15°C/hr. The environmental heat load is influenced by the ambient temperature, relative humidity, and degree of exposure to sunlight. For example, direct sunlight can result in a heat gain of 150 kcal/hr.

The body has four means of dissipating heat:

1. *Radiation.* The simple physical transfer of heat from the body to the surrounding environment is called radiation. This mechanism is generally the most effective and accounts for approximately 65% of heat transfer under moderate climate conditions. To facilitate this mechanism, peripheral blood flow can increase by a factor of 20 in response to heat.

2. *Convection.* Wind currents that disturb the insulating layer of warmth that surrounds the body are responsible for 12% to 15% of heat loss.

3. *Conduction.* Direct contact with a cooler environment accounts for a small proportion of heat loss under normal circumstances. However, immersion in cool water can enhance heat loss through this mechanism by a factor of 32 when compared with air.

4. *Evaporation.* For every 1.7 ml of sweat evaporated, one kcal of heat is dissipated. A conditioned athlete can produce up to 3000 ml of sweat per hour. Under normal temperate conditions evaporation accounts for about 25% of heat loss. However, if the temperature is high and the humidity is low, evaporation will account for the majority of the heat loss (up to 1000 kcal/hr). Relative humidity of greater than 85% causes evaporation to be ineffective.

Acclimatization is the process by which the body adapts to extremes of heat. This process takes 3 to 4 weeks. The main adaptive changes occur in the cardiovascular and metabolic systems, with additional changes occurring in the endocrine system and the sweating response.

PREHOSPITAL CARE

A rescue squad usually does not have the capability of determining body temperature in the field, but heat illness may still be suspected and preliminary treatment begun when patients in a hot environment have muscle cramps, headache, weakness, syncope, or near-syncope.

History

The following questions are asked by the prehospital personnel:
1. What is the exact nature of the problem for which the patient summoned help?
2. What was the ambient temperature and relative humidity in the immediate environment?
3. What level of physical activity was the patient involved in?
4. How much liquid had been consumed immediately before and during this episode? What type of liquid was it?

Physical Examination

1. What are the vital signs?
2. What is the patient's skin color and temperature?
3. Is there evidence of sweating?

Intervention

1. Cardiopulmonary evaluation is followed by stabilization as needed.
2. If heat illness is suspected, cooling measures are initiated. These include moving the patient to the coolest environment available, removing excess clothing, moistening the skin with water, and fanning the patient to expedite evaporative heat loss. In severe cases, placement of ice packs in the groin and axillae can be helpful.

3. Fluids are replaced in alert patients by giving them cold liquids by mouth; in those with a depressed level of consciousness an intravenous (IV) line is initiated and an isotonic crystalloid is administered.

PROBLEM 3 This patient collapsed during vigorous exercise and was unconscious. Regardless of the cause, the unconscious patient has a potentially life-threatening condition, and the ABCs of resuscitation are instituted immediately. Further history was unavailable owing to the patient's condition, but his skin was very warm and moist.

The paramedics have been instructed to do the following:
1. Start an IV line and give a 250-ml bolus of normal saline.
2. Place the patient on a cardiac monitor.
3. Start oxygen by nasal cannula at 3 liters/min.
4. Give 50 ml of 50% dextrose and 100 mg thiamine IV.
5. Give 2 mg of naloxone IV.
6. Cool the patient by undressing him, splashing him with water, and fanning.
7. Transport the patient to the emergency department for further evaluation and treatment.

Although this patient received the comprehensive initial treatment indicated for any comatose patient, the setting and skin signs raised the possibility of heat illness. The rescue squad has appropriately instituted cooling measures.

INITIAL APPROACH IN THE EMERGENCY DEPARTMENT

Patients identified as having heat illness present to the emergency department in various ways. Those with serious disturbances in heat regulation have signs and symptoms of central nervous system pathology—headache, syncope or near-syncope, disorientation, or coma. Such patients are immediately evaluated for the need for prompt intervention.

1. The need for airway support or ventilation is quickly assessed, and supplemental oxygen is begun.
2. IV fluids are started or maintained and hypotension is treated if present. Cardiac monitoring is also maintained.
3. The paramedics' history is confirmed.
4. Vital signs are reassessed. Temperature is usually not determined until initial evaluation and stabilization have been completed. However, when patients are known to have developed problems while in hot environments or during vigorous exercise, or when the patient's skin feels very warm, temperature is measured early, since a markedly elevated temperature requires immediate reduction in order to minimize the ill effects of hyperthermia. Only a core or rectal temperature will be accurate in these circumstances. It is important to note that many standard hospital thermometers register to 107.6°F (42°C). It may be necessary to use a thermometer capable of registering a higher temperature.
5. The patient is undressed, and temperature reduction is begun using tepid water misting and an electric fan. This is a very effective method of cooling. More aggressive cooling measures, including cold water immersion, are seldom needed.
6. Infusion of fluid should proceed cautiously, giving normal saline in 200- to 250-ml boluses. The patient's response is monitored watching for signs of fluid overload such as pulmonary edema, new S_3 sounds, or distended neck veins.

PROBLEMS 2 AND 3 The body temperature of the patient in Problem 2 was 103°F (39.4°C), and the patient in Problem 3 had a rectal temperature of 108°F (42.2°C). The latter patient required rapid cooling measures. External cooling measures were begun, using tepid misting and fans. This is generally sufficient. Close monitoring of temperature response is important. More aggressive cooling measures should be employed if temperature reduction is not promptly noted. In the patient with the temperature of 103°F (39.4°C), fluid replacement and evaluation can be started in a less emergent manner. In the critically ill patient, volume replacement is initiated immediately.

DATA GATHERING

The history with supporting physical findings is the basis for the diagnosis of heat illness.

History

Alert patients who are suspected of having heat illness usually come to the emergency department with symptoms of muscular cramping, weakness, nausea, vomiting, headache, or syncope. The following questions are asked:

1. *What are the symptoms and over what time frame did they develop?*
2. *What was the ambient temperature and relative humidity in the environment at the time?*
   Vigorous activity in a hot environment is the most common predisposing situation, but elderly or debilitated patients can suffer adverse effects from heat with no activity at all owing to inadequate means for dissipating body heat.
3. *What types of fluids have been ingested and how much has been ingested?*
   Replacement of fluid losses with hypotonic solutions such as water can lead to heat cramps or, if carried much further, to serious reductions in the serum sodium concentration. Curiously, conditioned athletes are more prone to develop these problems, probably owing to their ability to sweat larger volumes.
4. *What risk factors for the development of heat illness are present (see Table 21–1)?*
5. *What previous medical problems are present that may influence current care or suggest causes other than heat illness for the patient's disorder?*
   a. *All debilitated patients* are at increased risk for heat illness owing to their inability to dissipate endogenous heat loads. Such patients who also have abnormal mental status may not be able to communicate their feeling of thirst and therefore are at even greater risk of heat illness.
   b. Patients with *previous episodes* of *serious heat illness* are prone to develop recurrences.
   c. Patients taking *diuretics*, which may cause dehydration, and *phenothiazines* or *tricyclic antidepressants*, which inhibit sweating, are at increased risk.
   d. Patients with a history of *drug abuse* (e.g., cocaine, amphetamines, or alcohol) may develop hyperthermia due to these drugs.

In patients who have a depressed level of consciousness, an accurate history is more difficult if not impossible to obtain. However, family, friends, and paramedics are usually able to supply a good deal of information about the events that led to the patient's present condition and the past medical history.

PROBLEM 1 The patient had mild residual cramping and related a previous similar episode. In such cases, simply removing the patient from the hot environment is a major component of the treatment.

PROBLEM 3 This patient was comatose. The history, therefore, was limited. However,

TABLE 21-1. Risk Factors for Development of Heat Illness

1. External heat load or climate
2. Internal heat load or exercise
3. Preexisting illness
    a. Cardiovascular compromise
        (1) Cardiac disease
        (2) Dehydration
    b. Spinal cord injury if associated with impaired sweating function
    c. Skin or sweat follicle abnormality
        (1) Burns
        (2) Cystic fibrosis
        (3) Ectodermal dysplasia (congenital absence of sweat glands)
        (4) Scleroderma
    d. Increased motor activity
        (1) Parkinsonism
        (2) Pheochromocytoma
        (3) Hyperthyroidism
    e. Obesity
4. Drugs
    a. Drugs that inhibit sweating
        (1) Anticholinergics-antihistamines, phenothiazines, tricyclic antidepressants
    b. Drugs that increase metabolic activity
        (1) Amphetamines, phencyclidine, LSD, cocaine
    c. Diuretics due to potential for dehydration
    d. Alcohol
5. Miscellaneous
    a. Previous history of heat stroke
    b. Lack of acclimatization
    c. Fatigue
    d. Lack of sleep
    e. Infection
    f. Constrictive clothing
    g. Extremes of age

there were other sources of historical information available. Attempts were made to speak directly to the drill instructor and fellow recruits because they might be able to give additional information such as seizure activity or unusual complaints verbalized by the recruit. Family was also contacted since they may have had important information about the past medical history (e.g., seizures, heart disease, diabetes, medications, allergies, and risk factors for heat illness). Heat stroke is a strong possibility in this patient; however, other possible problems must still be considered.

Physical Examination

Analysis of vital signs and physical findings is helpful in establishing a correct diagnosis and guiding treatment.

Vital Signs

Blood Pressure. Changes in blood pressure may range from orthostatic changes that respond promptly to fluid therapy to frank hypotension, which is due either to pump failure (cardiac microinfarcts and petechial hemorrhages), volume depletion from sweat losses, or vasodilation.

Respiratory Rate. Respirations are frequently increased as an accessory mechanism for dissipating heat, but the increase can result in cramps from hypocapnia.

Pulse. Tachycardia usually is compensatory for hypovolemia.

Temperature. It is important to obtain and monitor the core temperature, usually by use of a rectal probe.

General Physical Examination

A thorough physical examination is helpful in providing confirmatory evidence that points to a primary heat injury or other illnesses in the differential diagnosis.

Cutaneous Signs. Skin temperature, presence of sweating, rashes, and tissue turgor are important signs to be noted. Muscular fasciculations and cramps may also be seen.

Cardiovascular System. A murmur, thrill, or lift, abnormalities in the pulse rate and regularity, and orthostatic changes may suggest a cardiovascular cause for syncope rather than primary heat illness.

Neurologic System. Focal deficits, neck stiffness, or Trousseau's or Chvostek's sign suggests alternative causes. Mental status changes are consistent with primary heat illness, however.

Endocrine System. In the presence of hyperventilation, the odor of acetone on the breath may suggest diabetic ketoacidosis. Hyperthyroidism is suggested by a goiter, skin and eye findings, and a hyperdynamic cardiovascular status.

DECISION PRIORITIES AND PRELIMINARY DIFFERENTIAL DIAGNOSIS

In addressing the patient with possible heat illness, the physician is faced with two sets of questions:

- Is this a heat-related illness? If so, which form?
- If this is not a problem related to heat regulation, what else is causing the patient's problem?

Primary heat illness is suspected when the presenting signs and symptoms and the situation in which they developed are consistent with that diagnosis. In a few instances, those factors, along with the rapid resolution of symptoms on removal to a cool environment, may be sufficient to justify the diagnosis. In general, however, other problems must be ruled out before a diagnosis of heat illness is confirmed. Therefore, the approach to possible heat illness is to determine the type of primary heat illness being considered (Table 21–2) and then work through the differential diagnosis for that specific illness (Tables 21–3, 21–4, and 21–5).

Primary Heat Illness

Although there are various types of heat illness, heat cramps, heat exhaustion, and heat stroke are the major forms encountered by emergency physicians.

Heat Cramps. Cramping of those muscles that are working the hardest occurs in heat cramps. The cause is dilutional hyponatremia, which usually occurs in conditioned athletes who replace fluid losses with water. Possible other causes such as hyperventilation, hypocalcemia, or hypokalemia are usually suspected on the basis of the history, particularly anxiety or use of diuretics (Table 21–3).

TABLE 21–2. Differentiation of Types of Primary Heat Illness

Condition	History	Temperature	Mentation	Skin Signs
Heat cramps	Muscle cramps	Normal	Normal	Sweating, muscle spasms
Heat exhaustion	Weakness Headache Syncope	102.2–106°F (39–41.1°C)	Normal	Profuse sweating
Heat stroke	Coma Seizures Confusion	106–108°F (41.1–42.2°C)	Impaired	Dry or sweating*

*Sweating is absent in classic heat stroke but it may be present or absent in exertional heat stroke.

TABLE 21-3. Heat Cramps: Differential Diagnosis[a]

Potential Diagnosis	Pertinent History	Pertinent Findings on Physical Examination	Pertinent Laboratory Findings
Hyperventilation	Stress Anxiety	Trousseau's sign[b] Chvostek's sign[c] Carpopedal spasm	ABG: decreasing P_{CO_2}, increasing pH
Hypocalcemia	Neck surgery Malabsorption symptoms	Trousseau's sign Chvostek's sign Tetany Convulsions Skeletal abnormalities	Hypocalcemia Soft tissue calcification on x-ray
Hypokalemia	Gastrointestinal losses Diuretic use Inadequate diet	Weakness Decreased or absent reflexes	Hypokalemia
Heat cramps	Conditioned athlete Exercise Sweat loss Access to water Previous similar illness	Muscle spasms Sweating Normal temperature	Hyponatremia

ABG = Arterial blood gas measurements.
[a]The table outlines the symptom complex represented in the patient in Problem 1—severe muscle cramps.
[b]Trousseau's sign is characteristic spasms of the hand stimulated by compressing the upper arm with a tourniquet or a blood pressure cuff.
[c]Chvostek's sign is unilateral spasm of the face following a tap over the facial nerve.

PROBLEM 1 On physical examination the patient exhibited muscle spasms, but there was no Chvostek's or Trousseau's sign, and no carpopedal spasms or reflex changes occurred. The remainder of the examination showed normal results. In addition, the patient seemed to improve with rest.

A diagnosis of heat cramps turned out to be most appropriate based on the history and physical examination. A conditioned athlete exercising strenuously in a hot environment sweats up to 3 liters/hr. In this case the history of replacing these fluid losses with water and then experiencing cramps in the muscles that were working hardest is consistent with a diagnosis of heat cramps. This diagnosis is primarily made by the history.

Heat Exhaustion. Dizziness, nausea, vomiting, fever, weakness, and occasionally syncope in a patient who is typically sweating profusely are characteristic of heat exhaustion. This is the most common form of heat illness, and it has a low morbidity and mortality.

Either water or salt depletion can be the cause. Salt depletion occurs when sweat losses are replaced only by hypotonic solutions, and symptoms are thought to be due to hyponatremia. Water depletion occurs when patients are unable to satisfy their thirst, and dehydration and hypernatremia result, a situation that often occurs in nursing home patients. In the salt-depletion type of illness, the temperature may be normal or elevated; in the water-depletion type the temperature is usually elevated, and the risk of progression to heat stroke is great.

PROBLEM 2 On reviewing this patient's history and physical findings, a diagnosis of heat exhaustion seems likely. However, this must be viewed as a diagnosis of exclusion. All the problems listed in Table 21-4 are considered and ruled out to a reasonable degree before the diagnosis of heat exhaustion is secure.

Heat Stroke. Heat stroke is the most severe form of heat illness, carrying a mortality of 17% to 80% and presenting with high fever and progressive neurologic deterioration, seizure, or coma. Heat stroke occurs when the body's heat loss mechanisms are overwhelmed. Its differential diagnosis is listed in Table 21-5.

TABLE 21–4. Differential Diagnosis of Heat Exhaustion—Symptom Complex: Weakness, Headache, Mild Disorientation, Syncope, or Near-Syncope

Potential Diagnosis	Pertinent History	Pertinent Findings on Physical Examination	Pertinent Laboratory Data
Head trauma	Injury, anticoagulant therapy	External trauma Focal neurologic deficit	Brain CT: hemorrhage
Subarachnoid hemorrhage	Sudden onset of severe headache during straining or exercise, family history, history of aneurysm	Variable level of consciousness, neck stiffness (Kernig's or Brudzinski's sign), retinal hemorrhages	Brain CT: hemorrhage Lumbar puncture (if CT negative): increased RBCs, xanthochromia
Aortic outflow tract stenosis (IHSS or congenital valve disease)	Murmur known, exertional syncope	Murmur, precordial thrill or lift	ECG Cardiac echocardiography Cardiac catheterization
Dysrhythmia	Sudden onset of lightheadedness, papitations, previous history	Abnormal heart rate, rhythm, and peripheral pulses, symptoms present during dysrhythmia	Cardiac monitor, ECG
Vascular dilatation	Postural symptoms, allergy (e.g., bee sting), drugs	Orthostatic changes, hives, wheezing	
Hypovolemia	Postural symptoms, fluid loss (e.g., sweat, blood, or GI loss)	Orthostatic changes, decreased tissue turgor, sweating, rectal blood	Hemoglobin/hematocrit: decreased BUN/creatinine: elevated
Diabetic ketoacidosis	Polyuria, polydipsia, polyphagia, family history	Fruity odor of breath, decreased tissue turgor, hyperventilation, orthostatic changes	Serum and urine ketones: elevated Arterial blood gases: metabolic acidosis
Poison/adverse medication	Exposure—skin, ingestion, and inhalation	Odor, toxidrome (e.g., anticholinergic syndrome)	Drug level Drug screen Arterial blood gases: acid/base abnormality Carboxyhemoglobin
Encephalitis/meningitis	Fever, prodromal illness, severe headache, chills	Temperature, neck stiffness (Kernig's and Brudzinski's signs)	Lumbar puncture: elevated WBCs, positive Gram's stain, cultures
Heat exhaustion	Hot environment, exercise, sweat loss	Temperature, sweating, orthostatic changes	Serum sodium: hyponatremia BUN/creatinine: elevated Aspartate aminotransferase (AST): slightly elevated

Classic heat stroke commonly occurs in the elderly and develops over a period of days. Dehydration leads to confusion, agitation, and lethargy. Usually the patient stops sweating and presents with a hot, dry skin.

Exertional heat stroke occurs in young, active, healthy individuals who overwhelm their body's heat dissipation capabilities. It can develop during a period of an hour or less. Signs of dehydration may or may not be present. Sweating is frequently still present in this subgroup.

Complications of heat stroke are common, especially if treatment is delayed, and are responsible for the high mortality (Table 21–6). Hypotension, rhabdomyolysis and renal failure, hepatic failure, and disseminated intravascular coagulation (DIC) are the most common complications. Rhabdomyolysis and renal failure are much more common (25%) in exertional heat stroke than in classic heat stroke (5%).

TABLE 21–5. Differential Diagnosis of Heat Stroke—Symptom Complex: Altered Mental Status, Hyperthermia

Potential Diagnosis	Pertinent History	Pertinent Findings on Physical Examination	Pertinent Laboratory Data
Encephalitis/meningitis	Fever, prodromal illness, severe headache, chills	Temperature, neck stiffness (Kernig's and Brudzinski's signs)	Lumbar puncture: elevated WBCs, positive Gram's stain, cultures
Malaria	Exposure, travel history, previous history	Fever pattern, confusion	Peripheral blood smear
Typhoid fever, typhus	Exposure, travel history	Fever pattern	Titers: Weil-Felix reaction, complement fixation
Sepsis	Fever, age extreme, immunocompromised	Fever, confusion, coma, focal infection	Chest x-ray; WBC: elevated; cultures: blood, urine, spinal fluid
Hypothalamic hemorrhage	Hypertension, anticoagulant therapy	Coma and fever, focal neurologic findings	Brain CT: hemorrhage
Thyroid storm	Preexisting hyperthyroidism (e.g., Graves' disease); risk factors include stress or surgery, trauma, infection, failure to take antithyroid medication	Goiter, tachycardia, seizures, hypotension	Thyroid function studies: T_3 and T_4
Malignant hyperthermia	Inhalation anesthetic, succinylcholine	Muscle fasciculations	Arterial blood gases: acidosis; Electrolytes: hyperkalemia, hypermagnesemia
Heat stroke	Risk factors (see Table 21–1), exposure to heat load, exercise	Hot, flushed skin, confusion, agitation, seizures, tachycardia, hypotension, vomiting, diarrhea, muscle tenderness	AST: elevated; WBC: elevated; Electrolytes: hyper- or hypokalemia, hyponatremia, hypocalcemia, hypophosphatemia; Arterial blood gases: metabolic acidosis; Urine: myoglobin; clotting factors: decreased; blood glucose: variable

DIAGNOSTIC ADJUNCTS

The diagnostic work-up is based on the patient's specific presentation and is aimed at confirming or ruling out diagnoses other than heat illness (Tables 21–3, 21–4, and 21–5). There is no single ancillary test that is specific for heat illness. Patients with heat cramps and mild heat exhaustion that rapidly resolves frequently require no ancillary testing. However, patients with more severe forms of the disorder require extensive evaluation to rule out other problems, and detect complications (Table 21–6).

TABLE 21–6. Heat Stroke—Poor Prognostic Factors

Temperature greater than 106°F (41.1°C)
AST (SGOT) greater than 1000 IU
Coma
Rhabdomyolysis
Renal failure
Hypotension

Laboratory Studies in Heat Stroke

Complete Blood Count with Differential Cell Count. The white cell count is usually elevated but is less than 20,000/mm³. A high percentage of immature neutrophils (bands) can be seen, but this is more common with underlying infection. The hemoglobin–hematocrit levels may be increased secondary to a depleted intravascular volume.

Electrolytes. The sodium level may be abnormal, and as rhabdomyolysis occurs potassium may become elevated.

Blood Urea Nitrogen–Creatinine. BUN and creatinine levels may be elevated owing to impaired renal function or dehydration.

Urinalysis. The urinalysis is used to monitor the hydration status and to detect the presence of rhabdomyolysis (the urine sample is positive for hemoglobin but negative for red blood cells).

Liver Enzymes. The liver is the organ that is perhaps most sensitive to heat stress. Elevation of transaminase levels can occur in heat exhaustion and is a common finding in heat stroke. These levels peak 24 to 48 hours after injury. The severity of illness correlates well with the magnitude as well as the duration of the aspartate aminotransferase (AST) elevation. AST levels in excess of 1000 IU predict severe illness with complications, especially renal failure.

Serum Glucose. Depending on the metabolic response of the body to an excessive heat load, the serum glucose can be high or low. It has no diagnostic value alone but does give information about the general metabolic status of the patient and the need for replacement.

Arterial Blood Gases. The PaO_2 is useful for assessing the systemic maintenance of oxygen at a time of high demand. The pH and $PaCO_2$ are necessary for calculating the degree of acid-base pathology. Lactic acidosis is commonly associated with the more severe heat-related illnesses as well as a number of diseases that mimic them.

Coagulation Profile. This test is reserved for patients with severe heat illness. It includes a platelet count, prothrombin time (PT), and activated partial thromboplastin time (PTT). Both severe heat illness and sepsis can trigger a disseminated intravascular coagulation syndrome.

Cultures. Heat stroke is significantly rarer than sepsis. Cultures of blood and urine are part of the evaluation to search for this common problem.

Radiologic Studies

A *chest radiograph* is part of the diagnostic search for infective sites while the diagnosis of moderate to severe heat illness is being considered.

Computed tomography (CT) is necessary in any patient with acutely altered mental status who does not rapidly improve with therapeutic intervention. Subarachnoid and intracranial hemorrhage can cause associated central elevations of temperature.

Electrocardiography

A 12-lead electrocardiogram is ordered in any patient considered to have moderate to severe heat illness. Increased metabolic demand and cardiovascular stress can predispose to myocardial ischemia or dysrhythmias.

PROBLEM 2 Because of the moderately severe heat illness and syncopal episode, a CBC, electrolytes, serum glucose, and AST measurements were ordered. All values were normal. The laboratory tests added significantly to the cost of the patient's care ($70 to $80). Unfortunately, the history and physical examination warranted this information to be gathered before the patient could be discharged. The waiting time needed for laboratory results can also be viewed as a "cost," but the need for treatment and observation negates this concern.

404 — TOXICOLOGIC/ENVIRONMENTAL DISORDERS

PROBLEM 3 In patients with heat stroke, extensive laboratory evaluation is necessary (Table 21–7). Results of laboratory tests not only assess the range of complications but also keep the physician thinking about diseases that mimic severe heat illness, particularly sepsis.

PRINCIPLES OF MANAGEMENT

Management principles for heat illnesses are:

1. Elimination of excess heat
2. Replacement of fluids and electrolytes
3. Treatment of complications

Elimination of Excess Heat

Elimination of excess heat may be accomplished through radiation, conduction, convection, or evaporation. Placing the patient in a cool environment will hasten heat loss through radiation, and the removal of clothing will enhance this as well as increase *convection* heat loss owing to wind currents contacting the skin. Fanning the patient will further enhance convection heat loss. Dissipation of heat by *conduction* can be accomplished by immersing the patient in cold water or placing ice packs in contact with the body. Ice can also cause vasoconstriction, which can retard heat loss, but this mechanism has not been shown to be clinically significant.

Evaporation is the most clinically useful mechanism, however. Spraying the skin with a mist and then fanning the patient is easily accomplished and highly effective. Other methods of cooling include ice water lavage of the stomach, bladder, or peritoneum and cardiopulmonary bypass, but these measures are rarely employed because simpler techniques are very effective. Aspirin is ineffective in patients with heat stroke, and acetaminophen is contraindicated owing to the risk of liver damage.

Whatever technique is used, active cooling should stop when the patient's temperature has reached 100°F (37.8°C), to avoid taking the patient into the hypothermic range.

Replacement of Fluids and Electrolytes

In patients with heat cramps or mild heat exhaustion, *replacement of fluids and electrolytes* can be accomplished by asking the patient to drink oral preparations such as Gatorade or Pedialyte. In patients with heat stroke or severe heat exhaustion, IV fluid replacement with isotonic crystalloid is appropriate. In water-depletion type illness, the fluid is switched to a hypotonic solution when the volume deficit has been replaced. The water deficit can be calculated as shown below:

TABLE 21–7. Laboratory Findings in Heat Stroke

CBC	WBC elevated (20,000–30,000)
Electrolytes	Hypokalemia, hyponatremia, hypophosphatemia, hypocalcemia, occasionally hyperkalemia from muscle breakdown
Arterial blood gases	Metabolic acidosis
Liver function	Elevated AST, lactic dehydrogenase, CPK
Glucose	Normal or low
Clotting	Picture of DIC may occur (decreased platelets, prolonged PT and PTT and increased fibrin split products)
ECG	Supraventricular tachycardia, nonspecific ST–T wave changes

CBC = Complete blood count; WBC = white blood cells; AST = aspartate aminotransferase; CPK = creatinine phosphokinase; DIC = disseminated intravascular coagulation; PT = prothrombin time; PTT = partial thromboplastin time; ECG = electrocardiogram.

Normal total body water (TBW) = $0.6 \times$ wt (kg)

$$\text{Abnormal TBW} = \frac{(\text{Normal Na}^+)(\text{normal TBW})}{\text{Observed Na}^+}$$

Water deficit = TBW − abnormal TBW

Example: 60-kg man with Na$^+$ of 160

Normal TBW = $0.6 \times 60 = 36$ liters

$$\text{Abnormal TBW} = \frac{140 \times 36}{160} = 31.5 \text{ liters}$$

Water deficit = 36 liters − 31.5 liters = 4.5 liters

Half of the calculated dose of a salt-free solution such as D/W 5% is given over 24 hours in addition to maintenance requirements and replacement of ongoing losses.

In patients with salt-depletion type illness, fluid is administered as normal saline at a rate of 250 to 500 ml/hr, and monitoring is accomplished by checking urinary output and, in severe cases, central venous or pulmonary artery pressure measurements. Salt tablets have been used for electrolyte replacement in the past but are no longer recommended because there is no way to gauge the appropriate dose. Hypernatremia as well as further fluid losses into the intestinal lumen can result.

Treatment of Complications of Heat Stroke

Shivering. During the cooling process, the patient may begin to shiver, therefore creating more heat. Diazepam 5 to 10 mg IV or chlorpromazine 12.5 mg IV can be used to control shivering.

Hypotension. Hypotension may be caused by volume depletion, vasodilation, or cardiac failure secondary to heat damage. Fluid replacement needs to be done cautiously in such cases to avoid overloading the patient in pump failure. Central venous monitoring is helpful in determining the cause of the hypotension and can guide fluid therapy. In elderly patients with preexisting heart disease, a pulmonary capillary wedge pressure monitor is a much better guide. Perfusion signs—blood pressure, heart rate, skin temperature, and urine output—need to be monitored carefully. Dobutamine may be effective treatment in the patient with cardiogenic hypotension.

Rhabdomyolysis. Rhabdomyolysis is more likely to occur in the exertional form of heat stroke than in the classic form. The cause is direct heat damage to muscle. If myoglobin is present in the urine, mannitol is administered (0.25 gm/kg) intravenously, and a urine output of 70 to 75 ml/hr is maintained. Administration of sodium bicarbonate is considered, as a brisk flow of alkaline urine will help to prevent precipitation of myoglobin in the renal tubules.

Renal Failure. Renal failure occurs in 25% of exertional heat stroke victims but in only 5% of patients with classic heat stroke. The cause is multifactorial—direct heat damage to the kidneys, dehydration, and myoglobin blocking the renal tubules. It should be recognized that renal failure is reversible and usually requires only temporary dialysis.

PROBLEM 2 This patient was treated with intravenous fluids, tepid misting, and fanning. The original temperature of 103°F (39.4°C) came down to 99°F (37.2°C). History, physical examination, and laboratory evaluation uncovered no additional abnormalities.

PROBLEM 3 This comatose patient with a temperature of 108°F (42.2°C) was at high risk of serious morbidity. No further history was available, and the physical examination revealed only a deeply comatose patient with no localizing neurologic signs and hot, moist skin. Laboratory studies showed a white blood cell count of 20,000/mm^3, AST of 1000 IU, and serum sodium concentration of 125 mEq/liter. Initial cooling by means of misting and fanning was successful in reducing the temperature. Once the temperature was reduced to 100°F (37.7°C), cooling measures were stopped. The temperature was carefully monitored for rebound. Fluid was administered as normal saline at a rate of 500 ml/hr, with close monitoring of vital signs, pulmonary status, and urine output. No evidence of myoglobinuria was detected.

These cases demonstrate the spectrum of severity of illness that is possible in patients with primary heat illness. The patient in Problem 2 needs no further immediate intervention, but the patient in Problem 3 requires continued intensive management and monitoring. Cardiac failure, rhabdomyolysis with myoglobinuria, renal failure, and disseminated intravascular coagulation are some of the complications that may develop.

SPECIAL CONSIDERATIONS

Hyperthermia in the Agitated, Intoxicated Patient

Temperature measurement is particularly important in patients who are agitated or intoxicated. It should be recognized that any preexisting physical or mental impairment that results in an inability to take the usual protective measures in response to heat (such as meeting the thirst need or moving to a cooler environment) predisposes the individual to heat illness.

Agitation can be either the result or the cause of heat illness. Agitation may be *caused* by a wide variety of conditions—primary metabolic disorders, primary neurologic disorders, sepsis, or drugs (e.g., phencyclidine [PCP], cocaine, or amphetamines). On the other hand, agitation *causes* heat illness by virtue of the tremendous internal heat load that results from increased muscular activity. The goals of therapy should include treating the primary disorder and cooling the patient.

Pediatric Patients

Two settings in which children are at particular risk for heat stroke include the febrile infant who is wrapped in excessive blankets and the small child who is left in an unattended car with the windows rolled up. Education is essential to eliminate these causes of heat stroke.

Geriatric Patients

Fever in the elderly is relatively common. Sepsis is a particularly common cause of fever in elderly persons who are debilitated or have other chronic illnesses that compromise the immune status. The usual sources of sepsis in the elderly are pneumonia, urinary tract infection, and skin infections. Heat illness as a cause for fever in the elderly is a diagnosis of exclusion. A high index of suspicion is appropriate, especially when environmental conditions are conducive.

The elderly are at high risk for heat illness based on several factors (see Table 21–1):

1. They are unable to take appropriate measures (drink fluids, move to a cooler environment) to protect against a hot environment owing to physical or mental impairment.

2. They are in poor physical condition.

3. They are unable to mount an adequate physiologic response to heat loads owing to impairment of sweating and cardiovascular responses.

4. They are commonly taking drugs that may predispose to heat illness.

DISPOSITION AND FOLLOW-UP

The disposition of patients with heat illness will vary from discharge from the hospital to intensive care unit admission, depending on the type and severity of the illness.

1. *Heat cramps* are self-limiting and are not associated with any serious sequelae. After resolution of the cramps, these patients are discharged home with instructions for fluid replacement and advice about prevention.

2. *Heat exhaustion* is a relatively benign condition that generally responds well to treatment in the emergency department. These patients can usually be discharged after treatment and 4 to 6 hours observation with instructions about fluid therapy and prevention. Patients with heat exhaustion who have even slight elevations in AST should refrain from any exercise and heat exposure for 48 to 72 hours despite an otherwise healthy appearance. These patients are at high risk for recurrent heat illness. Admission is considered when the patient has continued symptoms such as vomiting or orthostatic hypotension or if other serious diagnoses have not been ruled out satisfactorily.

3. *Heat stroke* victims require admission to a critical care unit. All patients with unexplained coma need critical care admission for aggressive monitoring of the patient's airway, neurologic status, cardiac rhythm, and vital signs. Factors indicating a poor prognosis in these patients are listed in Table 21–6.

Prior to discharge, victims of heat illness should be advised of *prevention tips*. The acclimatization process takes 2 to 3 weeks. During this time it is advisable to take frequent breaks to cool down and replenish fluid losses (beyond thirst). Gradually increasing exercise time and wearing light-colored, lightweight clothing will also help.

PROBLEMS 1 AND 2 These patients were discharged home with instructions for prevention of heat cramps or heat exhaustion.

PROBLEM 3 This patient had a great likelihood of developing life-threatening complications and was admitted to an intensive care unit for continued fluid management, temperature regulation, and monitoring for complications.

DOCUMENTATION

1. Risk factors: Heat load (ambient temperature, relative humidity), preexisting illness, drugs.
2. Physical examination: Temperature, level of consciousness, skin moisture.
3. Laboratory findings: Elevated AST or myoglobin level.
4. Therapeutic measures: Cooling methods and response (serial temperatures), preventive recommendations.
5. Flow sheet monitoring of vital signs, laboratory findings, and response to treatment.

SUMMARY AND FINAL POINTS

- The common forms of heat illness are heat cramps, heat exhaustion, and heat stroke.
- Heat cramps are benign and self-limited.
- Heat exhaustion usually responds readily to cooling and fluid replacement.
- Heat stroke is a serious illness that has significant mortality and requires aggressive therapy to reduce complications, morbidity, and mortality.
- Heat illness is preventable. Public education efforts continue to be necessary.

BIBLIOGRAPHY

Text

1. Yarborough B, Hubbard R: Heat-related illnesses. In Auerbach P, Geehr E (eds): Management of Wilderness and Environmental Emergencies. St. Louis, C.V. Mosby, 1989.

Journal Articles

1. Bark NM: Heatstroke in psychiatric patients: Two cases and a review. J Clin Psychiatry 43(9):377–380, 1982.
2. Clowes G: Heat stroke: Current concepts. N Engl J Med 21(11):564–567, 1979.
3. Exertional heat injury. Med Letter Drugs Ther 27(690):55, 1985.
4. Kew M, Bersohn I, Seftel H, et al: Liver damage in heat stroke. Am J Med 49:192, 1970.
5. Kilbourne EM, Choi K, Jones TS, et al: Risk factors for heat stroke. A case control study. JAMA 247(24):3332–3336, 1982.
6. Knochel JP: Environmental heat illness, an electric review. Arch Intern Med 133:841–864, 1974.
7. Leads from the MMWR: Illness and death due to environmental heat. Georgia and St. Louis, 1983. JAMA 252(1):20–23, 1984.
8. Pattison ME, Logan JL, Lee SM, et al: Exertional heat stroke and acute renal failure in a young woman. Am J Kidney Dis 11:184, 1988.
9. Roberts P, Hubbard R, Kerstein M: Serum glutamic-oxaloacetic transaminase (SGOT) as a predictor of recurrent heat illness. Mil Med 152:408, 1987.
10. Smith NJ: The prevention of heat disorders in sports. Am J Dis Child 138(8):786–790, 1984.
11. Stewart CE: Preventing progression of heat injury. Emerg Med Reps 8(16):121–128, 1987.
11. Stine RJ: Heat illness. JACEP 8(4):154, 1979.
13. Treatment of heat stroke. Med Letter Drugs Ther 23(17):76, 1981.

CHAPTER 22

HYPOTHERMIA

MARY ANN COOPER, M.D.
DANIEL F. DANZL, M.D.

PROBLEM 1 A 73 year old woman was found in her apartment. The rescue squad was called by concerned neighbors, who had not seen her for 3 days. The heat had been turned off, and the apartment was very cold. Her pulse rate was 60 beats/min and very weak, blood pressure 90/50 mm Hg, respiratory rate 6/min and shallow.

PROBLEM 2 A 4 year old who had chased a pet out onto an icy pond fell through the ice. He was under the ice for at least 20 minutes before being rescued. No vital signs were obtainable at the scene. The child's pupils were dilated and unreactive.

QUESTIONS TO CONSIDER

1. How is hypothermia defined?
2. What is the difference between primary and secondary hypothermia?
3. What are the common mechanisms of heat loss?
4. What organ systems have pathophysiologic derangements caused by temperature depression?
5. Which patients are predisposed to the development of hypothermia?
6. What are the common presenting symptoms and signs suggesting hypothermia?
7. How is the severity of hypothermia related to selecting the best rewarming technique in the emergency department?
8. What common complications are encountered during the rewarming and resuscitation of cold patients?
9. How can understanding the pathophysiology of heat loss help prevent hypothermia?

INTRODUCTION

Hypothermia is defined as a core temperature of less than 95°F (35°C). It is either accidental (primary) or secondary to other disease processes. The development of complications is dependent upon many factors. The most important is the degree of hypothermia. Age, concomitant injury, preexisting or predisposing illness, localized hypothermia, immersion in water, and intoxication are additional factors that may affect morbidity and mortality.

Well-publicized accounts of accidental hypothermia due to mountaineering accidents and submersion in cold water—accidents that are often survived—have brought the subject of hypothermia to the attention of the lay public. Far more common though less recognized are the cases of hypothermia that develop more subtly in urban settings. Severe cold and prolonged exposure are not necessary for a person to develop hypothermia. Six to ten percent of cases of mild to moderate hypothermia occur in warm seasons and may be unrecognized. Essentially all of these people come first to the emergency department.

Pathophysiology

Normal body temperature varies over a narrow 1°C range. Initially, exposure to cold stimulates the skin receptors, resulting in peripheral vasoconstriction and conservation of heat. As the temperature of the blood declines, the preoptic anterior hypothalamus is stimulated. Heat production is then increased by shivering and by metabolic and endocrinologic means of thermogenesis (Fig. 22–1).

There are five mechanisms of heat loss that threaten thermostability:

1. *Radiation.* Radiation accounts for 55% to 65% of heat loss and is modified by insulation (clothing, subcutaneous fat layer) and skin blood flow.
2. *Conduction.* Conduction is normally not a major source of heat loss, but conductive heat loss increases five times in wet clothing, 25 to 30 times in cold water.
3. *Convection.* Wind currents and body motion markedly increase heat loss. The windchill effect significantly increases the likelihood of hypothermia developing at a given temperature.
4. *Evaporation.*
5. *Respiration.* These last two mechanisms account for 20% to 30% of the heat loss in dry, windy conditions.

Hypothermia affects the entire body, and the major signs and symptoms are due to involvement of the cardiovascular, central nervous, respiratory, renal, and gastrointestinal systems.

Cardiovascular Effects. After an initial tachycardia, the heart rate decreases as the temperature falls. The "normal" heart rate is reduced by half at a body temperature of 82.4°F (28°C). The mean arterial pressure decreases progressively, and the cardiac output drops to 45% of normal at 77°F (25°C).

Atrial arrhythmias commonly appear at temperatures below 90°F (32.2°C) and are innocent. In contrast, ventricular ectopy is often initially suppressed by the cold until the body reaches a temperature of 86 to 82.4°F (30 to 28°C). At these temperatures, electrical conduction through the myocardial muscle fibers is faster than that through the His-Purkinje system. This greatly increases the risk of ventricular fibrillation.

A J wave (Osborn wave or hypothermic hump) may be present at the junction of

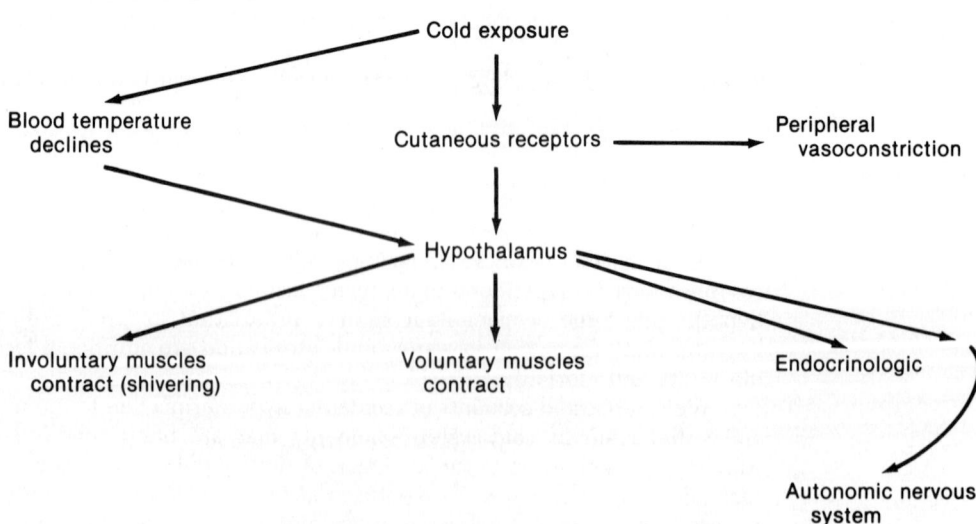

FIGURE 22–1. Physiologic responses in hypothermia.

the QRS complex and ST segment. Although the J wave is *not* prognostic or pathognomonic, it can be diagnostic (Fig. 22–2).

Core temperature *afterdrop* is a term referring to the continued drop in temperature after rewarming is started. Afterdrop results from simple temperature equilibration and circulatory changes. Cold acidotic hyperkalemic blood returns to the core when heat is applied directly to the extremities and vasoconstriction is reversed.

Central Nervous System Effects. There is a progression of changes in the brain as the temperature falls. Enzyme systems become less functional, and there is a linear decrease in cerebral metabolism. Cerebral perfusion is maintained until vascular autoregulation becomes ineffective at 77°F (25°C). At 68°F (20°C), the electroencephalogram shows a flat line.

Common neurologic findings include dysarthria, hypesthesia, hyporeflexia, and ataxia. Psychiatric symptoms range from a peculiar "flat" affect to impaired judgment, e.g., paradoxical undressing.

Respiratory Effects. Cold initially stimulates the respiratory drive. Later, as metabolism slows, there is a progressive depression of the respiratory minute volume. Bronchorrhea, brought on by the inhalation of cold air, can be severe, simulating pulmonary edema.

Renal Effects. The kidneys respond rapidly to hypothermic fluid sequestration. Although renal blood flow drops progressively, there is a large diuresis of dilute glomerular filtrate resulting from an initial central hypervolemia caused by vasoconstriction in the extremities. Ethanol can double the amount of volume loss. Cold water immersion may increase this diuresis by three and a half times.

Gastrointestinal Effects. Hypothermia decreases gastrointestinal motility. Gastric dilatation, ileus, constipation, and poor rectal tone commonly result. Though the precise cause is unknown, inflammatory changes in the pancreas and hyperamylasemia are often found in the hypothermic patient.

PREHOSPITAL CARE

A high index of suspicion is often required to diagnose hypothermia in the field, since these patients present in a variety of settings. Hypothermia in summer and in southern locales is not rare and can easily go unrecognized.

History

1. Where was the patient found? What was the ambient temperature? If the patient was found in water, what was the water temperature?
2. What type of clothing was the patient wearing?
3. Is the patient taking any medications? Were any medications found in the area?

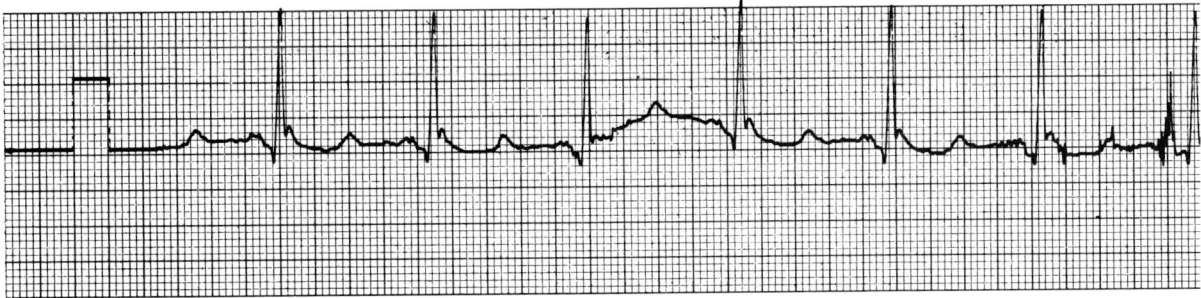

FIGURE 22–2. Example of a J wave in the 73 year old woman in Problem 1.

Physical Examination

1. What are the vital signs? Is ventilation adequate? In patients with severe hypothermia, palpation of a peripheral pulse is difficult. Femoral or carotid pulses are more reliable in the very cold patient.
2. What does the cardiac monitor show? Cardiopulmonary resuscitation (CPR) is not started if there is any sign of perfusion. Iatrogenic ventricular fibrillation *may* result if external chest compressions are inadvertently applied in a patient who is *not* in cardiac arrest.
3. Is there evidence of trauma or medical illness? Patients may become hypothermic after they collapse for other reasons. A rapid physical assessment may reveal signs of other problems such as gastrointestinal hemorrhage, myocardial infarction, or head trauma.

Intervention

1. The hypothermic patient is placed in a warm, protected environment. Wet clothes are removed, and dry blankets are used to cover the patient. A patient may become hypothermic during prolonged extrication efforts in a cold environment. A person who is wet, even in the summer, is predisposed to the development of hypothermia. Trauma victims who are routinely undressed and given cold resuscitation fluids are at similar risk.
2. If the patient is apneic or unable to protect the airway, oxygen administration and ventilatory support are given, followed by endotracheal intubation. The hypothermic patient may develop cardiac dysrhythmias if any stimulation is used. Interventions that are needed to stabilize the patient are not withheld, but are carried out as gently as possible.
3. Cardiopulmonary resuscitation is initiated only when there is cardiac monitor evidence of asystole or ventricular fibrillation. "Pulselessness" may be due simply to marked vasoconstriction and slowed cardiac activity.
4. In the patient with altered mental status, 50% dextrose (25 to 50 gm), thiamine (100 mg), and naloxone (2 mg) are administered intravenously as empiric treatment for coexisting hypoglycemia or opioid intoxication.
5. Concomitant trauma or medical illness may require other specific management.

PROBLEM 2 At the scene, the child was flaccid, cyanotic, and had no spontaneous respirations or palpable apical pulse. The cardiac monitor revealed no electrical activity. The paramedics initiated CPR and called the base station. They were instructed to:
1. Continue CPR and cardiac monitoring.
2. Insert a #5 endotracheal tube and ventilate with 100% oxygen.
3. Attempt to start an IV during transport.
4. Insulate the child in warm blankets.
5. Transport the child to the emergency department for rewarming.

Before the child arrived in the emergency department, personnel and equipment were assembled for active core rewarming.

INITIAL APPROACH IN THE EMERGENCY DEPARTMENT

There is no consistent presentation of hypothermia. Whenever it is suspected, or whenever the oral temperature reading is 95°F (35°C), a confirmatory core temperature measurement is obtained. An indwelling rectal thermometer probe or an infrared tympanic reading is the most practical technique for measuring temperature.

The ABCs of resuscitation do not change in patients with hypothermia. Obtunded patients without protective airway reflexes require endotracheal intubation after preoxygenation. A Doppler ultrasonic stethoscope may be necessary to detect pulses. Intravenous lines are started, and cardiac monitor leads are applied. CPR is started if the monitor shows ventricular fibrillation or asystole.

History

The exposure history is reconfirmed with the rescue squad. Additional history of the present illness or past medical history is obtained from family, friends, or even bystanders. When none of these sources is available, medical records, medic-alert tags, or contents of purses, pockets, or wallets may be of assistance.

Physical Examination

All clothing is removed from the patient, and an examination is conducted searching for evidence of trauma or medical illness. Insulation with blankets is provided.

Intervention

After initial stabilization and a directed examination to determine the presence of concomitant medical or traumatic conditions are accomplished, the following interventions are appropriate:

1. A flow sheet is initiated for following the patient's vital signs, mental status, and urinary output.

2. A urinary catheter is inserted to assist in monitoring urinary output.

3. A nasogastric tube is inserted because gastric dilatation and ileus are frequent complications.

4. A fluid challenge with 200 to 300 ml of isotonic crystalloid heated to 104°F (40°C) is appropriate unless there is evidence of congestive heart failure. Replacement of fluid lost as a result of the initial "cold diuresis" is continued, guided by the vital signs, urinary output, and pulmonary status.

5. Administration of 50% dextrose (25 to 50 mg), preceded by thiamine 100 mg intravenously, will ensure that a concomitant hypoglycemia will not remain untreated. An alternative approach is to check the blood glucose concentration at the bedside with a glucose oxidase reagent strip before deciding on dextrose therapy. This is not always accurate.

6. Naloxone 2 mg IV is administered in patients with depressed mental status as a specific antidote to narcotic intoxication. It also has nonspecific activity against ethanol, barbiturates, propoxyphene, benzodiazepines, and phenothiazines.

7. In moderate to severe cases of hypothermia, active rewarming is started as soon as possible. Heated, humidified oxygen and heated intravenous fluids are used from the beginning of treatment. More invasive rewarming techniques are discussed under Management (Table 22–1).

PROBLEMS 1 and 2 The rectal temperature of the 73 year old patient in Problem 1 was

TABLE 22–1. Core Rewarming Options

Heated humidified oxygen	Peritoneal dialysis
Tube	Extracorporeal
Mask	Hemodialysis
Heated IV fluids	Cardiopulmonary bypass
Irrigation	Diathermy
Bladder	
Stomach	
Colon	
Mediastinum	

90°F (32.2°C). The 4 year old child in Problem 2 had a rectal and esophageal temperature of 77°F (25°C). The first patient was placed on a monitor, and heated, humidified oxygen was delivered through a face mask. Warm blankets were used to cover the patient.

The 4 year old was placed in the code room, and CPR continued. Initial rewarming was performed with heated, humidified oxygen at 40 to 45°C, given through the endotracheal tube, and heated nasogastric, bladder, and peritoneal lavage. Active external rewarming efforts were begun while equipment and personnel for extracorporeal rewarming were being mobilized.

Although passive and truncal active rewarming methods are appropriate in mild to moderate cases of hypothermia, more severe cases require core rewarming techniques to avoid either "rewarming collapse" or "core temperature afterdrop" shock.

DATA GATHERING

The information gathered during this process will help to establish the underlying medical status of the patient before hypothermia occurred. This information is important in prognosis.

History

The hypothermic patient is often unable to give an adequate history owing to unconsciousness, confusion, or intoxication. Other sources are used as necessary.

1. What were the *circumstances surrounding the exposure? Where* did it occur? What was the *ambient temperature*? Was *submersion in water* involved? Was the patient's *skin or clothing wet* for other reasons?
2. *How long was the patient exposed* to these conditions?
3. Has the patient or family noted *mental status change* or *incoordination*?
4. Has there been any *trauma*? The origin of the exposure must be explained. Trauma is a common antecedent of hypothermia episodes.
5. Was the patient *acutely ill before the onset* of the current problem? Is he taking *any prescribed medications*?
6. Does the patient have any *chronic medical problems*? Is there a history of *alcohol or drug abuse*?
7. *Factors that may predispose patients to the development of hypothermia* are listed in Table 22–2. These are quickly explored during the history.

PROBLEM 1 The patient mumbled incoherently. Paramedics reported that neighbors believed that the apartment had been unheated for a week. Empty bottles labeled digoxin and amitryptyline were found on the bed.

The history of the duration and type of exposure is critical. Chronic hypothermia results in fluid sequestration and is more difficult to treat.

Physical Examination

The key physical findings in patients with hypothermia and the temperature level at which they occur are depicted in Table 22–3.

Vital Signs. The core temperature defines the severity of hypothermia. Pulse, blood pressure, and respiratory rate are correspondingly depressed. The pulse rate decreases by 50% at a body temperature of 82.9°F (28°C). Tachycardia in the setting of significant hypothermia suggests concomitant problems such as sepsis, hypoglycemia, hypovolemia, or drug ingestion.

TABLE 22–2. Common Factors that Predispose to Hypothermia

Decreased Heat Production	Increased Heat Loss
Insufficient fuel	Environmental exposure
Hypoglycemia	Lack of acclimation, immersion, drowning
Starvation	Dermatologic abnormalities
Major exertion	Burns
Endocrinologic failure	Erythrodermas
Thyroid	Iatrogenic
Adrenal	Cold fluid infusions
Pituitary	Neonatal resuscitations or deliveries
Neuromuscular	Prolonged extrications
Age extremes	**Miscellaneous**
Inactivity	Sepsis
Impaired Thermoregulation	Multisystem organ failure
Centrally	Hypovolemia
Pharmacologic, e.g., anticholinergics	Gastrointestinal hemorrhage
Toxicologic, e.g., opiates	Myocardial infarction
Traumatic	
Peripherally	
Spinal cord injury	
Diabetes	

General Appearance. Initially, the patient will shiver, a reaction that is maximal at a temperature of 95°F (35°C). Shivering ceases by the time the temperature has fallen to 87.8°F (31°C). The skin is typically cold, firm, pale, or mottled. Localized cutaneous damage due to frostbite may be present.

Neurologic Examination. Early signs of hypothermia may be vague and include disorientation, moodiness, apathy, poor judgment, slurred speech, and ataxia. By the time the body temperature falls to 80.6°F (27°C), the patient is usually comatose, unresponsive to pain, and without reflexes. The Glasgow Coma Scale (Chap. 45) can serve as a means of tracking the patient's mental status. Focal neurologic deficits may be present due to hypothermia alone.

Complete Physical Examination. Because the effects of hypothermia involve multiple systems, cardiovascular, pulmonary, abdominal, rectal, and extremity examinations can demonstrate significant findings. Signs of trauma or concomitant or predisposing medical illness is also often noted. The abdominal examination is particularly unreliable in hypothermic patients because of cold-induced ileus and spasm of the rectus muscles. This examination is repeated as the patient's body temperature improves.

PROBLEM 1 The 73 year old female had a score on the Glasgow Coma Scale of 9. The only other abnormalities noted included rales in the right lung base, some rigidity in the extremities, and cold skin.

TABLE 22–3. Pathophysiologic Changes During Hypothermia

Centigrade	Fahrenheit	Findings
37.6	99.6	Normal rectal temperature
37	98.6	Normal oral temperature
35	95.0	Maximal shivering; increased metabolic rate
33	91.4	Apathy, ataxia, amnesia, dysarthria
31	87.8	Progressive decrease in level of consciousness, pulse, blood pressure, respiratory rate. Shivering stops
29	85.2	Dysrhythmias may occur, insulin not effective, pupils dilated; poikilothermia
27	80.6	Reflexes absent, no response to pain, comatose
25	77	Cerebral blood flow one-third normal, cardiac output one-half normal, significant hypotension
23	73.4	No corneal reflex, ventricular fibrillation risk is maximal
19	66.2	Asystole, flat electroencephalogram
16	60.8	Lowest temperature survived from accidental hypothermia
9	48.2	Lowest temperature survived from therapeutic hypothermia

PROBLEM 2 The 4 year old was flaccid and cyanotic and had a Glasgow Coma score of 3. Pupils were fixed and widely dilated at 8 mm.

If the Glasgow Coma score is not consistent with the degree of hypothermia noted, CNS trauma, drug overdose, or hypoglycemia is suspected. Likewise, a relative tachycardia suggests hypovolemia or a drug overdose. If the patient is hyperventilating, diabetic ketoacidosis (DKA) or lactic acidosis is considered.

DECISION PRIORITIES AND PRELIMINARY DIFFERENTIAL DIAGNOSIS

In caring for the hypothermic patient, several key questions need to be addressed:

1. *How severe is the hypothermia?*
   The patient who is only mildly hypothermic (temperature above 90°F [32°C]) is not likely to develop complications and may be warmed slowly by passive external rewarming measures. With a body temperature below this level, dysrhythmias may occur, and rewarming should be more aggressive using active core rewarming techniques.
2. *Is the patient's hemodynamic status appropriate for the level of temperature depression?*
   Unexpectedly elevated or disproportionately depressed vital signs raise the question of concomitant disorders such as trauma, hypovolemia, or endocrine disorders.
3. *Is the hypothermia due to primary exposure or is it secondary to another medical problem?*
   Primary hypothermia, even when relatively severe, has a good prognosis when it is aggressively and appropriately treated. Secondary hypothermia is likely to be more difficult to treat and to respond more slowly. Treatment must include the underlying problem, as well as rewarming therapy. Extensive diagnostic testing is often necessary to diagnose or confirm the underlying problem.

PROBLEM 1 Although hypothermia in this patient was not severe, there was a high probability that it was secondary to underlying disease. Full laboratory and radiologic evaluation is necessary.

DIAGNOSTIC ADJUNCTS

The extent of ancillary testing depends on the degree of hypothermia, associated conditions, and response to rewarming. Mild accidental cases of hypothermia (95 to 90°F, 35 to 32.2°C) usually require no diagnostic tests. On the other hand, secondary hypothermia and patients with a core temperature below 90°F (32.2°C) require extensive evaluation. All ten of the laboratory tests listed below, the radiologic studies, and the electrocardiogram would be ordered for a patient in the second category.

Laboratory Studies

Arterial Blood Gases

Oxygen. Oxygenation is impaired during hypothermia. There is decreased tissue perfusion, and the oxyhemoglobin dissociation curve is shifted to the left, leading to further impairment of oxygen release at the tissue level (Fig. 22–3). Some authorities have recommended correcting blood gas results for the body temperature. Correction actually leads to a false elevation of the Po_2. Therapeutic decisions are best based on the measured (uncorrected) Po_2 value.

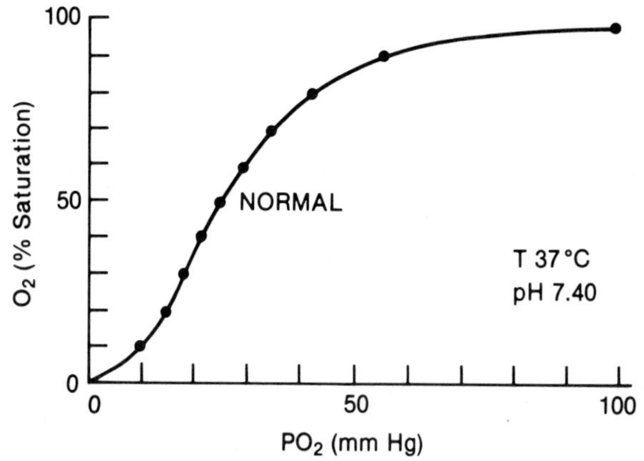

FIGURE 22-3. The normal oxyhemoglobin dissociation curve at 37°C (98.6°F). Hypothermia shifts the curve to the left, as with alkalosis, and impairs oxygen release.

pH and P_{CO_2}. The buffering capacity of cold blood is markedly reduced. As an example, a P_{CO_2} change of 10 mm Hg at 82.4°F (28°C) reduces the pH by approximately 0.16, whereas at normal body temperature the pH would change by only 0.08.

Complete Blood Count

Hemoglobin–Hematocrit. The hemoglobin may be decreased owing to chronic blood loss or illnesses such as malnutrition, leukemia, or uremia. The hematocrit increases 2% for each 1°C drop in temperature. In severe cases, the increased hematocrit can interfere with the diagnosis of acute blood loss or chronic anemia.

White Blood Cell Count. The WBC count is reduced by sequestration and bone marrow depression during hypothermia. Even in the presence of serious infections, leukocytosis may not be seen.

Serum Electrolytes. Temperature has no consistent effect on sodium, chloride, or potassium concentrations. Serial measurements are needed during the rewarming process to assess the need for intervention. The serum potassium level is followed closely because hypokalemia is the most common finding. It is frequently due to inappropriate antidiuretic hormone secretion, ethanol abuse, or hypopituitarism. If hyperkalemia is identified, the patient is evaluated for evidence of renal failure or rhabdomyolysis.

Blood Urea Nitrogen, Creatinine. Renal function test results may be abnormal because of preexisting renal disease or dehydration. They are poor indicators of fluid status in hypothermic patients; however, these tests are useful in establishing baseline renal function because acute tubular necrosis is not uncommon after rewarming, especially in patients suffering from chronic hypothermia.

Serum Glucose Concentrations

Hyperglycemia. Acute cold exposure elevates the serum glucose because of catecholamine-induced breakdown of glycogen. An additional cause is the inactivity of insulin below 28 to 30°C. Persistently elevated glucose levels suggest pancreatitis or DKA.

Hypoglycemia. Hypoglycemia usually results from glycogen depletion in the elderly, malnourished, or alcoholic patient.

Hemostasis Profile. Hemostatic studies including prothrombin time, partial thromboplastin time, platelet count, and fibrinogen level are performed in all patients with moderate to severe hypothermia. Cold induces thrombocytopenia, and clotting times are very prolonged in patients with core temperatures below 68°F (20°C). With rewarming, the results of the coagulation profile usually return to normal. Persistent changes suggest development of disseminated intravascular coagulation.

Serum Amylase and Lipase. Pancreatitis may be preexisting or may develop secondary to hypothermia. Because the abdominal examination is unreliable in the hypothermic patient, serum amylase or lipase elevation may be the only clue to the presence of pancreatitis. Hyperamylasemia has been shown to correlate with poor outcome in the hypothermic patient.

Toxicologic Studies. A full toxicologic screen is considered when there is a history suggestive of ingestion. Ethanol intoxication is one of the most common predisposing sources of hypothermia.

Urinalysis. The specific gravity is low (less than 1.010) owing to cold-induced diuresis. There are no other consistent findings, but occult trauma or urinary tract infection is suggested by the finding of red blood cells or white blood cells and bacteria, respectively.

Cultures. Cultures of urine, sputum, and blood are indicated in all moderate to severe cases of hypothermia. Cultures from other body sites may also be indicated as suggested by the history and physical examination results. Sepsis is a common cause of hypothermia and may also develop as a complication of accidental hypothermia.

Radiologic Imaging

Plain Films. *Cervical spine films* are considered in the patient in whom trauma is suspected, for example, the hypothermic, nearly drowned patient who has had a diving accident. A *chest radiograph* is necessary because pulmonary edema may develop during rewarming. Aspiration is relatively common in people with depressed mental status. In addition, pneumonia and pneumothorax may be difficult to diagnose in hypoventilating patients. An *abdominal series* may be useful in that it may demonstrate pancreatic calcifications, pneumoperitoneum, ileus, or gastric dilatation.

Computed Tomography. Cranial CT scanning is considered if the mental status does not improve during rewarming or if there is evidence of head trauma.

Electrocardiography

A 12-lead electrocardiogram (ECG) is ordered in any patient with a temperature below 90°F (32.2°C). Atrial and ventricular arrhythmias are common in such patients, as is silent myocardial ischemia. A J or Osborn wave may be present if the core temperature is below 90°F (32.2°C). The J wave is a hump at the junction of the QRS complex and the ST segment that typically enlarges as the temperature falls (Fig. 22–2).

PROBLEM 1 Because of the patient's age, medical history, and chronic exposure to cold, the following laboratory tests were performed: arterial blood gases, CBC, electrolytes, glucose, BUN, creatinine, digoxin level, and toxicologic screen. An ECG, chest radiograph, and urinalysis were also ordered. The majority of patients who are hypothermic secondary to other causes will require extensive laboratory, radiologic, and electrocardiographic testing.

PROBLEM 2 Extensive laboratory evaluation including screening for disseminated intravascular coagulation (DIC) and rhabdomyolysis was indicated. Appropriate radiologic studies and cultures were obtained later.

Diagnostic testing in the hypothermic patient is used to determine the cause of hypothermia as well as to detect complications. All patients with moderate and severe hypothermia from primary causes require an extensive diagnostic work-up.

PRINCIPLES OF MANAGEMENT

Management principles for hypothermia include:
1. Prevention of further heat loss.

2. Initiation of life-support techniques.
   3. Rewarming the patient.

Prevention of Heat Loss

After the core temperature is known, clothing is cut off without manipulating the patient, who is then covered with dry blankets. Respiratory heat loss is prevented by administering heated humidified oxygen.

Advanced Life Support

The recommendations for advanced life support (ALS) in hypothermic patients continue to evolve. It has been suggested that endotracheal intubation can precipitate ventricular fibrillation in the hypothermic patient. Although the cold myocardium is susceptible to fibrillation, hypoxia, acidosis, and electrolyte disturbances are more common causes of ventricular fibrillation than mechanical stimulation. Because airway protection is critical, preoxygenation followed by careful intubation is recommended in cases of severe hypothermia.

Cardiopulmonary resuscitation is begun when asystole or ventricular fibrillation is diagnosed by cardiac monitor. The cold myocardium is resistant to defibrillation as well as to pharmacologic agents. After initial defibrillation with 2 wsec/kg, CPR is resumed, and the patient is rewarmed to at least 86°F (30°C) before defibrillation is repeated. Many patients spontaneously convert to an organized cardiac rhythm at a core temperature of between 90 and 95°F (32.2 to 35°C).

The lower the temperature, the greater the protein-binding of drugs. Therefore, most drugs will not be effective at normal doses. If large doses are used, toxicity can develop after rewarming. Generally, pharmacologic attempts to alter the pulse or blood pressure with vasopressors and cardiac medications are to be avoided. Sodium bicarbonate is rarely indicated. Lidocaine and procainamide are largely ineffective at cold temperatures, but bretylium has demonstrated some beneficial actions at low temperatures.

Rewarming Techniques

The critical initial decision in rewarming the patient is determining the need for active versus passive rewarming. Patients with core temperatures of above 90°F (32.2°C) are candidates for passive external rewarming, whereas those below 90°F require active rewarming.

Passive External Rewarming

Previously healthy patients who are only mildly hypothermic (95 to 90°F [35 to 32.2°C]) usually reheat themselves safely in a warm environment if they are covered in dry insulating materials. This technique is termed passive external rewarming (PER); it is simple and noninvasive and can produce rewarming at a rate of 0.5 to 1.0°C/hr.

Candidates for PER must be able to generate sufficient endogenous heat. A variety of associated conditions can render patients poikilothermic—that is, unable to rewarm themselves spontaneously (Table 22–4).

TABLE 22–4. Conditions Requiring Active Rewarming

Cardiovascular instability	Spinal cord injury
Core temperature below 90°F	Vasodilatation—pharmacologic, toxicologic
Extremes of age	CNS disorders—cerebrovascular accident, trauma,
Fuel depletion—glycogen, fat, blood sugar	degenerative disease
Endocrinologic insufficiency	Failure to rewarm passively

TABLE 22–5. External Rewarming Options

Passive	Active
Elimination of ongoing heat loss	Hot packs
Dry blankets in warm environment	Electric blankets
	Immersion

Active External Rewarming

There are a variety of active external rewarming (AER) techniques (Table 22–5). Direct application of heat to the extremities can be dangerous, particularly in elderly and chronically hypothermic patients in whom acute peripheral dilatation can result in rewarming shock. Core temperature afterdrop develops as the cold peripheral blood is shunted centrally. AER of the trunk only is less likely to produce rewarming shock.

Use of AER is generally limited to young, previously healthy, acutely hypothermic patients. Rewarming baths and heating pads are the most commonly used techniques. Baths make monitoring and resuscitation difficult and defibrillation impossible. Heating pads are used with great care because cold, vasoconstricted skin is highly susceptible to thermal injury. Because of these problems, active core rewarming is used in most cases of hypothermia requiring active intervention.

Active Core Rewarming

The techniques for active core rewarming (ACR) are listed in Table 22–1. *Heated humidified oxygen* (40 to 45°C) will transfer more heat when administered through an endotracheal tube than through a mask. Either way, further respiratory heat loss is prevented. As an additional advantage, supplemental oxygen is supplied. This technique is useful alone in mild cases of hypothermia and is combined with other techniques in severe cases.

Intravenous fluids are *heated* to 40 to 42°C. The heat transferred by this means becomes significant only when large volumes of fluid are required.

Heat transferred by means of *irrigation* of the stomach, bladder, and colon is limited. Mediastinal and thoracostomy tube irrigations are very invasive options. Peritoneal lavage with heated fluid is probably the preferred method of irrigation for rewarming. Delivery of heat by means of a 40 to 45°C dialysate is expedited when two catheters and suction are used. Rewarming by means of peritoneal lavage is indicated in severe cases of hypothermia and in hypothermic patients with cardiac arrest prior to the availability of extracorporeal rewarming.

Extracorporeal rewarming (ECR) is the most rapid method of rewarming. But even in those facilities possessing the equipment and personnel for this technique, time is required to mobilize the resources. Ideal candidates are patients with hypothermic cardiac arrest and patients with completely frozen extremities.

PATIENT 1 This patient's temperature rose to 95°F (35°C) with use of PER and heated humidified oxygen administered through a face mask. She became much more alert. Clinical and laboratory findings included hypokalemia, a subtherapeutic digoxin level, pyuria, and a right lower lobe infiltrate.

This patient responded well to rewarming with noninvasive techniques. This response may reflect a less serious underlying problem, but the evaluation continued.

PATIENT 2 In addition to all the other forms of ACR being used, extracorporeal rewarming through hemodialysis was initiated in the emergency department. One attempt to defibrillate with 2 wsec/kg was unsuccessful at a core temperature of 86°F (30°C). The core temperature reached 90°F (32.2°C).

A slow junctional rhythm was established spontaneously, and pulses became palpable.

This patient requires continued aggressive rewarming and intensive care. Cerebral and pulmonary edema, DIC, acute renal failure, and sepsis are all possible complications.

SPECIAL CONSIDERATIONS

Cold Water Drowning

Victims of drowning in water that is at or below 60°F (16°C) are far more likely to respond to resuscitative efforts than victims who have been drowned in warm water. The protective effect of hypothermia is even more pronounced in children, one of whom reportedly recovered without neurologic sequelae after 66 minutes of immersion in icy water. Both the brain and the heart are protected by the cold. The mammalian diving reflex, often very effective in children, results in bradycardia and shunting of blood to the central circulation, both of which provide further protection.

In victims of cold water drowning, rewarming takes place in concert with other resuscitative maneuvers. Prolonged resuscitation efforts are indicated until the body temperature can be brought to near normal. Return of effective cardiac rhythm and recovery without neurologic sequelae may occur even after prolonged cardiac arrest.

Pediatric Hypothermia

The most common form of hypothermia in children is neonatal hypothermia. The newborn, if unprotected, has very high conductive and convective heat losses owing to a large body surface area compared to weight. Large evaporative heat losses also occur if the newborn's skin is not promptly dried of its covering of amniotic fluid. When childbirth occurs in emergency situations, attention to heat conservation is essential to prevent hypothermia. Radiant warmers are ideal for this purpose because they prevent heat loss without restricting access to the neonate.

Beyond the neonatal period, sepsis is the most common cause of hypothermia in infants. The finding of a low body temperature should prompt a thorough evaluation for a source of infection and early initiation of broad-spectrum antibiotics.

In older children, hypothermia is rare. Causes of hypothermia are similar to those seen in adults, the most common nonaccidental cause being malnutrition.

Local Hypothermia and Frostbite

Localized injury to the skin and underlying structures is commonly referred to as frostbite. Exposure to cold produces intense vasoconstriction in the cutaneous vessels, leading to impaired tissue perfusion. Persistent ischemia results in necrosis. Ice may form in the tissue as well, disrupting cell membranes and leading to further tissue destruction.

Localized hypothermia is described pathophysiologically in terms similar to those used for burns. Mild, first-degree frostbite is limited to the superficial epidermis. Erythema and mild edema occur and resolve without sequelae. Second-degree frostbite results in deeper epidermal involvement and presents with large, clear bullae. Third-degree injury is due to full-thickness skin injury. In very severe cases, muscle, bone, and tendon injury may also occur.

The treatment for localized hypothermia is rapid rewarming. Thawing in circulating lukewarm water (40 to 42°C) is the preferred technique. Reperfusion can be quite painful, but complete thawing is essential to minimize tissue loss. Narcotic analgesics may be required during rewarming. Rewarmed body parts are highly susceptible to refreezing, leading to even greater tissue loss. If reexposure is anticipated, it is better not to thaw the tissue. In mild cases, topical ointments and nonsteroidal anti-inflammatory agents are adequate treatment. In severe cases, prostaglandin inhibitors can be used to decrease dermal ischemia. Topical aloe vera cream (Dermaide) is applied, and ibuprofen is given (400 mg by mouth every 12 hours). The need for tetanus and streptococcal prophylaxis is also considered.

After localized hypothermia has occurred, it is very difficult to determine the viability of the involved tissue. Debridement is best delayed, sometimes for weeks, in order to preserve as much tissue as possible. Most patients are admitted for continued treatment and pain control.

DISPOSITION AND FOLLOW-UP

Admission

Patients presenting with moderate or severe hypothermia (core temperature of less than 90°F [32.2°C]) require admission to a monitored bed if:
1. There is cardiovascular instability.
2. There are predisposing factors (Table 22-2).
3. Metabolic or toxicologic abnormalities are identified.
4. The rate of rewarming is inadequate. This is influenced by the rapidity of the patient's cooling. Those with gradual induction (usually the secondary causes) are rewarmed more slowly, 1° to 1.5° per hour, because of dehydration and fluid sequestration problems.

Most with more severe secondary hypothermia will need to be admitted for further workup and care.

Immediate transfer to a tertiary care facility is indicated only when the need for extracorporeal rewarming is anticipated. Examples are impending cardiac arrest in profoundly hypothermic patients and patients with completely frozen extremities.

Discharge

Patients with mild primary accidental hypothermia (core temperature of 95 to 90°F, 35 to 32.2°C) can be safely rewarmed in the emergency department and discharged to a warm environment if they have no significant underlying disease.

Caution is then necessary to ensure that the patient is not discharged to return to the same environment that caused the hypothermia. Admission may be necessary while a safe disposition is worked out for the patient.

PROBLEM 1 This 75 year old patient was admitted to an unmonitored bed and received empiric antibiotic coverage pending culture results. Intravenous hydration and potassium supplementation were continued. The social service department was consulted about the home environment.

PROBLEM 2 This child was admitted to the pediatric intensive care unit for hemodynamic and intracranial pressure monitoring.

DOCUMENTATION

1. Site, duration, and details of exposure.
2. History of associated trauma, immersion, submersion, frostbite.
3. Medications and significant past medical illnesses.
4. Predisposing factors (Table 22-2).

5. Prehospital treatment including rewarming methods.
6. Physical findings and description of clothing.
7. A complete vital sign flow sheet including the hourly rate of rewarming, Glasgow Coma Score, and cardiac monitor strips.
8. Results of diagnostic testing.
9. Method of rewarming used and response to it.

SUMMARY AND FINAL POINTS

- Endotracheal intubation is not contraindicated in patients with hypothermia. It is preceded by preoxygenation and performed gently.
- Cold hearts fibrillate easily. Hypothermic patients are handled as gently as possible, but indicated procedures *are not* withheld.
- Pulses may be very difficult to palpate. An ultrasonic stethoscope is often required to detect blood flow. Chest compressions are started only after the cardiac monitor has documented asystole or ventricular fibrillation.
- Defibrillation of a cold heart is rarely successful in patients with a core temperature below 86°F (30°C). Defibrillation is indicated when ventricular fibrillation is recognized but *is not* repeated until rewarming is in progress.
- Most patients with a body temperature of 90°F (32.2°C) will benefit from a 250- to 500-ml fluid challenge of heated 5% dextrose in isotonic crystalloid.
- Passive external rewarming is ideal for most healthy patients with mild hypothermia (95 to 90°F, 35 to 32.2°C).
- Active rewarming is necessary when the core temperature is below 90°F (32.2°C) and whenever thermogenesis is insufficient.
- Active external rewarming of the extremities may result in core temperature afterdrop.
- With hypothermia, drug binding to protein increases, and target organs become unresponsive. Pharmacologic therapy is frequently ineffective until rewarming is achieved.

BIBLIOGRAPHY

Texts

1. Danzl DF, Pozos RS, Hamlet MP: Hypothermia. In Auerbach P, Geehr E: Management of Wilderness and Environmental Emergencies. St. Louis, C. V. Mosby, 1989.
2. Lloyd EL: Hypothermia and Cold Stress. Rockville MD, Aspen Systems Corporation, 1986.
3. Pozos RS, Wittmers LE: The Nature and Treatment of Hypothermia. Minneapolis, University of Minnesota Press, 1983.

Journal Articles

1. Althaus U, Aegerhard P, Schupbach P, et al: Management of profound accidental hypothermia with cardiopulmonary arrest. Ann Surg 195:492–495, 1982.
2. Bolte RG, Black PG, Bowers RS, et al: The use of extracorporeal rewarming in a child submerged for 66 minutes. JAMA 260:377–379, 1988.
3. Cohen D, Cline J, Lepinski S, et al: Resuscitation of the hypothermic patient. Am J Emerg Med 6:475–478, 1988.
4. Danzl DF, Hedges JR, Pozos RS, et al: Hypothermia outcome score: Development and implications. Crit Care Med 17:227–231, 1989.
5. Danzl DF, Pozos RS, Auerbach P, et al: Multicenter hypothermia survey. Ann Emerg Med 17:1042–1045, 1988.
6. Delaney KA, Howland MA, Vassallo S, et al: Assessment of acid-base disturbances in hypothermia and their physiologic consequences. Ann Emerg Med 18:72–82, 1989.
7. Harnett RM, Pruitt JR, Sias FR: A review of the literature concerning resuscitation from hypothermia: Part II—Selected rewarming protocols. Aviat Space Environ Med 54:487–495, 1983.
8. Hayward JS, Steinman AM: Accidental hypothermia: An experimental study of inhalation rewarming. Aviat Space Environ Med 46:1236–1240, 1975.
9. Reuler JB: Hypothermia: Pathophysiology, clinical settings and management. Ann Intern Med 85:519–527, 1978.
10. Solomon A, Barish RA, Browne B, et al: The electrocardiographic features of hypothermia. J Emerg Med 7:169–173, 1989.
11. Zell SC, Kurtz KJ: Severe exposure hypothermia: A resuscitation protocol. Ann Emerg Med 14:339–345, 1985.

CHAPTER 23

COCAINE

JAMES DOUGHERTY, M.D.

PROBLEM 1 A 26 year old unemployed male landscaper presented to the emergency department complaining of fleeting lightheadedness and palpitations approximately 30 minutes after smoking some "crack." He also mentioned vague left-sided chest pain radiating to the neck.

QUESTIONS TO CONSIDER

1. What is the pharmacology of cocaine?
2. What are the typical features of cocaine intoxication?
3. What are the complications of cocaine usage and how are they treated?
4. What are the psychobehavioral aspects of cocaine use?
5. Does cocaine abuse require a detoxification program? If so, when is it indicated?
6. Are there identifying factors that correctly raise one's suspicion of cocaine or other drug abuse?

INTRODUCTION

According to the Drug Abuse Warning Network, by 1986 cocaine had become the drug most frequently responsible for emergency department patient visits related to drug abuse. Between 1976 and 1986, there was a 15-fold increase in emergency department visits attributed to cocaine abuse, in cocaine-related deaths, and in admissions to public treatment programs for cocaine. The National Institute on Drug Abuse estimates that 3 million people abuse cocaine regularly, more than five times the number addicted to heroin. Cocaine currently ranks third, behind heroin and alcohol-drug combinations, as a cause of drug-related deaths. The number of acute complications associated with its use continues to increase.

Cocaine is the principal alkaloid of the coca shrub (*Erythroxylon coca*). It has been recognized since the early 1900s as a dangerous drug capable of being abused and producing dependence. It was erroneously classified as a narcotic and included in the Harrison Act of 1914, which regulated the use of addicting drugs. Its use declined during the next 50 years until its stimulatory and euphoric effects were "rediscovered" in the mid 1970s. By 1980, cocaine had become a favorite drug of all socioeconomic classes.

Cocaine is commonly available in two forms: a water-soluble hydrochloride salt, usually consumed by sniffing or injection, and as a chemically altered alkaloid ("freebase") that is soluble in acetone and alcohol. The alkaloid melts at 98°C and can be smoked in a pipe. Preprocessed freebase (crack) is a solid that vaporizes at high temperatures, producing a popping or cracking sound. Freebasing has the "rush" equivalent of intravenous (IV) cocaine without the necessity of a needle. Crack, or "rock," is readily available on the street and sells for as little as $5 or $10 per chunk, making it affordable to all.

The drug is rapidly absorbed from all mucosal membranes. A subjective "high" occurs within minutes after being taken by all routes. Compared with "snorting," smoking cocaine produces more rapid and intense drug effects. The rush or high includes feelings of euphoria, exhilaration, and energy. The user experiences a surge of excitement, a feeling of power, and a sense of heightened perception and alertness. This intense burst of excitement is the main attraction of cocaine.

The primary pharmacologic effects of cocaine are local anesthesia and intense stimulation of the sympathetic nervous system. The local anesthetic effect is due to binding and blocking within the sodium channel of the neural axon membrane. This prevents propagation of the nerve impulse. The autonomic effect occurs as cocaine stimulates the release of adrenergic neurotransmitters, e.g., norepinephrine, while blocking their re-uptake. This blockade floods the intrasynaptic junction with neurotransmitter and causes sustained stimulation of the postsynaptic receptors. This pharmacologic effect is responsible for many unpleasant side effects such as vasoconstriction, tachycardia, hypertension, and CNS excitation (Table 23–1). Peak heart rate and blood pressure elevation occur approximately 10 minutes after drug use.

PREHOSPITAL CARE

Involvement of prehospital personnel usually occurs as a result of three cocaine-related complications: acute chest pain, syncope, or acute behavioral emergency manifested by extreme agitation with psychotic and, particularly, paranoid features. The prehospital management of these situations is covered in other chapters (Chaps. 10, 12, and 52). Apart from suspicion and recognition of cocaine as a possible causal agent, there is no field care available that is specific to the drug.

INITIAL APPROACH IN THE EMERGENCY DEPARTMENT

Because of the number of complications associated with cocaine use, the initial approach to the patient is dictated by the presenting complaint. Initial assessment and stabilization are first directed at the clinically manifested pathology, and then at considering and confirming drug abuse. Many patients in the emergency department do not volunteer critical information, and illicit drug users are no exception.

Regardless of the chief complaint, the airway, breathing, and circulation must be stabilized. Altered mental status is treated with 2 mg of intravenous (IV) naloxone, and thiamine, 100 mg IV or intramuscularly (IM), is given to any alcoholic or malnourished patient. A bedside measurement of blood glucose is done to assess glucose levels, and 25 to 50 gm of 50% dextrose (1 to 2 ampules) is administered intravenously as necessary.

History

Cocaine must be suspected in appropriate situations. In one recent study, most patients with cocaine involvement presented with a single major sign or symptom. In order of frequency, these were altered mental status, chest pain, syncope, suicide attempt,

TABLE 23–1. The Major Pathophysiologic Effects of Cocaine*

Central Nervous System	Cardiac System	Respiratory System
Euphoria	Tachycardia	Tachypnea
Agitation	Hypertension	Dyspnea
Seizures	Dysrhythmia	Pulmonary edema
Hyperthermia	Ischemia	Increased oxygen consumption

*Most are dose related.

palpitations, and seizures. In these situations, the emergency physician must directly question the patient about previous drug use and ask whether drugs may be causing the presenting complaint. The questioning specifically refers to "coke, crack, blow, or cocaine." Serial repetition of this line of questioning may be necessary throughout the course of care. Friends and family are asked the same questions. They are more likely to share this information, particularly if they understand that it may benefit the patient.

Physical Examination

Because the major effects of cocaine resemble the "fight, flight, or fright" reaction, remembering this simple metaphor can help to identify the patient who may have used cocaine.

Intervention

It is common to establish intravenous access, give the patient supplemental oxygen, and monitor the cardiac rhythm. The aggressiveness of intervention varies with the condition of the patient.

Clinical situations in which cocaine may be suspected are listed along with the key elements of stabilization in these situations.

Clinical Situation	Stabilization
Acute ischemia, myocardial infarction, or sudden cardiac arrest in patient under 40 years old	Oxygenation, dysrhythmia therapy, analgesics, and volume repletion given as necessary
Acute seizure activity without a prior history of seizures	Airway protection, seizure control with diazepam, patient and staff protection from injury
Hypertensive crisis	Blood pressure decreased 10–20% during first hour
Acute behavioral emergency, e.g., violence, anxiety attack	Control is established, patient physically restrained as necessary; haloperidol given as necessary. Other nondrug or nonpsychiatric causes are considered

There is no specific antidote for cocaine, although extreme sympathomimetic side effects may be lessened by use of beta-blocking medications, e.g., propranolol.

PROBLEM 1 The patient was quickly triaged to the cardiac area. His vital signs were blood pressure 170/110 mm Hg, heart rate 130 beats/min, respirations 30/min, and temperature 98.6°F (37°C). The patient stated, "I feel like something real bad is happening to me, doc."

Any patient with a history of chest pain, palpitations, and lightheadedness is assumed first to have a problem of cardiac origin. Appropriate triage, oxygen by nasal cannula, intravenous access, and cardiac monitoring are necessary. A calm, reassuring manner can help a patient who is sensing loss of control or impending catastrophe. Caring for the immediate presenting complaints can establish a trusting relationship before a possible drug-related history is explored.

DATA GATHERING

A difficult obstacle to data gathering is the frequent denial of substance abuse by the patient. Many signs and symptoms of cocaine and other substance use are nonspecific, and only when they are seen together do they form a diagnostic pattern. The presence of several of the findings or historical points listed below should cause the emergency physician to seriously consider the possibility of cocaine or other substance abuse:

- Disheveled, unkempt appearance
- Altered mental status, particularly a heightened affect
- Rapid mood shifts
- Stigmata of ethanol abuse
- Drug paraphernalia found by family, friends, or paramedics
- Uncharacteristically expensive clothing for environment, e.g., $600 shoes
- Evasive or inconsistent answers
- Highly manipulative activity
- Family expresses concern about a recent change in "friends"
- Chronic lack of money
- Needle marks, multiple tattoos, burn marks or calluses on index finger and thumb
- Job-related problems or instability
- Wearing of a remote pager by an "unemployed" patient

History

Data gathering is relatively straightforward once cocaine use is suspected. The goal is to obtain the patient's admission of cocaine use in a nonthreatening, nonpunitive manner. The importance of confirming suspicions through a friend, relative, or paramedic cannot be overemphasized. Key questions include:

1. *Have you used any drugs? If so, when and how much?*
2. *How were these drugs taken? Intravenously, by mouth, "snorting," smoking?*
3. *Were these agents mixed with any other drugs including alcohol?*
   Up to 30% of cocaine-intoxicated patients state that they have combined the drug with something else, most often opiates or ethanol.
4. *What are the symptoms and when did they begin?*
5. *Are the symptoms becoming worse or improving?*
6. *What symptom(s) prompted the trip to the emergency department?*
7. *Have these symptoms ever been present before when using drugs? If not, do you have a new source?*

Since there are both physical and psychological effects of cocaine use, at some point during the patient's care a brief review of the drug's impact on the patient's health beyond the immediate complaint is necessary. Table 23–2 lists the physical and psychological effects of cocaine abuse and can serve as a guide for questioning.

The physician must be very wary of accepting a potential drug abuser's history at face value. At least 50% of patients either omit, misidentify, or fail to quantitate the amount and type of drug ingested and the time at which it was consumed. No single table can summarize all the "typical" features of cocaine abuse. The easy availability of the drug, its strong psychological dependence, and the relatively low cost of crack have allowed widespread use of cocaine across all levels of our society.

Physical Examination

Knowledge of the major pharmacologic effects of cocaine provides the basis for identifying findings that suggest the diagnosis. Extreme adrenergic stimulation causes cardiovascular excitation, resulting in hypertension and tachycardia. Sympathetic stimulation also may

TABLE 23–2. Less Acute Physical and Psychological Effects of Chronic Cocaine Abuse (Percent of Patients Experiencing)

Physical Effects		Psychological Effects	
Sleep problems	82%	Depression	83%
Chronic fatigue	76%	Anxiety	83%
Headaches	60%	Irritability	82%
Nasal bleeding	58%	Apathy, laziness	66%
Chronic cough	46%	Paranoia	65%
Nausea, vomiting	39%	Difficulty concentrating	65%
		Memory problems	57%
		Sexual disinterest	53%
		Panic attacks	50%

cause mydriasis, increased body temperature, tremor, seizure activity, and altered mental status. The key areas to be examined include those listed below. Common causes of the finding are added parenthetically.

Vital Signs. Blood pressure and heart rate are both elevated, sometimes to extreme levels. Fever is rare.

Nose. Nasal septal perforations or chronic rhinitis may be seen with cocaine sniffing.

Eyes. Mydriasis is common. Changes resulting from acute hypertension, arteriolar spasm, and flame hemorrhage may be seen on funduscopic examination.

Chest. Absent or decreased breath sounds (pneumothorax), subcutaneous emphysema (pneumomediastinum, pneumothorax), localized rales or rhonchi (pneumonia), or diffuse inspiratory rales (pulmonary edema) should be identified.

Cardiac Symptoms. The patient is examined for murmurs (endocarditis), S_4 or S_3 heart sounds (cardiomyopathy, acute myocardial ischemia, congestive heart failure), or irregular rhythm (dysrhythmia).

Abdomen. Signs of hepatomegaly (hepatitis, congestive heart failure) and abdominal pain (intestinal ischemia) are sought.

Extremities. Needle tracks, cyanosis (cardiovascular or pulmonary failure), edema (cardiovascular or renal failure), rash or petechiae (endocarditis, sepsis with bacteremia) may occur.

Neurologic System. A fine tremor is commonly seen. Focal findings are rare.

Psychiatric Signs. Patients may present with suicidal or homicidal tendencies, auditory or visual hallucinations, paranoid ideation, or flight of ideas. Further examination often reveals signs of depression: weight loss or gain, sleep derangements, anorexia, frequent crying spells, loss of sexual function or interest.

PROBLEM 1 The patient complained of increasing chest pain, palpitations, shortness of breath, and anxiety. The pain became worse with deep breathing and coughing. His blood pressure remained elevated at 180/120 mm Hg, and the heart rate was 120 beats/min. The cardiac monitor showed frequent unifocal premature ventricular contractions (PVCs). The patient admitted to frequent cocaine abuse by multiple routes and noted recently his crack had come from a new source.

Physical examination showed an anxious male with needle tracks in both antecubital fossae. There was a healing ulcer in the nasal septum. The lungs were clear. Examination of the heart showed rapid irregular rhythm without murmur or extra sounds. The liver was 3 cm below the costal margin and slightly tender. On mental status examination the patient was anxious, alert, and oriented to person, place, and time, and had no hallucinations.

Although this patient's symptoms may be due to myocardial ischemia, the pain on deep inspiration suggests a pleuritic or pulmonary origin. The hypertension, PVCs, and tachycardia may be due to the hyperadrenergic effects of the ingested cocaine or may be secondary to an underlying cardiac or pulmonary disorder.

DECISION PRIORITIES AND PRELIMINARY DIFFERENTIAL DIAGNOSIS

The priorities in diagnosis are directed toward two questions:

1. *Is cocaine involved?*
   If the history or other supporting information suggests that it is involved, the physician moves toward laboratory confirmation and assessment of the complications.
2. *If the role of cocaine is unclear, what else might cause the presenting signs and symptoms?*

The signs and symptoms seen with acute cocaine intoxication are nonspecific and are not unique to cocaine. Hence, a broad differential of possible causes is entertained until a confirmatory diagnosis is made (Table 23–3). The symptoms of cocaine ingestion are frequently indistinguishable from those of other stimulant ingestions such as amphetamines, phenylpropanolamine, or methylphenidate. The "sympathetic storm" seen with cocaine intoxication also occurs in alcohol withdrawal, with marked tremors, hallucinations, and seizures as presenting complaints. Acute myocardial ischemia in a person under 40 may mimic acute intoxication or may be caused by it. Other important possibilities include acute schizophrenia, sepsis, and thyrotoxicosis.

Certain features may help to differentiate these entities from cocaine ingestion. For example, heat stroke usually occurs under appropriate environmental circumstances. First-time psychiatric disorders, especially schizophrenia, rarely occur for the first time after age 30, and thyrotoxicosis usually has a more prolonged history of symptoms including weight loss, tremulousness, heat intolerance, and gastrointestinal symptoms such as nausea, vomiting, cramps, and diarrhea. Other ingestants may be diagnosed with appropriate laboratory testing, since the effects of cocaine intoxication are not always due to cocaine alone. Cocaine is commonly "mixed" with other drugs such as heroin, marijuana, barbiturates, and benzodiazepines. Alcohol is used most often to attenuate the hyperstimulatory effects.

PROBLEM 1 This patient readily admitted to cocaine abuse and related it to his symptoms. The concern was whether cocaine abuse was the only cause of the symptoms or whether other problems existed, including complications of abuse. On reviewing the list in Table 23–3, it is apparent that both polydrug ingestion

TABLE 23–3. Differential Diagnosis of Acute Cocaine Intoxication

Primary Cardiac Disorders	**Systemic Diseases**
Acute myocardial infarction	Thyrotoxicosis
Acute dysrhythmia of other etiology	Malignant hypertension
Alcohol Related	Sepsis
Ethanol withdrawal	**Pharmacologic Effects**
Ethanol intoxication	Amphetamines
Hyperthermia Syndromes	Hallucinogens
Classic heat stroke	Theophylline
Malignant hyperthermia	Methylphenidate
Neuroleptic malignant syndrome	Tricyclic antidepressants
Psychiatric Illnesses	Phencyclidine
Acute schizophrenia	Phenylpropanolamine
Acute mania	
Acute anxiety/panic attack	

and panic attack combined with an acute cardiothoracic event rank as high probabilities and known complications of cocaine abuse.

DIAGNOSTIC ADJUNCTS

The following tests are indicated in the patient with acute cocaine intoxication. Other ancillary tests are also selected as appropriate to assess the presenting complaints or findings.

Laboratory Studies

Urine Toxicology Screens. Urine toxicology screens are performed in patients with an admitted ingestion or in a high-yield situation, e.g., patients younger than 35 years old with acute central nonmuscular chest pain. They are useful for confirming cocaine ingestion and identifying other concomitantly ingested drugs. Cocaine is often "cut" with a variety of materials such as procaine, lidocaine, quinine, phencyclidine, or talcum powder to increase the volume and thereby value of the drug.

The screen can confirm the presence of cocaine or its metabolites taken within 3 days of presentation. Unfortunately, the results are rarely available sooner than 4 hours after being ordered and are positive in only 60% to 70% of cases. The half-life of a single dose of cocaine is approximately 50 minutes for an IV dose and 2.5 hours for intranasal ingestion. The short half-life and rapid metabolism of cocaine by plasma cholinesterase render blood levels of cocaine impractical and of no value in the emergent setting.

In no circumstances should negative results of a drug screen be accepted as "ruling out" drug ingestion. The accuracy of drug screening tests is highly variable and depends on the type of the drug ingested, the qualifications of the laboratory and personnel performing the test, and the amount of time that has elapsed from ingestion to sample collection. The patient, not the laboratory report, is the best guide to therapy.

Creatinine Phosphokinase. Creatinine phosphokinase (CPK) isoenzymes can be useful. They are measured in patients suspected of having myocardial infarction related to cocaine usage. The CPK-MB fraction is helpful in diagnosing myocardial injury, but the value of a single measurement in the emergency department has not yet been determined. An availability within 2 hours is preferable, but turn-around time varies among hospitals.

Other Laboratory Tests. Complete blood count, urinalysis, and electrolyte measurements may be ordered as part of the medical evaluation of patients suspected of having endocarditis. As a general rule, these tests are necessary to evaluate potential complications of cocaine or other substance abuse.

Arterial Blood Gases. Arterial blood gases are useful in any patient with suspected pulmonary insufficiency due to pulmonary edema, pneumonia, pulmonary embolus, or other causes of hypoxemia. In addition, blood gas measurements are valuable in any patient with an altered sensorium or with dyspnea or tachypnea without a good medical explanation.

Liver Function Tests. Liver function studies are obtained in any patient with clinical findings suggestive of hepatitis. These tests are not ordered as screening tests in patients with suspected cocaine abuse because they do not give a sufficient yield of positive results even in this preselected population.

Cultures. Blood cultures are obtained in any cocaine-intoxicated patient with suspected sepsis or endocarditis. Two sets of blood cultures collected 30 minutes apart will identify bacteremia in 90% of cases. Unless the patient is febrile, appears septic, or has a new onset of a nonfunctional cardiac murmur, blood cultures are usually not indicated.

Radiologic Imaging

1. Chest series. A standard chest radiographic series is indicated for any patient with signs or symptoms consistent with pneumothorax or pneumomediastinum, pneumonia, or pulmonary edema.

2. Computed tomography (CT) of the head is indicated in cocaine-intoxicated patients with a first-time seizure, or in suspected intracranial hemorrhage, or in any patient presenting with focal neurologic findings.

Electrocardiogram

A 12-lead electrocardiogram (ECG) is obtained in any patient with a history of cocaine use who presents with chest pain, syncope, or palpitations. The usual ECG findings are nonspecific or normal, and sinus tachycardia is common. The ECG contributes to the diagnosis only if positive for ischemia, infarction, or dysrhythmia. A negative ECG rules out very little.

PROBLEM 1 The 12-lead ECG was interpreted as showing frequent unifocal PVCs without any other evidence of myocardial ischemia. A portable chest film was taken in the emergency department because of the possibility of acute myocardial infarction. It showed a 20% pneumothorax of the left lung and a prominent pneumomediastinum.

In patients with substance abuse one must continually ask what else other than the drug being considered might cause these symptoms. What are the known complications of the drug being considered that might cause these symptoms? In this case, complications of substance abuse, i.e., pneumothorax and pneumomediastinum, rather than the abuse itself were contributing to the patient's complaints.

REFINED DIFFERENTIAL DIAGNOSIS

Once cocaine is identified as a contributing factor in the patient's presenting complaint, a search for the complications associated with its use is made. Questions based on the symptoms listed in Table 23–2 are asked, and the physical examination and laboratory studies are redirected toward assessing the major complications of cocaine intoxication listed in Table 23–4.

PRINCIPLES OF MANAGEMENT

Once the patient's complaint is identified as being cocaine-related, management is divided between treating any abnormal hyperadrenergic signs and symptoms involving one or more organ systems, and treating any complications listed in Table 23–4.

General Treatment

Most patients with cocaine intoxication do not require treatment with specific medications in the emergency department. Reassurance and protection of the patient from injury to self or others are the basic principles of supportive therapy. Other resuscitative measures were described earlier in the section Initial Approach in the Emergency Department.

Specific Treatment Methods

Specific drugs and treatment regimens are available to treat the effects of cocaine and hypersympathetic stimulation on one or more organ systems as listed in Table 23–5.

TABLE 23-4. Reported Complications of Cocaine by Organ System

Central Nervous System 　Cerebral infarction 　Cerebral vasculitis 　Headache* 　Intracranial hemorrhage 　Seizures 　Syncope 　Transient sensory loss 　Tremors* **Cardiovascular System** 　Aortic rupture 　Cardiac dysrhythmias* 　Cardiomyopathy 　Hypertension* 　Myocardial infarction 　Myocardial ischemia **Pulmonary** 　Chronic cough* 　Hypersensitivity lung reaction 　Pneumomediastinum 　Pneumothorax 　Pulmonary edema **Renal** 　Renal infarction 　Rhabdomyolysis-induced renal failure	**Ear, Nose, Throat** 　Hoarseness 　Nasal septal necrosis* 　Rhinitis* 　Sinusitis **Psychiatric** 　Paranoia, suicide 　Severe depression* 　Violent behavior* **Obstetric** 　Congenital malformation 　Neonatal behavioral 　Placental abruption 　Spontaneous abortion **Immunologic or Infection** (due to IV use) 　AIDS 　Endocarditis 　Tetanus 　Viral hepatitis* **Gastrointestinal** 　Hepatitis 　Intestinal ischemia

*Indicates a common complication.
From Brody SL, Slovis CM: Recognition and management of complications related to cocaine abuse. Emerg Med Rep 9(6):41–48, 1988. Used with permission.

PROBLEM 1 Once the pneumothorax and pneumomediastinum were discovered, a No. 28Fr chest tube was inserted in the left fifth midaxillary line. The patient's chest pain and shortness of breath improved dramatically, his PVCs resolved, and his blood pressure and heart rate fell to 140/95 mm Hg and 90 beats/min, respectively. No other drug therapy was necessary. Serial cardiac isoenzyme measurements and ECGs were ordered to identify an atypical myocardial infarction. Even though the patient's condition improved, a continued search for complications of cocaine or other drugs is necessary.

SPECIAL CONSIDERATIONS

"Body Packers"

PROBLEM 2 A 30 year old male was brought in by police from a nearby international airport. He was suspected of carrying drugs. Shortly before his arrest, he was seen to swallow several small bags in a men's rest room. Five minutes after being brought to the emergency department he developed grand mal seizure activity. This required large amounts of diazepam and ventilatory support for control. An x-ray film of the abdomen showed multiple sacks of semiopaque material throughout the colon.

This case is an example of a "body packer" or "body stuffer" syndrome. In order to smuggle cocaine across international borders, a body packer or "mule" will carry 50 to 200 discreetly and tightly wrapped condoms or latex bags filled with cocaine in the gastrointestinal tract by swallowing them before the journey. A similar situation can occur when a desperate person swallows a bag or bags of cocaine just prior to being arrested. Loosely bound bags can rupture or leak, causing massive cocaine toxicity with seizures,

TABLE 23–5. Specific Drugs for Organ-Specific Problems Related to Cocaine Intoxication and Hyperadrenergic Stimulation

System	Problem	Drug	Dosage	Comment
Cardiovascular	Tachycardia, hypertension	Diazepam	2.5–5 mg IV q 5 min	Useful if patient is agitated or extremely anxious
	Tachycardia, hypertension	Propranolol	0.5–1 mg IV q 5 min	Mild sensation Not often necessary
	Hypertensive crisis (diastolic BP > 130 mm Hg with end-organ damage)	Labetalol	10–20 mg IV total; 2.5 mg IV q 5 min	Rarely necessary Some controversy about degree of alpha receptor-blocking ability
	Myocardial ischemia	Nitrates (glycerol trinitrate)	0.3 or 0.4 mg given sublingually or as infusion	May cause significant hypotension by relaxation of capacitance vessels
	Ventricular dysrhythmias	Lidocaine	1 mg/kg, then 2–4 mg/min drip	Ventricular extrasystolic or ventricular tachycardia most often treated. Sinus tachycardia resolved without therapy
		Propranolol	0.5–1.0 mg IV q 5 min	
Central nervous system	Seizures	Diazepam Phenytoin	2.5–5 mg q 5 min 18 mg/kg slow IV	Single, short-lived seizure may not need treatment. May be repetitive and refractory
	Psychosis	Haloperidol	2.5 mg IV q 5 min	Aggressive therapy necessary if medical clearance given in selected situations
	Anxiety	Diazepam	2.5–10 mg IV or IM	
	Malignant hyperthermia	Dantrolene	1 mg/kg IV q 6 hr	Very rare
	Tremor, agitation	Propranolol	0.5–1.0 mg IV q 5 min	Rarely necessary but usually effective
Renal	Renal failure from rhabdomyolysis	Crystalloids, diuretics, alkalinization	Given to maintain 2–3 ml/hr/kg urine output; urine pH > 6	Rarely necessary but usually effective treatment of a complication that may have a hyperadrenergic basis

acute hypertensive crisis, and fatal cardiac dysrhythmias. The diagnosis is confirmed by abdominal radiographs. A urine toxicologic screen showing positive results for cocaine or its metabolites indicates possible intestinal leakage. If the patient is asymptomatic, conservative therapy consists of rectal suppositories and mild cathartics such as mineral oil and careful observation. Charcoal with sorbitol 20% offers the advantage of intestinal catharsis, charcoal binding of intraluminal cocaine, and a "marker" that shows when the gastrointestinal tract is evacuated along its full length. Serious complications that are refractory to medical management may require urgent abdominal laparotomy for removal of the toxic substance.

Sudden Cardiac Death

PROBLEM 3 A 38 year old real estate developer was involved in a minor motor vehicle accident in which his car swerved off the road and struck a small tree and a picket fence. He got out of the car and collapsed. The paramedics found him unresponsive with agonal respirations and a slow pulseless rhythm. After 40 minutes of resuscitative efforts, he was pronounced dead. Postmortem toxicology studies by the coroner's office revealed evidence of cocaine, alcohol, and diazepam.

Sudden cardiac death is a real and tragic consequence of cocaine ingestion. The lethal dose of cocaine in humans is unknown. Users may consume 3 to 5 gm IV during 6- to 12-hour "runs" or smoke more than 4 to 9 gm during 6 to 24 hours. Yet death has been reported with as little as 20 mg. Although the heart is the target organ, the precise cause of this lethal disorder is unknown. It is thought to result from the combined effects of enhanced dysrhythmogenicity, coronary artery vasospasm, sudden increase in myocardial oxygen demands associated with increased sympathetic stimulation, and catecholamine-associated increased platelet thrombogenicity. Cocaine is considered in any sudden cardiac death, myocardial infarction, or dysrhythmia that occurs in an otherwise young, healthy individual.

DISPOSITION AND FOLLOW-UP

Decisions regarding admission or discharge of these patients are based on a number of factors: the severity of the illness induced by cocaine, the presence of complications resulting from cocaine or other substance abuse, and the response of the patient to treatment in the emergency department.

Admission

Any patient who presents with the following symptoms is admitted for observation and treatment:

1. Acute severe chest pain of unknown origin that is unresolved in the emergency department
2. Seizure activity
3. Acute hypertension requiring medication
4. Suicide attempt thought to be of high risk
5. Suspected "body packer" with symptoms or cocaine metabolites in urine
6. Altered mental status of a persistent nature
7. Severe headache that does not resolve in the emergency department

Any patient in whom the following disorders are diagnosed is also admitted:

1. Acute myocardial ischemia or infarction
2. Depression with somatic complaints
3. Suicidal or homicidal intent
4. Pulmonary complications, e.g., pneumothorax, pneumomediastinum, pneumonia
5. Systemic infection, e.g., endocarditis
6. True syncope without a readily explained cause, e.g., vasovagal syncope
7. Cerebrovascular ischemia or hemorrhage
8. Rhabdomyolysis with or without altered renal function

Many patients are unwilling to be admitted for fear of being cut off from their suppliers, loss of money, possible collusion between physicians and police, and many other reasons. Explanation of the circumstances to the patient and family may help, but restraint and hold procedures following correct legal guidelines may be necessary. These patients can be extremely difficult to convince and are highly manipulative. Having them sign a form testifying that they are leaving against medical advice offers little legal protection, particularly because of their "drug-altered" condition. Evaluation of the patient's decision-making ability and the use of restraints are discussed in Chapters 62 and 64.

Discharge

The large majority of patients presenting to the emergency department with cocaine intoxication do not require admission. Two to four hours of observation with cardiac monitoring is usually adequate to identify those patients who are recovering sufficiently to be discharged. The patient must be alert, oriented, ambulatory, capable of understanding discharge instructions, and free of medical complications that might warrant admission. Most patients who admit to drug use accept the fact that their presenting complaint was drug-related. If the complaint is drug-related, they are informed of the findings during their evaluation and the cause of the concern that brought them to the emergency department is explained. Some perspective on the hazards of drug abuse is given, and an attempt is made to persuade them to refrain from further drug usage. The latter attempt may not result in any significant change in behavior, but it is an important responsibility for the physician. If there is a social service or drug detoxification consultative program available, referral to it can be made to assist the patient in obtaining drug counseling. Most communities have either paid or volunteer drug abuse counseling groups, and these can be included in the discharge instructions. Medical complications of cocaine or other substance abuse that do not require admission can be followed up by a primary physician.

A special situation occurs with the cocaine-dependent patient who comes to the emergency department requesting admission "for detox." Presenting to the emergency department for cocaine detoxification is often an insincere act that occurs when the patient has run out of money or a place to stay. Because outpatient treatment is regularly successful and stimulants such as cocaine produce no medically dangerous withdrawal symptoms, hospitalization is seldom necessary as a first treatment option. The role of the emergency physician in this circumstance is to exclude life-threatening complications, explore the possibility of a mixed dependency with a drug that might require inpatient care, treat the patient symptomatically, and provide the patient with referral to local facilities designed to handle cocaine detoxification.

Drug Testing and Medical Confidentiality

Increasingly, employers are requiring their employees to submit to drug testing under certain work-related circumstances. Frequently, the emergency department is thought to be the appropriate site for this purpose. Although required by law to report all physical assaults to the local authorities, reporting of even self-admitted drug use is *not* required by law and represents a breach of the confidentiality between patient and physician. The results of any drug tests, history, or chart reports of known drug usage cannot be released without the patient's written consent. In the treatment of the cocaine-intoxicated patient, the emergency physician's primary role is medical, not judicial.

PROBLEM 1 This patient was admitted because of the pulmonary complications. In view of the fact that he was no longer symptomatic, admission to a cardiac care unit or acute care ward is probably not necessary. If available, a "step down" or telemetry unit bed would be advisable to monitor the patient's rhythm for the next 12 to 24 hours.

While hospitalized, he is at risk for withdrawal symptoms from the drugs of abuse and may attempt to continue his addiction through "friends."

DOCUMENTATION

1. Chief complaint
2. The time, method, and approximate amount of drug ingested
3. Additional drugs used including alcohol

4. Pertinent past medical history, e.g., previous complications of drug use

5. Any pertinent findings specific to the chief complaint or supportive of possible substance abuse on physical examination

6. Identification and treatment of complications resulting from cocaine use

7. Evaluation of the patient through the course of care in the emergency department through serial examinations and frequent documentation of vital signs

8. Any contact with friend, family, police officer, or social service organization as part of the confirmation of drug abuse or disposition effort

9. An admitting or discharge diagnosis, with appropriate follow-up plans

PROBLEM 1 The patient was admitted to a telemetry floor, an acute myocardial infarction was ruled out, and the chest tube was removed in 48 hours. He met once with a substance abuse counselor but was not interested in stopping his drug use. He was discharged from the hospital on the third day with a referral to a substance abuse center and the general surgery clinic. Two weeks later he was brought to the emergency department in cardiac arrest and could not be resuscitated. During the resuscitation effort he was found to have a single small-caliber gunshot wound to the right fifth intercostal space medial to the scapula. An autopsy revealed a penetrating cardiac injury to the right and left ventricles and the pulmonary hilum. Later that night, police commented that he was shot "in a drug deal that went bad."

The emergency physician must recognize and be able to manage not only the serious consequences of cocaine ingestion but also the subtle manifestations, both clinical and psychobehavioral, that are associated with its use. Not every case will be a success. Some will be permanent "saves," others just temporary. Unfortunately, the widespread use of cocaine continues and results in many patients being seen in emergency departments with problems related to its use.

SUMMARY AND FINAL POINTS

- Cocaine is a drug of abuse that commonly causes or complicates the complaints of a number of patients presenting to the emergency department
- The diagnosis of cocaine abuse is particularly likely in patients (particularly those under 40 years old) with acute onset altered mental status, chest pain, palpitations, or syncope
- An active search is made for the complications of substance abuse in these patients
- An assumption is made that more than one drug has been ingested with or without the patient's knowledge
- Cocaine has no specific antidote. Treatment is directed toward its manifestations and complications.
- Cocaine detoxification is an outpatient process

BIBLIOGRAPHY

Text

1. Perry S: Substance-induced organic mental disorders. In Hall RE, Yadofsky CS (eds): Textbook of Neuropsychiatry. Washington, DC, American Psychiatric Press, 1987.

Journal Articles

1. Brody SL, Slovis CM: Recognition and management of complications related to cocaine abuse. Emerg Med Rep 9(6):41–48, 1988.
2. Cregler LL, Mark H: Medical complications of cocaine abuse. N Engl J Med 315:1495–1500, 1986.
3. Deriet RW, Albertson TE: Emergency department presentation of cocaine intoxication. Ann Emerg Med 18:182–186, 1989.
4. Frishman WH, Karpenos A, Molloy TJ: Cocaine-induced coronary artery disease: Recognition and treatment. Med Clin North Am 73(2):475–486, 1989.
5. Gawin FH, Ellinwood EH: Cocaine and other stimulants. N Engl J Med 318(18):1173–1182, 1988.
6. Smith HWB, Liberman HA, Brody SL, et al: Acute myocardial infarction temporarily related to cocaine abuse. Ann Intern Med 107:13–18, 1987.
7. Tarr JE, Macklin M: Cocaine. Pediatr Clin North Am 34(2):319–331, 1987.
8. Treatment of acute drug abuse reactions. Med Letter 29(748):83–86, 1987.

SECTION EIGHT

HEMATOLOGIC DISORDERS

CHAPTER 24

THE PATIENT WITH ABNORMAL BLEEDING

CLIFTON A. SHEETS, M.D.

PROBLEM 1 A 32 year old white female had epistaxis for 4 hours. The bleeding was not severe and persisted as a steady ooze. She had noted recent frequent epistaxis, easy bruising, and menorrhagia. Persistent bleeding after a tooth extraction prompted her last emergency department visit 2 months ago.

PROBLEM 2 A 56 year old black male suffered a syncopal episode at work. He had had coronary artery bypass surgery 1 year ago. His medications included propranolol and a "blood thinner." A rescue squad on the scene found him pale and anxious with a blood pressure (BP) of 90/60 mm Hg and a heart rate of 100 beats/min.

QUESTIONS TO CONSIDER

1. What questions provide the most important information necessary to discover a potential bleeding disorder?
2. How can historical information help differentiate between a platelet disorder and a coagulation disorder?
3. Can physical findings help differentiate between platelet and coagulation disorders?
4. What laboratory studies are useful for evaluating the patient with a suspected bleeding disorder?
5. What are the potentially life-threatening major bleeding disorders, and how are they diagnosed?
6. How is blood component therapy helpful in the management of a patient with a bleeding disorder?
7. What are the criteria for admission or discharge of a patient with a bleeding disorder?

INTRODUCTION

The hemostatic system is often neglected in the emergency management of the acutely ill or injured patient. Errors of omission can be fatal. It is important for the emergency physician to understand the common presentations, evaluation, and treatment of hemostatic disorders.

Hemostasis occurs in four phases. These are useful in classifying hemostatic disorders: the vascular phase, platelet or primary hemostasis, coagulation or secondary hemostasis, and fibrinolysis. The vascular phase begins with the disruption of the vessel wall. Initially, reflex vasoconstriction restricts hemorrhage. Vessel endothelial release of von Willebrand's factor and prostaglandin I_2 (PGI_2) helps trigger the hemostatic cascade. The platelet phase begins within 3 to 10 seconds of vessel injury. Platelet adhesion occurs in the presence of von Willebrand's factor. Platelets degranulate and release calcium, adenosine diphosphate (ADP), and serotonin, promoting platelet aggregation. These platelets then form a "plug" that occludes the disruption and creates a receptive surface for the coagulation phase.

The coagulation phase is a series of steps that transforms procoagulant factors and forms a fibrin clot. There are two separate mechanisms to activate coagulation: the intrinsic pathway and the extrinsic pathway. In the intrinsic pathway, all the components needed for activation are contained within the circulation. The extrinsic pathway is activated as a result of tissue damage. Both pathways culminate in the activation of common pathway factors. This coagulation cascade is best remembered as a "Y" and is illustrated in Figure 24–1. The final step of hemostasis is fibrinolysis. Fibrin is cleaved by plasmin, resulting in dissolution of the fibrin clot and production of fibrin split products.

When the intricate complexities of the four hemostatic phases remain in balance, the human body possesses a finely tuned and highly efficient mechanism for hemorrhage control. Disruptions can occur at each phase, and any change in function may result in inadequate hemostasis.

Vascular disorders seen in the emergency department are typically acquired, e.g., from trauma, sepsis, steroids, or aging. Congenital vascular disorders are rarely seen. Platelet disorders are common and are usually acquired, e.g., from aspirin use or idiopathic thrombocytopenia (ITP). Defects in the coagulation cascade are either congenital or acquired. Congenital defects stem from isolated deficiencies of clotting factor function or production, e.g., hemophilia A, or von Willebrand's disease. Acquired coagulation disorders can result from use of drugs such as heparin, warfarin (Coumadin),

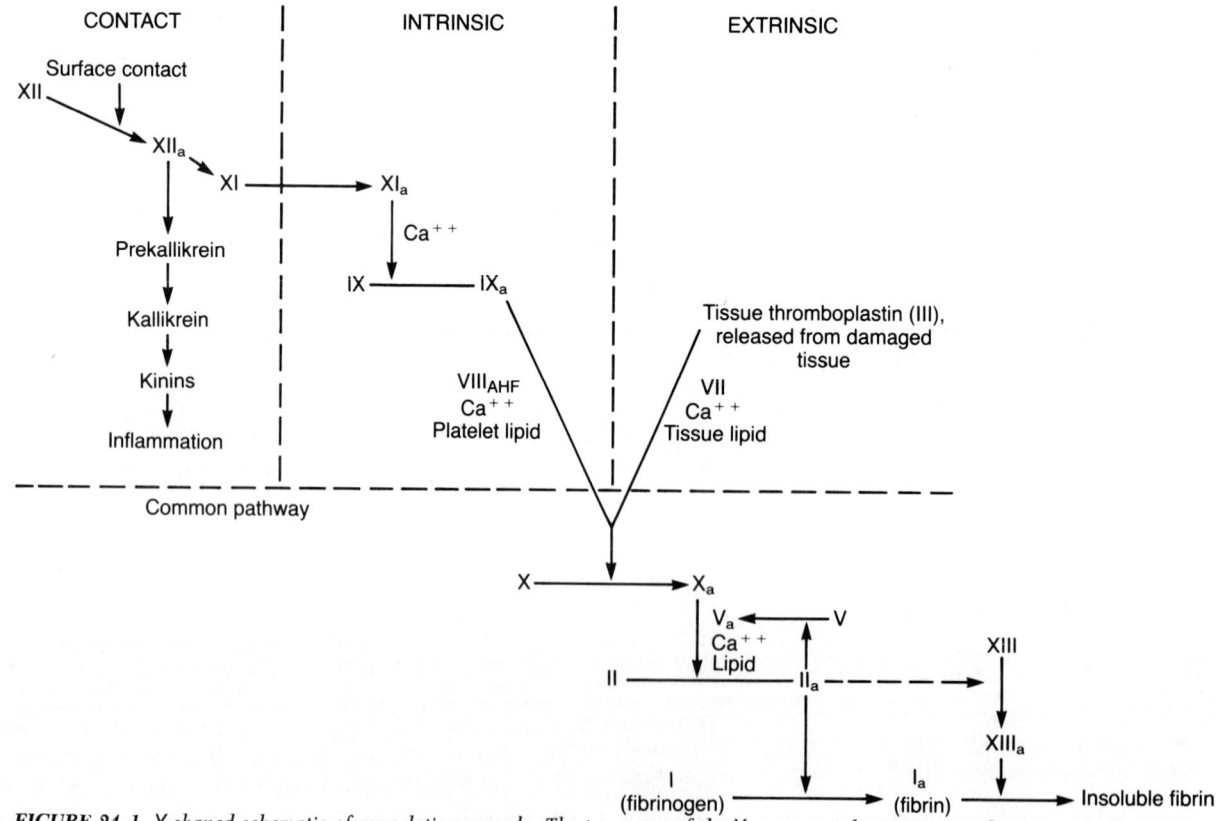

FIGURE 24–1. Y-shaped schematic of coagulation cascade. The two arms of the Y represent the intrinsic and extrinsic pathways. The stem is the common pathway. (Reproduced by permission from Hamilton GC: Disorders of hemostasis and polycythemia. In Rosen P, et al (eds): Emergency Medicine: Concepts and Clinical Practice. St. Louis, 1988, The C. V. Mosby Co.)

and certain antibiotics, or from hepatic dysfunction. Most defects in the fibrinolytic phase of hemostasis are acquired, e.g., disseminated intravascular coagulation (DIC) syndrome.

The number of patients presenting to the emergency department with hemostatic disorders is difficult to estimate. The congenital causes of bleeding such as Ehlers-Danlos syndrome, hemophilia, and von Willebrand's disease are relatively rare. Most acquired causes of disordered hemostasis such as anticoagulant or aspirin use, trauma, or sepsis are common. For example, each year more than 500,000 Americans begin anticoagulant therapy. Bleeding disorders are best considered a significant potential problem. They are considered in each patient with active bleeding or who has a clinical presentation that may stress the hemostatic system.

PREHOSPITAL CARE

Patients with bleeding disorders commonly seek access to emergency medical services. Clues to the etiology of the bleeding disorder are subtle and are recognized only by the sophisticated prehospital personnel. When confronted with problems of this nature, prehospital care providers should supply the following information:

History

Bleeding History. The length of this episode, an estimate of blood loss, and a history of bleeding problems are noted.

Other History. Any medications, especially aspirin and anticoagulants, being taken by the patient are important.

Physical Examination

Vital Signs. An abnormally low blood pressure or an unusually high heart rate is considered a sign of significant or continuing blood loss until proved otherwise.

General Assessment. The patient's tolerance of blood loss, particularly mentation, is noted.

Blood Loss. The site and estimated rate (oozing versus rapid flow) of blood loss are important.

Intervention

Control of Bleeding. Generally, direct pressure over a bleeding site will stop most bleeding. Pressure dressings, point pressure over a proximal pulse, or a blood pressure cuff tourniquet may be necessary.

Oxygen. Supplemental oxygen is considered if the patient is not tolerating blood loss well.

Volume Resuscitation. The amount of volume replacement is directed by the patient's clinical condition, vital signs, and complicating illnesses.

Reassurance. The benefits of patient reassurance can be significant.

PROBLEM 1 The 32 year old female with acute epistaxis activated the Emergency Medical Services (EMS) system by calling 911. Paramedics on the scene were unable to control her bleeding with direct pressure. The patient had stable vital signs and was in no distress. The squad called on telemetry to identify their transport status as nonemergent and estimated an arrival time of 15 minutes.

PROBLEM 2 The 56 year old black male was reassured by the rescue personnel but failed to calm down. They supplied oxygen at 6 liters/min via nasal cannula, established a large-bore intravenous line with normal saline, running as a 500 ml bolus over 10 minutes. They called on the radio and gave a brief history and physical findings. Their transport status was identified as critical, and the estimated arrival time was 3 minutes.

One of the primary goals of the EMS system is to identify patients with life-threatening illnesses and injuries. The patient in Problem 2, based on his vital signs, was appropriately placed in an urgent category of treatment and transport. The intravenous flow rate initiated by the paramedics was described as "wide open." Considering the short transport time, this is reasonable. The patient in Problem 1 is transported safely in a less urgent mode. Her vital signs were stable and she was in mild distress.

INITIAL APPROACH IN THE EMERGENCY DEPARTMENT

Most patients with bleeding disorders are taken immediately to the acute care area. Initial assessment of the patient's condition is performed quickly because rapid deterioration of the patient's condition can occur without warning. The following steps are performed during triage or the initial physician evaluation:

History

Basic confirmation of the rescue squad's information is obtained.

Physical Examination

1. Repeat vital signs are obtained and compared with those obtained by the rescue squad.
2. A rapid screening physical examination is performed, focusing on the location, nature, and extent of bleeding. Overt hemorrhage, petechiae, and purpura are sought. Hemorrhage may be "hidden" in closed spaces such as the chest, intestines, or pelvis. The physician also assesses how well the patient is tolerating the hemorrhage and estimates the loss (Chapter 4). Estimates of blood loss must take ongoing losses into consideration.

Intervention

1. Volume resuscitation is initiated when it is clinically indicated or when a high-risk situation exists based on the history. Any abnormal bleeding places the victim at risk for volume loss, hypoxia, and subsequent death. It is best to anticipate a potential problem. When giving IV orders, the physician should remember to specify blood tubing, 14- to 16-gauge catheters, and blood-compatible crystalloid solutions (normal saline, Plasmalyte, Normosol). This will save time should blood product administration be required later.
2. Life-threatening hemorrhage is controlled. Direct pressure is the first maneuver attempted. Blood exposure precautions must be remembered! Ice, elevation, and pneumatic tourniquets may be beneficial in patients with difficult-to-control bleeding from an extremity. Despite these efforts, bleeding may continue, especially if the patient is taking anticoagulants or suffers from a coagulation disorder. These patients require blood component therapy to reverse their blood deficit.
3. Because much of the diagnosis of abnormal bleeding rests with the laboratory, screening tests (Table 24–1), including blood typing, are performed early and on a priority basis.

PROBLEM 2 The patient taking propranolol and a "blood thinner" arrived in the

TABLE 24-1. Ancillary Testing

Test	Cost	Ordering Rationale	Sample	Range	Interpretation	Comments
Complete blood count with peripheral smear*	$30.00	Determines baseline hemoglobin, white cell count may indicate infection	Purple-top tube 10 ml (EDTA)	Hgb 14–16 gm/dl men; 13–15 gm/dl women	Schistocytes on peripheral smear indicate red cell destruction through microangiopathic-hemolytic anemia. If this is associated with low platelet count, suspect DIC or TTP	In acute hemorrhage, hemoglobin values may be normal. These values cannot be relied on to assess severity of bleeding
Platelet count*	$19.00 (estimate usually included with CBC)	A relative count of circulating platelets	Purple-top tube (EDTA)	150,000–400,000/mm^3	Increased bleeding risk occurs with counts below 50,000/mm^3. Spontaneous hemorrhage may occur below 20,000/mm^3. Dependent on platelet function	Not an indicator of platelet function. May be normal in spite of prolonged bleeding time
Prothrombin time (PT)*	$16.00	Ascertains function of extrinsic and common pathways	Blue-top tube (citrate); tube needs to be filled	12–15 sec compared with controls	Elevation of PT values more than 2 sec over control value is clinically significant and indicates less than 40% normal activity. Small reductions in activity beyond this point result in marked elevations in PT values	Isolated prolongation of PT suggests use of coumarin anticoagulants, vitamin K deficiency, or acquired or congenital coagulation disorders
[Activated] partial thromboplastin time (aPTT)*	$14.00	Ascertains integrity of intrinsic and common pathways	Blue-top tube (citrate)	25–29 sec	Reduction of 40% or more in clotting factors is needed to see elevation in value	Isolated prolongation of this value suggests heparin therapy or deficiencies in factors VIII, IX, or XI
Ivy bleeding time*	$16.00	Measures platelet function	Epidermal incisions on volar forearm under 40 mm Hg pressure from blood pressure cuff	4–8 min	A bleeding time of 10 min is considered abnormal	Bleeding time is independent of coagulation pathways. A platelet count less than 100,000/mm^3 correlates with platelet number as well as function
Fibrinogen	$22.00	Ascertains availability of thrombin precursors	Blue-top tube (citrate)	200–400 mg/dl	Indicates a steady state balance between production and consumption	Ordered in the evaluation of DIC, though values in this disorder vary widely
Thrombin time	$26.00	Measures isolated function of common pathway factors	Blue-top tube (citrate)	Within 5 sec of control	Useful as a screen for abnormalities of fibrinogen and fibrinogen inhibitors such as heparin and fibrin split products.	Measures conversion of fibrinogen to fibrin. Bypasses intrinsic and extrinsic pathways

* = Part of screening battery; DIC = disseminated intravascular coagulation; TTP = thrombotic thrombocytopenic purpura.

emergency department. He admitted to no previous episodes of bleeding and except for his heart disease was without underlying illness. During the interview, he vomited copious bright red blood. The patient's vital signs were BP 90/40 mm Hg, heart rate 100 beats/min and thready, respirations 24/min, temperature 98.6°F. His sclera were pale, and there was a large ecchymotic area on the volar forearm where the rescue squad had attempted intravenous access. He was anxious. Results of the remainder of the screening examination were normal.

Two 16-gauge peripheral intravenous (IV) lines were established, and 2 liters of Normosol were infused under 300 mm Hg pressure. The patient was given 6 liters of oxygen by nasal cannula, and a large-bore nasogastric tube was advanced, returning copious amounts of bright red blood. Stat prothrombin time (PT), partial thromboplastin time (PTT), platelets, and a bleeding time were ordered as well as a complete blood count (CBC) and blood type and a cross-match for 6 units of packed red blood cells and 2 units of fresh frozen plasma. Old medical records were summoned, and the surgeon on call was paged.

This patient's hemodynamic status requires aggressive fluid resuscitation and plans for early blood component therapy. His vital signs are complicated by the fact that his normal sympathetic vascular response was being blocked by propranolol. Without the drug, his heart rate would most likely be much faster. Because gastrointestinal hemorrhage is often concealed and his physiologic response was blunted, fluid resuscitation is assumed to be well behind blood loss until proven otherwise. Suspicions of a bleeding disorder either causing or complicating the gastrointestinal bleeding are supported by the history of anticoagulant use and the ecchymosis that occurred after the intravenous access attempt. Early surgical consultation is indicated because this patient may require a laparotomy to control his hemorrhage.

DATA GATHERING

History

Historical data are gathered to assist in separating acquired disorders from congenital disorders, and platelet abnormalities from coagulation and mixed disorders. Key historical points include:

1. *Nature* of the *bleeding*: petechiae, purpura (immediate or delayed), significant bleeding episodes
2. *Sites* of *bleeding*: mucosal, gastrointestinal, genitourinary, intracranial, hemarthrosis
3. *Pattern* of *bleeding*: recent versus lifelong, frequency, severity, response to challenge such as tooth extraction
4. *Medications*: especially anticoagulants and aspirin
5. *Associated diseases*: alcoholism, liver disease, uremia, infection, malignancy
6. *Previous transfusions*: including any transfusion reactions to anticipate delays in obtaining blood
7. *Family history*: hemostatic problems. If present, the history is repeated to clarify the type of bleeding.

Physical Examination

The physical examination rarely provides the diagnosis in patients with hemostatic problems. It does give insight into the severity of blood loss and suggests underlying illnesses or complications.

1. The vital signs indicate the degree of volume loss, compensation, and tolerance.
2. The skin is examined for evidence of petechiae, ecchymosis, or purpura.
3. The mucosae are examined for oral or nasal oozing.
4. Lymphadenopathy, especially of the supraclavicular and inguinal nodes, may be present. Lymphadenopathy is suggestive of underlying infection, lymphoma, or AIDS.
5. Examination of the abdomen may show hepatomegaly or splenomegaly. An enlarged liver may indicate an infiltrative process, and splenomegaly is consistent with hypersplenism, myeloproliferative disorders, or lymphoma.
6. The joints are examined for recent or remote evidence of hemarthrosis.
7. Potential concealed sites may be revealed on pelvic or rectal examinations as indicated; a urinalysis is performed to look for hematuria.

DECISION PRIORITIES AND PRELIMINARY DIFFERENTIAL DIAGNOSIS

After data gathering, two questions are asked.

1. *What is the estimated amount of blood loss and how is the patient tolerating it?* How this estimation is made and the appropriate interventions are discussed in Chapters 4 and 6.

2. *Does the patient have a platelet disorder, coagulation disorder, or mixed disorder?* Table 24–2 shows a comparison of the major differentiating points for each category.

Platelet disorders are usually acquired and have a pediatric and female predominance. Bleeding in these disorders is usually mild and occurs in mucosal areas as well as in the gastrointestinal and genitourinary tracts. Petechiae are the physical hallmark of these disorders and may appear spontaneously, after trauma, or after a procedure. Splenomegaly may indicate sequestration of platelets and other blood products.

Primary coagulation disorders are most often congenital but may occur with anticoagulant therapy. The congenital disorders have a male predominance owing to X-linked inheritance patterns. Bleeding is moderate to profuse and is often delayed 6 to 12 hours after injury. Significant bleeding episodes such as intracranial bleeding and hemarthrosis are common. The physical examination may reveal signs of purpura, ecchymosis, deep muscle and joint involvement, and signs of liver failure such as jaundice, telangectasia, and hepatosplenomegaly. In addition, lymphadenopathy may indicate the presence of lymphoma, leukemia, or infectious diseases such as acquired immune deficiency syndrome (AIDS) that may directly or indirectly affect liver function.

Mixed platelet and coagulation disorders are almost all acquired and show no sex- or age-related predominance. One exception is von Willebrand's disease. The most common acquired mixed disorder is disseminated intravascular coagulation syndrome. Its common initiating factors include trauma, sepsis, obstetric hemorrhage, transfusion reactions, and snake bite envenomations. Signs of multiple organ failure, unusual bleeding

TABLE 24–2. Major Features of the Three Categories of Bleeding Disorders

	Etiology	Population	Nature	Conditions	Physical Findings
Primary platelet disorders	Mostly acquired	Children and women predominantly	Mild hemorrhage	Post-traumatic or postprocedural or spontaneous	Petechiae Purpura Mucosal bleeding
Primary coagulation disorders	Mostly congenital	Male predominance	Moderate to profuse hemorrhage	Post-traumatic or spontaneous	Deep muscle, joint, urinary tract, and intracranial hemorrhage
Mixed platelet and coagulation disorders	Acquired	Varies	Varies	Trauma, sepsis, obstetric hemorrhage, transfusions, insect or snake bites, others	Signs of multiple organ failure, purpura, bleeding tendencies

tendencies, and purpura are all seen in mixed platelet and coagulation disorders. Clinical pictures that do not comfortably fit either pure platelet or pure coagulation patterns are categorized as mixed disorders until proved otherwise.

PROBLEM 1 The patient with epistaxis arrived in the emergency department. Direct pressure by rescue personnel had slowed the hemorrhage but not controlled it. Additional history obtained at this time revealed that three recent episodes of spontaneous epistaxis had occurred, though none had required emergency care. She was taking no medications except birth control pills. She did remember taking two Anacin tablets the day before for menstrual cramps. Her menses had been heavier than usual lately, which she attributed to a change in her birth control pill prescription. There was no history of any significant childhood bleeding disorder or any familial bleeding tendencies. She denied a history of transfusion, trauma, alcoholism, liver disease, or serious medical illnesses.

Physical examination showed several small ecchymotic areas on the forearms and thighs of various ages. Nasal speculum examination revealed a steady capillary ooze of blood from the right anterior septum. There was no lymphadenopathy or clinical evidence of deep muscle or joint hemorrhage. Vital signs were within normal limits.

Information provided by this patient points to an acquired platelet defect in an adult female. The bleeding is characterized as mucosal and petechial. It may have been exacerbated by aspirin use, but the underlying primary defect is unlikely to be induced by medication alone. There is no evidence of the serious bleeding episodes expected in a primary coagulation or mixed disorder.

PROBLEM 2 After 2 liters of crystalloid were infused, the patient's vital signs improved to BP 110/60 mm Hg, heart rate 100 beats/min, respirations 20/min. His nasogastric tube continued to return blood, but the flow appeared to be slowing. He had no prior history of major bleeding episodes. Three months ago a gastric ulcer was diagnosed, and he was placed on antacid and cimetidine therapy. He continued to use antacids for pain control but had discontinued the cimetidine because of its expense. His past history was positive for hypertension but negative for alcoholism, liver disease, or cancer.

Physical examination revealed an anxious black male with pale sclerae and nailbeds. Large ecchymoses were noted in the area of the IV access attempts. There was no hepatosplenomegaly or evidence of hemarthrosis. The rectal examination was notable for heme-positive brown stool. Otherwise the physical examination results were normal.

This patient most likely has an acquired bleeding disorder. Peptic ulcer disease is the likely source of the hemorrhage. The "blood thinning" medication is a probable contributor to the severity and continued nature of the hemorrhage. Every attempt should be made to identify this medication. Potential sources of information include family, pill bottles (a staff member may need to call home to check these), medical records, the EMS run sheet, and the patient's primary physician(s). The volar arm subcutaneous bleeding after attempts at intravenous access and the severity of the hemorrhage point to a coagulation defect as the primary defect in hemostasis. Platelet involvement, and therefore a mixed disorder, remains a possibility.

ANCILLARY TESTING

In the emergency setting, the laboratory evaluation of hemostasis is accomplished by tests that are available within 2 hours. These criteria limit the truly useful studies to

TABLE 24-3. Usual Findings on Screening Tests in Common Hemostatic Disorders

	Bleeding Time	Platelets	PT	PTT
Primary platelet disorders				
Platelet dysfunction	inc	nl	nl	nl
Thrombocytopenia—idiopathic (autoimmune), or thrombotic thrombocytopenic purpura	inc	dec	nl	nl
Primary coagulation disorders				
Hemophilia A	nl	nl	nl	inc
von Willebrand's disease	inc	nl	nl	inc
Vitamin K deficiency, Coumadin use, liver disease	nl	nl	inc	nl/inc*
Heparin or Coumadin overdose	nl	nl	inc	inc
Common pathway abnormality	nl	nl	inc	inc
Mixed platelet and coagulation disorders				
Disseminated intravascular coagulation	inc	dec	inc	inc

*PT increases first, then PTT. inc = increased, dec = decreased, nl = normal.

those summarized in Table 24-1. For most patients, a screening battery consisting of a prothrombin time, an activated partial thromboplastin time (aPTT), a platelet count, and an Ivy bleeding time will isolate the hemostatic defect (Table 24-3). Bleeding times are useful in patients suspected of having Von Willebrand's disease or those with platelet disorder presentations but normal platelet counts. This screening battery, along with a CBC, costs less than $100 and is ordered for any patient with an unknown bleeding disorder. If the patient suffers from a known condition such as hemophilia, more selective and cost-effective laboratory testing is appropriate.

PROBLEM 1 The patient with epistaxis required anterior nasal packing for hemorrhage control. Results of hemostasis screening were as follows: PT, 13 sec, 12 sec control; aPTT, 27 sec, 26 sec control; platelet count, 20,000/mm^3; bleeding time, 12 min; HgB, 14 gm/dl.
The thrombocytopenia and elevated bleeding time point toward either a primary platelet disorder due to thrombocytopenia or a mixed disorder. Normal coagulation studies (PT and aPTT) rule against a mixed disorder.

PROBLEM 2 Medical records indicated that the patient had been taking Coumadin, 5 mg/day since his bypass surgery. His screening battery returned from the laboratory with the following results: PT, 20 sec, 12 sec control; aPTT, 28 sec, 26 sec control; platelet count, 150,000/mm^3; HgB, 6.9 gm/dl.
This patient was exhibiting the classic hemostatic derangement found with coumarin anticoagulants. He had a marked elevation in prothrombin time and a mild PTT elevation, whereas his platelet count and bleeding time remained within normal limits. He also had a severe anemia.

REFINED DIFFERENTIAL DIAGNOSIS

Once the diagnosis is defined as a platelet disorder, coagulation disorder, or mixed disorder, the next step is to further define the underlying etiology. A brief discussion of the different pathologies and major diseases seen in the emergency department follows.

Primary Platelet Disorders
Thrombocytopenia

Less than 100,000 platelets per cubic millimeter defines this relatively common disorder. There are basically four mechanisms by which thrombocytopenia occurs. These are:

Decreased Bone Marrow Production. Decreased platelet production occurs in response to drugs such as alcohol, heparin, insecticides, heroin, chloramphenicol, and amrinone; following radiation, malignant infiltration of the bone marrow, folate or vitamin B_{12} deficiencies, or infection; as a result of aplastic anemia or pancytopenia, or congenital defects such as Wiskott-Aldrich syndrome or Fanconi's syndrome.

Increased Destruction. Increased platelet destruction may be immunologic in origin as in hepatitis, post-transfusion, idiopathic thrombocytopenic purpura (ITP), leukemia, or lymphoma; or mechanical or toxic as in DIC, vasculitis, thrombotic thrombocytopenic purpura (TTP), or infection.

Dilutional. This mechanism of thrombocytopenia occurs as the result of hemorrhage, massive blood transfusion, hypersplenism, or hypothermia.

Combination. A combination of factors such as increased destruction and decreased production may occur, as in liver disease.

Thrombotic Thrombocytopenic Purpura

Classically, TTP presents as a microangiopathic hemolytic anemia, thrombocytopenic purpura, fever, renal failure, and fluctuating neurologic symptoms. The initiating event in TTP is unclear, although platelet aggregation plays a central role. Although TTP may affect any patient, the majority are 10 to 40 year old females. The peripheral smear shows schistocytes (broken cells) and a low platelet count. TTP is a medical emergency. If it remains untreated, its mortality is 80% in 3 months. The therapy of TTP continues to evolve. Corticosteroids, exchange transfusions, splenectomy, and plasmapheresis have all been used. Due to the high morbidity and mortality, early consultation with an experienced hematologist is indicated.

Idiopathic (Autoimmune) Thrombocytopenic Purpura

ITP may be considered early, but it is diagnosed only when all other causes have been excluded. The initiating event is undetermined but results in the production of an IgG antiplatelet antibody. The acute forms occur most commonly in children 2 to 6 years old and are preceded by a viral prodrome. In children the disease is self-limited and has a 90% rate of spontaneous remission. Treatment of the acute form is supportive, although platelet counts may fall below 5000/mm^3.

Chronic ITP is an adult form of the disease that is three times more common in women. The onset is insidious, and the disease has an unpredictable course. Corticosteroids, splenectomy, and immunosuppression have all been used with some success in treating ITP. Platelet transfusions are reserved for patients with life-threatening hemorrhage.

Primary Coagulation Disorders

Hemophilia A (Classic Hemophilia)

Hemophilia A is a sex-linked recessive bleeding disorder that results from an abnormal function within clotting factor VIII. It is the predominant form of hemophilia, although factor IX (hemophila B) and factor XI (hemophilia C) deficiencies exist. Hemophiliacs are always male and often have a lifelong history of deep muscle, joint, urinary tract, and intracranial bleeding. Epistaxis and gastrointestinal hemorrhage are rare except in the presence of aspirin or ulcers. Trauma is a common initiator of bleeding, although hemorrhage may be delayed up to 48 hours. Most hemophiliacs are well educated about their disease and care for themselves at home. They present to the emergency department primarily for complications of trauma. The severity of hemophilia is directly related to factor VIII-ahf (antihemophilia factor) activity. People with severe forms of the disease have less than 1% activity of this factor and are prone to spontaneous hemorrhage. For those with factor activity in the 1% to 5% range, spontaneous bleeding is rare; however, trauma and surgery may pose serious threats to hemostasis. Patients with greater than 5% activity have little risk of spontaneous bleeding, although trauma and surgery are still risks. Hemophilia is treated with factor VIII-ahf (Factorate). Cryoprecipitate is an acceptable alternative. Both of these blood products carry risks of hepatitis and AIDS. Hemophiliacs represent a small but significant portion of today's AIDS population. Hemophilia B and C are managed in a similar fashion. Specific attention is given to replacing the missing factors.

Table 24–4 shows a comparison of the sites and nature of bleeding in hemophiliacs and their recommended treatment. Generally, the dose of factor VIII is 12.5 units/kg for those with a mild bleeding risk; 25 units/kg for patients with moderate risk of bleeding; and 50 units/kg for patients with severe disease. Because intracranial hemorrhage is a major cause of death, 50 units/kg are given in cases of potentially serious head trauma.

Von Willebrand's Disease

Von Willebrand's disease is an autosomal dominant disease that results from a diminished level and function of factor VIII-vwf (von Willebrand's factor). Interestingly, factor VIII-

TABLE 24–4. Recommended Treatment of Potential Bleeding Sites in Hemophilia A

Type of Bleeding	Initial Dosage	Duration	Comment
Skin			
Abrasion	None	None	Treat with local pressure and topical thrombin
Laceration	Usually none; if necessary treat as minor	None	Local pressure and anesthetic with epinephrine may benefit; watch 4 hours after suturing, reexamine in 24 hours
Superficial			
Deep	Minor bleed (12.5 mg/kg)	Single dose coverage	May need hospitalization for observation
Nasal			
Epistaxis	Usually none; may need to be treated as mild to moderate bleeds	None	Uncommon; consider platelet inhibition; treat in usual manner
Spontaneous			
Traumatic		Up to 5–7 days	Trauma-related bleed can be significant
Oral			
Mucosa or tongue bites	Usually none; treat as minor if persists	Single dose	Commonly seen
Traumatic (laceration) or dental extraction	Moderate (25 units/kg) to severe (50 units/kg)	Single dose; may need more	Saliva rich in fibrin lytic activity; oral ϵ-aminocaproic acid (Amicar) may be given 100 mg every 6 hours for 7 days to block fibrinolysis. Check contraindications; hospitalize patients with severe bleeds
Soft tissue/muscle hematomas	Moderate (25 units/kg)	2–5 days	May be complicated by local pressure on nerves or vessels
Hemarthrosis			
Early	Mild (12.5 units/kg)	Single dose	Treat at earliest symptom (pain)
Late or unresponsive cases of early	Mild to moderate (25 units/kg)	3–4 days	Arthrocentesis rarely necessary, and only with 50% level coverage; immobilization is a critical point of therapy
Hematuria	Mild (12.5 units/kg)	2–3 days	Urokinase, the fibrinolytic enzyme, is found in urine; with persistent hematuria an organic cause should be ruled out
Major bleeding			
Gastrointestinal severe bleeding	(50 units/kg)	7–10 days or 3–5 days after bleeding ceases	In head trauma, therapy may be given prophylactically
Retroperitoneal			
Intra-abdominal			
Major trauma			
Head injury			
Surgical procedure			
Central nervous system bleed			

Reproduced by permission from Hamilton GC: Disorders of hemostasis and polycythemia. In Rosen P, et al (eds): Emergency Medicine: Concepts and Clinical Practice. St. Louis, 1988, The C. V. Mosby Co.

ahf is also diminished in this disease owing to decreased production. The characteristic history is one of mucosal and cutaneous bleeding; menorrhagia and gastrointestinal bleeding are common. In actuality, the disease is similar to hemophilia A with an added defect in platelet function. The diagnosis is indicated by an increased bleeding time, normal platelet count, and increased PTT. Cryoprecipitate, 10 units/kg is usually sufficient to treat adults, although more may be required.

Acquired Coagulation Defects

Primary coagulation defects may appear when liver function is reduced to less than 15% of normal. Clinically, liver disease may result from alcoholism, cancer, hepatitis and other infections as well as from medications and toxins. All clotting factors except von Willebrand's factor are produced in the liver. Of these, factors II, VII, IX, and X are vitamin K dependent. Vitamin K acts as a cofactor for the vitamin K–dependent factors. In the presence of this vitamin, the cofactors are able to bind with calcium and become activated. Depletion of vitamin K (seen in malnourished individuals such as the elderly, those on hyperalimentation, and newborns) or interference with vitamin K binding (seen with use of the coumarin anticoagulants [warfarin, Coumadin]) results in prolongation of PT, mainly through reduction of factor VII levels.

Factor VII has the shortest half-life of all the coagulation factors, and therefore circulating levels of factor VII are the first to drop below required minimums in the presence of liver malfunction. Clinically, decreased levels of factor VII result in a prolonged prothrombin time (extrinsic pathway). Severe or advanced disease involves the other factors and also prolongs the PTT (intrinsic pathway). Overdose of coumarin anticoagulants or severe vitamin K deficiency eventually leads to prolongation of both the PT and PTT.

Treatment of acquired coagulation disorders centers on correcting the underlying pathology and, in mild cases, administration of vitamin K (Aquamephyton). The onset of action of vitamin K occurs in 4 to 8 hours. In severe cases, fresh frozen plasma is the treatment of choice.

Combined Platelet and Coagulation (Mixed) Disorders
Disseminated Intravascular Coagulation

Disseminated intravascular coagulation is a result of an imbalance in the control of coagulation and fibrinolytic pathways initiated by a pathologic process. The process is usually related to trauma or infection but may be caused by obstetric problems, cancer, transfusion reactions, or environmental injury (Table 24–5). In DIC, platelets and coagulation factors are consumed, and fibrin is deposited in the small vessels of multiple organs. In its extreme form, bleeding occurs owing to the loss of platelets, clotting factors, and fibrinolysis, and mechanical red blood cell destruction and small vessel occlusion result from fibrin deposition. DIC is suspected in any patient who presents with purpura, a bleeding tendency, and signs of multiple organ injury. DIC is suspected when the clinical hemostatic defect does not fit neatly into the picture of a primary platelet or coagulation disorder.

DIC is a clinical syndrome that is supported by characteristic laboratory values. The pattern most often seen comprises an increased PT, PTT, and thrombin time (TT) with decreased platelets and fibrinogen. Schistocytes are often seen on the peripheral smear. Fibrin split products are dependent on secondary fibrinolysis and may be nearly absent or present in large amounts.

The treatment of DIC is based on treating the underlying pathology while replacing the blood elements being consumed. Blood component therapy with packed red blood cells, platelets, and coagulation factors (fresh frozen plasma) is recommended if hemorrhage predominates. Heparin is used selectively when fibrin deposition and thrombosis predominate—e.g., in patients with fulminating purpura or obstetric sources of bleeding.

TABLE 24–5. Etiologies of Disseminated Intravascular Coagulation

Infections	**Obstetric**
Gram-positive sepsis	Amniotic fluid embolism
Gram-negative sepsis	Abruptio placentae
Rocky Mountain spotted fever	Dead fetus
Chlamydia	Toxemia of pregnancy
Mycoplasma	**Shock states**
Typhoid	Severe hemorrhage
Influenza	Anaphylaxis
Measles	Cardiac arrest
Others	**Miscellaneous**
Trauma	Aortic aneurysm
Head injury	Diabetic ketoacidosis
Heat stroke	Snake bite
Crush injury	Vasculitis
Hematologic or oncologic	
Metastatic carcinoma	
Acute promyelocytic leukemia	
Sickle cell disease	
Transfusion reactions	

PRINCIPLES OF MANAGEMENT

Managing the patient with a bleeding disorder in the emergency department is primarily evaluative. Many patients may be diagnosed and admitted but require no therapy, e.g., a patient with thrombocytopenia who is not bleeding. If intervention is necessary, the principles of management are (1) stop active hemorrhage; (2) treat the underlying cause; (3) give blood component therapy when indicated. The remainder of this section is on the use of blood component therapy.

Blood component therapy has several benefits:
1. The patient receives only the components that are needed.
2. The risk of transfusion reactions is lower.
3. It is economical because by separating the components, blood banks can serve more patients with fewer units of blood.
4. There is a decreased risk of transmitting disease.
5. Banked whole blood loses clotting factors and platelets rapidly. Therefore, most banked whole blood is useless in treating platelet and coagulation disorders.

Common blood replacement components include:

Packed Red Blood Cells. Packed red blood cells (PRBCs) are given to replenish lost red cell mass. PRBCs are given as uncross-matched low-titer ABO blood, as type-specific blood, or fully cross-matched.

Fresh Frozen Plasma. Fresh frozen plasma (FFP) is the fluid portion of one unit of human blood that has been centrifuged, separated, and frozen solid at $-18°C$ within 6 hours of collection. FFP is indicated for the replacement of isolated factor deficiencies (factors II, V, VII, IX, X, and XI) when specific components are unavailable, for reversal of coumarin anticoagulant therapy, for massive blood transfusions (more than the patient's total blood volume given within 4 hours), as part of the treatment of TTP, and in the treatment of antithrombin III deficiency or immunodeficiencies in infants.

Platelets. Platelets are preserved in type-specific "packs," which contain enough platelets to increase platelet counts by 8000 to $10,000/mm^3$. The number of packs given a patient depends on the hemostatic challenge and the functional state of the patient's platelets. Generally, 35% to 40% of platelets will remain after the entire blood volume has been replaced once. Most patients who receive two times their blood volume rapidly do not develop microvascular bleeding. Therefore, platelets are reserved for patients with thrombocytopenia of less than $50,000/mm^3$ and clinically abnormal bleeding.

Cryoprecipitate. Cryoprecipitate is the fraction of fresh frozen plasma that is insoluble at 4°C. It contains 80 to 100 IU of factor VIII-ahf and also contains von Willebrand's factor and fibrinogen.

Factor VIII-ahf (Factorate). Factorate is fractionated freeze-dried factor VIII-ahf; it contains 300 to 1500 IU per packet. Heat-treated (pasteurized) forms have been found to be free of hepatitis and human immunodeficiency virus (HIV). Ultrapure forms from monoclonal antibody sources remain expensive, and recombinant-DNA preparations are being investigated clinically.

PROBLEM 2 The black male with upper gastrointestinal bleeding continued to produce bright red blood through the nasogastric tube. His vital signs were unchanged after he had received 3 liters of crystalloid. The blood bank called and indicated that 6 units of PRBCs and 2 units of FFP were available; they wanted to know which should be sent first.

Reversal of coumarin anticoagulants is an indication for FFP therapy. Although vitamin K is also effective, its onset of action is delayed several hours, and it is not helpful alone. This patient has ongoing hemorrhage with severe anemia and will not tolerate much more blood loss. Although FFP will reverse the coagulation defect, the top priority is red blood cell mass. Therefore, the PRBCs are given first and the FFP next as a concomitant infusion.

SPECIAL CONSIDERATIONS

Pediatric Patients

The evaluation and treatment of bleeding disorders in children are identical to those in adults. The best history possible is obtained from the parents, and special attention is paid to a family history of bleeding tendencies that may suggest a sex-linked disease such as hemophilia. The history of birth and pregnancy may give clues to underlying diseases and should be sought when available.

Geriatric Patients

In the over-65 age group, the incidence of medical problems such as cancer, immunologic disease, and heart disease rises dramatically. The number of medications taken also increases. Antiplatelet drugs such as aspirin, nonsteroidal anti-inflammatory agents and dipyridamole, or blood thinners such as Coumadin should raise one's suspicions. Many drugs interfere with platelet or coagulation factors. When medication has been ruled out as an offending agent, other acquired causes such as sepsis are suspected.

DISPOSITION AND FOLLOW-UP

Disposition decisions are based on the category of hemostatic disorders and the patient's tolerance of the illness.

Platelet Disorders

Platelet disorders can be considered mild if bleeding is controlled and the platelet count is above 50,000/mm^3 or at baseline for that particular patient. Patients with mild disease can generally be sent home with follow-up scheduled in 1 to 2 days. They are advised to avoid antiplatelet drugs such as dipyridamole, aspirin, and nonsteroidal anti-inflammatory drugs. Patients with new-onset platelet disorders, uncontrolled hemorrhage, or platelet counts of less than 50,000/mm^3 are candidates for admission. Tolerance of low platelet counts will depend heavily on platelet function (check this with bleeding time) and the age and general health of the patient.

Coagulation Disorders

Coagulation defects are considered mild if bleeding is controlled and there is little risk of recurrent bleeding—for example, a hemophiliac who has received a factor VIII-ahf transfusion. These patients are generally rechecked in several days and repeat laboratory studies performed in 1 week. Patients with coagulation defects due to ongoing disease processes such as active hepatitis B infection require close (if not daily) follow-up to monitor hemostatic and liver function. Patients with new-onset coagulation defects should be admitted if the PT is greater than 20 seconds, if the aPTT is greater than two times control, or if the clinical diagnosis is confusing or uncertain. Any hemophiliac with significant head trauma who has a factor VIII level of less than 1% or in whom the factor VIII level of activity is unknown is admitted for observation, replacement therapy, and computed tomography of the head.

Mixed Platelet and Coagulation Defects

Mixed platelet and coagulation defects represent serious derangements of the hemostatic system. As such, patients with such defects should all be admitted, preferably to an intensive care unit. The underlying causative agent should be aggressively sought. Early consultation with an internist or intensive care specialist is a must.

PROBLEM 1 Based on the emergency department evaluation, a presumptive diagnosis of ITP was made. Although hemorrhage was controlled, this patient was admitted because her disorder was of new onset. A full hematologic work-up failed to reveal a cause of the thrombocytopenia. Discharge diagnosis was idiopathic thrombocytopenia.

PROBLEM 2 A total of 6 units of PRBCs and 2 units of FFP were given to this patient in the emergency department. The PT corrected to 13 sec/12 sec control after administration of the FFP. The patient's gastroenterologist performed an emergent endoscopic examination; a 3-cm gastric ulcer was identified as the source of hemorrhage. The patient was admitted to the ICU and during the next 10 days recovered without the need for surgery. Discharge diagnoses were gastrointestinal hemorrhage, gastric ulcer, bleeding diathesis from Coumadin, chronic hypertension, coronary artery disease.

DOCUMENTATION

    1. History, including the nature, sites, and pattern of prior episodes of bleeding, medications, and family history. (This detail is reserved for patients with serious abnormal bleeding or a known hemostatic disorder.)
    2. Physical examination, including notes on vital signs, skin, lymphadenopathy, liver and spleen size, and joints.
    3. Laboratory test results
    4. Response to therapy including any adverse reactions
    5. Presumptive diagnosis supported by the above documentation
    6. Disposition and follow-up arrangements

SUMMARY AND FINAL POINTS

- Using a careful history and physical examination, the etiology of a bleeding disorder can usually be classified as a platelet disorder, coagulation disorder, or mixed disorder.

- Using a screening battery of four readily available tests—the PT, PTT, platelet count, and bleeding time—most bleeding disorders are readily isolated.
- Although bleeding disorders may be mild, some are fatal if untreated. These include thrombotic thrombocytopenic purpura and disseminated intravascular coagulation.
- Treatment of bleeding disorders centers on hemorrhage control, treatment of the underlying cause, and blood component therapy.
- Patients with mild platelet disorders can generally be sent home, but patients with most other hemostatic problems require admission.
- Prompt recognition of bleeding disorders is essential for proper evaluation and treatment. Recognition depends on observation, awareness of the problem, and a clear approach.

BIBLIOGRAPHY

Texts

1. Jandl JH: Blood: Textbook of Hematology. Boston, Little, Brown & Co., 1987.
2. Rappaport SI: Introduction to Hematology (2nd ed). Philadelphia, J.B. Lippincott, 1987.
3. Thompson AR, Harkness LA: Manual of Hemostasis and Thrombosis (3rd ed). Philadelphia, F.A. Davis, 1984.

Journal Articles

1. Alpern JB: Coagulopathy caused by vitamin K deficiency in critically ill, hospitalized patients. JAMA 258(14):1916–1917, 1987.
2. Angleos MG, Hamilton GC: Coagulation studies: Prothrombin time, partial thromboplastin time, bleeding time. Emerg Med Clin North Am 4(1):95–113, 1986.
3. Brannan PP, Guthrie TH: Idiopathic thrombocytopenic purpura in adults. South Med J 81(1):75–80, 1988.
4. Bray GL, Luban NLC: Hemophilia presenting with intracranial hemorrhage: An approach to the infant with intracranial bleeding and coagulopathy, Am J Dis Child 141:1215–1217, 1987.
5. Carr ME: Disseminated intravascular coagulation: Pathogenesis, diagnosis and therapy. J Emerg Med 5:311–322, 1987.
6. Consensus Conference: Platelet transfusion therapy. JAMA 257(13):1777–1780, 1987.
7. Crain SM, Choudhory AM: Thrombotic thrombocytopenic purpura: A reappraisal. JAMA 246(11):1243–1246, 1981.
8. Hamilton GC: Platelet count. Emerg Med Clin North Am 4(1):75–85, 1986.
9. Lind S: Prolonged bleeding time. Am J Med 77:305–312, 1984.
10. McMillan R: Chronic idiopathic thrombocytopenic purpura. N Engl J Med 304(19):1135–1146, 1981.
11. Murphy S: Thrombocytosis and thrombocythemia. Clin Hematol 12(1):89–106, 1983.
12. Rose M, Eldor A: High incidence of relapse in thrombotic thrombocytopenic purpura. Am J Med 83:437–444, 1987.

CHAPTER 25

SICKLE CELL DISEASE

ROBERT L. ZURCHER M.D.
GLENN C. HAMILTON, M.D.

PROBLEM A 22 year old black male with sickle cell disease (SCD), who was well known to the emergency department personnel, arrived by emergency squad with a complaint of "chest pain for the last week."

QUESTIONS TO CONSIDER

1. What are the three major types of sickle cell crisis?
2. What are the key historical and physical findings that help determine the type of crisis that is present?
3. Which organ systems are evaluated as possible sites of sickle cell complications?
4. Which laboratory tests are ordered in every patient? Are there other tests to assist in the diagnosis and treatment of complex cases?
5. What sickle cell disease-associated conditions require emergent treatment?
6. How is pain managed in an uncomplicated vaso-occlusive crisis?
7. What special factors are considered in managing infants and children with sickle cell anemia?
8. What are the criteria for admission? What follow-up plans are made if the patient is discharged?

INTRODUCTION

A hemoglobinopathy is an inherited disease caused by the presence of one or more abnormal hemoglobins. Normal hemoglobin is composed of four polypeptide chains and four heme groups. The polypeptide chains consist of two alpha (α) and two other chains. The nonalpha chains are beta (β), gamma (γ), and delta (δ). Hemoglobin A ($\alpha_2\beta_2$) comprises 96% of adult hemoglobin.

Sickle cell anemia is characterized by the presence of hemoglobin S. This hemoglobin results from a single point mutation in the gene for the β chain. Specifically, there is a substitution of valine for glutamic acid in the sixth position of the β chain. The abnormal β globin chain then complexes with α chains to form the sickle hemoglobin, HbS ($\alpha_2\beta_2S$).

When combined with oxygen, HbS shows near-normal solubility. When the molecule gives up its oxygen (deoxy S), it tends to polymerize into tubelike fibers (tactoids), which induce erythrocyte sickling. Factors that promote hemoglobin S deoxygenation and consequent erythrocyte sickling include hypoxemia, acidosis, high 2,3-diphosphoglycerate (DPG) levels, and red blood cell (RBC) dehydration. Sickled cells are less deformable and increase the viscosity of blood. This causes obstruction or sludging in the capillary circulation, resulting in local tissue hypoxia. Local hypoxia promotes more deoxygenation and sickling. The red cell sickling can be reversed to a degree with reoxygenation. Repetitive sickling and unsickling damages the cell membrane, making it less deformable.

Organs with extensive capillary beds (i.e., spleen and kidney) may have multiple infarctions during sickle cell crises. As a result, most patients are functionally asplenic by 2 years of age and are highly susceptible to infection. The kidney develops an impaired ability to concentrate urine owing to damage of the countercurrent exchange system. All patients with sickle cell disease suffer from chronic hemolytic anemia. The life span of the RBC is reduced from 120 days to as short as 20 days.

Sickle cell disease usually occurs in individuals who are homozygous for the sickle cell gene (SS). The disease occurs in the heterozygous state when hemoglobin S is paired with other abnormal hemoglobins, such as hemoglobin C (SC) or β-thalassemia (S β-thal). Sickle cell trait is the heterozygous or carrier state and is generally considered a clinically benign condition.

Hemoglobin S has its highest incidence in individuals of African descent. It is estimated that 8% of American blacks are heterozygous for HbS. Individuals who are homozygous for HbS are estimated to comprise 0.15% to 0.2% of the black population, or approximately 50,000 people.

During their first decade of life, almost all patients with sickle cell disease suffer from frequent crises. These crises occur in three physiologic systems that may overlap:

1. Hematologic crises usually involve decreased red cell mass due to increased destruction and occasional acute decreased production.
2. Infectious crises result particularly from encapsulated bacteria, *Streptococcus pneumoniae* and *Hemophilus influenzae*.
3. Vaso-occlusive crises result in ischemia to a variety of organs, usually those with high blood flow, e.g., heart, lung, brain.

After the first decade, two distinct groups of patients emerge. The first group, consisting of 10% to 15% of patients with sickle cell disease, continues to have frequent crises requiring hospital admission. The second and larger group rarely requires admission.

The prognosis in terms of mortality is not well known. However, the first decade appears to be the critical period. After the first decade, mortality decreases markedly and is spread evenly over the next four decades. The majority of deaths result from complications of infectious disease.

PREHOSPITAL CARE

History

The differential diagnosis and proper care of the patient with sickle cell crisis is a difficult task, even for an experienced emergency physician. The rescue squad should not spend time on a thorough history and physical examination but should concentrate instead on communicating a brief directed history of the present illness including length of the pain episode and location of pain.

Physical Examination

The physical examination is limited to the vital signs, respiratory status, and tolerance of pain.

Intervention

Depending on the level of the squad's skills and training, preliminary treatment can include:

1. Establishing intravenous (IV) access if necessary. The majority of these patients do not need parenteral fluids in the prehospital setting unless their vital signs are unstable. If hypotension is present, isotonic crystalloid is the fluid of choice. It is

frequently difficult to start an IV in patients who have had previous venipunctures. This procedure may need to be performed in the receiving hospital by an experienced person.

2. Oxygen should be given *only* to patients with documented respiratory distress. Usually 4 to 6 liters/min by nasal cannula is adequate.

3. Cardiac monitoring is initiated as indicated.

PROBLEM This was the fourth time in the last 6 months that this squad had been called to this patient's home. His initial vital signs were respiratory rate 28, pulse 110 beats/min, blood pressure 130/90 mm Hg. They did not establish an IV line, but placed the patient on a cardiac monitor. Oxygen was administered at a rate of 4 liters/min by nasal cannula. During transport to the hospital the patient repeatedly demanded narcotics for his pain.

Emergency squads that frequently transport patients with sickle cell anemia may become frustrated because they feel that their services are being abused. However, it must be stressed to the medics that every patient with sickle cell anemia is potentially critically ill and deserves attentive and courteous care.

INITIAL APPROACH IN THE EMERGENCY DEPARTMENT

Sickle cell anemia is the most common hemoglobinopathy encountered by the emergency physician. It is a complex and frustrating illness for both the patient and the physician. Although a small subgroup of patients often make multiple visits to the emergency department, complacency in evaluating their complaints will certainly lead to disaster.

The three major types of crises in sickle cell disease have specific pathologic processes that can be life-threatening. Any or all of these processes may be active in the patient.

1. Hematologic pathology. In children under 5 years old, acute anemia from *splenic sequestration* can occur. In any age group, *aplastic anemia* may result from suppression of bone marrow activity.

2. Infectious pathology. *Septic shock* associated with functional asplenia and meningitis are immediate concerns.

3. Vaso-occlusive pathology. Acute *ischemia* to the *brain* or *myocardium* requires early intervention.

Evaluation of the patient with sickle cell anemia first identifies the major crisis type present and searches for an underlying life-threatening process. Early treatment is directed toward relief of symptoms and reducing the risks to life and limb.

The management principles followed when the patient with sickle cell anemia arrives at the emergency department are:

1. Every patient with sickle cell anemia, regardless of presenting complaint, requires a rapid evaluation of vital signs and level of consciousness. Patients with hypotension, fever, or altered mental status are seen immediately by an experienced physician. Signs of the potential life-threatening illnesses listed above are actively sought during the assessment.
2. Early treatment proceeds concomitantly with evaluation.
3. Initial management includes the following steps:
   a. If the patient has tachycardia or hypotension, an IV line is established for venous access and possible hydration. Because of the possibility of congestive heart failure, 0.45% normal saline given at one and a half times the maintenance dose is a good initial choice of fluids.
   b. An assessment of pain is made, and adequate analgesia is provided.
   c. Controversy exists about the use of oxygen in sickle cell crises because some experts feel that it may decrease erythropoiesis. However, any sickle cell patient in respiratory distress or with documented hypoxia is given oxygen.
   d. Cardiac monitoring is continued.

4. Patients with stable vital signs and no neurologic symptoms usually do not require immediate treatment. They may be triaged for urgent evaluation.

PROBLEM *Note:* This problem is given to review important elements of care *and* potential pitfalls. This was this patient's twelfth visit to the emergency department in the last 6 months. He was considered by the staff to be highly manipulative and was suspected of being a drug abuser. The patient's repeated vital signs taken by the triage nurse were BP 120/40 mm Hg, pulse 110 beats/min, respiratory rate 26/min, temperature 101.2°F. The nurse "knew" this patient and believed that he did not appear ill despite his abnormal vital signs and complaint of chest pain. Oxygen was maintained, and he was triaged to a bed for routine evaluation.

Although this patient does not look ill, his elevated temperature and tachypnea indicate a potentially serious problem. By triaging the patient to a routine bed instead of requesting immediate physician evaluation, a common error has been committed. Patients who frequently visit the emergency department are often labelled "abusers" and are treated casually. This ill-advised approach eventually leads to critical errors.

DATA GATHERING

Patients with sickle cell disease are usually well aware of their diagnosis. The history and physical examination focus on determining whether a crisis exists, its nature, and the chronic effects of the disease. Evaluating the potential for drug-seeking behavior is a necessary goal of data gathering.

History

History of Present Illness

Three major areas of questioning reflect the pathophysiologic high-risk areas.

Pain. Pain is the most common presenting complaint in sickle cell crisis. It is also the hallmark of vaso-occlusive crisis. The quality, location, and character of the pain need to be explored carefully because the pain pattern of vaso-occlusion tends to repeat itself. The pain history is fully explored—what makes it better or worse, associated symptoms, onset, evolving history, and what the patient has done to treat it. If the patient describes something new about the pain, the physician needs to consider the possibility of another disease process occurring, e.g. myocardial infarction, pulmonary infarction, or osteomyelitis.

Neurologic Symptoms. Patients presenting with new-onset lateralizing weakness or altered mental status are managed aggressively. The loss of oxygen-carrying capacity due to anemia must be included in the differential diagnosis.

Pallor, Weakness. These are nonspecific symptoms that may indicate increasing anemia.

Precipitating Factors

Vaso-occlusive crises occur when sickled cells cause sludging in the microvasculature. Factors that promote the sickling of HbS and subsequent RBC sludging include exposure to cold, high altitude, dehydration, and stress such as infection. Whenever a patient presents with vaso-occlusive crisis, a careful search is made for a precipitating event, especially infection. In adults, the triggering event is seldom identified. In children, acute viral illness precedes more than 80% of vaso-occlusive crises.

Complications of Sickle Cell Disease

One of the most devastating aspects of sickle cell disease is the chronic damage done to organs. The physician must consider high-yield areas for complicating damage because positive findings may alter the treatment plan. Table 25-1 outlines an organ systems approach to common complications.

Past Medical History

1. Medical history. Past crises are characterized by type and severity. The patient may know his or her "normal" hemoglobin or hematocrit.

2. Surgical history. The surgical history may assist in the diagnosis of the painful abdomen.

3. Medications. Medications taken prior to arrival in the emergency department are explored. The physician must establish what type of analgesics are available to the patient. Are there distinct preferences?

4. Family history. The family history may be the key in making the initial diagnosis of sickle cell disease.

Physical Examination

A focused physical examination is essential for the proper evaluation of the patient with sickle cell disease. By using a systems approach, the physician can organize the search for signs identifying the presence of a crisis and its type (Table 25-1). Finding the chronic complications of the disease completes the total assessment of the disease.

DECISION PRIORITIES AND PRELIMINARY DIFFERENTIAL DIAGNOSIS

There are few diseases, if any, that mimic the total body involvement of sickle cell disease. The emergency physician rarely establishes the presence of sickle cell anemia but primarily determines whether a crisis is occurring and, if so, what type. Identifying a crisis is not easy. Unless the patient is new and without a known diagnosis of sickle cell disease, or the potential for drug-seeking behavior is very high, it is best for the physician to assume that the "crisis" is real and focus on identifying the type. This process is simplified by placing the patient in one of three crisis categories—hematologic, infectious, or vaso-occlusive. New patients or those without a prior history are initially treated as having acute pain, usually abdominal in origin.

There are two types of *hematologic crises*: splenic sequestration and aplastic crisis. Splenic sequestration occurs primarily in children. It occurs when sickled cells obstruct the splenic outflow, leading to a massive accumulation of unsickled cells in the spleen. This may result in the rapid appearance of profound hypovolemic shock. In patients with sickle cell anemia the bone marrow is usually operating at its upper limits of RBC production to keep up with the ongoing destruction of sickled cells. Aplastic crisis occurs when erythropoiesis is slowed, leading to a decrease in the patient's hemoglobin as destruction outpaces production. The most common cause of aplastic crisis is viral infection. Other frequent causes are folate deficiency and bone marrow toxins, e.g., phenylbutazone.

Infectious crisis refers to the propensity for patients, especially children younger than 5 years old, to be rapidly overwhelmed by bacterial sepsis. It is the complication that most commonly results in hospitalization and is the most frequent cause of death in all age groups. During the first 5 years of life, *Streptococcus pneumoniae* is the dominant pathogen. The source of the infection may be occult. However, the middle ear and lungs are frequently the primary sites of infection. Infectious crises manifest also as specific sites of involvement. High-risk areas are the central nervous system (meningitis), lung (pneumonia), and bone (osteomyelitis). Infecting agents are commonly encapsulated bacteria. *Salmonella* is a unique but infrequent cause of osteomyelitis in sickle cell disease.

Vaso-occlusive crisis is the most common reason for emergency department visits. It is often the most difficult type of sickle cell crisis to diagnose. There are seven common anatomic sites of vaso-occlusive crisis: abdominal, bone and joint, cerebrovascular,

TABLE 25–1. Organ Systems Approach to the Physical Examination and Complications of Sickle Cell Disease

System	Specific Component	Physical Finding	Known Complications
Vital signs	Temperature	Fever in children may indicate infectious disease. In adults low-grade fever often accompanies vaso-occlusive crisis. Elevations greater than 101°F should be considered secondary to infection	Relative immunosuppression, especially against encapsulated bacteria
	Blood pressure	Hypotension could result from splenic sequestration or septic shock	Relative immunosuppression, as above
	Heart rate	Tachycardia may indicate fever, sepsis, impending shock	Relative immunosuppression, as above
	Respiratory rate	Tachypnea may indicate pulmonary disease or acute anemia	Relative immunosuppression or aplastic crisis; pulmonary embolism, infarct, or infection
Head, eyes, ears, nose, and throat	Ears, throat	Signs of otitis media, upper respiratory infection	Common source of encapsulated bacteria
	Eyes	Decreased visual acuity, funduscopic examination that is "blurry" or shows retinal damage	Retinal hemorrhages are common
		Pale conjunctiva	Suggests severe anemia
	Neck	Meningeal signs	Meningitis is 600 times more common in children with sickle cell disease
Cardiac		S_3 gallop, rub, or ischemic murmurs	Congestive heart failure, myocardial infarction
Pulmonary		Rales, pleural rub, decreased breath sounds with dull percussion from effusion, signs of consolidation	Intrapulmonary shunting, embolism, infarct, infection
Gastrointestinal		Guarding and rebound are common in abdominal crisis. Presence of bowel sounds is best physical finding consistent with crisis rather than with acute surgical abdomen. Enlarged spleen in children may indicate splenic sequestration	Hepatitis, liver infarcts. Bilirubin gallstones are common. Mesenteric infarcts. Splenic sequestration. Abdomen is common site of painful "crisis" without obvious site of injury
Genitourinary	Kidney	Costovertebral angle tenderness	Hyposthenuria, hematuria, papillary necrosis, urinary tract infections
	Genitalia	Complete exam warranted particularly in abdominal crisis or priapism	Impotence, priapism, decreased fertility
Skeletal	Hands and feet	Painful swelling of dorsa of hands and feet	Hand and foot syndrome
	Joints and long bones	Painful swollen joints, point tenderness on a long bone	Osteomyelitis, infarction, septic necrosis of hips
Central nervous system		Focal defect or altered mental status	Meningitis and cerebrovascular accident type is more frequent in sickle cell disease
Skin		Pretibial or malleolar ulcers, signs of cutaneous infection	Stasis ulcers

priapism, hand and foot, pulmonary, and renal. These crisis sites frequently coexist and are discussed later in the section on Refined Differential Diagnosis.

By asking the following questions, the physician may be able to identify which major crisis category predominates in the patient's complaint.

1. *Is the predominant complaint pain? If so, where is it located?*
   The hallmark of vaso-occlusive crisis is pain. The location and associated findings are usually sufficient to identify this category.
2. *Does the patient have neurologic symptoms?*
   Neurologic crisis is the only type of vaso-occlusive crisis that is painless.
3. *Do the patient's vital signs indicate hypovolemic shock or impending shock?*
   Splenic sequestration usually presents as hypovolemic shock. Dehydration due to viral illness may combine with an aplastic crisis to present as shock. Complicating sepsis may present similarly.
4. *Does the patient have a fever?*
   Infection can be rapidly overwhelming and requires assessment and therapy.

A frequently confusing issue in the differential diagnosis is the fact that a patient may have more than one type of crisis at a time. The coexisting crises may occur in any combination. Two of the more common combinations include aplastic crisis with an infection, and vaso-occlusive crisis in two sites, e.g., abdomen and bone.

If answers to the above questions do not identify one of the three major crises, the physician needs to reexplore the possibility of manipulative or drug-seeking behavior. Sickle cell disease can certainly be quickly identified by the laboratory if the patient is unknown. If the patient is known to have sickle cell disease, and the complaints are supported by physical findings, it is better to err on the side of treatment, even if the potential for analgesic abuse is high. It is appropriate in this situation to request hemotologic consultation, if available.

PROBLEM Forty-five minutes after arrival, the patient was evaluated by a physician. He was complaining of fatigue, dyspnea, cough, and pleuritic chest pain. He appeared younger than his stated age of 22 and was in moderate respiratory distress. Vital signs were BP 120/90 mm Hg, pulse 110 beats/min, respirations 26/min, temperature 101.2°F. Pertinent physical findings included pale conjunctiva, inspiratory crackles in the left lung fields, abdomen soft without organomegaly, and a normal neurologic examination.

The patient complained of chest pain. Vaso-occlusive disease may be present, but the physical findings of fever and inspiratory crackles support a preliminary diagnosis of infectious pulmonary problems. The complaints of fatigue and dyspnea are nonspecific and could be secondary to infectious pulmonary disease. They also raise the possibility of acute hematologic crisis due to aplastic anemia. Confirmation of these suspicions awaits laboratory results.

DIAGNOSTIC ADJUNCTS

Use of the clinical laboratory is a routine aspect of evaluating the patient with sickle cell disease. At a minimum, a complete blood count is determined. Other tests are selected as the patient's condition warrants.

Laboratory Studies

Patients with sickle cell anemia usually have a predictable range of values for hemoglobin, hematocrit, and reticulocytes (Table 25–2). There are patients with sickle cell variants that may have essentially normal hemogram values. The patient is usually aware of this condition. The patient's recollection and old chart are valuable sources for comparison.

Complete Blood Count
Hemoglobin–Hematocrit. These levels are evaluated in all patients with suspected sickle cell crisis. The results are routinely checked against the patient's previous recorded

TABLE 25–2. Mean Values and Ranges for Patients with Sickle Cell Anemia

	Mean	Range
Hemoglobin	7.5 gm/dl	5.5–9.5 gm/dl
Hematocrit	22%	17.0–29.0 gm/dl
Reticulocyte count	12.0%	5.0–30.0%
White blood cell count	13,000/mm^3	12,000–15,000/mm^3

values. A drop of more than 2 gm/dl in hemoglobin or 4% to 6% in hemotocrit indicates the presence of either aplastic crisis, splenic sequestration, or a different complicating etiology of anemia, e.g., blood loss.

White Blood Cell Count. This value is usually elevated in all sickle cell crises. However, a count greater than 15,000 with a left shift raises the suspicion of a bacterial infection.

Reticulocyte Count

Some physicians order a reticulocyte count routinely. A helpful and cost-efficient rule is to order a reticulocyte count if the patient's hemoglobin level has decreased by more than 2 gm/dl. This test result may differentiate aplastic crisis from other causes of active anemia. In aplastic crises, a decrease in erythropoiesis is reflected by a reticulocyte count less than 3.0%, or lower than the patient's usual value.

Electrolytes

Measurements of electrolytes are not routinely ordered. Patients with sickle cell disease frequently have renal complications. If significant IV rehydration is planned, electrolytes can be helpful in selecting the type of fluid to use.

Urinalysis

A urinalysis is ordered in any patient with a fever or dysuria. White cells, red cells, bacteria, or tissue is sought. The latter may be seen in papillary necrosis. Poor concentrating ability (isothenuria) is usually noted. Specific gravity is usually in the 1.010 to 1.012 range. If the urine is concentrated, the diagnosis is questioned. Sickle cell trait may be present, and the patient may be seeking narcotics.

Arterial Blood Gas

Arterial blood gas analysis is requested in any patient with respiratory distress. At sea level, a Pao$_2$ of less than 60 mm Hg in adults and 70 mm Hg in children may indicate potentially life-threatening disease.

Radiologic Imaging

Radiographs are ordered selectively in patients with sickle cell crises. The indications, listed below, are usually clear.

1. *Chest radiographs* are needed in any patient with pulmonary signs or symptoms.
2. *Bone radiographs* are indicated in any patient with bone and joint pain with well-localized point tenderness. Unfortunately, the early changes of osteomyelitis and infarction are difficult to differentiate, and the radiograph is often normal in early osteomyelitis.
3. In patients with right upper quadrant abdominal pain and tenderness, gallbladder *ultrasonography* can help to rule out cholecystitis.
4. The possibility of osteomyelitis in the patient with bone pain is a frequent diagnostic dilemma. The best method for evaluating this possibility is a *bone scan*, which usually shows positive signs of osteomyelitis in the early stages (1 to 3 weeks).

PROBLEM The results of the patient's laboratory studies returned: hemoglobin 5.5 gm/dl (patient's baseline was 8.8 gm/dl), reticulocyte count 5% (baseline 10%), WBC 17,000 with numerous sickled cells and 65% segmented neutrophils, 15% bands. Arterial blood gas measurement while the patient was receiving 4 liters of oxygen was pH 7.45, Pco$_2$ 35 mm Hg, and Pco$_2$ 65 mm Hg. The chest film demonstrated a right middle lobe infiltrate. Sputum Gram's stain showed multiple WBCs and gram-positive diplococci.

The patient's low hemoglobin and low reticulocyte count confirmed the initial impression of aplastic crisis. The radiographic findings and sputum Gram stain supported the possibility of pneumococcal pneumonia. Blood, urine, and sputum cultures were collected.

REFINED DIFFERENTIAL DIAGNOSIS

Once one or more of the three major crisis categories (hematologic, infectious, vaso-occlusive) has been identified, it is often necessary to search further for subsets of disease. Vaso-occlusive crisis is most common and each of its major sites warrants an expanded description. Table 25-3 can assist the physician in pursuing the refined differential diagnosis of the subsets in vaso-occlusive sickle cell crisis. Hematologic and infectious crises are less common; they are described in the sections on Decision Priorities and Preliminary Differential Diagnosis and Special Considerations—Pediatrics. The clinician should *always* remember that the patient may have a medical illness that represents a complication of sickle cell disease and that two crises may coexist.

PROBLEM By using Table 25-3 to create a refined diagnosis for this patient, the symptoms do not perfectly fit a diagnosis of either pneumonia or infarct. However, the purulent sputum, abnormal chest x-ray, and fever of 101.2°F support a diagnosis of pneumonia. This is not unusual in clinical medicine.

PRINCIPLES OF MANAGEMENT

General Principles

The majority of therapies in sickle cell disease are directed toward general supportive care. A few therapies are listed here for specific complications. Each crisis type requires specific management. Certain actions can be taken in all patients while diagnostic efforts proceed. As noted earlier under Initial Approach in the Emergency Department, analgesia, hydration, and supplemental oxygen establish the basis for care in patients with sickle cell disease.

Analgesia. Many physicians worry about creating or supporting drug dependency in patients with painful crises if they prescribe narcotics for pain. This should not be a concern. Prescribed drugs are rarely a major factor in narcotic addiction; instead, psychological, social, and economic factors are the determining forces.

Instituting a protocol for the treatment of painful crises has been shown to improve patient-physician rapport and lessen patient manipulation. The following guidelines are suggested:

1. Narcotic analgesia is provided based on an accurate assessment of the severity of the pain. Meperidine (Demerol), 50 to 75 mg with promethazine (Phenergan), 25 to 50 mg intramuscularly, is an often-used first-dose combination. Oral analgesics such as acetaminophen with codeine (Tylenol No. 3), 2 tablets, or Percodan, 2 tablets, are preferred in many medical centers. The important elements are consistency and the knowledge by the patient that a protocol is being followed. This protocol decreases the wide variety of analgesics prescribed by physicians, including placebo dosing with normal saline.

2. The patient is observed for 2 to 3 hours after the medication is given. At this time a second dose may be given if warranted by symptoms. If the patient is comfortable after one or two doses, discharge is arranged and a prescription written for a small number of oral analgesics. If significant pain persists, the patient is admitted.

Hydration. Most sickle cell patients are volume depleted by 1 to 2 liters at presentation. Oral repletion is preferred in cooperative patients. Patients who cannot or

TABLE 25–3. Subsets of Vaso-occlusive Crises

Subset	Frequency	Supporting History	Physical Examination	Diagnostic Tests	Differential Diagnosis	Comment
Abdominal	Common	Relatively acute onset, diffuse, poorly localized visceral pain. Repetitive pattern from crisis to crisis. Occasionally more typical of cholecystitis, hepatitis	Signs of peritoneal irritation are uncommon. Occasionally localized to organ involved, particularly gallbladder	Interpretation of complete blood count difficult. No other characteristic test, though gallbladder ultrasound useful	Mesenteric infarction, cholecystitis, appendicitis, pancreatitis, hepatitis, pelvic inflammatory disease	30% of patients have pigmented gallstones by age 10, 70% by age 30. Less than 10% are symptomatic. Acute hepatic crises with sinusoidal sickling may imitate acute cholecystitis
Bone and joint	Most common presenting complaint in emergency department	Patient usually >2 years old. Rapid onset of deep aching pain; once it peaks, it tends to remain at that level. Repetitive pattern from crisis to crisis. Frequency varies by individual	Occasionally local tenderness. More often, deep bone pain without physical findings	Radiographs are seldom diagnostic unless there are chronic changes of osteomyelitis. Bone scan may be useful early in course	Osteomyelitis, septic arthritis, rheumatic fever, gout	The slow sinusoidal circulation of the bone marrow is a common site for sickling
Cerebrovascular	Common—occurs in up to 26% of patients with symptomatic disease	Acute onset of any neurologic symptom: aphasia, headache, hemiparesis, cranial nerve palsy, altered mental status, seizure. Cerebrovascular accident more common in children and young adults. Mean age of onset is 10 years. Intracranial hemorrhage more common in older group	Consistent with type of process and location of injury	Computed tomography necessary in emergency department. If normal, follow with lumbar puncture to assess possible subarachnoid hemorrhage. Angiography may be necessary. Contrast material can cause sickling	Subarachnoid hemorrhage, intracerebral hemorrhage	Represents 16% of all causes of death in children with sickle cell disease. Tendency to recur
Hand and foot syndrome	Most common initial presentation of sickle cell disease in infancy, rare thereafter	Usually occurs in children <3 years old. One to four extremities may be affected	Painful nonpitting edema of dorsa of hands and feet	Radiologic changes of periosteal elevation and/or bone necrosis may not appear for 1 week or longer	Osteomyelitis, septic arthritis, rheumatic fever	Etiology is microinfarction of carpal and tarsal bones

Table continued on following page

will not drink are given fluid intravenously. The volume and rate of crystalloid administration are determined by the initial estimate of volume loss and the response to therapy. Because these patients are at risk for congestive heart failure, a conservative, closely monitored volume replacement regimen is recommended.

Oxygen. Supplemental low-flow oxygen is often given. Whether its beneficial effect on the crisis offsets the hazard of suppressing erythropoiesis is unknown. Any patient

TABLE 25–3. Subsets of Vaso-occlusive Crises *Continued*

Subset	Frequency	Supporting History	Physical Examination	Diagnostic Tests	Differential Diagnosis	Comment
Priapism	Rare as complaint in emergency department, though reported to occur in up to 30% of men	Painful prolonged nonsexual penile erection persisting more than several hours. Seventy-five percent of cases occur between 12 and 6 AM. Increases in frequency and severity with advancing age. Some degree of impotence in 25% of cases	Painful erection may be partial	None	None in sickle cell disease, though can be seen in leukemia and hyperviscosity syndromes	A more common form is "stuttering priapism"—painful reversible erection. This may precede more severe form. Normal sexual function may remain in 40% to 60% of men
Pulmonary	Common—occurs in up to 50% of patients	Acute onset pleuritic chest pain, cough, and dyspnea. Often preceded by other vaso-occlusive crises	Fever associated more often with infectious cause. Often tachypnea. Occasionally pleural rub, signs of consolidation	Chest film usually normal at onset of symptoms. Infiltrate appears at 2–3 days. Multilobe involvement suggestive of pneumonia. Arterial blood gases are compared with patient's baseline, not "normal range." Lung scan interpretation is confusing. Angiography rarely necessary, and contrast material may induce more sickling	Rib infarction, embolism, pneumonia, ischemic heart disease	Accounts for 15% of admissions of sickle cell patients. Underlying pathology is pulmonary infarction secondary to vascular occlusion. Can be complicated by pneumonia
Renal	Common	Often asymptomatic. May have acute back pain or ureteral colic due to papillary necrosis	Costovertebral angle tenderness	Concentrating defect on specific gravity, hematuria, tissue in urine. Intravenous pyelogram may show irregular renal papillae	Glomerulonephritis, nephrotic syndrome, urinary tract cancer	Loss of concentrating function occurs early. Increases obligatory urine losses. Hematuria from sickling occurs in vasa recta

who has respiratory distress or documented hypoxia is given oxygen, usually 2 to 4 liters/min by nasal cannula.

Specific Management Principles

Some of the more common crises require specific management techniques. Splenic sequestration and infectious crises are addressed under Special Considerations—Pediatrics.

Bone and Joint and Abdominal Vaso-occlusive Crises. These crises are the most common types and may occur together. Once more serious underlying disease has been ruled out, each type is treated with hydration and analgesia.

Pulmonary Crisis. Because it is frequently difficult to differentiate infarction from pneumonia, these patients are usually started on broad-spectrum antibiotics covering *Hemophilus influenzae, Streptococcus pneumoniae,* and *Mycoplasma pneumoniae.* Appropriate choices include amoxicillin or a cephalosporin such as cefotaxime or cefuroxime. In addition, erythromycin is usually given either IV or orally to cover for mycoplasma.

Exchange transfusion may be necessary in patients with rapidly progressing disease, respiratory insufficiency, or multiple lobe involvement. It is not an emergency department procedure.

Aplastic Crisis. Red blood cell transfusion may be required but only after consultation with a hematologist. Transfusion may actually slow the recovery of erythropoiesis. A careful search for an underlying cause for aplastic crisis must be made. Folate is given because it is a correctable cause of aplastic crisis.

Priapism. The goal of management of these patients is to decrease pain and prevent impotence. Initial management includes emptying the bladder, massaging the prostate, providing hydration, and pain relief. If after about 2 to 3 hours these treatments fail, the patient should have an exchange transfusion. Most experts recommend surgical therapy if detumescence has not begun within 24 to 48 hours of transfusion. Without intervention, the severe form results in impotence in 80% of patients.

Neurologic Crisis. This is a true emergency, and treatment must proceed rapidly. An emergency computed tomographic scan is necessary to localize any surgically correctable lesion. The patient requires emergent exchange transfusion to decrease the level of hemoglobin S to below 30%. This treatment has been shown to prevent progression and recurrence of the cerebrovascular accident. It may be initiated in the emergency department after discussion and agreement with a hematologist.

SPECIAL CONSIDERATIONS

Pediatric Patients

Sickle cell disease is often considered a disease of children because of its high early mortality. Children in high-risk groups may present first to the emergency department. Hand and foot crisis is the most common initial presentation of sickle cell disease.

Splenic sequestration from obstructed splenic outflow may be the initial presentation in up to 20% of patients less than 3 years old. Because a large proportion of the circulating blood volume is trapped in the spleen, it usually causes symptoms of increasing anemia and hypovolemic shock. Treatment needs to be immediate and aggressive because these patients can deteriorate and die in minutes. An adequate airway is established, and intravascular volume is restored as rapidly as possible. Crystalloid solution is not adequate alone. The patient will require red blood cells as soon as possible. Splenic sequestration is very rare after 3 years of age because most patients are functionally asplenic by that age.

All patients with sickle cell disease are susceptible to infection with polysaccharide encapsulated organisms, especially *S. pneumoniae.* Because of their functional asplenia and immunologic dysfunction, children less than 5 years old are particularly prone to a rapidly overwhelming sepsis, which is the most common cause of death in sickle cell patients in this age group.

Because of the rapid progression, bacteremia must be recognized and treated immediately and aggressively. Any toxic-appearing child or one with a temperature of 102°F (38.9°C) or more needs to have cultures taken immediately and antibiotics administered. The choice of antibiotic varies, but coverage for *S. pneumoniae* and *H. influenzae* is essential. Good initial choices include amoxicillin or a cephalosporin such as cefotaxime or cefuroxime.

In uninfected patients, antipneumococcal and *H. influenzae* vaccines have demonstrated some protective value. Penicillin prophylaxis is used as appropriate in children between the ages of 6 months and 5 years.

DISPOSITION AND FOLLOW-UP

Once the type of crisis has been diagnosed, the decision to admit or discharge the patient is usually straightforward.
1. Patients with splenic sequestration, neurologic crisis or infectious crisis require emergent treatment and admission to the intensive care unit (ICU).
2. A patient with aplastic crisis usually requires admission. If stable, such a patient can go to an unmonitored bed. If unstable, or if there is coexisting illness, the ICU is appropriate.
3. Patients with pulmonary problems require admission. If there is respiratory distress, multiple lobe involvement, or hypoxia, the patient is admitted to the ICU.
4. Patients with vaso-occlusive crisis who fail the analgesic management protocol outlined earlier require admission for pain management. This decision is made after 4 to 6 hours of observation.
5. If a patient with vaso-occlusive crisis is discharged home, certain preparations are made:
    a. Instructions about maintaining adequate oral hydration are given.
    b. A prescription is given for 2 to 3 days of adequate pain medication, usually following a protocol.
    c. The patient is instructed to return if fever of over 100.4°F (38°C), increased pain, vomiting, or changes in symptoms occur.
    d. Preferably, children are reevaluated in 12 to 24 hours and adults in 24 to 48 hours. A long-term relationship with a primary or consulting physician knowledgeable and interested in patients with sickle cell disease is strongly recommended for each patient.

PROBLEM The patient was admitted to the ICU with a working diagnosis of aplastic crisis and pneumococcal pneumonia. He was started on IV penicillin G for the pneumonia and folate for the aplastic crisis. A bone marrow biopsy was performed and showed active erythropoiesis. No transfusion was given.

This patient's disposition to the ICU was appropriate because he had aplastic anemia with a coexisting pneumonia and hypoxia. Most experts now agree that transfusion during aplastic crisis is guided by bone marrow biopsy. If the biopsy reveals the return of active erythropoiesis, no transfusions are necessary. They may even be harmful because the additional RBCs may slow erythropoietic recovery.

DOCUMENTATION

1. Characterization of the chief complaint—specifically, details about the pain.
2. Any precipitating features and associated symptoms.
3. Vital signs and findings on focused physical examination, particularly neurologic, chest, abdomen, and musculoskeletal signs.
4. Results of hemoglobin–hematocrit and other diagnostic adjuncts. Any significant changes from previous visits.
5. Patient's response to therapy in the emergency department.
6. Discharge instructions and follow-up arrangements.

PROBLEM The patient responded to the care given in the ICU and was transferred to the floor on the third day of hospitalization. He was discharged on day 10 with a hemoglobin of 7.1 gm/dl and a clearing chest x-ray.

This case could easily have ended in disaster. Happily for all, the physician who finally evaluated this patient was thorough and discovered two coexisting and potentially life-threatening disease processes. This case illustrates some important potential pitfalls in the care of these patients. *At every visit to the emergency department, the patient with sickle cell disease deserves a complete evaluation, during which the physician is always searching for more than one potential problem.*

SUMMARY AND FINAL POINTS

- Sickle cell crisis encompasses many different disease entities. A careful history and directed physical examination usually determine the type of crisis. Separating these types into three main categories—vaso-occlusive, hematologic, and infectious—assists the physician in making management decisions. Overlapping crises commonly occur.
- There are four true emergencies in sickle cell disease: splenic sequestration, sepsis, aplastic crisis, and neurologic crisis.
- Analgesia, hydration, and oxygenation continue to constitute the core of care in acute sickle cell crises.
- An established protocol for the administration of analgesia between the emergency physician and the patient lessens cheating by both parties and facilitates quality care.
- Complacency in the care of these patients will lead to diagnostic and therapeutic errors.

BIBLIOGRAPHY

Texts

1. Cline MJ: The hemoglobinopathies and thalassemias. In Stein J (ed): Internal Medicine. Boston, Little, Brown, 1983.
2. Huntsman RG: Sickle Cell Anemia and Thalassemia. Newfoundland, Canadian Sickle Cell Society, 1987.
3. Nagel RL: Pathophysiological Aspects of Sickle Cell Vaso-Occlusion. Vol. 24. Progress in Clinical and Biological Research. New York, Alan R. Liss, 1986.
4. Wintrobe MM: Hemoglobinopathies S, C, D, E, and O, and associated diseases. In Wintrobe MM (ed): Clinical Hematology. Philadelphia, Lea & Febiger, 1985.

Journal Articles

1. Bainbridge R, Higgs DR, Maude GH, et al: Clinical presentation of homozygous sickle cell disease. J Pediatr 106:881, 1985.
2. Barrett-Connor E: Pneumonia and pulmonary infarction in sickle cell anemia. JAMA 224:997, 1973.
3. Carache S, Lubin B, Reid CD (eds): Management and Therapy of Sickle Cell Disease. Washington DC, NIH Publication No. 85-2117, Sept. 1985.
4. Davie SC, Brozovic M: The presentation, management, and prophylaxis of sickle cell disease. Blood Rev 3:29-44, 1989.
5. Gaston MH: Sickle cell disease: An overview. Sem Roentgenol 22:150, 1987.
6. Galloway SI, Harwood-Nuss AL: Sickle cell anemia—a review. J Emerg Med 6:213-226, 1988.
7. Payne R: Pain management in sickle cell disease. Rationale and techniques. Ann NY Acad Sci 565:189-206, 1989.
8. Powers DR: Natural history of sickle cell disease: The first ten years. Sem Hematol 12:267, 1975.
9. Russell MO, Goldenberg HI, Reis L, et al: Transfusion therapy for cerebrovascular abnormalities in sickle cell disease. J Pediatr 88:382, 1976.

SECTION NINE

HORMONAL, METABOLIC, AND NUTRITIONAL DISORDERS

CHAPTER 26

METABOLIC COMPLICATIONS OF DIABETES MELLITUS

CARL M. FERRARO, M.D.
GARY R. STRANGE, M.D.

PROBLEM A rescue squad was called to the home of a 37 year old diabetic woman. Her husband stated that she had been vomiting and became increasingly sleepy through the day.

QUESTIONS TO CONSIDER

1. What metabolic abnormalities in diabetes mellitus may present with an altered level of consciousness?
2. What findings from the history and physical examination can be used to help differentiate the causes of an altered level of consciousness in a diabetic?
3. What rapid determinations must be made on presentation of the patient to guide immediate therapy?
4. What further laboratory determinations may be helpful?
5. How are patients with hypoglycemia, diabetic ketoacidosis, and hyperosmolar coma managed in the emergency department?

INTRODUCTION

Diabetes mellitus is a common disease affecting approximately 1% of the general population. Over 11 million Americans are diabetic. The underlying metabolic defect is a deficiency of insulin, either absolute or relative. In type 1 diabetes, often referred to as insulin-dependent, there is an absolute deficiency of insulin. Type 1 diabetes usually begins during childhood, and patients are prone to develop ketosis. It is felt that this type of diabetes results from autoimmune destruction of the insulin-producing pancreatic islet cells, thereby leading to a decreased synthesis of insulin. Type 2 diabetes, known as noninsulin-dependent or maturity-onset diabetes, is characterized by a relative lack of insulin and a resistance to ketosis. The actual level of circulating insulin may be normal or low, and defective insulin receptors lead to a relative ineffectiveness of the circulating insulin. Although there is no known cure for this disease, medications are available that can control the blood glucose level in an effort to prevent the neural, renal, and vascular complications of the disease.

Metabolic complications from diabetes are common and frequently present as an altered level of consciousness. Approximately 10% of all hospital admissions for diabetes will be for altered mentation. Hypoglycemic states, diabetic ketoacidosis, and hyperosmolar hyperglycemic nonketotic coma (HHNC) are the common causes of these mental changes.

Hypoglycemia is an extremely common problem and is considered in *all* patients who are in coma. For many diabetics, hypoglycemia is a frequent event. The blood glucose concentration can fall owing to an excess of insulin, a lack of substrate (glucose or glycogen), an overabundance of an oral hypoglycemic agent, or the action of other drugs. Ethanol predisposes to the development of hypoglycemia because of its inhibitory effect on glycogen storage and gluconeogenesis. Early signs and symptoms accompanying hypoglycemia result from sympathetic catecholamine release. They consist of tachycardia, diaphoresis, and anxiety. More subtle symptoms, such as hyperactivity, sleeplessness, or psychotic behavior, may be present in up to 25% of cases. Seizures occur in 10% of episodes. If the patient is on beta-adrenergic blocking agents, coma may develop without premonitory symptoms.

Diabetic ketoacidosis (DKA) is characterized by hyperglycemia, ketonemia, and acidemia. It results from hormonal imbalance involving both insulin lack and an excess of a group of counterregulatory hormones: glucagon, growth hormone, catecholamines, and cortisol. A complex interrelated metabolic cascade triggered by an insulin deficit occurs, leading to hyperglycemia, ketoacidosis, dehydration, and, if unchecked, to shock and ultimately death (Fig. 26–1).

Hyperosmolar coma occurs in the setting of a relative insulin lack in which hyperglycemia may exist without concomitant ketosis. The extreme hyperosmolality accompanying this condition often becomes manifest as neurologic deficits more commonly than DKA. Mortality is high and is often due to myocardial infarction or cerebrovascular accidents.

The initial diagnosis and management of the diabetic with an altered mental status in the emergency department is critical in determining the outcome. An early diagnosis with appropriate therapy can be lifesaving, whereas failure to differentiate the cause and initiate proper therapy may lead to significant morbidity or death.

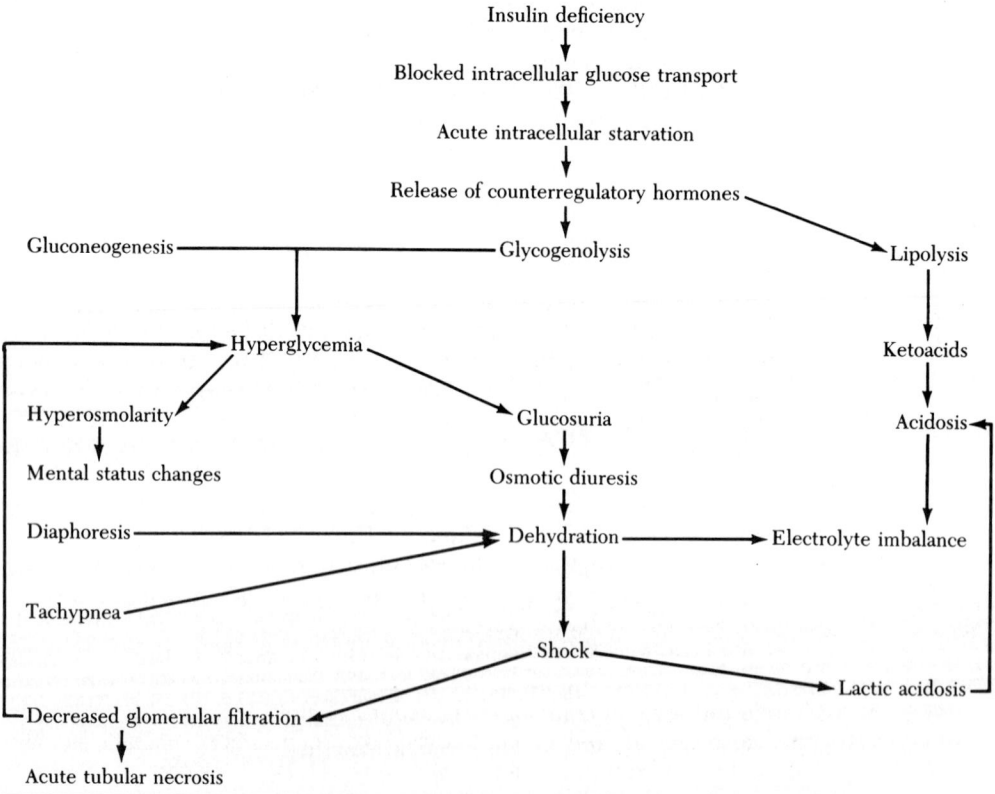

FIGURE 26–1. Pathophysiology of diabetic ketoacidosis.

PREHOSPITAL CARE

The information requested by the rescue squad is limited to that necessary to determine proper field management. The known diabetic is approached in the same manner as any patient presenting with an altered level of consciousness (see Chap. 45).

History

1. What are the patient's complaints?
2. How long has the patient been ill?
3. Were there any preceding illnesses?
4. Are there associated symptoms such as nausea, vomiting, or fever?
5. Is there a past history of diabetes, and what are the current medications? The squad should bring the medications in.

Physical Examination

1. What are the vital signs?
2. Is the airway patent, and is there adequate ventilation?
3. What is the level of consciousness?

Intervention

Airway. Patients in deep coma may require support of their airway and ventilation. Initially, ventilation is supported with a bag-valve-mask device and enriched oxygen supply. If there is no improvement in the ventilatory status after subsequent interventions, endotracheal intubation is indicated.

Oxygen. Supplemental oxygen is supplied by nasal cannula or mask to all patients.

Intravenous Access. An intravenous line is established, and isotonic crystalloid is begun.

Glucose Level. Blood is obtained for a rapid glucose determination using a glucose oxidase reagent strip. Optimally, a sample is saved for serum glucose measurement at the hospital.

If the glucose level is determined to be low, 50% dextrose in a dose of 1 to 2 ampules (25 to 50 gm) is administered. Many authorities recommend giving at least 1 ampule in any diabetic patient with altered mental status, as many rescue squads do not carry reagent strips and problems with accuracy have been reported.

If the glucose concentration is determined to be high (>250 mg/dl), the patient usually has concomitant significant dehydration. Isotonic crystalloid is administered at relatively rapid rates as long as the lungs are clear and there is no history of cardiac problems. An approximate rate of 500 ml/hr is appropriate during transport.

PROBLEM The rescue squad was met by a very anxious husband. The patient was responsive to verbal stimulation but gave no coherent answers to questions. The husband stated that his wife had not been feeling well for a week or more. Yesterday she complained of abdominal pain and began to vomit. These complaints continued through today. She was a lifelong diabetic and took daily NPH insulin in a dose of 25 units each morning. There were no other medications, nor were there medical complications from the diabetes. The patient's vital signs included a pulse rate of 120 beats/min, a respiratory rate of 36/min, and a blood pressure of 100/60 mm Hg. Respirations were deep, and there appeared to be adequate ventilation. The glucose reagent strip revealed a glucose level of 180 to 240 mg/dl. The squad was instructed to give the patient oxygen and start an intravenous line of normal saline at a rate of 500 ml/hr.

Glucose reagent strips are very useful for estimating the blood glucose concentration but cannot be relied on conclusively. In the field, where these strips are more likely to be exposed to excess heat and moisture, the possibility of an error is significant. Administration of 50 ml of 50% dextrose will result in an increase of 75 to 100 mg/dl in the serum glucose level. Even in the hyperglycemic patient, this is unlikely to cause additional problems. Therefore, some physicians will elect to administer dextrose empirically to all patients with a significantly altered level of consciousness. In this case, the rescue squad has decided against supplemental dextrose because the history and physical findings are also consistent with a diagnosis of hyperglycemia as the origin of this patient's problem.

INITIAL APPROACH IN THE EMERGENCY DEPARTMENT

The patient with a significantly altered level of consciousness will obviously require immediate evaluation by the emergency physician. Ambulatory diabetic patients who present with nonspecific complaints such as dizziness, fever, or vomiting may also have major metabolic disturbances that require prompt intervention. Triage personnel should be aware of the need to obtain rapid assessment for diabetic patients.

The following activities are indicated during the initial assessment:
1. The status of airway patency and protection as well as the adequacy of respirations is evaluated. Airway and ventilatory support are rarely needed in patients with complications of diabetes, but prompt identification of the need for intervention is essential.
2. Supplemental oxygen is provided to all patients with significant alteration in mental status.
3. The adequacy of circulation is evaluated. Hypotension requires immediate intervention with rapid administration of isotonic crystalloid. Existing intravenous lines are checked for patency, and new lines are placed as needed.
4. Blood specimens are obtained and prepared for the laboratory. A glucose oxidase reagent strip is checked. Even if the glucose level was determined in the field, a recheck is indicated.
5. Dextrose 50%, 1 to 2 ampules (25 to 50 gms), is administered intravenously. If the glucose oxidase reagent strip indicates hyperglycemia, dextrose may be held. However, administration of dextrose even to a patient in DKA is not likely to cause significant harm. On the other hand, withholding dextrose in a setting of hypoglycemia can cause substantial cerebral damage. Knowledge obtained from the glucose oxidase strip is preferred, but many physicians use dextrose for all patients presenting with altered level of consciousness.
6. A cardiac monitor is placed, and the rhythm is assessed. The height and configuration of the T wave is specifically noted because this observation will be useful in guiding initial electrolyte replacement if the patient proves to have DKA.
7. Naloxone, 2 mg, may be administered empirically to avoid missing an occult opioid intoxication.
8. Arterial blood gas measurements and venous blood determinations are ordered for patients who have not responded to the preceding interventions by an improvement in the level of consciousness. Serum electrolytes, blood urea nitrogen, creatinine, glucose, ketones, osmolality, and a complete blood count are important and are ordered early.
9. A urine sample is obtained, glucose and acetone concentrations are determined by dipstick, and a urinalysis is requested. In patients with significantly depressed mental status, minicatheterization is usually necessary. This procedure carries a slight risk of infection in diabetics, but it is offset by the need for information. The patient with DKA and HHNC will continue to produce large amounts of urine even during

moderate hypotension. Glucosuria and the subsequent osmotic diuresis will maintain urine production until shock leads to decreased glomerular filtration. In unstable, unconscious patients, an indwelling catheter is useful to monitor the patient's urinary output.
10. The initial level of consciousness is assessed and recorded in terms that are descriptive and understandable by subsequent care providers. The Glasgow Coma Scale, as described in Chapter 45, is a widely accepted system of grading the level of consciousness objectively.
11. A flow sheet is initiated for serial recording of vital signs, urine output, fluid intake, mental status, and biochemical parameters.
12. The results of certain diagnostic tests are generally available during the initial assessment phase and will guide the initial therapy of the patient.
    a. **Reagent Strip Blood Glucose Determination.** Commercially available reagent strips are based on the glucose oxidase reaction. The color change produced with varying levels of blood glucose can be discerned by the naked eye, but more accuracy can be obtained by observing it with a light meter. Because reagent strips are sensitive to light, heat, and moisture, great care must be exercised to ensure that they are properly stored and not left open to the environment.

    Accuracy of reagent strips is better in the hypoglycemic range than in the hyperglycemic range. This is not a problem because strips are used only to obtain a rough estimate of the blood glucose level, and laboratory determination of the exact blood glucose always follows the bedside estimate.

    b. **Urine Glucose and Acetone Concentrations.** Urine glucose and acetone levels are determined using Clinitest and Acetest tablets or Chemstrips bG. Glycosuria results when the kidney is presented with a large glucose load. The level of glucose in the urine cannot be directly correlated with the serum glucose concentration, but the presence of glycosuria is supportive evidence for hyperglycemia as measured by the reagent strip. Similarly, ketonuria is supportive evidence for the presence of ketonemia, and in the diabetic it suggests DKA.

    c. **Arterial Blood Gases.** Arterial blood gas (ABG) results, including the arterial pH, are usually available rapidly. A pH below 7.30 is suggestive of DKA. The P_{CO_2} is usually decreased and represents respiratory compensation (see Chapter 30).

    d. **Electrocardiogram.** In the presence of DKA, the serum potassium value will usually be normal to high, but it falls precipitously when treatment is started. To avoid hypokalemia, potassium supplementation is started as early as possible. The T wave of the electrocardiogram (ECG) is a fair gauge of the serum potassium level, and if the T waves are normal or small, early potassium supplementation is considered. In the presence of tall, peaked T waves, which are consistent with hyperkalemia, potassium is held until the level is known (see Chapter 28).

    The ECG may also be helpful in recognizing acute injury patterns that may be a precipitating factor in the development of DKA or the result of the metabolic stress. The ECG is also helpful in diagnosing silent myocardial infarction, which occurs more frequently in diabetics. In diabetic patients presenting with nonspecific complaints such as dizziness, shortness of breath, or weakness, an ECG should be ordered.

PROBLEM The patient was rapidly transported to the emergency department, where she was evaluated immediately. She remained responsive to verbal stimulation but was incoherent. Repeat vital signs were pulse 128 beats/min, respirations 36/min, and blood pressure 90/50 mm Hg. Oxygen was continued at 10 liters/min by mask. The falling blood pressure was of great concern, and an additional large-bore intravenous line was initiated. Both lines were allowed to run wide open. Blood was obtained for laboratory studies, and the blood glucose level was rechecked at the bedside. The reagent strip gave a reading of 180 to 240 mg/dl. Arterial blood gas results revealed a pH of 7.10, and urine obtained by catheterization revealed 4+ glucose and 2+ acetone.

Because the reagent strip reading was elevated, the physician decided against dextrose administration. Although administration of dextrose will not cause significant harm metabolically, there are potential problems with it due to the hypertonicity of the solution. If 50% dextrose is administered into the subcutaneous tissue by error, a large area of skin may slough. An intravenous line should be specifically checked for patency before 50% dextrose is administered through it. The rest of the treatment and rapid focus on the complications of diabetes are appropriate.

DATA GATHERING

History

A history is obtained from all available sources with emphasis on a few key points:

1. *Is the patient a known diabetic?*
   Knowing that a patient is diabetic is helpful, but lack of such knowledge does not preclude a complication of diabetes as the initial presentation of the disease.
2. *Has the patient experienced problems from hypoglycemia or hyperglycemia previously? How frequently?*
3. *What type and how much insulin does the patient usually take, or what type and dose of oral hypoglycemic agent is used? Has the patient altered the dose recently?*
   Hypoglycemia is not uncommon when a patient's dose of insulin or oral agent is increased. Also, when a patient takes the regular dose but fails to eat, hypoglycemia may follow. On the other hand, a reduction in doses of medication or increases in dietary intake may result in hyperglycemia.
4. *Has the patient's food intake been less than usual?*
5. *Is the patient taking a beta-adrenergic blocking agent?*
   The beta-adrenergic blocking agents mask the signs of sympathetic release that are the warning signs for the development of hypoglycemia. Patients taking these agents may therefore slip into coma without premonitory signs or symptoms.
6. *Does the patient take or have access to drugs that may cause alterations in level of consciousness?*
   Diabetics are frequently taking other medications that can result in alterations of level of consciousness. Sedative-hypnotics and tricyclic antidepressants are common agents that may be responsible for a diabetic's change in mental status.
7. *Has the patient been more active than usual?*
   Exercise increases glucose requirements.
8. *What are the events leading to the patient's presentation?*
   The classic triad of polyuria, polyphagia, and polydipsia strongly suggests hyperglycemia but is present in less than half of cases of DKA.
9. *What is the patient's usual mental status? Over what time course did changes develop?*
   Hypoglycemia may cause subtle forms of mental status change such as personality changes or lassitude. True coma may follow. Coma is common in hyperosmolar coma but occurs in only 10% of patients with DKA and does not correlate with the degree of metabolic disturbance. The altered level of consciousness due to hypoglycemia usually occurs abruptly, whereas hyperglycemic coma has a gradual onset.
10. *Has the patient had any gastrointestinal complaints?*
    Patients may complain of anorexia, nausea, vomiting, abdominal pain, or hunger

with either high or low blood glucose levels. In patients with DKA, abdominal pain secondary to the metabolic acidosis may be severe, leading the physician to suspect intra-abdominal problems such as pancreatitis or appendicitis. Gastroenteritis is a common misdiagnosis in early DKA as well.

11. *Has the patient been exposed to specific stresses?*

Any stress may lead to an alteration in insulin or glucose metabolism. Recent infections of the respiratory, genitourinary, or gastrointestinal tracts are frequently implicated. Recent trauma (accidental or surgical) may also be a cause.

12. *Does the patient have known complications of diabetes?*

These include neuropathy, retinopathy, nephropathy, and vascular disease.

Physical Examination

The physical examination can provide useful clues to the etiology and severity of a diabetic's altered mental status and can be used to assess the end-organ damage due to vascular changes resulting from diabetes.

General Appearance. Does the patient appear to be in shock, pale, or diaphoretic? Is the skin dry or lacking in turgor? In hypoglycemia, sympathetic release may result in pallor and diaphoresis. DKA and hyperosmolar coma are both associated with significant dehydration, which can progress to hypovolemic shock.

Vital Signs. What are the pulse rate, respiratory rate, blood pressure, and temperature levels? Tachycardia is a manifestation of stress and is present in all forms of diabetes-related coma. Tachypnea is present in patients with DKA as a compensatory mechanism for the metabolic acidosis. Rapid, deep, sighing respirations, termed Kussmaul respirations, are very suggestive of the presence of DKA, and the fruity odor of ketones may also be noted. Hyperventilation may also be caused by respiratory infection and by some toxic ingestions such as salicylates. Hypoventilation may be present with severe hypoglycemia.

Blood pressure is often elevated owing to stress early in all forms of diabetic coma. As the dehydration of DKA and HHNC progresses, however, hypotension and shock may ensue.

Elevated temperature is uncommon in the setting of DKA, even in the presence of serious infection. Infection is a common predisposing factor for HHNC, and associated elevated temperature will require a thorough search for a focus of infection. Hypoglycemia is not commonly associated with temperature changes.

Level of Consciousness. Is the patient alert? Does he respond to verbal or painful stimuli? Are responses appropriate? The Glasgow Coma Scale (Chap. 45) is an excellent means of quantitating and following the patient's mental status.

Head, Eyes, Ears, Nose, Throat. Are there signs of head trauma? As with any patient, head injury may be responsible for the change in mental status, and external signs may be subtle. Falls due to "dizziness" from metabolic disturbances may lead to combined metabolic and traumatic abnormalities.

Is any evidence of infection found? Infection is a common predisposing condition for the development of DKA. Some rare ear, nose, and throat infections occur almost exclusively in poorly controlled diabetics. Malignant otitis externa is a rapidly progressive, life-threatening condition that requires early diagnosis and aggressive therapy. Does the patient have a stiff, rigid neck? Meningitis must be considered in any patient with an altered level of consciousness.

Do the fundi show diabetic changes? The retinal vessels are an externally visible reflection of the degree of end-organ damage due to diabetes. The most common changes seen are increased width and tortuosity of vessels, microaneurysms, hemorrhages, and exudates. Diabetic retinopathy may be graded based on these observations to correlate with the severity of end-organ damage throughout the body.

Cardiovascular Signs. Is there adequate perfusion? Both DKA and HHNC are associated with severe dehydration that can progress to shock. Is there evidence of a primary cardiac problem? DKA may result from the stress of acute myocardial infarction in a diabetic, and either hypoglycemia or hyperglycemia can result in myocardial infarction. Signs of congestive heart failure are sometimes seen in HHNC patients; such patients require close monitoring during fluid replacement.

Pulmonary Signs. Is there adequate air exchange? Is there evidence of consolidation or infiltration? Pulmonary infection may be a predisposing condition for the development of DKA or HHNC. Hypoglycemia is not uncommonly associated with aspiration.

Abdomen. Is the abdomen distended? Distention from ileus or obstruction may be present. Are bowel sounds present? Electrolyte disturbances, especially hypokalemia, may result in diminished bowel sounds. Are peritoneal signs present? Patients with DKA may have abdominal pain, but careful examination should reveal an absence of peritoneal signs such as guarding and rebound. Is there rectal tenderness or blood? Gastrointestinal bleeding can occur in conjunction with hyperglycemic states.

Extremities. Is capillary refill adequate? Is skin turgor good? Poor peripheral perfusion and turgor are indicators of severe dehydration.

Neurologic Signs. Are there any focal deficits or lateralizing signs indicating an intracranial event? Cerebrovascular accidents occur with increased frequency in diabetic patients and may be solely responsible for a change in mental status.

PROBLEM The initial information supplied by the patient's husband was all that was readily obtainable. He had been married for only a short time and had no knowledge of previous similar episodes. Physical examination revealed a young woman without external evidence of trauma who was responsive to verbal stimulation with incoherent mumbling. Her skin was pale and dry. The oral mucosa was dry and cracked, and there was a strong fruity odor on the breath. Cardiac and lung examination revealed no abnormalities. The abdomen was soft and nontender. There were no focal neurologic findings.

DECISION PRIORITIES AND PRELIMINARY DIFFERENTIAL DIAGNOSIS

After completion of the history and physical examination two questions are addressed:

1. *Do the history and physical examination suggest a cause of altered level of consciousness unrelated to diabetes?*

   Common causes of coma that may occur in any patient, including diabetics, are head trauma, drug ingestion, meningitis, and cerebrovascular accidents. The diagnosis and initial management of these problems are discussed in Chapter 45.

2. *Is the altered mental status due to a metabolic derangement caused by diabetes? If so, what specific metabolic derangement is present?*

   Altered level of consciousness from diabetes is differentiated as depicted in Figure 26–2.

   Early in the approach to the patient, the glucose concentration is measured at the bedside by reagent strip testing. If the blood sugar level is low, hypoglycemia is diagnosed. If it is high, a hyperglycemic problem exists. The next step is to determine the acid-base status of the patient by assessing the arterial blood gas values. A normal blood pH in the presence of significant hyperglycemia indicates HHNC. A low blood pH indicates metabolic acidemia. The nitroprusside test is then used to assess the presence of serum ketones. If ketones are present in a dilution of 1:2 or greater, DKA is diagnosed. A commonly used working definition appropriate for most patients with DKA is:

   a. Blood glucose level in excess of 300 mg/dl.
   b. Ketonemia with serum ketones present in a dilution of 1:2 or greater.
   c. Acidemia with a blood pH of less than 7.30 or a serum bicarbonate concentration of less than 15 mEq/liter.

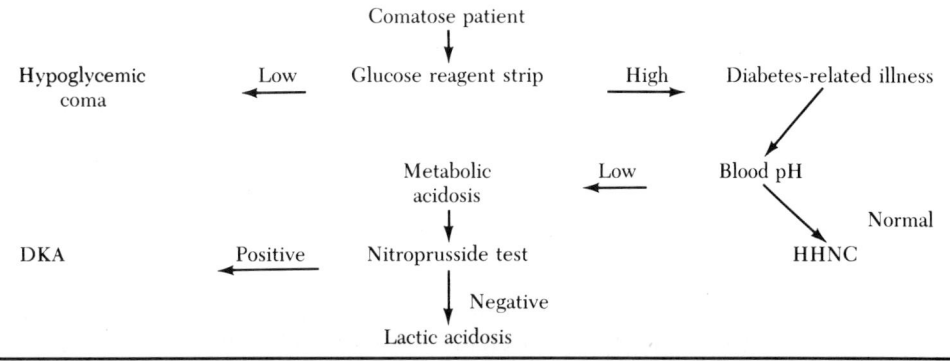

FIGURE 26-2. *Decision tree for diabetic coma.*

PROBLEM The history and physical examination revealed no evidence of nondiabetes-related problems. The blood glucose value was high, the patient was dehydrated, and ketones were noted to be present.

The history and physical examination failed to suggest causes of coma unrelated to diabetes, and the bedside glucose screening test revealed a modest elevation of the blood glucose level. The findings of hyperventilation, dehydration, and fruity odor of the breath were very suggestive of DKA. Arterial blood gas measurements will confirm the suspicion of acidosis, and a rapid check of the urine for glucose and acetone provided further support to this preliminary diagnosis.

DIAGNOSTIC ADJUNCTS

Laboratory Studies

Laboratory diagnostic tests that are useful in evaluating diabetes-related coma are numerous. They can be grouped into two categories: those for which results are immediately available and those for which results are often delayed for 60 minutes or more. All tests are ordered immediately, but results become available at different times.

The tests for which results are available immediately and are therefore used to guide initial therapy are the reagent strip blood glucose concentration, urine glucose and acetone levels, arterial blood gases, and electrocardiogram. The use of these tests was discussed in the section Initial Approach in the Emergency Department, above. From these tests, insight is gained into the degree of hypoxemia, acidemia, and osmolality that is present. Initial therapy is started on the basis of these test results while awaiting the following test results, which may modify the treatment course:

Complete Blood Count and Differential. Even in the absence of infection, the white blood cell count is usually 15,000 to 20,000/mm^3 in patients with DKA. The white blood cell count correlates more closely with the severity of DKA than the presence of sepsis. A left shift of the differential cell count is suggestive of an infectious process. The hemoglobin and hematocrit values are elevated if there is significant dehydration.

Serum Electrolytes. Sodium deficit in DKA is approximately 6 mEq/kg. In addition, the measured sodium level may be spuriously lowered by hyperglycemia. To obtain a true value, 1.6 mEq/L is added to the measured value for every 100 mg/dl of blood glucose over 100 mg/dl. Therefore, a highly elevated glucose concentration with a normal sodium level may represent a hypernatremic condition.

The potassium deficit averages 5 mEq/kg in patients with DKA. The initial level is usually normal to high owing to the extracellular shift that occurs as a compensatory mechanism for acidosis. With fluid and insulin administration, the level falls precipitously.

To anticipate the amount of change, one should estimate that for every 0.1 change in pH, there is a 0.6 mEq/liter change in potassium in the opposite direction.

Chloride loss in patients with DKA averages 4 mEq/kg. Replacement is easily accomplished with isotonic saline. In fact, over-replacement is common, leading to hyperchloremic acidosis.

Renal Function Tests. Blood urea nitrogen is elevated above the usual 10:1 ratio with creatinine owing to dehydration. The serum creatinine level may be spuriously elevated owing to interference in testing by ketonemia.

Blood Glucose and Acetone Levels. Blood glucose determination is essential to confirm the results of urine and blood reagent strip estimates. Serum acetone and acetoacetate are measured by means of the nitroprusside reaction, which causes a color change when acetoacetate is present in the specimen. Acetoacetate usually exists in a 1:3 ratio with beta-hydroxybutyrate. The equilibrium is shifted toward beta-hydroxybutyrate in the presence of severe acidosis. Because beta-hydroxybutyrate is not measured by the nitroprusside reaction, measured ketones may be spuriously low or absent in patients with severe DKA and may actually "appear and increase" as treatment takes effect.

Serum Osmolality. Serum osmolality is measured and followed during therapy of patients with DKA and HHNC to prevent a rapid decrease, which may be responsible for the development of cerebral edema. If measurements are unavailable, serum osmolality may be calculated as follows:

$$\text{Serum osmolality} = 2(\text{Na}) + \frac{\text{glucose}}{18} + \frac{\text{BUN}}{3}$$

The normal range is 285 to 295 mOsm/liter. Significant hyperosmolarity exists at levels greater than 320 mOsm/liter.

Urinalysis. Urinalysis may reveal glycosuria and ketonuria. Proteinuria and hyaline casts may also be present owing to dehydration. White blood cells and bacteria may be present indicating urinary infection, which is common in diabetics and may be a predisposing factor in the development of DKA.

Other Tests. Serum magnesium and phosphorus levels may be followed in patients with DKA. Changes in these cations parallel those for potassium. Serum calcium levels are followed if phosphate is administered because hypocalcemia can result in this situation. Cultures of urine, blood, and cerebrospinal fluid may be indicated based on historical, physical examination, or laboratory evidence of infection.

Radiologic Imaging

Chest radiographs are used in the search for a common source of infection in patients with DKA or HHNC. If the patient has been unconscious, the possibility of aspiration is assessed. *Computed tomography* of the head is considered if the altered mental status is possibly due to a CNS disorder.

PROBLEM Test results that were immediately available revealed estimates of a bedside glucose concentration at 180 to 240 mg/dl, urine glucose of 4+, urine ketones of 2+, arterial pH of 7.10, and a normal electrocardiogram with no T-wave abnormalities.

During the next 30 minutes to 1 hour, additional test results became available. They showed a blood glucose level of 540 mg/dl, serum ketones present in a 1:8 dilution, and serum electrolytes measured as follows: sodium 140 mEq/liter, potassium 4.0 mEq/liter, and chloride 100 mEq/liter. BUN was 30 mg/dl and creatinine 1.8 mg/dl.

Treatment should proceed based on the immediately available test results. Even when laboratory results are rapidly available, the delay is too great to allow initial therapy to be postponed pending their arrival.

Interpreting the laboratory test results provides the following information.

1. For every 100 mg/dl above 100 mg/dl of glucose, the serum sodium level falls 1.6 mEq/liter owing to osmotic dilution. At 500 mg/dl, the serum sodium concentration should be $140 - (1.6 \times 4) = 133.6$ mEq/liter. In this patient it is 140 mEq/liter, and therefore she is in a hyperosmolar condition. This can be confirmed by substituting in the osmolality equation (see earlier section Diagnostic Adjuncts—Serum Osmolality)

$$2(140) \text{ mEq/liter} + \frac{540}{18} + \frac{30}{3} = 329 \text{ mOsm/liter}$$

This is significant hyperosmolality.

2. It may be useful to estimate what the potassium level would be if the pH were normal. To correct the pH to 7.4, the present 7.1 value needs to have 0.3 pH units added to it. Because potassium moves 0.6 mEq/liter in the opposite direction for each 0.1 change in the pH, the serum potassium would decrease $3 \times -0.6 = -1.8$ mEq/liter. Therefore, the present serum potassium of 4.0 mEq/liter would fall to 2.2 mEq/liter if the pH were corrected without supplemental potassium. This is a dangerously low level and can be avoided by the addition of a potassium supplement.

PRINCIPLES OF MANAGEMENT

There are several aspects of management to be considered for each diabetic state. Although the following principles may not apply in every situation, each is included when formulating a plan for the emergency department care of the diabetic with hypoglycemia, DKA, or HHNC. The principles are:

1. Restoration of circulating volume.
2. Normalization of blood glucose.
3. Clearance of ketones.
4. Correction of acidemia or acidosis.
5. Correction to and maintenance of normal serum electrolyte concentrations.
6. Gradual restoration of the equilibrium of the serum osmolality.
7. Close clinical and laboratory monitoring.

Hypoglycemia

Patients who are hypoglycemic are usually not hemodynamically unstable and have an adequate intravascular volume. In the awake patient who is not at risk for aspiration, orally administered glucose is sufficient to reverse hypoglycemia. The initial dose should be followed by a meal containing some protein to ensure that continued glucose metabolism will occur.

If the patient is unable to ingest oral glucose, administration of intravenous dextrose is necessary. If intravenous access cannot be obtained, intramuscular injection of glucagon can stimulate gluconeogenesis provided the patient's liver glycogen stores are not depleted.

In hypoglycemia there are no significant ketones to clear, and rarely are there electrolyte abnormalities. The patient's clinical response must be monitored to ensure resolution of lethargy or coma and maintenance of an alert state. A repeat blood glucose measurement is obtained to verify adequate glucose levels.

Diabetic Ketoacidosis

Restoration of Circulating Volume. Fluid administration is the most important component of therapy. Intravenous fluids not only restore circulating volume but also help to lower the blood glucose level and clear free fatty acids. The adult patient in diabetic ketoacidosis has an average fluid deficit of 6 liters. If the patient is hemodynamically unstable, 2 liters of isotonic crystalloid are given at a rapid rate while monitoring the patient's response. In the patient whose blood pressure does not respond adequately or whose clinical condition worsens after fluid administration, invasive hemodynamic monitoring is indicated. In the stable patient in diabetic ketoacidosis, fluid is given as 1 liter of normal saline during the first 30 minutes. The second liter is given over 1 to 2 hours. At this point, fluids are changed to one-half normal saline and are given at a rate that ensures adequate urine output, typically 300 to 500 ml/hr.

Normalization of Blood Glucose Concentration. The administration of normal saline alone may account for a 15% to 20% decrease in blood glucose in the first hour. The goal of therapy is to reduce blood glucose by 100 mg/dl/hr. Insulin administration is not always necessary during this first hour of fluid therapy and may lower blood glucose too rapidly, predisposing the patient to cerebral edema and hypoglycemia. The recommended method of insulin administration and the amount given vary. Most often an insulin-loading dose of 0.1 unit/kg is given by intravenous push during the first hour of fluid administration. It is followed by a continuous infusion of 0.1 unit/kg/hr. When a blood glucose level of 250 to 300 mg/dl is attained, the insulin infusion is reduced to 0.05 mg/dl/hr, and dextrose is added to the fluids. The insulin infusion is continued until acidosis and ketonemia are resolved. Correction of serum glucose to a normal range is usually completed outside of the emergency department.

Clearance of Ketones. Fluid administration aids in the clearance of free fatty acids, the precursors of ketone bodies. The administration of insulin is important to halt intracellular starvation and leads to a decrease in the counterregulatory hormones and cessation of lipolysis and ketogenesis. Fluids and insulin are usually sufficient to effect clearance of ketones.

Correction of Acidemia. Bicarbonate therapy for acidemia is controversial and may be associated with the development of cerebral edema, alkalosis, and paradoxical cerebrospinal fluid acidosis. Its use is limited to patients in a severely acidemic state (pH less than 7.0 or bicarbonate concentration of less than 10) and it is given slowly as an infusion (1 to 2 mEq/kg over 2 hours).

Maintenance of Normal Serum Electrolytes. Administration of potassium should proceed in the patient who has urinary output and in whom there is no electrocardiographic evidence of hyperkalemia (peaked T waves). Potassium, 20 to 40 mEq, may be added to the second liter of fluid. One regimen is to give it half as potassium chloride and half as K_3PO_4. Except in patients with extreme hypokalemia, it is administered at a rate not to exceed 10 mEq/hr. Further potassium therapy is guided by serum levels obtained hourly.

Replacement of magnesium in the patient who is hypomagnesemic may be accomplished by adding 4 gm of magnesium to each liter of fluid after the initial rapid infusions are completed.

Close Clinical and Laboratory Monitoring. Hourly laboratory values are obtained in a patient with diabetic ketoacidosis until improvement is noted. These include (1) glucose, (2) electrolytes, (3) osmolality, and (4) arterial blood gases.

A flow sheet will aid in organizing the data and allow for easy recognition of trends. Vital signs obtained frequently and assessment of the patient's sensorium and handling of fluid load are invaluable in assessing response to therapy. A discrepancy between the laboratory data and an unchanging clinical status of the patient mandates a search for additional problems, e.g., sepsis, meningitis, ingestion, head trauma.

Hyperosmolar Hyperglycemic Nonketotic Coma

Restoration of Circulating Volume. Normal saline is administered until hemodynamic stability is achieved. Fluids are then changed to one-half normal saline. Because of large fluid shifts and the frequency of associated disease, hemodynamic monitoring is frequently required.

Normalization of Blood Glucose Level. Again the goal of therapy is to lower blood glucose by 100 mg/dl/hr. In patients in HHNC fluid administration can lower the blood glucose level by 25% to 30% during the first hour. Because there is a relative insulin lack, patients in HHNC may be sensitive to insulin administration, and therefore an insulin dose of 0.02 to 0.05 units/kg/hr given by infusion is begun initially. This is especially true when the blood glucose concentration is more than 1000 mg/dl.

Clearance of Ketones and Correction of Acidemia or Acidosis. These patients are not ketotic (or are only mildly so) by definition.

Maintenance of Serum Electrolytes. As in patients with DKA, dehydration and fluid shifts will result in electrolyte imbalances. Potassium is administered as soon as urine flow is established, and true hyperkalemia is ruled out.

Close Clinical and Laboratory Monitoring. A flow sheet is used to follow hourly observations of

- Glucose level
- Electrolytes
- Osmolality
- Mental status
- Vital signs
- Urine output

The high association between HHNC and other serious illnesses may make additional specific management necessary and may require modification of the treatment regimen outlined.

PROBLEM Because of the patient's fall in blood pressure, 2 liters of normal saline were administered during the first 30 minutes in the emergency department. Blood pressure promptly responded to 110/60 mm Hg. Normal saline was continued, the third liter being given during the next hour. The patient had a normal ECG (normal T waves) and was producing copious urine. Potassium chloride 20 mEq and K_3PO_4 20 mEq were added to the third liter of normal saline.

Insulin was started through a second IV line after the first liter of fluid had been given. This 50-kg woman was given a loading dose of 5 units of regular insulin and was started on an infusion at 5 units/hr. After one hour of insulin therapy and 1 1/2 hours of fluid therapy, the blood glucose was 400 mEq/dl, pH 7.12, potassium 3.5 mEq/liter, and bicarbonate 14 mEq/liter.

Slow resolution of the metabolic derangement is preferable. A general guide for the desired change in blood glucose concentration is a decrease of 10% per hour of therapy. Rapid falls predispose the patient to development of hypoglycemia, electrolyte disturbances, and cerebral edema. The potassium level in this patient, which was initially normal, became low normal with therapy in spite of potassium supplementation. This change was anticipated by earlier calculations. Early potassium replacement is essential to prevent hypokalemia because the level will fall with therapy.

SPECIAL CONSIDERATIONS

Pediatrics

Metabolic complications of diabetes mellitus are not uncommon in children. Hypoglycemia is extremely common in critically ill children, and screening or empiric treatment with dextrose is indicated in all neonates and infants who present with critical illness or altered mental status. The lack of significant glycogen reserves leads to hypoglycemia in the presence of a wide variety of stresses.

Ninety-seven percent of children with diabetes have type 1 disease and are therefore ketosis prone. An episode of diabetic ketoacidosis is the initial presentation of this disease in approximately 10% of cases. The diagnosis of DKA in children is achieved in essentially the same fashion as for adults but the management varies considerably. Rapid shifts in osmolality lead to the complication of cerebral edema more frequently in children than in adults, and many children will die when cerebral edema develops. Therefore, every effort is made during treatment to bring the serum glucose level down gradually in an effort to prevent this dreaded complication.

Fluid resuscitation is begun with normal saline given at a rate of 20 ml/kg over the first hour (more rapidly if there are signs of shock). Insulin is administered as a continuous infusion at a rate of 0.1 unit/kg/hour. No loading dose is recommended in order to provide a more gradual, linear decline in the serum glucose level.

Geriatrics

Maturity-onset (type 2) diabetes mellitus is extremely common in the geriatric population. These patients are frequently adequately treated with proper diet and an oral hypoglycemic agent. DKA is rare in this population but HHNC is not uncommonly seen.

Geriatric diabetic patients are likely to have a host of vascular complications of this disease. Proper evaluation and management require a high index of suspicion of peripheral vascular disease, renal failure, coronary artery disease, and cerebrovascular accidents.

DISPOSITION AND FOLLOW-UP

Hypoglycemia

Patients Requiring Admission. The patient who fails to respond to initial therapy, who has an inadequate oral intake, or who relapses into a hypoglycemic state is admitted. The patient who has taken a long-acting hypoglycemic agent (long-acting insulin or one of the oral agents) is admitted.

Patients Requiring Intensive Care Unit (ICU) Admission. Patients with profound hypoglycemia unresponsive to therapy, usually in the setting of a massive overdose with a hypoglycemic agent, require intensive care.

Patients Who Can Be Discharged. After the patient's blood glucose level is normalized, the hypoglycemic patient must be fully awake and alert before discharge is considered. If the cause of the patient's reaction is not clear, admitting the patient to investigate possible causes is recommended.

Hyperglycemia (DKA and HHNC)

Patients Requiring Admission. If a patient cannot tolerate oral fluids (i.e., has continuous vomiting) or has moderate to severe diabetic ketoacidosis or HHNC, admission is arranged. If the patient cannot monitor blood glucose closely at home or cannot administer the appropriate insulin dose, in-hospital therapy and education are advised.

Patients Requiring ICU Admission. Although all patients admitted for DKA or HHNC are considered for ICU admission, some guidelines that mandate intensive care are:
1. Age less than 2 or greater than 60 years
2. pH less than 7.0
3. Serious concurrent illness

If a separate metabolic unit is not available in the hospital, all patients with moderate to severe DKA or HHNC should be monitored in the ICU for the first 24 hours.

Patients Who Can Be Discharged. An alert patient with mild symptoms, mild ketoacidosis without vomiting, reasonable intelligence, and accessibility to the hosptial may be treated as an outpatient. If vomiting persists despite initial therapy, the patient is admitted.

PROBLEM Although this patient's metabolic disturbance was not too great, her initial cardiovascular instability and her mental status made intensive care unit admission advisable. The clinical findings, including mental status, did not correlate with the degree of metabolic disturbance found. Disposition decisions should take both of these aspects into consideration.

DOCUMENTATION

1. Vital signs.
2. Current therapy. The patient's current drug regimen, current diet, and recent activity are recorded.
3. Level of consciousness.
4. Hydration status.
5. Initial blood glucose level, electrolyte measurements, and acid-base status.
6. Response to initial therapy.
7. Repeat vital signs, mental status check, and biochemical parameters for patients with DKA or HHNC. These data are best recorded on a flow sheet.

SUMMARY AND FINAL POINTS

- Patients with derangements in glucose metabolism most frequently present to the emergency department with a depressed level of consciousness.
- Rapid determination of blood glucose level is essential in the initial approach to all patients with an altered level of consciousness.
- Administration of dextrose may be used empirically because it will do no harm even in the hyperglycemic patient.
- In hypoglycemic patients an adequate blood glucose level must be ensured before disposition is decided on. Long-acting agents may result in recurrent episodes of coma.
- In hyperglycemic states, adequate fluid and insulin administration with careful monitoring of acid-base status and electrolytes are the *mainstays* of therapy.
- The dehydrated patient who is still voiding has DKA until proved otherwise.
- A discrepancy between the laboratory findings and clinical status should lead the emergency physician to consider other complications.

BIBLIOGRAPHY

Texts

1. Becker DJ, Drash AL: Diabetic ketoacidosis. In Dickerman JD, Lucey JF: Smith's The Critically Ill Child (3rd ed). Philadelphia, Saunders, 1985.
2. Brownlee M: Handbook of Diabetes Mellitus (Vol 5). New York, Garland Press, 1981.
3. Marks V, Rose FC: Hypoglycemia (2nd ed). Oxford, Blackwell, 1981.

Journal Articles

1. Casparie AF, Elving LD: Severe hypoglycemia in diabetic patients. Diabetes Care 8:141–145, 1985.
2. Cheeley RD, Joyce SM: Clinical comparison of the performance of four blood glucose reagent strips. Am J Emerg Med 8(1):11–15, 1990.
3. Collier H, Steedman DJ, Patrick AW, et al: Comparison of intravenous glucagon and dextrose in treatment of severe hypoglycemia in an accident and emergency department. Diabetes Care 10(6):712–715, 1987.
4. Foster DW, McGarry JD: Metabolic derangements and treatment of diabetic ketoacidosis. N Engl J Med 309(3):159–169, 1983.
5. Gerich JE: Glucose counterregulation and its impact on diabetes mellitus. Diabetes 37:1608–1617, 1988.
6. Kitabchi AE, Matler R, Murphy MB: Optimal insulin delivery in DKA and HHNC. Diabetes Care 8:141–145, 1985.
7. Lindsay R, Bolte RG: Use of an insulin bolus in low-dose insulin infusion for pediatric diabetic ketoacidosis. Pediatr Emerg Care 5(2):77–79, 1989.
8. Morris LR, Murphy MB, Kitabchi AE: Bicarbonate therapy in severe diabetic ketoacidosis. Ann Intern Med 105:836–840, 1986.
9. Slovis CM, Mork VGC, Slovis RJ, et al: Diabetic ketoacidosis and infection. Am J Emerg Med 2(1):1–5, 1987.
10. Sperling MA: Diabetic ketoacidosis. Pediat Clin North Am 31:591–610, 1984.

CHAPTER 27

HYPONATREMIA

GARY R. STRANGE, M.D.

PROBLEM A 69 year old female was brought by ambulance to the emergency department after having a seizure at home. She had no previous history of seizures but had not been feeling well for the past 2 to 3 days and had been sleeping excessively. Her family stated that she had had nausea and vomiting, and her diet had been limited to clear liquids. She was taking hydrochlorothiazide for hypertension.

In the emergency department she had a second generalized seizure and then remained unconscious. Vital signs were blood pressure 102/60 mm Hg, pulse 110 beats/min, respirations 18/min, temperature 99°F (37.2°C). A complete physical examination revealed no significant findings except for dry mucous membranes and dry skin with poor turgor.

Laboratory tests were ordered. The serum electrolyte values were sodium 115 mEq/liter, potassium 2.8 mEq/liter, chloride 95 mEq/liter, and bicarbonate 18 mEq/liter.

QUESTIONS TO CONSIDER

1. What are the causes of hyponatremia?
2. At what serum sodium level may signs and symptoms of hyponatremia appear?
3. Which patients are at risk for developing hyponatremia?
4. How can the clinical volume status of the patient be used to classify the causes of hyponatremia?
5. What treatment is given a patient with symptoms related to a low serum sodium concentration?

INTRODUCTION

The serum sodium concentration is determined by the ratio of sodium to water within the body. In patients with hyponatremia, there is excess water relative to the total body sodium level. The total body sodium level can be normal, high, or low regardless of the serum level measured. The amount of sodium and water is usually represented clinically by the volume status of the patient, i.e., low total body sodium indicated by volume depletion and high total body sodium seen as volume overload. Using the volume status of the patient to estimate the total body sodium concentration is an important concept in the assessment of hyponatremia. Most patients with hyponatremia seen in the emergency department will be relatively volume depleted.

The major regulator of total body sodium and water balance is the kidney. A small amount of sodium is also excreted in sweat and feces. The amount of sodium filtered by the kidneys is determined by the plasma volume as sensed by the arteriolar baroreceptors. The renin-angiotensin-aldosterone sequence and antidiuretic hormone (ADH) secretion are additional mechanisms of renal control of sodium and water balance. Hyponatremia is most often caused by disorders of renal diluting ability. Most are associated with secretion of ADH despite hyposmolality of the serum, impaired reabsorption of chloride in the ascending loop of Henle, or factors that decrease the amount of fluid available to the distal diluting segments of the nephron, e.g., a decrease in glomerular filtration rate (GFR).

Excess water in relation to sodium results in dilution of the extracellular fluid and hyposmolality of the blood. The central nervous system (CNS) is affected by this condition because the osmotic gradient in the CNS favors accumulation of intracellular water. Cerebral edema is the basis for many of the clinical manifestations of hyponatremia.

The normal range of serum sodium concentration is between 135 and 145 mEq/liter. The symptoms produced by sodium levels that are significantly outside this range are highly dependent on the rate of change to that level. Most symptomatic patients seen in the emergency department have serum sodium levels of less than 125 mEq/liter. Hyponatremia is a challenging problem because its presentation is nonspecific, and the causes are diverse. It is a laboratory finding that requires a search for its cause. Although it is not always necessary or possible for the emergency physician to identify the specific cause, identifying the metabolic abnormality and initiating therapy are important to prevent further deterioration.

INITIAL APPROACH IN THE EMERGENCY DEPARTMENT

The initial approach varies with the patient's presentation. Many patients present early in the evolution of hyponatremia with nonspecific complaints or concerns specific to an organ system, e.g., congestive heart failure. In these patients, the history, physical examination, and laboratory evaluation are performed in the traditional sequence. Other patients, who may have delayed seeking care or who have experienced a precipitous fall in sodium level, require therapy concomitant with diagnosis. Most symptomatic patients present with hemodynamic instability due to a volume deficit, altered mental status, or seizure activity.

Volume Deficit

Regardless of the cause, the patient with hyponatremia and signs of volume depletion will benefit from fluid replacement with normal saline. Restoration toward normal body volume can begin before the serum values are known. Even some patients who appear euvolemic but have histories suggestive of volume loss will benefit from early conservative fluid replacement. Hemodynamic monitoring is considered in elderly and cardiac patients to avoid fluid overload.

Altered Mental Status

Patients with depressed level of consciousness will first receive naloxone 2 mg intravenously, measurement of serum glucose by means of glucose oxidase test strip followed by 25 to 50 ml of 50% dextrose as necessary, thiamine 100 mg intravenously as appropriate, and oxygen supplementation. The possible causes of altered mental status are assessed as described in Chapter 45. Serum sodium levels are measured in all of these patients unless a very obvious explanation is available.

Seizures

Seizure activity is evaluated and treated as described in Chapter 48. In most patients with seizure activity, particularly very young children, suspected or known alcoholics, patients taking diuretics, patients with psychiatric histories, and the elderly, the serum sodium level is measured. Exceptions may occur when an obvious explanation for the seizure exists.

PROBLEM (*Note:* Evaluative or management errors exist in this case as a means of reinforcing specific points.) The patient was clinically dehydrated, relatively hypotensive, and tachycardic. Her recurrent seizures and progressive loss of responsiveness indicated central nervous system pathology. Efforts to stabilize her condition included administration of dextrose, thiamine, naloxone, and later phenytoin. No intervention was made initially to treat her volume deficit.

It is easy to focus on the more dramatic elements of a patient's presentation, e.g., seizures. The stabilization effort in this case was appropriate, although the underlying volume deficit and hyponatremia should have been treated simultaneously by giving normal saline.

DATA GATHERING

Most patients with hyponatremia are asymptomatic. Because this condition is usually not suspected, the initial history and physical examination are guided by the presenting complaint, not by suspicion of this biochemical abnormality. Once hyponatremia is diagnosed, data gathering has two goals: (1) To determine the presence of symptoms due to hyponatremia, and (2) to assess the volume status of the patient. Most of these symptoms occur in the gastrointestinal tract and central nervous system. The serum sodium level and the symptoms have a crude relationship that is highly dependent on the rate of change of the serum sodium level (Table 27–1). Categorizing the patient by volume status can greatly narrow the diagnostic possibilities.

Patients with renal disease, those on diuretics, and psychiatric patients constitute the three groups of patients at highest risk of hyponatremia. Young children and the elderly are most likely to have symptoms.

History

Gastrointestinal Symptoms. Gastrointestinal symptoms occur early in the development of hyponatremia but are often overlooked or attributed to other causes.
1. Has the patient noticed a decreased *sense of flavor* or *taste*?
2. Has there been *anorexia, nausea,* or *vomiting*?
3. Has the patient noticed *excessive thirst*?
4. Has there been *abdominal cramping*?

Neurologic Symptoms. Neurologic symptoms do not correlate well with the degree of hyponatremia and are dependent on the rate of decline in the sodium level. With a gradual decrease, signs and symptoms may not appear until the level is as low as 110 mEq/liter. Most patients with seizures or coma have serum sodium concentrations of below 120 mEq/liter.

TABLE 27–1. Signs and Symptoms of Hyponatremia*

Serum Sodium Level (mEq/liter)	Signs and Symptoms
130–135	Decreased taste
125–130	Thirst
	Anorexia, nausea, vomiting
	Muscular cramping
120–125	Weakness
	Lethargy
	Restlessness
	Confusion
Below 120	Delirium
	Coma
	Seizures

*Signs and symptoms are closely related to the rate of development of the disorder.

1. Have there been complaints of *weakness* or *lethargy*?
2. Has the patient been *confused*?
3. Has the patient been *agitated*?

Past Medical History. A previous history of *malignancy* or *renal, endocrine, cardiac, hepatic,* or *psychiatric problems* may suggest specific etiologies. Each is a known risk factor in the development of hyponatremia.

Medications. *Loop diuretics* (furosemide) and *thiazide diuretics* are frequent causes of hyponatremia. The loop diuretics decrease sodium chloride resorption in the ascending loop of Henle. The thiazide diuretics are the most common offenders because they also decrease the dilution of tubular fluid in the distal nephron, thereby diminishing the urine concentrating ability of the kidney. Intravascular volume depletion associated with diuretic use is a secondary cause because the fall in GFR increases sodium and water resorption in the proximal tubule.

Other drugs reported to cause hyponatremia include ADH analogs, chlorpropamide, vincristine, haloperidol, amitriptyline, acetaminophen, and nonsteroidal anti-inflammatory drugs (NSAIDs).

Physical Examination

During the clinical examination one assesses the patient's tolerance of the underlying condition and establishes the initial volume status category for the differential diagnosis. An attempt is made to classify the patient as volume depleted, euvolemic, or volume overloaded. Attention is given to the following areas:

Volume Status. Signs of dehydration, including relative or orthostatic hypotension, resting tachycardia, dry mucous membranes, decreased urinary output, and poor skin turgor may point to a volume-depleted state. A hypervolemic condition may present as increased abdominal girth or frank ascites, the patient noting significant weight gain, lower extremity or sacral edema, an S_3 gallop on cardiac examination, or rales on auscultation of the lung. The body can vary from plus or minus 5% to 10% of its weight in water without significant physical findings. Therefore, a euvolemic state is often apparent despite a relative hypervolemia or hypovolemia.

Skin. Skin changes suggestive of endocrine or renal disorders may be detected, e.g., myxedema, hyperpigmentation of Addison's syndrome, or the sallow, slightly yellow-tinged color of chronic renal failure. As noted above, poor skin turgor may be a sign of dehydration, but it is less reliable in older patients because of changes in tissue elasticity.

Cardiopulmonary Signs. Examination of the heart and lungs may reveal evidence of congestive heart failure, left ventricular enlargement, chronic pulmonary disease, or pulmonary tumors.

Neurologic Signs. Neurologic examination often reveals abnormalities and may provide specific clues to the cause of hyponatremia. The level of consciousness is usually altered in patients with a sodium level below 120 to 125 mEq/liter. Exceptions can occur if there is a very slow rate of change from normal to abnormal. True muscle weakness and some muscular twitching may be seen. Although lateralized findings suggest structural CNS pathology, hemiparesis may be present owing to hyponatremia alone. Plantar reflexes are frequently abnormal, and ambulatory patients may exhibit ataxia.

DECISION PRIORITIES AND PRELIMINARY DIFFERENTIAL DIAGNOSIS

Once hyponatremia is diagnosed, two questions will direct the rest of the evaluation.

1. *Is it real?*
   Until recently, this question held more importance than it does now because flame photometry measurements were subject to error with high levels of triglycerides and proteins. With ion-selective electrode measurement, the osmotic

effect of a high serum glucose level is the major source of pseudohyponatremia. Artifactual hyponatremia due to hyperglycemia will be obvious once the glucose level is known. For every 100 mg/dl increase in glucose over 100 mg/dl, the serum sodium measurement decreases by approximately 1.6 mEq/liter.

2. *What is the clinically estimated volume status?*

The volume status is applied to determine the major diagnostic categories of hyponatremia (Fig. 27–1): volume depleted—low total body sodium concentration (deficit of total body water but larger deficit of total body sodium); euvolemic—normal total body sodium (excess total body water); hypervolemic—excess total body sodium with a larger excess of total body water.

PROBLEM The patient was quickly categorized into the volume-depleted category representing a low total body sodium level. The glucose level was then evaluated to determine its potential role in the patient's serum sodium level.

DIAGNOSTIC ADJUNCTS

Laboratory Studies

The clinical laboratory is most important in assessing the patient with hyponatremia. Each of the first seven tests below is recommended as appropriate laboratory testing in the hyponatremic patient.

Serum Electrolytes. In addition to sodium, serum potassium levels are also measured. Diuretic-induced hyponatremia is usually associated with hypokalemia. It is also found in patients with fluid loss from the gastrointestinal tract. Hyponatremia due to adrenal insufficiency is usually associated with hyperkalemia. The serum chloride levels usually follow the changes in serum sodium level. The serum bicarbonate concentration is measured to check the acid-base status. Hyponatremia can occur with either metabolic acidosis or metabolic alkalosis.

Glucose Concentration. Glucose is a major determinant of serum osmolality, and significant elevations can artifactually lower sodium levels. An associated osmotic diuresis can also promote a hypovolemic hyponatremia.

Serum Osmolality. This value is often helpful in evaluating the hyponatremic patient. It may be measured but is more often calculated by the following formula:

$$\text{Serum osmolality} = 2[\text{Na}^+] + \frac{\text{Glucose}}{18} + \frac{\text{BUN}}{2.8}$$

Normal osmolality ranges between 285 and 295 mOsm/kg of H_2O. A normal value in the presence of hyponatremia indicates artifactual hyponatremia or the presence of osmotically active substances other than sodium. A discrepancy between the measured and calculated values may also indicate the presence of unmeasured osmotically active substances such as mannitol, methanol, or ethylene glycol. Urinary osmolality may be elevated appropriately in hypovolemic patients or inappropriately as in syndrome of inappropriate ADH secretion (SIADH).

Urinalysis. The specific gravity of urine from a normal functioning kidney provides an estimate of the patient's volume status. Levels greater than 1.020 suggest renal concentration. A level of 1.010 represents maximal dilution or an inability of the kidney to concentrate urine. Proteinuria and glycosuria may reflect associated renal problems. In most patients, glucose is not found in the urine until levels have exceeded 200 mg/dl. The pregnant patient is a common exception.

Urinary Electrolytes. Urinary sodium levels are infrequently measured in the emergency department but are easy to obtain and are important in narrowing the diagnostic possibilities (Fig. 27–1). A urinary sodium level of less than 10 mEq/liter implies a non–renal-mediated cause of hyponatremia, whereas levels greater than 20 mEq/liter suggest sodium loss from the kidney. These are "spot" measurements, not collections taken over a period of time. They may be falsely elevated by an increased sodium load or by use of a diuretic in the previous 24 to 48 hours.

Renal Function Tests (Blood Urea Nitrogen [BUN], Creatinine). These measurements are usually elevated in patients with renal failure. Renal salt-wasting due to polycystic kidney disease or chronic interstitial nephritis may occur without causing significant renal insufficiency. Because of the difference in absorption and secretion by the nephron, the BUN will rise faster than the creatinine in volume-depleted patients, and therefore the usual 10:1 ratio will be exceeded.

Complete Blood Count with Differential Cell Count. This test may be useful in identifying occult hemorrhage or in supporting a suspicion of an intra-abdominal inflammatory process with third-spacing of fluid.

Serum Amylase. This test is selected when pancreatitis is suspected. It is not diagnostic but may confirm one's suspicion.

Other Laboratory Tests. Other tests may be selected when clinically indicated to evaluate liver, thyroid, and adrenal function.

Radiologic Imaging

Anteroposterior and lateral radiographs of the chest may show inflammatory or neoplastic disease of the lung or cardiac disease. Any of these may be associated with hyponatremia.

Computed tomography (CT) of the head is usually reserved for patients with signs of an intracranial mass lesion, patients with acutely altered mental status, and patients with severe hyponatremia who do not improve with treatment.

Electrocardiography

The electrocardiogram is indicated when evaluating a patient with new onset of congestive heart failure or pulmonary edema. It is nondiagnostic in patients with hyponatremia but may be altered by concomitant changes in serum potassium (see Chap. 28).

PROBLEM The patient's laboratory values were: serum sodium 115 mEq/liter, serum potassium 2.8 mEq/liter, serum glucose 180 mg/dl, BUN 28 mg/dl, and creatinine 2.1 mg/dl. Other values, including measurements of urinary electrolytes, were still pending. Based on these values, the patient's serum osmolality was calculated as:

$$2[Na^+] + \frac{glucose}{18} + \frac{BUN}{2.8}$$

$$2(115) + \frac{180}{18} + \frac{28}{2.8}$$

$$230 + 10 + 10 = 250 \text{ mOsm/liter}$$

This value represents marked hyposmolality. The measured serum osmolality should agree with the calculated value, plus or minus 10 mOsm/liter. If there is a discrepancy, with the measured value being more nearly normal, artifactual hyponatremia or unmeasured osmotically active agents such as ethanol may be present.

REFINED DIFFERENTIAL DIAGNOSIS

When the results of the history, physical examination, and selected diagnostic tests are available, the etiology of hyponatremia may be determined or the differential diagnosis significantly narrowed.

Hypovolemic Patients

In hypovolemic patients, ADH release is stimulated and water is retained, even when hyposmolality develops in the blood. The major sources of sodium and water losses are the kidney, gastrointestinal tract, and "third space" losses into interstitial tissues. The urinary sodium level will differentiate between renal and nonrenal losses, and other readily available tests will confirm the specific cause (Fig. 27–1 and Table 27–2). Levels between 10 and 20 mEq/liter may result from mixed etiologies but are most often of renal origin.

Euvolemic Patients

Clinically, euvolemic patients with hyponatremia fall into four etiologic groups:
1. Artifactual disorder
2. Diuretic use with water replacement
3. Thyroid or adrenal insufficiency
4. Syndrome of inappropriate ADH secretion

Artifactual causes were considered in the earlier discussion of Preliminary Differential Diagnosis. The history and physical examination will reveal those patients who use diuretics and may have replaced fluid loss with water. They usually have a deficit of both sodium and potassium. History, physical examination, and laboratory studies may lead the physician to suspect hypothyroidism or hypoadrenalism. Thyroid or adrenal function tests can subsequently confirm this suspicion. These tests may be ordered in the

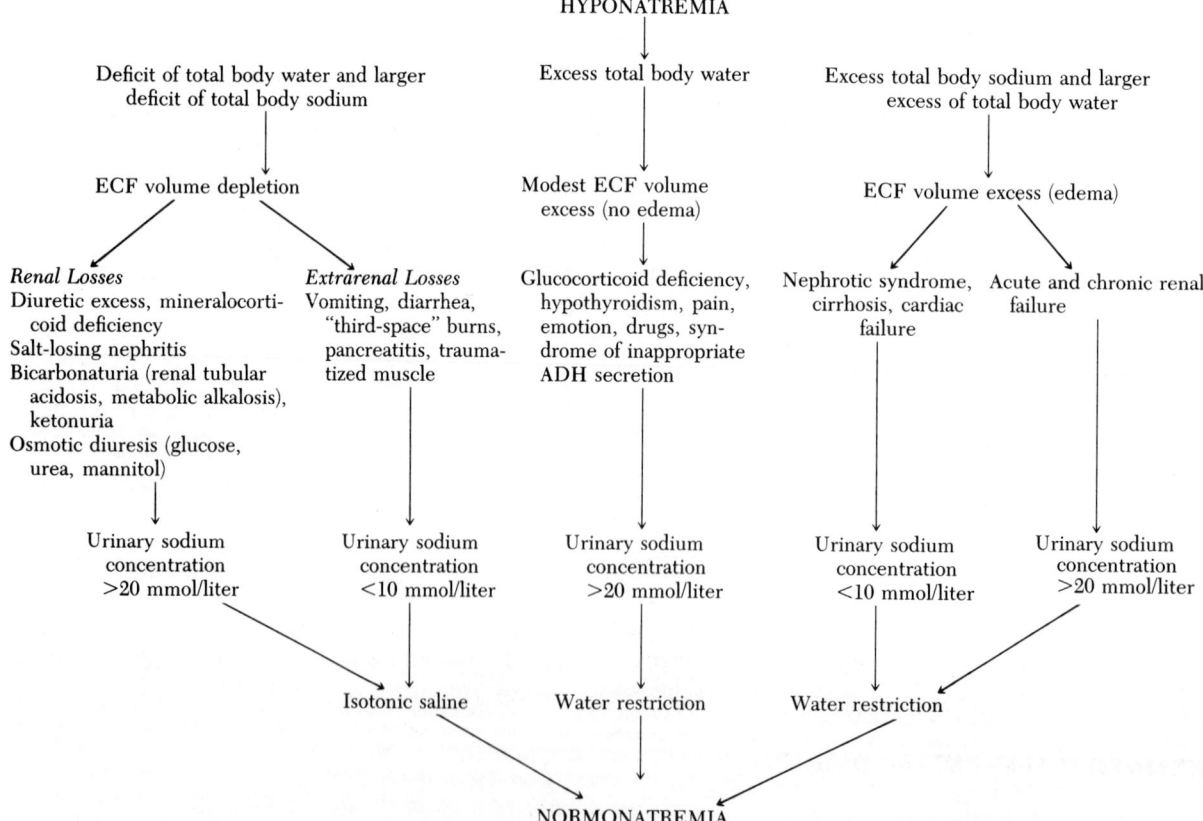

FIGURE 27–1. *Diagnostic and therapeutic approach to the hyponatremic patient. (From Berl T, Anderson RJ, McDonald KM, et al: Clinical disorders of water metabolism. Kidney Int 10:117, 1976. Reprinted from* Kidney International *with permission.)*

TABLE 27–2. Etiology of Hypovolemic Hyponatremia Based on Spot Urinary [Na+] Values

Causes	Confirmatory Data	Comments
Renal causes (>20 mEq/liter)		
Diuretics	History, hypokalemia, hypochloremia, alkalosis	These agents cause ADH release by hypovolemia and decrease renal diluting capacity. Hyponatremia is more commonly seen with thiazide diuretics. Sometimes these patients have retained enough water to alter the physical findings of volume depletion, but they still have relative decreased intravascular volume as perceived by the kidneys and arteriolar baroreceptors
Osmotic diuresis	History of mannitol or urea therapy; hyperglycemia	May result in volume depletion through sodium and water loss. Ketonuria also increases obligate sodium loss. Hyperglycemia and mannitol increase fluid shift into the intravascular space, accentuating hyponatremia
Renal insufficiency with salt restriction, diuretic use, vomiting, or diarrhea	History, BUN, creatinine	Kidney is not able to conserve sodium and water in response to extrarenal losses
Salt-wasting nephropathy	History, BUN, creatinine, urinary electrolyte measurements	Seen in severe chronic renal failure, polycystic kidney disease, analgesic nephropathy, and proximal renal tubular acidosis. There may be varying degrees of salt wasting and different responses to changes in sodium intake
Adrenal insufficiency	History and physical findings, hyperkalemia, hypoglycemia, prerenal azotemia, serum cortisol levels	There is decreased urinary potassium excretion—therefore, hyperkalemia is usually seen in patients with mineralocorticoid deficiency. The glucocorticoid deficiency influences suppression of ADH and permeability of the collecting duct
Nonrenal causes (<10 mEq/liter)		
Hemorrhage with water replacement	Hemoglobin, hematocrit, rectal examination	Isotonic crystalloid is the correct replacement fluid. There may be some decrease in sodium level due to fluid shifts into intravascular space
Gastrointestinal tract losses	History of vomiting, diarrhea	Urinary sodium level may be as low as 1–2 mEq/liter. Exception occurs if bicarbonate level is >28 mEq/liter in serum and bicarbonaturia occurs. Sodium is an obligate cation accompanying bicarbonaturia, and therefore the urinary sodium level is elevated. In this case, urinary chloride is measured. This condition may also occur with ketonuria due to diabetes mellitus or starvation
Third-space losses	History; physical evidence of burns, muscle trauma, abdominal processes; complete blood count; amylase; creatine phosphokinase; urinary myoglobins. Supine and upright abdominal radiographs are taken to detect signs of obstruction	These losses may be a subtle phenomenon with gastrointestinal disease and muscle injury

emergency department, but the results are seldom available to contribute to the diagnostic effort of the emergency physician.

The syndrome of inappropriate antidiuretic hormone secretion is associated with benign and malignant disorders, a number of pharmacologic agents, and even prolonged pain or emotional states. Most patients with this disorder have a defect in the osmoregulation of vasopressin. It is basically a diagnosis of exclusion and usually requires further observation and testing outside the emergency department. To make the diagnosis, hypovolemia, hypervolemia, endocrine dysfunction, renal insufficiency, and the presence of certain drugs must be excluded. Classic findings are a urinary osmolality that is inappropriately high in the presence of a low serum osmolality. The urinary sodium level is generally greater than 20 mEq/liter because the patients are slightly volume overloaded. If patients are placed on a low-sodium diet or become volume depleted, the urinary sodium level will fall to less than 10 mEq/liter. SIADH is usually associated with carcinomas (bronchogenic, gastrointestinal, pancreatic, genitourinary), pulmonary disorders (pneumonia, tuberculosis, aspergillosis, cystic fibrosis), central nervous system disorders (encephalitis, meningitis, trauma, brain abscess), and drugs (chlorpropamide, vincristine, vasopressin, amitriptyline, NSAIDS). The most productive diagnostic tests are the chest radiograph (to rule out oncologic and inflammatory lung disease) and the CT scan of the head (to diagnose CNS lesions, or pituitary tumor).

Hypervolemic Patients

Hypervolemic hyponatremic patients are usually sorted into etiologic categories based on results of the history, physical examination, and readily available diagnostic tests (Table 27–3). Because these diseases are often treated with diuretics, it may be a diagnostic dilemma to determine whether the hyponatremia was caused by the primary disease or the diuretic therapy.

PROBLEM This patient was clinically hypovolemic. Her history supplied at least three

TABLE 27–3. Etiology of Hypervolemic Hyponatremia

Cause	Confirmatory Tests	Comments
Congestive heart failure	History, physical examination, chest radiograph, electrocardiogram	Hyponatremia is mediated by both a "relative" decrease in GFR and increased release of vasopressin
Hepatic failure or advanced cirrhosis with ascites	History, physical examination, liver function tests	The classic explanation is the "relative" decrease in intravascular volume as perceived by the kidney
Nephrotic syndrome	History, physical examination, urine protein levels	Hyponatremia is less common in this group. It may be due to a combination of decreased intravascular volume and elevated vasopressin levels
Severe renal failure	History, physical examination, BUN, creatinine	The impaired kidneys may have difficulty in excreting enough sodium to offset sodium intake. Owing to smaller amounts of filtrate, the kidneys' water-handling ability is also less
Severe polydipsia	History, diagnosis of exclusion	Though difficult to achieve, the water-handling ability of the kidney may be overwhelmed by pathologic water drinking. SIADH may have a role in the process because it can be present in psychosis

GFR = glomerular filtration rate; BUN = blood urea nitrogen; SIADH = syndrome of inappropriate antidiuretic hormone secretion.

potentially contributing factors—diuretic use, vomiting, and volume replacement with clear liquids. The accompanying hypokalemia supported the roles of the diuretic and vomiting in this case. Although the urinary sodium level was not measured, we would expect it to have been elevated above 20 mEq/liter, indicating a renal source of the loss of sodium. There was no evidence from the history, physical examination, or laboratory tests to suggest hemorrhage, third-space fluid, osmotic diuresis, renal insufficiency, salt-wasting nephropathy, or adrenal insufficiency.

PRINCIPLES OF MANAGEMENT

The therapeutic approach to the hyponatremic patient is guided by the clinical assessment of the volume status. The goal is to restore total body sodium levels to normal and promote the excretion of excessive water (see Fig. 27–1). The rate of correction depends on the patient's symptoms. Even in the most urgent situation (the patient with neurologic findings), a correction rate of less than 2.5 mEq/liter/hr is recommended because faster rates have been associated with central pontine myelysis. The target level is determined by the resolution of symptoms. In most patients, symptomatic improvement is noted at levels between 118 and 125 mEq/liter. No effort is made to correct the serum sodium rapidly to the normal range. There are four major treatment modalities.

1. Volume-depleted patients are treated primarily by *rehydration* and *sodium replacement*.
2. Euvolemic patients are treated by *water restriction or excretion* and some degree of *sodium replacement*.
3. Volume-overloaded patients are treated with *sodium* and *fluid restriction* or *excretion*.
4. All patients receive definitive therapy directed toward the *underlying cause* of the hyponatremia.

Volume Depletion with Decreased Total Body Sodium

Volume repletion with normal saline is the most important step in managing hypovolemic hyponatremic patients. The amount and rate of administration depend on the severity of the deficit. An initial starting rate is 10 to 15 ml/kg/hr. The serum sodium concentration is monitored by frequent measurements. Regardless of the specific etiology, this treatment will ensure hemodynamic stabilization while the associated symptoms are corrected. In elderly patients, those with cardiac disease, or otherwise cardiovascularly unstable patients, rehydration is guided by hemodynamic monitoring.

Euvolemic Patients

Patients with symptomatic euvolemic hyponatremia, which usually correlates with serum sodium levels of 115 mEq/liter or less, require sodium replacement and water restriction or excretion in the emergency department. A loop diuretic, e.g., furosemide, is used to increase urine flow, and the electrolytes lost in the urine are replaced with hypertonic saline (3% normal saline = 500 mEq/liter).

Assuming that there are no volume deficits, furosemide 1 mg/kg is administered intravenously and repeated as needed to achieve a urine output of 200 to 300 ml/hr. Urine losses are calculated as 0.45% normal saline (about 75 mEq/liter) until actual urinary sodium levels are measured. Therefore, 2 liters of urine output would be replaced by about 300 ml of 3% normal saline. Another method is to calculate fluid replacement as a fraction of the output to be replaced, using the following formula:

$$\frac{\text{Serum [Na}^+\text{]}}{\text{Infusate [Na}^+\text{]}} = \text{fraction of output to be replaced}$$

The 3% normal saline is used to replace these losses with an equivalent amount of sodium. In this fashion, correction of the sodium level to about 125 mEq/liter is obtained in 4 to 6 hours or until the symptoms resolve. Another "guestimate" method using 3% saline is to give 3 ml/kg/hr. Potassium replacement is usually necessary as well. Hourly monitoring of electrolyte levels and the patient's hydration status will prevent overcorrecting the sodium deficit.

Asymptomatic patients are treated with fluid restriction and assessed for an underlying cause, including SIADH. This work-up is seldom done in the emergency department. Patients with a mild to moderate depression of serum sodium level (more than 120 mEq/liter) usually do well with fluid restriction alone. Medications used to treat ADH-induced water retention, such as lithium or demeclocycline, are not part of the initial therapy.

Hypervolemic Patients

In patients with acute neurologic symptoms, treatment consists of both water and sodium restriction. In severe cases, the use of a diuretic and hypertonic saline is used as described above. Occasionally, in severe conditions, smaller volumes of 7.5% saline are recommended. Eventually both water and sodium must be removed in a manner appropriate for the underlying disease process, e.g., dialysis in patients with severe renal insufficiency or aldosterone blockade in those with cirrhosis with ascites. Close attention is paid to the acid-base balance, renal function, and potassium status in these patients.

Definitive Therapy

Medications that may have contributed to the hyponatremic state are discontinued. Specific therapy is given for the underlying disease states.

PROBLEM Unfortunately, this patient had no fluid or electrolyte replacement while her work-up progressed. Rehydration therapy was necessary to correct her fluid deficit. It would have been appropriate to start this process with normal saline after the initial evaluation. She weighed 50 kg; therefore, a rate of 500 to 750 ml/hr was used. After 2 hours of therapy, her blood pressure was 126/80 mm Hg, pulse 90 beats/min, and the respiratory rate and bibasilar rales were increased. There was only slight improvement in mental status. Repeat serum sodium level was 116 mEq/liter.

Assuming hyponatremia is the patient's primary problem, normal saline could be continued, or, if there are concerns about hypervolemia, 3% saline and furosemide could be considered. Fluid replacement with 3% saline can be initiated at 3 ml/kg/hr or more precisely calculated as a fraction of the output to be replaced:

$$\frac{\text{Serum [Na+]}}{\text{Infusate [Na+]}} = \text{fraction of output to be replaced}$$

$$\frac{116 \text{ mEq/liter}}{513 \text{ mEq/liter*}} = 0.23 \text{ (23\% of output)}$$

Because of the change in respiratory rate and rales, furosemide was used; it achieved an output of 345 ml in the first hour. Replacement of 23% of the output (i.e., 345 ml ×

---

*3% NaCl contains 513 mEq/liter of sodium.

0.23 = 80 ml) as 3% saline continued to normalize the serum sodium level. Two hours later, the serum sodium concentration was 120 mEq/liter, and the patient responded to verbal commands. The potassium level dropped to 2.0 mEq/liter. It is important to monitor both sodium and potassium concentrations hourly and replace potassium as needed.

SPECIAL CONSIDERATIONS

Pediatric Patients

Infants and small children with vomiting and diarrhea can develop hyponatremia and other electrolyte disorders much more rapidly than adults. This is especially true when fluid losses are replaced with hypotonic solutions such as water or D/W 5%. The dehydrated child who presents with seizures and a history of gastrointestinal losses of fluid from vomiting or diarrhea that were replaced with dilute liquids can be presumed to be hyponatremic. Fluid and electrolyte replacement in such patients is started immediately, usually as a 10 ml/kg bolus of normal saline.

DISPOSITION AND FOLLOW-UP

Admission

Symptomatic patients and those with very low serum sodium levels require close monitoring of fluid, electrolyte, and mental status. They are best managed in an intensive care unit.

Patients with mild symptoms and moderate depressions of serum sodium (120 to 125 mEq/liter) who are otherwise stable may be admitted to a general medical floor. Even patients with mild depressions of sodium concentration may be admitted for observation and further evaluation if the cause is unclear.

Discharge

Asymptomatic patients with mild depressions of serum sodium (over 125 mEq/liter) due to an easily remediable cause, such as diuretic overuse or mild congestive heart failure, may be evaluated in the emergency department, instructed about changes in medication or fluid restriction, and discharged for appropriate early follow-up on an outpatient basis.

Consultation

Many asymptomatic or mildly symptomatic patients can be diagnosed and treated without consultation other than planned follow-up. Problems related to symptomatic patients are best discussed with an internist or nephrologist prior to or at the time of initiating therapy and planning admission.

PROBLEM Although this patient's condition improved, she still required intensive care unit monitoring of her fluid status and electrolyte replacement. A review of the potential causes of her altered mental status and hyponatremia is important prior to transferring her from the emergency department.

DOCUMENTATION

1. Pertinent history, specifically risk factors for hyponatremia
2. Vital signs

3. Mental status

4. Flow sheet. It is practically impossible to document fluid and electrolyte replacement adequately as well as *serial electrolyte measurements* without the aid of a chronologically recorded flow sheet. Findings on repeated assessments are included.

5. Differential diagnosis. As with any complicated medical problem, a brief discussion of the diagnostic possibilities is recorded. A supplemental record is added as necessary.

6. Disposition or discussion with consultant

SUMMARY AND FINAL POINTS

- The hyponatremic patient presents with nonspecific signs and symptoms and a myraid of potential causes for the biochemical abnormality.
- The patient's fluid status, history, other physical findings, and selected laboratory test results are used to narrow the diagnostic possibilities.
- Evaluation of volume status is central to classifying the hyponatremic patient.
- Not all hyponatremic patients require administration of normal saline.
- Treatment is linked to the volume status of the patient on presentation.
- Sodium replacement is done with careful monitoring of volume status and electrolyte levels.
- The speed at which the serum sodium level is corrected depends on the severity of the symptoms on presentation. A rate of less than 2.5 mEq/liter/hr is considered optimal.

BIBLIOGRAPHY

Texts

1. Schrier R, Berl T: Disorders of water metabolism. In Schrier R (ed): Renal and Electrolyte Disorders (3rd ed). Boston, Little, Brown, 1986.
2. Schrier R, Leaf A: Effects of hormones on water, sodium and potassium metabolism. In Williams R (ed): Textbook of Endocrinology. Philadelphia, Saunders, 1981.

Journal Articles

1. Ayus JC, Krothapalli RK, Arieff AI: Treatment of symptomatic hyponatremia and its relation to brain damage. N Engl J Med 317(19):1190–1195, 1987.
2. Berl T, Anderson R, McDonald K, et al: Clinical disorders of water metabolism. Kidney Int 10:117–132, 1976.
3. Chung HM, Kluge R, Schrier RW: Clinical assessment of extracellular fluid volume. Am J Med 83(5):905–908, 1987.
4. Janz T: Sodium. Emerg Med Clin North Am 4(1):115–130, 1986.
5. Miller M: Fluid and electrolyte balance in the elderly. Geriatrics 42(11):65–68, 1987.
6. Sterns R: Severe symptomatic hyponatremia: Treatment and outcome. Ann Intern Med 107(5):656–664, 1987.
7. Wilson P: A severe case of hyponatremia. Arch Emerg Med 5(2):125–126, 1988.
8. Votey SR, Peters AL, Hoffman JR: Disorders of water metabolism. Emerg Med Clin North Am 7(4):749–769, 1989.

CHAPTER 28

HYPERKALEMIA

MARCUS L. MARTIN, M.D.
TIMOTHY C. EVANS, M.D.

PROBLEM A 66 year old male presented to the emergency department with a 3-day history of malaise, anorexia, mild nausea, and diffuse weakness. The weakness had progressed during the last 24 hours to the point where the patient was having difficulty walking. The patient stated that he had been in good health except for mild hypertension, for which he took a "water pill." He denied taking any other medications.

On examination the patient appeared well and was alert and cooperative. Blood pressure was 130/80 mm Hg, pulse 84 beats/min, respirations 20/min, and oral temperature 36.7°C (98°F). Motor strength was assessed as equally diminished in the upper and lower extremities. Deep tendon reflexes were also symmetrically diminished. The remainder of the physical examination was unremarkable.

After obtaining intravenous access and sending blood to the laboratory for analysis, an electrocardiogram (ECG) was done (Fig. 28–1); it revealed a regular ventricular rhythm with a QRS duration of 0.20 second. The P–R interval was also prolonged, and the T waves appeared tall. The physician suspected hyperkalemia.

QUESTIONS TO CONSIDER

1. What patients are considered at risk for hyperkalemia?
2. What are the common signs and symptoms of hyperkalemia?
3. What emergency department tests may help in evaluating this problem?
4. When does hyperkalemia require immediate intervention?
5. What are the treatment modalities for the various degrees of hyperkalemia?
6. When should a hyperkalemic patient be admitted to the hospital, and what follow-up arrangements should be made for those discharged to home?

INTRODUCTION

Potassium is the major intracellular cation in the body. Ninety-eight per cent of potassium is intracellular, and only 2% is extracellular. In the healthy adult, total body potassium approximates 50 mEq/kg body weight, of which 75% is found in muscles. Normal extracellular concentrations range from 3.8 to 5.0 mEq/liter in the adult and child, and 5.0 to 7.5 mEq/liter in the newborn. Intracellular concentrations are 150 mEq/liter in tissue and 105 mEq/liter in red blood cells. Serum potassium levels above 5.0 mEq/liter constitute hyperkalemia. The appearance of symptoms and their severity generally correspond to the level of increased potassium.

A large potassium gradient across cell membranes is critical for normal neuromuscular

500 — HORMONAL, METABOLIC, AND NUTRITIONAL DISORDERS

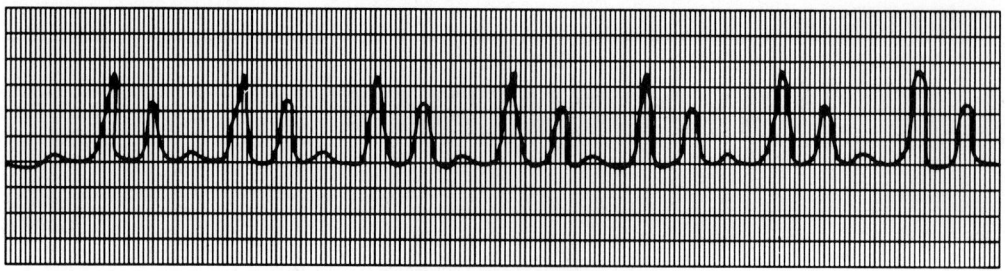

Lead II rhythm strip

FIGURE 28–1. Initial electrocardiogram.

and cardiac conduction. Maintenance of this gradient depends on the Na$^+$–K$^+$ ATPase pump system plus other physiologic factors. The major influences on potassium homeostasis are intake, output, and transcellular shifts. Daily oral intake for the average adult ranges from 50 to 150 mEq, of which 80% to 90% is excreted by the kidney. Approximately 10 mEq/day of potassium is lost through fecal excretion, and 10 to 20 mEq/liter lost in sweat daily. Variations in dietary intake have a proportionate influence on the excretion rate. In response to low dietary intake of potassium, sodium delivery to the distal nephron, aldosterone secretion, anion excretion, and renal cellular potassium concentration are all decreased. Ammonia production is increased. High dietary intake of potassium influences these mechanisms in an opposite manner and also enhances potassium-stimulated exchange for sodium in the distal nephron.

Exogenous sources of potassium include oral and intravenous supplements, high potassium-containing salt substitutes, medications such as potassium penicillin (1.7 mEq potassium per million units penicillin), and banked blood. Endogenous sources of potassium are erythrocyte and tissue breakdown (rhabdomyolysis, burns, tumor dissolution, and massive gastrointestinal bleeding).

Transcellular shifts of potassium occur in response to acid-base changes. In alkalosis hydrogen moves from the cell into the extracellular fluid, and potassium moves into the cell to maintain electrical neutrality. Acidosis causes a shift of potassium from the intracellular to the extracellular compartment, resulting in hyperkalemia. Roughly, a 0.1 change in pH results in a potassium change of 0.6 in the opposite direction. Glucose and insulin therapy and beta-adrenergic agonists can cause potassium to move intracellularly, reducing serum potassium. Intravenous calcium directly antagonizes the neuromuscular membrane depolarizing effects of elevated serum potassium.

Hyperkalemia is less commonly encountered in the emergency department than hypokalemia, but it can be a very serious condition. Although dietary excess and transcellular ion shifts can result in hyperkalemia, the majority of cases are due to decreased excretion resulting from renal failure or the effects of hormones or drugs on the kidneys.

INITIAL APPROACH IN THE EMERGENCY DEPARTMENT

Patients at greatest risk for acute hyperkalemia are those with underlying renal disease. Next to clinical suspicion, the 12-lead electrocardiogram (ECG) is the most useful diagnostic measure readily available to the emergency physician (Fig. 28–2). True "stat" laboratory testing, in which results of serum potassium and arterial blood gas analysis are available in 10 minutes or less, are very valuable in cases of suspected hyperkalemia.

If laboratory values are not available but characteristic ECG changes are present, suspected hyperkalemia is treated. The aggressiveness of treatment depends on the severity of the condition. Mild hyperkalemia is generally not accompanied by ECG changes, and the expected potassium level in such cases is below 6.5 mEq/liter. Moderate

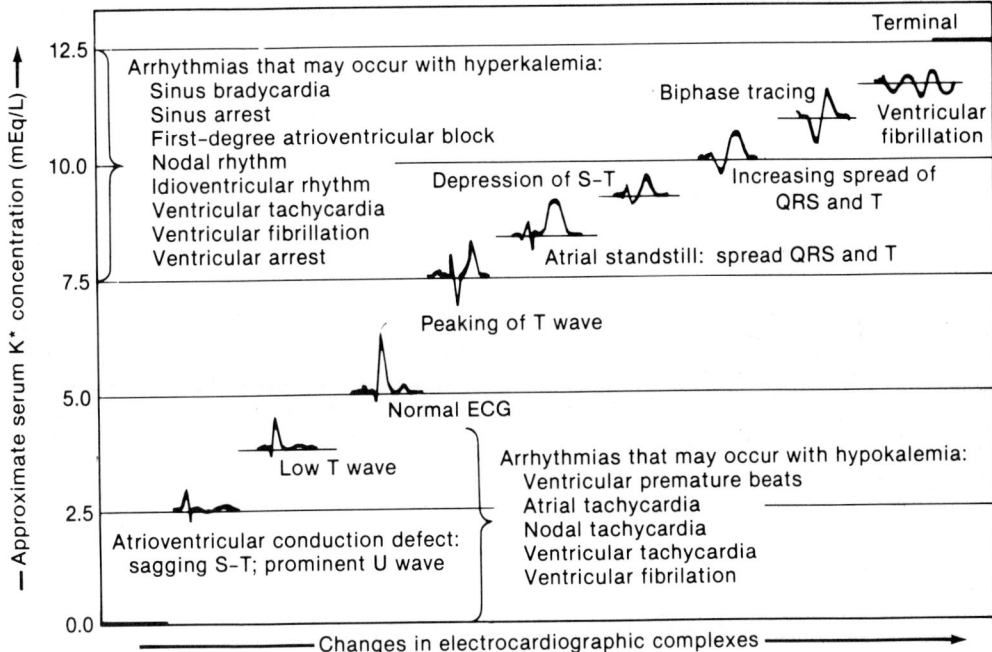

FIGURE 28–2. Correlation of serum potassium concentration and electrocardiogram (provided there is no parallel change in sodium and calcium). (Reproduced with permission from Krupp MA, Chatton MJ: Current Medical Diagnosis & Treatment. Copyright 1974, Lange Medical Publications.)

hyperkalemia (potassium concentration of 6.5 to 8.0 mEq/liter) and severe hyperkalemia (potassium levels above 8.0 mEq/liter) generally produce ECG abnormalities. These patients should have continuous cardiac monitoring and are treated as discussed under Principles of Management.

PROBLEM Shortly after the ECG was performed, the patient became diaphoretic, vomited once, and then lost blood pressure and pulse. Ventricular fibrillation was noted on the monitor. Serial defibrillations with 200, 300, and 360 watt-seconds failed to convert the rhythm.

The condition of this patient had rapidly deteriorated to a life-threatening condition unresponsive to conventional life-support techniques. The only test result available was the abnormal ECG rhythm strip (see Fig. 28–1). While preparations were under way to administer epinephrine to the patient, the physician's own levels of endogenous catecholamines were rapidly rising.

DATA GATHERING

The clinical signs and symptoms of hyperkalemia primarily involve the gastrointestinal, neuromuscular, and cardiovascular systems.

History

Gastrointestinal Symptoms. Has the patient experienced *anorexia, nausea, vomiting,* or *abdominal pain?*

Neuromuscular Symptoms. Has the patient experienced *paresthesias* or *muscular weakness?* Ascending muscular weakness can progress to flaccid quadriplegia and respiratory paralysis.

Cardiovascular Symptoms. Has the patient experienced *palpitations?* Abnormalities of cardiac rate and rhythm are common in patients with hyperkalemia and can lead to hemodynamic compromise.

General Information. What are the patient's *current medications?* Specific questioning about the use of nephrotoxic agents, potassium-sparing diuretics, and oral or intravenous potassium supplements is indicated. What are the patient's *past medical problems?* Specific inquiries about renal disease, dialysis, or recent blood transfusions may reveal aspects of the history that general questioning misses. Are there any *known allergies?*

Physical Examination

The physical examination is directed not only toward discerning the manifestations of hyperkalemia (as noted above) but also toward eliciting the cause of the hyperkalemia. This examination should emphasize

1. A search for evidence of tissue destruction or rhabdomyolysis is included.
2. Evaluation of the skin may reveal the malar rash of systemic lupus erythematosus or the bronze pigmentation of Addison's disease.
3. Special attention should be paid to the cardiac (including vital signs) and the neurologic systems. Testing for symmetrical proximal weakness and decreased reflexes is carefully performed.
4. Evaluation of the patient's vasculature. For example, palpating for an abdominal aortic aneurysm that may be impairing renal blood flow or for an arteriovenous fistula, which may be the only clue that the patient has renal failure and is on dialysis.
5. Pelvic and rectal examinations are performed to exclude obstructive uropathy.

DIAGNOSTIC ADJUNCTS

Electrocardiography is the most readily available and helpful diagnostic adjunct initially. The laboratory is important in documenting and quantitating the suspected hyperkalemia as well as in assisting in the search for the cause of the disturbance.

Electrocardiography. The most serious problem induced by hyperkalemia is cardiotoxicity, which is primarily manifested by ECG abnormalities (see Fig. 28–2). When the serum potassium concentration increases above 5.6 mEq/liter, tall peaked T waves in the precordial leads may be observed. As potassium levels rise past 6.5 mEq/liter, prolongation of both the P–R and QRS intervals can occur. As the potassium level exceeds 8 mEq/liter, the ventricular rhythm may become irregular, P waves may be absent, the QRS complex may widen, and the S and T waves may merge. Terminal arrhythmias are associated with potassium concentrations above 10 to 12 mEq/liter. Wide, complex, pulseless tachycardias or classic "sine wave" patterns should be treated as acute hyperkalemia, particularly in the patient with known renal insufficiency. If hyperkalemia occurs without ECG changes, pseudohyperkalemia is suspected.

Laboratory Tests. The following tests are routinely ordered as part of the assessment of hyperkalemia.

1. Serum potassium level. Laboratory determination of the potassium level is essential. A variety of laboratory techniques are used to measure potassium. All are considered accurate and precise.
2. Renal function tests. Elevations of the blood urea nitrogen (BUN) and creatinine levels will be present in patients with renal failure, and the BUN–creatinine ratio will help to distinguish intrinsic renal disease from extrinsic causes of the failure.
3. Hemoglobin–hematocrit. Anemia may be present in patients with both acute and chronic renal failure.
4. Urinalysis. Examination of the urinary sediment can be useful in the differential

diagnosis of acute renal failure. Crystals, casts, and red and white blood cells may point to the underlying source of the failure.

5. Other blood chemistries. Hyperphosphatemia, hypocalcemia, hypermagnesemia, and hyperuricemia are usually present in patients with renal failure. Serum levels are measured for each electrolyte disorder. Arterial blood gases are routinely measured because metabolic acidosis regularly accompanies acute renal failure and may cause hyperkalemia itself.

PROBLEM While resuscitation efforts continued, the patient's electrolyte measurements returned from the laboratory. A nonhemolyzed sample revealed values as follows: sodium 132 mEq/liter, potassium 9.7 mEq/liter, chloride 95 mEq/liter, carbon dioxide 19 mEq/liter, BUN 43 mg/dl, and creatinine 5.2 mg/dl.

These values revealed severe hyperkalemia and a BUN–creatinine ratio of less than 10:1, indicating azotemia of renal origin. The patient had no previous history of renal failure or electrolyte imbalance. He had taken a diuretic, but this more commonly leads to potassium depletion. In fact, the clinical manifestations of both hypokalemia and hyperkalemia are remarkably similar, and both are part of the differential diagnosis at the beginning of the case.

DECISION PRIORITIES AND DIFFERENTIAL DIAGNOSIS

The etiologies of hyperkalemia can be derived by answering the following questions:

1. *Could the serum potassium level be falsely elevated (pseudohyperkalemia)?*
Artifactual hyperkalemia (pseudohyperkalemia) or normokalemia masking true hypokalemia may occur when samples are improperly obtained. This results in potassium release from erythrocytes, leukocytes, or platelets. Red blood cells have a potassium concentration 20 times that of plasma, and platelets contain a similarly high concentration. Traumatic hemolysis by mechanical forces of aspiration may cause spurious elevations of potassium. Opening and closing the hand to make a fist with a tourniquet in place can cause a 10% to 20% rise in serum potassium values. Potassium released from platelets during blood clotting in the specimen tube may cause a falsely elevated serum potassium level, especially if the platelet count exceeds $10^6/mm^3$. Extreme leukocytosis with counts exceeding $600,000/mm^3$ can cause pseudohyperkalemia and is thought to be the result of leakage or lysis of cells, typically in specimens that have been allowed to stand more than 30 minutes after venipuncture. Prompt separation of serum from cells is important to deter falsely elevated potassium levels.

2. *Did the patient have some form of excessive potassium intake?*
Excessive intake of potassium rarely causes hyperkalemia in healthy people because the normal kidney readily excretes the increased potassium load. Oral or intravenous potassium supplements, salt substitutes, potassium-containing drugs, or transfusion of hemolyzed blood may induce hyperkalemia in patients with renal insufficiency.

3. *Does the patient have a disease process that causes decreased excretion of potassium?*
Patients in renal failure may present with hyperkalemia due in part to impaired renal excretion and in part to an accompanying metabolic acidosis. Nephrotoxicity due to analgesics is well known, and causative drugs include acetaminophen, phenacetin, salicylates, and nonsteroidal anti-inflammatory drugs (NSAIDS). Although only a small number of patients using NSAIDS develop acute renal failure, the widespread use of these agents makes them increasingly important as possible causes.

Other causes of renal failure include small vessel and glomerular diseases, large vessel disease, obstructive uropathy, and ischemic and hypersensitivity disorders. Obstructive uropathy is a postrenal cause of azotemia and renal failure and may stem from obstruction at the level of the kidney (papillae, pelvis), ureter (retroperitoneal fibrosis, calculi, injury), bladder (tumor, bladder neck contracture), or urethra (prostate hypertrophy, carcinoma, stricture).

Potassium-sparing diuretics such as triamterene, spironolactone, and amiloride may induce hyperkalemia by decreasing distal tubular potassium secretion. Addison's disease or adrenal insufficiency may result in hyperkalemia owing to a deficiency of mineralocorticoid. Isolated hypoaldosteronism with normal cortisol secretion may result in urine sodium wasting and decreased potassium excretion.

4. *Is there a pathologic condition causing a transcellular flux of potassium?*
Transcellular shift of potassium out of the cells in exchange for hydrogen ions occurs in some patients with acidosis, especially in cases of untreated or complicated diabetic ketoacidosis. Conditions causing tissue destruction may release large amounts of potassium from the cells. Normally, this potassium load is rapidly excreted, but severe hyperkalemia can occur if there is underlying renal insufficiency. Myoglobinuria should alert one to the possibility of hyperkalemia, and serum potassium is measured in such cases. Hyperkalemic periodic paralysis is an uncommon disorder inherited as an autosomal dominant trait in which transient attacks of weakness occur with an attendant extracellular flux of potassium.

The causes of hyperkalemia can be placed in one of the four categories above and are listed in Table 28–1.

PROBLEM During the resuscitation effort, a nurse left the room to talk with the patient's

TABLE 28–1. Causes of Hyperkalemia

1. Spurious (pseudohyperkalemia)
    a. Laboratory error
    b. In vitro hemolysis
    c. Venipuncture technique
    d. Leukocytosis or thrombocytosis
    e. Abnormal erythrocytes
2. Excessive intake
    a. Oral or IV potassium supplementation
    b. Potassium-containing drugs
    c. Transfusion of hemolyzed blood
3. Decreased excretion of potassium
    a. Acute or chronic renal failure
        (1) Nephrotoxic agents
        (2) Ischemic disorders
        (3) Small vessel and glomerular diseases
        (4) Large vessel diseases
        (5) Obstructive uropathy
    b. Potassium-sparing diuretics—triamterene, spironolactone, amiloride
    c. Primary hypoaldosteronism
    d. Hyporeninemic hypoaldosteronism
    e. Addison's disease
    f. Congenital adrenal hypoplasia
    g. Sickle cell disease
    h. Systemic lupus erythematosus
    i. Amyloidosis
    j. Inadequate distal sodium delivery and decreased distal tubule flow
    k. Renal transport disorder
4. Transcellular flux
    a. Acidosis
    b. Tissue destruction, rhabdomyolysis, tumor destruction, burns, gastrointestinal bleeding
    c. Hyperkalemic familial periodic paralysis
    d. Drugs—digitalis, arginine, succinylcholine, glucagon

wife. She learned that for the past several weeks the patient had been taking over-the-counter ibuprofen for "some bursitis in his shoulder."

Nonsteroidal anti-inflammatory medications are an important cause of acute renal failure, which may be the result of the development of interstitial nephritis or secondary to the inhibition of prostaglandin synthesis. When renal prostaglandins are important in the maintenance of renal perfusion, e.g., in patients with prerenal conditions leading to a reduction in renal blood flow, the reduction in prostaglandin synthesis may precipitate overt renal failure. Patients at greatest risk for this adverse reaction are those with impaired renal function, heart failure, or liver dysfunction, those taking diuretics, and the elderly. The exact mechanism by which hyperkalemia occurs in the setting of near-normal kidney function is not fully elucidated, but it is clear that inhibition of prostaglandin synthesis has a role.

PRINCIPLES OF MANAGEMENT

Emergency treatment of the patient with hyperkalemia depends on the severity of the presentation, ECG findings, and serum potassium levels when available. ECG monitoring is instituted whenever hyperkalemia is suspected, and therapy begun on the basis of the ECG findings even before laboratory confirmation is available. The different modalities for treatment include antagonizing potassium directly, influencing potassium to shift intracellularly, increasing potassium excretion, and decreasing potassium intake. The first two modalities are used when response is needed rapidly (within 10 minutes); the last two act more gradually.

Immediate Response—Antagonizing Potassium and Producing Intracellular Shifts

All patients with moderate hyperkalemia (6.5 to 8.0 mEq/liter) are continuously cardiac monitored while in the emergency department. Cardiotoxic effects may occur more quickly in patients with acute hyperkalemic states (i.e., acute renal failure) than in those with chronic conditions. Therefore, patients with characteristic ECG changes suggestive of moderate or severe hyperkalemia deserve immediate treatment.

Calcium. Intravenous (IV) calcium is the most rapid means of antagonizing the neuromuscular effects of hyperkalemia. Calcium gluconate (10 to 30 ml of 10%) may be administered over 2 to 5 minutes. Although the effect is immediate, it is also transient and does not result in reduction of total body potassium.

Bicarbonate. Sodium bicarbonate in a dose of 50 to 150 mEq (1 to 3 amps) results in an intracellular shift of potassium. The onset of action takes 20 to 30 minutes, and the effect persists for several hours. Sodium bicarbonate has known hypernatremia and hyperosmolarity hazards. These are anticipated and tracked by serial laboratory measurements.

Glucose and Insulin. Glucose and insulin administered together, or glucose and then insulin but not vice versa, also result in an intracellular shift of potassium. Treatment regimens vary, but the addition of 10 to 20 units of regular insulin per 100 gm of infused glucose is generally advocated. An IV bolus of 50 ml of 50% dextrose or an infusion of 500 ml of 10% dextrose is given along with 10 to 20 units of regular insulin. Some physicians prefer to administer a mixture of 10 to 20 units of regular insulin in 1000 ml of 10% dextrose in water with the addition of 1 to 2 amps of bicarbonate for an augmented effect. Onset of action occurs in 30 minutes and lasts for 4 to 6 hours.

Delayed Response—Reducing Total Body Potassium

After directly antagonizing the membrane effects of potassium and shifting potassium intracellularly, efforts must be made to remove potassium from the body. Reducing total body potassium is required in all patients with hyperkalemia and must be accomplished rapidly in all those with cardiac manifestations.

Diuretics. In patients who are nonoliguric, the loop diuretics increase the renal excretion of potassium. A forced saline diuresis (e.g., 40 mg of furosemide administered intravenously, matching urine outputs with intravenous saline) will lower potassium levels. However, this method has the disadvantage of a slow onset of action and can potentially cause the loss of other electrolytes (e.g., magnesium).

Kayexalate. Cation exchange resins such as sodium polystyrene sulfonate (Kayexalate) may begin to affect potassium levels in 1 to 2 hours. Kayexalate may be administered orally by mixing 15 to 30 gm of Kayexalate in 50 to 150 ml of 50% sorbitol solution. Sorbitol increases the amount of fluid entering the intestinal tract and facilitates ion exchange while preventing constipation. Kayexalate may also be administered rectally by adding 25 to 50 gm to 100 ml of 50% sorbitol solution in 200 ml of tap water. The enema must be retained for 30 to 45 minutes and may be administered hourly as needed. A single enema may deplete the plasma potassium by as much as 0.5 to 2.0 mEq/liter. Kayexalate releases 2 to 3 mEq of sodium per gram. Therefore, it is used with caution in patients with congestive heart failure or hypertension.

Dialysis. In very severe cases of hyperkalemia, dialysis may be used. Hemodialysis is extremely effective and removes potassium at a rate of 25 to 50 mEq/hr. Peritoneal dialysis is less effective, removing 10 to 15 mEq of potassium per hour. These methods are preferred in patients who cannot tolerate the high sodium load that results from Kayexalate administration. Unfortunately, both techniques require invasive procedures and may not be available in some facilities. Therefore, all patients with significant hyperkalemia are treated first with the methods previously described.

Reduced Intake. Reducing intake by stopping potassium supplements and reducing dietary intake is also important. Medications containing potassium (e.g., penicillin-VK) and potassium-sparing diuretics are also discontinued.

PROBLEM The patient was rapidly given intravenous calcium gluconate, sodium bicarbonate, glucose, and insulin, and the rhythm converted in a few minutes to sinus tachycardia. A repeat serum potassium level was 7.2 mEq/liter.

The above medications act rapidly to antagonize the membrane effects of potassium and increase the transport of potassium intracellularly. However, they are only temporary measures. Additional doses of these drugs may be necessary as the definitive therapy to remove potassium from the body is readied.

DISPOSITION AND FOLLOW-UP

All patients with moderately or severely elevated serum potassium levels are admitted to a monitored bed. Any patient with electrocardiographic evidence of hyperkalemia requires cardiac monitoring until therapy has reduced the serum potassium level to noncritical levels. This monitoring should continue during dialysis if this modality is selected.

Patients with mild hyperkalemia need not be admitted if it is possible to identify and correct an underlying cause. Examples include dialysis patients who are referred for timely dialysis and patients taking potassium-sparing diuretics who are referred to their primary physicians after the medication has been stopped.

PROBLEM The patient was transported to the intensive care unit for placement of a Quinton catheter in the right subclavian vein and hemodialysis at the bedside with continuous cardiac monitoring. He also received several doses of Kayexalate. During the course of therapy his metabolic abnormalities and his symptoms resolved. He was advised to avoid nonsteroidal anti-inflammatory medications in the future and was discharged after 6 days of hospitalization.

This case demonstrates several important points: first, a precipitous cardiovascular deterioration can result from hyperkalemia; second, the importance of continuous cardiovascular monitoring if potassium disorders are suspected; and finally, the potential complications implicit in the use of certain medications and the importance of obtaining a thorough history, making use of all sources available.

DOCUMENTATION

1. Associated symptoms.
2. Past medical history, medications, and allergies.
3. Physical examination, particularly heart and neuromuscular findings.
4. ECG findings.
5. Laboratory values, particularly potassium levels.
6. Treatment rendered.
7. Response to treatment.
8. Fluid intake and output.
9. Disposition (admission, arrangements for dialysis or other postemergency department treatment, discharge).

SUMMARY AND FINAL POINTS

- Patients with hyperkalemia may present with nonspecific symptoms of malaise, anorexia, and generalized weakness, and paresthesias, paralysis, and cardiotoxicity can occur.
- The etiology of hyperkalemia may belong to one of four categories: (1) spurious (pseudohyperkalemia), (2) excessive intake, (3) decreased excretion, and (4) transcellular shift.
- The severity of hyperkalemia usually correlates with ECG findings and serum potassium levels.
- Clinical suspicion and use of the ECG are relied on in the immediate assessment of hyperkalemia.
- In the patient presenting with acute renal failure and hyperkalemia with no clear-cut cause, one should be suspicious of a nephrotoxic agent.

BIBLIOGRAPHY

Texts

1. Cohen JJ, Gennari FJ, Harrington JT: Disorders of potassium balance. In Brenner BM, Rector FC (eds): The Kidney. Philadelphia, Saunders, 1981.
2. Epstein M, Oster JR: Disorders of potassium homeostasis. In Halstead JA, Halstead CH (eds): The Laboratory in Clinical Medicine: Interpretation and Applications (2nd ed). Philadelphia, Saunders, 1981.
3. Gabow PA, Peterson LN: Disorders of potassium metabolism. In Schrier RW (ed): Renal and Electrolyte Disorders (3rd ed). Boston, Little, Brown, 1986.
4. Tannen RL: Potassium homeostasis. In Massry SG, Glassock RJ (eds): Textbook of Nephrology. Baltimore, Williams & Wilkins, 1983.

Journal Articles

1. Clive DM, Stoff JS: Renal syndromes associated with nonsteroidal anti-inflammatory drugs. N Engl J Med 310:563–572, 1984.
2. Cox M: Potassium homeostasis: Symposium on body fluid and electrolyte disorders. Med Clin North Am 65:363–384, 1981.
3. Defronzo RA, Bia M, Smith D: Clinical disorders of hyperkalemia. Ann Rev Med 33:521–554, 1982.
4. Knochel JP: Neuromuscular manifestations of electrolyte disorders. Am J Med 72:521, 1982.
5. Levinsky NG: Management of emergencies VI: Hyperkalemia. N Engl J Med 174:1076–1077, 1966.
6. Marasco WA, Gikas PW, Azziz-Baumgartner R, et al: Ibuprofen-associated renal dysfunction: Pathophysiologic mechanisms of acute renal failure, hyperkalemia, tubular necrosis and proteinuria. Arch Intern Med 147:2107–2116, 1987.
7. Martin ML, Hamilton R, West MF: Potassium. Emerg Med Clin North Am 4:131–144, 1986.
8. Schwarz A, Krause PH, Keller F, et al: Granulomatous interstitial nephritis after non-steroidal antiinflammatory drugs. Am J Nephrol 8:410–416, 1988.
9. Stillonan MT, Schlesinger PA: Non-steroidal antiinflammatory drugs nephrotoxicity. Should we be concerned? Arch Intern Med 150:268–270, 1990.
10. Surawicz B, Chlebus H, Mazzoleni A: Hemodynamic and electrocardiographic effects of hyperpotassemia: Differences in response to slow and rapid increases in concentration of plasma K. Am Heart J 73:647–654, 1967.

CHAPTER 29

HYPERCALCEMIA

JOHN P. RUDZINSKI, M.D.

PROBLEM A 58 year old female with a history of depression was brought to the emergency department with a complaint of chest pain. Her family had noted progressive confusion and decreased appetite during the past several days.

Physical examination revealed a thin white female who appeared confused and dehydrated. Vital signs were remarkable: blood pressure 90/60mm Hg, pulse 120 beats/min, respirations 24/min. Initial examination showed normal findings except that the mucous membranes and axillae were dry to the touch; the right costal margin was tender to palpation without crepitus or ecchymosis; bowel sounds were hypoactive; and deep tendon reflexes were slow but symmetric. The patient was uncooperative with the staff, muttering unintelligibly.

The patient was given supplemental oxygen and placed on a cardiac monitor. A large-bore intravenous line was started, and 1000 ml of normal saline was given during the first half hour. Laboratory studies were ordered, and results became available during infusion of the first liter of fluid. Complete blood count revealed a mild anemia with a normal leukocyte count. Urinalysis and serum electrolytes were within normal limits. The serum calcium level was elevated at 15 mg/dl.

QUESTIONS TO CONSIDER

1. What is the spectrum of symptoms and signs seen in the hypercalcemic patient?
2. What are the possible causes of hypercalcemia, and which of these are most common?
3. By what mechanisms is the level of serum calcium regulated?
4. What diagnostic tests are of use in evaluation of the patient with possible hypercalcemia?
5. How can significant hypercalcemia be treated in the emergency department?

INTRODUCTION

One to two kilograms of calcium are present in the average adult, making it the most abundant mineral. Ninety-nine percent of total calcium is in bone; of the 1% in the circulation, 40% to 45% is bound to proteins (mainly albumin), 5% to 10% is complexed with anions (chiefly phosphate and citrate), and 45% to 50% is free in the physiologically ionized state.

Calcium homeostasis is tightly controlled over a narrow range by the interaction of parathormone (PTH), vitamin D, and calcitonin. These substances influence calcium obtained through dietary intake, intestinal absorption, skeletal resorption, and renal reabsorption. Close regulation is critical because calcium is essential for:

1. Excitation-contraction coupling in the muscle cell.

2. Depolarization of the cell membrane.
3. Neurotransmitter release in the central and peripheral nervous systems.
4. Secretion of numerous hormones.
5. Function of leukocytes.
6. Aggregation of platelets and completion of clot formation.

The clinical presentation of patients with hypercalcemia depends on the rate and extent of the rise in serum calcium and ranges from chronic, nonspecific complaints to sudden, life-threatening crises.

Four primary organ systems demonstrate pathologic changes as the calcium concentration rises:

Gastrointestinal System. Nonspecific gastrointestinal symptoms are common, probably due to increased gastric acid secretion and chronic dehydration.

Neurologic System. Impairment in neurotransmitter release, both centrally and peripherally, commonly leads to neurologic involvement.

Cardiovascular System. Calcium ions are essential for cellular depolarization and mechanical contraction. Altered contractility and impaired conduction result from elevations of calcium levels.

Renal System. In the kidneys there is impaired concentrating ability, and precipitation of calcium salts may result in nephrolithiasis or nephrocalcinosis.

Several disease processes affect calcium control sites under the influence of vitamin D or parathormone and may result in rise of the serum calcium level (Fig. 29-1).

DATA GATHERING

Because the signs and symptoms of hypercalcemia are nonspecific, lengthy delays before patients come to medical attention or before a correct diagnosis is rendered are common. This multisystemic disease process may be very confusing in its presentation.

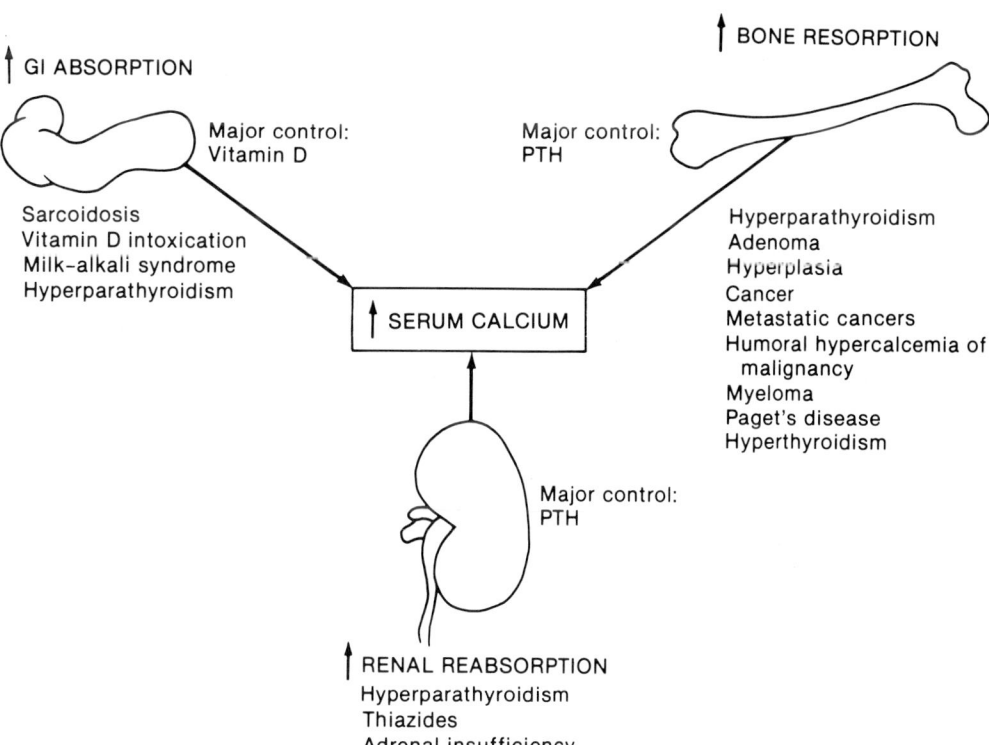

FIGURE 29-1. Calcium regulation. (From SCIENTIFIC AMERICAN Medicine Section 3, Subsection VI. © 1988 Scientific American, Inc. All rights reserved.)

History

The chief complaint in a hypercalcemic patient is likely to be gastrointestinal or neurologic.

Gastrointestinal Symptoms

1. Has the patient experienced *constipation, anorexia, nausea,* or *vomiting*?
2. Is there *associated abdominal pain*? Diffuse abdominal pain is common, and hypercalcemia can precipitate acute pancreatitis.
3. How *long* have these *problems* been *present*? Chronic hypercalcemia is associated with peptic ulcer disease and pancreatitis.

Neurologic Symptoms. Has the patient been *lethargic, depressed,* or *confused*? Depression of mental status is almost always present even with mild elevations of the serum calcium level. As the level rises, however, irritability or psychotic behavior may occur. At very high levels, coma may develop.

Cardiac Symptoms

1. Has the patient *perceived* a *rapid* or *irregular heartbeat*?
2. Is the patient taking a *digitalis preparation*? Dysrhythmia may be directly related to the calcium ion or to increased sensitivity to digitalis preparations.

Renal Symptoms

1. Has the patient noticed *polyuria* or *nocturia*? These symptoms are related to impaired concentrating ability.
2. Is there *flank pain* or *hematuria*? Calcium salts may be precipitated out in the renal tubules, resulting in nephrolithiasis.
3. Has the patient noticed *oliguria* or *anuria*? In some instances, renal failure may develop, pushing calcium levels even higher and leading to other electrolyte imbalances.

Other Symptoms

1. Has the patient experienced *bone pain*? Such pain is commonly present in the hypercalcemic patient owing to hormonal overactivity, but metastatic lesions are also a possibility.
2. Has the patient experienced *visual disturbances*?
3. Has *weakness* or *dizziness* been noted? Weakness may be due to the neuromuscular effects of hypercalcemia, but anemia is a frequent concomitant factor.

Physical Examination

Physical signs may be due directly to hypercalcemia or may be related to the underlying disease process. Because malignancy or endocrine disorders may be present, a careful, thorough examination is important.

General Appearance. These patients most commonly appear lethargic and chronically ill. Skin and mucous membrane signs of dehydration are also common.

Vital Signs. Pulse irregularity may result from dysrhythmias, and sinus tachycardia may be present owing to dehydration or stress. Blood pressure may be depressed due to dehydration, but hypertension may result from chronic hypercalcemia.

Chest. Auscultatory findings may suggest malignancy or granulomatous disease.

Cardiac Signs. Abnormal rate or irregularity may be found secondary to dysrhythmia.

Abdomen. Distention may be present owing to constipation. Diffuse mild tenderness is a nonspecific finding, but tenderness localized to the epigastrium or left upper quadrant is suggestive of acute pancreatitis. Masses suggest malignancy or benign tumors such as pheochromocytoma. Costovertebral angle tenderness may be present with nephrolithiasis. Rectal examination with a check for occult blood in the stool is important in the search for malignancy as well as for associated peptic ulcer disease.

Neurologic Examination. Mental status is often depressed, but irritability and psychotic behavior are possible. Some degree of disorientation is likely. Deep tendon reflexes are depressed. Coordination is impaired. Focal deficits suggest the possibility of malignancy involving the central nervous system.

Extremities. Generalized bony tenderness is frequently present. Localized tenderness suggests malignancy or Paget's disease.

DIAGNOSTIC ADJUNCTS

Although hypercalcemia may be suspected on clinical grounds, laboratory tests are necessary for confirmation, and laboratory, radiologic, and electrocardiographic data are all important in the search for complications of hypercalcemia and its cause.

Laboratory Studies

Serum Calcium. Hypercalcemia is defined as a *serum calcium* concentration elevated above 10.5 mg/dl; a level of 12 mg/dl or less is considered mildly elevated, whereas a level of 14 mg/dl or greater is usually associated with significant symptoms. Levels are commonly determined by flame emission spectrophotometry, which measures total serum calcium levels. Ionized calcium levels are available at specialized facilities.

Serum Protein. Additional necessary laboratory data include serum protein and albumin levels because they affect the amount of calcium that is free in the physiologically ionized state. For every 1 gm/dl change in serum protein, serum calcium is corrected by a factor of 0.8 mg/dl.

Complete Blood Count. A complete blood count is performed because anemia, impaired leukocyte function, and thrombocytopenia are common. Incidental findings such as the rouleaux formation characteristic of multiple myeloma may also be of value.

Other Tests. Renal function may be impaired, so urinalysis, blood urea nitrogen (BUN), creatinine, and serum electrolyte measurements are routinely sought. Abnormalities of electrolytes including potassium, sodium, chloride, and phosphorus are common, as are acid-base abnormalities. A hyperchloremic metabolic acidosis suggests primary hyperparathyroidism as the underlying cause. Magnesium and calcium regulation are intertwined, and magnesium levels may be lowered by the treatment of hypercalcemia. A serum PTH level may be sought, and the serum amylase concentration may indicate an associated pancreatitis.

Radiologic Tests

Plain Film. A chest radiograph is helpful in determining the presence of malignancy or bony metastases as well as serving as a baseline guide prior to beginning fluid therapy. Specific areas of pain or tenderness may be examined radiographically to look for bone disease (as in skull metastases in the patient with multiple myeloma or hand abnormalities in the patient with hyperparathyroidism).

Electrocardiography

Cardiac studies should include a 12-lead electrocardiogram (ECG) and rhythm monitoring, because bradycardia, heart block, sinus arrest, and dysrhythmias may occur. Additionally, shortening of the QT segment is common.

PROBLEM The electrocardiogram revealed the presence of a sinus tachycardia at 120 beats/min with a left bundle branch block. The chest radiograph revealed pathologic fractures and osteolytic lesions of the right sixth and seventh ribs. A mild anemia was present with normal platelets and leukocytes. The urinalysis and serum electrolyte measurements were within normal limits. The measured calcium level was 15 mg/dl, with a serum albumin level of 2.0 gm/dl. Using a corrective formula, the corrected calcium is 16.6 mg/dl.

Corrected calcium (mg/dl) = measured calcium (mg/dl) + (4 − albumin (gm/dl)) × 0.8

The left bundle branch block could be a direct effect of the elevated calcium level, and more significant conduction disturbances could ensue. The osteolytic lesions in the ribs indicate metastatic lesions, prompting an intensive search for a primary malignancy.

DECISION PRIORITIES AND PRELIMINARY DIFFERENTIAL DIAGNOSIS

When the emergency physician is presented with a patient with a significantly elevated serum calcium level, two questions are considered.

1. *Is the reported value accurate?*
   Correcting the value for the serum protein is accomplished as described above. If the clinical presentation does not correlate with the reported level, a repeat measurement is considered.
2. *Does the patient have a malignant or nonmalignant cause for the calcium elevation?*
   The physical examination will often suggest one category or another, but extensive evaluation is necessary to ensure that treatable disorders are diagnosed.

There are many causes for hypercalcemia (Table 29–1), but approximately 90% of cases are due to either primary hyperparathyroidism or malignancy.

Hyperparathyroidism

In the general population, the leading cause of hypercalcemia is hyperparathyroidism. This disorder is often asymptomatic and is picked up incidentally on routine chemistry screening. Typically, calcium levels are mildly elevated (less than 12 mg/dl), and chronic, nonspecific complaints are present. Hyperparathyroidism can, however, progress to hypercalcemic crisis.

Malignancy

Among hospitalized patients, malignancy is clearly the disease process most responsible for hypercalcemia. It is estimated that 10% to 20% of cancer patients will develop hypercalcemia at some point. It is common in patients with breast, lung, and kidney tumors as well as in those with multiple myeloma and has been reported with almost all types of malignancy. Malignancy-related hypercalcemia may result from multiple mechanisms including direct bony resorption, excess prostaglandin synthesis, ectopic PTH secretion, and osteoclast-activating factor. These patients may present to the emergency department in a toxic and critically ill condition. Usually the history is one of short duration and rapid acceleration of symptoms. Dehydration may be profound owing to gastrointestinal losses and renal concentrating defects. Neuromuscular findings of severe weakness and altered mentation are common. Calcium levels are often higher than they are with other causes of hypercalcemia.

TABLE 29–1. Causes of Hypercalcemia

Malignancy	Granulomatous disease
Primary hyperparathyroidism	Sarcoidosis
Secondary hyperparathyroidism	Tuberculosis
Acute renal failure	Coccidioidomycosis
Drugs	Hypervitaminosis A
Thiazide diuretics	Hypervitaminosis D
Lithium	Idiopathic hypercalcemia
Calcium carbonate	Immobilization
Familial hypocalciuric hypercalcemia	Milk-alkali syndrome
	Paget's disease
	Pheochromocytoma

PROBLEM After initial stabilization, a more thorough examination was performed. The right nipple was noted to be retracted, and there was a palpable 3 × 5 cm hard mass in the right breast. Several hard, fixed lymph nodes were also felt in the right axilla. The patient was unable to tolerate oral fluids because of nausea. She was still confused, unable to recognize family members in the emergency department.

The findings indicating a primary malignancy and metastatic lesions in this patient establish the probable cause of her hypercalcemia. Acute treatment of the hypercalcemia as well as arrangement for more definitive management of the malignancy is indicated.

PRINCIPLES OF MANAGEMENT

Although mild, asymptomatic elevations of serum calcium (less than 12 mg/dl) require no immediate intervention, patients with levels above 14 mg/dl or with significant central nervous system or cardiac changes are started on therapy in the emergency department. The principles of management include:
1. Expansion of the extracellular fluid volume.
2. Removal of calcium ion from the body.
3. Increase of calcium stores in bone.
4. Intravascular sequestration of calcium ion.
5. Definitive care of the underlying problem.

Expansion of Extracellular Fluid Volume (Rehydration)

Since most hypercalcemic patients are significantly dehydrated, the mainstay of therapy is rehydration using isotonic fluids. Rapid rehydration with intravenous fluid rates of up to 1 liter/hr, in association with diuretic therapy, is employed. A urinary catheter will be needed to monitor output, and central venous or pulmonary artery pressure monitoring may be required to guide fluid administration.

Removal of Calcium from the Body

Diuresis. Along with rapid rehydration, a brisk diuresis on the order of 500 ml/hr is sought using intravenous diuretics. Hourly administration of a loop diuretic (20 to 100 mg furosemide, for example) is most commonly used. The combination of aggressive rehydration and diuretic therapy will result in a rapid lowering of serum calcium. Electrolyte abnormalities (hypokalemia and hypomagnesemia) may result; therefore, serial electrolyte determinations are needed.

Hemodialysis. In the setting of renal failure or immediately life-threatening symptomatology, such as cardiac dysrhythmias, hemodialysis offers a rapid and effective alternative to diuresis.

Increase of Calcium Stores in Bone

Corticosteroids are particularly useful in certain malignancies, granulomatous disease, or hypervitaminosis D. The mechanism of action is not well understood, but it has been proposed that they suppress bone resorption and may decrease intestinal absorption of calcium. Because the effect of steroids will not be seen for several days, they are often started on initial diagnosis of hypercalcemia. *Mithramycin* also suppresses bone resorption. It is used as a second-line treatment in patients who are unresponsive to saline diuresis within 12 to 24 hours. Onset of action occurs within 24 hours, but the agent can be associated with serious side effects. Other agents that act in a similar manner are *calcitonin* and *diphosphonates*. Oral or intravenous *phosphates* also suppress resorption but in addition cause deposition of calcium in bone and soft tissues. Side effects limit the use of phosphates.

Intravascular Sequestration of Calcium Ion

Intravenous sodium-EDTA acts as a chelating agent, binding calcium. The chelated complex is then excreted in the urine. Nephrotoxicity of the agent limits its use to cases with life-threatening dysrhythmias and severe hypercalcemic crisis.

Definitive Care

The final step in management is arranging for specific treatment of the underlying disease process.

PROBLEM After 1000 ml of IV fluid had been administered, the pulse slowed to 100 beats/min, and the blood pressure rose to 110/70 mm Hg. A urinary catheter and central venous pressure monitor were placed, and a second liter of normal saline was started. Furosemide 40 mg was administered intravenously. As treatment proceeded, the patient became more responsive and complained of chest pain. The patient's physician was contacted about admission to the ICU and the family informed of the patient's diagnosis and condition.

DISPOSITION AND FOLLOW-UP

Admission

All patients with symptomatic or severe hypercalcemia (greater than 14 mg/dl) should be hospitalized and admitted to an intensive care setting, where appropriate cardiac and electrolyte monitoring is available. If facilities for such monitoring or other therapeutic modalities (e.g., hemodialysis) are not available, patient transfer to an appropriate facility may be necessary.

Discharge

Patients with mild hypercalcemia (less than 12 mg/dl) in whom the diagnosis is incidental or is associated with chronic and mild symptoms may be discharged to pursue an outpatient workup under the direction of their primary physician or internist. A follow-up visit is arranged within 1 week.

DOCUMENTATION

1. Duration and intensity of symptoms.
2. Findings on physical examination (especially neurologic and cardiopulmonary status).
3. Serum calcium level.
4. Hydration status prior to initiation of diuresis therapy.
5. Consultation with primary care physician or specialist.
6. Condition of patient on emergency department discharge.

SUMMARY AND FINAL POINTS

- Hypercalcemia is a relatively uncommon disease with a broad spectrum of clinical presentations. Since it often presents with nonspecific signs and symptoms, a high index of suspicion must be maintained.

- Common organ systems involved include the gastrointestinal, neuropsychiatric, cardiovascular, and renal systems.
- Ninety percent of all cases of hypercalcemia are due to hyperparathyroidism and malignancy.
- Patients with malignancy-associated hypercalcemia often present with significant signs and symptoms and a very high calcium level.
- A thorough history, physical examination, and laboratory evaluation are needed to fully assess the multisystemic involvement of this disease process.
- Rapid hydration followed by saline diuresis is the cornerstone of treatment.
- Patients with symptomatic and severe hypercalcemia will require rapid consultation and admission to an intensive care setting.

BIBLIOGRAPHY

Texts

1. Fields ALA, Josee RG, Bergsagel DE: Metabolic emergencies in cancer. In DeVita VT, Hellman S, Rosenberg SA (eds): Principles and Practice of Oncology. Philadelphia, J. B. Lippincott, 1982, pp. 1594–1604.
2. Papontzer M, Knochel J: Disorders of calcium, phosphorus vitamin D and parathyroid hormone activity. In Schrier R (ed): Renal and Electrolyte Disorders. Boston, Little, Brown, 1986, pp. 25–329.

Journal Articles

1. Bone HG III, Snyder WH III, Pack CYC: Diagnosis of hyperparathyroidism. Ann Rev Med 28:111–117, 1977.
2. Fitzpatrick LA, Bilezikian JP: Acute primary hyperparathyroidism. Am J Med 82:275–282, 1987.
3. Ginsberg H, Schwartz KV: Hypercalcemia and complete heart block. Ann Intern Med 88:57–58, 1978.
4. Lee DBN, Zawada ET, Kleeman CR: The pathophysiology and clinical aspects of hypercalcemic disorders. West J Med 129:278–320, 1978.
5. Olinger ML: Disorders of calcium and magnesium metabolism. Emerg Med Clin North Am 7(4):795–822, 1989.
6. Orwoll ES: The milk-alkali syndrome: Current concepts. Ann Intern Med 97:242–248, 1982.
7. Singer FR, Fernandez M: Therapy of hypercalcemia of malignancy. Am J Med 82(2A):34–41, 1987.

CHAPTER 30

ACUTE METABOLIC ACIDOSIS AND METABOLIC ALKALOSIS

DIETRICH JEHLE, M.D.
FRED HARCHELROAD, M.D.

PROBLEM 1 A 35 year old man was escorted to the emergency department by the police for medical clearance prior to incarceration for public intoxication. The patient stated that he had no medical problems and had been drinking alcohol. He complained of vague abdominal pain.

The patient appeared intoxicated. He had slurred speech and a wide-based gait. Vital signs were blood pressure 120/70 mm Hg, pulse 112 beats/min, respirations 22/min, and oral temperature 37.0°C (98.6°F). Physical examination was unremarkable except for mild, nonspecific abdominal pain. The patient was discharged to police custody. He returned to the emergency department 12 hours later, poorly responsive and hypotensive.

PROBLEM 2 A 60 year old woman was brought to the emergency department by her husband because of persistent nausea and vomiting of 5 days' duration. She had become increasingly weak during this period. She appeared moderately ill. Her blood pressure was 110/70 mm Hg, pulse 66 beats/min, respirations 14/min, and oral temperature 37.7°C (99.9°F).

INTRODUCTION

Disturbances in acid-base equilibrium are common findings in the practice of emergency medicine. In every seriously ill patient, the presence and influence of an acid-base imbalance must be considered. The problem-solving approach in these disorders is usually different from that used in "symptom-oriented" presentations. Initial decision priorities and the preliminary differential diagnosis are established after laboratory test results have returned. This chapter is arranged to reflect this difference. After a review of basic pathophysiology, an approach to deciphering the laboratory results is given. This is followed by the differential diagnosis of metabolic acidosis and alkalosis.

The normal blood pH ranges between 7.36 and 7.44. The suffix *–emia* refers to blood pH; acidemia indicates a pH of less than 7.36, and alkalemia signifies a pH of greater than 7.44. There are two basic types of acid-base disturbances, metabolic and respiratory. Respiratory disorders primarily alter the P_{CO_2}, whereas metabolic disorders are characterized by changes in the plasma bicarbonate concentration. The compensatory process is a normal physiologic response triggered by the primary acid-base disturbance. It attempts to move the plasma pH closer toward normal. If the source of the primary disorder is removed or resolved, compensation is often followed by "correction." This is the definitive process of returning the acid-base balance to normal. Acidosis and alkalosis refer to primary processes, which, if unopposed, result in a decrease and an increase in pH, respectively. Acidosis occurs secondary to the addition of acid or loss of bicarbonate. Alkalosis results from the addition of bicarbonate or loss of acid. A simple acid-base disorder is a single primary disturbance accompanied by its compensatory process. A mixed disorder implies the coexistence of two or more primary processes. The remainder of this chapter is devoted to simple metabolic processes and their causes.

Physiology

Diagnosis and management of these disorders require an understanding of normal acid-base physiology, which involves generating hydrogen (H^+) and bicarbonate (HCO_3^-) ions, handling and eliminating these ions, and responding to excess ion loads from endogenous and exogenous sources.

Oxidative metabolism of carbohydrates and fats results in the generation of carbon dioxide ("volatile" acid) and water. Every day approximately 15,000 mM of carbon dioxide gas is generated. Most of the carbon dioxide is transported from the tissues to the lungs in the form of plasma bicarbonate (HCO_3^-) and hemoglobin-bound carbamino groups. In the lungs, the transport forms are converted back into carbon dioxide and eliminated by normal ventilation. Approximately 200 ml/min of carbon dioxide is removed from the tissues at rest. During physical exertion up to 2000 ml/min is expired.

Dietary proteins and incompletely oxidized carbohydrates and fats are metabolized to "fixed" acids. The metabolism of protein results in approximately 1 mEq of fixed acid for each gram of protein ingested, or about 75 to 100 mEq/day in the average American diet. This fixed acid is usually in the form of sulfuric or phosphoric acid. These new acids are chemically buffered by HCO_3^- to maintain pH within the narrow range required for the optimal performance of the body's numerous enzyme systems. To sustain acid-base equilibrium, the kidney compensates by secreting the fixed acid load and regenerating the bicarbonate previously consumed by the buffering process. Disruption of this finely integrated balance between production, buffering, and compensation results in a metabolic acid-base disturbance.

In acid-base physiology not only does the bicarbonate ion serve as a transport form of carbon dioxide, but also the bicarbonate-carbonic acid buffer system is quantitatively the most important of the body's buffers. The system operates through the chemical equation:

$$CO_2 + H_2O \rightleftharpoons H_2CO_3 \text{ (carbonic acid)} \rightleftharpoons HCO_3^- + H^+$$

This buffer system is unique because it is open-ended, since the lung constantly excretes carbon dioxide, and is self-regulating because the kidney excretes, reabsorbs, and regenerates bicarbonate.

Renal reabsorption of bicarbonate in the proximal tubule normally averages 80% to 90% of the filtered load. The fraction of reabsorbable bicarbonate is relatively constant over a wide range of glomerular filtration rates and bicarbonate concentrations. The reabsorption of bicarbonate by the proximal tubule may be altered by extracellular volume, carbon dioxide tension, serum calcium, potassium level, and parathyroid hormone. For example, the existence of significant extracellular volume contraction or hypokalemia causes an increase in proximal tubular bicarbonate reabsorption and may result in a metabolic alkalosis.

Within the distal nephron, i.e., the distal convoluted tubule and collecting ducts, bicarbonate is also reabsorbed to the extent that no bicarbonate escapes into the urine during systemic acidosis. As shown in Figure 30–1, distal H^+ secretion not only mediates reabsorption of remaining HCO_3^-, but the decreased tubule fluid pH causes the existing cellular NH_3 and nonbicarbonate buffers to be trapped in the luminal fluid as NH_4 and titratable acid. The excretion of H^+ in these forms combined with regenerated bicarbonate keeps the body in pH balance. Facilitation of bicarbonate excretion occurs in response to extracellular volume expansion. However, other factors including primary hyperaldosteronism, hypokalemia, and increased nonreabsorbable anion delivery, may independently enhance distal hydrogen ion secretion, thus preventing HCO_3^- excretion.

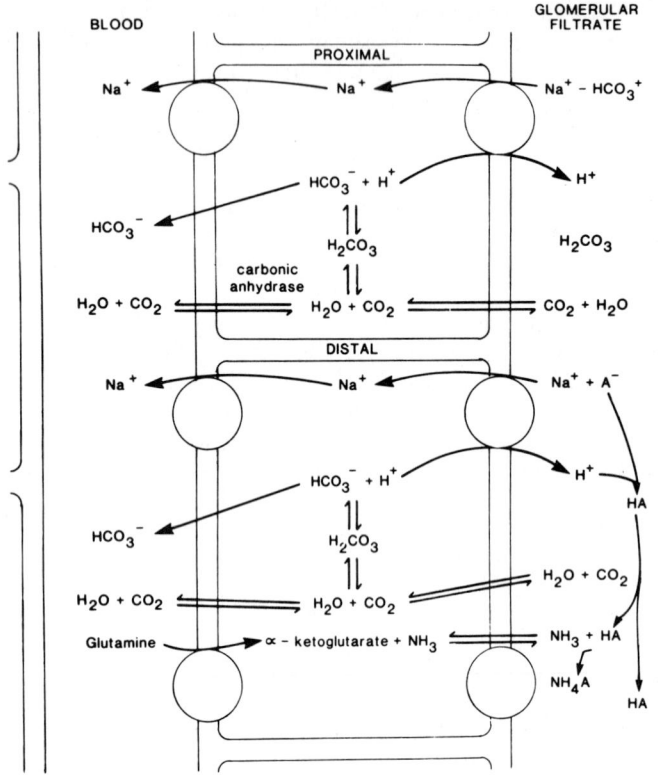

FIGURE 30–1. Renal control of bicarbonate. In the proximal tubule, most H^+ is actively secreted into the glomerular filtrate by a Na^+–H^+ exchange. It reacts with the filtered HCO_3^- to form carbonic acid (H_2CO_3). Carbonic anhydrase in the brush border of the luminal cell membrane rapidly catalyzes its breakdown to H_2O and CO_2, and a hydrogen ion gradient is not established. Water and carbon dioxide diffuse into the cell, where H_2O is split to H^+ and OH^-. The OH^- combines with CO_2 to form HCO_3^- in another carbonic anhydrase–facilitated reaction. This HCO_3^- then moves with Na^+ into the blood, and the H^+ moves into the lumen to react with another filtered HCO_3^-.

The distal tubule has carbonic anhydrase only within the cell. This allows a hydrogen gradient to become established. In the distal tubule, the rest of the HCO_3^- is reclaimed, and the tubular fluid is acidified. This added H^+ to the lumen results in a newly generated HCO_3^- moving into the blood. This balances the new "fixed" acid created in protein metabolism. The H binds with ammonia, sulfate, or phosphate and is excreted. This process is influenced by urinary Na^+, intracellular K^+, aldosterone, and the HCO_3^- load reaching the distal nephron. (From Jehle D, Harchelroad FP: Bicarbonate. Emerg Med Clin North Am 4(1):150, 1986.)

Pathophysiology

Metabolic Acidosis

Metabolic acidosis is an acid-base disturbance created by a primary reduction in bicarbonate concentration with a consequent fall in pH. It may be caused by one of three mechanisms: increased production or addition of acids, decreased renal excretion of acids, or loss of alkali through the kidneys or gastrointestinal tract. This decrease in HCO_3^- is first limited by buffers such as hemoglobin and phosphate. Respiratory compensation follows. Central chemoreceptors respond to the fall in pH by stimulating the respiratory center and causing alveolar hyperventilation. This lowers the P_{CO_2} in an attempt to return the pH closer to normal.

Metabolic Alkalosis

The hallmark of metabolic alkalosis is the primary elevation of the plasma bicarbonate concentration, with a subsequent increase in pH. The compensatory response is alveolar hypoventilation. This process is limited to increasing the P_{CO_2} to 55 mm Hg. The development of metabolic alkalosis requires two physiologically distinct processes. Initially, there is loss of acid or addition of alkali to generate the metabolic alkalosis. Under normal circumstances, the efficiency with which bicarbonate can be excreted by the kidneys is so great that it is difficult to induce more than a mild alkalosis even when 24 mEq/kg/day of $NaHCO_3$ is ingested. Thus, to maintain a metabolic alkalosis, enhanced renal reabsorption (or regeneration) of bicarbonate must be present. Factors causing this include volume depletion, chloride deficiency, mineralocorticoid excess, and hypokalemia.

INITIAL APPROACH IN THE EMERGENCY DEPARTMENT

Suspicion of a metabolic disorder depends on recognizing the clinical settings in which it may occur. The patients at greatest risk for metabolic acidosis are those with altered mental status, diabetes mellitus, alcoholism, toxic ingestion, and renal or gastrointestinal disturbances. Patients with a metabolic acidosis often present with nonspecific symptoms. Its clinical effects are often overshadowed by the signs and symptoms of the underlying disorder. Frequently the only clue to the presence of a metabolic acidosis is an abnormality in the vital signs. Any patient with hyperventilation, altered mental status, and hemodynamic instability may be suspected of having a potentially significant decreased pH.

Metabolic alkalosis may occur in patients with prolonged vomiting, significant dehydration, or diuretic use. There are no specific signs or symptoms of metabolic alkalosis; thus laboratory studies play an essential role in its assessment.

PROBLEM 1 On reexamination, the patient was now poorly responsive with vomitus around his mouth. Vital signs were blood pressure 100/50 mm Hg, pulse 120 beats/min, respirations 40/min, and temperature 36.0°C (96.8°F). Initial stabilization included endotracheal intubation, ventilation with 100% oxygen, and intravenous access. After checking for normal breath sounds, 1 liter of isotonic crystalloid was given over 15 minutes. The glucose oxidase test strip measured 120 mg/dl, and intravenous glucose was not given. Naloxone 2 mg and thiamine 100 mg were administered intravenously. Following the initial resuscitation, the patient's blood pressure was 80 mm Hg/palpation, pulse 120 beats/min. The skin was mottled and cold. He made no spontaneous noise and withdrew symmetrically from painful stimuli without posturing. His pupils were 8 mm bilaterally and were sluggishly reactive. Papilledema was noted on funduscopic examination. There was no evidence of trauma. A cardiac monitor, nasogastric tube, and indwelling urinary catheter were placed. Samples were sent for laboratory studies.

The only information available is that the patient had been "medically cleared" 12 hours earlier. He gave a history of alcohol intake and vague abdominal pain. He was tachycardic and tachypneic during the prior evaluation and became increasingly lethargic over the intervening hours. The medics reported that the patient was in a cell alone. There were no signs of trauma, and the possibility of drug ingestion in this setting is slight. Because of the altered mental status and unstable vital signs, metabolic acidosis may have a role, either as a cause or a complication. The primary goal is to stabilize the patient.

DATA GATHERING

There may be historical points or findings on physical examination suggestive of acid-base metabolic disorders. This information is often gathered after the laboratory results have identified the problem.

History

The history is directed to uncover high-risk settings in which a metabolic disorder is known to occur.

Metabolic Acidosis

1. Are there clinical *manifestations* that are *suggestive* of *diabetes mellitus*, including polyuria, polydipsia, and polyphagia?

2. Are there *gastrointestinal complaints*, especially abdominal pain or vomiting? These are frequently seen in diabetic, alcoholic, and starvation ketoacidosis.

3. Is there a history of *depression, suicidal ideation*, or *drug/alcohol abuse?* These may suggest a possible ingested poison.

4. Is there a history of *renal insufficiency?* Oliguria and pruritus are late manifestations.

Metabolic Alkalosis

1. Are there symptoms consistent with *volume depletion?* These include thirst, dry mouth, dizziness or syncope (often orthostatic), and decreased urine output.

2. Is there persistent or prolonged *vomiting* or *diarrhea?* This is one of the most common histories in patients with metabolic alkalosis.

3. Is the patient taking *diuretics?* This medication, particularly thiazide or loop diuretics, is most often associated with an elevated HCO_3^-.

4. Does the patient complain of *physical weakness* or *muscle cramps?* These can be seen in patients with changes in potassium, magnesium, or calcium.

Physical Examination

The major goal of the physical examination is to identify further the presence and etiology of the metabolic process. The vital signs and general appearance may indicate the body's response to a metabolic acidosis. Specific signs are few (Table 30–1). Findings in metabolic alkalosis are limited to those of dehydration or secondary complications, such as muscle weakness from hypokalemia or muscle irritability from hypocalcemia.

PROBLEM 1 The physical examination findings that hint at an underlying metabolic acidosis are limited: alteration in vital signs (especially increased respiratory rate), depressed mental status, and peripheral skin changes consistent with a hyperadrenergic state. Papilledema may be an early indication of increased intracranial pressure. In the setting of metabolic acidosis, it also suggests a specific ingested toxin. Confirmatory laboratory testing is necessary to make the diagnosis of a metabolic acidosis.

PROBLEM 2 The patient and her husband stated that her nausea began after 1 day of general malaise. It had no association with abdominal pain, chest pain, or diarrhea. Her past medical history included hypertension, for which she was taking a beta-blocking agent and a thiazide diuretic. She continued to take her medications throughout this illness. The patient had had a total hysterectomy and bilateral oophorectomy 25 years ago. Orthostatic blood pressure and pulse: blood pressure 110/70 mm Hg, pulse 66 beats/min supine; blood pressure 80/60 mm Hg, pulse 72 beats/min standing, with symptoms of "lightheadedness." The patient had dry mucous membranes.

Ordinarily, a patient with evidence of dehydration on history and physical examination (persistent vomiting and dry mucous membranes) exhibits some level of tachycardia. This patient's vital signs are altered by her medication. Her beta-blocker is preventing a normal physiologic response to hypovolemia. Hypertension and premature menopause are risk factors for coronary artery disease. Some thought can be given to a primary cardiac event causing the nausea, but the time course over 5 days is inconsistent. Certainly, obtaining an electrocardiogram is appropriate. Volume depletion and continued use of a thiazide diuretic is a common situation in which to find a metabolic alkalosis.

TABLE 30–1. Physical Examination Findings in Metabolic Acidosis (Nonspecific)

Examination Area	Components	Comments
Vital signs	Heart rate	Tachycardia common secondary to acidosis-induced epinephrine release
	Blood pressure	Decrease in myocardial contractility is balanced by positive inotropic effect of acidosis-induced epinephrine release. If pH < 7.20, there is progressive loss of catecholamine responsiveness, and myoinhibitory effects dominate
	Respiratory rate and depth	Tachypnea is compensatory respiratory response to metabolic acidosis. Hyperventilation (Kussmaul respiration) may be pronounced in acute metabolic acidosis, pH < 7.20. In chronic metabolic acidosis, the increased ventilatory rate may not be clinically apparent. However, tachypnea is not a specific sign of metabolic acidosis
	Temperature	Fever points to an infectious process contributing to the acidosis
General appearance	Skin	Evidence of poor perfusion and/or hydration; alcoholic liver disease or inadequate diet (palmar erythema, ecchymosis, or perifollicular hemorrhage); renal disease or infection. Signs of diabetes, e.g., necrobiosis
Eyes	Tearing; funduscopic examination	Hydration. Papilledema or erythema may be present with toxic ingestions, e.g., methanol. Vascular changes may suggest diabetes, e.g., cotton wool spots, hemorrhage, neovascularization
Mouth	Breath	Smell for ketosis, wintergreen (methyl salicylate), cyanide
Lungs	Percussion and auscultation for signs of pneumonia	Infectious process may cause sepsis and metabolic acidosis
Cardiac	Auscultation	Murmurs may suggest a hyperdynamic state, valvular heart disease, or endocarditis. S_3 gallop present with congestive heart failure
Abdomen	Inspection, auscultation percussion, palpation	Presence of diffuse pain common in diabetic ketoacidosis and toxic ingestion. Appropriately localized pain may give evidence of pancreatic or small bowel fistula
Neurologic	Altered sensorium	Common in all types of severe acidosis. May reflect toxic ingestion or coexistent hyperosmolar state

DIAGNOSTIC ADJUNCTS

Laboratory Studies

The laboratory identifies and diagnoses acid-base disorders. In any patient suspected of metabolic acidosis or alkalosis, the following tests are ordered:

Sodium (Na^+). This may give information on the origin of a change in volume status. Hyponatremia also causes an altered mental status.

Potassium (K^+). The serum level is influenced by cellular shifts in both acidemia and alkalemia. An important ion to monitor in all cases.

Chloride (Cl^-). In most cases, chloride moves in the direction opposite that of HCO_3^-. It is useful as part of the anion gap equation.

Bicarbonate (HCO_3^-). Elevations and decreases of this ion are important in identifying metabolic disorders. Isolated values may be confusing because of mixed acid-base disturbances.

Glucose. Important because of the high incidence of metabolic problems associated with diabetes and hyperosmolar states.

Blood Urea Nitrogen (BUN) and Creatinine (Cr). It is important to assess renal function. An elevated BUN to Cr ratio (> 10:1) may indicate dehydration.

Arterial Blood Gases (ABG). This test is essential to determine the pH, P_{O_2}, and P_{CO_2}. All influence acid-base balance. There may be other useful information in the ABG report. The HCO_3^- level may be correlated with the serum level, if it is not a calculated value. The measured percent hemoglobin (Hb) saturation may indicate a variance from the expected Hb saturation at the measured P_{O_2}. This can occur if the hemoglobin is dysfunctional, e.g., carbon monoxide poisoning, methemoglobinemia, sulfhemoglobinemia.

Venous pH. Can be used to measure pH and HCO_3^-, if oxygenation is not a major concern. It is drawn without a tourniquet from an unexercised arm. These limitations may preclude its availability if central access is not established.

Urinalysis. The specific gravity helps gauge dehydration and kidney function. Dipstick testing is valuable for measuring the urinary pH, presence of ketones, and urinary glucose. The microscopic evaluation may be diagnostic in urinary infections or certain ingestions, e.g., calcium oxalate crystals in ethylene glycol poisoning.

Other Tests. Other tests are selected on the basis of the foregoing values and the clinical setting. They include:

1. Urinary electrolytes (Na^+, K^+, Cl^-). The ^uCl is particularly useful in distinguishing "saline-responsive" from "saline-resistant" alkalosis.

2. Serum and urine osmolality. These may be valuable in hyperosmolar states and specific ingestions, e.g., alcohols.

3. Calcium, phosphate, magnesium. These serum levels should be evaluated in rhabdomyolysis, chronic alcoholism, starvation, or metastatic carcinoma.

4. Measures of specific endogenous or exogenous acids or toxins, when suspected: lactic acid, salicylic acid, serum ketones, alcohols (ethanol, methanol, ethylene glycol, isopropanol), and serum iron.

Radiologic Imaging

There is no specific role for imaging in acid-base disorders. The abdominal plain film may be useful in identifying an ingested substance, e.g., iron tablets, or a gastrointestinal problem causing or complicating the acid-base imbalance, e.g., bowel obstruction, dead bowel.

Electrocardiogram

Cardiac monitoring is often useful. The ion changes accompanying acid-base disorders can have significant dysrhythmogenic effects. The 12-lead ECG is usually reserved for (1) clarification of the dysrhythmia, (2) monitoring changes due to elevated or decreased potassium, and (3) assisting in the diagnosis of ischemic heart disease in patients with nausea, vomiting, or epigastric pain.

DECISION PRIORITIES AND PRELIMINARY DIFFERENTIAL DIAGNOSIS

Once the laboratory values are available, and assuming they are accurate, five steps are followed in all metabolic acid-base disorders. These steps identify the process as acidosis or alkalosis, assess whether it is a simple or mixed acid-base disorder, and begin to differentiate between causes.

1. *What is the pH?*
   Though HCO_3^- is the major ion altered in the primary process, the P_{CO_2} will change as part of compensation or another primary process. The pH measures the blood as acidemic or alkalemic. This specifies the primary process, since compensatory mechanisms do not overcorrect.
2. *What is the physiologic compensation?*
   Since this chapter is about metabolic acid-base disorders, the compensatory response is respiratory.

   If the primary process is metabolic acidosis (HCO_3^-), the normal compensatory response (hyperventilation) will lower the P_{CO_2} to equal $1.5 \times$ (measured HCO_3^-) $+ 8 \pm 2$. If the observed P_{CO_2} is not within this range, then a respiratory disorder coexists. The limit of compensation for the P_{CO_2} is 10 mm Hg.

   If the primary process is metabolic alkalosis, the response (hypoventilation) will raise the P_{CO_2} to equal $0.9 \times$ (measured HCO_3^-) $+ 9 \pm 2$. If not in this range, a problem with respiration again coexists. The compensatory hypoventilation will not allow the P_{CO_2} to rise above 55 mm Hg in the person without chronic pulmonary disease.
3. *What is the anion gap?*
   This is an estimate of the unmeasured anions that may be contributing to the disorder. It is most useful in determining the cause of metabolic acidosis. The gap originates as bicarbonate is consumed to buffer organic acids and anions in the blood. Its usual calculation is $Na^+ - (HCO_3^- + Cl^-)$. The anion gap has historically been reported as less than 16 mEq/L, although recent work suggests that most normal individuals have an anion gap below 12 mEq/L. The normal gap does not misrepresent electrical neutrality, as the 12 mEq/L is made up of anions, such as albumin (the major contributor), phosphate, and sulfates. An elevated gap suggests an organic acidosis, a mixed acid-base disorder, or a severe alkalemia. The gap may be influenced by plasma proteins, magnesium, calcium, or lithium.
4. *If a primary metabolic acidosis leading to acidemia is present, the differential diagnosis is categorized as "increased" anion gap or "normal" anion gap in nature.*
   Most acidoses are "increased" anion gap in origin, meaning endogenous or exogenous acid has been added. Most normal gap acidoses result from bicarbonate being lost from the kidney or gastrointestinal tract. Electrical neutrality is maintained by the addition of Cl^-, and the calculated gap remains normal.
5. *If a primary metabolic alkalosis leading to alkalemia is present, the differential is categorized as "saline-responsive" or "saline-resistant."*
   Most disorders are saline responsive and may be differentiated by the patient having volume depletion and a urinary chloride of less than 10 mEq/L.

An alternative method of assessing metabolic disorders involves using the acid-base map (Fig. 30–2). This nomograph is used by plotting two of three parameters (HCO_3^-, P_{CO_2}, pH) to identify the type of acid-base disorder. Simple acid-base disturbances will plot within the labeled areas. Mixed acid-base disorders usually plot outside these regions.

Two other important questions must be asked:

1. *What is the potassium level in relation to the abnormal pH?*
   Metabolic disorders may lead to cardiac dysrhythmias. One source of these abnormal rhythms is hyper- or hypokalemia. Because of intracellular shifts with H^+, K^+ moves in the opposite direction to the pH. That is, as the pH decreases, the serum potassium increases, and vice versa. It is helpful to calculate a "corrected" serum potassium level to determine approximately what $[K^+]$ will be at a normal pH. This may be estimated with this formula: For each 0.1 change in the pH, the K^+ changes 0.6 mEq/L in the opposite direction.

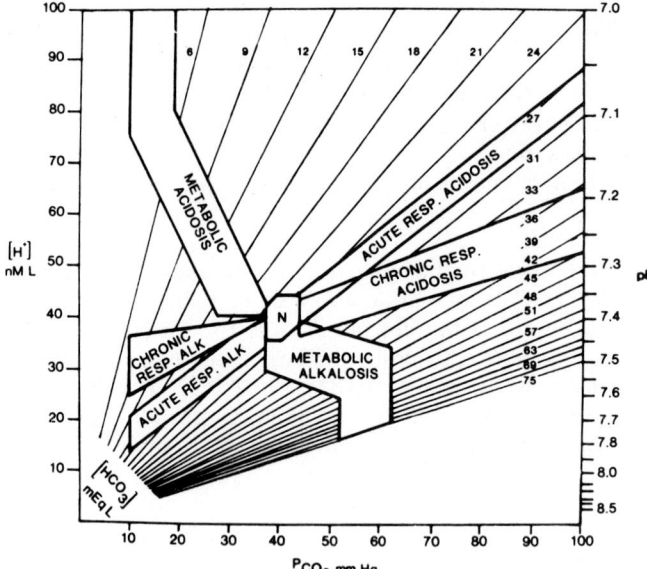

FIGURE 30-2. Acid-base nomogram. A point plotted within the labeled area usually represents a simple acid-base disorder. Following the five steps listed in the text is preferred, as it promotes a clearer understanding of the process. (From Jehle D, Harchelroad FP: Bicarbonate. Emerg Med Clin North Am 4(1):151, 1986.)

2. *What is the calculated serum osmolality?*

If the sodium, glucose, and blood urea nitrogen levels are all elevated, or if one level is particularly high, it is advisable to calculate the estimated osmolarity with the formula: Calculated osmolality = 2 (Na^+) + glucose/18 + BUN/3. If the result is elevated beyond the normal range of 285 to 295 mOsm/L, a serum osmolality is ordered to check its accuracy and to calculate the osmolal gap: Measured mOsm/L − calculated mOsm/L. An osmolal gap of greater than 15 to 20 mOsm/L is significant and represents low molecular weight osmotically active substances, circulating in the blood. In patients with metabolic acidosis, methanol and ethylene glycol are possible causes. Metabolic acidosis and a widened osmolal gap require a search for these toxins.

PROBLEM 1 At this time, laboratory test results began arriving. Arterial blood gas (taken soon after intubation) values showed a pH of 6.95, Pco_2 14 mm Hg, and Po_2 350 mm Hg. Electrolytes: Sodium 136 mEq/L; potassium 6.0 mEq/L; chloride 100 mEq/L; bicarbonate 3 mEq/L. Glucose was 120 mg/dl, and BUN 21 mg/dl.

Following the steps for analyzing the laboratory data:

1. A pH of 6.95 is an obvious acidemia.
2. The physiologic respiratory compensation range is Pco_2 = 1.5 × 3 (measured HCO_3^-) + 8 ± 2 = 10.5 to 14.5 mm Hg. The measured Pco_2 of 14 mm Hg falls in the range; therefore, this is a simple, but severe, metabolic acidosis.
3. The anion gap is 136 mEq/L − (100 mEq/L + 3 mEq/L) = 33 mEq/L. This is an increased anion gap and places the origin of the acidosis as an added endogenous or exogenous acid. The BUN of 21 mg/dl makes renal failure unlikely, but the full urinalysis is not available.

This is an "elevated anion gap" simple metabolic acidosis. The patient's low pH with almost maximal respiratory compensation places him at great risk. Early replacement of HCO_3^- is necessary, and hyperventilation is maintained. To answer the other two important questions:

1. The potassium is 6.0 mEq/L with a pH of 6.95. Increasing the pH 0.4 (4 × 0.1) to 7.35 would decrease the K^+ 2.4 (4 × 0.6) mEq/L to 3.6

mEq/L. The elevated K⁺ is consistent with the severity of acidemia. A slightly low normal K⁺ is anticipated as the pH is corrected.

2. The calculated osmolality is

$$2(136 \text{ mEq/L Na}^+) + \frac{120 \text{ mg/dl G}}{18} + \frac{21 \text{ mg/dl BUN}}{3} = 285.7 \text{ mOsm/L}$$

This is within the normal range. By itself this gives no indication of the actual osmolal status.

The patient was treated with 3 mEq/kg of sodium bicarbonate by intravenous bolus. Additional specimens were sent to the laboratory for determination of serum ketones, osmolality, lactate, toxicology screen, and urine analysis.

PROBLEM 2 Laboratory studies disclosed: sodium 148 mEq/L; potassium 3.1 mEq/L; chloride 91 mEq/L; bicarbonate 38 mEq/L; glucose 126 mg/dl; BUN 30 mg/dl; and creatinine 1.2 mg/dl. Because of the marked elevation of bicarbonate, an arterial blood gas was obtained on room air: pH 7.52; P_{CO_2} 46 mm Hg; P_{O_2} 100 mm Hg; and HCO_3^- 36 mEq/L. Urinalysis: specific gravity 1.033, moderate ketones, otherwise unremarkable. An electrocardiogram and abdominal radiographs were ordered.

Analyzing the laboratory data:
1. A pH of 7.52 is an alkalemia.
2. The appropriate respiratory compensation range is P_{CO_2} = (0.9 × 38 (measured HCO_3^-)) + 9 ± 2 = 41.2 to 45.2 mm Hg. A measured P_{CO_2} of 46 mm Hg is close enough to designate this a simple metabolic alkalosis.
3. The anion gap is 148 mEq/L − (91 mEq/L + 38 mEq/L) = 19 mEq/L. This is slightly increased. Significant alkalemia can raise the anion gap by facilitating endogenous organic acid production (unmeasured anions).

The combination of a metabolic acidosis with a relative hypokalemia and hypochloremia is typical of "saline-responsive" alkalosis. It is often caused by diuretics or prolonged vomiting. Other laboratory data support the clinical finding of dehydration. The urine specific gravity of 1.033 represents an almost maximally concentrated urine. The BUN (30 mg/dl) to creatinine (1.2 mg/dl) ratio exceeds 10, which suggests a decreased glomerular filtration rate from hypovolemia. The answer to the other questions:

1. The potassium level is 3.1 mEq/L with a pH of 7.52. Calculating a pH decrease of 0.1 (to fall in the normal range) would result in the K⁺ increasing 0.6 mEq/L to 3.7 mEq/L. This corrected K⁺ is in the normal range.
2. The calculated osmolality was

$$2(148 \text{ mEq/L Na}^+) + \frac{126 \text{ mg/dl G}}{18} + \frac{30 \text{ mg/dl BUN}}{3} = 313 \text{ mOsm/L}$$

This is slightly elevated and consistent with the patient's volume-depleted state, particularly without water replacement because of the vomiting.

REFINED DIFFERENTIAL DIAGNOSIS
Metabolic Acidosis

The differential diagnosis of metabolic acidosis is classified according to the amount of unmeasured anions (Table 30–2). The normal gap (hyperchloremic) acidoses may be

TABLE 30–2. Differential Diagnosis of Metabolic Acidosis

Normal Anion Gap (Hyperchloremic)	Increased Anion Gap
Gastrointestinal loss of HCO_3^-	Ketoacidosis
Diarrhea	Diabetic
Small bowel or pancreatic fistula	Alcoholic
Ureterosigmoidostomy	Starvation
Ileal loop (obstructed or too long)	Renal failure
Anion exchange resins	Lactic acidosis
Ingestion of $CaCl_2$, $MgCl_2$	Exogenous toxins
Renal loss of HCO_3^-	Ethylene glycol
Renal tubular acidosis	Ibuprofen
Carbonic anhydrase inhibitors	Iron
Tubulointerstitial renal disease	Isoniazid (INH)
Hypoaldosteronism—deficiency or drug inhibition	Methanol
	Paraldehyde
Hyperparathyroidism	Salicylates
Addition of hydrochloric acid	Miscellaneous
Ammonium chloride	Nonketotic hyperosmolar coma
Arginine HCl	Inborn errors of metabolism

divided further into three pathogenic categories: (1) gastrointestinal loss of bicarbonate, (2) renal loss of bicarbonate, and (3) addition of hydrochloric acid equivalents. This group tends to be less severe, with HCO_3^- levels rarely less than 12 mEq/L.

Diarrhea is the most common cause of normal anion gap acidosis and is always included in the differential diagnosis. HCO_3^- concentration in diarrhea exceeds that of plasma. Potassium depletion is a frequent accompaniment. Small bowel or pancreatic drainage has an increased HCO_3^- concentration. Fistulas lead to a steady loss of HCO_3^- and metabolic acidosis.

The kidney is a less common source of bicarbonate loss. In renal tubular acidosis (RTA) there is defective handling of H^+ or HCO_3^-. In proximal RTA, the defect is in proximal reabsorption of HCO_3^- and other filtered substances, such as glucose and uric acid. In distal RTA, the problem is in secreting adequate H^+ to maintain acid balance. Both are commonly associated with significant hypokalemia. An exception is hypoaldosteronism (RTA type IV) that results in a hyperkalemic distal RTA. Carbonic anhydrase inhibitors (acetazolamide) inhibit the hydrolysis of luminal carbonic acid to H_2O and CO_2. This impairs HCO_3^- reabsorption, resulting in a normal anion gap metabolic acidosis.

Elevated anion gap acidoses may be separated into five categories: (1) ketoacidosis, (2) lactic acidosis, (3) renal insufficiency, (4) exogenous toxins, and (5) miscellaneous. These acidoses are often seen in the emergency department. Table 30–3 outlines the pathogenesis and clinical manifestations of these common disorders.

Ketoacidosis

The production of ketones (β-hydroxybutyrate, acetoacetate, and acetone) is the hallmark of diabetic, alcoholic, and starvation ketoacidosis. Ketoacids rapidly dissociate into hydrogen ions and ketones (unmeasured anions), resulting in an anion gap acidosis. The diagnosis of ketoacidosis is based on finding a metabolic acidosis and serum ketones. The severity of the ketoacidosis cannot be followed by serum ketone measurements because β-hydroxybutyrate is not measured by the laboratory or bedside test. In addition, the ratio of β-hydroxybutyrate to acetoacetate increases in conditions causing hypoxia or tissue ischemia. Paradoxically, when the patient begins to improve clinically and these conditions are reversed, an increase in measured ketones may be noted despite clinical improvement. This is from the conversion of β-hydroxybutyrate to measurable acetoacetate.

Diabetes mellitus is the most common cause of ketoacidosis. It usually occurs in juvenile-onset diabetics with little if any endogenous insulin. The lack of insulin causes an overproduction and undermetabolism of glucose and ketoacids. A history of chronic

TABLE 30–3. Common Anion Gap Metabolic Acidoses: Anions Involved and Diagnosis

Disorder	Anion	Diagnosis
Ketoacidosis		
Diabetic	Acetoacetate (AcAc)	Elevated glucose (less than 350 mg/dl in 10–15% of cases)
	β-hydroxybutyrate (βHB)	Decreased pH, ketones—βHB to AcAc ratio up to 8:1
Alcoholic	Predominantly βHB, smaller amount AcAc	Alcoholism, binge drinking, starvation, decreased pH, ketones—βHB to AcAc ratio up to 14:1
Starvation	AcAc, βHB	Decreased intake, $HCO_3^- \geq 18$
Lactic Acidosis	Lactic acid	Clinical setting with or without hypoxia
Renal Failure	Sulfates, phosphates, other organic acids	Usually Cr > 4 mg/dl; acidosis may be more severe in acute renal failure due to increased catabolic rate
Toxins		
Salicylate	Salicylate, lactate, ketones	Mixed acid-base, salicylate level
Methanol	Formate	Intoxicated, visual and gastrointestinal symptoms, optic nerve swelling and erythema, osmolal gap
Ethylene glycol	Glycolate	Intoxicated
	Glyoxalate	Osmolal gap (serious disease can occur without gap)
	Oxalate	Calcium oxalate crystals in urine
Paraldehyde	Unknown	Characteristic breath, sedation
Miscellaneous		
Hyperosmolar coma	Unknown	Increased glucose, absent or small amount of ketones

excessive alcohol intake, abdominal pain, and protracted vomiting is elicited from most patients with alcoholic ketoacidosis. Ethanol inhibits gluconeogenesis and promotes lipolysis. This process, in association with decreased caloric intake and a secondary lowering of the insulin level, promotes accelerated ketogenesis. Alcoholic ketoacidosis can be associated with lactic acidosis and metabolic alkalosis, from vomiting and volume depletion, to create a complex mixed acid-base disorder. Almost one-half of these patients present alkalemic. Prolonged starvation in the nonalcoholic patient results in a mild ketoacidosis. The plasma HCO_3^- is usually above 18 mEq/L.

Lactic Acidosis

The most common form of elevated anion gap metabolic acidosis is lactic acidosis. Lactate is a metabolic end product of anaerobic glycolysis. It is in equilibrium with pyruvate. The major determinants of lactate concentration are the redox state of the cell and the pyruvate concentration. A presumptive diagnosis of lactic acidosis is made when serum lactate concentrations of greater than 4 mM are found in association with acidemia. Causes of lactic acidosis can be divided into those with overt tissue hypoxia (type A) and those with clinically inapparent tissue hypoxia (type B). These are listed in Table 30–4.

Renal Insufficiency

Early in renal failure, there is a hyperchloremic metabolic acidosis secondary to impaired ammonia excretion and a variable deficiency in bicarbonate reabsorption. As failure advances, there is impaired phosphate, sulfate, and organic anion excretion leading to an increased anion gap. Generally, the anion gap does not begin to rise until the glomerular

TABLE 30–4. Causes of Lactic Acidosis

Type A: Overt Tissue Hypoxia	Type B: Inapparent Tissue Hypoxia
Shock states	Ischemic bowel
Congestive heart failure	Diabetes mellitus
Hypoxia	Uremia
Anemia	Hepatic failure
Carbon monoxide poisoning	Seizures
	Leukemia
	Hereditary metabolic defects
	Drugs*

*Phenformin, ethanol, fructose, streptozotocin, isoniazid, iron, cyanide, nitroprusside.

filtration rate drops to below 20 ml per minute and the creatinine is greater than 4 mg/dl. The bicarbonate level is usually lowered into the 16 to 20 mEq/L range.

Exogenous Toxins

Ingested toxins are often causes of metabolic acidosis. (See Chapters 19 and 20.) Salicylate intoxication may occur secondary to attempted overdose or as a side effect of therapy for rheumatologic disorders. Levels above 30 mg/dl are toxic but correlate poorly with symptoms. In children, metabolic acidosis develops early and is the major acid-base disorder. In contrast, adults exhibit a mixed acid-base disturbance, with respiratory alkalosis predominating. Early symptoms include nausea, vertigo, and tinnitus.

Methanol is found in windshield wiper solution, fuel line de-icer, paint thinners, and an assortment of industrial solvents. It is occasionally substituted for ethanol in illicit alcohol production. It is metabolized by alcohol dehydrogenase to its toxic metabolites formaldehyde and formic acid. Clinical manifestations include abdominal pain, nausea, vomiting, and visual disturbances ranging from blurred vision to blindness. The appearance of symptoms may have a latent period of 12 to 72 hours due to the timelag in metabolism. Simultaneous ingestion of ethanol will delay the onset of toxicity, as both methanol and ethanol are metabolized by alcohol dehydrogenase.

Ingestion of ethylene glycol, present in antifreeze and lacquer, is associated with central nervous system dysfunction, cardiovascular collapse, respiratory failure, severe metabolic acidosis, and renal failure. Toxicity is from its metabolites, glycolic and glyoxylic acids. As in methanol poisoning, the initial degradation by alcohol dehydrogenase can be slowed by ethanol. A clue to the diagnosis of ethylene glycol poisoning is the presence of monohydrate and dihydrate calcium oxalate crystals in the urine of 50% to 75% of patients. Methanol and ethylene glycol are among the rare causes of an anion gap above 50 mEq/L.

Metabolic Alkalosis

It is useful to divide the causes of metabolic alkalosis into two major subgroups: saline-responsive and saline-resistant (Table 30–5), based on history, volume status, and response to therapy. Urine chloride concentrations are required only occasionally in the diagnostic evaluation.

Saline-Responsive

A saline-responsive metabolic alkalosis is maintained by volume and chloride deficits. Intravascular volume depletion is such a powerful stimulant that the kidneys sacrifice acid-base homeostasis to maintain plasma volume. Reduction of extracellular volume results in avid renal sodium conservation. Sodium is transported with bicarbonate because of the relative unavailability of chloride, accelerating the rate of bicarbonate reabsorption, thereby sustaining the alkalosis. In saline-responsive conditions, the urinary chloride

TABLE 30–5. Classification of Metabolic Alkalosis

Saline-Responsive (uCl<10 mEq/L)	Saline-Resistant (uCl<10 mEq/L)
Gastrointestinal disorders	Mineralocorticoid excess
Vomiting	Hyperaldosteronism
Nasogastric suctioning	Cushing's syndrome
Chloride diarrhea	Licorice ingestion
Villous adenoma	Bartter's syndrome
Diuretic therapy	Severe hypokalemia
Cystic fibrosis	
Posthypercapnic	
Alkali administration	
Nonreabsorbable anion	
Refeeding alkalosis*	
Hypercalcemic/hypoparathyroid*	

*Classified as saline-resistant by some workers despite extracellular volume contraction.

concentration remains less than 10 mEq/L, unless diuretic action is still present. Sodium chloride replacement corrects the metabolic alkalosis.

Gastrointestinal disturbances can produce metabolic alkalosis either by loss of gastric contents or by diarrhea that is unusually rich in chloride. Vomiting or nasogastric suction can result in significant H^+, chloride, and volume losses. The loss of H^+ is not offset by HCO_3^- elimination, because of volume depletion. Chloride diarrhea is a rare congenital syndrome arising from a defect in intestinal chloride reabsorption, resulting in volume depletion and significant chloride losses. Occasionally, villous adenoma will result in a diarrhea with elevated chloride concentrations and secondary metabolic alkalosis, although diarrhea-induced metabolic acidosis is more common in this disease. All diuretics, except those that specifically block bicarbonate reabsorption (acetazolamide) or acid excretion (spironolactone and triamterene), can result in a metabolic alkalosis. This is due to renal $NaCl^-$ loss, enhanced acid excretion secondary to increased delivery of sodium to the distal tubule, and volume depletion. Cystic fibrosis can produce significant volume and chloride losses in the patient's sweat. Posthypercapnic alkalosis occurs as a consequence of delayed renal adjustment to the abrupt respiratory correction of chronic hypercapnia. Administration of the nonreabsorbable anions carbenicillin or penicillin to volume-depleted patients can produce an alkalosis secondary to enhanced distal renal acidification. In addition, hypercalcemia without hyperthyroidism increases renal HCO_3^- reabsorption. The mechanism underlying the elevation of HCO_3^- seen during carbohydrate feeding after starvation has been uncertain, although metabolism of ketones to bicarbonate and extracellular volume contraction play an important role.

Excessive bicarbonate administration can result in a metabolic alkalosis, if there is volume depletion with diminished renal reabsorption of bicarbonate, or renal failure. It may occur from oral antacid therapy or parenteral administration of the citrate anticoagulant in transfused blood. Milk-alkali syndrome occurs in patients ingesting large amounts of calcium-containing antacids. In time, mild renal failure develops, limiting bicarbonate excretion and promoting the maintenance of the metabolic alkalosis. In these disorders, removal of the bicarbonate load is usually curative.

Saline-Resistant

Maintenance of metabolic alkalosis in the saline-resistant disorders is due to mineralocorticoid-induced stimulation of distal tubular acid secretion and the regeneration of bicarbonate. A similar process can occur with severe hypokalemia (less than 2 mEq/L). Increased ammoniagenesis and chloruresis result in regeneration of bicarbonate. Patients with saline-resistant disorders are neither volume nor chloride deficient; consequently, urinary chloride concentrations remain greater than 10 to 20 mEq/L, and therapy with sodium chloride is ineffective. Significant potassium depletion occurs in both the saline-responsive and saline-resistant disorders.

Primary hyperaldosteronism, Cushing's syndrome, and licorice ingestion produce metabolic alkalosis, hypokalemia, and hypertension secondary to excessive mineralocorticoid activity. The glycyrrhizic acid in licorice has a mineralocorticoid action. Bartter's syndrome is a rare condition found in children, characterized by increased renin and aldosterone production owing to hyperplasia of the juxtaglomerular apparatus. The increased secretion of aldosterone results in a metabolic alkalosis, yet hypertension is usually absent. Profound hypokalemia can produce a metabolic alkalosis with increased urinary chloride concentrations, without evidence of increased mineralocorticoid effect.

PROBLEM 1 The patient remained poorly responsive. Vital signs: blood pressure 90 mm Hg/palpation and pulse 115 beats/min. The additional laboratory data returned: BUN 9 mg/dl; creatinine 0.8 mg/dl; glucose 100 mg/dl; serum osmols 340 mOsm/L; ethyl alcohol 0 mg/dl; ketones none detectable. Urine analysis is unremarkable. Lactate level and complete toxicology screen pending. An electrocardiogram showed a sinus tachycardia without acute ischemic changes.

The extremely high measured serum osmolality cannot be overlooked, and must be compared with a calculated osmolality. In this case, the calculated osmolality is 286 mOsm/L. The osmolal gap is 340 − 286 = 54 mOsm/L. The osmolar gap is greater than 20 mOsm. Therefore, some substance is creating an anion gap metabolic acidosis, as well as a significant osmolal gap. The two most common causes of this are methanol and ethylene glycol.

PROBLEM 2 The patient's ECG and abdominal films were completed. Electrocardiogram showed a normal sinus rhythm with prolonged QT interval. The abdominal films showed a nonspecific ileus.

Of major concern is this patient's history of abdominal surgery and her persistent nausea and vomiting. She is at risk for abdominal adhesions causing an intestinal obstruction. The radiographs of her abdomen demonstrated a nonspecific ileus consistent with gastroenteritis. The two processes responsible for her metabolic alkalosis are vomiting and diuretic therapy. They result in loss of acid to generate a metabolic alkalosis and induce volume depletion, which maintains the alkalotic state. Her clinical history, physical examination, and laboratory results pointed to a saline-responsive metabolic alkalosis. Urine chloride measurements were not required in the diagnostic evaluation of this patient.

PRINCIPLES OF MANAGEMENT

Treatment of acidosis and alkalosis is directed toward the underlying causative disorder and correction of the patient's acid-base disturbance. General principles of management include replacement of electrolyte and water deficits. This may often be sufficient for correction or improvement of the acid-base disturbance.

Metabolic Acidosis

If the acidemia is causing serious organ dysfunction, the patient's acidosis warrants correction. Bicarbonate therapy is reserved for severe organic acidoses or those not easily reversed. Lactic or toxic acidemia generally requires treatment when the pH drops below 7.20 or the HCO_3^- falls below 10 mEq/L. In contrast, patients with ketoacidosis may not require bicarbonate therapy unless the metabolic acidosis is extremely severe with pH less than 7.1 or HCO_3^- less than 6 mEq/L, assuming there is no compromise of cardiac function. As the ketosis is reversed, the patients metabolize ketones to endogenous alkali, rapidly correcting their acid-base disorder. Chronic metabolic acidosis, e.g., in renal failure, is usually treated with supplemental bicarbonate when the HCO_3^- drops below 17 mEq/L, to prevent skeletal demineralization.

1. The goal of therapy in acidemia is to raise arterial pH above 7.2. Unfortunately, there is no perfect formula for estimating bicarbonate doses. One commonly used formula is:

$$NaHCO_3 \text{ dose in mEq} = (\text{desired } [HCO_3^-] - \text{observed } [HCO_3^-]) \times 50\% \text{ of body weight in kg}$$

   The desired HCO_3^- is usually in the 12 to 15 mEq/L range. This target avoids alkalemia during correction, from organic anions being metabolized into HCO_3^- and persistent compensatory hyperventilation. One-half of this dose is given initially (full dose for cardiac arrest), and further replacement is based on repeat laboratory testing. The formula is a rough guideline and tends to underestimate bicarbonate replacement in severe acidosis, i.e., pH less than 7.1, $HCO_3^- < 5$ mEq/L. In this case, 80% of body weight is used to estimate the bicarbonate space in the calculation.

2. Bolus therapy is recommended only for those with severe acidosis or when there is hemodynamic compromise. Patients with less life-threatening acidosis may be treated with an intravenous bicarbonate infusion. Two to three ampules of $NaHCO_3$ can be added to 1 liter of D_5W. Hypernatremia, hyperosmolality, volume overload, hypokalemia, and post-treatment alkalosis can complicate treatment of metabolic acidosis with HCO_3^-. A 50-ml ampule of $NaHCO_3$ has 50 mEq of sodium. This is a sodium concentration of 1000 mEq/L. Normal saline has 150 mEq/L. Symptoms of hypocalcemia may occur secondary to a reduction in the ionized calcium fraction, although the total serum calcium level will remain unchanged. Paradoxical cerebral spinal fluid acidosis after HCO_3^- administration exists but does not influence therapeutic decisions.

3. Specific therapy is directed to the underlying pathologic process.
   For example:
   a. Diabetic ketoacidosis is treated with insulin, volume repletion, and electrolyte replacement, especially potassium. (See Chapter 26.)
   b. Alcoholic ketoacidosis is treated with volume, glucose, and phosphate repletion. (See Chapter 20.)
   c. Methanol or ethylene glycol poisoning is treated with ethyl alcohol to block conversion to toxic metabolites. (Specific treatment guidelines are given in Chapters 19 and 20.)
   d. Severe persistent lactic acidosis may require hemodialysis against an HCO_3^- dialysate.

Metabolic Alkalosis

Therapy of metabolic alkalosis is directed at the primary problem and the subsequent process maintaining the disorder.

   1. The saline responsive disorders are treated with saline (0.9 NS) volume replacement.
   2. The saline-resistant disorders, with excessive mineralocorticoid activity, can be treated with aldosterone antagonists, spironolactone (300 to 600 mg/day), or triamterene (200 to 300 mg/day).
   3. Potassium depletion is almost universally present in both forms. Supplements are administered as the chloride salt.
   4. Persistent gastric acid losses can be diminished by the use of H_2-antagonists.
   5. In patients in renal failure with neuromuscular irritability or cardiotoxicity, a pH of greater than 7.55 is treated with dialysis with a low HCO_3^- bath or acid administration. Parenteral HCl may be administered via central vein as a 0.1 to 0.2 M solution, infusing up to 20 mEq per hour. Ammonium chloride administration may result in ammonium

toxicity, and arginine chloride can cause significant hyperkalemia. These acidifying agents are used infrequently.

6. In life-threatening situations caused by severe alkalemia (pH > 7.6), the P_{CO_2} may be allowed to rise if ventilatory control is established and oxygenation is adequate. This may be accomplished by volume repletion, sedation, and, if necessary, paralysis and mechanical ventilation.

PROBLEM 1 The nurse at last was able to contact the patient's family by phone. They had been looking for him, and were concerned for his welfare because he had been seen drinking some gasoline "drying agents" with his beer a day earlier. He had been hospitalized for a methanol ingestion about a year ago.

Laboratory investigation confirmed the suspicion of a metabolic acidosis and directed the differential diagnosis to a severe, elevated anion gap, nonketotic, osmolal gap metabolic acidosis with an entirely normal urine analysis. Combined with the initial history of alcohol ingestion, abdominal pain, and papilledema, it appeared the patient's problems were secondary to methanol ingestion. This was supported by the phone conversation with the family. The ethanol ingestion by the patient had been metabolized by the time he returned to the emergency department. The time lag in onset of severe symptoms may have been extended due to the initial ingestion of both methanol and ethanol. The preferential degradation of ethanol over methanol served as a temporary protective mechanism, inhibiting the formation of methanol's toxic metabolites.

The laboratory confirmation of methanol ingestion at a cost of several hundred dollars was somewhat more expensive than the cost of the phone call. After immediate supportive care had been accomplished, it was necessary to correct the acidosis and to prevent the production of additional acids.

DISPOSITION AND FOLLOW-UP

Admission

Essentially all patients with significant acid-base disorders are admitted for further evaluation and treatment.

Admission to Critical Care Unit

Many patients admitted to the hospital will be monitored and have serial laboratory and clinical assessments in a critical care unit. Conditions appropriate for this setting include, but are not limited to:

1. Any finding of organ dysfunction, causing or resulting from the acid-base imbalance—for example, altered mental status, hemodynamic instability, or renal insufficiency.
2. Extremes of age.
3. Initial laboratory values of pH less than 7.1, more than 7.6, or HCO_3^- less than 10 mEq/L. Elevated HCO_3^- levels are usually the result of chronic compensation for P_{CO_2} retention. Acute increases of HCO_3^- over 35 to 40 mEq/L are appropriate for admission. These increases are almost always due to vomiting.
4. Patients with ingested exogenous toxins.

Discharge

Rarely, a patient with a known underlying disorder causing a recurrent acid-base imbalance may be treated and discharged from the emergency department. This might include a patient with a mild (pH > 7.2) diabetic ketoacidosis or alkalosis associated with diuretic use requiring volume and potassium repletion only.

At the time of discharge, such patients should have:

1. Their primary physician contacted and an appointment made for follow-up care.
2. A basic understanding of what happened and how their medications may help or hurt them.
3. A support system that can check on their status between the time of discharge and the primary physician appointment.

PROBLEM 1 An ethanol bolus and infusion are started, and the nephrologist is contacted for dialysis plans. A methanol level of 50 mg/dl was received after the patient had been transferred to the intensive care unit.

The delay in therapy began with an inadequate history during the first visit to the emergency department. The setting of chronic alcoholism plus police custody may result in a less than complete evaluation. Unfortunately, these patients are the ones requiring the most attention, including outside phone calls for additional information. The care during the second visit was appropriate though the ethanol infusion may have been started earlier. The severity of the acidosis and history pointed to a metabolized toxin causing the problem. Methanol and ethylene glycol were the most likely sources.

PROBLEM 2 This patient was admitted for inpatient hydration after 3 hours in the emergency department when 2 liters of isotonic fluid and 40 mEq of KCl intravenously failed to entirely resolve her symptoms. One day later she was no longer vomiting, and electrolytes measured sodium 140 mEq/L; potassium 3.5 mEq/L; chloride 102 mEq/L; bicarbonate 24 mEq/L; BUN 12 mg/dl; and creatinine 1.2 mg/dl.

DOCUMENTATION

1. History to include problems that initiated and maintained the acid-base imbalance.
2. Pertinent past medical history.
3. Medications.
4. Physical findings, particularly related to volume status.
5. Laboratory results.
6. Course of care, e.g., fluid and volume given, electrolyte replacement. Response to treatment, including repeated vital signs. Repeat laboratory values.
7. Diagnosis.
8. Disposition/follow-up.
9. Consultations.

SUMMARY

- Patients with acid-base disorders often present with nonspecific symptoms. Frequently, the only clue to the presence of an acid-base disturbance is an abnormality of the vital signs.
- The diagnosis of an acid-base disturbance depends on recognition of the clinical settings in which it may occur. Confirmatory laboratory studies are then required to support the clinical impression.
- A consistent step-wise analysis of the laboratory data is the best method for understanding these disorders.

- The adequacy of respiratory compromise in metabolic acidosis can be evaluated using the formula:

$$\text{Expected } P_{CO_2} = [1.5 \times (HCO_3^-) + 8] \pm 2$$

- The limit of respiratory compensation is approximately 10 mm Hg.
- The differential diagnosis of metabolic acidosis can be divided into groups based on the state of unmeasured anions (normal or elevated). The anion gap equation is:

$$\text{Anion gap} = Na^+ - (Cl^- + HCO_3^-)$$

- The influence of alkalemia or acidemia on the potassium level must be anticipated as corrective therapy is initiated.
- Small-molecular-weight, nonpolar toxins, such as methanol and ethylene glycol, result in an elevated anion gap, osmolal gap metabolic acidosis.
- Potassium depletion is almost universally present in metabolic alkalosis, and supplements should be administered as the chloride salt.
- When treatment is indicated in metabolic alkalosis, the saline-responsive disorders require saline and the saline-resistant disorders need to be treated with aldosterone antagonists.

BIBLIOGRAPHY

Texts

1. Cogan MG, Rector FC Jr: Acid-base disorders. *In* Brenner BM, Rector FC Jr (eds): The Kidney (3rd ed). Philadelphia, Saunders, 1986.
2. Maxwell M, Kleeman L, Narins RG: Clinical Disorders of Fluid and Electrolyte Metabolism (4th ed). New York, McGraw-Hill, 1987.
3. Schrier RW: Renal and Electrolyte Disorders (3rd ed). Boston, Little, Brown, 1986.

Journal Articles

1. Arbus GS: An in vivo acid-base nomogram for clinical use. Can Med Assoc J 109:291, 1973.
2. Du Bose TD: Clinical approach to patients with acid-base disorders. Med Clin North Am 67(4), 799, 1983.
3. Emmett M, Narins RG: Clinical use of the anion gap. Medicine 56:38, 1977.
4. Jacobsen D, McMartin KE: Methanol and ethylene glycol poisonings—mechanism of toxicity, clinical course, diagnosis and treatment. Med Toxicol 1(5):309, 1986.
5. Jehle D, Harchelroad FP: Bicarbonate. Emerg Med Clin North Am 4(1):145, 1986.
6. Kreisberg RA: Lactate homeostasis and lactic acidosis. Ann Intern Med 92:227, 1980.
7. Lawson NW, Butler CH III, Ray CT: Alkalosis and cardiac arrhythmias. Anesth Analg 52:951, 1973.
8. Narins RG, Cohen JJ: Bicarbonate therapy for organic acidosis: The case for its continued use. Ann Intern Med 106:615, 1987.
9. Winter SD, Pearson JR, Gabow PA, et al: The fall of the serum anion gap. Arch Intern Med 150:311, 1990.

SECTION TEN

DISORDERS OF THE HEAD AND NECK

CHAPTER 31

EPISTAXIS

STEVEN M. JOYCE, M.D.

PROBLEM 1 A 70 year old male arrived in the emergency department complaining of recurrent nosebleeds. At first the bleeding had been controlled by direct pressure, but by the time of arrival the bleeding was copious.

PROBLEM 2 A 17 year old female had been injured in a motor vehicle accident. She arrived by ambulance supine on a backboard with a cervical collar in place. Her face was swollen and her nose asymmetric. Bright red blood was being suctioned from her nose and mouth.

QUESTIONS TO CONSIDER

1. Is the patient's airway threatened by the bleeding? If so, how should it be managed?
2. Is the blood loss significant? Does it require immediate treatment?
3. What initial measures are necessary to control bleeding prior to performing a detailed history and physical examination?
4. What is the sequence for examining the nasal cavity and identifying the bleeding site?
5. What are the causes of epistaxis, and how is the differential diagnosis attained quickly?
6. Is there a sequence to optimize treatment?
7. What are the possible complications of treatment, particularly nasal packing?
8. What are the indications for hospitalization?

INTRODUCTION

Epistaxis presents a difficult challenge for the emergency physician. If severe, it can lead to hypovolemia and shock. The patient is usually very anxious and may be orthostatic from blood loss or nauseated from swallowed blood. Examining a small cavity that is difficult to access must be performed expeditiously. The process is time consuming in a time-limited setting. Fortunately, most epistaxis is neither severe nor difficult to treat, but the emergency physician must always be prepared for the worst.

The exact incidence of epistaxis is uncertain, and only about 6% of patients with epistaxis seek medical attention. One estimate is that 15% of the population experiences epistaxis each year. It is more common in the winter months and is often associated with upper respiratory infection. About 10% of maxillofacial injuries are accompanied by epistaxis. Most nosebleeds are isolated incidents, but about 4% of the population has recurrent episodes in a given year. Death from epistaxis is rare. Most cases are treated with local pressure, and only a few require immediate operative intervention.

Proper management of epistaxis requires knowledge of basic nasal vascular anatomy. The blood supply to the nose originates from branches of both the external and internal carotid arteries (Fig. 31–1). The mucosa of the anterior-inferior portion of the nasal septum is the site of an anastomotic plexus of vessels supplied by the nasopalatine, descending palatine, and anterior and posterior ethmoidal arteries. This location is known

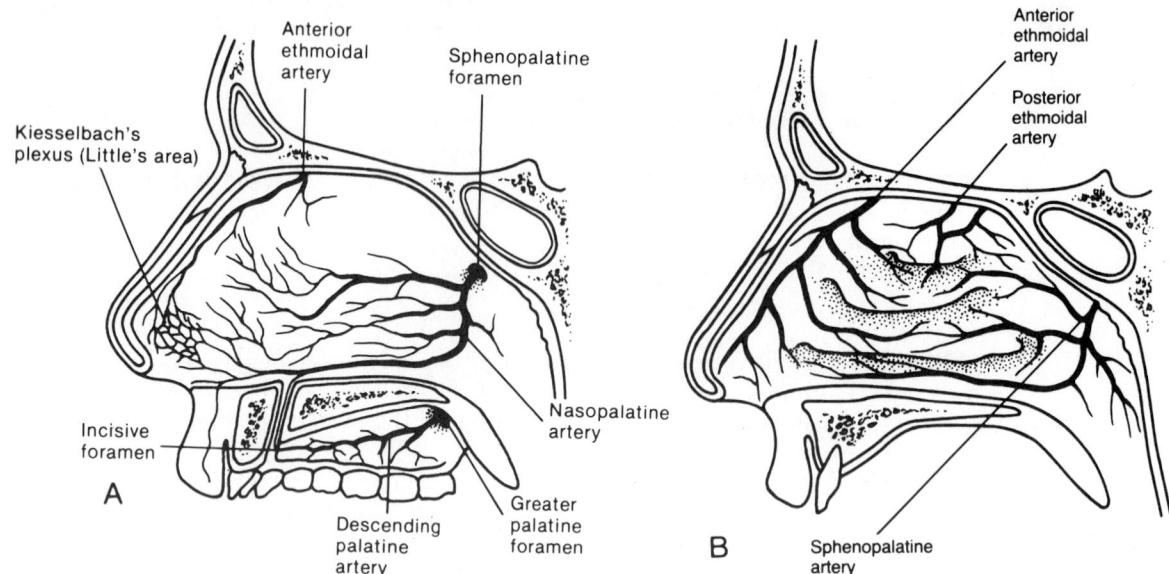

FIGURE 31–1. A, Arterial blood supply to the nasal septum. B, Arterial blood supply to the lateral wall of the nose. (From Peretta LJ, Denslow BL, Brown CG: Emergency evaluation and management of epistaxis. Emerg Clin North Am 5(2): 265–277, 1987.)

as Kiesselbach's plexus or Little's area, and it is the site of 90% of anterior nosebleeds. Venous drainage parallels the arterial supply in this area. A venous plexus at the posterior portion of the inferior turbinate is a common site of posterior epistaxis. The fleshy portion of the nose beyond the nasal bones is compressible by external pressure. The posterior portion of the nasal cavity is not, making bleeding control difficult in this area.

PREHOSPITAL CARE

Assessment of airway and hemodynamic status, volume resuscitation as necessary, external compression of the nose, and reassurance of the patient are the major goals of prehospital care of a patient with epistaxis. Many patients may be asked to travel by private car to the hospital depending on their condition.

INITIAL APPROACH IN THE EMERGENCY DEPARTMENT

Most patients with epistaxis are alert and able to protect their airway by expectorating blood, and they do not have significant blood loss. However, some patients are unstable and need immediate attention. The nurse and physician will intervene when the patient arrives. Their activity includes the following:

    1. History. What is the length and severity of the episode? Are there any underlying bleeding disorders?

    2. Airway assessment. Is the patient able to protect the airway? Airway management progresses as necessary. Is the airway compromised by pharyngeal clots? Clots may be removed manually, by suction, or by forceps.

    3. Circulation. Incipient hypovolemic shock may be recognized by evaluation of the vital signs, mental status, skin color, and capillary refill. If the vital signs are stable and the patient can tolerate it, orthostatic pulse and blood pressure are measured. Signs of hypovolemia mandate immediate placement of an intravenous line and crystalloid infusion (see Chap. 4). Blood for hemoglobin, hematocrit, and transfusion cross-matching is sent to the laboratory at this time.

4. Bleeding control. In most cases, patients are stable hemodynamically on arrival. They may become unstable if the bleeding is not controlled. Anterior bleeding is best controlled by having the patient sit upright and apply manual squeezing pressure to the entire fleshy part of the nose for 10 to 15 minutes. This maneuver allows time for equipment to be set up and in some cases stops the bleeding.

Bleeding that is not controlled by this simple maneuver may be posterior in origin. A decision is necessary at this juncture: Is the bleeding severe enough to require immediate control, or can a quick inspection for the bleeding site be made? If the former, a nasal catheter with 30-ml balloon (Epistat) is placed to control the bleeding while the patient's condition is stabilized (Fig. 31-2).

5. Cervical spine. Patients presenting with epistaxis from trauma are evaluated for cervical spine injury. Cervical immobilization is applied if the mechanism of injury or symptoms warrant it.

The above measures will be necessary in only a few situations. Because patients are often anxious, they may not accurately estimate the amount of blood loss. Early assessment of the patient's respiratory and cardiovascular status will prevent subsequent interruption of the nasal inspection and treatment procedures by a patient who is too dizzy to sit up or cooperate. Such assessment and reassurance also establish the necessary rapport to allow a complete and sometimes uncomfortable inspection of the patient's nasal cavity.

PROBLEM 1 The 70 year old patient was not orthostatic; his blood pressure was 180/120mm Hg, pulse 110 beats/min, and respirations 24/min. He was sitting in the examination chair, pinching his nose as instructed. He reported that he could feel blood "running down the back of his throat" and proved this by periodically spitting blood into an emesis basin.

The patient is hypertensive and tachycardic. This may be due to anxiety. Emergency airway or hemodynamic support is not necessary at this point. Efforts directed toward calming the patient will be well rewarded.

DATA GATHERING

History

Present Illness. Was the epistaxis *spontaneous* in *onset*, or was it induced by some *mechanical trauma*? Common causes of mechanical disruption of the nasal mucosa include drying from upper respiratory infection or low humidity, fingernails or other foreign bodies, increased vascular pressure from sneezing, or a direct blow to the nose. Is this

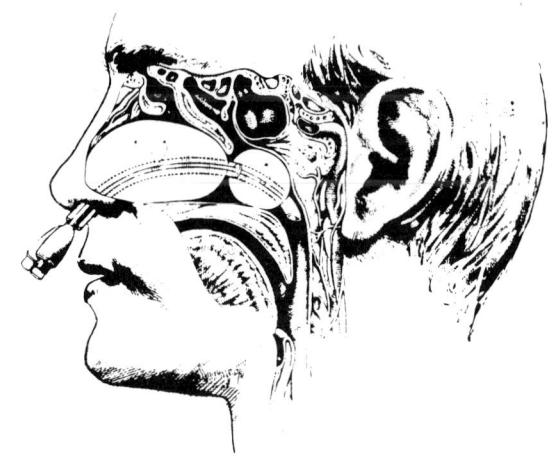

FIGURE 31–2. The balloon tamponade device serves as both an anterior and posterior pack. It is easily inserted and is often successful for the temporary control of posterior epistaxis in the emergency department. The balloon shown here is the Epistat balloon. (Courtesy of Xomed Inc, Jacksonville, FL. Reproduced with permission from Abelson TI, Witt WJ: Otolaryngologic procedures. In Roberts JR, Hedges JR (eds): Clinical Procedures in Emergency Medicine. Philadelphia, W.B. Saunders, 1985.)

an *isolated incident*, or does the patient suffer from *recurrent epistaxis*? What *treatment*, if any, was tried at *home*?

Past Medical History. Is there a history of *blood dyscrasias, bleeding disorders,* or *easy bruising* or *bleeding? Recent illnesses,* especially upper respiratory infections, may be relevant.

Medication or Drug Use. Queries should be made about *medications* that may affect hemostasis, such as aspirin, other platelet inhibitors, anticoagulants, or alcohol. Cocaine may alter the structural integrity of the nasal mucosa.

Physical Examination

General Findings. A directed physical examination is done to search for signs of bleeding disorders—specifically, mucosal or cutaneous purpura or petechiae, lymphadenopathy, or hepatosplenomegaly.

Head, Eyes, Ears, Nose, and Throat. In cases of epistaxis caused by facial trauma, careful palpation of the orbital rims, nasal bridge, and cheekbones is performed. Extraocular muscle function and facial symmetry are assessed. Findings may suggest nasal bone fractures or other injuries such as orbital floor blowout, tripod, or LeFort fractures.

Nasal Examination. All the equipment needed to identify the bleeding site is readied before beginning the examination including:

1. Protective coverings for both the physician and the patient. The nasal examination of a patient with epistaxis involves exposure to at least two body fluids. Thus, full blood precautions are indicated including gown, gloves, a mask, and eye shield (see Chap. 18). The patient's clothes may be protected with a hospital gown, towels, or protective drape.
2. Equipment for inspection of the nasal cavity. The minimum equipment needed includes:
   a. Headlamp or head mirror with light source
   b. Nasal speculum of appropriate size
   c. 5 to 8 Fr suction tip connected to suction at midrange
   d. Bayonet forceps
   e. Vasoconstrictor and anesthetic
      (1) 4% to 5% cocaine topical solution on cotton pledget *or*
      (2) 4% lidocaine topical solution with 1:1000 epinephrine or 0.5% to 1.0% phenylephrine added
3. Technique
   a. The patient is positioned sitting with the emesis basin held below the chin; the face is elevated to the examiner's eye level providing that the patient can tolerate sitting upright and the cervical spine is stable.
   b. The nose is emptied of clots using suction or forceps or by having the patient blow and then inhale through the nose. The "sniff" may move a clot into the oropharynx and cause gagging. The patient is warned of this happening, and an emesis basin is readily available (in the patient's lap).
   c. Using the nasal speculum, the nasal septum is observed for the presence of a septal hematoma. In external nasal trauma, the nasal bones including the septum may be fractured, causing not only epistaxis but occasionally accumulation of blood beneath the mucosa. Pressure from the hematoma may result in septal necrosis and nasal deformity if it is not recognized and drained.
   d. An attempt is made to see the bleeding site by suctioning blood while holding the nostril open. The nose is examined for bleeding from the anterior septum, roof, and floor of the nasal cavity. One starts on the side from which the bleeding may have originated, but both sides are inspected.
      Often this examination will reveal a discrete bleeding site within reach of the catheter tip. If so, treatment may begin. If a discrete bleeding site is not found, a

diffuse or posterior bleed must be suspected. One method of differentiating a posterior bleed from an anterior bleed is to have the patient blow his nose, sit forward, and apply manual pressure to the nostrils while the examiner observes for blood running down the back of his pharynx. Continued bleeding in the posterior pharynx with adequate anterior pressure indicates a posterior bleed.

e. Vasoconstrictor and anesthetic solution saturated on cotton pledgets is applied against the suspected bleeding site. The solution decreases the bleeding, shrinks the nasal mucosa, and decreases the discomfort of the examination. Pledgets are inserted deeply into the nasal cavity, and additional pledgets are placed over them to maintain their position. The patient is asked to pinch the nose for 5 to 10 minutes.

Cocaine, epinephrine, and phenylephrine may be absorbed to some degree, and the patient's blood pressure is checked during this time. If a dangerous elevation in blood pressure occurs, the pledgets are removed, and the blood pressure is measured again. Nasal packing is appropriate if the bleeding continues after the blood pressure has come down.

f. After 5 to 10 minutes, the pledgets are removed. Often the bleeding has ceased. The nose is reexamined to confirm the suspected bleeding site, usually a small defect or papule in Kiesselbach's plexus (Fig. 31–1). Foreign bodies, tumors, and mucosal defects due to fractures are more easily visualized at this time. If the bleeding is not stopped, reapplication of pledgets, nasal packing, or balloon tamponade may be considered.

PROBLEM 1 The 70 year old patient was found to have a small defect in the septal mucosa that was actively bleeding. After a 10-minute application of 5% cocaine-soaked pledgets, the site was visible as a 2-mm papule.

PROBLEM 2 The 17 year old trauma victim was having a difficult time. Bleeding was brisk from both nares, and it was difficult to keep the patient from aspirating. Bilateral balloon nasal catheters were placed to control the bleeding. Fortunately, the rest of the physical examination showed only minor abrasions and contusions, and the patient's cervical spine radiographs were normal. When the nasal balloon catheters were cautiously removed, a nonbleeding mucosal laceration high in the left nasal cavity was visible. This was most probably associated with a fracture and appeared to be too extensive to be treated by cautery.

DECISION PRIORITIES AND PRELIMINARY DIFFERENTIAL DIAGNOSIS

1. *Is the site of bleeding located anterior or posterior?*
   Up to 90% of cases of acute epistaxis originate from the anterior nasal septum. The source of bleeding is usually visible. When the source is unclear after inspection, hematologic disorders or posterior bleeding are more likely. Posterior bleeding may be due to tumor, elevated venous pressure, or possibly hypertension or arteriosclerosis. Different researchers have found varying degrees of correlation between the presence of hypertension and the incidence of epistaxis, varying from none to significantly high.

2. *What is the most likely local cause of the bleeding?*
   Table 31–1 lists the causes of epistaxis. Mechanical and traumatic causes predominate in emergency department patients. Irritation of the mucosa from drying due to low humidity or high altitude, inflammation caused by upper respiratory infection, accidental scratches from a fingernail (epistaxis digitorum), and external blows to the nose with or without fracture are frequently seen. Altered anatomy of the septum is a common cause of recurrent epistaxis.

TABLE 31–1. Causes of Epistaxis*

I. Traumatic or Mechanical
   A. Digital (epistaxis digitorum)*
   B. External blow (with or without nasal or facial fracture)*
   C. Desiccation (winter, deviated septum)*
   D. Inflammation (upper respiratory infection, allergic rhinitis)*
   E. Foreign body (children)
   F. Septal perforation (cocaine abuse, repeated cautery, submucosal hematoma)
   G. Barotrauma (diver's squeeze, rapid altitude gain)
   H. Elevated venous pressure (sneezing, Valsalva maneuver, congestive heart failure, mitral stenosis)*
II. Tumor (juvenile angiofibroma, sinus tumors)
III. Hematologic or vascular disorders
   A. Vascular
      1. Telangiectasia
      2. Vitamin deficiency (scurvy)
      3. Hypertension or arteriosclerosis
   B. Disorders of hemostasis
      1. Thrombocytopenia (drug-induced, malignancies, other)
      2. Platelet inhibition (aspirin, NSAIDs, Von Willebrand's disease)
      3. Coagulopathy (hereditary, anticoagulants, liver or renal disease)
IV. Other
   A. Endometriosis
   B. Idiopathic (accounts for about 10% of cases of epistaxis)

*Denotes a common cause.

3. *Is this a sign of an underlying systemic problem? Especially, a hemostatic disorder?*

Hematologic disorders comprising a deficit in primary hemostasis, such as thrombocytopenia or impaired platelet function, usually cause diffuse, bilateral mucosal bleeding. Hematologic disorders are considered in persistent or recurrent epistaxis.

DIAGNOSTIC ADJUNCTS

Laboratory Studies

Hematocrit and Hemoglobin. These are measured if the history of blood loss is significant, if signs or symptoms are suggestive, or if a hematologic disorder is suspected.

Transfusion. Samples for blood type and cross-match are sent immediately when significant blood loss is either observed or suspected by hypotension, orthostasis, or falling hematocrit. Although transfusion is seldom necessary, anticipating its need will prevent unnecessary delays. An acute drop in hematocrit below 30% suggests the need for transfusion.

Clotting Studies. When diffuse or severe nasal bleeding occurs or when a hematologic disorder is suspected, a platelet count, prothrombin time, and partial thromboplastin time are indicated.

Radiologic Imaging

Plain Films. *Nasal or facial bone radiographs* may be indicated in patients with external trauma but may be delayed pending control of significant bleeding. In cases of suspected simple nasal fractures without asymmetry or obstruction, repair is often not necessary, and films may not be indicated. Complex facial fractures are sometimes best diagnosed by tomography or CT scan.

PRINCIPLES OF MANAGEMENT

The management of epistaxis is based on a logical progression of maneuvers designed to stop the bleeding quickly with the least invasive method possible in a given situation.

Often bleeding is controlled with one or two simple maneuvers. Treating the underlying cause helps prevent recurrence. In all but the simplest cases, this requires cautery of the bleeding site or some method of tamponade. Exploring the medical basis for bleeding, e.g., hypertension or hematologic disorders, is an essential part of the management plan. It cannot be forgotten after the bleeding has stopped.

Steps to control bleeding from epistaxis may be undertaken in the following order. In cases of severe and probable posterior bleeding, starred steps (*) may be skipped in favor of expedient control.

Manual Pressure. Squeezing the fleshy part of the nose against the septum while sitting upright for 10 to 15 minutes will often control simple nosebleeds at home. Recurrence after two trials warrants examination by a physician.

Application of Topical Vasoconstrictors and Anesthetics. These may actually stop the bleeding, but this effect is usually temporary. If a mucosal bleeding site can be identified, cautery is done. If not, packing is usually necessary before the effect of the drug wears off.

Cautery. Silver nitrate is the compound most commonly used for cautery. Electrocautery is another method, but it is seldom available in the emergency department. Once hemostasis is obtained by application of topical vasoconstrictors, the bleeding point may be cauterized by touching the silver nitrate applicator to it for a few (up to 20) seconds. Some authors have recommended additional cautery of the surrounding mucosa. Overzealous cautery is avoided, however, because it may lead to septal perforation, especially after multiple applications on both sides of the septum. Any form of cautery is not applied without prior anesthesia because it is painful and may induce sneezing. Cautery is contraindicated when a tumor is suspected because it may cause continued bleeding. It has little use in patients with epistaxis due to nasal fractures.

Anterior Packing. When the above measures do not control bleeding and an anterior site is suspected, the nasal cavity may be packed under experienced supervision to tamponade the bleeding site. Several materials are available:

Vaseline-Impregnated One-Half Inch Gauze. Vaseline gauge should be placed using the bayonet forceps, starting at the floor of the nasal cavity and layering superiorly until the cavity is filled (Fig. 31–3).

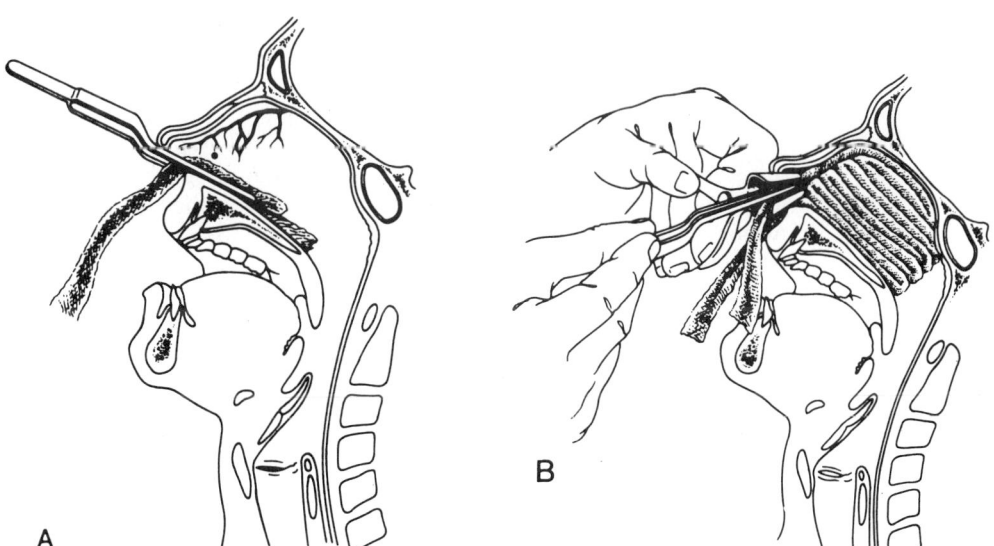

FIGURE 31–3. A, Incorrect method for placement of an anterior nasal pack. Note that one end of the nasal packing remains inside the nasal cavity. B, Correct method for the placement of a layered nasal pack. (From Peretta LJ, Denslow BL, Brown CG: Emergency evaluation and management of epistaxis. Emerg Clin North Am 5(2): 265–277, 1987.)

Absorbable Hemostatic Agents. Avitene, Oxicel, Gelfoam, Surgicel, and other similar products stimulate coagulation and are absorbable. They are especially useful in patients with diffuse epistaxis that is due to disorders of hemostasis. The mechanical irritation of gauze packing or its removal may cause recurrent hemorrhage.

Balloon Nasal Packs. Nasal packs are available commercially (e.g., Epistat) and are easily and quickly placed in position. They are not always effective. They should be coated with antibiotic ointment to make removal less traumatic (see Fig. 31–2).

Nasal packing occludes paranasal sinus ostia and may predispose to sinusitis. Prophylactic oral antibiotics, e.g., ampicillin, may be prescribed until the pack is removed in 48 to 72 hours. Some authorities recommend packing both sides of the nose to prevent septal displacement and loss of effective tamponade. This is an individual choice and not a medical standard.

Posterior Packing. When bleeding is posterior or cannot be controlled by anterior packing, the entire nasal cavity may be packed from posterior to anterior using one of several techniques.

Conventional Gauze Nasal Packs. This pack is made from a rolled gauze tampon that is drawn into the posterior nasopharynx through the mouth by means of attached silk sutures that have been tied to catheters previously passed through the nose into the pharynx. Once in place, bilateral anterior gauze packs are placed as previously described, and the sutures are secured over padding at the nostrils. The technique is somewhat cumbersome and time-consuming and is uncomfortable for the patient.

Foley Catheter Balloon Pack. A 16-Fr Foley catheter with a 30-ml balloon is passed into the pharynx, inflated with about 10 ml of saline, and withdrawn against the posterior opening of the nasal cavity. Bilateral balloons are placed for posterior epistaxis. Anterior gauze packs are placed as previously described, and the catheters are secured over padding at the nares.

Balloon Nasal Packs. Epistat, Nasostat, and others tamponade the posterior and anterior nasal cavities, some with separate balloons. They are easily and quickly placed and are thus useful in patients with severe bleeding. Supplementation with gauze packing in the roof of the nasal cavity may be necessary.

The same precautions regarding prophylaxis for sinusitis apply to posterior packs as to anterior packs. In addition, posterior packs have been associated with a high rate of complications, especially hypoventilation and hypoxemia. All patients requiring posterior packing are admitted to the hospital.

Septal Hematoma. A septal hematoma must be drained by an experienced physician. If it is left untreated, pressure on the septum may result in necrosis.

Refractory Epistaxis. When bleeding cannot be controlled despite appropriate trial of the methods described above, operative arterial ligation may be necessary. Other invasive methods such as arterial embolization have also been described. Persistent bleeding from nasal fractures may require reducing the fracture to resolve the bleeding. Admission to the otorhinolaryngology (ENT) service is mandated to stabilize the patient prior to operation.

SPECIAL CONSIDERATIONS IN PEDIATRIC PATIENTS

Nasal foreign bodies are a common cause of epistaxis in toddlers. Beads, toy parts, or beans may be found. A vasoconstrictor such as phenylephrine is applied. If able, the patient gently blows the nose with the other nostril occluded. If unsuccessful, a lubricated pediatric Foley catheter with a 5-ml balloon may be passed beyond the foreign body and the balloon gently inflated until resistance is met. The catheter is then gently withdrawn, bringing the foreign body out of the nostril. This method is probably less traumatic than the use of bayonet or "alligator" forceps and avoids the problem of aspiration if the foreign body is pushed into the pharynx. This technique, however, is used only by a physician familiar with it.

DISPOSITION AND FOLLOW-UP

Discharge

Patients with uncomplicated epistaxis that has been controlled by direct pressure, vasoconstrictors, or cautery can be sent home after a short (20- to 30-minute) period of observation. Patients are warned not to mechanically irritate the nose by rubbing or blowing it for 24 hours. If drying is the suspected cause of anterior bleeding, the patient is given a petrolatum-based ointment and instructed to apply it gently inside the nares every 12 hours for 1 to 2 days. A home humidifier may be helpful in preventing recurrence.

Patients with first-time epistaxis treated with anterior packs are referred for follow-up in 24 to 48 hours. Packs are removed in 48 to 72 hours. Antibiotic coverage is maintained while the pack is present. Patients who have recurrent nosebleeds requiring anterior packing are treated in consultation with a specialist.

Consultation

Displaced nasal fractures may be reduced by an experienced physician within 1 hour of occurrence. Alternatively, the patient may be referred to an otorhinolaryngologist for subsequent reduction within 5 to 7 days after the swelling has subsided.

Facial fractures associated with significant epistaxis merit otorhinolaryngologic consultation in the emergency department. These patients may be admitted or scheduled for later reduction, depending on the nature and severity of the fractures.

Hospitalization

Hospital admission is indicated for the following types of patients:

1. Patients who have lost enough blood to require transfusion until the hematocrit is stabilized.
2. Patients who develop epistaxis owing to hematologic or coagulation disorders. Definitive diagnosis and blood product therapy should be initiated as indicated (see Chap. 24).
3. Patients with epistaxis that is refractory to nonoperative methods of treatment of underlying disorders.
4. Patients with posterior packs, who are observed for hypoventilation and hypoxia.

PROBLEM 1 Silver nitrate cautery was applied to the bleeding site on the patient's septum. After 20 minutes of observation, no recurrence of bleeding was noted, and the blood pressure was 150/90mm Hg. The patient was discharged with instructions to avoid nose blowing or mechanical irritation of the nose and to begin application of a petrolatum-based ointment with a cotton swab after 24 hours.

PROBLEM 2 This patient's problem was a little more complex. An otorhinolaryngologist was consulted, who recommended packing the lacerated area with an absorbable hemostatic gel. This was done, and the patient was discharged, only to return in 4 hours with recurrent epistaxis from the same site. At this point, the anterior nasal cavity was packed with vaseline gauze, ampicillin was started, and the patient was instructed to return for removal of the packing in 3 days. Removal was uneventful, and ENT follow-up resulted in repair of a displaced septal fracture several days later.

DOCUMENTATION

1. *Historical details*—specifically trauma, recent infections, medications, bleeding disorders, and estimated blood loss.
2. *Physical findings* recorded should include vital signs (including orthostatic measurements), signs of abnormal bleeding, and findings on nasal examination (bleeding site).
3. *All treatment modalities* used should be recorded, specifically intravenous fluids, blood products, topical and injected medications, any foreign bodies removed, cautery, packing method, and response to treatment.
4. *Discharge and follow-up instructions* should be clearly recorded, including packing removal appointment, prophylactic antibiotic use, precautions to be used against rebleeding, and specialty referral.

SUMMARY AND FINAL POINTS

- Epistaxis is a common problem that is often managed in the emergency department.
- The most frequent causes are trauma and mechanical factors.
- Most epistaxis originates from the anterior nasal septum.
- An ordered approach to diagnosis and treatment begins with ensuring the patency of the airway and cardiovascular stability and proceeds through identification of the bleeding site(s) and application of the least invasive treatment modality needed to achieve hemostasis.
- It is invaluable to have all the necessary equipment for diagnosis and treatment at hand before attempting management.
- Systemic causes of epistaxis, particularly disorders of hemostasis, are always considered in the differential diagnosis.

BIBLIOGRAPHY

Texts

1. Friedman WH, Rosenblum BN: Epistaxis. In Goldman JL (ed): Principles and Practice of Rhinology. New York, Wiley, 1987.
2. Lucente FE, Sobol SM: Essentials of Otolaryngology (2nd ed). New York, Raven Press, 1988.

Journal Articles

1. Chait RH, White JD: Emergency management of epistaxis. Emerg Med Serv 16(9):55–85, 1987.
2. Cook PR, Renner G, Williams F: A comparison of nasal balloons and posterior gauze packs for posterior epistaxis. Ear, Nose, Throat J 64:446–449, 1985.
3. Jacobs JR, Levine LA, Davis H, et al: Posterior packs and the nasopulmonary reflex. Laryngoscope 91:279–284, 1981.
4. Perretta LJ, Denslow BL, Brown CG: Emergency evaluation and management of epistaxis. Emerg Med Clin North Am 5(2):265–277, 1987.
5. Petrusen B: Epistaxis. Acta Otolaryngol 317(Suppl):6–66, 1974.
6. Yonkers AJ (ed): Epistaxis. Ear, Nose, Throat J 60(10):442–471, 1981.

CHAPTER 32

ACUTE SORE THROAT

STEVEN M. JOYCE, M.D.

PROBLEM 1 An 18 year old college student came to the emergency department complaining of a sore throat of one day's duration. It hurt to swallow, and the pain was keeping him awake. He requested "a shot of penicillin to get rid of this," since he had an important test coming up.

PROBLEM 2 Because of a worsening sore throat, a 7 year old child was brought to the emergency department by her parents. She had been seen the day before by her pediatrician, who prescribed erythromycin for "strep throat." She did not want to drink liquids because of the pain. Her parents reported that her voice seemed "muffled."

QUESTIONS TO CONSIDER

1. Are there potential life-threatening problems in the patient presenting with an acute sore throat?
2. What elements of the history and physical examination are important to rule out these problems?
3. What clinical findings can help determine the likely etiology of pharyngitis?
4. Are laboratory tests available to identify the patient with streptococcal pharyngitis in the emergency department?
5. What is appropriate management for patients with a complaint of sore throat? Specifically, which patients should receive antibiotics?
6. What are the noninfectious causes of sore throat?

INTRODUCTION

Virtually everyone is bothered by sore throat at some time. Studies estimate an office visit rate of over 15 million patients in a single year in the United States for pharyngitis, with an annual cost of over $300 million. Sore throat is a common problem seen frequently by emergency physicians. The pain and discomfort in swallowing interfere with the daily activities of eating and sleeping, and patients come seeking relief. Unfortunately, many have the impression that an antibiotic will effect a quick cure: This is true in only a small percentage of cases. There are life-threatening complications of sore throat, and it is necessary to consider them in each patient who presents with this common complaint.

The sensory innervation of the throat is important for an understanding of the sources of throat pain. The ninth and tenth cranial nerves innervate the pharynx, larynx, middle ear, and auditory canal. Throat pain may be referred to or originate in the anatomic area ranging from the ears to the upper thorax. The pharynx has sensory fibers capable of distinguishing between sharp, burning, and scratchy discomfort.

Though acute sore throat may be caused by trauma or a number of inflammatory conditions, it is most often the result of infection. Table 32–1 lists the common infectious

TABLE 32-1. Infectious Causes of Acute Pharyngitis

Etiology	Syndrome/Disease	Estimated Importance*
Viral		
Rhinovirus	Common cold	20
Coronavirus	Common cold	≥5
Adenovirus	Pharyngoconjunctival fever, acute respiratory disease	5
Herpes simplex 1 and 2	Gingivitis, stomatitis, pharyngitis	4
Parainfluenza virus	Common cold, croup	2
Influenza virus A and B	Influenza	2
EB virus	Infectious mononucleosis	<1
Cytomegalovirus	Infectious mononucleosis	<1
Bacterial		
Streptococcus pyogenes	Pharyngitis/tonsillitis	15–35
Chlamydia trachomatis	Pharyngitis, pneumonia	0–20
Mycoplasma pneumoniae	Pneumonia, bronchitis, pharyngitis	5
Mixed anaerobic infections	Gingivitis, pharyngitis (Vincent's angina), peritonsillitis/peritonsillar abscess (quinsy)	<1 <1
Neisseria gonorrhoeae	Pharyngitis	<1
Corynebacterium diphtheriae	Diphtheria	<1
Corynebacterium hemolyticum and *C. ulcerans*	Pharyngitis	<1

*Estimated percentage of cases of pharyngitis due to indicated organism in civilians of all ages. (Modified from Gwaltney JM: Pharyngitis. *In* Mandell GL, Douglas RG, Bennett JE: Principles and Practice of Infectious Disease (3rd ed). New York, Churchill Livingstone, 1990.)

etiologies of acute pharyngitis and their relative incidences. Streptococcal infection ("strep throat") is responsible for only 15 to 35% of acute pharyngitis. The incidence of streptococcal pharyngitis is highest in children aged 5 to 15 years, with boys and girls equally affected. Carriage rates may be up to 20% in this age group. Transmission is by oral droplets. Streptococcal pharyngitis assumes importance because of the potentially disastrous sequelae of rheumatic fever. This inflammatory syndrome is thought to be precipitated by immunologic cross-reactivity between streptococcal membrane antigens and human tissue antigens, particularly in myocardial sarcolemma. This complication may occur in up to 3% of patients with streptococcal infection during epidemics.

Sore throat can also be a secondary finding in systemic diseases, such as infectious hepatitis, leukemia, and severe neutropenia.

INITIAL APPROACH IN THE EMERGENCY DEPARTMENT

In a busy emergency department, a patient with the chief complaint of a sore throat may wait until more acutely ill patients are treated. However, patients with certain complaints or signs should alert the staff to the possibility of airway compromise. These are *stridor or labored respirations, inability to swallow secretions* resulting in drooling, inability to open or close the mouth completely *(trismus)*, and *changes in the voice* (muffling or "hot potato voice"). All these findings may be caused by swelling of the tissues of the pharynx or larynx. Airway obstruction may be imminent, and immediate attention is required (see Chap. 2).

In most cases, these findings are absent. The patient may present with fever and a hoarse, scratchy voice but no apparent respiratory distress.

DATA GATHERING

The history seeks the course and severity of the disease process. The physical examination emphasizes the anatomic location and searches for potential complications, especially airway compromise and systemic disease.

History

1. *Present illness*
   a. What is the *duration* and *severity* of the sore throat? The duration may indicate whether a deep infection, such as peritonsillar abscess, has had time to evolve. This usually takes 48 to 72 hours.
   b. Are there accompanying *upper respiratory tract symptoms*, such as rhinorrhea or coryza? Upper respiratory tract symptoms are most common with viral infections. Streptococcal infections tend to localize to the oropharynx with or without systemic symptoms.
   c. How did the *symptoms begin?* A gradual onset of scratchy sensation evolving to pain is consistent with a spreading viral disease. Pain related to trauma is not always spontaneously mentioned.
   d. Are there *systemic symptoms*, such as fever, headache, weakness, abdominal pain, or trouble breathing? Asking about these findings keeps the physician from focusing too narrowly on the throat and may help gauge systemic toxicity.
   e. Are there any *household* or close *contacts* with similar symptoms? This information supports an infectious source, but both viral and bacterial causes have similar patterns.
   f. Has "*strep throat*" been *diagnosed* by laboratory methods in the past? Streptococcal infection has a recurrent pattern in some patients.
   g. Is there *genital discharge?* This may be difficult to address in the context of "sore throat," but a history of gonorrhea in sexual contacts, or recent orogenital sex, is important to obtain tactfully in sexually active patients.
2. *Medications.* Is the patient *taking* or *allergic* to any *medication?* Many patients take antibiotics on their own in advance of visiting the physician. This may limit the usefulness of cultures.
3. *Past medical history.* Does the patient have a history of any immunocompromising condition (e.g., diabetes mellitus, splenectomy, neoplastic disease), rheumatic fever, or valvular heart disease?
4. *Immunization history.* Has the patient received *diphtheria* immunizations? This is usually part of the diphtheria-pertussis-tetanus series (DPT).

Physical Examination

During the physical examination, there is more to do than simple inspection of the throat. In fact, in children with suspected epiglottitis or retropharyngeal abscess, such a maneuver may precipitate occlusion of the airway and is relatively contraindicated. Usually, these are children in the 3- to 6-year age group who present with fever, stridor, trismus, and drooling. The approach to these patients is discussed under the disease entities.

Vital Signs. These may reveal the presence of fever and tachycardia. They are nondiagnostic but demonstrate the degree of systemic effect of the illness.

General Inspection. A general inspection is necessary to assess the patient's "toxicity" or distress. In talking with the patient, any hoarseness or muffling of the voice or significant difficulty in swallowing is noted.

Lymph Nodes. The neck is palpated for the presence of enlarged or tender anterior and posterior cervical lymph nodes. If there is presumptive evidence for mononucleosis, AIDS, or malignancy, axillary and inguinal nodes are examined, as is the spleen.

Pharynx. A good light and a tongue depressor are usually sufficient for an adequate examination. Some patients are unable to open their mouths fully and may be helped by a topical anesthetic spray to the oropharynx. The famous "ahhh" elevates the uvula and soft palate, giving a clearer view of the pharynx. The tissues of the pharynx may vary in appearance from normal to swollen and erythematous. Varying amounts of exudate may be present on the mucosa of the pharynx and extending from the crypts of the tonsils.

The mucosa of the hard palate, soft palate, pharynx, and tonsillar pillars is examined for petechiae, vesicles, or ulcerations. The size, position, and symmetry of the uvula and tonsils are noted, with particular attention to airway patency. The peritonsillar area may be palpated for induration or fluctuance if a peritonsillar abscess is suspected. The presence and color of any pseudomembranes are noted, as well as their adherence to the underlying mucosa.

Otolaryngologic Examination. The otolaryngologic examination is completed by observing the nasal passages, external auditory canal, and tympanic membranes, and palpating the sinuses for tenderness.

Lungs and Abdomen. Depending on associated symptoms, the lungs and abdomen are examined.

PROBLEM 1 The student had been ill for one day. He denied fever, chills, coryza, or cough but complained of a mild bilateral earache. Other students in his dormitory had colds and sore throats. None had "strep throat" to his knowledge. He had no known allergies, no cardiac risk factors, and no recent antibiotic use. The patient was in no distress. Vital signs were normal, except for an oral temperature of 38°C (100.4°F). He spoke normally but appeared uncomfortable when swallowing. Examination revealed several mildly enlarged and tender anterior cervical lymph nodes without other adenopathy, atrophied tonsils, and a beefy red pharyngeal mucosa with whitish exudate. The exudate was easily dislodged without bleeding. The tympanic membranes were normal. The spleen was not palpable.

The patient's low grade fever, tender cervical adenopathy, and exudative pharyngitis are consistent with an infectious etiology of the sore throat. There are no signs or symptoms of airway compromise.

PROBLEM 2 According to her parents, the child had all her childhood shots and was allergic to penicillin. She was unable to swallow anything but her first dose of erythromycin. Recurrent sore throats had been a problem, and many children at her school had "strep throat." She had not been drooling, nor complaining of difficulty breathing. On examination, the child appeared ill, and her breath was foul. Her temperature was 39°C (102.2°F), pulse 120 beats/min, and respirations normal. She was unable to open or close her mouth completely and spoke with a muffled voice. Several anterior cervical nodes were enlarged and tender. Other nodes and the spleen were normal. Inspection of the pharynx showed swelling of both tonsils, most marked on the left, with deviation of the left tonsillar pillar and uvula toward the right.

This patient is toxic. Her muffled voice and the deviated tonsils and uvula are significant. She has no respiratory difficulty, nor other signs indicative of epiglottitis.

DECISION PRIORITIES AND PRELIMINARY DIFFERENTIAL DIAGNOSIS

Following the history and physical examination, the physician begins to formulate a differential diagnosis and prioritized approach based on the following questions:
1. *Does the patient have a potentially life-threatening disease?*
   Before considering the "uncomplicated" sore throat, the emergency physician must rule out potentially life-threatening problems that may occur. The three most important are epiglottitis, retropharyngeal abscess, and severe tonsillar or uvular edema. Each will be further discussed in the Refined Differential Diagnosis, but there are important precautions for the emergency physician to take if any of the three are suspected.
   Epiglottitis. When the diagnosis is suspected but immediate respiratory

obstruction does not appear likely, arrangements are made to confirm the diagnosis and secure the airway under controlled conditions. The patient is either accompanied to radiology by a physician with equipment for ventilation and intubation, or films are obtained in the emergency department. A soft tissue lateral radiograph of the neck usually confirms the diagnosis, and the patient is taken to the operating room or ICU for endotracheal intubation under light anesthesia. Emergent cricothyrotomy or tracheostomy may be necessary if intubation is impossible.

If respiratory obstruction seems imminent in the emergency department, cautious laryngoscopy and orotracheal intubation are attempted, with provision for surgical or needle cricothyrotomy if the intubation is not successful. In a young child, bag-valve-mask insufflation may produce adequate respiration until the airway is definitively managed. Under no circumstances should the patient be left by the physician until the airway is secured.

Retropharyngeal abscess. Since the presentation is similar to that of epiglottitis in children, the diagnosis is confirmed by lateral soft tissue neck radiography. Unless immediate airway management is required, inspection and palpation are limited to the operating room. Intravenous antibiotics are given early.

Severe tonsillar or uvular edema. This situation is most commonly encountered in the tonsillitis that accompanies mononucleosis. Stridor, drooling, and vocal changes are present. Inspection shows bilateral swollen tonsils that meet in the midline, obscuring the pharynx and potentially threatening to obstruct the upper airway. These patients may be admitted for treatment with systemic steroids and close observation for imminent airway obstruction.

2. *Does the patient have an infectious etiology of pharyngitis? Is it group A beta-hemolytic streptococcus (GABS) infection?*

Once serious complications are ruled out, the emergency physician can address the etiology of the sore throat. The majority of sore throats are infectious in origin (see Table 32–1). At this stage, the most important decison is whether this may be a GABS infection.

Group A beta-hemolytic streptococcus (S. pyogenes, GABS) is the most common bacteria cultured. It is the major cause of pharyngitis and tonsillitis for which antibiotic treatment is indicated to prevent sequelae such as rheumatic fever or peritonsillar abscess. The "strep throat" may vary in appearance from mildly inflamed mucosa to the "classic" exudative tonsillitis and pharyngitis, with a beefy red mucosa, anterior cervical adenopathy, and high-grade fever. This "classic" appearance has generated a variety of adult and pediatric scoring systems to support the diagnosis of GABS. These may be used in making treatment decisions also. Table 32–2 and Table 32–3 are adult and pediatric examples. The predictive value for GABS-positive throat cultures of these scoring methods ranges from 30% to 50%.

3. *Does the patient have a noninfectious cause of the sore throat?*

TABLE 32–2. Adult Scoring System for GABS

Risk Factors
1. Pharyngeal exudate
2. Anterior cervical adenopathy
3. Fever
4. Absence of cough

Decisions
1. The presence of two or more risk factors suggests the validity of empiric oral antibiotic therapy.
2. The presence of three or more risk factors supports the use of empiric parenteral penicillin therapy on a cost-effective basis.

Modified from Wigton RS, et al: Arch Intern Med 146:81–83, 1986. Copyright 1986, American Medical Association.

TABLE 32–3. Pediatric Streptococcal Scorecard*

Month			
Feb, Mar, Apr	_____(4 points)		
Jan, May, Dec	_____(3 points)		
June, Oct, Nov	_____(2 points)		
July, Aug, Sept	_____(1 point)		
Age (years)			
5 through 10	_____(4 points)		
4 or 11–14	_____(3 points)		
3, 15, or older	_____(2 points)		
2 or younger	_____(1 point)		
WBC			
<8500	_____(1 point)		
8500–10,400	_____(2 points)		
10,500–13,400	_____(3 points)		
13,500–20,400	_____(5 points)		
>20,400	_____(6 points)		
Not done	_____(3 points)		
Clinical Findings			
Fever 38°C or more	_____(4 points)	_____(2 points)	_____(2 points)
Sore throat	_____(4 points)	_____(2 points)	_____(2 points)
Cough	_____(2 points)	_____(4 points)	_____(4 points)
Headache	_____(4 points)	_____(2 points)	_____(2 points)
Abnormal pharynx	_____(4 points)	_____(1 point)	_____(3 points)
Adenopathy	_____(4 points)	_____(2 points)	_____(3 points)

*Consider the score positive for streptococcal pharyngitis when the total is 30 or more. (From Breese BB: A simple scorecard for the tentative diagnosis of streptococcal pharyngitis. Am J Dis Child 131:514, 1977. Copyright 1977, American Medical Association.)

These etiologies are extremely uncommon and often are suggested by the history or lack of physical findings. They are listed in the Refined Differential Diagnosis.

Unfortunately, the "classic" appearance of the pharynx seen in each specific etiology is often the exception rather than the rule. Diagnosis of the cause of pharyngitis by clinical means can be notoriously inaccurate. Laboratory assessment can be an important complement to the history and physical examination.

PROBLEM 1 This patient's findings were suggestive, but not diagnostic, of a bacterial infection. In the adult GABS scoring system he had all four risk factors.

PROBLEM 2 The patient had a peritonsillar cellulitis or abscess. The latter usually takes 48 hours or more to form. Concern about the status of her airway continued.

DIAGNOSTIC ADJUNCTS

Laboratory Studies

A number of laboratory tests are useful in diagnosing pharyngitis, depending on the suspected etiologic agent. Almost all the work is done in the bacteriology laboratory. Hematology and chemistry tests are of limited benefit, unless a specific disease is being considered, such as leukemia. Because rheumatic fever can be prevented by treatment within 9 days of onset, it is very important to identify those patients with pharyngitis and tonsillitis infected with group A beta-hemolytic streptococci.

Pharyngeal Swab Gram Stain. This study is useful in identifying patients with a high probability of streptococcal pharyngitis. A stained smear from the area of pharyngeal inflammation is examined under oil-immersion. In areas where polymorphonuclear leukocytes are noted, gram-positive ovoid cocci in pairs or singly signify a high likelihood of streptococcal infection. Other etiologic agents, such as *C. diphtheriae*, may also be identified by the Gram stain.

Rapid Latex Agglutination Test. Another useful tool in identifying streptococci in pharyngitis patients. It is based upon isolation of the group A antigen from the throat swab. Several tests are commercially available, with sensitivities of 60 to 95%, specificities of 94 to 100%, and a reasonable cost per test. Results are available in under 10 to 15 minutes for most products. These tests identify only the presence of streptococcal antigen, not active infection. Some patients treated on the basis of this test will be streptococcal carriers, with other causes of their acute pharyngitides. To many physicians, this "overtreatment" is acceptable.

Throat Culture. It remains the "gold standard" for identification of GABS in patients with acute sore throat. The specimen is collected using a dry swab in the area of inflammation and transported for plating onto blood agar for incubation. Beta-streptococcus is identified by its hemolysis pattern and group A by bacitracin inhibition. This "strep screen" throat culture has many limitations. If improperly collected, transported, plated, or read, false-negative results may occur. Partially treated streptococcal infection may yield a negative culture. The false-negative rate for culture is estimated at 5 to 10%. If GABS is present in a carrier state, the patient may be treated for the wrong infection. These false-positive carriers account for 15 to 20% of patients cultured. Results are not available for 48 hours, allowing continued patient discomfort and risking development of complications like peritonsillar abscess, spread to other family members, and loss of treatment opportunity due to attrition. Finally, other organisms that may cause sore throat may not be identified by blood agar cultures. Figure 32–1 is an algorithm for guiding throat culture selection in the patient with acute sore throat.

Other Tests. The preceding discussion has dealt with the identification of GABS pharyngitis. Many other infectious organisms can cause pharyngitis. Identification and specific treatment are indicated for some of these agents because of their potential for causing complications.

1. *Diphtheria*, suspected because of a poor immunization history and presence of the characteristic pseudomembrane, may be identified by smears stained by *Gram's* method, *methylene blue*, or *fluorescein-labeled antitoxin culture* on Loeffler's medium.

2. *Gonococcal pharyngitis* may be cultured by using a swab or synthetic material (not cotton) to collect the sample, which is then incubated in a high CO_2 atmosphere on Thayer-Martin (chocolate) agar. Culture of the urethra or cervix by the same method is useful in these patients.

3. *A peripheral blood smear* may reveal a relative lymphocytosis or more than 10% atypical lymphocytes in infectious mononucleosis. The heterophil antibody test usually is not positive until one to two weeks of illness have elapsed. Epstein-Barr virus (EBV)–specific antigen may add to the diagnosis. Its use may be restricted to these cases.

Radiologic Imaging

A *soft tissue lateral view of the neck* is most useful in the diagnosis of epiglottitis and retropharyngeal abscess. It is ordered when signs or symptoms of either disease process are present and airway obstruction is not imminent. The patient is always accompanied by a physician skilled in airway management.

REFINED DIFFERENTIAL DIAGNOSIS

Potentially Life-Threatening Diseases

Epiglottitis is a relatively uncommon acute bacterial infection of the laryngeal and pharyngeal mucosa, resulting in edema and occasionally upper airway obstruction. Although it is most often seen in children 3 to 6 years old, epiglottitis has been reported in adults over 60 years old. Pediatric epiglottitis is almost always caused by *Haemophilus influenzae* type B. Adult epiglottitis is also usually caused by *H. influenzae*, although

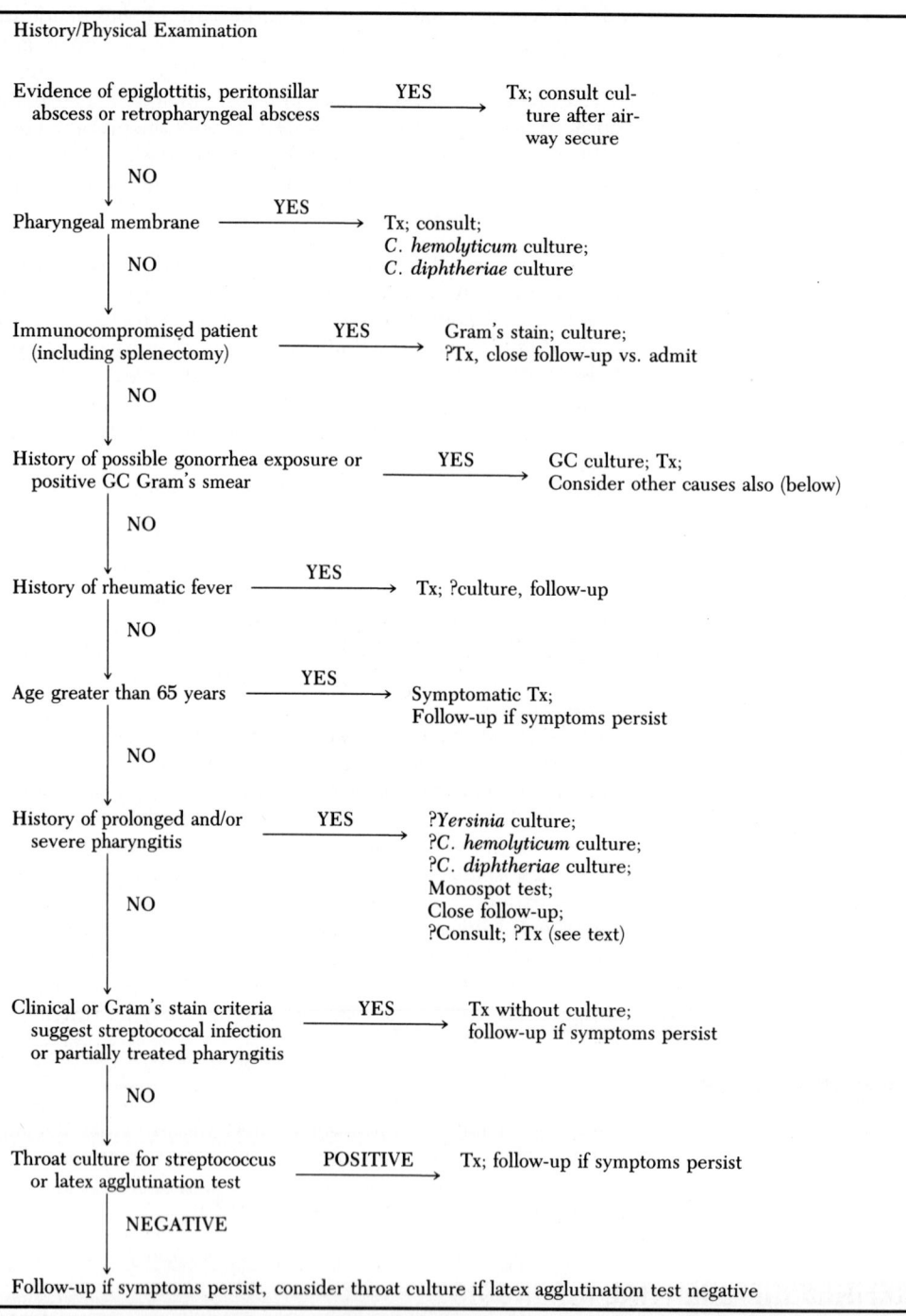

FIGURE 32–1. Suggested algorithm for guiding throat cultures in the patient with acute pharyngitis. Treatment (Tx) is dependent upon many variables. Potential need for throat cultures (?culture), potential need for treatment (?Tx), and the potential need for specialty consultation (?consult) also are dependent upon patient population. (Modified from Hedges JR, Lowe R: Sore throat: to culture or not to culture. Ann Emerg Med 15(3):123–127, 1986, with permission.)

other bacteria, including streptococci, pneumococci, and staphylococci, have been implicated.

Symptoms of epiglottitis usually develop rapidly, especially in children. It begins as a localized sore throat with pain on swallowing. The supraglottic laryngeal edema prevents normal swallowing, causing the patient to lean forward and drool. The speech is muffled by loss of hypopharyngeal resonance ("hot potato voice") and trismus is evident as the edema spreads. The most striking and worrisome development is imminent upper airway obstruction, as evidenced by inspiratory stridor and intercostal retractions. In addition to airway management, all patients are given intravenous antibiotics.

Adults with epiglottitis may not often present with such a rapid progression of symptoms. Pain out of proportion to that explained by the pharyngeal examination, dysphagia, and a subjective feeling of airway tightness may be more typical in adults. If the adult patient is not in extremis, cautious indirect laryngoscopy may be attempted. Rapid endotracheal intubation may be required.

Peritonsillar abscess may occur as tonsillitis extends to the surrounding tissues as cellulitis, then as an abscess. Abscess development usually takes more than 48 hours of infection. The patient presents with progressive dysphagia, trismus, drooling, and, if untreated, potentially airway compromise or deep neck infection. Pain may radiate to the ear. The abscess usually causes high fever and a toxic-appearing patient. Inspection shows bulging of the tonsillar pillar with deviation of the uvula to the opposite side (Fig. 32–2). Palpation of the pillar with a gloved finger confirms a tender, sometimes fluctuant mass. To confirm a suspected diagnosis of abscess, a careful needle aspiration medial to the carotid/jugular sheath is performed by an experienced physician. After topical anesthesia, a 20-gauge needle, taped or guarded to prevent penetration beyond 1 cm or so, is introduced into the fluctuant area medial to a perpendicular line imagined from the base of the tonsillar pillar, and below the level of base of the uvula. If purulent material is aspirated, the diagnosis of abscess is confirmed, and surgical drainage is indicated.

If no purulent material is present, the diagnosis of peritonsillar cellulitis is made, and antibiotic treatment with parenteral penicillin is given. The patient should be re-examined in 12 to 24 hours to ensure that an abscess has not developed.

Retropharyngeal abscess is similar in evolution to peritonsillar abscess. This purulent infection develops in the retropharyngeal soft tissues following an upper respiratory infection in children less than 3 years of age or at any time following a foreign body

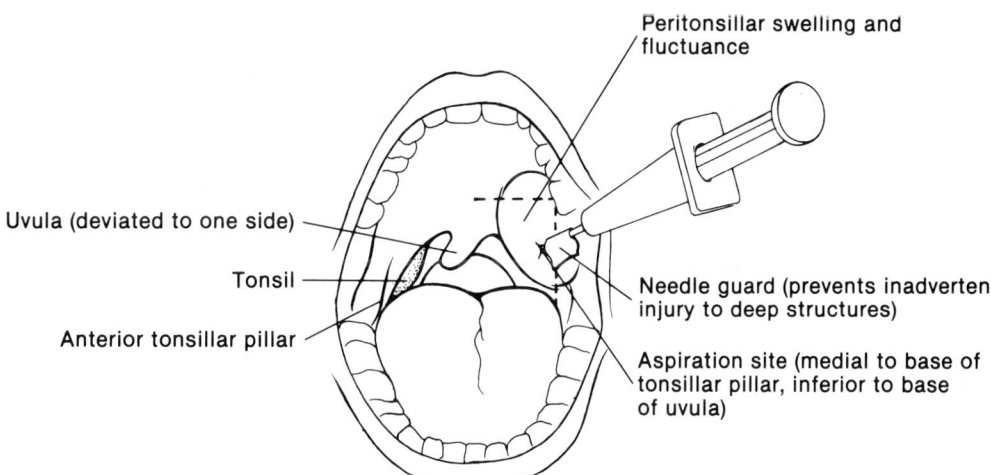

FIGURE 32–2. Pharyngeal structures in peritonsillar abscess. Purulent aspirate confirms diagnosis. Incision and drainage follow (from same site). Dashed line denotes border of area for aspiration site.

penetration of the posterior pharyngeal mucosa. Findings include sore throat, fever, inspiratory stridor, drooling, and voice changes. The neck is often stiff and held extended.

Diphtheria, while uncommon, may be re-emerging as an etiologic agent in sore throat, because of failure of some parents to immunize their children. A low-grade fever is usually present, and systemic symptoms may be mild. Sore throat is a symptom in most of the patients. Cough, hoarseness, and dysphagia are noted in about 25% of patients. Cervical lymph nodes are often tender and enlarged. The finding of a thick, gray pseudomembrane, which is tightly adherent to the pharyngeal mucosa, is "classic" for the disease, although it may be absent. Pseudomembranes also may be found in mononucleosis and staphylococcal and other pharyngitides. Complications of diphtheria include acute upper airway obstruction from dislodgement and aspiration of the pseudomembrane, myocarditis, and severe peripheral neuritis. The latter two complications are caused by the diphtheria toxin.

Infectious Causes

Viral upper respiratory infection (URI) is probably most common (about 40%) even though the exact virus is not identified in many cases in epidemiologic studies. Most of these infections affect other areas of the upper airway mucosa, causing conjunctivitis, rhinorrhea, sneezing, and laryngotracheitis in addition to the sore throat. Systemic symptoms such as headache, fever, and myalgias are usually present but mild. Adenovirus may cause an exudative pharyngitis.

Both Epstein-Barr virus and cytomegalovirus (CMV) may cause *mononucleosis*, an uncommon illness that often presents as persistent pharyngitis and markedly edematous tonsils. Generalized lymphadenopathy and splenomegaly are seen in EBV, but not in CMV forms.

Chlamydia and mycoplasma have a greater role in causing sore throat than was previously suspected (5 to 25%). Empiric treatment is not widely practiced, since these infections are self-limited and generally uncomplicated.

Gonococcal pharyngitis is rare, but should be sought in those who practice orogenital sex or in patients with genital gonorrhea. It may range in presentation from asymptomatic to exudative pharyngitis.

Candida pharyngitis (thrush) is noted in immunocompromised patients. It may prompt a search for AIDS or neoplastic disorders when the etiology is not otherwise evident in an adult patient. White patches of exudate over shallow mucosal ulcerations are noted in the oral cavity and throat. Thrush is fairly common in immunologically normal infants whose formula or breast-milk diet enhances yeast growth.

Noninfectious Causes

Trauma by sharp objects, such as bones, usually causes localized pain and dysphagia. Penetrating injuries may lead to retropharyngeal abscess.

Burns may be caused by hot liquids, by thermal inhalation, and frequently by chemicals. The mucosa may appear hyperemic and edematous, and upper airway obstruction is a concern. Coagulative or liquefactive necrosis may occur with various chemicals. Heavy smokers may have an irritated mucosa that is chronically sore.

Neoplastic disorders may cause pain in the throat as a direct result of the tumor, e.g., tonsillar or nasopharyngeal carcinoma; diffuse mucosal infiltration, e.g., leukemia; or immunosuppression with overgrowth and mucosal invasion by oral flora, e.g., fusobacteria and spirochetes.

Subacute thyroditis is rare, usually presents as a prolonged or recurrent sore throat, and is suggested by the findings of a normal-appearing throat and tender thyroid.

Glossopharyngeal neuralgia is an extremely rare cause of throat pain, again with normal findings.

Psychogenic disorders may be accompanied by the complaint of chronic sore throat or nagging cough, with normal findings on examination.

PRINCIPLES OF MANAGEMENT

The management of patients with pharyngitis involves decisions regarding analgesia and antibiotics.

Analgesics. Patients are often uncomfortable when swallowing. Those patients with mild to moderate discomfort may be treated with anesthetic lozenges and sprays or salt water gargles. Viscous lidocaine can be used for temporary relief in patients, but it may decrease the gag reflex through sensory anesthesia. Systemic oral analgesics such as codeine or derivatives may be necessary in selected patients with severe pain. Analgesia and reassurance that the symptoms will resolve in 5 to 7 days are the basis of therapy for viral pharyngitides.

Antibiotic Therapy. Therapy is guided by the initial clinical impression and ancillary testing:

1. *Streptococcal pharyngitis.* Patients are given antibiotics because purulent complications can be prevented by prompt treatment. Spread of infection to family members and other close contacts may also be decreased. Most important, however, proper treatment of streptococcal pharyngitis prevents rheumatic fever and its sequelae of carditis, chorea, and chronic valvular cardiac disease. So, though the attack rate of rheumatic fever even in epidemic streptococcal pharyngitis is less than 3%, antibiotic treatment is mandatory when the disease is suspected.

The GABS scoring systems have been used to aid decision making (Tables 32–2 and 32–3). In the adult example, two or more risk factors suggest the need for empiric antibiotic therapy. Additionally, various algorithms have been proposed for the approach to and treatment of pharyngitis, with an emphasis on screening for streptococcal pharyngitis (see Fig. 32–1). Most authorities agree that in the absence of an epidemic streptococcal pharyngitis outbreak or a previous history of rheumatic fever (both of which warrant empiric treatment), patients are treated for GABS infection when clinical scores or rapid screens so indicate. The remaining patients are cultured for GABS or other organisms, if indicated, and treatment is based upon culture results. This seems to be the most cost-effective approach to identifying and treating the great majority of streptococcal infections.

Penicillin is the treatment of choice in nonallergic patients. Although more expensive than oral therapy, parenteral benzathine penicillin G is appropriate, since rheumatic fever prophylaxis is assured when definitive treatment is given within 9 days of onset of the illness. Patients weighing over 60 pounds receive 1.2 million units intramuscularly; smaller patients, 600,000 units of benzathine penicillin. If treatment is delayed pending culture results or the patient prefers oral treatment, a full 10-day course of penicillin V, 500 mg b.i.d. for adults or 250 mg b.i.d. for children under 12 years, is given. The latter dose is adjusted by weight in infants. In allergic patients, erythromycin in like doses for a 10-day course is the drug of choice. Trimethoprim-sulfamethoxazole and tetracycline are relatively ineffective against streptococci and may not be adequate prophylaxis for rheumatic fever. Compliance with oral therapy remains a serious problem.

2. Although uncomplicated genital gonorrhea can be treated with oral antibiotics, *gonorrheal pharyngitis* is best treated parenterally. Ceftriaxone, 250 mg IM, is the drug of choice in adults. Alternative regimens include IM procaine penicillin plus probenecid or oral trimethoprim/sulfamethoxazole. Compliance may be poor with oral treatment regimens.

3. When *Mycoplasma* or *Chlamydia* is suspected, symptomatic treatment is probably acceptable, since the infections are self-limited. Empiric antibiotic treatment with erythromycin may create problems with streptococcal resistance to the drug.

4. *Diphtheria*, as mentioned, is an emergency problem requiring admission, isolation,

airway protection, parenteral penicillin or erythromycin, and specific antitoxin therapy. Close contacts may be treated with active immunization boosters or antitoxin as the situation warrants.

Treatment of Infectious Mononucleosis Pharyngitis. This is a self-limited viral syndrome. No specific treatment is available. However, patients are counseled that malaise, easy fatigability, and adenopathy may persist for weeks or months. In addition, patients with splenomegaly should avoid strenuous activity or contact sports until it resolves, usually 6 to 12 weeks. Steroid treatment can reduce severe tonsillar edema in mononucleosis.

PROBLEM 1 The patient's clinical appearance fulfilled the GABS scoring criteria for the empiric use of antibiotics. The reason for giving the penicillin, other than "patient request," was explained to the patient. He was informed and counseled about the small likelihood of a penicillin reaction or hypersensitivity. He was not encouraged to expect a miraculous recovery, although evidence suggests that treatment of streptococcal pharyngitis may shorten symptoms by hours to days. Following the algorithm in Figure 32–1, treatment was given without a throat culture.

PROBLEM 2 The diagnosis of peritonsillar abscess was confirmed upon aspirating 3 ml of purulent material. An otolaryngologist was consulted, and the child was taken to the operating room for drainage under light sedation. She was admitted for intravenous antibiotic therapy, oral suctioning, and observation for signs of airway compromise. She was discharged after 3 days to complete a full course of oral penicillin for streptococcal pharyngitis.

SPECIAL CONSIDERATIONS

Age

Generally, infectious pharyngitis becomes less frequent with age.

1. Streptococcal pharyngitis has its peak incidence in the 5- to 15-year age group. Its incidence decreases in adulthood, as does the carrier state.

2. Viral pharyngitides are the most common cause of acute sore throat in all age groups.

3. A persistent pharyngitis without obvious physical findings in an elderly patient should prompt a search for leukemia or other neoplasm. The incidence of noninfectious causes increases with age.

4. Gonococcal pharyngitis is most common in sexually active adults, although it has been found in sexually abused children.

Immune Status

1. Splenectomized patients may be especially susceptible to streptococcal sepsis. Only mildly symptomatic patients who are reliable and close to a hospital for careful, close follow-up are treated as outpatients.

2. Leukopenic or leukemic patients are evaluated for adequate granulocyte counts before outpatient treatment is considered. Close follow-up is essential.

3. Diabetic patients and steroid-dependent patients may require close supervision during any intercurrent illness, and admission is a viable option.

4. Oral candidiasis is the most common pharyngeal infection in patients with AIDS. This finding may suggest this underlying disease in patients who are at risk.

Previous Rheumatic Fever

These patients are susceptible to relapses when exposed to streptococcal infection. Since the morbidity of recurrent rheumatic fever is potentially high, anyone with a prior history who presents with pharyngitis is treated with parenteral penicillin, regardless of the results of screening tests.

DISPOSITION AND FOLLOW-UP

Admission

Admission to the hospital is appropriate for:
1. Patients at risk for airway compromise.
2. Patients who simply cannot take in adequate fluids and risk becoming volume-depleted.
3. Patients who are immunocompromised and require parenteral antibiotic therapy.
4. Patients in whom the pain cannot be adequately controlled by oral analgesia. These are a rarity.

Consultation

In cases of suspected airway compromise, epiglottitis, peritonsillar abscess, retropharyngeal abscess, or severe pain of unknown origin, an otolaryngologist is consulted to assist in airway management and inpatient care. Unless the need for airway stabilization is an emergency, definitive airway management is best accomplished in the operating room.

Discharge

Symptomatic treatment as described under Analgesia may be applied to sore throat of any etiology. Unless the airway is threatened or surgical drainage is indicated, most patients are sent home. When antibiotic treatment is delayed pending culture results, the patient must be available by telephone. The importance of follow-up cannot be overstressed. It is often prudent to parenterally treat patients who may be unreliable or otherwise lost to follow-up. A 10-day course of oral antibiotics is often difficult to finish, even for compliant patients.

DOCUMENTATION

1. Background history of the illness.
2. Airway patency status is clearly described (presence or absence of stridor, drooling, voice changes, or signs of peritonsillar or retropharyngeal abscess).
3. Medication, allergies, and immunization status.
4. A history of rheumatic fever, exposure to known etiologic agents (especially GABS), and any immunocompromising conditions.
5. The rationale for decision to treat or to withhold treatment pending culture results.
6. Treatment given and follow-up instructions.

SUMMARY AND FINAL POINTS

- Evaluation and management of acute sore throat is a complicated decision process. A basic understanding of the various etiologies and familiarity with one or more suggested algorithms for treatment are essential.

- Although not the most common cause of sore throat, *group A beta-hemolytic streptococcus* commands attention because of its potential for complications, most notably pharyngeal abscesses and rheumatic fever.
- When other treatable etiologies are unlikely, GABS should be ruled in or out using clinical scoring, rapid screening tests, and/or cultures as described. Treatment with antibiotics is guided by these diagnostic schemes.
- Regardless of etiology, airway compromise in patients with sore throat mandates swift action by the emergency physician. Such patients may be stabilized by endotracheal intubation and/or admission for specific treatment and observation.

BIBLIOGRAPHY

Texts

1. Lucente FE, Sobol SM: Essentials of Otolaryngology, 2nd ed. New York, Raven Press, 1988.

Journal Articles

1. Guroy ME, Murray HW: Management of pharyngitis. Emerg Decisions Jan:25–31, 1986.
2. Hedges JR, Lowe RA: Sore throat—to culture or not to culture. Ann Emerg Med 15:312, 1986.
3. Hedges JR, Lowe RA: Streptococcal pharyngitis in the emergency department: Analysis of therapeutic strategies. Am J Emerg Med 4:107, 1986.
4. Hedges JR, Lowe RA: Approach to acute pharyngitis. *In* Stair T (ed): Emerg Med Clin North Am 5:335, 1987.
5. Taylor RB, Werman HA, Rund DA: Streptococcal pharyngitis—emerging concepts. Am J Emerg Med 6:306, 1988.

CHAPTER 33

EARACHE

NICHOLAS BENSON, M.D.

PROBLEM 1 A 30 month old boy was brought to the emergency department at 2:00 AM by his parents. They gave a 2-day history of runny nose, low-grade fever, and dry cough. Since midnight that night the child had been awake and screaming.

PROBLEM 2 A 66 year old woman was brought by her daughter to the emergency department. She stated that her mother had had intense pain in her left ear for several hours and was "not acting right."

PROBLEM 3 A mother brought in her 6 year old daughter because she had noticed a foul-smelling, creamy colored fluid coming out of the child's left ear for the past 2 days. The child said that her ear hurt "a little."

QUESTIONS TO CONSIDER

1. What are the common diseases that can present as earaches in the emergency department?
2. What are the most frequent etiologies of ear pain in infants? In young children? In young adults?
3. What aspects of the history and physical examination can assist in delineating the cause of pain in patients with earache?
4. What is the role of the pneumatic otoscope in evaluating patients presenting with earache?
5. In what clinical situations may earache represent a potentially lethal problem?
6. What is the management of patients presenting with otitis media? Otitis externa?
7. What is the appropriate disposition and follow-up for patients with otitis media? Otitis externa? Referred pain?

INTRODUCTION

Earache is a common complaint of patients coming to the emergency department. It can originate from a variety of sites in and around the ear. Otogenic causes include problems with the mastoid, middle ear, or external canal, although involvement of the temporal bone or inner ear also occurs. The ear is innervated by sensory branches of the vagus nerve (cranial nerve X), glossopharyngeal nerve (IX), auriculotemporal branch of the trigeminal nerve (V), facial nerve (VII), and branches of cervical nerves 2 and 3. Pathologic conditions, including infection and malignancy, of the upper respiratory or digestive tract (oropharynx, larynx, hypopharynx) and the teeth or mandible can cause referred pain to the ear.

The ear canal and temporal bone surrounding the middle and inner ear structures provide a relative barrier against infectious agents and trauma. Most infectants arrive by means of the communication between the middle ear and the posterior pharynx through the eustachian tube. The tympanic membrane is the boundary between the middle and the external ear. It is made up of squamous, fibrous, and mucosal layers. Each layer may be involved in pathology specific to its cell type, although most problems are either infectious or secondary to rapid shifts in air pressure between the external and middle ear. The external canal, lined with squamous epithelium and open to the environment, is vulnerable to all forms of dermatitis and environmental pathogens.

Most earaches are caused by an acute infection of the middle ear (otitis media) or the external ear canal (otitis externa). Otitis media is the most common cause of ear pain seen in the emergency department. It occurs most commonly in infants and young children, with peak incidences occurring between 6 and 24 months of age and between 4 and 6 years of age. At least 15% to 20% of all infants will develop acute otitis media. Although these infections can occur year round, the incidence is highest in the winter and early spring.

Acute otitis externa occurs in all age groups and in a wide variety of conditions. Certain conditions predispose to its development. They include exposure of the external ear canal to water, as with swimming, hair washing, or irrigating the canal; trauma to the canal, usually self-inflicted during attempts to remove cerumen; and a congenitally small external auditory meatus. Otitis externa lasting longer than 2 months is called chronic external otitis.

INITIAL APPROACH IN THE EMERGENCY DEPARTMENT

Patients with earaches are triaged to the nonacute section of the emergency department. In the great majority of cases, this placement is completely appropriate. However, the triage nurse and physician must be alert for the patient complaining of an earache who may have a serious condition associated with or causing the pain. Most of these causes are not otic in origin.

History

1. Pain. The rapidity of onset and severity of pain are assessed.
2. Associated symptoms. Particular attention is given to complaints of shortness of breath, headache, or systemic malaise.

Physical Examination

1. General appearance. The purpose is to sort out the patient with high fever, toxic appearance, or respiratory compromise.
2. Mouth and throat. If respiratory compromise is suspected, the oropharynx is examined for signs of a retropharyngeal abscess or a peritonsillar abscess.
3. Neck. The neck is checked for suppleness or a finding of meningismus.

Intervention

1. Any patient with a high fever (over 103°F [39.4°C]), toxic appearance, or respiratory compromise is moved to the acute care area.
2. If the patient has not taken antipyretics within the last 3 hours, acetaminophen is administered for temperature greater than 103°F (39.4°C).
3. Airway management equipment is moved near the patient if there is respiratory distress.

Patients with diabetes mellitus and those who are immunosuppressed are considered at risk for malignant otitis externa. This is an invasive infection that begins in the ear canal and spreads to the adjacent soft tissue, bone, nerves, vessels, and central nervous system. The signs of extensive inflammation are obvious.

PROBLEM 2 The patient was extremely uncomfortable from the ear pain and had to rely on her daughter to answer many of the questions. She was an insulin-dependent diabetic and was recently discharged from the hospital with a diagnosis of pneumonia.

This woman's recent hospitalization for a major infection is strong evidence that her diabetes mellitus and perhaps other problems place her in the immunosuppressed category. To compound the situation, she may have been exposed to nosocomial pathogens during her hospital stay. Finally, the mild alteration in her mental status, evidenced by her reliance on her daughter during the history taking, suggests a systemic disease. She was moved to an acute care area of the emergency department.

DATA GATHERING

History

The history is directed toward the details of the pain, any associated complaints, and predisposing factors to ear, neck, or mouth problems. Due to the pediatric prevalence among patients with this complaint, the source of the history is often someone other than the patient. This "one step removed" information is interpreted cautiously because the observations are less accurate.

1. *Pain*
   a. *Onset* and *duration*. Most ear pain is acute in onset, although a dull pressure often precedes the increase in pain due to infectious causes. Most patients do not wait a long time (less than 24 hours) before coming to the emergency department.
   b. *Location*. Most earache is unilateral; bilateral ear pain points to an infectious etiology.
   c. *Pattern* of pain. Constant pain is consistent with pain of ear origin; intermittent pain or pain with highly variable intensity more often arises from extraotic sites. A sudden decrease of pain is typical of tympanic membrane rupture.
   d. *Character* or *quality*. Most ear pain is sharp or stabbing with associated pressure and throbbing. Dull aching pain is uncommon in patients who present with acute pain.
   e. *Severity*. Interpreting severity may be impossible in children. In adults, pain of infectious origin is usually intense and moderately severe. The phrase, "the worst pain I've had in my life" is not usually heard.
   f. *Factors* that *relieve* or *worsen* pain. Pain that increases with biting or chewing may arise from the teeth, temporomandibular joint, or external canal.
2. Associated *symptoms*
   a. Effect on *hearing*. Otitis externa can cause a significant decrease in acuity by blocking the canal, whereas otitis media usually "muffles" the sound.
   b. *Discharge* or *drainage*. Discharge or drainage is characteristic of otitis externa or otitis media with tympanic membrane rupture.
   c. *Upper respiratory* symptoms or *sore throat*. These symptoms are common with middle ear infections. Referred pain from an oropharyngeal lesion should also be considered, e.g., peritonsillar abscess.
   d. Extra *sounds*. Ringing is rare, but crackling or popping is common.
   e. *Dizziness* or *vertigo*. Dizziness is a rare symptom in otitis media and suggests inner ear involvement. Labyrinthitis or a deep temporal bone infection is considered in such cases.

3. *Precipitating* factors
    a. Exposure to *barotrauma*. Questions about recent airplane flights, underwater diving, or possible trauma from a blow or a slap on the ear are in order.
    b. Blunt *trauma*. Blunt trauma often occurs from attempts to "clean" the ear.
4. *Past medical history*
    a. Inquiries are made about any previous history of *ear problems*, particularly infections, and any treatment received.
    b. Any underlying *medical problems*, especially diabetes mellitus, are clarified.
    c. Queries about recent *travel* or vacation may point toward possible barotrauma.
5. Queries specific to patients who cannot give their own history
    a. Is there a *change* in *affect*, mood, or attention?
    b. If the patient is an infant, has *ear pulling* been noted?

Physical Examination

Physical examination is done to (a) assess the general status of the patient; (b) identify potential sites of referred pain, such as the mouth, throat, teeth, and temporomandibular joint; and (c) assess the status of the ear.

Vital Signs. Tachycardia may be a sign of significant pain, high fever, hypoxia, or septicemia. High fever is much more common in patients with otitis media than otitis externa.

General Appearance. Patients with uncomplicated infections do not look toxic. In infants it is best to assess alertness serially as treatment progresses. The status of the infant who presents with lethargy, high fever, and ear pain should improve as the fever comes down. Sepsis or meningitis is considered if the child does not become more alert and interact more with the surrounding environment as the fever declines.

A "muffled" voice suggests the presence of a retropharyngeal or peritonsillar abscess.

External Ear Examination. The external ear and periauricular area are inspected, looking for drainage, trauma, or edema. Gentle pressure on the tragus is painful in patients with external otitis but should not cause any pain in those with otitis media.

The Ear Canal. The largest-sized speculum that will fit easily in the canal is inserted. Traction on the external ear in the superior and posterior directions will straighten out the canal. In infants, traction in the inferior direction may provide better results. If insertion of the speculum causes pain, acute otitis externa is suggested. The entire canal is inspected for erythema, edema, bleeding, discharge, and foreign bodies.

Cerumen in the canal can limit the examination of the canal and drum. Careful removal of any obstructing material with either a cerumen spoon or gentle irrigation is very helpful. Removal may be aided by instilling a topical solution of benzocaine, antipyrine, and glycerin (Auralgan).

The Tympanic Membrane. After the canal has been inspected, the tympanic membrane is examined. The normal eardrum has a characteristic topography and is shiny with a pearly gray color. Specific pertinent findings relative to the eardrum are listed here:

1. Serous fluid in the middle ear can cause the membrane to be yellow or amber in color.
2. Blood in the middle ear is seen as a blue or purple membrane.
3. Purulence in the middle ear causes a white or chalky appearance.
4. Erythema of the membrane is often seen in infants who have a high fever or are crying and resisting examination. Erythema in a quiet infant with ear pain and a mild fever is highly suggestive of otitis media.
5. With serous otitis, the membrane can appear dull and retracted.
6. Numerous prior ear infections may cause fibrotic white membranes.
7. A bullous lesion on the eardrum is often due to an infection with either *Hemophilus influenzae* or *Mycoplasma pneumoniae*.

8. Visualizing a perforation of the eardrum requires a close examination, especially in the posteroinferior corner.

Pneumatic Otoscopy. An often neglected but important examination is a test of the mobility of the tympanic membrane with the pneumatic apparatus of the otoscope (Fig. 33–1). Loss of or limited movement is an early sign of otitis media and is often the only finding in serous otitis. It is useful in assessing a reddened tympanic membrane in the crying or febrile infant. Scarring from multiple infections may decrease mobility.

Hearing Acuity. In general, attempts to test hearing acuity will be successful only with cooperative adults. Most children are unable or unwilling to truly discriminate with which ear they hear something. Both otitis media and otitis externa may produce a conductive hearing loss.

A tuning fork can be used for the Weber's and Rinne's test. They can differentiate between hearing loss due to disorders of the middle and external ear and disorders of the neural apparatus. In the Weber test the sound radiation from a tuning fork placed on the patient's forehead is toward the ear with a conductive hearing loss and away from one with a sensorineural loss. The Rinne test assesses air conduction versus bone conduction by comparing sound transmitted through the mastoid process to sound transmitted through air. In otitis media, bone conduction may be longer than air conduction.

The Extraotic Examination. Even if the source is "obvious," it is best to examine quickly other sites that might explain the patient's ear pain.

1. The preauricular and postauricular (mastoid) areas are palpated for lymph node swelling and tenderness.
2. The temporomandibular joint is checked for soreness and trismus.
3. The neck is palpated to determine if there are inflamed lymph nodes.
4. The tonsils and pharynx are examined for erythema, edema, and exudates.

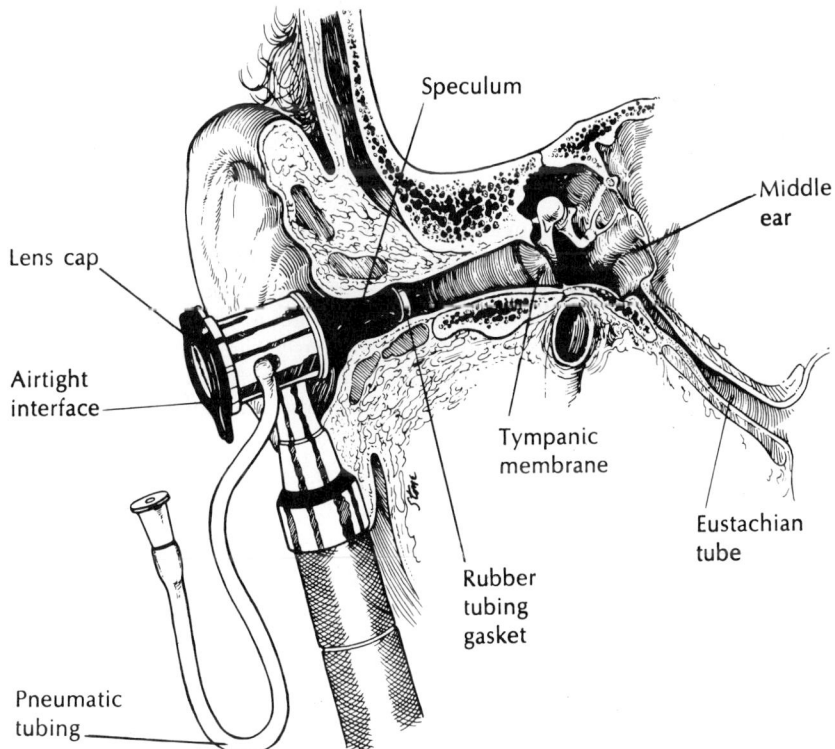

FIGURE 33–1. Pneumatic otoscopy. (From Schwartz RH: New concepts in otitis media. Am Fam Phys 19(5):91–98, 1979. Published by the American Academy of Family Physicians.)

5. The teeth, sinuses, and salivary glands are examined for occult infections or inflammation.

PROBLEM 1 The child's mother stated that he had been seen that day by the pediatrician. She was told that it was "a cold" and was given a decongestant. The child had been pulling his right ear. He had had one previous ear infection. The toddler's rectal temperature was 103.4°F (39.7°C). His nose and posterior pharynx were mildly erythematous but showed no exudate. He cried and moved away when the right anterior cervical lymph nodes were palpated. The ear canals were clean. The tympanic membranes were both moderately red. The pneumatic otoscope showed normal mobility of the left membrane and decreased mobility of the right membrane.

The child's history is consistent with the rapid onset of pain that occurs in otitis media. The upper respiratory symptoms are also supportive of this diagnosis. The pediatrician is not to be faulted for "missing the problem" because it was most likely not apparent earlier in the day. The difference in mobility of the membranes raises the physician's confidence in diagnosing acute otitis media.

PROBLEM 2 The daughter stated that her mother had had ear pain and drainage from the ear for the last 3 days. The pain had increased significantly that day. She said that her mother "didn't seem right" and noted "a lot of redness" around her left ear. The patient was in fair health and took 60 units of NPH insulin daily. Vital signs were blood pressure 170/100 mm Hg, heart rate 100 beats/min, respirations 20/min, temperature 102°F (38.9°C). Cellulitis and granulation tissue was noted around the opening of the left ear canal. The tympanic membrane could not be visualized. The patient had some "droop" in the left side of her face, including her eyelid.

The history and physical findings are consistent with a rapidly spreading infectious process that most likely has extended beyond the external auditory canal. The patient's slightly altered mental status and seventh cranial nerve involvement point to a very serious disease.

PROBLEM 3 On examination, the little girl had no tenderness when her outer ear was moved. However, she strongly resisted efforts to look inside the canal of her left ear with an otoscope. With her mother's assistance, she was held still. Otoscopy showed a moderate amount of purulent fluid and a shiny bright, red, round object about halfway down the canal.

Children frequently put things in their ears, nose, and any other opening available to them. These foreign objects can cause local irritation and infection. The physician, faced with an uncooperative child who has all the symptoms of an acute infectious otitis externa, may acquiesce and treat the patient without completing the physical examination. The presence of a foreign object cannot be ruled out unless the canal is well visualized.

DECISION PRIORITIES AND PRELIMINARY DIFFERENTIAL DIAGNOSIS

At this point in the assessment, the physician generally has enough information to answer three questions.

1. *Is a serious disease process present?*
    The patient's level of consciousness and vital signs supply major clues about the possibility of the presence of a serious disease. If the patient is alert and oriented, the fever is under control, and the airway is safe, then the risk of life-threatening

disease is very small. If there is any doubt, steps are taken at once to place the patient in an environment where close observation is guaranteed and aggressive airway interventions can be instituted in case the airway should suddenly become occluded or the child should have a febrile seizure. In the group at risk, malignant external otitis has potentially life-threatening complications. It is a diagnosis not to be missed.

2. *Is the earache of otic origin or is it referred pain from another source?*
The basic physical examination of the external canal and tympanic membrane, coupled with the initial information obtained from the history, should give enough data to confirm or refute the presence of otogenic disease. Focal causes of ear pain are more common in children. The incidence of referred pain increases with age.

3. *Does the patient have one of the three most common causes of ear pain?*
The three common causes of pain of otic origin are otitis media, otitis externa, and a foreign body in the external canal. Although they have been introduced earlier in this chapter, Table 33–1 lists their distinguishing points.

TABLE 33–1. Three Common Causes of Otogenic Ear Pain

Diagnosis	Prevalence	History	Physical Examination	Comments
Otitis media	Most common in children; first peak occurs at 6–36 months, second peak at 7 years. Sixty-seven percent of children have one episode by age 2. More common in males, Caucasians, lower socioeconomic levels, premature infants, and those who are bottle fed	Prior URI, often prior infections, usually rapid onset of sharp throbbing pain without major associated symptoms. Sense of pressure, "fullness" in ear, and decreased hearing	Patient is usually febrile; experiences no pain on movement of ear lobe. Depending on stage, TM may be slightly red with poor movement to very red and bulging. If condition is superimposed on a scarred, retracted TM, it may be difficult to diagnose. Canal has purulent drainage if there is spontaneous perforation. Occasionally mastoid tenderness occurs	Usually there is extension of viral infection through eustachian tubes. Common bacteria are *Streptococcus pneumoniae* and *Hemophilus influenzae*. May spread to mastoid, intracranial area, and soft tissues of neck
Otitis externa (external otitis)	Most common cause in adults	Varies from mild itching to severe pain with purulence. Sense of congestion and often decreased hearing	Erythematous canal, drainage or debris. Movement of auricle (ear lobe) painful, often out of proportion to findings. Canal may be edematous and swollen shut	Originates from damage to protective waxy coating by dryness, wetness, or treatment. Organisms: *Proteus, Staphylococcus, Streptococcus*. Extreme form, malignant otitis externa, occurs in elderly diabetics. *Pseudomonas* invades deep tissue
Foreign body	More common in children. Beads, pebbles, beans, and paper are common. In adults, insects such as cockroaches are most frequent	Children: ear pain, which may be more chronic; drainage, foul odor. Adults: acute onset of pain, fullness, and altered hearing acuity. If TM is perforated, bleeding, marked hearing loss, and vertigo may be present	Children: Foreign body is usually more difficult to locate because children are less cooperative. Adult: Foreign body is usually easily seen, next to TM. May need to anesthetize or suffocate live insect. Check hearing status	An otic microscope may be necessary for removal. After removal, re-examine patient for injury to canal or TM. About 10% of foreign bodies will not be removable in emergency department. Limit the time devoted to the procedure

URI = upper respiratory infection; TM = tympanic membrane.

PROBLEM 1 Acute otitis media was the diagnosis in this patient. It is important to maintain suspicion about other possible causes of the patient's fever and crying, as well as the complications of otitis media, while planning therapy.

PROBLEM 2 It was readily apparent that this patient was seriously ill and at high risk for malignant otitis externa. Early consultation with an otolaryngologist was necessary while the patient was being more extensively evaluated.

PROBLEM 3 In this case, diagnosis of the foreign body was easy. The hard part was removal.

DIAGNOSTIC ADJUNCTS

In most patients with earache, diagnostic adjuncts are unnecessary. Few ancillary tests are useful for reaching a diagnosis. However, in the patient with a severe middle ear or external ear infection, and in the diagnosis of referred pain, testing is often beneficial.

Laboratory Studies

Complete Blood Count. A complete blood count (CBC) with white cell differential cell count, although not diagnostic, may assist the physician in confirming the toxic state of the patient.

Serum Glucose. Even a random sample taken for serum glucose determination may add to the suspicion of underlying diabetes mellitus in the patient with a severe infection.

Cultures. In patients with resistant or frequent otitis media and in neonates or immunosuppressed patients with middle ear infections, tympanocentesis may be helpful in obtaining fluid for Gram stain and culture. This procedure is performed by an experienced physician with a 20-gauge spinal needle and a tuberculin syringe after the ear canal has been carefully suctioned and cleansed with an antibacterial solution. In general, cultures of middle ear fluid in patients with acute suppurative otitis media will grow *Streptococcus pneumoniae* or *Haemophilus influenzae*. Pneumococcus is the most common agent, causing up to 50% of cases. *H. influenzae* is the second most common agent, especially in infants and young children. *Streptococcus, Mycoplasma pneumoniae*, and *Branhaemella catarrhalis* account for most of the others.

In patients with both acute and chronic otitis externa, cultures of the exudate of the canal tend to grow *Staphylococcus aureus, Pseudomonas aeruginosa*, or both. Fungus is recovered from the canal less often than bacteria. Cultures are needed in patients with resistant infection or suspected malignant otitis externa to guide antibiotic therapy.

Radiologic Imaging

Diagnostic imaging techniques are rarely needed in the work-up of a patient with an earache. However, in unusual instances they may be helpful.

Plain Films. Plain films of the ear canal and mastoid may demonstrate a radiopaque foreign body in the canal (in the rare case in which uncertainty remains after the physical examination) or clouding of the mastoid air cells, which can be a complication of acute otitis media in children. A lateral soft-tissue film of the neck may demonstrate disease in the retropharyngeal soft tissue space. Temporomandibular joint views may show joint erosion indicating temporomandibular disease.

Computerized Tomography. Patients with malignant otitis externa or suspected bony spread of otitis media may require CT or tomography of the temporal bone. Consultation is advised.

Nuclear Medicine. Bone scan or gallium scan may be indicated in patients with malignant otitis externa. These tests can monitor the efficacy of the treatment.

Audiometric Testing

Evaluation of a patient's hearing may play a role in the diagnosis and management of resolving or chronic otitis but is usually not available in the emergency department. Simple bedside hearing tests with a wristwatch or Rinne's and Weber's tests are sufficient for testing hearing acuity.

PROBLEM 3 The little girl finally remembered that she did stick "something" into her ear 3 days ago but could not remember what it was. The emergency physician was concerned about the unknown foreign body and considered ordering soft tissue radiographs to determine its size and shape.

Although it is good to recognize that all of the information concerning the nature of this foreign body is not available, it is appropriate to attempt simple methods of removal before obtaining radiologic studies. A radiograph is of questionable utility and significantly adds to the cost of the visit.

REFINED DIFFERENTIAL DIAGNOSIS

Less common causes of otogenic ear pain are considered if the patient does not readily fit into the diagnosis of otitis media, otitis externa, or foreign body in the external canal. Table 33-2 lists these diseases with their typical characteristics.

When the ear canal and tympanic membrane are normal, referred pain is the most likely cause of earache. Due to the extensive nerve supply to the ear, pain may radiate to the ear from a number of structures in the head and neck. These patients are usually older, and about 80% of the complaints are caused by cervical spine lesions, dental pathology, or temporomandibular joint dysfunction. Table 33-3 lists the most common causes of referred pain and their characteristics.

PRINCIPLES OF MANAGEMENT

Therapy for acute otitis media centers around antibiotic therapy, decongestants, and pain relief. Otitis externa is managed with topical therapy and analgesia. Appropriate methods of removal of foreign bodies are reviewed below.

Otitis Media

Antibiotics. Although antibiotics have been the cornerstone of treatment for acute otitis media for many years, some studies have suggested that treating children with uncomplicated acute otitis media with nose drops and analgesics is adequate. Until this conservative therapy is accepted, emergency physicians are advised to employ antibiotics as soon as the diagnosis is made.

There is a broad choice of antibiotics for acute otitis media (see Table 33-4). The usual medication is ampicillin or amoxicillin. For patients who are allergic to penicillin and its derivatives, a combination of erythromycin ethylsuccinate and sulfisoxazole acetyl or trimethoprim-sulfamethoxazole is often used. In the past few years, the use of cefaclor has dramatically increased as penicillin-resistant strains of *H. influenzae* have emerged. Although some physicians reserve it for resistant cases, cefaclor may be more successful than amoxicillin in eradicating middle ear effusions. Recently, amoxicillin with clavulanate potassium has been shown to be as successful as cefaclor in treating acute otitis media with effusion.

Since cost is an important issue, ampicillin or amoxicillin is recommended, with erythromycin-sulfisoxazol or trimethoprim-sulfamethoxazole reserved for penicillin-allergic patients. Cefaclor may be used in areas with a high incidence of beta-lactamase-producing *H. influenzae*.

TABLE 33–2. Less Common Causes of Otogenic Ear Pain

Diagnosis	Pathophysiology	History	Physical Examination	Comments
Aerotitis	Sustained pressure imbalance between middle ear and environment. Often due to eustachian tube blockage secondary to URI	Previous URI, associated with recent descent from altitude or underwater diving. Pain is severe, persistent, with associated "popping" and internal pressure. May be temporarily decreased by yawning or blowing nose	TM retracted, may be hemorrhage behind drum or in canal. Poor TM mobility	Suggest patient prevent condition with nasal spray before descent if URI is present
Bullous myringitis	Reaction of epithelium to viral or *Mycoplasma* infection	Acute onset pain, similar to that of otitis media	Hemorrhagic or serous blebs on TM and in auditory canal. Hearing is not impaired	Blebs resolve with treatment. Needs to be distinguished from herpes zoster otitis
Trauma	Direct injury from ear picking, attempts to "clean out ear." Hemotympanum from head injury and basal skull fracture. Blunt trauma to mandible can directly injure ear canal. TM ruptures with blow to external ear	"Cleaning out" ears. Trauma to face, head, mandible, or ears. "Slap" on ear or side of head	Ranges from minor abrasion and excoriation to disruption of external canal and tympanic membrane. Other signs of head and mandibular trauma are present	Minor trauma far more common. Ear examination part of all head and facial trauma assessment. If TM perforation covers more than 20% of surface, referral is necessary. Significant hearing loss or vertigo is uncommon; if present, it points to more serious injury
Impacted cerumen	Direct pressure on TM by inspissated cerumen	Occurs more often in elderly. Associated with attempts to "clean out wax" while actually impacting it. Symptoms may range from severely to slightly decreased hearing. Usually a long-standing recurrent problem	External canal occluded by cerumen, which may be almost black in color. TM not visible. Increased pain occurs with attempts to remove outer layers manually	Prior softening may be necessary before removal is possible
Herpes zoster oticus (Ramsey Hunt syndrome)	Herpes zoster infection of geniculate ganglion	Prodrome of malaise and fever. Deep severe ear pain	Vesicular rash in ear canal. Facial paralysis	Treatment is supportive and symptomatic
Cholesteotoma	Cyst of squamous epithelium within middle ear cleft	Progressive hearing loss	Mass in middle ear	Bony destruction may occur. Prompt surgical intervention is indicated

URI = upper respiratory infection; TM = tympanic membrane.

Although antibiotic therapy has traditionally been given for approximately 10 days, recent studies have suggested that therapy for as little as 5 days is effective. If the eardrum is perforated, then 10 days of therapy is appropriate. If the patient does not show improvement as evidenced by decreased fever or pain in 48 hours, the antibiotic may be changed on the assumption that the infecting agent is resistant.

Decongestants. In the past, physicians routinely prescribed decongestants along with antibiotics. The theory was that the decongestant would reestablish the function of the eustachian tube. More recently, this adjunctive treatment has fallen into disfavor because decongestants have not been demonstrated to be efficacious in the treatment of ear infections.

Analgesia. Most patients will benefit from analgesics. Aspirin or acetaminophen with codeine in tablet or liquid form is beneficial for the first 24 to 48 hours. The mild sedation is also useful. A slightly warmed topical anesthetic is sometimes used to assist in pain relief, especially in infants. The most common preparation is a solution of the anesthetics antipyrine and benzocaine with glycerin (Auralgan).

Outcome. Treated properly, about 50% of patients have no effusion at 2 weeks, and

TABLE 33–3. Common Causes of Pain Referred to the Ear

Diagnosis	Nerve Supply and Pathophysiology	History	Physical Examination	Comments
Cervical spine lesions	Cervical nerves 2 and 3. Rarely arises from disk, more often bony impingement	Pain is often chronic and may be severe, with continual aching or burning. May worsen with neck flexion	Usually normal. Pain may increase with neck flexion	Radiographs may be inconclusive. Referral necessary
Sinusitis	Cranial nerve V. Infection of maxillary sinus	URI symptoms, dull facial pain. Increased pressure when leaning head forward. Nasal congestion	Tenderness over sinus. Opacification of sinus on transillumination	Radiograph may confirm. Often overdiagnosed
Dental pathology 1. Impacted third molars (wisdom teeth)	Cranial nerve V. Third molar lodges against second molar. Inflammation may occur in gingiva	Common in the 15–30 yr age group	Partial eruption may be visible. Gingiva may be red and tender	May be accompanied by pericoronitis, an inflammation of gingiva surrounding the crown. Dental radiographs may confirm diagnosis
2. Dental caries/ Periapical abscess of mandibular or maxillary molars	Cranial nerve V. Destruction of enamel; process extends into dentine	Pain may not be apparent at tooth. May worsen with biting on hot or cold foods	Caries are usually visible. Tapping suspected tooth may induce pain	
Temporomandibular joint dysfunction	Damaged articular surface due to malocclusion, teeth grinding, or arthritis	Pain is intermittent, may be worse in AM or PM depending on timing of bruxism (teeth grinding). May be associated with vertigo, tinnitus, headache, and jaw click	Joint may be tender or click with chewing. Trismus or muscle pain while biting may be seen	Evaluation is complex and referral necessary
Retropharyngeal abscess	Cranial nerve X. Infection of retropharyngeal space	Occurs more often in children. Usually accompanied by fever, sore throat	Erythema, fullness in oropharynx	Airway at risk. Early consultation
Peritonsillar abscess	Cranial nerve IX. Complication of tonsillitis, primarily *Streptococcus*	Occurs at any age. Sore throat, odynophagia, "hot potato" voice	Usually obvious swelling to side of tonsil, pushed toward midline	Airway seldom at risk. May aspirate or treat with close follow-up
Malignancy of oropharynx and larynx	Cranial nerves VII, IX, X. Cancerous involvement of nerves supplying involved organ	Usually occurs in elderly. May have dysphagia, hoarseness, odynophagia, or mass sensation. Systemic symptoms rare	Suspicion requires full examination including palpation and laryngoscopy	Patient is usually referred, and extensive radiologic assessment is necessary

the tympanic membrane is normal in 1 to 2 months. A failure rate of 5% to 10% is frequent after a 10-day course of antibiotics. When this occurs, a different antibiotic should be used for a second 10-day course. Culture of the middle ear is considered when choosing the appropriate antibiotic for the second round of treatment.

Inadequate therapy may lead to complications that include rupture of the eardrum, cholesteatoma formation, acute mastoiditis, facial nerve damage, and meningitis. When a serous effusion is allowed to linger in the middle ear for prolonged periods, a permanent hearing loss can result.

Otitis Externa

For patients with acute external otitis, treatment consists of removing debris, reducing edema, and treating inflammation and infection. Debris may be suctioned from the canal.

TABLE 33-4. Oral Antibiotic Therapy for Acute Suppurative Otitis Media*

Drug	Dosage Child	Dosage Adult	Number of Doses per 24 hr
Ampicillin	50–100 mg/kg/24 hr	250–500 mg/dose	4
Amoxicillin	20–40 mg/kg/24 hr	250–500 mg/dose	3
Erythromycin-sulfisoxazole	50 mg/kg/24h + 150 mg/kg/24 hr (maximum 6 gm/24 hr)		4
Erythromycin		250–500 mg/dose	4
Trimethoprim-sulfamethoxazole	8 mg/kg/24h + 40 mg/kg/24 hr	160 mg + 800 mg (one double-strength or two single-strength)	2
Cefaclor	40 mg/kg/24 hr	250–500 mg/dose	3

*Consult the PDR for full prescribing information.
From Reich JJ: Ear infections. Emerg Med Clin North Am 5(2):227–241, 1987.

If suction is not completely effective, irrigation of the canal or manual removal of debris with a cerumen spoon is performed. Irrigation requires an intact tympanic membrane, whereas use of a cerumen spoon requires care and adequate lighting and visualization.

Once the canal is clean, ear drops containing a combination of antibacterial, antifungal, and steroid preparations (Table 33–5) are instilled every few hours for a week to 10 days. If the canal is so swollen that the debris cannot be removed or the drops are not guaranteed to reach the medial end of the canal, a wick of cotton or narrow gauze is inserted carefully and allowed to remain for 12 to 24 hours. The combination ear drops are then placed on the wick. If there is suspicion that the tympanic membrane is perforated or if ventilation tubes are in place, a suspension is used instead of the weak acid solution. Patients with cellulitis or systemic signs are given both topical and systemic antibiotics. Otitis usually clears in 10 to 14 days. Recurrence may be avoided by avoiding further trauma or exposure to wetness.

Foreign Body

A foreign body lodged in the canal is removed expeditiously to ease pain and to prevent the external otitis that often accompanies it. All methods of removal are variations on either suction, irrigation, or direct instrumentation. The technique used depends on the physician's experience and equipment. The least invasive technique, irrigation, is tried first unless a perforated tympanic membrane is suspected. If the foreign body in the ear canal is made of vegetable material, irrigation is not recommended because the fluid may cause the object to swell and become harder to extricate. If the object is an insect and the tympanic membrane is intact, mineral oil or 2% lidocaine solution can be placed in the ear to kill the insect before it is removed. Lidocaine is preferred.

All patients who have foreign bodies removed are presumed to have an early,

TABLE 33-5. Commonly Used Otic Drops*

Preparation Name	Principal Agents	Dosage
Coly-Mycin S Otic	Colistin Neomycin Hydrocortisone	3–4 drops 3–4 times/day
Cortisporin otic solution	Polymyxin B	3–4 drops
Cortisporin otic suspension	Neomycin Hydrocortisone	3–4 times/day
Otic domeboro	Acetic acid in aluminum acetate	4–6 drops q 2–3 hr
VoSol otic	Acetic acid in propylene glycol	5 drops 3–4 times/day
VoSol HC otic	Acetic acid hydrocortisone in propylene glycol	5 drops 3–4 times/day

*Consult the PDR for full prescribing information.
From Reich JJ: Ear infections. Emerg Med Clin North Am 5(2):227–241, 1987.

unrecognized otitis externa and are started on a combined antibiotic-corticosteriod ear drop. It is very unusual for the object to get caught in the canal and subsequently be removed without inducing some degree of damage to the canal epithelium.

If attempts to remove a foreign body in the emergency department are unsuccessful, the patient is referred to an otolaryngologist within 24 hours. Appropriate warnings are given to the patient and family in an attempt to prevent a recurrence.

SPECIAL CONSIDERATIONS

Patients who wear a hearing aid and develop an external otitis due to the hearing aid mold are treated and referred to an otologist for further care because of the need to optimize their ability to use the hearing aid.

DISPOSITION AND FOLLOW-UP

Discharge

The patient with a routine ear infection can be sent home with treatment and can be followed by a primary care physician in several days. The patient is instructed to seek care sooner if the symptoms fail to resolve in 24 to 48 hours. Patients with small eardrum perforations require close follow-up, generally by a specialist, although most such problems heal over time without any difficulty.

Routine follow-up in 2 weeks is important in any patient with acute otitis media in order to make sure that any middle ear effusion is gone. A lingering effusion can signal a latent infection that may cause damage if allowed to smolder. Patients with an underlying chronic illness, recurrent ear disease, or resistant ear infections should be seen either by their primary care physician or by a specialist within 48 to 72 hours of the emergency department visit. Patients whose ear pain is unexplained after a careful history and physical examination are referred for reexamination within 3 to 5 days.

Consultation/Admission

Consultation with an otolaryngologist while the patient is still in the emergency department is indicated if any of the following signs or symptoms are present: excruciating pain, significant bloody discharge, granulation tissue in the ear canal, complete absence of hearing, vertigo, or other unusual problems. Patients with disruption of greater than 20% of the surface area of the tympanic membrane or with significant hearing loss or vertigo are discussed with a specialist prior to discharge. Whenever the emergency physician has a suspicion of malignant otitis externa, the patient should be seen by an otologist in the emergency department.

DOCUMENTATION

1. Description of pain and associated symptoms, including fever, discharge, vertigo, and altered hearing
2. Existence of any prior ear problems
3. Appearance of the patient and specific findings including the appearance of the external ear, ear canal, and tympanic membrane
4. The character of any discharge present
5. The mobility of the tympanic membrane
6. Results of the examination of the temporomandibular joint, teeth, and neck
7. Results of any tests performed

8. Any treatment given, including antipyretics or cerumen removal
9. The patient's disposition and plans for further care

SUMMARY AND FINAL POINTS

- The history will provide the bulk of the diagnostic information.
- The physical examination almost always allows the cause of the pain to be classified as otic or nonotic.
- Regional structures are examined to include sources of pain referred to the ear.
- Most otogenic earache is due to otitis media, otitis externa, or a foreign body.
- Most nonotogenic earache originates from either temporomandibular joint dysfunction, dental problems, or cervical spine problems.
- Foreign bodies of the ear canal can be missed unless the examiner specifically looks for them.
- Elderly patients with diabetes mellitus and all patients with immunosuppression are at risk for a potentially lethal malignant infection of the external ear.

BIBLIOGRAPHY

Texts

1. DeWeese DD, Saunders WH: Textbook of Otolaryngology (6th ed). St. Louis, Mosby, 1982.
2. Lucente FE, Sobol SM: Essentials of Otolaryngology (2nd ed). New York, Raven Press, 1988.

Journal Articles

1. Bell DN: Otitis externa: A common, often self-inflicted condition. Postgrad Med 78(3):101–105, 1985.
2. Bluestone CD, Shurin PA: Middle ear disease in children: Pathogenesis, diagnosis, and management. Pediatr Clin North Am 21:379, 1974.
3. Cohen D, Friedman P: The diagnostic criteria of malignant external otitis. J Laryngol Otol 101:216–221, 1987.
4. Fritz S, Kelen GD, Sivertson KT: Foreign bodies of the external auditory canal. Emerg Med Clin North Am 5(2):183–192, 1987.
5. Hawke M, Wong J, Krajden S: Clinical and microbiological features of otitis externa. J Otolaryngol 12(5):289–295, 1984.
6. Hendricksee WA, et al: Five vs. ten days of therapy for acute otitis media. Pediatr Infect Dis J 7:14–23, 1988.
7. Odio CM, Kusmiesz H, Shelton S, et al: Comparative treatment trial of augmentin versus cefaclor for acute otitis media with effusion. Pediatrics 75(5):819–826, 1985.
8. Reich JJ: Ear infections. Emerg Med Clin North Am 5(2):227–241, 1987.
9. Van Buchem FL, Peeters MF, Van'T Hof MA: Acute otitis media: A new treatment strategy. Br Med J 290:1033–1037, 1985.

CHAPTER 34

THE RED PAINFUL EYE

DAVID S. HOWES, M.D.

PROBLEM 1 A 30 year old male presented to the emergency department with a feeling of left eye irritation and redness that had lasted for 1 day.

PROBLEM 2 A 50 year old woman complained of an eye that had been red and painful for 1 week.

QUESTIONS TO CONSIDER

1. How does one determine that a patient presenting with a painful red eye has a condition that needs immediate treatment?
2. What are conjunctivitis, keratitis, and uveitis?
3. How do the history and physical examination help differentiate among common diseases presenting as a painful red eye?
4. What ancillary tests are useful in distinguishing between these common diseases?
5. What is the appropriate management of patients with conjunctivitis, iritis, corneal injury, and acute glaucoma?
6. What is the appropriate disposition and follow-up of patients with a painful red eye?

INTRODUCTION

The eye has only a few ways of responding to noxious stimuli, infection, or vascular or neurologic insult. It can become painful, the vision can be disturbed, or the conjunctiva can become red. A red and painful eye constitutes one of the most common eye complaints seen in the emergency department setting. Many conditions are responsible for these ocular findings. Some are relatively innocuous, whereas others endanger visual function. Almost all are based on inflammation of one or more of the anatomic structures of the eye.

The *sclera* or "white of the eye" is covered by a thin, translucent mucous membrane called the *bulbar conjunctiva*. The palpebral conjunctiva lines the inner aspect of the eyelids. Conjunctival inflammation, conjunctivitis, is characterized by vasodilation (redness), fluid exudation (swelling), and cellular migration (discharge). Conjunctivitis is the most common etiology of the red eye. It is not associated with disturbance of vision or significant ocular pain.

The *cornea* has well-developed sensory fibers. It responds to infectious, inflammatory, or traumatic injury with intense pain. Corneal edema often accompanies this process and results in blurred vision. Corneal inflammation, keratitis, is a common cause of acutely symptomatic red eyes. An intense foreign body sensation differentiates keratitis from other causes of the painful red eye.

Between the cornea and the iris is the *anterior chamber*. The posterior chamber is the space just behind the iris that ends with the crystalline lens and ciliary body. The ciliary body secretes the aqueous humor, which flows into the anterior chamber through the pupillary opening. The anterior chamber drains through Schlemm's canal in the limbic area. In addition, the ciliary muscle allows accommodation of the lens. The choroid is the vascular layer of the posterior three-fifths of the eye that nurtures the adjacent retina. The uvea consists of the iris, ciliary body, and choroid.

The *iris*, ciliary body, and anterior choroid share a common blood supply and therefore tend to be involved in the same inflammatory processes, broadly termed uveitis. The patient will experience blurred vision due to aqueous flare or increased protein and photophobia due to the presence of cells in the aqueous humor with accompanying ciliary body spasm. Pupil size and response to light are affected because of involvement of the iris.

The more posterior elements of the eye include the *vitreous humor*, a transparent medium that occupies the interior of the eye, thereby allowing light transmission to the photosensitive *retina*. Disorders of these structures produce visual disturbance, usually without eye pain or redness. Figure 34–1 is an overview of the anatomy of the surrounding tissues and globe of the eye.

INITIAL APPROACH IN THE EMERGENCY DEPARTMENT

Ocular emergencies must be promptly recognized to preserve visual function successfully. The following patient problems are brought to the immediate attention of the emergency physician:
1. Sudden visual loss
2. Chemical eye injury
3. Severe eye trauma

Visual Loss

Sudden onset of visual loss is a true ocular emergency. It is of the utmost concern in an older patient presenting with painless loss of vision without complaint of eye redness or a history of trauma. Questioning is limited to asking about the patient's usual visual acuity and determining the timing and nature of onset of the visual loss. In this type of patient visual acuity is likely to be poor. The patient may be able to count fingers or perceive light, or he may be completely blind. The pupil will react to consensual light stimulus but reacts minimally or not at all to direct light.

Central retinal artery occlusion is an uncommon but treatable lesion in these patients. This time-dependent ischemic insult is graphically apparent on funduscopic examination. The retina appears very pale with few or no retinal arteries visible. Other findings include an intact fovea, which allows the choroid vessels to be seen, presenting a "cherry-red spot" on funduscopy. Occasionally, one notes a retinal artery with a "boxcar" appearance in which there are segments of blood interspersed with atheromatous material within the vessel. When involvement is limited to a branch of the retinal artery, the corresponding findings on physical examination and loss of vision reflect the distribution of that branch.

The most important aspect of management of the patient with painless loss of vision is prompt recognition. Immediate therapy of the patient with central retinal artery occlusion centers on efforts to promote cerebral vasodilation. This is readily accomplished by having the patient rebreathe his expired air by means of a paper bag for 20 minutes each hour. When available, Carbogen R (95% oxygen, 5% carbon dioxide) is used in the same manner. To lower the intraocular pressure oral osmoglyn, timolol eye drops, and intravenous acetazolamide are administered rapidly. Intermittent gentle massage of the globe may be helpful.

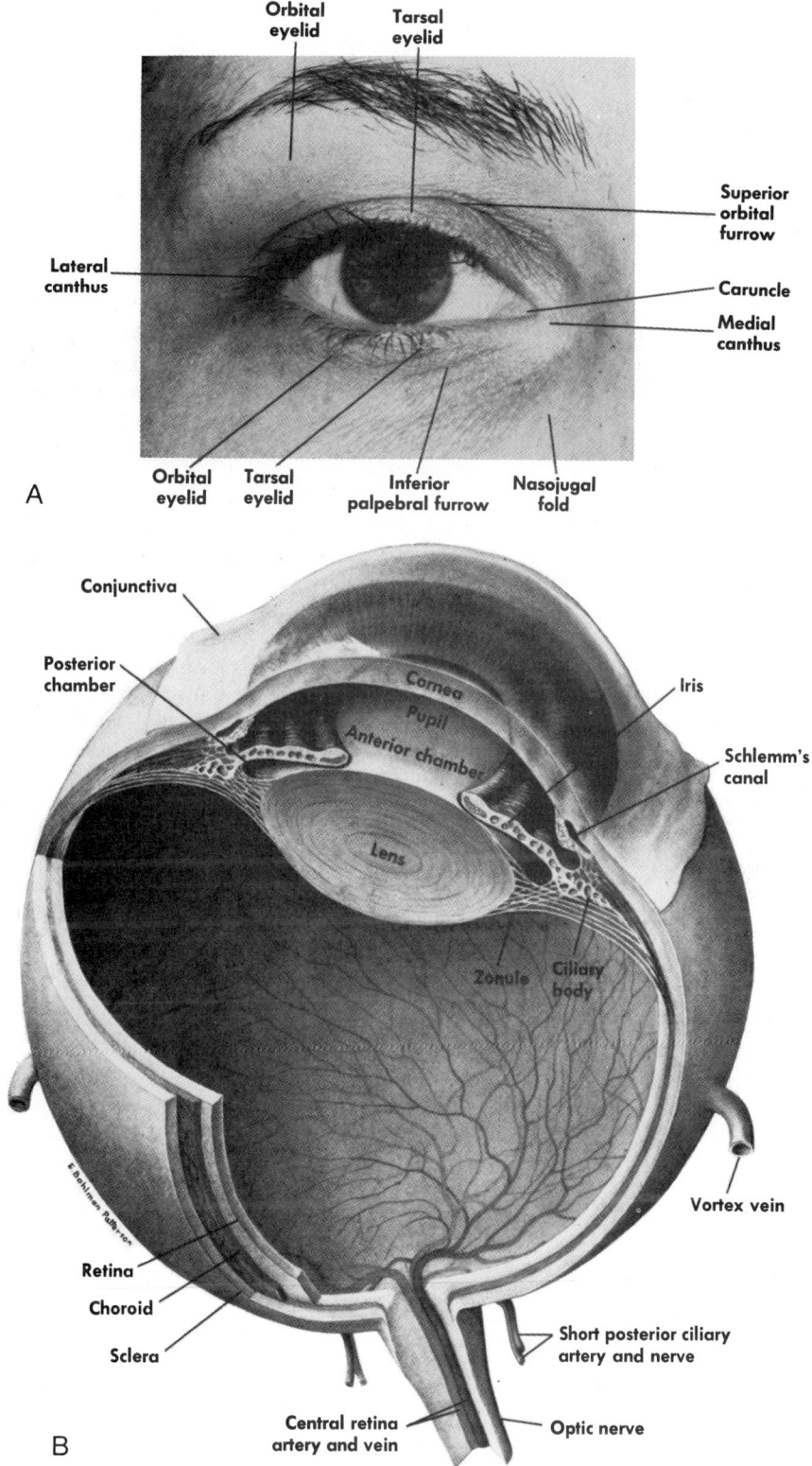

FIGURE 34–1. A, B, *Ocular anatomy. (From Newell FW: Ophthalmology: Principles and Concepts (6th ed.). St Louis, C.V. Mosby, 1986.)*

Chemical Burn

The patient with a chemical burn is self-identified by the chief complaint. Further evaluation, including evaluation of visual acuity, is delayed until initial therapy is accomplished. This includes immediate irrigation with copious amounts of fluid. Anesthetic eye drops may facilitate this treatment. Further management concerns are reviewed in Chapter 35.

Severe Eye Trauma

The patient with a severely traumatized eye is brought to the emergency physician's attention promptly. Nursing and ancillary staff are instructed to handle the severely injured eye in a gentle manner to prevent further injury. The eye with evidence of extensive bruising and soft tissue swelling or obvious penetrating injury is a potentially disrupted globe. Never bring pressure to bear on such an eye. Simply place a shield over the eye to protect it until a physician with more experience in eye care is able to examine the patient. Chapter 35 reviews the management of this problem.

Visual Acuity Testing

Apart from these emergent concerns, visual acuity testing is done in all patients with eye symptoms when they are initially evaluated. The Snellen eye chart is generally used to evaluate visual acuity. If eye glasses are normally worn, the test is conducted with them in place. If glasses are not available, a pinhole occluder may be used to approximate the lens correction. Although a Snellen eye chart is preferable, any printed material will do as long as the examiner documents the nature of the testing material, such as large newsprint at two feet. The patient with a severe visual deficit may be unable to read printed material. In this case, perception of fingers at a noted distance or perception of light may be all that can be recorded.

Visual acuity may be difficult to ascertain initially because of many factors, several of which can be eliminated by the use of a topical anesthetic. Intense pain due to foreign bodies, corneal abrasions, keratitis, or penetrating trauma can cause severe tearing and lid spasm. Not only does anesthesia allow the best possible assessment of visual acuity, it helps gain the patient's cooperation for the remainder of the examination.

PROBLEM 2 The 50 year old woman complained of blurry, painful vision in the right eye for one week. There was no history of acute visual loss, chemical injury, or eye trauma for one week. She would not cooperate with the initial visual acuity testing because of the associated pain. Following instillation of a topical anesthetic, her visual acuity was found to be 20/80 in the right eye and 20/20 in the left eye.

This patient does not need immediate treatment. The emergency physician was concerned about her intense pain and visual disturbance and appropriately relieved her main symptoms.

DATA GATHERING

By means of the history and physical examination the physician attempts to determine the degree of visual loss and the symptoms surrounding the chief complaints.

History

Background. What are the *circumstances* surrounding the *complaint*? A brief background of the problem is necessary. This includes timing and speed of onset of the problem, and therapies used to date.

What is the *occupation* or *avocation* of the patient? Has he been hammering or striking metal objects to metal objects, grinding metallic or granular surfaces, or working with overhead objects that may shed particulate matter? Exposure to the ultraviolet radiation of arc welding is an obvious problem, but it should not be forgotten that reflected sunlight, for example, with skiing in snow, prolonged time on the beach, or use of a sunlamp may also be a cause of significant injury. A history of *contact lens use* is sought.

Visual History

1. Has the patient sustained *visual impairment*? If so, what is its *character*? Blurred vision that does not improve with blinking implies a serious disease, e.g., keratitis, glaucoma.

2. Was this a *sudden, dramatic loss*, a *progressive loss*, or does the *vision wax* and *wane*?

3. Is the *whole visual field* affected or are there *specific areas of loss*?

4. Are *one* or *both eyes affected*?

Pain History

1. What is the *severity, duration*, and *progression of ocular pain*?

2. Does the discomfort feel *superficial* or is there a *deep* ocular lesion? The gritty, scratching, or burning sensation of conjunctivitis is more superficial in nature than the deep, burning, severe eye discomfort of acute narrow angle closure glaucoma. Because of the pain fibers, even minor irritation of the cornea can be very painful.

3. Is there *photophobia*? This is an abnormal sensitivity to light that accompanies iritis. Although many patients complain of sensitivity to light, few have true photophobia. A distinction is made between those patients who find light uncomfortable and those who find light unbearable.

Appearance

1. Is there *redness*? When did it appear in the context of other symptoms? The most common change in appearance of an eye is redness.

2. Is there *swelling*? Patients may feel a "sense of fullness" with significant physical findings. The bulbar and palpebral conjunctiva are primary sites.

3. Is there *exudate* or *"matter"*? Eye secretions can be characterized as scant, copious, watery, or frankly purulent. Often on waking, the patient's eyelids are stuck together owing to the discharge drying overnight.

Trauma History (see Chap. 35)

1. Is there *trauma associated* with the redness or pain? The patient who presents with a swollen "black eye" usually can relate the mechanism of injury. Trauma to the eye can be sustained from less obvious causes. A dust-filled environment or a windy day can be the cause of a foreign body in the eye.

2. Does the traumatic event carry a *high risk for penetrating the globe*? Penetrating injuries can be catastrophic to the eye. This must be considered in the traumatic setting, even from a more subtle cause such as a grinding wheel spark.

Systemic Complaints. Are there *associated systemic complaints* such as fever, arthritis, skin eruption, upper respiratory infection, urethritis, or neurologic deficit?

Eye History. Has the patient ever had *previous symptoms* or *complaints* similar to those of the current problem? Is there a history of *prior eye disease* or *ocular operation*?

Ocular Medications. Were any *medications* put in the eye for *relief of symptoms*? This should include previously prescribed medications, borrowed eye medications, and over-the-counter preparations.

Past Medical History. Are there *underlying medical illnesses*, such as diabetes mellitus, collagen vascular disorder, hypertension, or conditions that would render the patient an immunocompromised host?

PROBLEM 1 The 30 year old male with left eye irritation and redness for one day also noted slight blurring of vision and photophobia. He was otherwise healthy and denied a history of trauma, foreign body sensation, or occupational or environmental exposure to injurious agents. He did not wear contact lenses and denied use of eye medications. This history does not point to an immediate eye-threatening condition.

Physical Examination

The patient with a painful red eye is given a complete ocular examination. This is accomplished by approaching the eye anatomically from anterior to posterior. Examination of the head and neck, as well as other areas of the body, is indicated by vital signs or other symptoms.

Eyelids and Adnexa. The eyelids and adnexa or surrounding structures of the eye are observed for symmetry, swelling, discharge, or erythema, followed by gentle palpation of the soft tissue of the orbit, lids, and zygoma.

The history of a foreign body sensation requires inspection of the lids; eversion of the upper lid is necessary. This can be accomplished by applying gentle upward and outward traction of the lashes while asking the patient to look downward. Foreign bodies such as soft contact lenses and organic materials can hide in the temporal cul-de-sac of the upper lid.

Expression of purulent material from the lacrimal sac located inside the lower inner orbital rim can establish a diagnosis of dacryocystitis. A well-circumscribed inflammation of the lid margin, especially when associated with a discharge of purulent material, is suggestive of a hordeolum (stye).

Redness, swelling, and tenderness of the lids involving the periorbital areas suggest periorbital cellulitis. This is often associated with paranasal sinus infection or previous trauma.

Pupils. The pupils are normally equal in size, round, and react briskly to direct and consensual light. Approximately 10% of the population have anisocoria or a difference in pupil size, typically 1 mm or less. A previous picture of the patient (e.g., a driver's license picture or a parent's wallet picture of a pediatric patient), when closely examined with an ophthalmoscope at the 20+ setting, may reveal preexisting inequality of the pupils.

In evaluating pupils of unequal size, it is helpful to remember that the abnormal pupil is less reactive to light. Mydriasis or pupillary extraocular muscle dysfunction may be due to pharmacologic agents placed in the eye.

The awake patient with a dilated pupil, drooping eyelid (ptosis) and extraocular motion abnormality is likely to have a third nerve palsy due to a space-occupying lesion, such as an intracranial aneurysm. The comatose patient with a suspected head injury with a dilated pupil needs immediate and aggressive intervention because this anisocoria may be a sign of third nerve compression due to cerebral herniation.

A small or miotic pupil is characteristic of iritis. Iritis can be a sequela of trauma or medical illness. The red painful eye of iritis remains uncomfortable even after the instillation of a topical anesthetic. A painful response to both direct and consensual light is characteristic.

Cornea. The cornea is an avascular structure that appears optically clear. Corneal abrasions and foreign bodies are the most common types of injuries seen in the emergency department. Fluorescein is a valuable agent in the diagnosis of foreign bodies, abrasions, and inflammations of the cornea (Fig. 34–2). Defects of the corneal epithelium may be demonstrated by instillation of a small quantity of fluorescein. Areas of disruption or retained foreign body stain a brilliant green color. It is best applied by wetting a dry fluorescein strip with an eye solution such as dacriose and dropping the formed bead into the lower conjunctival sac. Fluorescein will stain soft contact lenses; they must be removed prior to instillation of this agent.

The cornea is a structure that is exquisitely sensitive to pain. Severe pain, lacrimation, and lid spasm (blepharospasm) are characteristic of severe or diffuse corneal injury.

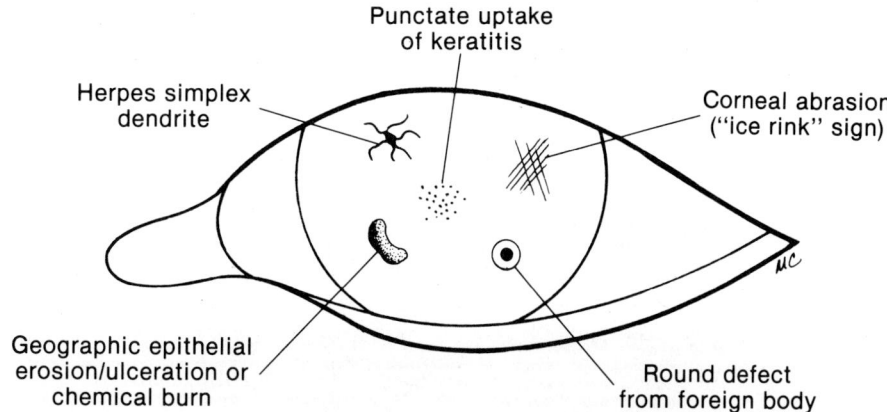

FIGURE 34–2. Identifying corneal epithelial staining defects. (Modified from Demartini DR, Vastine DW: Corneal abrasion and burn. In Callaham M. (ed): Current Therapy in Emergency Medicine. Toronto, B.C. Decker, 1987, 243.)

Visual inspection of the cornea reveals a smooth, regular, and mirrorlike surface. Corneal edema produces a diffuse groundglass appearance. In the patient with a red painful eye, blurred vision, and a poorly reactive pupil with a hazy cornea, acute narrow angle closure glaucoma is to be highly suspected.

Anterior Chamber. The anterior chamber is a space that extends from the cornea to the iris and is an optically clear zone. Blood present in this chamber (hyphema) will layer out and cause a meniscus in the upright patient that is usually identifiable by direct inspection. A large number of inflammatory cells that layer out in a similar fashion is termed a hypopyon, which is generally caused by inflammation of the uveal tract.

The slit lamp is a binocular microscope that has approximately the same power as a laboratory dissecting microscope. The light source projects a slit of light that illuminates a thin section of the cornea and lens. When the light source is placed at an angle to the microscope, the examiner can recognize the depth at which abnormalities occur.

The slit lamp is a helpful tool for evaluating corneal abrasions and for detecting foreign bodies of the lid conjunctiva, bulbar conjunctiva, and corona that may be overlooked on visual inspection.

If iritis or uveitis is suspected, the anterior chamber should be examined with a slit lamp for the presence of "flare and cell." The "flare" is caused by the release of rich plasma protein into the anterior chamber and appears as a solid beam of light extending from the back of the cornea to the iris. The "cell" is caused by the release of white blood cells into the anterior chamber and appears as tiny floating specks within the beam. The appearance of flare and cell is similar to that caused by a beam of sunlight coming into a dark, dusty room (Fig. 34–3).

Lens. The lens is rarely considered in the general examination of the eye. In general, it becomes apparent only by its absence, as when a sudden dramatic change in visual acuity occurs due to a lens subluxation. Ophthalmoscopy reveals a distant-appearing retina such as one would find in the aphakic patient who has had a cataract extraction.

Vitreous. The vitreous is a gel-like substance that fills the space between the retina and the lens. Spontaneous hemorrhage may occur owing to abnormal vasculature or retinal detachment in patients with diabetes mellitus, sickle cell disease, or hypertension. The patient complains of diminished vision. Dark red or black spots and the absence of the red reflex when the fundus is viewed with an ophthalmoscope are characteristic of vitreous hemorrhage.

Retina. Most causes of the red painful eye will not include disease of the retina. However, a complete examination of the eye includes evaluation of the fundus with

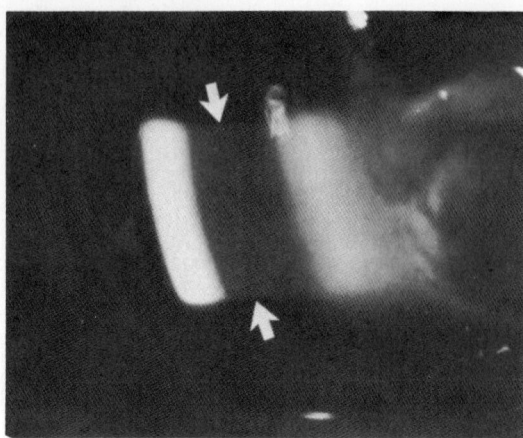

FIGURE 34–3. *A short, narrow slit beam illuminates the flare and cell of acute iritis (arrows). (From Lubeck, D, Greene JS: Corneal injuries. Emerg Med Clin North Am (1):80, 1988.)*

attention paid to the optic nerve, arteries, and veins as well as to the background appearance of the retinal surface. The typical findings of central retinal artery occlusion have been previously discussed. Retinal vein occlusion produces a "blood and thunder" fundus due to the extensive engorgement of the venous system and frank hemorrhage.

The diabetic patient is likely to exhibit abnormal findings on funduscopy. Although up to 70% of all diabetics have some form of retinopathy, only about 2% develop significant visual loss. This is usually due to frank retinal hemorrhage in an area of neovascularization or proliferative new blood vessel formation.

Retro-orbit and Optic Nerve. This area is assessed indirectly by the position of the eye in the orbit (endophthalmos versus exophthalmos), the range of extraocular motion, and the visual field testing. The conduction of the prechiasmal portion of the optic nerve is specifically tested using the "swinging flashlight" or Marcus-Gunn pupil test.

General Physical Examination

Systemic diseases cause a red painful eye. The exophthalmic ocular "stare" of hyperthyroidism is best appreciated from a distance. Joint pains or skin rashes may identify collagen vascular or rheumatic diseases. A latent or even active urethritis may not be volunteered by an embarrassed patient who feels that this has nothing to do with his red painful eye.

Special Tests

1. Marcus-Gunn pupil test (see Chap. 35).
2. Use of fluorescein (see Chap. 35).
3. Response to topical anesthetic. A few drops of topical anesthetic can serve as a reliable diagnostic aid to differentiate between superficial (corneal and conjunctival) and deeper sites of pain. An almost total absence of pain with a topical anesthetic denotes the former kind of pain.
4. Tonometry. Tonometry allows the emergency physician to measure the intraocular pressure of the globe. In patients with ocular pain, nausea, vomiting, photophobia, and a poorly reactive midpoint or larger pupil the intraocular pressure is measured to diagnose or rule out acute glaucoma. Pressures may be measured with a Schiotz or applanation tonometer. The Shiotz tonometer is more readily available in the emergency department. After the instillation of topical anesthesia, the tonometer is gently applied to the cornea to measure the eye pressure. Normal intraocular pressure is 10 to 20 mm Hg. Patients with acute glaucoma may have readings greater than 60 mm Hg. Tonometry is not performed in patients in whom perforation or keratitis is present.

5. **Mydriasis.** Dilation of the iris is rarely part of an ocular examination in the emergency department. Mydriasis and cycloplegia are commonly done as part of management (see Principles of Management, further on).

PROBLEM 1 The patient's visual acuity was 20/50 in the affected eye and 20/20 in the other. He described normal vision on a recent eye examination done for employment screening. Diffuse conjunctival injection that was especially striking around the cornea was noted. The left pupil was 2 mm smaller than the right, and both direct and consensual light responses were painful for the patient. The cornea was clear, fluorescein staining was negative for abrasion, and there was no foreign body. The fundus was normal. No pain relief occurred on instillation of a local anesthetic.

The fact that the local anesthetic did not relieve the pain indicates intraocular pathology that is deeper than the cornea and conjunctiva. The conjunctival injection around the cornea is consistent with a *limbic flush* found with deeper eye inflammation.

DECISION PRIORITIES AND PRELIMINARY DIFFERENTIAL DIAGNOSIS

Following the history and physical examination, the emergency physician can classify the painful red eye into emergent, urgent, and nonurgent categories.

1. *Emergent* conditions are marked by sudden visual loss, chemical eye injury, or severe eye trauma. These entities are reviewed in the earlier section on Initial Approach in the Emergency Department.

2. *Urgent* conditions are characterized by decreased visual acuity and moderate to severe pain. Acute glaucoma, keratitis, and uveitis are diseases that deserve prompt attention.

3. *Nonurgent* conditions are characterized by normal visual acuity and mild ocular discomfort. Conjunctivitis and hordeolums are nonurgent causes of a painful red eye.

PROBLEM 2 The 50 year old woman had been an insulin-dependent diabetic for 10 years. She had had a gradual onset of eye symptoms for 1 week, and 3 days ago had borrowed a friend's eye medication because she could not afford to come to a doctor. Her symptoms worsened during the last 2 days. Ophthalmologic examination revealed a diminished corneal blink reflex and erosions of the central cornea, which took up fluorescein dye. Fundus examination showed mild diabetic retinopathy. The patient's symptoms improved greatly with use of the local anesthetic.

This patient's history and physical examination point to an urgent condition with decreased visual acuity and moderate to severe pain.

DIAGNOSTIC ADJUNCTS

Laboratory Studies

Cultures. Not all cases of suspected external ocular infection require a culture. The great majority of bacterial and viral infections are self-limiting. Cultures are indicated, however, if there is clinical evidence of corneal involvement, if symptoms are prolonged, or if initial antimicrobial therapy has failed.

A Gram stain of the exudate is especially important in identifying the acute, severe, purulent conjunctivitis caused by *Neisseria gonorrhoeae*. This infection occurs in newborn infants who are infected during passage through the birth canal and in adults contaminated from acute gonorrheal urethritis. Microscopic examination reveals gram-negative intracellular diplococci. Confirmatory culture is important.

Chlamydia Testing. Use of newer immunofluorescent antibody tests are helpful for identifying chlamydial conjunctivitis. One such commercially available system (Syva MicroTrak Chlamydia Trachomatis Direct Specimen Test) is useful for identifying the organism obtained from any appropriate body site and includes specific directions for obtaining conjunctival specimens.

Eosinophils. Ocular exudate may be examined for the presence of eosinophils. A finding of one or more eosinophils on material prepared with Wright's stain or a simple wet prep examination that demonstrates dark or green granulated white blood cells is considered highly suggestive of allergic conjunctivitis.

Radiologic Imaging

In general, radiography is not helpful in the evaluation of the patient with visual loss, chemical injury, or a nontraumatic cause of a red, painful eye. However, special circumstances necessitate the use of radiographs. The patient with suspected orbital cellulitis may benefit from a computed tomogram of the orbit. Plain radiographs are useful in the localization of penetrating foreign objects.

Other Laboratory Tests

Other laboratory tests are rarely of use in management of eye problems. One important exception might be the use of the erythrocyte sedimentation rate (ESR) in patients with loss of vision. Among the causes of amaurosis fugax are the vasculitis syndromes, including temporal arteritis. This treatable cause of visual loss is suggested by an elevated ESR.

REFINED DIFFERENTIAL DIAGNOSIS

Following a thorough history, physical examination, and performance of diagnostic adjuncts, a diagnosis can be reached in most patients. This chapter will focus on the six most serious and common causes of a painful red eye: infectious and allergic conjunctivitis, iritis, keratitis, herpetic infection, corneal abscess, and acute glaucoma. Table 34–1 highlights key differential points in making the diagnosis. Subconjunctival hemorrhage is a common cause of painless red eye. Unless severe or recurrent, it is a benign condition. More complex causes include hypertension and hemostatic disorders (Fig. 34–4A).

Infective Conjunctivitis

The most common etiology of the red eye is conjunctivitis. This condition is not associated with marked ocular pain or disturbance of vision. It may be due to bacterial or viral

TABLE 34–1. Features That Differentiate Causes of the Red Painful Eye

	Acute Conjunctivitis	Iritis, Uveitis, Iridocyclitis	Corneal Trauma and Inflammations	Acute Glaucoma
Incidence	Common	Common	Common	Uncommon
Pain	None–moderate	Moderate	Moderate–severe	Severe
Vision affected	No	Slight	Moderate–severe	Severe
Discharge	Yes	No	Yes	No
Photophobia	No	Moderate	Moderate	Severe
Injection	Diffuse (+lid)	Circumcorneal	Diffuse	Diffuse
Cornea	Clear	Clear	Abrasion, foreign body, ulceration, punctate stain	Cloudy
Pupil: size, response	Normal / Normal	Small / Poor to normal	Normal / Normal	Large / Poor
Intraocular pressure	Normal	Normal	Normal	Elevated

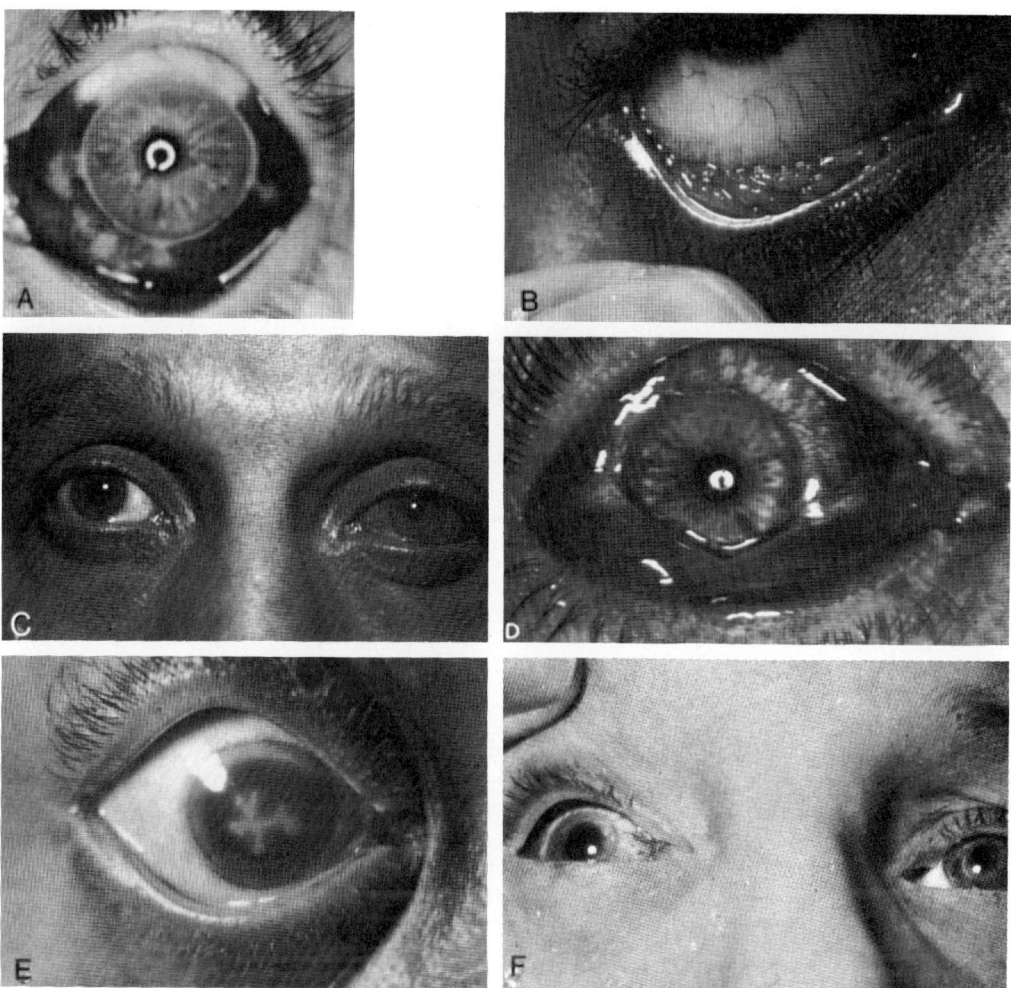

FIGURE 34–4. *External signs of eye pathology. (A) Subconjunctival hemorrhage. (B) Ocular allergy, enlarged lid follicles. (C) Acute iritis. (D) Acute epidemic keratoconjunctivitis showing corneal infiltrates and chemosis. (E) Herpes simplex (dendritic keratitis). (F) Narrow angle-closure glaucoma showing dilated pupil, loss of corneal luster, and red eye. (See color plate at the front of this book.) (From Scheie HG, Albert DM: Textbook of Ophthalmology, 9th ed. Philadelphia, W.B. Saunders, 1977.)*

infection, and the two are often difficult to distinguish on examination. The presence of a purulent discharge with crusting of the lid margin suggests bacterial infection. However, on awakening, the patient with a viral infection may also find himself prying open an eye closed by dried secretions.

Obtaining a culture is normally not necessary because conjunctivitis is a self-limited illness that responds to a broad range of topical antibiotics. Exceptions include conjunctivitis in the neonate, for which gonococcal or chlamydial etiology is considered. The former is marked by a hyperacute conjunctivitis with profuse purulent exudate. Gonorrhea may also cause a severe hyperacute, painful conjunctivitis in the adult patient.

Conjunctivitis due to *Chlamydia trachomatis* is increasingly recognized. Newborns are infected in the birth canal and develop an acute conjunctivitis after an incubation period of 5 to 14 days. Infants who have received appropriate antichlamydial prophylaxis at birth may later become infected from mothers who have chlamydial cervicitis and practice poor hygiene in relation to the neonate's care.

Adult inclusion conjunctivitis due to *Chlamydia* begins as an acute disease that is often indistinguishable from viral infection. It is most common in young adults in the sexually active years and may occur in combination with other types of venereal disease. Up to 60% of men will report associated genitourinary symptoms. Findings suggestive of chlamydial infection include association with venereal symptoms and a history of chronic conjunctivitis that is unresponsive to topical antimicrobial therapy.

Allergic Conjunctivitis

Ocular allergy is a common cause of conjunctivitis. Patients may be allergic to many substances, including airborne allergens, drugs, cosmetics, and contact lens products. In many cases the causes are never identified. Redness is the most reliable sign, and itching is the most reliable symptom of ocular allergy. Itching is not a prominent feature of other ocular diseases.

The pale pink conjunctivae typical of ocular allergy may be accompanied by localized swelling or angioneurotic edema; this chemosis may assume alarming proportions. The lids may swell as well. If the presentation is uniocular, one should consider a reaction to insect protein as in gnats and other flying insects that lodge as conjunctival foreign bodies. This is a common problem in the summer months.

A recurrent bilateral hypersensitivity often found in children with a history of family atopy is vernal conjunctivitis. This typically occurs in the spring or fall and is characterized by huge cobblestone papillae under the upper lid (Fig. 34–4B). The discharge is characteristic in that several times a day the child may pull a ropy, thick strand of yellow material from beneath the eyelids.

Iritis

The patient with acute iritis usually presents with monocular pain, redness, and photophobia. There is no discharge as with conjunctivitis, and the inflammation typical of iritis is much deeper, especially around the limbus. The pain is usually described as a deep ache like that of a toothache. The globe itself is sore to the touch. Iritis can be a recurring condition; thus, the patient may relate similar experiences in the past.

The pupil in patients with iritis is small (miotic) and is poorly reactive to light (Fig. 34–4C). The intraocular pressure is low and a careful examination, including fluorescein staining, will confirm the absence of foreign body or corneal abrasion as a cause of the patient's symptoms. As previously discussed, a slit lamp examination reveals cells and protein exudation (flare) in the anterior chamber. Pupillary dilatation and ciliary muscle relaxation with a mydriatic-cycloplegic medication often decrease the pain significantly.

Keratitis

Corneal injury, whether due to trauma or infection, may also present with accompanying conjunctival injection (Fig. 34–4D). This is why the cornea is carefully examined in all cases of red eye. The corneal nerve endings are quite sensitive; therefore, injury due to a variety of causes will present with moderate to severe pain, depending on the amount of epithelial disruption present. Vision is affected variably following corneal injury. A small central corneal abrasion or mild corneal swelling due to overwear of a contact lens may reduce visual acuity dramatically. In contrast, a more peripheral corneal injury may affect vision minimally except for blurriness due to increased lacrimation.

Increased tearing is a reflex caused by the irritated corneal nerve endings, as is blepharospasm. Photophobia may also occur following corneal injury. Disruption of the optical surface causes light to be scattered within the eye. This causes bright light sources to create glare and discomfort. In addition, deep corneal injury may inflame the iris sphincter; this mild iritis leads to pain and aversion to light. These responses occur to varying degrees with most corneal injuries and further reduce vision as well as limit the ease of examination.

Occasionally symptoms of keratitis occur in the absence of an identified insult. This may be due to corneal erosion and represents spontaneous loss of corneal epithelium. This sloughing of epithelium in an area of previous abrasion or injury is probably due to a lack of complete, tightly adherent healing of the epithelium to the underlying layers of the cornea.

A similar condition occurs in the contact lens wearer who leaves the lens in place for excessively long periods. The drying effect of this overuse causes lens adherence to the cornea and subsequent removal will cause extensive corneal damage. The patient typically awakens with severe eye pain several hours after removal. Infection secondary to contact lenses may also cause keratitis.

Excessive exposure to ultraviolet light sources such as sunlight, a sunlamp source, or an arc-welding instrument may cause diffuse corneal injury. This may be demonstrated as fine punctate fluorescein staining of the cornea that is best appreciated by slit lamp examination and is suspected based on the history.

Herpetic Infection

Symptoms of herpetic infection of the cornea may mimic those of corneal abrasion. Therefore, it is necessary to check corneal sensation if there is doubt about the cause of injury. Gentle stroking of the cornea with a drawn-out cotton swab may reveal a diminished response and may suggest herpetic infection. In early herpetic infection, superficial punctate erosions or a single vesicle of the cornea may be all that is apparent. Eventually, a typical dendritic or branching pattern of the corneal injury will be apparent on fluorescein staining (Fig. 34–4E). An early herpetic infection can sometimes be mistaken for conjunctivitis, corneal abrasion, iritis, or even allergic conjunctivitis.

Other infectious organisms capable of causing corneal injury include herpes zoster virus and gonorrhea. Typically, bacteria invade the cornea of the immunocompromised host. Zoster infection is characterized by typical lesions in the distribution of the trigeminal nerve. Involvement of the tip of the nose (nasociliary nerve) suggests corneal involvement.

Corneal Abscess

The patient with prolonged eye redness and discharge who presents with ocular pain and diminished vision may develop an invasive corneal infection. A flocculent area of corneal exudate that cannot be removed by means of irrigation suggests that ulceration has occurred. Slit lamp examination will reveal the depth and extent of corneal injury.

Acute Glaucoma

An acute narrow angle closure glaucoma attack is a relatively uncommon problem. It must be considered in the patient with a red, painful eye who complains of poor vision. Vision may be described as increasingly foggy with associated halos surrounding light sources. Classically, the patient complains of a deep, severe, boring type of globe pain and appears acutely ill. Constitutional symptoms of headache, nausea, and vomiting often accompany this condition. In contrast to the small pupil seen in iritis, the pupil in the patient with acute glaucoma is usually mid-dilated and nonreactive. There is a loss of corneal luster; it may appear quite hazy (Fig. 34–4F). The globe itself feels very hard to palpation, and this strongly suggests the diagnosis if there is a marked difference between the two eyes. The diagnosis of acute glaucoma is made by the finding of an elevated intraocular pressure by tonometry.

PROBLEM 1 In the young man with blurry vision, eye redness, a small pupil, and photophobia findings on physical examination suggested iritis. Slit lamp examination demonstrated the classic flare and cell findings associated with this disorder.

PROBLEM 2 The emergency physician considered allergic and infectious causes of this patient's condition. He was concerned about the medication the patient had been putting into her eyes during the last few days. The corneal involvement and diminished blink reflex pointed to a herpetic infection, even though she did not have the classic "dendritic" pattern of corneal defects. If her friend's medication contained steroids, it may have worsened her infection.

PRINCIPLES OF MANAGEMENT

The general management of patients with a red painful eye includes relief of pain and inflammation.

Pain Control

Ocular pain may be controlled with local anesthetics, mydriatics, cycloplegics, and oral analgesics. Topical anesthetics such as 0.5% proparacaine are frequently applied during the physical examination. Relief of superficial ocular pain occurs immediately but wears off in 15 minutes. Repeated use of local anesthetics can retard healing and cause corneal injury. Therefore, local anesthetics should not be given to patients for home use. Table 34–2 lists the characteristics of commonly used anesthetics.

Muscle spasm is thought to play a role in the ocular pain of many conditions. Mydriatics paralyze the pupillary constrictor muscle, causing dilation, whereas cycloplegics affect the ciliary muscle. Combinations of cycloplegics and mydriatics are frequently used for relief of ocular pain. Since pupillary dilation occurs, the patient is warned about driving an automobile or going out in the sunlight without eye protection. Mydriatics and cycloplegics are contraindicated in patients with known narrow-angle glaucoma. Table 34–3 lists the characteristics of common mydriatics and cycloplegics.

TABLE 34–2. Topical Anesthetics*

Drug	Concentration (%)	Onset	Duration	Reactions	Comments
Cocaine	2–10	Immediate	20 min	Possible local ischemia, tachycardia, hypertension, restlessness. Excitation infrequent	Mydriatic (rarely used in emergency department)
Benoxinate hydrochloride (Dorsacaine)	0.4	1–2 min	10–15 min	Infrequent side effects	Compatible with fluorescein
Proparacaine hydrochloride (Ophthaine)	0.5	20 sec	10–15 min	Transient local symptoms, allergic reactions rare	Least irritating and toxic; anesthetic of choice
Tetracaine hydrochloride (Pontocaine, Ancel)	0.5	4 min	30–40 min	Drowsiness	Stings on instillation

*One or two instillations of these medications can be used for short-term examination and procedures. Prolonged use may delay healing.
From Zun L, Mathews J: Formulary of commonly used ophthalmologic medications. Emerg Med Clin North Am 6(1):121, 1988.

TABLE 34-3. Mydriatics/Cycloplegics

Drug	Concentration (%)	Duration	Effects/Uses	Contra-indications	Adverse Reactions	Notes
Mydriatic						
Phenylephrine hydrochloride (Neo-Synephrine)	2.5–10.0 (solution)	2–3 hr	Pupillary dilation, treatment of uveitis, decongestant, vasoconstriction, refraction	Narrow-angle glaucoma; hypertensive, cardiac, or patients with aneurysms	Pain on instillation, blurred vision, glare in sunlight; possible cardiovascular collapse with large dose	No cycloplegic effect; sensitive to air, heat, and light
Mydriatic/cycloplegic						
Atropine sulfate	0.25–2.00 (solution) 0.5–1.0 (ointment)	2 wk	Long duration, pupillary dilation. Use for treatment of uveitis	Narrow-angle glaucoma, hyper-sensitivity	Possible systemic absorption, photophobia, dry mouth, loss of accommodation	Produces mydriasis and cycloplegia for refraction
Cyclopentolate hydrochloride (Cyclogel)	0.5–2.0 (solution)	24 hr	Pupillary dilation for refraction and funduscopy	Narrow-angle glaucoma	Anticholinergic behavioral changes in older adults and children	
Homatropine hydrobromide	2–5 (solution)	10–48 hr	Long duration, pupillary dilation. Use for treatment of uveitis and for refraction in children	Narrow-angle glaucoma	2–4 day loss of accommodation, dry mouth, and photophobia	Anticholinergic. Moderate to long-acting sensitivity. Side effects are rare. Drug of choice in emergency department
Scopolamine hydrobromide (Hyoscine)	0.25 (solution)	2–7 days	Cycloplegia, treatment of uveitis, refraction in children. Use in postoperative cataract patients	Narrow-angle glaucoma	Dizziness and disorientation in elderly; tachycardia	Effective cycloplegic. Rarely used in emergency department
Tropicamide (Mydriacil)	0.5–1.0 (solution)	6 hr	Papillary dilation, cycloplegia, uveitis, refraction, fundus examination	Narrow-angle glaucoma	Loss of accommodation, photophobia, dry mouth, behavioral disturbances; cardiorespiratory collapse reported in children	Most useful for ophthalmoscopy. Weak cycloplegic, effective mydriatic

From Zun L, Mathews J: Formulary of commonly used ophthalmologic medications. Emerg Med Clin North Am 6(1):122, 1988.

Patients with moderate to severe ocular pain may require oral or parenteral narcotic analgesics for relief of pain.

Relief of Inflammation

Topical vasocontrictors and decongestants are used by some physicians to help control the inflammatory symptoms of conjunctivitis. They are especially useful for the treatment of allergic symptoms. Ophthalmic steroids *are not* given unless the emergency physician has consulted an ophthalmologist.

Specific Conditions

The specific management of the painful red eye depends on the diagnosis made. Table 34–4 summarizes the management of specific conditions.

Infective Conjunctivitis. Conjunctivitis is the most common cause of a red eye and is not associated with visual disturbance or significant eye discomfort. Differentiating bacterial from viral etiology is not essential in most cases because these are self-limited infections. Treatment in either instance consists of a brief course (5 to 7 days) of a topical antibiotic such as 10% sulfacetamide (Sulamyd). Table 34–5 lists the characteristics of available topical antibiotics. The preferred antibiotics for initial therapy are erythromycin, sulfacetamide sodium, and sulfisoxazole. If chlamydial infection is suspected, confirmatory immunofluorescent testing is performed. A prolonged course of oral and topical therapy with erythromycin is given for these infections.

Allergic Conjunctivitis. Ocular allergy is best treated by removing the offending agent, especially inappropriately self-prescribed eye drops. Topical or oral antihistamine or decongestant medications such as the combination product of naphazoline and antazoline (Vasocon-A) may be given for symptomatic treatment. Although corticosteroid eye drops are extremely effective for allergic conditions, their use is deferred to the ophthalmologic consultant. Treating an unsuspected herpetic infection with steroids can have a devastating effect on the patient's outcome.

Iritis. The therapy for acute iritis is directed at dilating the pupil. This promotes comfort by paralyzing the ciliary body, thus eliminating the painful ciliary spasm. A listing of mydriatic and cycloplegic agents is provided in Table 34–3. Homatropine is the drug of choice prior to referral. Because iritis is an inflammatory condition, a corticosteroid may be necessary. It is prescribed by the ophthalmologic consultant after confirmation of the diagnosis.

Acute Glaucoma. In acute angle-closure glaucoma, the goal of therapy is to constrict the iris away from its point of contact with the peripheral portion of the cornea. In this position, it occludes the normal drainage mechanism for the aqueous humor. This is best accomplished by constricting the pupil with a miotic agent such as 1% pilocarpine. Unfortunately, even short periods of increased intraocular pressure cause ischemia of the iris and render it unresponsive to stimulation. Therefore, medication is given to lower the intraocular pressure, thus restoring circulation to the sphincter muscle so that a miotic agent will work. The first line drug is the beta-adrenergic blocker, Timolol 0.5%. It reduces the production of aqueous humor. If therapy fails, a hyperosmotic agent is given to increase the osmolarity of the intravascular compartment. Increased osmolarity leads to a bulk flow of water from the extravascular compartment (including the eye), thereby reducing the volume of fluid inside the eye and the intraocular pressure. Oral glycerol will suffice unless the patient is nauseated or vomiting; in this instance, mannitol is given intravenously. In addition, some authors recommend acetazolamide given parenterally to further reduce the pressure. This drug can cause severe potassium loss, so close monitoring is necessary. The most important treatment from the patient's perspective is adequate analgesia. Parenteral narcotics are commonly employed.

As the intraocular pressure falls, the iris sphincter will respond to the miotic agent; the peripheral iris will be stretched sufficiently to pull it away from the chamber angle. Usually this medication approach successfully terminates an attack. As the intraocular pressure falls, the corneal edema will resolve within several hours. It is emphasized that an ophthalmologist should be contacted early in the treatment phase. In addition to assisting in medical management of the attack, the ophthalmologist may perform a laser iridectomy immediately after resolution of the acute event.

Invasive Keratitis. When corneal invasion due to infection is suspected, immediate consultation with an ophthalmologist is necessary. All patients are given intense topical antibiotic therapy. Patients with suspected gonorrheal infection or evidence of abscess formation are admitted to the hospital. These patients will require intensive ocular

TABLE 34-4. Management of the Red Painful Eye

	Acute Conjunctivitis	Iritis, Uveitis	Corneal Trauma	Corneal Infection	Acute Glaucoma
Initial emergency department phase	*Infectious Causes* Topical antibiotics Oral erythrocin or tetracycline (not in children) for *Chlamydia* *Allergic Causes* Antihistamine-decongestant, PO or topical	Cycloplegics Corticosteroids may be necessary but should be given by eye consultant	Foreign body removal Consider cycloplegic if lesion is deep or extensive Topical antibiotics Patching	Topical antibiotics Penicillin or cephalosporin IV for gonorrheal infection Topical antiviral agents for herpetic infection	Timolol, a topical beta-blocking agent Hyperosmolar agents: (a) glycerol PO, (b) mannitol IV Acetazolamide IM or IV (optional) Miotic agent, pilocarpine 2% drops Pain relief, usually systemic narcotics
Acute consultant intervention	None	Telephone consultation	None (unless perforation is suspected)	Corneal abscess requires immediate intervention by consultant	Consultant should assist in management begun by emergency department personnel
Disposition and follow-up	If not improved in 48 hours	Arranged with eye consultant in 24-48 hours	Arrangement is made for prompt removal by consultant if necessary Otherwise, follow-up is dependent on severity of injury	Hospitalization for abscess or gonorrhea Prompt referral for remainder of cases	Per consultant's direction

TABLE 34–5. Topical Ophthalmic Antibiotics

Drug*	Preparation	Use	Comment
Bacitracin	500–1000 μ/gm ointment	Most gram-positive organisms	Limited ophthalmic uses. Combined with polymyxin as Polysporin
Chloramphenicol (Chloromycetin, Chloroptic, Econochlor, Ophthochlor)	0.5% solution, 1% ointment	Gram-positive and some gram-negative and anaerobic organisms	Bacteriostatic. Aplastic anemia has been reported from topical usage
Erythromycin (Ilotycin)	0.5% ointment	*Chlamydia* and *Staphylococcus*	Chlamydial infections need topical and oral treatment for at least two weeks
Gentamicin sulfate (Garamycin, Genoptic)	3 mg/ml solution 3 mg/gm ointment	Gram-negative organisms	Indicated for serious ocular infections and corneal ulcers
Neomycin	2.5 mg/ml solution 5 mg/gm ointment	Limited number of gram-negative and gram-positive organisms	About 6% of the North American population is allergic to neomycin. Usually combined with polymyxin and bacitracin as Neosporin
Sulfacetamide sodium (Bleph 10, Cetamide, Sulamide, Vasosulf)	10–30% solution 10% ointment	Gram-positive and gram-negative organisms	Initial therapy for conjunctivitis; low cost, low allergenicity. Stinging on instillation
Sulfisoxazole (Gantrisin)	4% solution 4% ointment	Same as for sulfacetamide sodium	Same as for sulfacetamide sodium
Tetracycline (Aureomycin)	1% solution and ointment	*Chlamydia*	Treatment of *Chlamydia* infections topically and systemically
Tobramycin (Tobex)	0.3% solution and ointment	Same as for gentamicin	Same as for gentamicin

*Erythromycin, sulfacetamide sodium, and sulfisoxazole are preferred for initial therapy.
From Zun L, Mathews J: Formulary of commonly used ophthalmologic medications. Emerg Med Clin North Am 6(1):123, 1988.

irrigation with frequent application of a topical antibiotic. In addition, intravenous antibiotic therapy may be directed by the consultant.

PROBLEM 1 The young man with iritis was given a mydriatic-cycloplegic, homatropine. It was decided not to give him steroids at this time because of the danger of undiagnosed early herpetic infection.

SPECIAL CONSIDERATIONS

Pediatric Patients

A reddened eye in a neonate or infant is always abnormal. It is usually caused by infection, and chlamydial conjunctivitis is of concern. Congenital glaucoma is also considered and may be difficult to diagnose; therefore, all patients less than 6 months of age need ophthalmologic follow-up.

Geriatric Patients

The older adult frequently has coexisting medical problems. Hypertension and atherosclerosis predispose to vascular catastrophe; diabetes mellitus may be the setting in which a simple conjunctivitis has progressed to an invasive infectious keratitis with corneal abscess formation. As with children, baseline visual acuity may be more difficult to assess, and the geriatric patient may have a less impressive inflammatory response.

DISPOSITION AND FOLLOW-UP

The following categories are useful guidelines for ophthalmologic consultation:

Immediate	Urgent	Follow-Up Examination Required
Acute glaucoma	Iritis	Conjunctivitis
Corneal abscess	Most keratitis, including superficial infections	Ocular allergy
Central retinal artery occlusion		
Perforation of globe		
Herpetic keratitis		

Most patients with acute conjunctivitis will improve regardless of the cause; thus acute consultant intervention is not necessary. It is important to emphasize to the patient that if the problem has not improved in 48 hours further ophthalmologic examination is necessary. This is especially important in the patient who has a loss of visual clarity or increasing eye pain during the follow-up period.

The management of patients with acute iritis or keratitis is discussed on the telephone with the ophthalmologist; arrangements for a follow-up visit within 24 to 48 hours should be made.

Patients with invasive corneal infection, acute glaucoma, central retinal artery occlusion, or perforation of the globe need to be seen immediately by an ophthalmologist. Prompt hospitalization is indicated in most instances.

PROBLEM 1 The patient was referred to the ophthalmologist, who saw him the next day.

PROBLEM 2 The ophthalmologist was called to see the patient in the emergency department. He agreed with the diagnosis of herpetic keratitis. Cultures were taken, and the patient was placed on an antiviral agent, idoxuridine. The consultant followed the patient's condition daily in his office.

DOCUMENTATION

1. Historical notes about pain, any alteration of vision, and the presence of traumatic or chemical injury.
2. Results of visual acuity testing.
3. Pupil equality and responses, extraocular motions, clarity of the cornea and anterior chamber, and results of fundus examination.
4. Results of fluorescein staining and examination of lid for foreign bodies.
5. Notes on phone consultation with ophthalmologist.
6. Medications given.
7. Discharge instructions.

SUMMARY AND FINAL POINTS

- The eye responds to noxious stimuli in three ways, resulting in redness, pain, or diminished vision.
- Sudden loss of vision indicates an emergent condition that needs immediate attention.
- Visual acuity is the best indicator of eye function and must be documented in all cases.
- Steroids are not given by the emergency physician unless the patient is evaluated by an ophthalmologist, and herpetic infection is ruled out.
- Pain that is relieved by local anesthetics generally indicates superficial inflammation.
- The main differential diagnoses concerned in the red painful eye are conjunctivitis, keratitis, herpes, iritis, trauma, and glaucoma.

BIBLIOGRAPHY

Texts

1. American Academy of Ophthalmology: Ophthalmology Study Guide for Students and Practitioners of Medicine (5th ed). San Francisco, American Academy of Ophthalmology, 1987.
2. Goldberg S: Ophthalmology Made Ridiculously Simple (3rd ed). Miami, Med Master, 1987.
3. Newell FW: Ophthalmology: Principles and Concepts (6th ed). St. Louis, C. V. Mosby, 1986.
4. Yanoff M, Fine BS: Ocular Pathology. Philadelphia, J. B. Lippincott, 1988.

Journal Articles

1. Abelson MB, Smith MR, Friedlaender MH: Effects of topically applied ocular decongestant and antihistamine. Am J Ophthalmol 90:254–257, 1980.
2. Friedlaender MH: Ocular allergy: Scratching the surface of the red eye. Postgrad Med 79:261–271, 1986.
3. Henderly DE, Gentsler AJ, Smith RE, et al: Changing patterns of uveitis. Am J Ophthalmol 103:131–136, 1987.
4. Howes DS: The red eye. Emerg Med Clin North Am 6:43–56, 1988.
5. Johnson DH, Brubaaker RF: Glaucoma: An overview. Mayo Clinic Proc 61:59–67, 1986.
6. Melamed MA: A generalist's guide to eye emergencies. Emerg Med 16:99–126, 1984.
7. Perkins ES: Intraocular inflammatory disorders: Uveitis. Primary Care 9:715–728, 1982.
8. Shingleton BJ: A clearer look at ocular emergencies. Emerg Med 21:52–69, 1989.
9. Yanofsky NN: The acute painful eye. Emerg Med Clin North Am 6:21–42, 1988.

CHAPTER 35

EYE TRAUMA

WARREN J. VENTRIGLIA, M.D.

PROBLEM 1 A 16 year old student was brought in by ambulance after he was struck in the right eye by a batted baseball.

PROBLEM 2 Police and rescue personnel were at the scene of a domestic argument during which drain-cleaning crystals were thrown into the eyes of a 32 year old female.

PROBLEM 3 A 43 year old auto mechanic felt some discomfort in his left eye just before his lunch break. He came to the emergency department after noting a gradual increase in pain after he had finished working.

QUESTIONS TO CONSIDER

1. What types of eye injury are seen in the emergency department?
2. In the prehospital setting, what immediate treatment is given to patients with eye injuries?
3. What are the key historical questions to ask patients who have sustained blunt, penetrating, chemical, or other types of eye trauma?
4. What constitutes an adequate physical examination of a patient with ocular trauma? What specific tests are important?
5. What is the appropriate emergency department management of eye injuries?
6. How is the eye patched correctly?
7. Which patients with eye trauma need immediate referral for ophthalmologic consultation?

INTRODUCTION

Eye trauma is a leading cause of visual impairment and blindness in the United States. More than 1000 eye injuries occur each day in the workplace, and millions of eye injuries require medical attention annually. Approximately 25% of all eye injuries related to sports and fireworks result in permanent visual impairment.

Eye trauma is a challenging problem for the emergency physician for several reasons. First, the dramatic presentation of many eye injuries may distract the physician from attending to more serious extraocular injuries. Second, severe eye injury may make assessment difficult owing to patient discomfort, thereby obscuring findings that may have prognostic implications. Third, physicians often have a limited understanding of ocular pathophysiology, thereby impeding discovery or delaying treatment. The emergency physician's major role is to anticipate, evaluate, and diagnose the presence and nature of injury to the eye. The range of treatment options is limited, and the timing of ophthalmologic referral is determined by both findings and suspicion.

A basic understanding of eye anatomy is necessary to translate data found on physical examination into potential pathophysiology. The eye is a relatively tough globe containing important structures that constitute the visual axis—the cornea, anterior chamber, lens, vitreous, and retina (Fig. 35–1A). The cornea, which is important for gross refraction (bending) of light prior to fine focusing by the lens, is thinner (0.5 mm) at the center and thicker (1.0 mm) near the margin (limbus). This anatomic fact is important when considering removal of a central corneal foreign body. Injury to the corneal surface causes light to be scattered instead of focused. Consequently, patients with corneal abrasions have an aversion to bright light. The cornea also contains sensory fibers and is a major source of pain felt in the eye.

The conjunctiva may respond to injury with engorged blood vessels and edema, causing an uncomfortable and ugly chemosis. Significant intraocular inflammation can be heralded by the presence of dilated vessels from the anterior ciliary artery around the margin of the cornea. This phenomenon is called a *limbic flush*. The conjunctival fornices extend superiorly, inferiorly, medially, and laterally from the easily visible portions of the eye and can serve as repositories for foreign bodies or caustic materials.

The eye is suspended in the orbit by connective tissue, fat, and the extraocular muscles (Fig. 35–1B). Swelling behind the eye due to edema or blood can push it forward from the orbit (exophthalmos). Loss of the substance behind the eye, e.g., from a "blowout" that forces the retrobulbar fat into a sinus, can cause the eye to sink into the orbit (enophthalmos). Extraocular muscle (EOM) injury can cause a variety of gaze disturbances, most commonly pain and double vision (diplopia), during testing of eye movement. A frequently seen problem is limited upward gaze due to swelling or entrapment of the inferior rectus muscle secondary to blunt trauma and injury to the

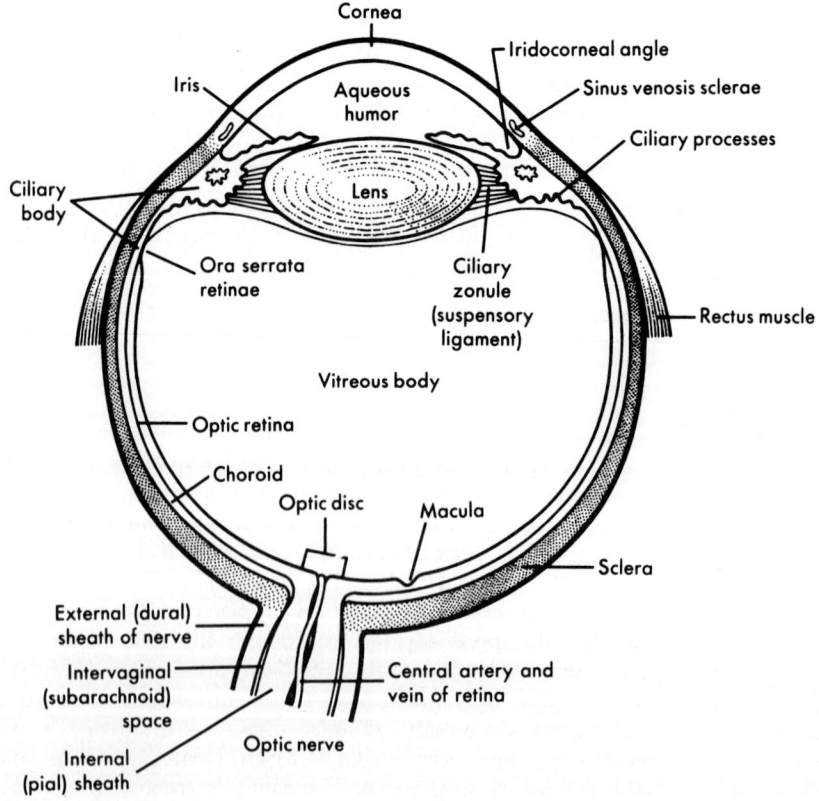

FIGURE 35–1. *A, Basic anatomy of the eye. (Reproduced by permission from Greene JS, Yanofsky NN: Common ophthalmologic problems. In Rosen P, et al (eds): Emergency Medicine: Concepts and Clinical Practice. St. Louis, The C.V. Mosby Co., 1983.)*

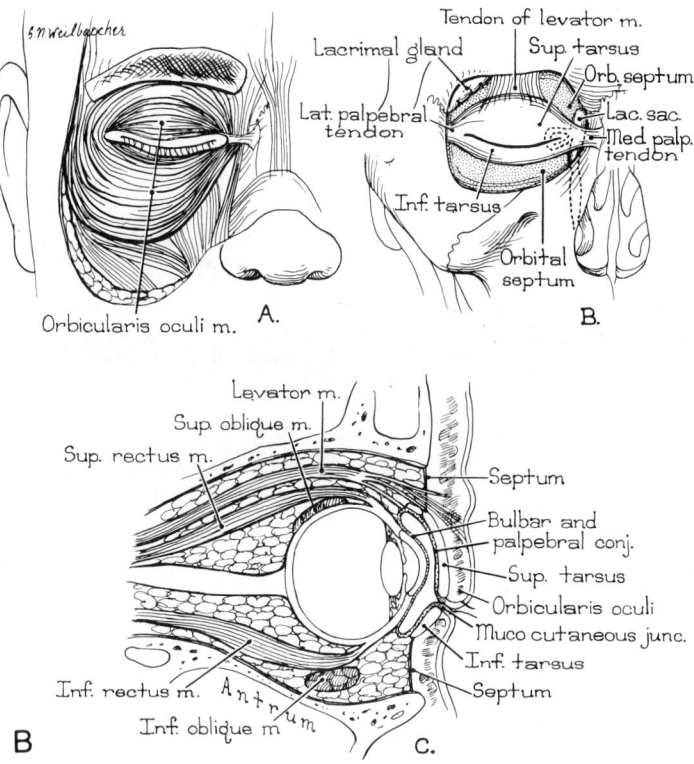

FIGURE 35–1 Continued B, Anatomy of the lids and orbit. (Reproduced by permission from Deutsch TA, Feller DB (eds): Paton and Goldberg's Management of Ocular Injuries. Philadelphia, W.B. Saunders, 1985.)

inferior bony support of the orbit. The bony orbit protects the eye fairly well. The medial and inferior walls are the weakest and are susceptible to fracture or blowout from the blunt injury. Blunt forces can also damage other structures, including the lens and supporting tissue, retina, insertions of the extraocular muscles, the choroid and limbus, and the insertion of the optic nerve.

Injuries to the lacrimal gland, lacrimal sac, and nasolacrimal duct can result in dysfunction of the lubricating mechanisms of the eye. A laceration through the mucocutaneous junction of the lid, called a *gray line laceration,* may heal improperly, resulting in problems with tearing or scar. The meticulous layered approximation of this wound is most often completed by a consultant. Ptosis of the upper lid may occur owing to injury to the levator muscle or its insertion on the upper tarsal plate.

Physiologically, the eye is protected by reflex mechanisms. The blink reflex rapidly closes the eyelids when impending trauma is perceived. When the eyelids close, the Bell's reflex causes the eye to rotate upward and out, moving the cornea under partial protection of the upper bony orbital rim. Thus, the inferior portion of the cornea and lower sclera are at greater risk of injury and must be carefully examined.

PREHOSPITAL CARE

Prehospital care of injury to the eye first excludes any other significant injury. Accordingly, careful assessment and monitoring of the airway, breathing, circulation, and stabilization of the cervical spine are primary considerations.

History

In attending to the eye, the rescue squad will determine (1) the mechanism of injury, (2) the status of vision prior to injury, (3) the presence of a coexistent medical illness, e.g., diabetes mellitus, hypertension, seizure disorder.

Physical Examination

Prehospital evaluation of eye trauma is limited.
1. Gross visual acuity is assessed by testing the patient's vision for perception of light, hand movement, or counting of fingers.
2. Gross inspection is made to look for obviously altered eye anatomy.
3. If ocular rupture or laceration is suspected, the eye is not manipulated.

Intervention

1. All chemical injuries are *immediately* irrigated with water or crystalloid.
2. The patient's head is elevated to decrease intraocular pressure.
3. The eye is covered with a shield, and no pressure is applied to the globe.
4. Activities that may cause the patient to blink vigorously or produce the Valsalva maneuver are avoided. These actions may extrude ocular contents if the sclera is ruptured.
5. If penetrating objects are still in place, they are not removed.
6. Time is taken to calm and reassure the patient.

PROBLEM 1 The rescue squad reported that the student misjudged a hit, and, although "stunned," he was not rendered unconscious. He walked to the dugout with some assistance. His neck was found to be nontender, and he appeared to be alert and could count fingers with the injured eye. The eye was reported to be "not looking normal." The patient's vital signs were normal. He was transported in a sitting position.

The reported history indicated no apparent neurologic deficits. As the patient was transported, the squad paid close attention to his level of consciousness. A gently applied eye shield minimized the possibility of further eye injury.

PROBLEM 2 The rescue squad reported that the patient was "hysterical." She stated that her husband had left immediately after throwing the crystals, but would soon return. The squad quickly explained to the patient the need to dilute the material in her eyes and began irrigating. After 2 to 3 minutes of irrigation with normal saline solution, the patient became calmer. She was able to count fingers, although she complained of burning and blurring.

Although normal saline solution is more "physiologic," any source of clean water can be used for irrigation, including a garden hose, shower, sink, or industrial eye wash station. Although rescue personnel at the scene of the domestic argument would like to expedite the patient's transfer from a "hostile" environment, *immediate* irrigation is indicated.

INITIAL APPROACH IN THE EMERGENCY DEPARTMENT

The evaluation of eye trauma requires an organized approach, which begins in the emergency department triage area. The initial assessment includes the following steps.
1. If warranted by the history, the physician continues to anticipate significant and potentially life-threatening traumatic processes elsewhere in the body.
2. The history obtained by the rescue squad is confirmed, and a brief history of the incident is obtained from the patient.

3. The benefit of any treatment instituted by the patient or rescue personnel is assessed.

4. After chemical injury, irrigation usually precedes formal visual acuity testing, although gross finger counting may be attempted while the equipment is being set up. Blepharospasm often impedes adequate irrigation, and topical anesthesia is necessary. Occasionally, opening the lids by using Desmarres retractors or a lid speculum may be necessary. Particulate debris is removed by gently sweeping the conjunctival fornices with a moistened cotton swab or flushing with a stream of irrigating solution. One liter is the usual volume used in noncaustic chemical injuries. Irrigating lenses are avoided initially because they may trap debris on the cornea, cause direct corneal trauma, and require frequent anesthetic use. After 300 to 500 ml of solution has been used in irrigation, they may be considered depending on patient tolerance. In the patient with a caustic injury, irrigation should be copious. At least 3 liters of saline solution are needed to neutralize the effects of alkaline burns. A nitrazine test strip can be used to test for a normalized pH after copious flushing. Early consultation is recommended in patients with these injuries.

5. The patient's vital signs and visual acuity are measured. The most important parameter to measure during examination of eye injuries is early, accurate visual acuity testing. Visual acuity testing specifically records the vital function of the eye. The need to document visual acuity before, and preferably after, treatment cannot be overemphasized. Measurement of visual acuity *prior* to any manipulation may protect emergency department staff from liability if poor visual outcome results. The only exceptions are the immediate irrigation needed for corneal chemical injuries and situations requiring a topical anesthetic before the patient will open the eye, e.g., ultraviolet light keratitis.

Most emergency departments use a Snellen eye chart to measure vision at 20 feet. A passing score is given if more than half of a line of symbols is correctly identified. Eyeglasses are worn, or, if glasses are damaged or are not available, vision may be tested looking through a small pinhole eyecover. Pinhole vision reduces the refractive error for patients who usually need corrective lenses. Each eye is tested separately, and the other untested eye is covered with an opaque eye cover. A significant visual acuity defect based in refractive error is a passing score of more than one or two lines difference between the visual acuity with and without the pinhole eye cover. An alternative method of visual acuity testing is use of a pocket near card, which can be used to screen acuity from a specified near distance. If vision is grossly impaired, the patient's ability to count fingers, detect hand motion, localize a light source, or perceive light, in that order, indicates decreasing visual ability. *Normal* visual acuity does *not* exclude significant injury. Visual acuity may be normal in a patient with a hyphema or penetrating injury.

DATA GATHERING

History

A thorough history and ophthalmologic examination are important for patients with acute eye injuries because treatment options are limited, and accurate communication with an ophthalmologic consultant is essential.

Mechanism of Injury. What was the possible speed of the injuring object? What material might it be made of? Hammering metal on metal, use of a pressurized air gun or sprayer, or injury associated with a sharp object are mechanisms that commonly penetrate the globe. The *"penetration potential"* of each mechanism must be considered because these injuries may not cause major symptoms.

In patients with chemical injuries identifying of the causal agent has prognostic importance. For example, acid causes protein precipitation, and damage is somewhat self-limited. Alkali exposure causes an aggressive coagulative necrosis that may penetrate the anterior chamber. Other irritants, such as detergents or solvents, usually cause less severe injury. Cyanoacrylate ("super" glue) often causes only a superficial corneal abrasion if it is removed gently.

Prolonged or incorrect use of contact lenses can result in minimal corneal abrasions or potentially devastating corneal ulcers. Inadvertent viewing of arc-welding light or tanning salon lamps cause superficial corneal damage. Thermal burns may result from contact with a hot object (such as a hair curling iron) or heated liquids. Protective eye reflexes usually limit thermal burn severity, but significant injury can still occur. Explosive injuries may result in deforming mechanisms to the globe, causing retinal or lens injuries. Blunt injury to the orbit, such as that caused by a fist or thrown object, can injure both the ocular globe and the orbital bones.

Timing of Incident. Patients usually come to the emergency department soon after an eye injury. Delays of more than 24 hours should raise the physician's concern about complications, such as rust ring, iritis, or infection.

Sensation of Pain. The *presence* of pain can be caused by significant or minor injuries to the eye. It must be assumed to be significant, and the source investigated thoroughly. The cornea has the most sensitive pain fibers in the eye and severe pain may be caused by corneal irritation only. Pain on illuminating the pupil may result from corneal defects or more significant intraocular damage. Pain felt in the affected eye with penlight illumination of the unaffected eye indicates at least a mild reactive iritis in the affected eye. The *absence* of pain does *not* mean that severe injury has not occurred. Penetration and perforation may not manifest pain immediately. Patients with global disruption due to blunt injury may not feel pain in proportion to the magnitude of the injury.

Visual Disturbance. Alteration in visual ability can provide a clue to the nature of the eye injury.

1. Total *visual loss* (the inability to perceive light) has a grave prognosis and may imply optic nerve damage, severe retinal injury, or opacification along the visual axis.

2. Binocular *diplopia* during eye movement often indicates extraocular muscle dysfunction. Diplopia on upward gaze can occur after blunt trauma because of orbital floor blowout fractures with extraocular muscle entrapment.

3. Severe *photophobia* can result from superficial corneal, iris, or ciliary body injury.

4. Visual *"flashes"* of light or the perception of a hazy area in the visual field may be symptoms of a retinal detachment.

5. A visual *field defect* (scotoma) can indicate injury anywhere along the visual axis, e.g., vitreous hemorrhage, retinal tear, optic nerve injury, optic tract injury, or other cause.

Other Historical Considerations

1. Was the patient *wearing eyeglasses* or *goggles* at the time of the injury? Many industrial and racket sport injuries result from lack of protective eyewear.

2. Does the patient have a *preexisting eye abnormality*, for example, diabetes mellitus with retinopathy, previous ocular trauma, history of eye surgery, or need for eyeglasses?

3. Did the patient *manipulate* the eye or *apply* any *medication after* the *injury* occurred? Improperly performed attempts to remove a foreign body can compound eye trauma.

4. Is the patient's *tetanus* immunization status up to date? Even "minor" eye trauma has been associated with fatal tetanus.

5. Does the patient have any *systemic disease* that may affect evaluation or impede resolution of injury, for example, alcoholism, diabetes mellitus, or sickle cell disease?

PROBLEM 2 The patient's caustic injury was continuously irrigated while en route to the hospital. A rapid vision screening test indicated that the visual acuity was approximately 20/50 in each eye. The patient reported that her eyes were starting to burn again.

Continous irrigation was indicated. There was a visual acuity defect, the symptoms were recurring, and the causative agent was known to cause coagulation necrosis.

PROBLEM 3 The auto mechanic told the triage nurse that he noted a sharp but brief pain in his eye when he was hammering out a bent tire rim. He had always had good vision and did not wear glasses. Visual acuity was recorded as OD (right eye) 20/15 (dominant uninvolved eye) and OS (left eye) 20/30. The patient said that he was in a hurry.

Because of the causative mechanism, this patient was at risk for an ocular perforation. The physician was obligated to make a vigorous search for a penetrating foreign body.

Physical Examination

A systematic approach to all eye injuries will ensure a complete assessment.

Gross Inspection. The pupil, eyelid, conjunctiva, iris, anterior chamber, lens, and adnexa are examined, and the bony orbit is palpated. Sites of potential penetration are sought. When the anterior chamber appears to be flattened, the globe may be ruptured, and ocular manipulation is to be avoided. A hyphema, in which blood collects in a layer in the anterior chamber, implies the existence of an iris root injury. Lacerations of the medial inferior eyelid can damage the canaliculus, an important structure for draining tears from the eye.

Lid Eversion. The palpebral and bulbar conjunctivae must be fully exposed and inspected for injury. The lower conjunctiva can be inspected by asking the patient to gaze upward and applying downward traction on the lower lid. The upper lid requires eversion using a cotton swab or lid retractor (Fig. 35–2). The patient is instructed to look

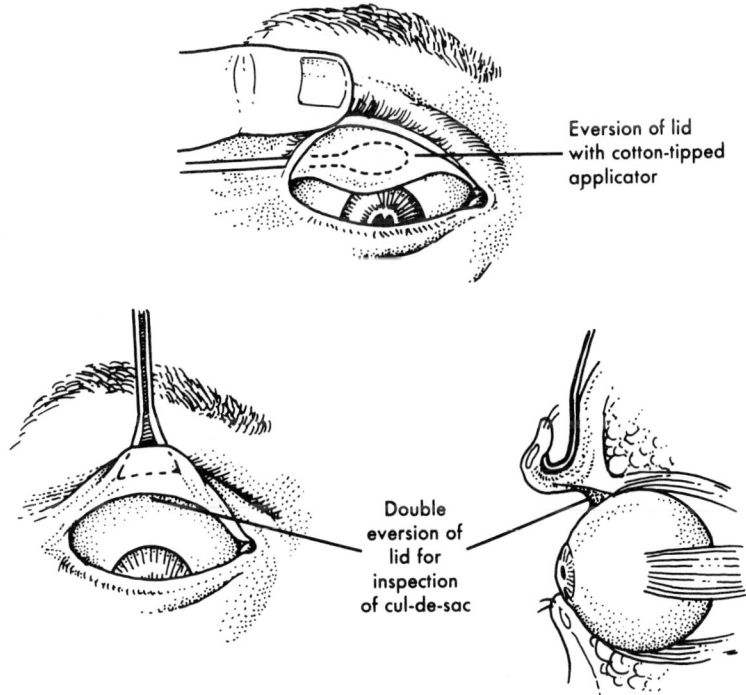

FIGURE 35–2. Techniques of single and double eversion of the upper eyelid. (Reproduced with permission from Clark RB: Common ophthalmologic problems. In Rosen P, et al (eds): Emergency Medicine: Concepts and Clinical Practice (2nd ed). St. Louis, The C.V. Mosby Co., 1988.)

down as the device is placed above the upper tarsal plate and the lid is everted. If a globe rupture is suspected, this procedure is deferred because of the potential for external pressure to extrude internal contents. The upper palpebral conjunctival area is a common site for ocular foreign bodies. The lower bulbar conjunctiva may be injured because of Bell's reflex.

Pupillary Size, Shape, and Reactivity. Pupillary dilation or irregularity can imply serious ocular, cranial nerve, or central nervous system injury. Both pupils should be approximately the same size and should constrict when light is shined in either eye. This dual response is the normal direct and consensual response. Decreased constriction response to light may represent local injury, an efferent pupillary defect commonly arising from an intracranially compressed third cranial nerve ("blown pupil"), or the less commonly diagnosed afferent pupillary defect. The latter is also called a Marcus-Gunn pupil and represents retinal or prechiasmal optic nerve injury. It is tested by placing the patient in a darkened room and shining a penlight into the unaffected eye. This should cause constriction of both pupils owing to direct and consensual effects. Swinging the light to the affected eye normally maintains the direct and consensual constriction. If the afferent tract is injured, the presence of light is not effectively transmitted, and the pupil in the affected eye dilates. The test is sufficiently sensitive to be positive in patients with near normal (20/30) visual acuity. The pupil with local damage or with an efferent defect does not respond to either direct or consensual reflexes. Findings in the normal eye and one with efferent and afferent defects are illustrated in Figure 35–3.

An irregular pupillary shape may indicate muscle injury, scarring, or spasm due to intraocular inflammation. A pointed "teardrop" pupil can be the clue to the presence of an ocular penetration injury. The point of the pupil is directed toward the site of entry because the iris is drawn to occlude the opening. After blunt injury, a slightly dilated, irregular, poorly reactive "traumatic mydriatic" pupil is often seen. It may resolve completely, but the finding often heralds significant ocular damage.

Funduscopic Examination. A normal red reflex usually indicates clarity of the

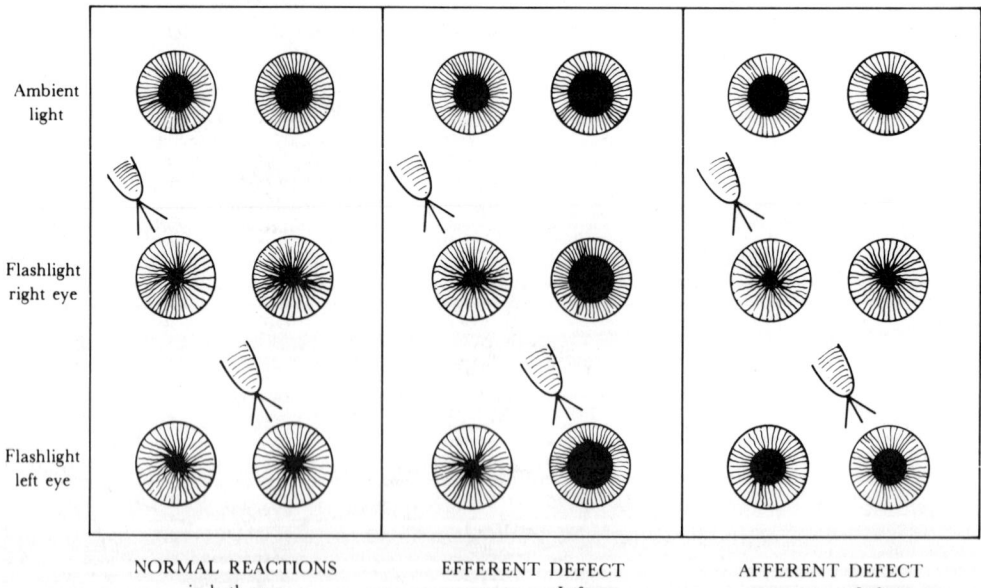

FIGURE 35–3. Pupillary reactions to penlight illumination. Note that an eye that has an efferent defect will not respond to either a direct or consensual light stimulus, whereas an eye with an afferent defect will constrict when the contralateral eye is illuminated and then dilates when the penlight is swung to the involved eye. (From American Academy of Ophthalmology: Ophthalmology Study Guide. San Francisco, American Academy of Ophthalmology, 1982.)

aqueous and vitreous media of the eye. Although ophthalmologists routinely dilate the pupil to obtain a complete view of the fundus, chemical dilation for examination is rarely necessary in the emergency department. If dilation is considered necessary, a pure mydriatic agent (phenylephrine) rather than a long-acting mydriatic-cycloplegic is used. This avoids the problem of precluding an accurate pupillary assessment for hours. Funduscopic inspection of the optic disk, macula, and retina is routinely performed. Visualization of a gray or blurry retina may indicate retinal detachment, although a peripheral detachment is difficult to see with an ophthalmoscope alone. Yellow exudates and flame hemorrhages can result from fat embolism due to long bone fractures.

Extraocular Muscle Testing. The extraocular muscles are examined by asking the patient to follow a light source through to the extremes of gaze in at least six positions. The patient is to report if more than one light is seen during the exercise. Visualization of two lights (diplopia) implies dysfunction of the cranial nerves or extraocular muscles. Monocular diplopia can result from a cataract or lens dislocation, although it is also described by the hysterical or malingering patient. Grossly limited extraocular muscle function along with proptosis or bulging of the eye from the orbit may indicate a retro-orbital hemorrhage. If there is enophthalmos, or if the eye seems "sunken" in the orbit, a blowout fracture of the orbital floor is suspected. This is often combined with a limited upward gaze due to entrapment of the inferior rectus or oblique muscle.

Peripheral Visual Field Testing. Visual fields are screened by confrontation testing. When facing each other, both the examiner and the patient should be able to see an object in various locations equidistant between them; the visual field of each eye should be tested separately. Visual field defects may result from injuries along the visual axis of the eye or in the optic nerve, optic tracts, or occipital lobe of the brain.

Specialized Ocular Examination Techniques

Topical Anesthetic Use. Two or three drops of a topical anesthetic may help differentiate pain due to superficial corneal injury from deeper ocular damage. If topical anesthesia completely eliminates any pain, deeper injury is less likely. A complete eye examination is still required to exclude a more serious process. Persistent pain implies a cause more extensive than a simple corneal abrasion or other superficial process.

Fluorescein Staining. Applications of a moistened fluorescein-impregnated strip to the lower conjunctiva and use of a cobalt blue light will reveal corneal defects where the chemical fluoresces. This is an important part of the routine examination of any patient with a traumatic eye injury. In a special examination, the Seidel test, fluorescein is applied to a suspected corneal laceration. If aqueous humor is leaking from the laceration, a stream of fluorescein will be noted. Note that a negative result on Seidel's test does not always exclude a corneal laceration because small lacerations may seal quickly.

Slit Lamp Examination. A slit lamp is a binocular ophthalmic examining microscope. It is especially useful for examining the cornea, anterior chamber, lens, and ocular adnexa. The slit lamp examination (SLE) is an important part of the complete eye assessment. The emergency physician must have ready access to this equipment and be familiar with its operation and interpretation of findings. Most slit lamps have both white and cobalt blue light sources so that fluorescein staining can be evaluated. Common findings include vertical linear fluorescein staining "scratches" due to an upper eyelid foreign body or diffuse corneal fluorescein stippling caused by chemical or ultraviolet light keratitis. The lamp can be used to inspect the lens for possible subluxation or lens opacification due to cataract formation. Also, the lamp can focus a small beam of light through the anterior chamber to search for "flare" (visualized as "smoke" or "headlights in the rain" light pattern along the beam's path). Flare occurs when leukocytes and protein are present in the aqueous humor owing to intraocular inflammation.

Tonometry. Schiotz tonometry is used to measure intraocular pressure, and the equipment is usually available in the emergency department. The weighted plunger is linked to a needle that lies along a scale. The higher the intraocular pressure in the globe, the less the needle moves on the scale. The use and interpretation of Schiotz tonometry are worthwhile skills for the emergency physician. This test should *not* be performed if there is suspected ocular rupture. Elevated intraocular pressure can result from an ocular process (acute glaucoma) or possibly from an extraocular process (retro-orbital hemorrhage). Decreased pressure can result from an ocular rupture or possibly from an iritis severe enough to decrease aqueous humor production.

PROBLEM 1 The ballplayer's visual acuity was OD 20/20, OS 20/20. Inspection revealed layering of blood in the anterior chamber and lower eyelid ecchymosis; crepitus was palpable in the lower lid. Extraocular muscle function testing revealed diplopia on upward gaze, and there was an area of hemorrhage on the inferior bulbar conjunctiva and sclera.

Hyphema usually results from an iris root injury, and the vertical diplopia is probably secondary to an orbital floor fracture with extraocular muscle entrapment. Both findings suggest significant blunt force injury. The examiner should also test sensation of the involved side malar area of the face to exclude infraorbital nerve injury. Scleral hemorrhage is usually benign, although circumferential subconjunctival hemorrhage may indicate a ruptured globe.

PROBLEM 2 The patient required an additional 5 liters of normal saline irrigation to decrease discomfort and return pH to approximately 7.4. There was injection of the conjunctivae, and the corneas appeared hazy. Repeat visual acuity testing now showed 20/70 in each eye.

Decreasing visual acuity implies worsening of corneal injury or possibly edema due to the chemical necrosis. The finding of corneal haziness necessitates admission and early consultation.

PROBLEM 3 The mechanic had a visual acuity of 20/30 in the involved eye. He had moderate discomfort on penlight illumination of either eye, and there was a limbic flush around the cornea. There appeared to be no scleral injury. Slit lamp examination revealed a reddish metallic foreign body on the cornea; otherwise, the anterior chamber was clear.

Corneal foreign bodies are best seen on slit lamp examination. Here the presence of bilateral photophobia and the limbic flush of vessels indicate an early reactive iritis. Despite finding a corneal foreign body, the examiner should still maintain a high degree of concern about a possible penetrating injury due to the high-velocity mechanism.

DECISION PRIORITIES AND PRELIMINARY DIFFERENTIAL DIAGNOSIS

At the conclusion of the history and physical examination, the clinician addresses the following questions:

1. *Is there an adequate explanation for any impairment of the patient's visual acuity?* Three elements must be accounted for in answering this question: (a) Visual acuity abnormalities due to a refractive error should correct with pinhole testing. (b) The clarity of the visual axis from cornea to fundus should be apparent. (c) Testing for a pupillary afferent defect (Marcus-Gunn pupil) is done to assess unseen optic nerve injury.
2. *Is there any suspicion or indication that penetration or rupture of the globe has occurred?*
3. *Is there any condition (such as possible penetration) that warrants further diagnostic testing?*

Most of these tests involve radiologic imaging.

Once these questions are answered, the physician can then move to more sophisticated testing or to refining the differential diagnosis.

DIAGNOSTIC ADJUNCTS

Most significant ocular injuries are anticipated by the history and proved on physical examination. Some diagnostic examinations will be confirmatory, such as a positive result on Seidel's test for a corneal laceration.

Radiologic Imaging

Several diagnostic adjuncts involving radiologic imaging may be indicated for further ocular injury evaluation. These modalities include:

1. *Plain film radiography.* Significant blunt injury or suspected radiopaque foreign body penetration is further evaluated by plain film radiologic study of the orbit and globe. Posteroanterior, Waters' (head tilt up), and Caldwell (head tilt down) views are used to examine the orbital rim and sinuses, searching for fracture, air-fluid level, or opacification. A soft tissue film of the globe is the first study advised when searching for intraocular foreign bodies.

2. *Computed tomography (CT) of the orbit.* Orbital CT in 1.5-mm axial and coronal sections can provide detailed imaging of the orbit, optic nerve, and retrobulbar space. It is particularly useful in locating sites of hemorrhage. Magnetic resonance imaging (MRI) also is potentially useful in defining the extent of injury to the orbit and its contents, especially the optic nerve.

3. *Ultrasonography.* Specialized ophthalmologic ultrasound techniques can help to locate intraocular foreign bodies as small as 1 mm^2 as well as vitreous hemorrhage, lens displacement, and retinal detachment.

Laboratory Studies

Laboratory tests are generally not indicated for patients with acute eye injuries. In patients who may have systemic diseases, such as diabetes or clotting disorders, laboratory tests are ordered that are specific for the disease.

REFINED DIFFERENTIAL DIAGNOSIS

Following the data-gathering process, the specific diagnosis is generally evident. Table 35–1 lists the major injuries to the eye classified by anatomic location. Trauma to the eye can result in numerous immediate and delayed effects, depending on the mechanism of injury. Traumatic hyphema, blowout injury to the orbit, chemical burns to the cornea, corneal foreign bodies, and corneal abrasions deserve more detailed consideration because they are the more commonly encountered traumatic ocular diagnoses.

Hyphema

Hyphema usually results from a blunt injury to the eye. As the globe deforms, blood vessels in the iris root avulse from their insertions, resulting in hemorrhage into the anterior chamber. Blood then layers out below the aqueous humor and appears as a bloody meniscus. If the entire chamber fills with blood, the phenomenon is known as an "eight-ball eye" or total hyphema. The blood will be absorbed, but if the red cells occlude the aqueous humor drainage from the anterior chamber, an acute increase in intraocular pressure will occur. This can result in acute glaucoma and corneal staining with hemoglobin. Rebleeding occurs in about one-third of cases, often between three

TABLE 35-1. Refined Differential Diagnosis of Major Injuries to the Eye, Orbit, and Adnexa

Diagnosis	Treatment Considerations	Treatment (Emergency Department)
Adnexal Injuries		
Eyebrow lacerations	R/O central nervous system, orbital, ocular injury; palpate for orbital fracture	Repair of wound *Note: Do not shave eyebrows*
Eyelid lacerations (simple)	R/O CNS or ocular injury; R/O tarsal plate or levator muscle injury	Repair of wound
Eyelid laceration involving "gray line"	Eyelid notching (coloboma), entropion or ectropion may result if incorrectly repaired	Specialized multilayer repair (refer immediately to ophthalmology or plastic surgery
Orbital ecchymosis	R/O perforation, blowout fracture of orbit, ocular rupture, other ocular injury	Ice, eye rest; lateral canthotomy may be indicated for retrobulbar hemorrhage
Eyelid foreign body	R/O corneal abrasion, perforation; check for "rust ring"	Careful removal of foreign body; antibiotics, patch
Orbital fracture	R/O corneal extraocular muscle entrapment, CNS injury	Antibiotics, decongestants; refer patient to ophthalmology
Eyelid burns	R/O upper airway burns, corneal injury	Occlusive dressing with antibiotic ointment; refer to plastic surgeon
Conjunctival Injuries		
Subconjunctival hemorrhage	R/O associated blunt or penetrating injury	No specific therapy, reassurance; resolves over 2–3 weeks
Conjunctival swelling	R/O scleral perforation, orbital fracture	Bland ointment for lubrication, referral
Corneal Injuries		
Chemical injuries	Promptly refer caustic (esp. alkali) injuries or injury with corneal opacification or increased intraocular pressure	*Irrigate!* Neutralize, give antibiotics; with or without patch vs. continued irrigation
Corneal abrasion	R/O perforation or associated injury; 40% or more of corneal injuries develop iritis; (repeat evaluation in 24 hours)	Antibiotics, with or without mydriatics, analgesics; eye patch and rest are mainstays
Ultraviolet keratitis	Counsel patients about prevention; R/O associated injury (e.g., foreign body). Continued ultraviolet light exposure results in cumulative injury	Eye patch and rest or dark glasses; analgesics since usually very painful
Thermal corneal injury	R/O perforation, adnexal or lid injury; refer if corneal opacification is present	Antibiotic/cycloplegics, with or without mydriatic, patch; analgesics, remove any eschar with moistened swab
Contact lens injury	Do not use fluorescein stain if lenses are still in (will stain soft lenses)	Remove lenses; treat as corneal abrasion
Corneal foreign body	R/O perforation; "rust" rings best removed by ophthalmologist 24–36 hr after injury	Remove foreign body with eye spud, 27-gauge needle, or ophthalmology drill, patch
Corneal ulcer	Will result in significant corneal damage	Immediate ophthalmology referral
Corneal laceration or perforation	Avoid manipulation; note that very small lacerations may be "self sealing." Iris may be included in "seal," resulting in teardrop-shaped iris	Immediate ophthalmology referral, consider IV antibiotics, antiemetics, mydriatics, eye shield
Anterior Chamber		
Hyphema	R/O associated injuries; inpatient vs. outpatient management is controversial; ophthalmology follow-up mandatory to evaluate for second-degree glaucoma, corneal staining	Bedrest, eye rest, cycloplegics, and possible antifibrinolytic therapy to prevent rebleeding (main complication or sequel)
Scleral Injuries		
Scleral rupture or laceration	Avoid manipulation of the eye, Valsalva maneuver, etc.	Immediate ophthalmology referral, eye shield
Subconjuctional hemorrhage	R/O scleral rupture, other ocular injury; R/O retrobulbar hemorrhage	If minor injury only, counsel patient about resolution
Retrobulbar hemorrhage	R/O central retinal artery occlusion, check intraocular pressure. Pressure from behind orbit may be transmitted to optic tract or globe	If intraocular pressure is >50, consider lateral canthotomy; if central retinal artery occlusion, consider rebreather, digital massage, mannitol, or paracentesis

TABLE 35–1. Refined Differential Diagnosis of Major Injuries to the
Eye, Orbit, and Adnexa *Continued*

Diagnosis	Treatment Considerations	Treatment (Emergency Department)
Extraocular Muscle Laceration	R/O CNS or other orbital or ocular injury; R/O other cause for diplopia	Ophthalmology referral
Iris Injuries		
Mydriasis	R/O CNS injury or pharmacologic cause	Refer for follow-up; counsel patient that lesion may persist
Iridodialysis (separation of iris from attachment)	R/O other ocular injury, hyphema	Refer for follow-up; no specific therapy unless associated with hyphema
Pointing "teardrop" iris	R/O perforation, avoid manipulation; consider x-ray or CT to locate foreign body	Immediate ophthalmology referral
Lens Injuries		
Traumatic cataract	More immediate treatment needed if lens capsule disrupted; R/O other blunt ocular injury	Refer for ophthalmology follow-up
Subluxation	R/O other blunt ocular injury, may manifest as abnormal tremulousness of iris on eye movement (iridodonesis)	Ophthalmology referral
Dislocation into vitreous	R/O other injury	Urgent referral
Anterior dislocation	R/O entrapment of lens in iris; R/O lens contacting corneal	Immediate ophthalmology referral
Implanted lens dislocation	R/O other ocular injury	Refer for ophthalmology follow-up
Vitreous Hemorrhage	R/O retinal detachment; R/O rupture or other blunt injury	Eye rest; elevate head; urgent referral
Ruptured Globe	R/O associated injuries	Immediate referral, eye shield, avoid manipulation, Valsalva maneuver
Optic Nerve Injury	R/O CNS injury; consider CT or MRI scan	Immediate referral (remote possibility of optic nerve decompression)
Ocular Perforation or Penetration	R/O CNS injury; note that vegetative material is extremely destructive	Immediate referral; eye shield, avoid manipulation
Retinal Injuries		
Retinal tear or detachment	R/O blunt injury to CNS, globe or orbit	Eye rest, bilateral patch; urgent referral
Retinal edema or hemorrhage	R/O associated injury	Urgent referral; eye rest, no specific therapy

R/O = rule out.

and five days after the initial injury. The long-term prognosis is best for small hyphemas that do not rebleed.

The presence of a hyphema should prompt immediate further examination for the presence of other blunt injury pathology, such as an iris or lens injury, vitreous hemorrhage, retinal tear, scleral rupture, or blowout fracture of the orbit. Note that a hyphema by itself does not cause an afferent pupillary defect (Marcus-Gunn pupil), although blunt trauma can cause a traumatic mydriasis that can persist for several days.

Blowout Fracture of the Orbit

Fracture of the orbit can result from direct bony injury, such as occurs with orbital rim fractures. Blunt injury to the globe, however, can cause transmission of force to the thin orbital walls, resulting in an orbital blowout fracture. The inferior and medial orbital walls are at the greatest risk of injury. Orbital fat and extraocular muscle tissue can prolapse through the fracture into the adjacent sinus, sometimes causing a gaze palsy. A common example is inferior rectus muscle entrapment resulting in impaired upward gaze. This can also be seen without fracture and is caused by tissue edema restricting muscle and globe movement.

Symptoms and signs of a blowout fracture include diplopia, hypesthesia of the ipsilateral nose and lower eyelid area (due to compression injury to the inferior orbital nerve), conjunctival crepitus, and subcutaneous emphysema. As with hyphema, the presence of a blowout fracture should alert the examiner to other injuries within the eye.

Surgery to correct orbital fracture defects is usually not needed, unless persistent diplopia or cosmetically unacceptable enophthalmos results. When operative repair is necessary, it is usually delayed for at least a week or more to allow local edema to subside. Retrobulbar hemorrhage following blunt injury may need emergent surgical decompression by means of a lateral canthotomy, however, and the clinician should observe the patient for proptosis, limited extraocular motion, pain, visual loss, elevated intraocular pressure, and an afferent pupillary defect to screen for this infrequent condition.

Chemical Injury to the Cornea

Of all eye injuries seen in the emergency department, chemical injury deserves the most immediate treatment. As emphasized previously, irrigation of the eye should precede evaluation by the physician; particulate debris may require mechanical removal. Continued chemical destruction can proceed from the epithelium through to the stroma and then to the endothelium unless it is halted by decontamination. Full-thickness corneal injury can result in corneal perforation, which can be refractory to corneal transplantation. Therefore, prognosis is inversely proportional to the delay between injury and successful decontamination. A normal "non-hazy" cornea after irrigation is a good prognostic sign.

Corneal Foreign Body

Sensory nerve supply to the cornea is provided by the fifth cranial nerve; sensation is intense, and any injury to the cornea results in discomfort that often is severe. The presence of a corneal foreign body virtually always results in gradually increasing pain, photophobia, blepharospasm, and lacrimation. A corneal foreign body may not always result in diminished visual acuity, however. The presence of secondary iritis is dependent on the degree and duration of the foreign body injury.

Corneal foreign bodies are a hazard with certain occupations, such as automobile mechanics and grinder operators, and they are more frequent on windy days. A high-velocity mechanism of injury should alert the examiner to possible ocular penetration.

The presence of a foreign body should prompt careful inspection of the depth of the injury; the thickness of the cornea diminishes at the center to approximately 0.5 mm. Penetration of the stroma of the cornea is termed a *corneal laceration*, either partial or full thickness. Full-thickness lacerations imply violation of the anterior chamber. In this circumstance, the foreign body is not removed, and the case is referred expeditiously to an ophthalmologist.

The objectives of treatment of a corneal foreign body are to remove the offending material and avoid further injury. The removal of most metallic foreign bodies leaves a residual area of oxidation, called a "rust ring." These rings are usually removed at a follow-up appointment in 24 hours. Ideally, all rust rings should be removed; otherwise a cosmetic and sometimes inflammatory deposition may persist. After the foreign body is removed, a corneal defect remains but usually heals rapidly. If foreign body removal is incomplete, the healing process is greatly delayed.

Contact Lens Injuries

One particular "foreign body," the contact lens, has caused a number of emergency department visits. Retained contact lenses can be removed using special suction devices or a pinching technique applied with the patient looking upward. Contact lenses can also make foreign body injuries worse by means of the pressure effect of the lens on the cornea. Prolonged contact lens use can cause hypoxic injury to the corneal epithelium, resulting in onset of pain several hours after removal of the lenses. Note that fluorescein can permanently stain "soft" contact lenses, and these lenses are removed before any staining is done. In general, patients should avoid using their contact lenses until they are reexamined by an ophthalmologist.

Corneal Abrasion

Corneal abrasions are the most frequently encountered ophthalmologic injury in the emergency department. Although very rapid, the blink reflex is insufficient to prevent all injuries to the cornea. The resulting defect in the epithelium allows the stroma to come into contact with toxic substances and microbes. It is this defect that allows the uptake of fluorescein, thus facilitating the diagnosis of a corneal abrasion.

The corneal defect can result from direct trauma to the cornea or from delayed sloughing of epithelial cells after nonmechanical trauma (as with prolonged contact lens wear or ultraviolet light keratitis), and it sometimes occurs spontaneously. This latter condition is known as a *corneal erosion*, and treatment is similar to that of a corneal abrasion.

Innervation of the corneal epithelium is extensive; most epithelial defects result in significant discomfort. Irritation of these corneal nerve endings cause lacrimation and blepharospasm. Visual acuity is variably affected, depending on the location, size of the defect, resultant corneal edema, tearing, and photophobia. Redness results from the dilation of blood vessels, which occurs as a response to the insult. Light sensitivity can occur owing to light scatter from the corneal defect itself or secondary to a reactive iritis.

The injured cornea heals very rapidly; most corneal abrasions of a few square millimeters will heal within 24 hours. Larger defects, or injuries that penetrate into the corneal stroma, take several days or longer to heal. Until the defect heals, the exposed stroma is vulnerable to toxins, bacteria, and other foreign material. Therefore, most corneal defects are treated with topical antibiotics and an eye patch. Full-thickness corneal injuries should be referred to an ophthalmologist immediately; although small corneal lacerations may seal spontaneously, risk of ocular infection is significant.

PROBLEM 1 Radiographic study of the baseball player's orbit appeared to be normal, although the Waters' view revealed an air-fluid level in the maxillary sinus.

The clinical findings of extraocular muscle entrapment and crepitus and radiographic evidence of a sinus fluid level indicated an orbital floor fracture. CT scanning confirmed this abnormality.

PROBLEM 3 The mechanic, anxious to get home, refused any radiologic study and wanted his injury taken care of "immediately."

A corneal foreign body was demonstrated on the slit lamp examination. Any consideration of foreign body perforation mandates a radiologic assessment. Penetration of the eye by metallic (nickel) or vegetative material (plant or wood fibers) can result in catastrophic ocular infection. If a patient clearly needs further evaluation and refuses it, the risks involved are carefully explained to the patient and family. This information is documented on the chart.

PRINCIPLES OF MANAGEMENT
General

The dictum "first do no harm" certainly applies to eye injuries. As described earlier, chemical injury requires urgent and copious irrigation *prior* to any extensive evaluation.

Conversely, no manipulation or examination is performed on any eye suspected of being ruptured. A penetrating object that is still in place is left in place until appropriate consultation is obtained. There are a number of basic management tools that are used repeatedly in caring for eye injuries.

Eye Irrigation. Irrigation is accomplished by using intravenous tubing with normal saline solution. The eyelids are retracted and all conjunctival fornices are irrigated as the patient looks up, down, medially, and laterally. Premedicating the patient with a topical anesthetic usually facilitates this procedure. Particulate debris can be gently removed from the fornices with an irrigating stream or a moistened swab.

Ophthalmic Medications

Topical Anesthetics. The most widely used and best tolerated topical eye anesthetic is 0.5% proparacaine (Ophthetic). It may burn slightly on initial administration, but onset of the topical anesthetic effect occurs within minutes. Tetracaine is also used, but it stings more than proparacaine on instillation. The medication is never given to a patient for home use, because prolonged use can result in corneal injury.

Mydriatics and Cycloplegics. Mydriatics dilate the pupil by paralyzing the pupillary constrictor muscle. Cycloplegics act on the ciliary muscle. Agents with both actions are used therapeutically to relieve pain and enhance eye rest in patients with iritis and other internal eye inflammatory disorders. These agents may also be used in patients with large corneal abrasions (covering more than 30% of the corneal surface area) because of the high incidence of subsequent secondary iritis with such lesions. The major concern when selecting one of these drugs is the duration of action.

Agent	Duration of Action
Mydriatics	
Phenylephrine—1.5%–2%	20–40 min
Hydroxyamphetamine—2.1%	20–40 min
Mydriatics/Cycloplegics	
Tropicamide—1%	6 hr
Cyclopentolate—2%	24 hr
Homatropine—1%	10–48 hr
Scopolamine—0.5%	2–7 days
Atropine—0.5%	10–14 days

Homatropine is recommended for most post-traumatic indications because it is of medium duration and systemic side effects are rare.

Antibiotics. The more commonly used topical ocular antibiotics, sulfacetamide and sulfisoxazole, are of low cost and relatively low risk. These sulfa agents are recommended as the first-line antibiotic of choice. Gentamicin and tobramycin are used if gram-negative organisms are suspected in serious corneal infections or ulcers. Tetracycline is used systemically and topically if *Chlamydia* is suspected. Chloramphenicol has been associated with aplastic anemia, and its use is deferred until after consultation with an ophthalmologist. The combination of polymyxin and bacitracin (Polysporin) is another good choice. Neomycin has been combined with it (Neosporin) although there is little added benefit, and the risk of a contact allergic reaction is increased. If an eye patch is used and if there is no deep penetrating injury, an ointment may be used. Otherwise, eye drops are preferred.

Steroids. Steroids may be indicated in patients with keratitis, allergic conjunctivitis, or deeper inflammation. They are administered and prescribed *only after consultation* with an ophthalmologist.

Eye Patching. Application of a semipressure patch is done as follows (Fig. 35–4). An eyepatch is folded in half and applied to the involved eye with the eyelid closed. Next, an unfolded patch is placed over the folded patch and taped into place. The tapes are placed diagonally from the forehead to the cheek and enough pressure maintained to

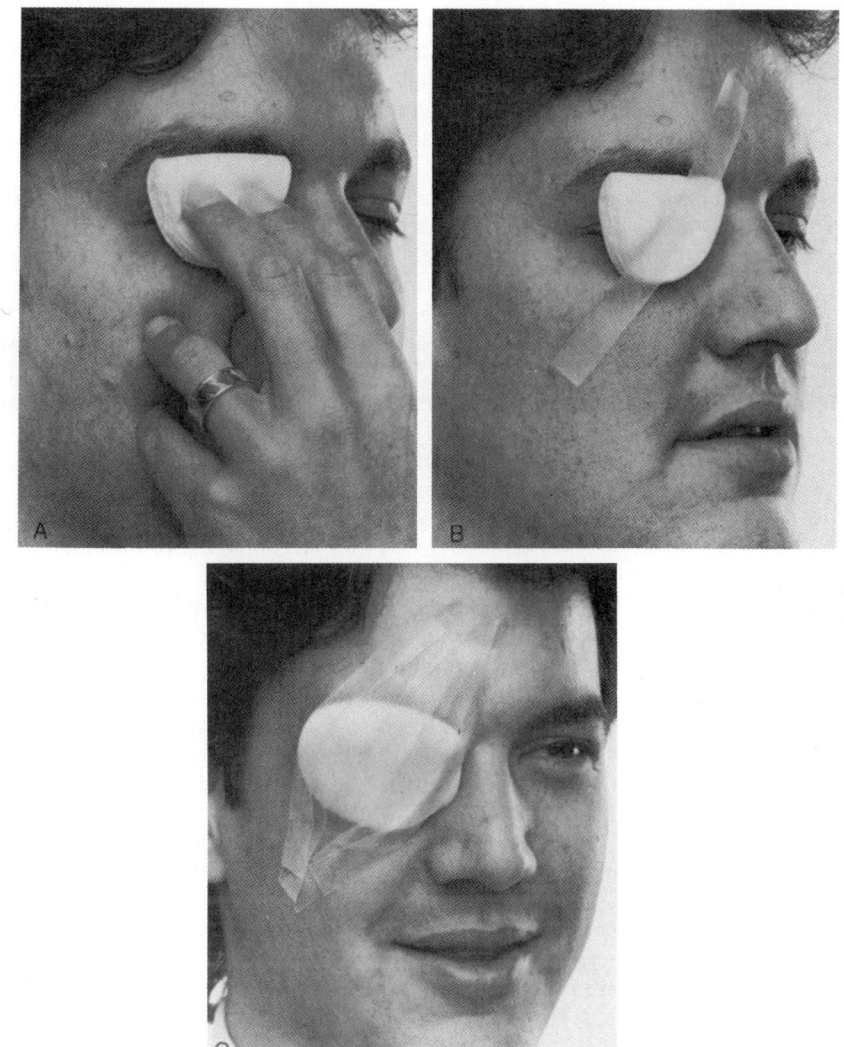

FIGURE 35–4. *Application of a semipressure patch. See text for details. (Reproduced with permission from Lubeck D, Greene J: Corneal injuries. In Mathews J, Zun L (eds): Ophthalmologic emergencies and ocular trauma. Emerg Med Clin North Am 6(1):93, 1988.)*

keep the eyelid closed but not so tight as to cause discomfort. A patient with an eye patch is cautioned not to drive because patching results in loss of depth perception.

Specific Eye Injuries

Hyphema. The management of hyphema remains controversial. Late sequelae of this injury are rebleeding, development of corneal staining, and secondary glaucoma. Inpatient versus outpatient management and the use of steroids versus antifibrinolytic therapy continue to be debated. The mainstay of care in the emergency department is bed rest with the patient sitting up at least at a 45-degree angle. This prevents the red blood cells from occluding the outflow tract of the anterior chamber (canals of Schlemm), causing acute glaucoma.

Blowout Fracture of the Orbit. Orbital blowout fractures are usually managed conservatively. The key to management is suspicion followed by diagnosis. Determining the presence of extraocular muscle entrapment is important and is often easier to diagnose. Broad-spectrum antibiotics (such as ampicillin or a first-generation cephalosporin) and decongestants may decrease the risk of orbital infection from bacteria that colonize the sinuses. Although opinions vary, many of these cases to not require surgery. Persistent diplopia usually requires surgical decompression and repair of the orbital floor.

Chemical Injury. As emphasized earlier, irrigation is the mainstay of treatment for chemical injuries. Minor chemical injury to the cornea can be managed on an outpatient basis if the involved cornea shows no opacification or blanching of the conjunctiva. Such injuries can be treated with a short-acting cycloplegic, a topical antibiotic, and patching.

Severe chemical and significant alkali burns to the eye require continued irrigation, further analgesia, and extended observation for 4 to 6 hours. These injuries may result in ulceration or corneal perforation, eyelid adhesions, glaucoma and other sequelae.

Corneal Foreign Bodies. Corneal foreign bodies are frequently removed in the emergency department. A stream of irrigating solution is used first to try to dislodge the object gently. If the foreign body is embedded, it is removed by carefully lifting or "teasing" it off the cornea. This is usually accomplished after topical analgesia has been applied. After careful patient preparation and preferably using a slit lamp, the physician chooses an eye "spud" or, if unavailable, a 27-gauge needle on a syringe. As little damage is done to the cornea as possible. If the foreign body is difficult to remove or is embedded deeply in the cornea, the aid of a physician experienced in corneal foreign body removal is recommended. Removal of metallic foreign bodies often leaves a "rust ring." This oxidized metal tissue ring is best removed with a small "burr" instrument after 24 to 48 hours, when the surrounding corneal tissue has softened. A corneal abrasion usually remains after foreign body removal.

Corneal Abrasion. The mainstay of treatment of corneal abrasion is protection by patching. The cornea reepithelializes rapidly and needs only an appropriate cover. An abrasion that extends beyond Bowman's membrane will usually heal with some scarring. In addition to the eyepatch, an antibiotic ointment may be used if the abrasion is not deep. If the abrasion is extensive (covering more than 30% of the corneal surface) or especially deep, or if reactive symptoms have begun, a mydriatic-cycloplegic is added to the regimen. Corneal abrasions are extremely painful and systemic analgesics ease this discomfort.

After the patch is removed in 12 to 24 hours, antibiotic drops are instilled every 3 to 4 hours until healing is complete. If a full-thickness laceration or perforation is suspected, an eye shield is applied, and immediate ophthalmology consultation is obtained.

PROBLEM 1 The ballplayer's injuries included a blowout fracture of the inferior orbit with extraocular muscle entrapment, a traumatic hyphema, and a small subconjunctival hemorrhage. He had a complete funduscopic examination, which was normal, and tonometry revealed a normal intraocular pressure.

The blunt injury may cause an orbital hemorrhage or post-traumatic glaucoma, two conditions that may require urgent intervention. Both are actively sought during the examination. The subconjunctival hemorrhage is managed with observation only because it will usually resolve over several weeks' time.

PROBLEM 3 The mechanic remained calm during the foreign body removal and understood the implication of a rust ring. He assented to eye patching but wanted to know when he could go back to work. An appointment was scheduled in the industrial clinic for one day later.

Although primary emergency department management is appropriate, the physician should stress that a follow-up examination is important prior to returning to work. The problem remains that penetration has occurred. The patient's unwillingness to allow the complete examination is documented and the industrial clinic contacted about the problem. This patient will leave the emergency department at considerable risk for a serious eye problem.

SPECIAL CONSIDERATIONS

Pediatric Patients

Pediatric patients pose special problems. Very young children cannot cooperate with visual acuity testing or describe the nature of their discomfort. They often frustrate the emergency physician by resisting examination. A patient and complete examination is nevertheless performed. Light response can be assessed by pupillary reflexes, and visual acuity can be roughly gauged by the child's tracking of an object. Children with a suspected serious injury are referred to an ophthalmologist. Eye patches are poorly tolerated by children and can worsen the discomfort of some injuries.

Geriatric Patients

Many geriatric patients have a preexisting impairment of vision due to, for example, diabetic retinopathy or previous cataract surgery. It is necessary to obtain information about the base line visual status from the patient or an old chart. As with children, early referral for any suspected serious problem may reduce morbidity in these patients. The elderly patient may already have difficulty performing activities of daily living, and visual loss can have a devastating effect.

Prevention

The emergency physician has a role in preventing eye injuries. Emergency physicians can educate patients by encouraging them to wear protective goggles and by instructing them to avoid potential causes of eye injury such as fireworks or careless use of caustic materials or power tools.

DISPOSITION AND FOLLOW-UP

Most patient injuries are managed on an outpatient basis. Ophthalmologic follow-up is indicated for persistent problems or any visual impairment. The following chart can help the emergency physician guide disposition in regarding ophthalmologic consultation.

I Immediate	II Urgent	III Follow-Up Examination
Ruptured globe	Hyphema	Minor chemical burns
Perforation or penetration	Blowout fracture	Corneal abrasions
Chemical burns with corneal opacification	Extraocular muscle lacerations	Corneal rust rings
Orbital hemorrhage	Gray line lacerations	Eyelid lacerations
Corneal laceration	Retinal injury	Blunt injury with normal findings on eye examination
Lens dislocation into anterior chamber	Lens dislocation into posterior chamber	Iris injuries

Ophthalmologists are called to see all patients in category I immediately in the emergency department. Telephone consultation with the ophthalmologist is indicated for patients with II (urgent) conditions. These patients are seen by the consultant within 12 to 24 hours.

All minor eye injuries (category III) require a follow-up examination within 2 to 4 days because some "trivial" injuries may develop unanticipated catastrophic end results. No patient should return to work without an appropriate follow-up examination.

PROBLEM 1 The patient was admitted for bilateral eye patching, pain management, and close observation. His symptoms resolved, and normal vision returned. Surgery to repair the orbital floor fracture was discussed, but a decision was deferred until a later outpatient evaluation.

Noncompliance with home bed rest and concern about patient welfare in regard to follow-up are relative considerations for admission.

PROBLEM 2 The patient was admitted to the hospital and had a prolonged bout with corneal ulceration and corneal damage. She was placed on a waiting list for a corneal transplant.

The earliest emergency management of this problem may have a significant impact on long term morbidity. All emergency department staff should immediately institute vision-saving irrigation therapy when a patient arrives with this type of injury.

DOCUMENTATION

1. Mechanism of injury.
2. Associated risk factors, e.g., tetanus status, preexisting visual impairment.
3. Visual acuity prior to treatment (except in the case of chemical injury).
4. Treatment rendered in emergency department, e.g., irrigation.
5. Clear documentation of physical findings, including slit lamp examination, fluorescein staining, and tonometry as indicated.
6. Visual acuity after treatment.
7. Clinical impression and diagnosis.
8. Ophthalmologic consultation (when indicated).
9. Discharge instructions, medications, patch instructions, and follow-up arrangements made with the patient.

SUMMARY AND FINAL POINTS

- Emergency physicians can help to improve the outcome of eye injuries by anticipating a number of problems based on the mechanism of injury and by following a thorough standardized examination.
- Caustic chemical exposures are treated by immediate and extensive irrigation.
- Visual acuity is recorded before and after therapy.
- The mechanism of injury is an important consideration, especially penetrating or blunt injury to the globe.
- Attention should be paid to subtle examination clues, such as pain on consensual illumination or the presence of a Marcus-Gunn pupil.
- Penetrating injuries, ruptures, major chemical burns, and other vision-threatening injuries are immediately referred to an ophthalmologist.
- Corticosteroids are not prescribed without consultation and agreement by an ophthalmologist.

BIBLIOGRAPHY

Texts

1. Cinotti A (ed): Handbook of Ophthalmologic Emergencies (3rd ed). New York, Medical Examination Publishing, 1985.
2. Deutsch T, Feller D: Paton and Goldberg's Management of Ocular Injuries (2nd ed). Philadelphia, Saunders, 1985.
3. Pavan-Langston D (ed): Manual of Ocular Diagnosis and Therapy (2nd ed). Boston, Little, Brown, 1985.
4. Wilensky J, Read J: Primary Ophthalmology. New York, Grune & Stratton, 1984.

Journal Articles

1. Bachynski B, Flynn J: Direct trauma to the superior oblique tendon following penetrating injuries of the upper eyelid. Arch Ophthalmol 103(10):1510–1514, 1985.
2. Barr C: Prognostic factors in corneoscleral lacerations. Arch Ophthalmol 101:919–924, 1983.
3. Brinley J: Emergency management of ocular trauma. Topics Emerg Med 6(1):35–44, 1984.
4. Cobb S, Yeakley J: Computed tomographic evaluation of ocular trauma. Computerized Radiol 9(1):1–10, 1985.
5. Epstein D, Paton P: Keratitis from misuse of corneal anesthetics. N Engl J Med 279(8):396–399, 1968.
6. Goldberg M, Tessler H: Occult intraocular perforations from brow and lid lacerations. Arch Ophthalmol 86:145–149, 1971.
7. Mathews J, Zun L (eds): Ophthalmologic emergencies and ocular trauma. Emerg Med Clin North Am 6(1):1–172, 1988.
8. Mono J, Hollenberg R: Occult transorbital intracranial penetrating injuries. Ann Emerg Med 15(5):589–591, 1986.
9. Packer A: Ocular trauma. Primary Care 9(4):777–792, 1982.
10. Searl S: Minor trauma, disastrous results. Surv Ophthalmol 31(5):337–342, 1987.

SECTION ELEVEN

DISORDERS PRIMARILY PRESENTING IN INFANCY AND CHILDHOOD

CHAPTER 36

FEBRILE INFANTS

SUCHINTA N. HAKIM, M.D.
DENISE J. FLIGNER, M.D.

PROBLEM 1 A 6 month old boy presented with a 12-hour history of high fever, irritability, and refusal to feed. On initial assessment the infant was difficult to arouse, warm to the touch, and had cool mottled extremities with delayed capillary refill.

PROBLEM 2 A 12 month old boy with a 3-day history of a runny nose, chest congestion, and cough had been crying excessively for the last 12 hours. One hour prior to arrival he had had a seizure. In the emergency department he was alert and crying vigorously.

PROBLEM 3 An 18 month old girl with a 1-day history of fever to 103.1°F (39.5°C) and mild rhinorrhea appeared happy and playful on arrival in the emergency department.

QUESTIONS TO CONSIDER

1. What constitutes a fever in an infant or young child less than 24 months of age?
2. What is the significance of fever in this age group?
3. When is fever treated? What interventions are used for treatment?
4. What are the infectious causes of fever in children? Which represent serious illness?
5. Which signs and symptoms indicate serious illness?
6. When is diagnostic testing necessary for febrile children and what are the appropriate tests?
7. How are seriously ill febrile children managed in the emergency department?
8. How is the febrile child who appears well and has no apparent source of infection managed?

INTRODUCTION

About 20% of all pediatric patients presenting to the emergency department have fever as a sign or symptom. Although most febrile illnesses in young children are self-limited and benign, the physician must rule out serious illness and identify those infections that are benefited by treatment.

Fever is defined as a rectal temperature of more than 100.4°F (38°C). Temperatures measured rectally or intra-aurally (tympanic membrane) are most reliable. Oral temperatures are not recommended in young children, and skin temperatures, e.g., axillary or forehead strips, are less reliable. Oral and skin temperatures are lower than rectal temperatures by 1°F (0.6°C) and 2°F (1.1°C) respectively. Temperature-sensitive pacifiers are unreliable and cannot be recommended.

Fever is most commonly seen in children as a response to infection. However, fever may be due to immune-mediated disease, collagen vascular disease, and environmental factors such as a hot environment or heavy exertion. Importantly, fever may be a side effect of drug ingestion. The most common example in children is salicylate toxicity.

During infection, moderate fever is probably beneficial because it enhances host defense reactions. Rapidly rising fevers and hyperpyrexia, defined as a core temperature of more than 106°F (41.1°C), are complicated by problems. Rapidly rising fever will precipitate febrile convulsions in approximately 5% of children. Hyperpyrexia may lead to central nervous system damage and rhabdomyolysis.

Fever in children has different implications depending on the age of the child. Neonates and young infants under 3 months of age are at high risk for serious bacterial illness. Clinical evaluation is unreliable in determining the cause of the fever or the severity of illness. In this age group, fever requires an aggressive approach and generally mandates hospital admission. In children over the age of 24 months, clinical assessment is increasingly reliable for localizing infection and determining the risk of serious bacterial illness, particularly bacteremia and meningitis.

The child with fever who is 3 to 24 months old presents a unique challenge to the physician. The clinical assessment for serious bacterial infection is unreliable in this age group. In addition, about 5% of infants with high temperatures and no other signs of infection will have positive results of blood cultures, a diagnosis termed occult bacteremia. This chapter is written about evaluating the infant 3 to 24 months old with fever.

PREHOSPITAL CARE

The rescue squad is rarely summoned for a complaint of fever alone. It may be requested for the child who has another and more urgent complaint in addition to fever. The rescue personnel must first determine whether a problem other than fever is present. Evaluation and intervention are then directed to the more serious complaint.

History

1. Does the child have any evidence of respiratory distress?
2. Was there a seizure? If so, has it stopped?

Physical Examination

1. Is the child alert?
2. What is the skin color and temperature?
3. Is capillary refill normal or delayed?
4. Are the heart rate and respiratory rate within normal limits? Accurate blood pressure measurements may be difficult to obtain in the field, and obtaining a temperature in a young child is time-consuming. Neither is necessary in the prehospital setting.

Intervention

The four problems that may accompany fever and require specific intervention by the rescue squad are respiratory distress, seizure, obtundation, and dehydration. Prehospital care as well as subsequent evaluation and management for each of these problems is discussed specifically in the indicated chapter of this text: stridor (Chap. 37), dehydration (Chap. 39), obtundation (Chaps. 45 and 47), seizures (Chap. 48), dyspnea (Chap. 55), and wheezing (Chap. 56).

Table 36–1 lists the specific findings that require prehospital intervention. The child

TABLE 36–1. Criteria for Prehospital Intervention in Febrile Children

Finding	Stable—No Intervention	Unstable—Requires Intervention
Level of consciousness	Alert	Lethargic, obtunded, or seizing
Color	Normal	Pale, cyanotic, mottled
Respirations	Normal	Rapid or labored
Capillary refill	Normal (<2 sec)	Delayed (>5 sec)

who is alert and has no problems other than fever may be transported to the hospital with the parent without further intervention.

INITIAL APPROACH IN THE EMERGENCY DEPARTMENT

The majority of children with fever are brought to the emergency department by their parents rather than the rescue squad. A small number of these children are critically ill. A brief initial assessment by the triage nurse will identify children who are at high risk for serious infection or complications of fever and determines the urgency with which the child needs evaluation. Only one question is addressed: Does the child appear "ill"?

The Yale Observation Scale (Table 36–2) is a rapid observational device used to score the probability of illness objectively. Children with a score of more than 16 on this scale have a 92% probability of being seriously ill, whereas children with a score of less than 10 have only a 2% to 3% chance of serious illness. Children who appear seriously ill on observation are brought directly into the treatment area for immediate evaluation and stabilization as follows:

1. Supplemental oxygen with an appropriate nonrebreathing mask and a reservoir bag is given at 10 to 15 liters/min.

2. Respirations are assisted by a bag-mask-valve (BMV) device if ventilation is inadequate.

3. Oropharyngeal secretions are suctioned as needed.

TABLE 36–2. Yale Observation Scale for Febrile Children

Observation Item	1 Normal	3 Moderate Impairment	5 Severe Impairment
Quality of cry	Strong with normal tone *or* Content and not crying	Whimpering *or* Sobbing	Weak *or* Moaning *or* High pitched
Reaction to parent stimulation	Cries briefly then stops *or* Content and not crying	Cries off and on	Continual cry *or* Hardly responds
(State variation)	If awake → stays awake *or* If asleep and stimulated → wakes up quickly	Eyes close briefly → awake *or* Awakes with prolonged stimulation	Falls to sleep *or* Will not rouse
Color	Pink	Pale extremities *or* Acrocyanosis	Pale *or* Cyanotic *or* Mottled *or* Ashen
Hydration	Skin normal, eyes normal *and* Mucous membranes moist	Skin and eyes—normal Mouth slightly dry	Skin doughy *or* Tented *and* Dry mucous membranes *or* Sunken eyes
Response (talk, smile) to social overtures	Smiles *or* Alerts (≤2 mo)	Brief smile *or* Alerts briefly (≤2 mo)	No smile Face anxious, dull, expressionless *or* No alerting (≤2 mo)

From McCarthy PL, et al: Observation scales to identify serious illness in febrile children. Reproduced by permission of Pediatrics, vol. 70, p. 802, copyright 1982.

4. The heart rate is monitored. Bradycardia is a sign of trouble.

5. An intravenous (IV) or intraosseous line is established. Intravenous access is often a problem. For the child who emergently requires fluids, intravenous access is attempted for no longer than 90 seconds, after which an intraosseous line is established.

6. A fluid bolus of 20 ml/kg of isotonic crystalloid is administered if there are signs of shock. Mottled extremities and delayed capillary refill are characteristic of shock.

7. Hypoglycemia (less than 50 mg/100 ml) is treated with intravenous 25% glucose (0.5 to 1.0 gm/kg).

8. Intravenous antibiotics are indicated for children who have serious bacterial illness, e.g., meningitis or sepsis (see Principles of Management).

9. Acetaminophen and tepid water sponging are indicated for children with a temperature of 104°F (40°C) or higher.

For patients outside this urgent category, initial measures include (1) recording an accurate temperature, (2) vital signs: respiratory rate and pulse rate, (3) a history of antipyretic use: the most recent dose and the time it was taken, and (4) acetaminophen administration as determined by recent use. Children with temperatures of 102.2°F (39°C) or more should receive acetaminophen if no antipyretic has been given within the last 3 hours. Children who have received less than 10 mg/kg of an antipyretic in the last 2 hours are given an additional dose of 10 mg/kg.

PROBLEM 1 On initial assessment in the emergency department the infant appeared seriously ill. His Yale score was 23. He was brought immediately to the treatment room. His skin color and responsiveness did not improve with oxygen, and there was delayed capillary refill. Two unsuccessful attempts were made to start peripheral IV lines. An intraosseous line was then inserted, and after a bolus of 20 ml/kg of Ringer's lactate, the infant appeared more responsive and peripheral perfusion seemed improved. After blood was drawn for culture and testing, he was given an IV antibiotic. These measures were appropriately aggressive and rapid responses for this very ill-appearing infant.

PROBLEM 2 Initial assessment revealed an alert boy, crying while sitting in his mother's lap, who struggled and cried vigorously while his temperature was being taken. His skin color and hydration appeared to be normal. His Yale score was 8, temperature 104°F (40°C), respirations 30/min, and heart rate 130 beats/min. No antipyretic had been given at home, so the child was given acetaminophen, 15 mg/kg, while awaiting evaluation.

History of the seizure in this patient should prompt early evaluation. At this point, however, the child appeared well. Most febrile seizures occur during periods of rapidly rising temperatures, often before the parent recognizes the fever. Evaluation is aimed at determining the cause of the fever.

DATA GATHERING

History

The history is taken from the person who knows most about the child, usually the mother. Observing the infant while taking the history is an essential technique for quantifying and clarifying the symptoms, which may have different meanings for the parent and the examiner. Occasionally, the primary care giver does not accompany the child. In this case, attempts are made to reach this person to confirm the history.

1. When did the *illness begin* and *what is its relationship to the fever?* Moderate fevers of short duration with mild or no symptoms are often self-limited and need only

supportive therapy. A fever that begins well after the start of an illness often indicates an extension of the primary infection with secondary bacterial infection.
2. *How high was the temperature* and *what has been used to treat it?* The incidence of bacterial disease increases with the height of the temperature. Measures used to control the fever such as antipyretic medication or sponging gauge the parents' knowledge of fever and may reveal inappropriate treatment, such as bundling a febrile child in warm clothes or sponging with alcohol.
3. How "*ill*" *does the child seem* to the care giver? Interest in feeding and playing, general activity, and overall well-being are sensitive indicators of the severity of illness. Lack of well-being may be described simply as "something wrong." Vague terms such as "irritable" and "lethargic" can be clarified by simultaneous observation of the infant.
4. What *other symptoms* has the child had? Associated symptoms may be either specific, suggesting a focus of infection, or nonspecific, associated with a variety of illnesses.
    a. *Upper respiratory symptoms.* The combination of mild rhinorrhea, cough, and pharyngitis suggest viral upper respiratory infection (URI). Acute otitis media is often superimposed on these symptoms. Older infants with otitis media may rub or pull the affected ear.
    b. *Respiratory difficulty.* Respiratory problems are often described as "chest congestion." Rapid, noisy, and difficult breathing are separate symptoms that can be quantified by simultaneous observation. Difficult breathing can be partially quantified by asking whether the infant can nurse or take a bottle in the usual way.
    c. *Vomiting* and *diarrhea.* Vomiting and diarrhea may be either specific symptoms of gastroenteritis or nonspecific symptoms associated with illness outside the gastrointestinal tract, particularly otitis media and urinary tract infection (UTI). Both vomiting and diarrhea are quantified as to frequency, number of episodes in a given period, and relation to feeding. Abdominal pain is not a common finding in gastroenteritis and a child who screams and draws up his legs is evaluated for other significant abdominal problems.
    d. *Hydration* and *intake.* Fluid intake is assessed for all febrile infants, not only those at obvious risk of dehydration from vomiting or diarrhea (Chap. 39). The amounts and type of fluid ingested are quantified by asking how many 4- or 8-ounce bottles the baby has drunk in the last 24 hours. The frequency of wetting of diapers can be used as an estimate of urine output, but this is not useful if the child has diarrheal stools with every diaper change.
    e. *Rash.* Typical exanthems confirm the clinical diagnosis of a number of childhood diseases. A petechial rash in a febrile child is considered meningococcemia until proved otherwise (see Chaps. 14 and 47).
    f. *Pain* and *swelling* in the *soft tissues or extremities.* Cellulitis of the face, orbit, or elsewhere is an obvious source of fever, whereas deeper soft tissue infections are often occult. A febrile infant who cries each time the diaper is changed or refuses to walk should be suspected of having bacterial arthritis (Chap. 40) or osteomyelitis of the hip or lower extremity.
5. Has the child been *exposed* to a *known illness?* Similar symptoms in household members or day care contacts may raise suspicion of a specific illness. Contact with confirmed *Neisseria meningitidis* or *Hemophilus influenzae* requires close evaluation and consideration of antibiotic prophylaxis.
6. What *medicines* is the child taking? Parents often independently start treatment with an antibiotic remaining from a previous illness. Current or recent antibiotic use may alter both the typical symptoms of illness and the sensitivity of bacterial organisms. Allergies and undesirable side effects, commonly rash and gastroenteritis, may be symptoms of antibiotic use rather than infection.
7. Are *immunizations* "up-to-date"? Immunization status is a general measure of the care giver's ability to provide for the child's basic health care. Immunizations may also be the cause of the "illness." Examples are fever within 24 hours of diphtheria-pertussis-

tetanus (DPT) injection and mild measleslike illness following measles-mumps-rubella (MMR) immunization.
8. Is the child *usually healthy?* Screening questions about other medical problems and previous overnight hospitalizations will quickly elicit this information. Chronically ill and immune-compromised children are at significantly greater risk of serious infection. A developmental history is generally not necessary in an otherwise normal child with an acute febrile illness. In children who appear to have chronic illness, questions about birth weight and number of days spent in the nursery will help to clarify their medical problems.

PROBLEM 1 Fever, irritability, lethargy, and refusal to feed are common symptoms of meningitis in children under 18 months, as is the rapid onset of severe illness.

PROBLEM 2 The onset of high fever following 3 days of URI symptoms suggests a secondary bacterial infection, most commonly acute otitis media. The mother of this child added that the child had just completed a 10-day course of amoxicillin for otitis media.

PROBLEM 3 The history elicited a report of mild rhinorrhea and two episodes of vomiting accompanying the fever. Otherwise, the child had been playing and taking fluids well.

Of these three problems, only the child in Problem 2 shows specific symptoms that suggest a focus of infection. Mild rhinorrhea and occasional vomiting may occur with any infection, whereas lethargy and irritability indicate the severity of illness, not necessarily a specific focus.

Physical Examination

The physical examination consists of a general assessment to determine the probability of serious illness and a detailed examination to detect a specific focus of infection. Of the two, the general assessment is more important in determining the course of action.

General Assessment. The Yale Observation Scale for febrile children (Table 36–2) is a useful guide for identifying children who appear ill. The items on this scale address the child's consolability and response to stimulation in addition to skin color and hydration.

The child is first observed in the company of the parent. If he or she is crying, the vigor of the cry and the response to the parent's attempts to console the child are noted. In children described as "irritable," maternal rocking and cuddling often calm the infant. However, in the presence of central nervous system inflammation, rocking the baby may result in increased (paradoxical) irritability, an observation that is highly sensitive for meningitis. In contrast, a "smiling and playful" child is probably not ill.

The physician must deliberately observe a sick infant's interest in drinking fluids, his interest (judged by eye contact and gestures) in interacting with his mother, and his curiosity about the environment. The infant's interest may be piqued with a bright finger puppet or penlight or by offering a tongue blade for him to hold. The same object can be used to persuade him to look down, checking for a supple neck, or to follow with his eyes.

Specific Examination for Focus of Infection. A detailed physical examination in a febrile infant is made in an attempt to determine the source of the fever. The information obtained in the history may be used to guide the examination, but all febrile infants require a complete examination. A thorough examination will prevent missing a focus such as otitis media, for which nonspecific symptoms such as vomiting or diarrhea might otherwise be attributed to gastroenteritis.

The approach to physical examination in the infant in flexible. Assessment and auscultation of the heart, lungs, and abdomen are best done when the child is quiet. Maneuvers that typically provoke crying, such as inspecting the ears and oropharynx, are done last.

Vital Signs. Normal values for age and weight are listed in Table 36–3.

Respirations. A slight increase in respiratory rate occurs with fever. Tachypnea is a very sensitive indicator of respiratory pathology and may be the only clinical sign in children with pneumonia. It is defined as a respiratory rate of more than 40/min in children older than 3 months. Recorded respiratory rates may be unreliable, and the physician should confirm the rate independently.

Heart rate. Fever causes tachycardia, which is well tolerated in infants. The cardiac output is dependent on the heart rate, and rates up to 200 per minute are not unusual. The expected heart rate is generally estimated to be four times the respiratory rate. Heart rates of more than 220/min are more likely to be due to cardiac pathology and may require treatment. Bradycardia signifies decompensation, most often due to hypoxia.

Blood pressure. Low blood pressure in the presence of tachycardia signifies shock secondary to volume depletion. The following guidelines can be used to estimate the normal lower limit for systolic blood pressure: newborn, 60 mm Hg; 1 to 12 months, 70 mm Hg; over 12 months, 80 mm Hg plus two times age in years.

Body weight. A measurement of body weight is essential to guide fluid therapy and drug dosages. When accurate comparisons are available, it is very sensitive for quantifying dehydration.

Head. The anterior fontanelle is assessed when the infant is quiet and is in a sitting position. A tense or bulging anterior fontanelle suggests meningitis, whereas a depressed fontanelle indicates dehydration. The fontanelle closes between 12 and 18 months of age.

Eyes. Conjunctival injection and discharge indicate conjunctivitis, either as an isolated finding or associated with upper respiratory tract findings. Periorbital redness or swelling suggests cellulitis.

Ears. Otitis media is a common diagnosis in the febrile infant regardless of other symptoms. Criteria for diagnosis are discussed in Chapter 33.

Nose. Mucosal edema and drainage signify upper respiratory involvement. Nasal flaring is a sign of respiratory distress.

Oropharynx. Swelling, inflammation, and mucosal lesions suggest specific infectious etiologies discussed in Chapter 32.

Neck. Stiffness and refusal to move the head and neck are significant signs when present, but their absence does not rule out meningitis in infants under 18 months of age. Active voluntary neck flexion is more reliable than passive flexion.

A few small, mobile, nontender lymph nodes in the anterior triangles of the neck are common. Large, tender anterior nodes and palpable posterior nodes indicate active infection. The axillary and inguinal areas are also palpated for nodes.

Chest. Signs of respiratory pathology include increased work of breathing (retractions) and abnormal breath sounds. Stridor (Chap. 37) occurs in an upper airway partial obstruction and suggests epiglottitis or croup, whereas wheezing (Chap. 56) is heard in bronchiolitis and asthma and indicates lower airway obstruction. Percussing the chest while listening with the stethoscope is more sensitive for determining an area of

TABLE 36–3. Normal Vital Signs for Age and Weight

Age	Weight (kg)	Respiratory Rate (per minute)	Pulse (beats per minute)	Systolic Blood Pressure (mmHg)
Newborn	2–4	30–60	100–160	50–70
1–6 Wk	2–4	30–60	100–160	70–95
6 Mo	6–8	25–40	90–120	80–100
1 Yr	10	20–30	90–120	80–100
3 Yr	15	20–30	80–120	80–110
6 Yr	22	18–25	70–110	80–110
10 Yr	30	15–20	60–90	90–120

pneumonic consolidation than are abnormal breath sounds. Rales are seldom heard in infants, even in those with well-documented pneumonia.

Abdomen. Very active bowel sounds are common in gastroenteritis. Tenderness is very difficult to assess or localize in infants. A rectal examination is essential for evaluating abdominal pain or blood in the stool. The inguinal, genital, and perianal areas are also assessed.

Skin. Mottling and poor capillary refill are evidence of poor circulation. Cellulitis and typical exanthems indicate a specific etiology (Chap. 14).

Extremities and Spine. Observation of the child's active use and range of motion of each extremity during crawling, walking, or reaching for objects can rapidly exclude significant pathology. Abnormal use of an extremity requires a detailed examination of the skin, soft tissues, and joints.

PROBLEM 1 Following initial stabilization, reassessment of the patient showed an infant who required prolonged stimulation to become aroused, had dull facies, and responded minimally to examination. The anterior fontanelle was bulging, and further detailed examination showed no focus of infection.

PROBLEM 2 General assessment confirmed the triage nurse's impression of a well-appearing child who was crying off and on. Detailed examination revealed signs of a mild URI and acute otitis media. The anterior fontanelle was flat, and the neck was supple during active motion.

PROBLEM 3 During examination the child was active and playful despite the fever. There was no apparent focus of infection. The examination was recorded as follows:

General Appearance: Active and playful
Vital Signs: Respirations 26/min, pulse 110 beats/min, temperature 103°F (39.5°C)
Skin: Color and hydration normal, no rash
Head, Eyes, Ears, Nose, Throat: Anterior fontanelle closed, tympanic membranes and oropharynx normal, nose—mild rhinorrhea
Neck: Supple with small anterior nodes bilaterally
Chest: Good breath sounds, no retractions, no rales or wheezing
Abdomen: Soft, nontender; genitals normal
Extremities: Full active range of motion in all extremities

DECISION PRIORITIES AND PRELIMINARY DIFFERENTIAL DIAGNOSIS

Following the initial assessment, history, and examination, the physician forms a preliminary differential diagnosis and develops management priorities by considering the following questions.

1. *Does the child appear ill?*
   The seriously ill-appearing child (Yale score of more than 16) is identified in the initial assessment. Following stabilization, these children require comprehensive testing with a presumptive diagnosis of sepsis.

   The child who does not appear seriously ill but is irritable or mildly lethargic (Yale score of 11 to 15) also requires diagnostic testing. A high temperature frequently results in this picture. Reassessment following lowering of the temperature may clarify the appearance as ill or well.
2. *Is there an apparent focus of infection?*
   The child may have an obvious focus of infection following clinical evaluation.

Further action is based on the severity of the infection and the probability that it is bacterial. Table 36–4 lists the common infections that are identified on clinical examination and their potential for serious sequelae. Although uncommon, a second site of infection, e.g., otitis and pneumonia, or extension of infection, e.g., otitis leading to meningitis, must be considered. Finding a site of infection does not preclude a complete assessment in the ill infant.

3. *If there is a focus of infection, is the infection viral or bacterial?*
   Infections identified on clinical examination that are clearly bacterial or viral require no further testing in the well-appearing child. The most common bacterial infection identified on clinical examination is acute otitis media. A number of infections may be either bacterial or viral, and specific diagnostic testing is necessary to identify bacterial cases.

4. *If there is no focus of infection, what is the highest temperature that has been recorded at home or in the emergency department?*
   Children with temperatures of 103°F (39.5°C) or higher have an increased likelihood of having significant bacterial disease, including occult bacteremia. The well-appearing child with no focus of infection or with only nonspecific symptoms should undergo further evaluation with diagnostic testing to search for a focus of infection not apparent on clinical evaluation.

PROBLEM 1 This child appeared ill, and the localizing signs (bulging fontanelle) suggested a diagnosis of meningitis with possible sepsis.

PROBLEM 2 This patient had a viral URI with acute bacterial otitis media. Usually no further diagnostic testing would be necessary. This case was complicated by the history of a febrile seizure; however, the work-up was properly directed primarily at determining the cause of the fever.

PROBLEM 3 The symptoms of rhinorrhea and occasional vomiting without any other signs were not sufficient to indicate any localized infection. The temperature of 103°F (39.5°C) in an otherwise well-appearing child prompted a search for a nidus of infection.

DIAGNOSTIC ADJUNCTS

Ancillary testing is commonly obtained in children with fever. Indications for each test are discussed below.

TABLE 36–4. Common Pediatric Infections Identified on Clinical Examination

System	Usually Mild	Serious
Central nervous		Meningitis
Respiratory	Upper respiratory infection	Epiglottitis
	Gingivostomatitis	Pneumonia
	Pharyngitis	
	Cervical adenitis	
	Acute otitis media	
	Croup (LTB)	
	Bronchiolitis	
Gastrointestinal	Gastroenteritis	Appendicitis
Skin and soft tissue	Viral exanthems	Cellulitis
	Scarlet fever	Meningococcemia
Musculoskeletal	Viral synovitis	Septic arthritis
		Osteomyelitis

Laboratory Studies

Complete Blood Count with Differential Cell Count. A complete blood count (CBC) is often ordered in the evaluation of young febrile children. If the child clearly has a viral illness (e.g., croup, bronchiolitis, viral exanthem) or an obvious bacterial illness (otitis media, UTI, or streptococcal pharyngitis), the results of the CBC will not alter the method of management. CBC is useful as a screening test when the clinical picture is not clear. If the white blood cell count (WBC) is clearly elevated (over 15,000 cells/mm^3) with a left shift, further tests such as a blood culture for suspected occult bacteremia or a chest radiograph to rule out pneumonia are indicated. A marked left shift without an elevated WBC count has the same significance as leukocytosis.

Sedimentation Rate. The erythrocyte sedimentation rate (ESR) is a nonspecific indicator of disease and in acute febrile illness does not add significant information to that obtained from the CBC. An ESR of more than 15 mm/hour is statistically related to an increased frequency of bacteremia.

Blood Culture. A blood culture is indicated in any patient who appears ill or has serious bacterial illness, such as meningitis, sepsis, pneumonia, arthritis, or facial cellulitis, and in children between the ages of 3 and 24 months who have a temperature of over 103°F (39.5°C). One blood culture is sufficient in most pediatric patients.

Urinalysis. "Bag" urine is adequate for a screening urinalysis. If the microscopic analysis is positive for leukocytes, a clean urine sample is obtained by either catheter or suprapubic aspiration and sent for culture. UTI may present as nonspecific gastrointestinal symptoms or fever only. A screening urine sample is indicated in the infant with vomiting, diarrhea, or fever without a focus of infection.

Rapid *Streptococcus* Screen. Clinical assessment of streptococcal pharyngitis is, at best, 50% accurate. *Streptococcus* screening is indicated for children with isolated pharyngitis, cervical adenitis, and scarlatiniform rashes and in infants under 36 months of age who present with upper respiratory tract symptoms. Positive results on the test form an adequate basis for antibiotic treatment. Negative results on the rapid test (which may include false-negative results) are confirmed with a throat culture specific for group A beta-hemolytic *Streptococcus* (Chap. 32).

Radiologic Imaging

Chest Radiograph. Pneumonias are often "silent" in young infants, that is, not evident on clinical examination. A chest radiograph is indicated for patients with clinical findings of tachypnea or lower respiratory tract involvement in addition to an ill appearance. A chest radiograph is considered in the well-appearing child with no focus of infection and a temperature of at least 103°F (39.5°C) or a WBC count of over 15,000.

Other Tests

Lumbar Puncture and Cerebrospinal Fluid Analysis. A lumbar puncture (LP) is indicated in any child who appears seriously ill, has meningeal signs, has a petechial rash, and in all febrile infants under 1 month of age. For the infant with an uncomplicated febrile seizure, the need for LP is controversial. A conservative approach is to perform an LP in all children under 12 months of age who have a febrile seizure. Older children may be evaluated by the same criteria used for any febrile child—i.e., ill appearance, the presence of a focus of infection, and the height of the temperature. If the seizure is focal, prolonged, or repetitive or if the child has been partially treated with antibiotics, an LP is indicated.

Young, ill children may become apneic when they are flexed and restrained for the lumbar puncture. LP is deferred until the child is stabilized. If a delay in obtaining the fluid is anticipated, it is prudent to start administering antibiotics following the initial resuscitation and before obtaining the cerebrospinal fluid (CSF). Cerebrospinal fluid studies and interpretation are given in Chapter 47.

Joint Aspiration and Synovial Fluid Analysis. Arthrocentesis is indicated in children with symptoms and signs of joint inflammation. The hip is the most common site of septic arthritis in young children, and arthrocentesis is performed in conjunction with orthopedic consultation. Synovial fluid studies and interpretations are discussed in Chapter 40.

PROBLEM 1 Blood was obtained for culture, CBC, and serum chemistries. The WBC count was 20,000 with a left shift. Catheter urine was sent for culture. A portable chest film was read as normal. The LP revealed cloudy, turbid CSF.

PROBLEM 2 After considering the febrile seizure, the patient's age, and his temperature, the physician chose to do an LP; the CSF proved to be normal.

PROBLEM 3 A bag urinalysis showed a specific gravity of 1.010, no leukocytes, and no bacteria. A CBC and one blood culture were ordered; the white blood cell count was 12,000 with a left shift. The physician decided not to order a chest radiograph because the WBC count was under 15,000 and tachycardia and respiratory signs were absent.

REFINED DIFFERENTIAL DIAGNOSIS

After diagnostic testing, the physician may have a firm diagnosis in mind (focus of infection) and enough evidence to categorize the infection as bacterial or viral. By combining clinical and diagnostic results, patients usually can be classified into one of three groups:

- "Ill" with presumed or documented bacterial disease.
- "Well" with a focus of infection, either minor bacterial or viral.
- "Well" with no focus of infection following both clinical and diagnostic evaluation.

The ill-appearing child, as identified previously, may not have a focus of infection following clinical examination and diagnostic testing. However, the child's ill appearance alone warrants a presumptive diagnosis of serious bacterial disease.

The child who appears well and has no focus of infection on clinical examination may now have an identifiable focus on diagnostic testing, most commonly pneumonia or UTI.

The last group of children are those who appear well and have no apparent focus of infection. The majority of these children will recover without further treatment. However, approximately 5% of all febrile children aged 3 to 24 months will have bacteremia on blood culture, and a smaller percentage will go on to develop a serious focal illness such as meningitis.

Occult Bacteremia

Bacteremia, defined as a positive blood culture, is an expected finding in invasive or deep bacterial infections such as meningitis, sepsis, epiglottitis, septic arthritis, osteomyelitis, and facial cellulitis. Bacteremia is less frequently found in well-appearing febrile children with no focus of infection. When bacteremia occurs in this setting, it is termed *occult*. The most common organisms isolated in unexpectedly positive blood cultures are *Streptococcus pneumoniae* (65%), *Hemophilus influenzae* (25%), *Neisseria meningitidis* (5%), and *Salmonella* species (5%).

All socioeconomic groups are equally affected. Children at greatest risk are those aged 3 to 24 months with temperatures of 102°F (38.9°C) or more. The height of fever has a positive correlation with the prevalence of occult bacteremia. WBC counts between 10,000 and 20,000 have the same predictive value as a temperature greater than 102°F

(38.9°C). WBC counts below 5000/mm³ are most commonly found with viral infection but are also associated with occult meningococcemia. A total polymorphonuclear count of more than 10,000, immature neutrophils (bands) amounting to more than 500/mm³, and an ESR of more than 15 mm/hour also correlate positively with bacteremia. However, the predictive value of these tests is no better than that of the combination of fever and WBC count (Table 36–5).

Conversely, occult bacteremia is very unlikely in a child who presents with a fever of less than 102°F (38.9°C), has no clinical focus for the fever, and does not appear toxic. A febrile child with a WBC count of between 5000 and 10,000/mm³ has a 99% chance of *not* having bacteremia.

There is no combination of laboratory tests and clinical observations that will reliably differentiate the child with bacteremia from one with a self-limited benign febrile illness. Diagnosis depends on positive results of a blood culture. A single blood culture is indicated in a child with a temperature of at least 103°F (39.5°C) who has no focus of infection. Using the WBC count as a screening test prior to the blood culture reduces the percentage of negative blood cultures obtained but will still miss up to 30% of children who are bacteremic but have normal WBC counts.

The natural history of pneumococcal bacteremia is benign, provided the spleen is functional, compared to that of *H. influenzae* or *N. meningitidis*. In the majority of children with pneumococcal bacteremia the organism is spontaneously cleared from the blood. The remainder continue with fever, and in 2% to 10% of all patients the illness progresses to meningitis. In contrast, focal infection and sepsis develop in 50% to 80% of children with *H. influenzae* bacteremia. Although spontaneous clearing of *N. meningitidis* has been documented, a high percentage of patients develop meningitis and sepsis.

Blood culture results are unfortunately not available for at least 24 hours. Empiric antibiotic treatment of patients at risk for occult bacteremia has been proposed to hasten recovery and prevent complications. However, there is no clear evidence that antibiotic therapy prevents the development of serious illness, especially meningitis. Negative aspects of antibiotic therapy include promotion of a false sense of security and undesirable side effects.

Sepsis

Sepsis is bacteremia with systemic toxicity (see Chap. 17). It is less common than bacteremia. The same organisms that predominate in bacteremia and meningitis are responsible for sepsis, although enteric bacteria may also be found in the immunocompromised host. Meningococcal sepsis (meningococcemia) often occurs in epidemics.

Sepsis should be suspected in the ill-appearing child, regardless of the temperature. The onset of sepsis may be insidious or acute. Tachypnea, tachycardia, hypotension, metabolic acidosis, hypoglycemia, and disseminated intravascular coagulation (DIC) are common features.

TABLE 36–5. Temperature and WBC Count Correlated with Prevalence of Bacteremia

Sign		Prevalence of Bacteremia
Temperature	≥102° F (38.9° C)	3%–5%
	≥104° F (40° C)	8%–10%
	≥106° F (41.1° C)	>20%
Temperature and WBC	≥102° F (38.9° C) and ≥15,000	8%–10%
Temperature and WBC	≤102° F (38.9° C) and 5,000–10,000	<1%

WBC = white blood cell.

PROBLEM 1 The results of the LP and the clinical picture confirmed the initial impression of sepsis, in this case associated with meningitis.

PROBLEM 2 The normal LP confirmed the clinical impression of an uncomplicated febrile seizure associated with otitis media.

PROBLEM 3 The laboratory results added no further information about a focus of infection; the diagnosis remained fever without localizing signs. Bacteremia cannot be excluded without the results of the blood culture.

PRINCIPLES OF MANAGEMENT

Immediate management of the seriously ill child was discussed earlier in the section Initial Assessment in the Emergency Department. General principles of management for the febrile child include fever therapy, hydration, and antibiotic therapy.

Management of Fever

Fever of 100.4°F (38°C) or more is uncomfortable. The primary aim of lowering fever is to increase patient comfort. Lowering the temperature also permits clinical observations when the child is most comfortable and may clarify the appearance of an "irritable" child. Treating the fever does not obscure disease processes. Fever is no more or less likely to decrease with antipyretic therapy in a mild than in a serious illness; therefore, defervescence cannot be used to judge the seriousness of the underlying illness.

Fever is treated primarily with acetaminophen. Aspirin is not given to children who have viral illnesses, especially influenza and chicken pox, because of the association between aspirin use and Reye's syndrome. Acetaminophen is administered every 4 hours at a dose of 15 mg/kg. Acetaminophen is available in the following preparations:

1. Pediatric infant drops (80 mg in 0.8 ml)
2. Pediatric elixir (160 mg in 5 ml (1 tsp)
3. Children's chewable tablets (80 mg)
4. Junior strength tablets (160 mg)
5. Adult strength tablets (325 mg)

Sponging the febrile infant in tepid water can be used in conjunction with acetaminophen therapy to lower the temperature. Tepid water sponging is most useful for rapidly decreasing very high temperatures of more than 105.8°F (41°C). For temperatures of less than 105.8°F (41°C) sponging is an optional measure and is guided by patient comfort. Alcohol and cold or ice-water sponging are never recommended; they may result in systemic toxicity and hypothermia, respectively.

Hydration

Fever increases fluid loss, and all febrile children are encouraged to increase their fluid intake above normal. Oral hydration is appropriate for all but very ill children. Parents are informed that lack of interest in eating is normal but that adequate fluid intake is essential.

Antibiotics

Antibiotic therapy for most childhood infections is based on the likely bacterial etiology rather than on the bacterial culture (Table 36–6). Choice of antibiotics depends on the child's recent antibiotic experience and the local sensitivities of various organisms.

PROBLEM 1 Early in his care, the patient was given an IV antibiotic, ceftriaxone. This was a good choice, and it was continued.

TABLE 36–6. Empiric Antibiotic Therapy for Children Over 3 Months

Infection	Organisms	Antibiotic
Otitis media	Hemophilus influenzae	Amoxicillin
	Streptococcus pneumoniae	Trimethoprim-Sulfamethoxazole (TMP-SMX)
		Erythromycin-Sulfasoxazole
		Cefaclor
Pneumonia	S. pneumoniae	Amoxicillin
	Mycoplasma pneumoniae	Erythromycin
UTI	Escherichia coli	Amoxicillin
		TMP-SMX
Pharyngitis	Streptococcus species	Penicillin
Facial and periorbital cellulitis	H. influenzae	Ceftriaxone or cefotaxime
Suspected occult bacteremia	S. pneumoniae	Ceftriaxone (50 mg/kg IM)
	H. influenzae	
	Neisseria meningitidis	
	Salmonella species	
Sepsis and meningitis	S. pneumoniae	Ceftriaxone or ampicillin and chloramphenicol
	H. influenzae	
	N. meningitidis	
Septic arthritis	Staphylococcus aureus	Nafcillin and ceftriaxone
	H. influenzae	

PROBLEM 2 In view of the history of recent failed amoxicillin therapy, an antibiotic effective against beta-lactamase-resistant *H. influenzae*, such as cefaclor, was chosen. Acetaminophen and increased fluids were advised as treatment for the fever in addition to the antibiotic.

PROBLEM 3 The physician considered the mother reliable and decided to withhold antibiotics pending the blood culture results.

Empiric antibiotic therapy for suspected bacteremia is controversial. Alternative choices are to give amoxicillin by mouth or ceftriaxone intramuscularly.

SPECIAL CONSIDERATIONS

Immunocompromised Children

Immunocompromised children are characterized by an (1) increased susceptibility to infectious agents, (2) inability to respond to infection, and (3) failure to develop typical signs and symptoms of infection. In the immunocompromised child signs of infection that would usually be considered trivial require aggressive evaluation, paying special attention to areas affected by opportunistic and unusual infections, such as the oral and perianal areas, joints, bone, and skin.

Sickle Cell Disease and Asplenia. Children under 5 years of age with sickle cell disease are extremely vulnerable to overwhelming sepsis (*S. pneumoniae, H. influenzae*). Surgical asplenia from trauma, hereditary spherocytosis, Hodgkin's disease, and idiopathic thrombocytopenia purpura result in similar risk. Fulminant sepsis can evolve over hours and carries a high mortality.

Cancer and Leukemia. Immune system compromise may be caused by the disease itself, by chemotherapy, or by steroid use. Serious infection occurs with the usual bacterial pathogens, usually benign viruses (varicella and rubella) or opportunistic organisms from endogenous skin and gut flora. The height of fever correlates with the severity of infection; children with temperatures of more than 102.2°F (39°C) have a 25%

incidence of positive blood cultures. Normal or low temperatures may, however, occur in the presence of sepsis. Neutropenia, an absolute neutrophil count of less than 500/mm^3, increases the risk of infection significantly.

Acquired Immune Deficiency Syndrome. Most infants with acquired immune deficiency syndrome (AIDS) present with a triad of hepatosplenomegaly, chronic interstitial pneumonia, and failure to thrive. In addition to opportunistic infections, the child with AIDS is also susceptible to recurrent infections with the common childhood bacterial organisms.

Steroid Therapy. Prolonged high-dose therapy (more than 4 weeks) increases the risk of both common and opportunistic infection. Importantly, steroid therapy may mask the usual signs of infection, especially fever, pain, and granulocytosis.

Age Less Than 3 Months. Neonates and young infants (especially premature infants) have immature immune systems and commonly fail to develop fever in response to bacterial infection. A fever of more than 100.4°F (38°C) in infants under 3 months old requires a thorough investigation.

Chronic Illness. Children with congenital heart disease, lung disease, cystic fibrosis, nephrotic syndrome, and other chronic illness are at increased risk of various infections.

DISPOSITION AND FOLLOW-UP

Admission

Which children are admitted to the hospital?
1. Children with documented serious bacterial disease.
2. The child who appears ill despite an unclear diagnosis.
3. Children who are immunocompromised or have a chronic illness.
4. Children who need therapy that cannot be provided at home, e.g., oxygen, intravenous fluids, or antibiotics.
5. Children who need diagnostic tests that are unavailable on an outpatient basis, e.g., hip arthrocentesis.
6. Children whose families cannot be relied on to observe the patient or return for repeat evaluation or therapy.

Admission to Intensive Care Unit

Which patients should be admitted to the intensive care unit?
1. Any child who requires high-flow oxygen, ventilation, or fluids for initial resuscitation or continued management of compromised vital functions.
2. Children with bacterial meningitis or sepsis.

Discharge

Which patients can go home?
1. The "well" febrile child who has a reliable care giver, clearly understood instructions for follow-up, available follow-up, ability to comply with the indicated therapy (oral antibiotics, fluids), and a system for blood culture follow-up.

The plan for the patient who goes home should include:
1. Acetaminophen for fever
2. Oral hydration
3. Antibiotics as indicated
4. Clear instructions on what to do if the illness becomes worse
5. Plan (and a place to go) for follow-up within 24 hours

PROBLEM 1 This patient was admitted to the intensive care unit with a diagnosis of sepsis and meningitis.

PROBLEM 2 The child was discharged on oral cefaclor, and instructions were given to the mother on maintaining hydration and fever control. He was to be seen by his pediatrician the next day.

PROBLEM 3 The physician documented the following: diagnosis—fever without localizing signs; rule out bacteremia. The mother understood that blood culture results were pending and promised to bring the child in for reassessment the following day or sooner if she became worse. No antibiotics were prescribed.

DOCUMENTATION

1. From whom the history was obtained.
2. Height and duration of temperature.
3. Specific symptoms, including pertinent negative symptoms.
4. Hydration status.
5. Exposure to illness.
6. Immunizations, medications, and allergies.
7. General assessment of "illness" or "wellness."
8. Results of physical examination including all positive and negative findings specific for focus of infection.
9. Results of any diagnostic tests and a list of cultures that are pending.
10. Response to therapy including oral hydration and acetaminophen.
11. Final diagnosis and whether it is presumptive or confirmed, and an appropriate differential for nonspecific clinical findings.
12. Instructions and follow-up arrangements for all patients who are not admitted to the hospital.

SUMMARY AND FINAL POINTS

- The goal in the initial approach to the febrile infant is to determine whether the child appears ill. Objective scales such as the Yale Scale can assist in this assessment.
- Febrile infants who are lethargic and poorly responsive are presumed to be septic, and intravenous antibiotics are administered early in their emergency department course.
- Simultaneous observation of the child while obtaining a history from the care giver allows the examiner to clarify the reported behavior and symptoms of the child.
- Physical examination will help to determine the probability of serious illness as well as detect a specific focus of infection.
- The general condition of the child (well versus ill), the presence of a specific focus of infection, and the height of the temperature determine the need for and type of diagnostic tests ordered.
- Blood culture is indicated for infants who appear ill or have deep bacterial infections and for those at risk for occult bacteremia (aged 3 to 24 months with a temperature over 103°F [39.5°C]).
- Evaluation of the child with a simple febrile seizure emphasizes determining the cause of the fever.
- Management of a febrile illness in children consists of providing therapy for the fever, hydration, and appropriate antibiotic therapy, which is usually based on the likely bacterial organism rather than on culture results.
- In a well-appearing child between 3 and 24 months of age who presents with a temperature of 103°F (39.5°C) or more, a screening blood culture may be ordered, and the child is discharged from the emergency department if the care giver is reliable and understands the importance of follow-up on the culture results.

BIBLIOGRAPHY

Texts

1. Barkin RL: The Emergently Ill Child: Dilemmas in Assessment and Management. Rockville, MD, Aspen Publishers, 1987.
2. Ludwig S: Pediatric Emergencies. New York, Churchill Livingstone, 1985.

Journal Articles

1. Bluestone CD: Management of otitis media in infants and children: Current role of old and new antimicrobial agents. Pediatr Infect Dis J 7:S129–S136, 1988.
2. Buck GE: Nonculture methods for detection and identification of microorganisms in clinical specimens. Pediatr Clin North Am 36:95–112, 1989.
3. Chamberlain JM, Gorman RL: Occult bacteremia in children with simple febrile seizures. Am J Dis Child 142:1073–1076, 1988.
4. Crocker PJ: Occult bacteremia in the emergency department. Ann Emerg Med 13:45–48, 1984.
5. Crocker PJ, Quick G: Occult bacteremia in the emergency department: Diagnostic criteria for the young febrile child. Ann Emerg Med 14:1172–1177, 1985.
6. Jaffe JM, Tanz RR, Davis AT, et al: Antibiotic administration to treat possible occult bacteremia in febrile children. N Engl J Med 317:1175–1180, 1987.
7. Klein JO, Feigin RD, McCracken GH, Jr: Report of the task force on diagnosis and management of meningitis. Pediatrics 78:959–982, 1986.
8. Lebel MH, Freji BJ, Syprogiannopoulos GA: Dexamethasone therapy for bacterial meningitis: Results of two double-blind, placebo-controlled trials. N Engl J Med 319:946–971, 1988.
9. McCarthy PL, Lembo RM, Baron MA, et al: Predictive value of abnormal physical examination findings in ill-appearing and well-appearing febrile children. Pediatrics 76:167–171, 1985.
10. McCarthy PL, Lembo RM, Fink HD, et al: Observation, history, and physical examination in diagnosis of serious illnesses in febrile children <24 months. J Pediatr 110:26–30, 1987.
11. McCarthy PL, Sharpe MR, Spiesel SZ, et al: Observation scales to identify serious illness in febrile children. Pediatr 70:802–809, 1982.
12. Powell KR, Mawhorter SD: Outpatient treatment of serious infections in infants and children with ceftriaxone. J Pediatr 110:898–901, 1987.
13. Roberts KB, Charney E, Sweren RJ, et al: Urinary tract infection in infants with unexplained fever: A collaborative study. J Pediatr 103:864–866, 1983.
14. Rosenberg NM, Bobowski T: Clinical indications for lumbar puncture. Pediatr Emerg Care 4:5–8, 1988.
15. Word BM, Klein JO: Current therapy of bacterial sepsis and meningitis in infants and children: A poll of directors of programs in pediatric infectious diseases. Pediatr Infect Dis J 7:267–270, 1988.
16. Yogev R, Shulman ST, Chadwick EG, et al: Once daily ceftriaxone for central nervous system infections and other serious pediatric infections. Pediatr Infect Dis 5:298–303, 1986.

CHAPTER 37

STRIDOR

HELENE CONNOLLY, M.D.
GARY R. STRANGE, M.D.

PROBLEM 1 A 3 year old boy was well until he awoke from sleep at 3 AM with a high fever. His mother brought him to the emergency department because he was unable to lie down, had noisy respirations, and was drooling saliva.

PROBLEM 2 A 10 month old boy was given an apple slice to eat by his 3 year old sister. He suddenly developed choking sounds and respiratory distress.

PROBLEM 3 A 2 year old girl with a 3-day history of a cold awoke at 11 PM with a cough and difficulty in breathing.

QUESTIONS TO CONSIDER

1. How is stridor recognized and what is its clinical significance?
2. How is the anatomy of the upper airway of the child different from that of an adult?
3. What problems may cause stridor in children?
4. How can the history, physical examination, and diagnostic adjuncts help to differentiate the causes of stridor?
5. What is the appropriate therapeutic approach for the three major causes of stridor?

INTRODUCTION

Stridor is a harsh, high-pitched, raspy sound made as air passes through a partially obstructed upper airway. It is heard best during inspiration, in which it signifies glottic or subglottic obstruction. If stridor is expiratory only, a ball-valve mechanism below the vocal cords is usually confirmed.

Upper airway obstruction in children may be due to infection, inflammation, foreign body, or congenital abnormality. Ninety percent of cases are due to infection. The same processes occur in the adult population but only rarely result in clinically recognizable obstruction, largely due to anatomic differences.

The pediatric airway (Fig. 37–1) differs in several important ways from that of the adult:

- The tracheal cartilage of the child is relatively soft and pliable. During inspiration, negative intratracheal pressure results in narrowing of the upper airway, whereas during expiration, the airway widens. Inspiratory stridor is therefore much more common than expiratory stridor.
- The epiglottis of the infant or small child is relatively long, and the aryepiglottic folds are redundant. The mucous membranes are softer and looser, and lymphoid tissue is abundant. Swelling of these tissues can be marked and may lead to obstruction.
- The epiglottis and larynx lie higher in the infant, at the level of C2 or C3. In the adult they are found at the level of C5 or C6. This more cephalad position of the glottic opening makes intubation of the infant more difficult.

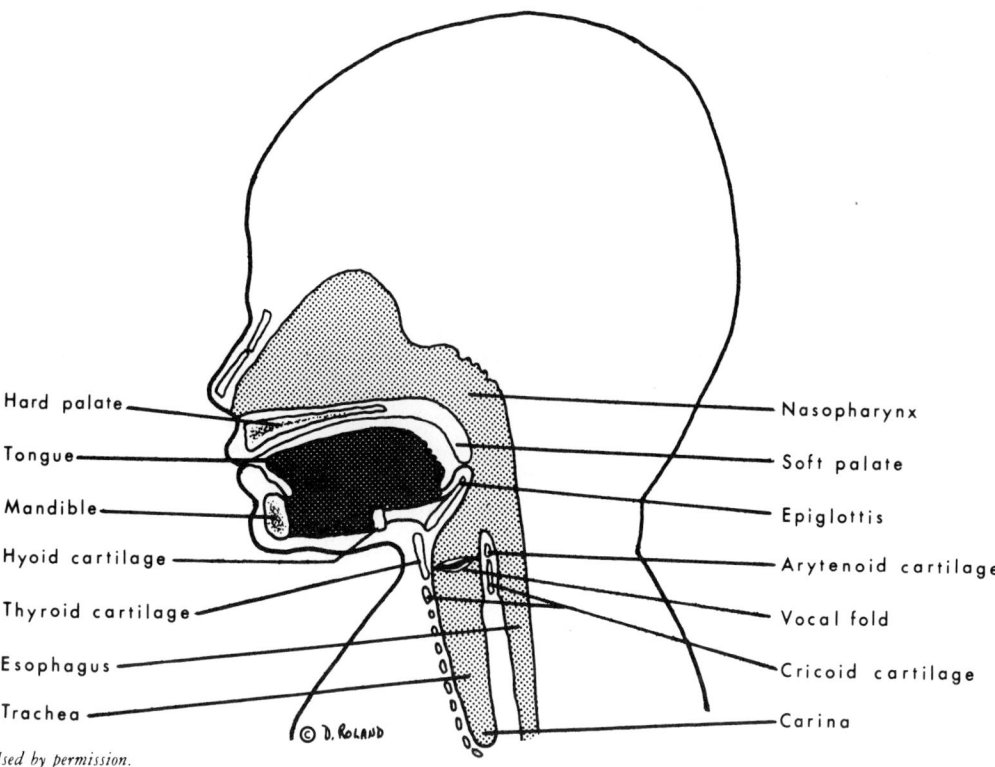

FIGURE 37–1. Anatomy of pediatric airway. (From Lumpkin JR: Airway obstruction. Topics Emerg Med 2(1):16, 1980.)

- The diameter of the trachea in the infant and child is far smaller than that in the adult (6 to 7 mm). Foreign bodies or edema that cause only partial blockage in the adult airway may result in complete obstruction in children. Airway resistance is inversely proportional to the fourth power of the radius. Therefore, a reduction in the radius of the trachea by half causes a 16-fold increase in resistance. Clearly, small amounts of edema can result in marked obstruction of air flow.
- The cricoid ring is the only circumferential support of the upper airway in the child, and it represents the narrowest portion. An endotracheal tube that fits through the glottic opening will be snug in the subglottic region. This obviates the need for cuffed endotracheal tubes in children below 8 years of age. Since the cricoid is the only circumferential support for the pediatric airway, injury to it by pressure from a cuffed tube or by surgical disruption during cricothyrotomy is to be avoided. For this reason, many authorities state that surgical cricothyrotomy is contraindicated in pediatric patients.

PREHOSPITAL CARE

The rescue squad is often called by parents who become concerned about noisy or difficult breathing in their child. On arrival, the child may be found to have complete obstruction with apnea, partial obstruction with imminent danger of complete obstruction, or mild obstruction with noisy but good air flow. Management of the completely obstructed airway is discussed in Chapter 2. Management in the field of partial airway obstruction varies with the severity of the obstruction. A few questions and physical observations will help the rescue squad to assess the degree of obstruction and therefore the best therapeutic approach.

History

1. What sort of breathing difficulty has the child been having and when did it begin?
2. Is he able to speak or cry? A child who is still phonating is moving air reasonably well.
3. Is he able to swallow? Has he been drooling? Supraglottic obstructions will lead to dysphagia and drooling. These are the most dangerous symptoms because upper airway obstruction can progress to complete obstruction very rapidly.
4. Is there possible or known foreign body aspiration?

Physical Examination

1. Does the child feel feverish or look toxic? High fever and toxic appearance are more consistent with supraglottic infections.
2. How is the child sitting or positioning himself? Most patients in respiratory distress maintain a sitting position, but those with supraglottic obstruction usually sit very upright and hold the head forward.
3. What are the airway sounds like? Stridor is to be differentiated from wheezes or rhonchi.
4. Is there drooling?
5. Are there intercostal or supraclavicular retractions? These indicate a significant obstruction to air flow, necessitating the use of accessory muscles for breathing.
6. Is the child cyanotic? Is he lethargic or poorly responsive? These observations suggest hypoxemia and the need for rapid intervention.

Intervention

1. As long as the child is moving air, quiet, efficient, and nonupsetting transport to the hospital is recommended.
2. Optimally, the child is allowed to sit on the mother's lap.
3. Oxygen is administered by "blow-by" technique—the mother holds a mask with high-flow oxygen near the child's face, not over it. If this process agitates the child, it is stopped.
4. Intravenous lines are not attempted.
5. Should complete obstruction develop, ventilation is attempted using an adult bag-valve-mask. Even in the presence of supraglottic obstruction, high pressures usually force adequate air into the lungs. If bagging is unsuccessful, endotracheal intubation is attempted, but it may be impossible owing to supraglottic edema. Without delay, needle cricothyrotomy is performed, and the child is ventilated with high-pressure oxygen. Although the rescue squad and the physician must be familiar with this procedure, this invasive airway maneuver is rarely necessary.

PROBLEM 2 The rescue squad arrived to find this 10 month old boy struggling to breathe. A history of a possible foreign body aspiration was obtained from the anxious mother. The child had marked inspiratory and expiratory stridor and demonstrated marked intercostal and supraclavicular retractions. His skin color was normal, and he was alert. Because the child was still moving air and was alert and noncyanotic, the squad was instructed to transport him to the emergency department. They were instructed to use chest thrusts if complete obstruction developed en route.

INITIAL APPROACH IN THE EMERGENCY DEPARTMENT

The first priority when presented with a stridorous child is to determine the adequacy of ventilation and oxygenation and therefore the need for respiratory support.

History

The history is as listed under Prehospital Care, plus asking about any home therapy and any change in status during the transport to the emergency department.

Physical Examination

Simple observation of the child while he is being held by the parent provides very useful information.

Position. The position the child assumes spontaneously is noted.

Respiratory Rate. As a rough approximation, respiratory rates above 40 are abnormal in infants, and those above 30 are abnormal in children. Specific age-dependent normal respiratory rates are given in Table 37–1.

Respiratory Effort. Use of accessory muscles, the presence of intercostal and supraclavicular retractions, and nasal flaring all indicate increased work of breathing.

Cyanosis. Central cyanosis indicates significant hypoxemia secondary to marked obstruction to air flow.

Lethargy or Unresponsiveness. Changes in mental status suggest marked hypercapnia or hypoxia due to respiratory failure.

Auscultation of the Chest. This reveals breath sounds that are characteristic of the level of obstruction.
1. Wheezing suggests small airway disease, as in asthma or bronchiolitis.
2. Stridor suggests upper airway disease. In the setting of an upper respiratory infection, the nares may have to be suctioned to eliminate transmitted sounds from the nasopharynx. High-pitched crowing is typical of subglottic obstruction, whereas low-pitched, muffled sounds are suggestive of supraglottic obstruction.

Vital Signs. Tachycardia out of proportion to the degree of fever is an important warning. However, trends are more helpful than the absolute value. Increasing tachycardia and tachypnea indicate increasing distress. As hypoxemia develops, however, bradycardia may ensue.

Recognition of Impending Respiratory Failure. If the child is in marked respiratory distress and there is frank or impending respiratory failure, ventilatory support is instituted immediately. Impending respiratory failure is recognizable when the following signs are observed:
1. Increased work of breathing with tiring.
2. Increasing tachypnea.
3. Increasing tachycardia.
4. Abrupt onset of bradycardia.
5. Cyanosis.
6. Marked lethargy or unresponsiveness.

Intervention

If the child is not in severe distress with impending respiratory failure, the following interventions are indicated, followed by a more complete history and physical examination.

TABLE 37–1. Normal Pediatric Respiratory Rates

Age	Rate (per minute)
Neonate	30–60
1–6 months	30–40
6–12 months	24–30
1–4 years	20–30
4–6 years	20–25
6–12 years	16–20
Over 12 years	12–16

1. Oxygen is given by blow-by technique or mask if tolerated. Oxygen flow is 6 to 8 liters/min.

2. The child is allowed to assume his position of comfort. He is not forced to lie down—complete obstruction may result.

3. All unnecessary disturbances are eliminated. No intravenous lines, arterial blood gases, or laboratory specimens are collected until absolute need is determined.

If the child is unable to move air effectively, ventilation with a bag-valve-mask unit and 100% oxygen is attempted. High pressures may be necessary to force oxygen past an upper airway obstruction, and these are best generated with an adult-sized bag. Endotracheal intubation is likely to be difficult, especially with supraglottic infections. If adequate ventilation is achieved by bagging, moving the child to the operating room for attempted intubation by an anesthesiologist, with a surgeon standing by to do a tracheostomy if intubation is unsuccessful, is the best approach. If inadequate ventilation is obtained with bagging, endotracheal intubation is attempted. If it is unsuccessful, needle cricothyrotomy and ventilation are performed.

PROBLEM 1 On arrival in the emergency department, this 3 year old boy was sitting upright with his neck extended and his head held forward. Saliva was drooling from his mouth, and he had quiet, muffled speech and a low-pitched stridor. He was alert, had good skin color, a respiratory rate of 30, and a heart rate of 140 beats/min.

This presentation is consistent with a supraglottic obstruction, and complete obstruction is possible at any time. Oxygen is administered by blow-by technique while the child is allowed to sit on his mother's lap. No venous or arterial punctures are done at this time, and the staff is instructed not to lay the child down or disturb him in any way.

PROBLEM 2 On arrival in the emergency department this child was in severe respiratory distress with loud expiratory and inspiratory stridor, marked retractions, and a respiratory rate of 40. He appeared lethargic and slightly cyanotic. The physician inverted the infant over his arm and applied four back blows with the heel of his hand between the infant's shoulder blades. No respirations were noted. The child was turned over, and four chest thrusts were administered by compressing the midsternum with the physician's index and long fingers. The child coughed, and a 2-cm by 1-cm chunk of apple was expelled, after which the child began to move air spontaneously.

This child has impending respiratory failure. Immediate intervention is essential. As long as adequate air is being moved by the child's respiratory efforts, intervention is inappropriate because a partially obstructed airway can be converted to a completely obstructed one. However, this child is tiring, developing cyanosis and lethargy. Further delay is not warranted.

PROBLEM 3 This 2 year old was alert with good skin color when she was seen. She had a frequent brassy cough and rather loud inspiratory stridor. There were mild intercostal retractions. When not coughing, she was playful and happy.

Based on these observations, a thorough history and physical examination is necessary and appropriate before deciding on therapy.

DATA GATHERING

The history and physical examination allow the causes of upper airway obstruction to be differentiated, thereby guiding proper management.

History

1. What *type of breathing difficulty* has the child been having? *When did it begin?* The parents' description of the problems and sounds they have observed will assist the physician in categorizing the problem.
2. Had the *child been well* before the onset of stridor? Had he had symptoms of an *upper respiratory infection* or *sore throat* prior to onset? Abrupt onset of stridor with maximal distress from the beginning suggests foreign body aspiration. Rapidly progressive distress is characteristic of epiglottitis, whereas slowly progressive or sputtering progression is consistent with viral laryngotracheobronchitis (LTB).
3. Has the child had *similar problems* before? Congenital airway problems can lead to recurrent episodes of distress.
4. Has the child had *pain on swallowing?* Has he been drooling? Supraglottic obstructions give rise to dysphagia.
5. Is there known or possible *foreign body aspiration* or exposure to *caustic agents?*
6. Has the child had a *cough* or *hoarseness?* A harsh, brassy cough, often described as a croupy cough, is suggestive of subglottic infection. Hoarseness results when there is interference with the precise, symmetric approximation of the vocal cords owing to pathology in the larynx.
7. Has the child been running a *fever?* What was the *temperature?* Although fever may be associated with any of the causes of stridor, high fever is more common with supraglottic infections.
8. Are the child's *immunizations* up-to-date? With aggressive immunization programs, diphtheria has practically disappeared. Sporadic resurgences do occur, however.
9. What is the child's *past medical history?* Is he taking any medications? Does he have any known allergies? Laryngeal edema and laryngospasm due to allergies present as stridor, which frequently develops very rapidly.
10. Has there been any *trauma* to the neck or any *inhalation* of smoke or chemical fumes? A fractured larynx or chemical inflammation also results in hoarseness and stridor.

Physical Examination

Initial Respiratory Assessment. The degree of respiratory distress is assessed as described under Initial Approach in the Emergency Department. Parameters to be considered are respiratory rate, respiratory effort, skin color, and mental status.

Vital Signs. Respiratory rate, pulse rate, and temperature are obtained. In addition to initial measurements of pulse and respirations, the trend in these parameters is followed closely because they correlate with the child's improving or deteriorating respiratory status. Table 37–1 lists the normal respiratory rates by age group for comparison.

The temperature is helpful in differentiating the causes of upper airway obstruction. A normal temperature is evidence, though not conclusive, against infectious causes. Foreign bodies of the upper airway are not associated with fever in the acute situation. Those that have passed the carina may present subacutely with atelectasis, infection, and fever. High fever and toxic appearance are highly suggestive of supraglottic infection in the stridorous child. Obtaining an oral or rectal temperature in this setting is contraindicated, but a tympanic temperature may be obtained if the procedure does not disturb the child.

Auscultation of the Chest. Breath sounds are assessed both in a quiet state and during crying, when this is possible. The forced air flow during crying may reveal abnormal sounds that are not appreciated when the child is quiet. In the infant the nose may be the source of loud transmitted air flow sounds. Suctioning the nares will facilitate assessment of air flow in the rest of the upper airway, but suction is not attempted if epiglottitis is suspected.

Body Position. The position the child assumes can be quite characteristic for the type of obstruction. Patients with respiratory distress often prefer the upright position. Subglottic obstruction (as with viral LTB) is an exception because position has minimal effect on the airway in this area. These patients frequently remain recumbent.

Supraglottic obstructions are greatly affected by position. Children with retropharyngeal abscess (RPA) often assume a position with their elbows on a table, head supported on their hands, and neck hyperextended. Infants with RPA tend to lie on their side with the neck hyperextended. The classic position of the child with epiglottitis is upright with mouth open and chin forward.

Visualization of the Pharynx and Epiglottis. Direct visualization of these structures may be diagnostic. Unfortunately, if the child has epiglottitis, visualization may precipitate a complete obstruction. The cephalad position of the epiglottis in the infant makes its visualization much simpler than it is in the adult. Successful visualization, by simply asking the patient to open his mouth and shining a light in, has been reported in up to 80% of cases of epiglottitis. The tip of the erythematous, edematous epiglottis is seen in these circumstances. The use of a tongue blade to depress the back of the tongue facilitates visualization but can force swollen tissue into the glottis or provoke laryngospasm. Direct visualization of the epiglottis with a laryngoscope is used in some centers, but, like use of the tongue blade, this can produce further airway compromise. If any instrumentation is considered, the physician must be prepared to secure the airway by endotracheal intubation and, if that is unsuccessful, by needle cricothyrotomy. In patients with suspected epiglottitis, instrumentation to improve visualization is not indicated.

In viral LTB, the mucous membranes are erythematous, with only slight edema, and the epiglottis, if visualized, is normal. Foreign bodies may be seen, but inability to visualize them directly does not rule out their presence. RPA may be visualized as a midline or unilateral erythematous swelling in the posterior pharynx.

Palpation of the Neck. The cervical lymph nodes are frequently enlarged and tender in patients with RPA. Tenderness evoked by external pressure on the larynx is seen with epiglottitis in older children and adults.

PROBLEM 1 No further pertinent history was obtained. Physical examination was limited to observation of the child's general appearance and respiratory status. The temperature, obtained tympanically, was 104°F (40°C). The emergency physician attempted to visualize the epiglottis by asking the child to open his mouth wide, but nothing was seen.

The guiding principle in the initial approach to the stridorous child is to avoid disturbing or upsetting the child. In most children with partial airway obstruction, particularly epiglottitis, the child is usually anxious but quietly concentrating on maintaining an open airway and breathing. Any disturbance can lead to marked worsening of this condition, even to inducing complete airway obstruction. Any manipulation of the upper airway, such as insertion of a tongue blade, is contraindicated.

PROBLEM 3 The mother confirmed that this 2 year old had had a mild cold for a few days. That night the child had awakened with noisy respirations. She had not had this type of problem before. She had had no problems with swallowing. A harsh cough had been noted for the last 24 hours. The child had no significant previous medical history. On physical examination she was alert and playful, with loud inspiratory stridor and slight intercostal retractions. Her temperature was 100.5°F (38°C) rectally. Her pharynx was clear on inspection, and the neck was supple without palpable nodes.

This child's presentation is consistent with a diagnosis of viral laryngotracheobronchitis. She was in mild distress.

DECISION PRIORITIES AND PRELIMINARY DIFFERENTIAL DIAGNOSIS

On completion of the history and physical examination, the physician will usually be able to answer these questions:

1. *Is stridor present?*
   Stridor is differentiated from other airway sounds, such as wheezing or rhonchi, on physical examination. The presence of stridor points to upper airway obstruction.
2. *If stridor is present, is the obstruction supraglottic or subglottic?*
   Subglottic obstruction results in a harsh stridor and is frequently associated with a similarly harsh cough. Supraglottic obstruction results in a softer stridor, which is associated with muffled voice and cough. Dysphagia is a prominent associated finding.
3. *What is the likely cause?*
   The most likely cause will have been determined in most cases after the history and physical examination. Table 37–2 outlines the causes of acute upper airway compromise in the pediatric age group.

If the diagnosis is clinically evident, the physician proceeds to specific management of the problem. For example, most children with viral LTB (croup) are diagnosed on the basis of evidence obtained from the history and physical examination and may be treated at this point. If the specific diagnosis is not clear, however, laboratory and radiographic evaluations are used to further refine the differential diagnosis.

PROBLEM 1 On comparing this patient's presentation with the criteria listed in Table 37–2, it was evident that acute epiglottitis was the most likely diagnosis. Further testing to confirm this diagnosis was not needed, and specific management was begun.

PROBLEM 2 The history and physical findings were consistent with foreign body

TABLE 37–2. Etiology and Treatment of Children with Stridor

	Epiglottitis	Viral Croup	Foreign Body	Retropharyngeal Abscess
Mechanism or organism	Bacteria: *H. influenzae*	Viral: parainfluenza, respiratory syncytial virus	Objects, peanuts, etc.	Mouth flora including *Staphylococcus aureus*
Age	Any: usually preschool or school age	Usually 6 months to 3 years	Any: usually toddler	Less than 6 years
Location	Supraglottic	Subglottic	Anywhere	Posterior pharynx
Onset	Abrupt: 1 hour	Gradual: days	Instantaneous or gradual	Usually gradual: days
Features	High fever Drooling Toxic appearance Apprehensive Position: sitting up with head forward Muffled stridor Dysphagia	Low-grade fever Loud stridor Barking cough	No fever Sometimes drooling May have dysphagia May have loud stridor Aphonia	Fever Drooling Dysphagia Odynophagia Upper airway obstruction
Treatment	Intubation or tracheostomy Antibiotics	Mist Racemic epinephrine Steroid Occasionally artificial airway	Back blow Chest thrust Intubation Cricothyrotomy Bronchoscopy	Incision and drainage Antibiotics
Course	A few days: swelling often gone by 3 days	Several days (5–7)	Until foreign body removed	A few days

Adapted from Ochsenschlager DW: Acute upper airway obstruction. In Ludwig S: Pediatric Emergencies. New York, Churchill-Livingstone, 1985.

aspiration, probably in the subglottic area. Specific management had been given, and diagnostic testing was not required.

PROBLEM 3 The history and physical examination were consistent with a diagnosis of viral LTB. Further testing was unnecessary prior to beginning treatment.

DIAGNOSTIC ADJUNCTS

Radiographic visualization of the upper airway is the most useful adjunct after the history and physical examination. Laboratory tests may be supportive of a specific diagnosis or can be used to evaluate the patient's clinical status and progress during treatment, but specimens are not obtained from the stridorous child until airway control is assured.

Radiologic Imaging

Soft tissue *neck radiographs* in the stridorous child are not always necessary. When the diagnosis is unclear, they can be very helpful. At no time should a stridorous child be sent to the radiology department unattended by a physician with proper equipment for airway management. The safest alternative is a portable upright film taken in the emergency department.

In patients with epiglottitis, the lateral neck x-ray reveals the enlarged epiglottis, thickened aryepiglottic folds, and ballooning of the hypopharynx (Fig. 37–2). In patients

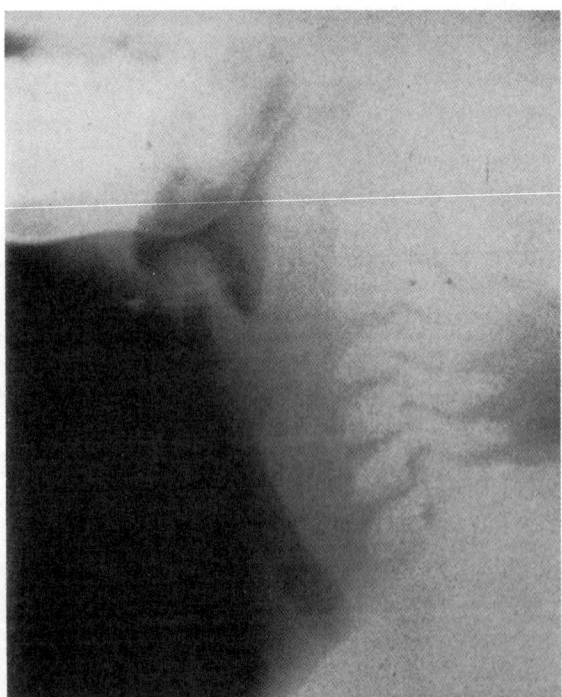
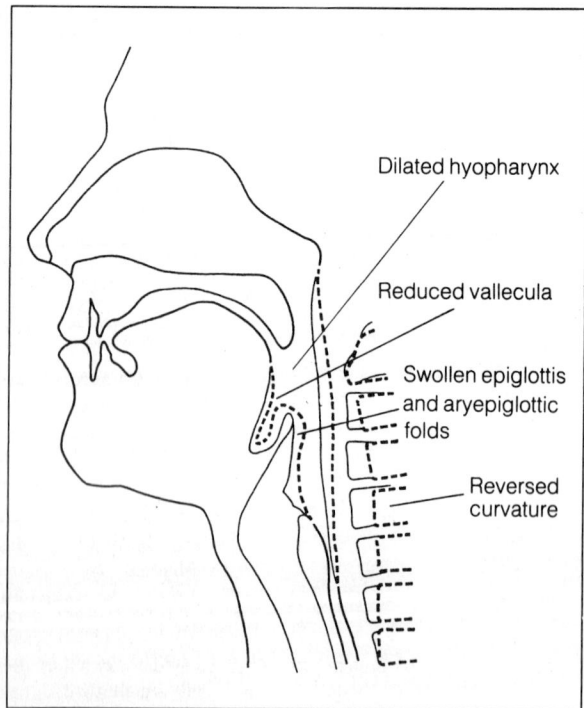

FIGURE 37–2. The classic "thumb sign" of an edematous epiglottis is evident in this lateral neck film. The schematic illustrates the findings to look for in a lateral film in a patient with suspected epiglottitis. Such films are superfluous in a child with the classic history, signs, and symptoms of epiglottitis; they can be tremendous help, however, in the diagnosis of mild or questionable cases—particularly when explaining to parents the need for aggressive treatment. (From Ashenoft C, Steele R: Epiglottitis. J Respir Dis 9(7):31, July 1988.)

with viral LTB, radiography is usually unnecessary. The lateral view is usually normal. An anteroposterior view may reveal subglottic narrowing. The trachea in this view has been described as having the appearance of a steeple.

Retropharyngeal abscess is a difficult clinical diagnosis to make, and the lateral neck film is often helpful. A bulging in the posterior pharynx is highly suggestive of RPA, but the physician must keep in mind that there is abundant prevertebral soft tissue in the child and that this tissue is even more prominent during expiration. Inspiratory views and fluoroscopy can be used when there is uncertainty.

Foreign bodies may be radiopaque and easily visualized (Fig. 37–3) or radiolucent and give rise only to secondary changes that allow their diagnosis. In addition to tracheal foreign bodies, esophageal foreign bodies can produce respiratory compromise by compressing the posterior tracheal wall. When a foreign body is suspected, lateral and anteroposterior views of the neck and chest are obtained. The patient's condition determines when and where these radiographs are taken.

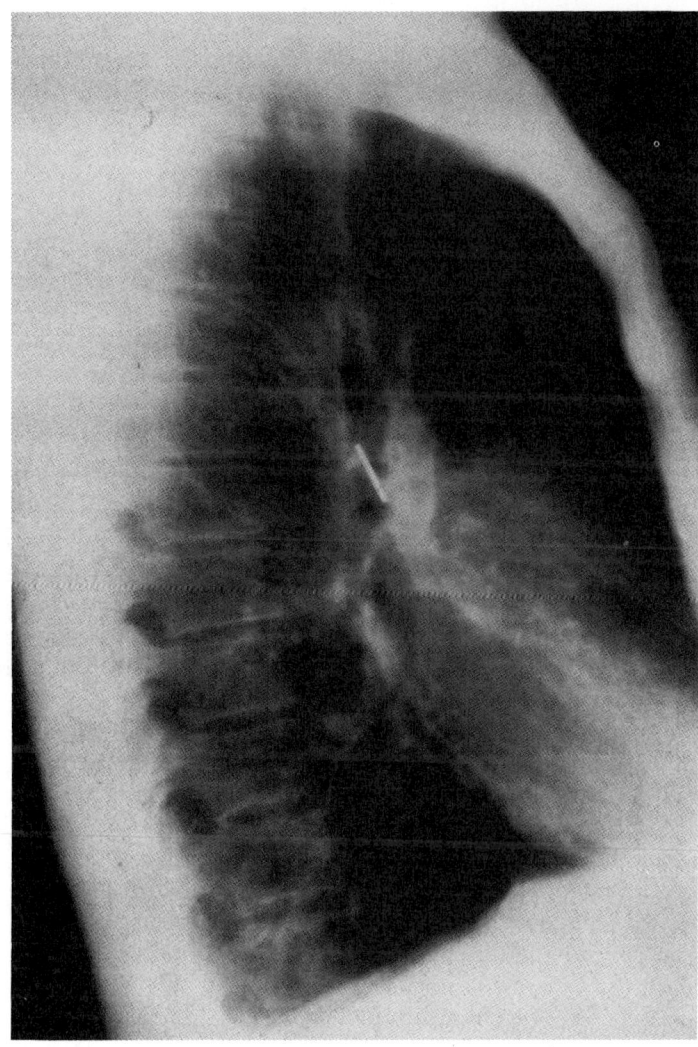

FIGURE 37–3. *Lateral x-ray study of chest showing aspirated coin in tracheal air column. (Reproduced by permission from Pons P: Foreign bodies. In Rosen P, et al (eds.): Emergency Medicine: Concepts and Clinical Practice (2nd ed.). St. Louis, The C.V. Mosby Co., 1988.)*

Laboratory Studies

Arterial Blood Gas Analysis. Arterial blood gases are not indicated early in the evaluation of patients with upper airway obstruction because the trauma of obtaining the specimen can precipitate struggling and further airway compromise. Furthermore, in this situation, the initial diagnosis of respiratory failure is made on clinical grounds. In severe cases and after initial diagnosis and management, arterial blood gases may be used to follow the patient's respiratory status.

Complete Blood Count and Differential. A complete blood count (CBC) may be useful in supporting the diagnosis made on clinical and radiographic grounds. A high white blood cell count with a shift to the left is consistent with a diagnosis of bacterial infection, e.g., epiglottitis or bacterial tracheitis. The white blood cell count with viral LTB and foreign bodies is usually normal.

Cultures. Specimens of blood or purulent drainage from the site of infection are obtained for culture. In children with epiglottitis, blood cultures are frequently positive for *Hemophilus influenzae*. In patients with RPA, cultures of blood, posterior pharyngeal secretions, or abscess are obtained. Both aerobic and anaerobic organisms are sought.

Special Tests

Pulse Oximetry. Pulse oximetry is a noninvasive tool that may be used for monitoring hypoxemia in the setting of upper airway obstruction.

REFINED DIFFERENTIAL DIAGNOSIS

With all the historical, physical, radiologic, and laboratory evidence at hand, the most likely specific diagnosis is selected, and specific management for that problem is started. The most commonly encountered problems are listed in Table 37–2 and discussed below. Table 37–3 lists less common causes of upper airway obstruction that are considered when the presentation is atypical and the diagnosis remains unclear.

Epiglottitis

Approximately 5% of children presenting with stridor have epiglottitis, which is due to infection of the epiglottis and surrounding tissues by *H. influenzae* in almost all cases. Epiglottitis can occur at any age, but the great majority of cases occur in children between 1 and 9 years of age (mean, 2 years 4 months). Chapter 32 includes a discussion of this problem in adults. Since the infection involves the aryepiglottic folds and cartilage and the surrounding pharyngeal tissue as well as the epiglottis, the term *supraglottitis* is more anatomically correct, although it is less commonly used.

TABLE 37–3. Uncommon Causes of Upper Airway Obstruction in Children

Congenital anomalies	Trauma
Vascular ring	Blunt laryngeal
Tracheoesophageal fistula	Penetrating neck
Tracheal web	Ingestions or inhalations
Tumors	Caustics
Subglottic hemangioma	Chemical fumes
Infections	Smoke inhalation
Bacterial tracheitis	Allergic laryngeal edema
Mononucleosis	
Cervical osteomyelitis	
Tetanus	
Botulism	
Diphtheria	

Epiglottitis is an especially important problem for the emergency physician because the natural history of the disease is acute onset with rapid progression to respiratory compromise. The initial complaint is usually sore throat and pain on swallowing. This is accompanied by fever and a markedly toxic appearance. As the edema and infiltration of the supraglottic structures increase, muffling of the voice, low-pitched stridor, and drooling of saliva develop. At this point, the child typically assumes an upright posture, holding the neck extended and the jaw forward. These patients are usually very apprehensive and fearful but sit quietly and give their full attention to holding the airway open and breathing. As the obstruction progresses, intercostal and supraclavicular retractions and use of accessory muscles are seen.

In infants under 2 years of age, this classic presentation is not seen. The progression of the disease in infants is not as rapid as that in older children, and frequently an upper respiratory infection has preceded it. Recumbency does not seem to produce the expected increase in respiratory obstruction, and drooling is rarely noted. A harsh cough may be present, making differentiation from croup even more difficult.

The diagnosis is confirmed by direct or radiographic visualization of the edematous epiglottis as described above.

Viral Laryngotracheobronchitis (LTB or Croup)

Approximately 90% of children presenting with stridor have croup. This is an infection of the subglottic trachea and, to a lesser extent, the bronchi by parainfluenza or respiratory syncytial viruses. It occurs in children younger than those affected by epiglottitis, most commonly between the ages of 6 months and 3 years.

There is usually a preceding upper respiratory infection, and the child will have been ill for several days before the onset of stridor. Fever may be present but is usually low grade. Due to the tracheal involvement, there is hoarseness, and the subglottic obstruction results in a characteristic barking cough as well as the higher pitched stridor. These children do not appear toxic and in spite of noisy respirations are often playful and active. Occasionally, viral LTB can be very severe and can result in significant respiratory compromise. Croup scores (Table 37–4) have been developed to assist the physician in determining the degree of compromise and therefore the need for intervention.

Foreign Bodies

Sudden onset of stridor and respiratory distress with no antecedent or associated signs or symptoms suggests the possibility of foreign body aspiration or ingestion. Approximately 2000 deaths occur yearly from this problem. It can occur in any age group but is most common in infants and younger children, who so frequently put any object they encounter in their mouths.

Large foreign bodies are most likely to lodge in the supraglottic area or to enter the

TABLE 37–4. Croup Score

	0	1	2	3
Stridor	None	Mild	Moderate at rest	Severe on inspiration and expiration
Retraction	None	Mild	Moderate	Severe
Air entry	Normal	Mild decrease	Moderate	Marked decrease
Color	Normal	Normal (0 score)	Normal (0 score)	Dusky, cyanotic
Level of consciousness	Normal	Restless when disturbed	Anxious, agitated, restless when disturbed	Lethargic, depressed

Score: 4–5 mild, 5–6 mild-moderate, 7–8 moderate, 8 severe (or any sign of severe).
From Davis HW et al: Acute upper airway obstruction, croup and epiglottitis. Pediatr Clin North Am 28:4, 1981.

esophagus, where they may result in compression of the posterior tracheal wall. Complete obstruction may result. Smaller foreign bodies may pass through the glottis and come to lie in the trachea (Fig. 37–3) or may pass into the bronchi. The child may be in marked distress and unable to speak in the former situation but may be surprisingly asymptomatic in the latter. Bronchial foreign bodies may exist for some time before they cause symptoms and may be diagnosed in the setting of unilateral atelectasis, hyperinflation, or pneumonia.

Retropharyngeal Abscess

Retropharyngeal abscess usually develops as an extension of a pharyngeal infection. However, penetrating trauma, iatrogenic instrumentation, and foreign bodies are other important causes. These are usually mixed aerobic and anaerobic infections, with group A streptococci predominating. This problem occurs most frequently in children under the age of 1 year and almost always before age 6.

Sore throat and fever have usually been present for a few days, at which time stridor, drooling, and respiratory distress develop. The presentation is very similar to that for epiglottitis except for a slower progression of disease and a younger age group. The cervical lymph nodes are usually tender and enlarged.

PRINCIPLES OF MANAGEMENT

The therapeutic approach to the pediatric patient with upper airway obstruction will vary depending on the precise etiology. The therapeutic principles that may be applied depending on the specific etiology are:
1. Mechanical maintenance of an open airway.
2. Provision of an enriched oxygen content for inhalation.
3. Provision of humidified oxygen or mist for inhalation.
4. Vasoconstriction and bronchodilatation through inhaled racemic epinephrine.
5. Antimicrobial therapy.
6. Endoscopic removal of foreign bodies.

Specific Therapy

Epiglottitis. The diagnosis of epiglottitis is confirmed by direct or radiographic visualization. When the diagnosis is clinically evident and the patient is maintaining air flow, the recommended approach is direct visualization by an anesthesiologist in the operating room. Following visual confirmation of the diagnosis, endotracheal intubation is attempted. If this is unsuccessful, an attending otolaryngologist performs a tracheostomy. Once the supraglottic obstruction is bypassed by either of these techniques, the patient will usually be able to ventilate adequately by himself. Sedation and restraints are necessary to prevent the patient from accidentally or intentionally removing the tube.

When the diagnosis is not so evident, radiologic visualization of the epiglottis is performed. Once the diagnosis is confirmed, the protocol outlined above is again recommended. In some centers, children with epiglottitis who are not in extreme distress are observed and given antibiotic therapy without intubation or tracheostomy. If this approach is elected, a physician experienced in pediatric airway control must be immediately available, and close intensive care unit monitoring of respiratory status is essential.

Antibiotic therapy is instituted as soon as possible. Intravenous ampicillin and chloramphenicol are recommended because ampicillin-resistant *H. influenzae* is present in up to 30% of cases. Second- and third-generation cephalosporins are alternatives. Steroid therapy is used by some, but there is no conclusive evidence of its benefit in epiglottitis.

Viral LTB (Croup). The management of viral croup is guided by the use of a clinical croup score like the one outlined in Table 37–4.

1. Patients with croup scores less than 6: Humidified oxygen/mist therapy.
2. Patients with croup scores of 7 to 8: Humidified oxygen/mist therapy, racemic epinephrine.
3. Patients with croup scores of more than 8: Racemic epinephrine; intubation is considered.

Humidified air or oxygen is the mainstay of treatment of croup. This may be achieved at home or in the emergency department using a cool mist humidifier. Humidified oxygen is used in more severely ill children. The mechanism of action is probably reduction of reflex tracheal spasm due to mobilization of secretions. Croup tents are effective in this respect but restrict observation of the patient. For this reason, their use is limited.

Racemic epinephrine is administered by diluting 0.5 ml (2% solution) in 2.5 ml of sterile water or saline and delivering this mixture by nebulizer. Its effects result from vasoconstrictive and bronchodilator actions. The duration of action is 2 to 4 hours, and recurrence of stridor is to be expected. Therefore, admission for observation is indicated even if a good response to racemic epinephrine is achieved.

Steroids are of potential use with viral LTB because they may block the inflammatory response at the cellular level, reducing capillary permeability. Further well-controlled studies of the use of steroids in LTB are needed to establish their role, but they are widely used with reported significant improvement in respiratory status.

Foreign Bodies. Management of patients with complete airway obstruction is outlined in Chapter 2. A patient with a partial obstruction is allowed initially to clear his airway by coughing. If this is not effective or if the patient's condition is deteriorating, abdominal thrusts are recommended in the adult and older child. In smaller children and infants, a combination of back blows and chest thrusts is recommended. If this is unsuccessful, direct laryngoscopy with removal of visualized foreign bodies using Magill forceps is recommended. For subglottic foreign bodies, bronchoscopy is necessary for removal.

Esophageal foreign bodies may result in airway obstruction by compressing the posterior tracheal wall. Endoscopy is the preferred technique for their removal.

Retropharyngeal Abscess. Retropharyngeal abscess is treated by incision and drainage and antibiotic therapy. It generally requires drainage in the operating room. Antistaphylococcal penicillins or cephalosporins are the preferred antibiotics.

PROBLEM 1 This patient was transported to the operating room, where an anesthesiologist and an otolaryngologist were standing by. The anesthesiologist visualized the epiglottis by direct laryngoscopy. It was fiery red and markedly swollen. The tissue was so swollen that the glottic opening could not be identified. Pressure on the chest caused some egress of air through this swollen tissue, but an attempt at intubation was unsuccessful. A tracheostomy was rapidly performed, and the patient was ventilated.

Even under the most controlled circumstances, intubation in the setting of epiglottitis may be very difficult. It is not attempted in the emergency department unless necessitated by patient decompensation.

PROBLEM 3 For this child with viral croup, a croup score was calculated as follows:

Stridor, moderate	2
Retractions, mild	1
Air entry, mildly decreased	1
Color, normal	0
Level of consciousness, normal	0
Croup score	4

Based on a croup score of 4, treatment was started with a cool mist humidifier placed in the child's room. After 1 hour, stridor persisted, without improvement. Treatment with nebulized racemic epinephrine was administered and achieved good response.

DISPOSITION AND FOLLOW-UP

Admission

The following patients are admitted for treatment or observation to a general pediatric floor:
1. Children with viral LTB who respond to racemic epinephrine.
2. Children from whom a foreign body has been removed when observation is indicated.
3. Children with RPA after drainage.

The following patients are admitted for monitoring in the intensive care unit:
1. Children with epiglottitis.
2. Those with viral LTB who do not respond to racemic epinephrine.
3. Children with a foreign body prior to removal.
4. Children with RPA prior to drainage.

Discharge

The following patients may be discharged with follow-up by their pediatrician or other primary care physician:
1. Those with viral LTB who respond to mist therapy alone.
2. Those with foreign body with uncomplicated removal.

On discharge, the parents are instructed in the use of humidification at home, if this is appropriate, and are given criteria for determining the need to return to the emergency department. Close observation for recurrence of respiratory distress is essential, and if the parents give any indication of inability to provide close monitoring, admission is recommended.

PROBLEM 1 After tracheostomy, intravenous ampicillin and chloramphenicol were administered, and the child was transported to the intensive care unit.

PROBLEM 2 After treatment, this child was admitted to the pediatric floor for observation. The child was stable but was at risk for sequelae. Follow-up chest radiographs are appropriate to ensure that smaller pieces of foreign material were not aspirated into the lower airways.

PROBLEM 3 This child was now breathing normally, but a recurrence of stridor was expected after 2 to 4 hours, when the effect of racemic epinephrine would wear off. Therefore, admission was considered.

Since this patient's obstruction was fairly minimal before racemic epinephrine was given, cool mist humidification was probably all that was indicated. The emergency physician decided to hold the patient in the emergency department for 4 hours, at which time she was in no distress and was discharged. The mother was instructed in the use of a humidifier at home and was told to return to the emergency department if respiratory distress recurred. Follow-up was scheduled with her pediatrician in 24 hours.

DOCUMENTATION

1. Patency of airway on arrival.
2. Serial observations of vital signs, work of breathing, skin color, and mental status.
3. Time and type of airway interventions.
4. Onset, progression, and nature of symptoms.
5. Position spontaneously assumed by the child.
6. Radiographs ordered and their interpretation.
7. Diagnostic conclusions.
8. Emergency department therapy provided.
9. Disposition and follow-up arrangements made if the patient is discharged.

SUMMARY AND FINAL POINTS

- Stridor is a high-pitched, raspy sound made as air passes through a partially obstructed airway.
- The pediatric airway is particularly susceptible to obstruction owing to its small diameter. Resistance to air flow is inversely proportional to the fourth power of the radius of the airway.
- Infection is the most common cause of upper airway obstruction in the pediatric age group, with viral laryngotracheobronchitis and epiglottitis accounting for 95% of cases.
- The onset and rapidity of progression of symptoms, and the prodromal and associated symptoms will help to differentiate the cause of the obstruction.
- The position spontaneously assumed by the child is also helpful in differentiating between the types of obstruction.
- When supraglottic obstruction is suspected, the patient is not disturbed and is allowed to stay upright, and no instrumentation of the mouth or pharynx is allowed until definitive airway control is readied.
- When viral LTB is treated with racemic epinephrine, improvement is temporary, and recurrence of obstruction after 2 to 4 hours is to be expected.
- An alert patient with a partially obstructed airway is allowed to continue to try to clear the airway by coughing before attempts are made to remove a foreign body.

BIBLIOGRAPHY

Texts

1. Barkin RM: The Emergently Ill Child. Rockville, MD, Aspen Publishers, 1987.
2. Barkin RM, Rosen P: Emergency Pediatrics. St. Louis, Mosby, 1986.
3. Ludwig S: Pediatric Emergencies. New York, Churchill-Livingstone, 1985.
4. American Academy of Pediatrics and American College of Emergency Physicians: Advanced Pediatric Life Support. 1989. Available from American College of Emergency Physicians, Dallas, TX.

Journal Articles

1. Barkin RM: Pediatric airway management. Emerg Med Clin North Am 6(4):687–692, 1988.
2. Brilli RJ, Benying G, Cotcomp DH: Epiglottitis in infants less than two years of age. Pediatr Emerg Care 5(1):16–21, 1989.
3. Brunette DB: Stridor in a toddler. Case Studies Emerg Med 5(7):1–4, 1989.
4. Davis HW, Gartner JC, Galvis AG, et al: Acute upper airway obstruction. Pediatr Clin North Am 28(4):859–880, 1981.
5. Glover DM, Wetson CB: Pediatric infections. Emerg Med Clin North Am 3(1):25–45, 1985.
6. Kimmitt TP, Defries HO: Pharyngeal emergencies. Topics Emerg Med 6(3):66–68, 1984.
7. Moazam F, Talbert JL, Rodgers BM: Foreign bodies in the pediatric bronchial tree. Clin Pediatr 22:148–193, 1983.
8. Postma DS, Jones RO, Pillsbury HC: Severe hospitalized croup: Treatment trends and prognosis. Laryngoscope 94:1170–1175, 1984.
9. Selbst SM: Epiglottitis. Am J Emerg Med 3:342–350, 1983.
10. Singer JI, McCabe JB: Epiglottitis at the extremes of age. Am J Emerg Med 6(3):228–231, 1988.
11. Strife JL: Upper airway and tracheal obstruction in infants and children. Radiol Clin North Am 26(2):309–322, 1988.

CHAPTER 38

SUSPECTED CHILD ABUSE

STEPHEN LUDWIG, M.D.
REBECCA R. S. SOCOLAR, M.D.

PROBLEM 1 A 4 year old boy was brought in with multiple bruises on the trunk, buttocks, and legs; he also had a cold and a cough. The triage nurse noted that he seemed withdrawn and unresponsive to questions. When the physician asked directly, "How did he get all of these terrible bruises?" the mother stated, "I'm just here for his cold."

PROBLEM 2 A 6 month old boy was brought to the emergency department for a severe diaper rash. The examiner noted a protuberant abdomen and wasted extremities. The child's birth weight was 7 pounds. At 6 months he weighed 8 pounds, 4 ounces. The mother placed him in the crib and fell asleep in the chair across the examining room.

PROBLEM 3 A 2½ month old male infant was brought in by the rescue squad with acute onset of seizures. There were no external signs of trauma.

PROBLEM 4 An adolescent girl was brought in by the police. She was found on a highway and was a known runaway. She was obviously pregnant.

QUESTIONS TO CONSIDER

1. What diverse forms of family behavior may constitute child abuse?
2. How can the emergency physician recognize clues from the history and physical examination that suggest abuse?
3. What constitutes appropriate documentation and reporting in cases of suspected abuse?
4. What constitutes an appropriate disposition for an abused child?
5. What mechanisms are in place to protect physicians from legal liability when they report suspected abuse?

INTRODUCTION

Child abuse and neglect are common problems of our society. Abuse can appear in varied guises. Many manifestations are subtle and difficult to detect. Whether the emergency department presentation is a medical or psychosocial emergency, it is necessary to maintain a heightened level of suspicion to diagnose the situation.

The incidence of child abuse is difficult to assess. In the United States, 1.5% of all children are reported each year to protective services because of suspicion of abuse or neglect. Unquestionably, this figure understates the true incidence. It is estimated that one-third of the victims of physical abuse are less than 1 year old, one-third are 1 to 6 years old, and one-third are older than 6 years. It is also estimated that 10% of children under 5 years of age who are brought to the emergency department with traumatic injuries are child abuse victims.

Abuse occurs when an individual caretaker loses control. Beyond the individual, major contributors to the problem can be familial, community, and societal factors (Fig 38–1). Even an emotionally "weak" adult can retain control when family, social, and financial supports are strong. When beset by multiple frustrating and stressful external factors, even relatively "strong" adults can begin to transfer these negative feelings by becoming abusive. The shame and guilt of having abused a child may lead to lowered self-esteem, further frustration and stress, and eventually to a vicious cycle of escalating abuse. Some personal situations that correlate with higher rates of child abuse are:

1. Parents who have recently experienced high levels of stress with little opportunity for stress release.
2. Previous family violence.
3. Low marital satisfaction.
4. Low income.
5. Social isolation.
6. Premature infants or children with prolonged neonatal hospitalizations.
7. Children with handicapping conditions.

PREHOSPITAL CARE

The prehospital care provider can often supply valuable information about the possibility that abuse has occurred. A view of the home environment and the reactions of family members to the situation while they are on their "own turf" is critical in some cases of abuse.

History

1. How did the paramedics find the child and parents?
2. Were their actions appropriate to the situation?
3. What are the child's living circumstances like?

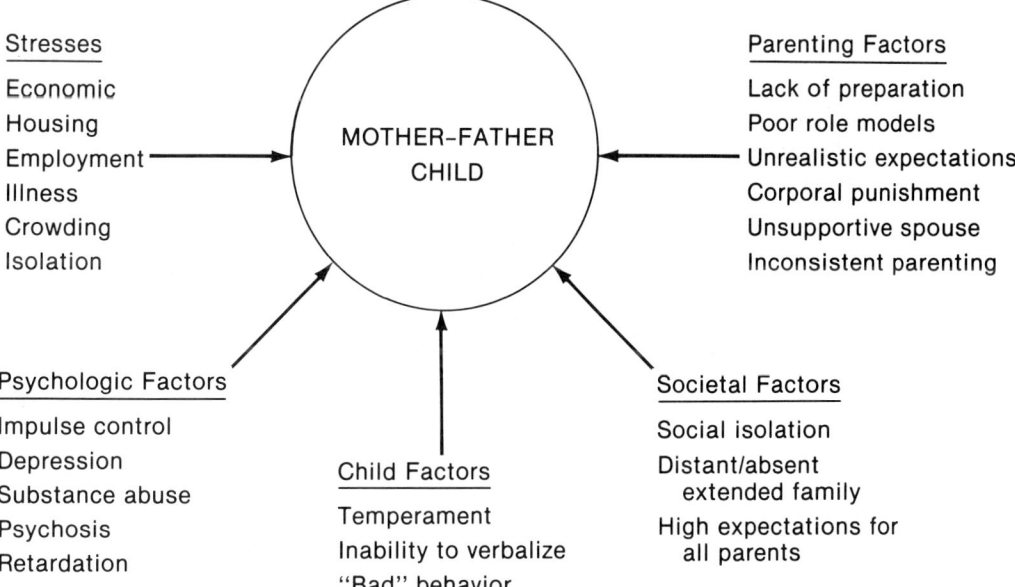

FIGURE 38–1. Factors that contribute to the dynamics of child abuse.

4. How did the parents act toward each other?

5. Were there helpful neighbors or other relatives nearby to help and support the family?

Physical Examination

1. Does the child appear clean and well cared for?
2. Does he or she seem well hydrated and well nourished?
3. What are the physical findings, e.g., burns, bony deformities, bruises, bites, strap marks? Do they seem reasonable given the history?

Intervention

The prehospital provider may report these findings to hospital personnel; in some states, state law requires that the paramedics themselves initiate a report of suspected abuse. The prehospital care provider should supply the emergency department with a written record of observations and suspicions because these may become criteria in subsequent legal management. Once abuse is suspected, every effort is made to remove the child from the abusive environment in order to ensure adequate medical evaluation and to prevent further abuse.

PROBLEM 3 The paramedics reported that when they arrived on the scene to evaluate this seizing patient, the parents were fighting. The mother had apparently just arrived home to find the baby in this condition. The father had been "babysitting." He did not come to the hospital and said nothing to the paramedics at the scene.

These simple observations may help the emergency department staff to focus initially on trauma as the cause of this child's problem rather than on sepsis or meningitis. Such clarity of focus and institution of proper therapy can be lifesaving.

INITIAL APPROACH IN THE EMERGENCY DEPARTMENT

The initial approach to the child should be directed toward the physical injuries and their treatment. This approach rightfully places the highest priority on the child's health. Evaluation and management of the traumatized patient are fully discussed in Chapter 4. During evaluation and initial management of specific injuries, the emergency department staff must remain open to the possibility of abuse and be vigilant for signs, symptoms, and telling interactions that may support the level of suspicion.

PROBLEM 3 As the rescue squad arrived in the emergency department with this seizing infant, overt seizure activity was limited to occasional "jerks," but the child remained unresponsive. He was intubated, ventilations were assisted with high-flow oxygen, and phenobarbital infusion was begun. Shortly after the infusion was started, the child developed decerebrate posturing, stopped breathing altogether, and went into asystole. Resuscitative attempts were unsuccessful.

During the resuscitation effort, a bulging fontanelle and bilateral retinal hemorrhages were noted. The rapid neurologic deterioration in this infant in association with these findings suggests intracranial hemorrhage. Even without external evidence of trauma, this serious problem can develop as a result of vigorous shaking of a child. Child abuse was therefore considered highly probable.

DATA GATHERING

The role of the history and physical examination in cases of suspected abuse is to define the child's medical problems and need for treatment and to ask questions and make observations that support the suspicion of abuse.

History

Sometimes the diagnosis of child abuse can be made on physical findings alone, but the history is usually helpful when the diagnosis is not obvious. Unfortunately, neither the parent nor the child may give a true account of the events that caused the injury. Answers to the following questions may assist the physician in ascertaining the plausibility of a given account:

1. *How did the injury occur?* Is the explanation adequate and does it fit the physical findings observed? Allegations of self- or sibling-inflicted injury raise the suspicion of abuse.

2. *When did the injury occur?* Delays in seeking treatment should heighten the suspicion of abuse or neglect.

3. *Has the child been injured before?* If so, is there a plausible explanation for these events?

4. *What is the child's daily routine?* Unpredictable schedules, inadequate or inappropriate supervision, varying caretakers, and parental absence all heighten the suspicion of abuse.

5. *What is the child's past medical history?* Has routine well-child care been obtained? Was the child premature or in a neonatal intensive care unit for an extended period? Failure to obtain routine care when available and seeming lack of knowledge or interest in the child's medical problems are reasons for increased suspicion. Prematurity and other reasons for lack of early bonding make subsequent abuse more likely.

While gathering this information, it is important for the physician to remain supportive of the family and focus his or her concern on the child. The physician's role is to gather information rather than to accuse. History-taking combined with implied accusations can prevent useful information from surfacing and hinder the ongoing doctor-family relationship.

Family Observation

In addition to collecting information by questioning, much can be learned by simple observation of the parent and child.

Is the child's behavior in the presence of the parent fearful, withdrawn, aggressive, destructive, or characterized by excessive crying?

Is the parental attitude toward the child underconcerned or overconcerned? Does the parent have an unrealistic view of the child's condition or unrealistic expectations of the child's behavior or development? Does he or she refuse to allow any diagnostic studies or refuse to allow admission to the hospital?

Are there findings suggestive of parental drug or alcohol abuse?

PROBLEM 1 This child was presented for care for a cold although multiple bruises were present. The physician's questioning was emotionally charged by being very direct and value-laden.

It is best not to approach the family in an accusatory, interrogative, or self-righteous manner. On some level most parents who abuse their children would like to be controlled. However, when confronted too early or accused too directly they will become defensive and argumentative and may even remove the child from care against medical advice. Raising the parents' level of fear or guilt will probably transform those emotions into anger.

656 — DISORDERS PRIMARILY PRESENTING IN INFANCY AND CHILDHOOD

Anger may be directed toward the physician or toward the child. It is important to avoid either situation. Remaining focused on the child with concern for his health and well-being will allow a common ground on which the parent will usually meet the physician.

PROBLEM 2 The parent of this malnourished child did not recognize the problem. She brought him to the emergency department for a diaper rash but had no recognition of the lack of weight gain. She fell asleep in the examining room, obviously not attentive to her small child. Lack of concern and seeming unawareness of obvious medical problems heightened the physician's suspicion of abuse or neglect.

Physical Examination

The physical examination may support a diagnosis of abuse, and the findings are correlated with the history that was given. Unexplained findings will heighten the suspicion of abuse.

1. **General appearance**
   a. Overall poor care or uncleanliness
      (1) Cradle cap
      (2) Severe diaper rash
   b. Growth failure as evidenced by measurements of weight, height, head circumference
   c. Developmental delay, especially in social areas and language
   d. Apathetic, dull facies
   e. Excessive self-stimulation
      (1) Rocking
      (2) Sucking
   f. Dehydration or malnutrition
      (1) Wasted extremities
      (2) Protuberant abdomen
2. **Bruises**
   a. Location. Bruises of the forehead and extremities are commonly accidental. Centrally located bruises, especially those of the genital area or buttocks, or extensive bruises increase the likelihood of abuse.
   b. Age. Bruises may be in different stages of healing. It is important to date any bruises and to compare this information with the history provided (Table 38–1).
   c. Patterns of bruising include:
      (1) Loop marks from cord or wire beating (Fig. 38–2)
      (2) Linear belt or strap marks (Fig. 38–2)
      (3) Hand prints
      (4) Bite marks
3. **Burns.** Burns constitute 5% to 10% of physical abuse cases. Whenever a burn is seen in a child, the physician compares the story with the physical evidence to determine whether they are congruous.

TABLE 38–1. Dating Bruises

Color	Age
Red	0–1 day
Blue, purple	1–4 days
Green, yellow	5–7 days
Yellow, brown	8–10 days
Cleared	1–3 weeks

Adapted from Wilson EF: Estimation of the age of cutaneous contusions in child abuse. Reproduced by permission of Pediatrics, vol. 60, p. 750, copyright 1977.

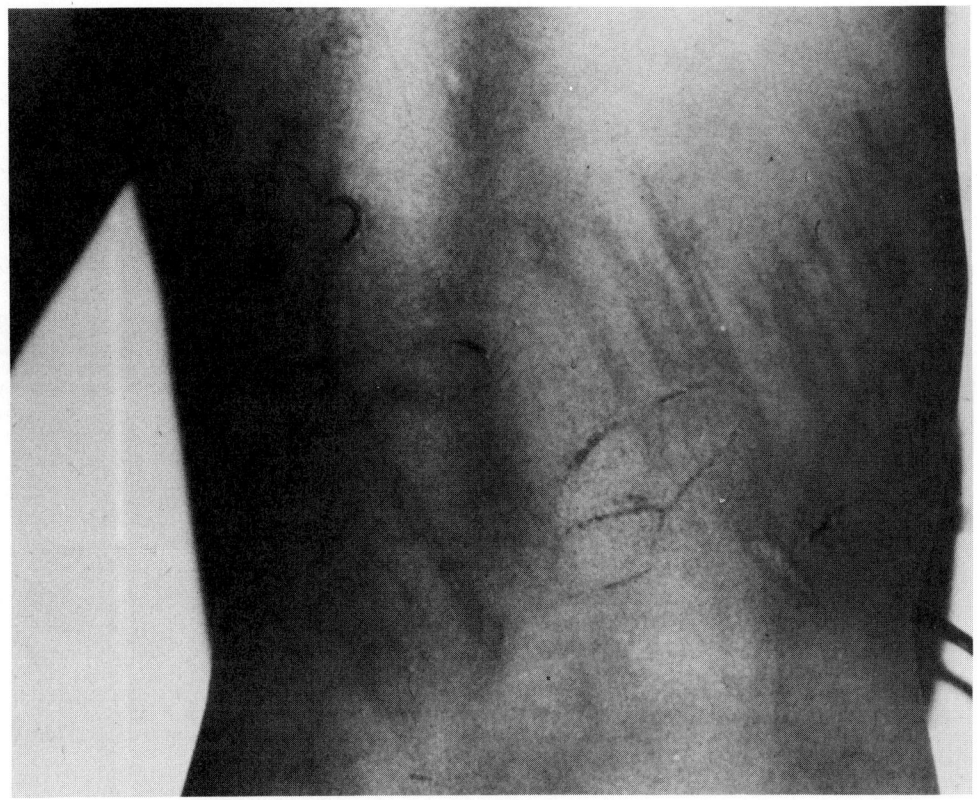
FIGURE 38–2. Multiple linear and loop-shaped contusions and abrasions inflicted by a belt. Note acute, subacute (scabbed), and chronic (hypopigmented) lesions.

    a. Hot water immersion is the most common type of burn inflicted (Fig. 38–3). Burns caused by hot water immersion are characterized by:
      (1) Distinct margins without splash marks
      (2) Unburned central area of skin resulting from the child being pressed to the cooler container bottom
      (3) Sparing of intertriginous areas
    b. Burns from hot objects include:
      (1) Cigarette burns
      (2) Burns from cigarette lighters, irons, hot plates, and other objects that may leave their imprint (Fig. 38–4)
4. **Evidence of skeletal injury**. Tenderness, swelling, deformity, and loss of function suggest fracture. Bone trauma is found in 10% to 20% of physically abused children. Clinical findings may disappear within a week in children under the age of 5. Radiographs will be necessary to diagnose these subacute injuries, and they should be obtained liberally.
5. **Neurologic examination**. Central nervous system injuries account for the greatest number of deaths due to abuse. These injuries may result from direct trauma when the child is struck or thrown or from vigorous shaking. Evidence of neurologic trauma includes:
   a. Scalp bruises
   b. Bulging fontanelle
   c. Retinal hemorrhage (Fig. 38–5)
   d. Lethargy, coma
   e. Seizures
   f. Head circumference greater than that in the ninetieth percentile

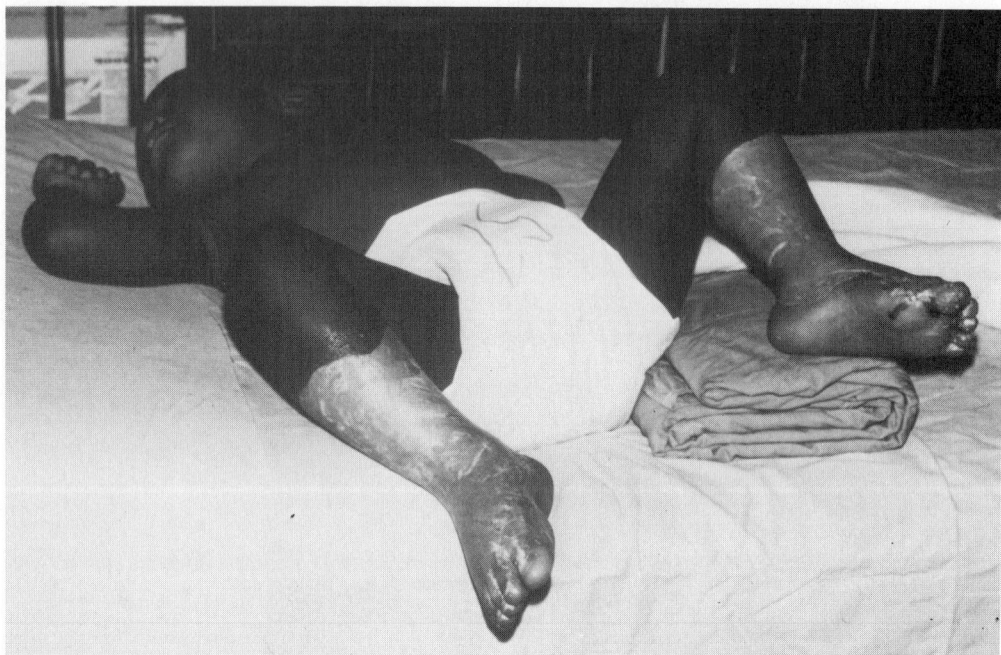

FIGURE 38–3. *Stocking distribution of second-degree burn of both lower extremities. This was caused by immersion in hot water following a toileting accident.*

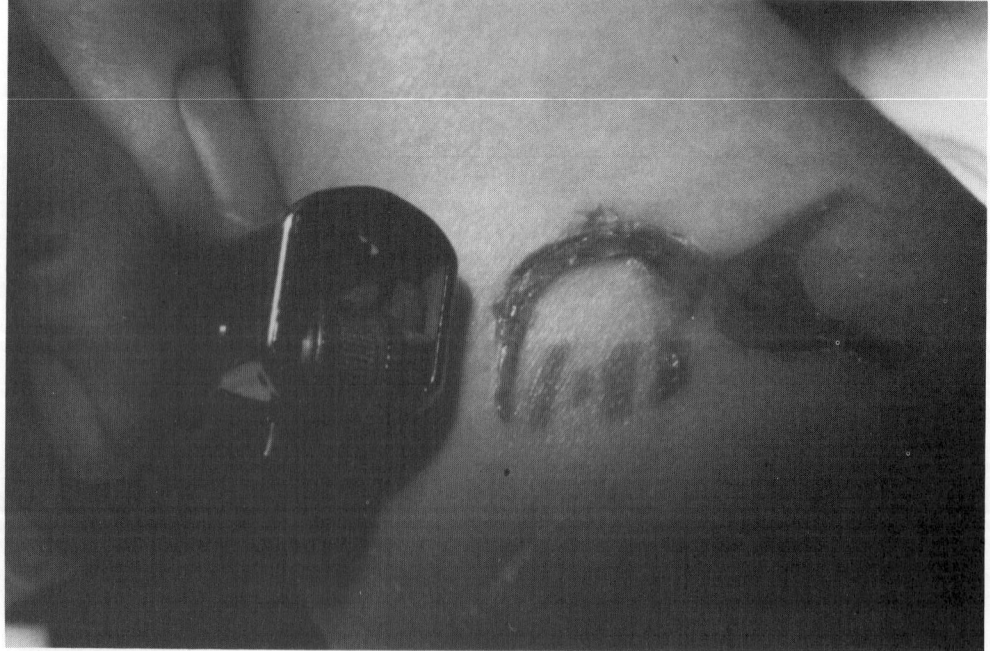

FIGURE 38–4. *Pattern burn on child's leg caused by branding from disposable cigarette lighter.*

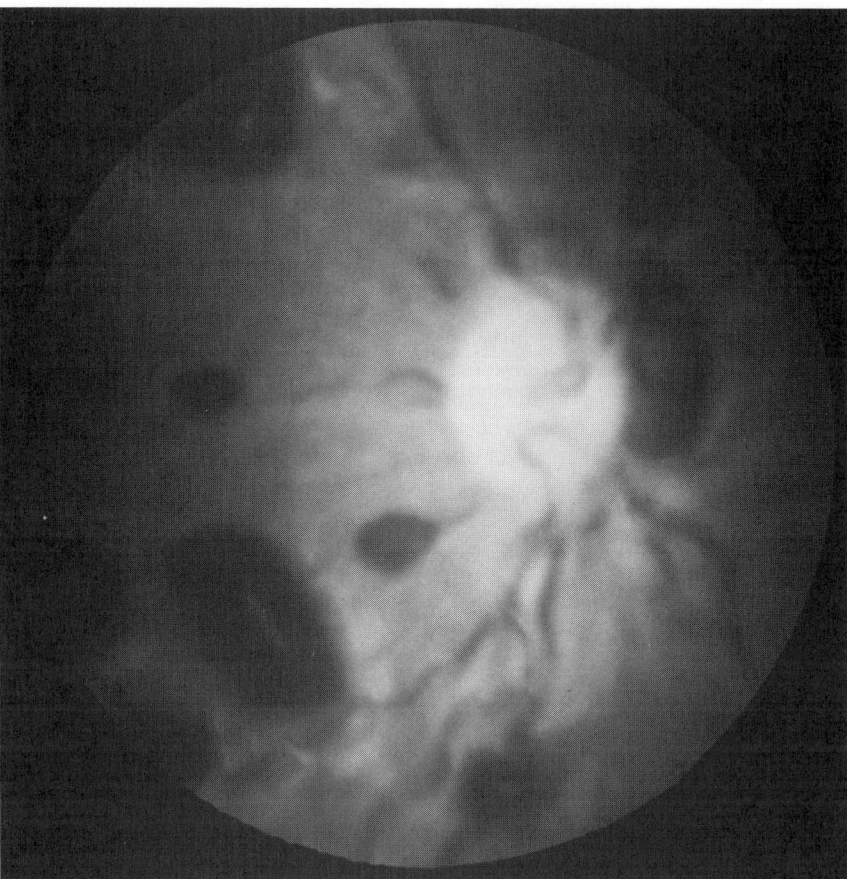

FIGURE 38–5. *Retinal hemorrhages following shaking injury of a 9 month old child.*

6. **Abdominal examination.** Abdominal injury ranks second to head trauma as a cause of abuse-related deaths. The abdominal organs most commonly injured by blunt trauma are the spleen, liver, and kidneys. Evidence of abdominal trauma includes:
   a. Abdominal tenderness
   b. Abdominal distention
   c. Hypotension, tachycardia, shock
7. **Genitourinary-perineal examination.** Findings may include:
   a. Penile or vulvar bruises or lacerations
   b. Buttock bruises

PROBLEM 1 Multiple bruises were noted on this child. This finding, when limited to the lower legs, is not uncommon due to the minor trauma incurred by a playful child. But bruises of the thighs, buttocks, and trunk are not usually incurred by minor bumps and falls. A history is obtained by means of nonjudgmental questioning, focusing on the health and well-being of the child, and this information is compared with the physical findings. Any discrepancy increases the suspicion of abuse.

The age of the bruises is also noted. In this child there were red marks (fresh injuries), bluish patches (1 to 4 days old), and greenish-yellow spots (5 to 10 days old). Multiple bruises at various stages of resolution markedly increase the suspicion of abuse. Reasonable suspicion is all that is required for reporting.

PROBLEM 2 This child showed a failure to thrive. Further work-up was needed to differentiate organic from nonorganic causes. However, the mother's lack of attention and concern as well as the severe diaper rash, which could have been due to inattention to routine care, strongly suggested a nonorganic etiology, and neglect was strongly suspected.

DECISION PRIORITIES AND PRELIMINARY DIFFERENTIAL DIAGNOSIS

Having taken a history, performed a physical examination, and observed the family interactions, the physician considers the possible problems leading to the child's presentation. The first question to be asked is, *Is the child's problem due to trauma?* Although rare, medical conditions can result in easy bruisability, fractures, and other findings that may initially appear to be due to trauma (Table 38–2).

If the child's condition is due to trauma, the next question is, *What is the likelihood of abuse?* The risk factors for abuse, ascertained from the history, physical examination, and observation of the family (Table 38–3), are considered together as the physician determines his level of suspicion of abuse. Certain diagnostic tests may support or confirm this suspicion.

DIAGNOSTIC ADJUNCTS

Radiologic Imaging

Standard Views. The history and physical findings will indicate the specific views to order. Extremity films are commonly needed, and skull films are recommended in any child less than 1 year old with a history of head trauma.

TABLE 38–2. Medical Conditions Simulating Trauma, Abuse, or Neglect

Physical Findings	Medical Condition	Diagnostic Adjuncts
Bruising	Hemophilia	Partial prothrombin time Thromboplastin time
	Von Willebrand's disease	Bleeding time
	Anaphylactoid purpura, purpura fulminans	Complete blood count, urinalysis, chest x-ray, lumbar puncture, cultures
	Ehlers-Danlos syndrome	Hyperextensibility
Dehydration, signs of malnutrition and failure to thrive	Organic versus nonorganic etiology	Complete blood count, serum electrolytes, BUN, creatinine, serum glucose, urinalysis
Abdominal tenderness	Infection, tumor	Complete blood count, urinalysis, serum amylase, abdominal ultrasound
Mental status changes, neurologic abnormalities	Aneurysm, tumor	Cranial CT scan
Fractures	Osteogenesis imperfecta	Radiographs, blue sclera
	Rickets	Nutritional history, radiographs
	Birth trauma	Birth history, radiographs
	Hypophosphatasia	Decreased alkaline phosphatase level
	Leukemia	Complete blood count, bone marrow biopsy
	Neuroblastoma	Bone marrow biopsy
	Postosteomyelitis or septic arthritis	History, radiographs
	Neurogenic sensory deficit	History, physical examination

TABLE 38–3. Risk Factors for Child Abuse

History	Physical Findings
Inadequate explanation	Poor care or uncleanliness
Alleged self-infliction	Growth failure
Alleged sibling infliction	Developmental delay
Delay in seeking care	Dull facies
Previous injuries	Excessive crying
Unpredictable routine	Self-stimulating activities
Inadequate supervision	Dehydration or malnutrition
Varying caretakers	Multiple bruises of varying age
Lack of well-child care	Centrally located bruises
Parental absence	Patterned bruises (cords, belts, bites)
Prematurity	Immersion burns
Neonatal intensive care ward	Cigarette burns
	Imprints of hot objects
Family Observation	Multiple fractures of varying age
Fearful, withdrawn child	Scalp bruises
Hyperactive, aggressive child	Retinal hemorrhages
Parental overconcern	Genital or perineal injuries
Parental underconcern	
Parental drug or alcohol abuse	
Unrealistic expectations	
Refusal of diagnostic studies	
Refusal of admission	

Skeletal Survey. In any child less than 5 years old in whom physical abuse is suspected, a roentgenologic skeletal survey is obtained, including films of the skull, thorax, long bones, and spine, because this by itself may confirm the diagnosis. Fractures in various stages of healing are also pathognomonic of abuse (Fig. 38–6). The type of

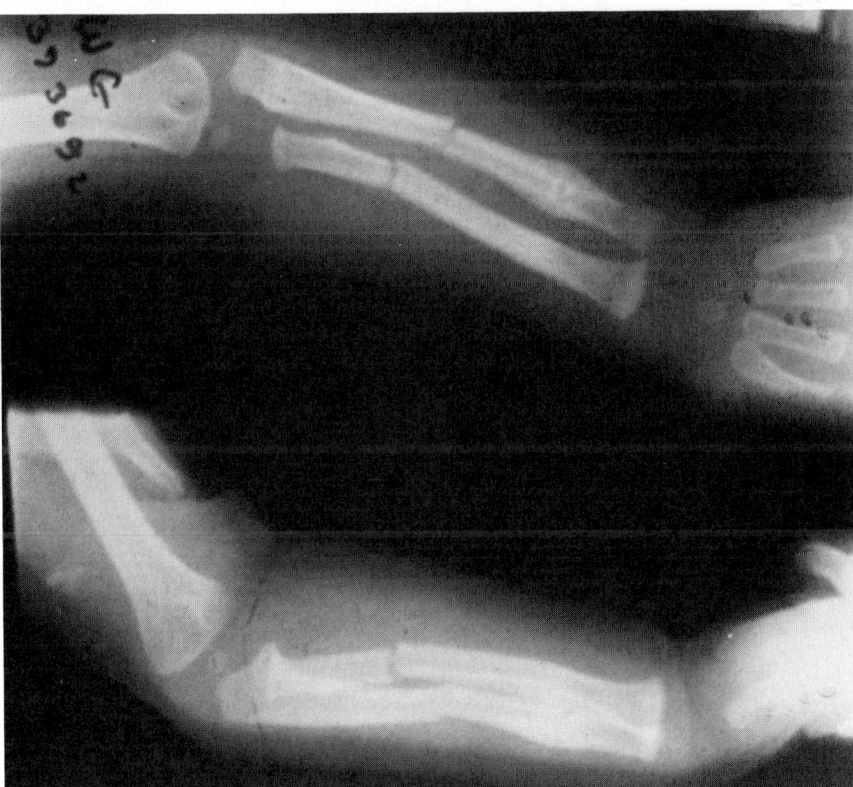

FIGURE 38–6. Radiograph (AP and lateral views) of radius and ulna showing acute fracture at proximal one-third point and healing fracture at distal one-third point.

fracture seen should be compared with the history to see if they are congruent. Unusual fractures are a cause for increased suspicion of abuse.

Computed Tomography of the Head. Cranial computed tomographic (CT) scans are ordered when the history and physical examination reveal mental status changes or focal abnormalities. Cerebral contusions or hemorrhages, subarachnoid hemorrhage, and epidural or subdural hematomas may be visualized (see Chap. 50).

Computed Tomography of the Abdomen. Abdominal CT scans are used to identify specific intra-abdominal pathology and to help assess the need for surgical intervention.

Laboratory Studies

Laboratory tests are of limited use in the evaluation of the possibly abused child. They are used primarily for evaluating possible etiologies other than trauma for the presentations described above (Table 38–2).

PROBLEM 1 A child with multiple, centrally located bruises in various stages of resolution whose mother gives no reasonable explanation is further evaluated radiographically. If there are specific findings, such as deformity or localized tenderness, specific views are ordered. When this is not the case a skeletal survey is done.

This child's skeletal survey revealed a skull fracture and two lower extremity fractures, one well-healed with considerable remodeling and the other relatively recent with early signs of healing. These injuries are pathognomonic of abuse and mandate protective custody of the child, reporting, and investigation.

PROBLEM 2 This malnourished, dehydrated infant required complete metabolic evaluation to diagnose the organic causes as well as the metabolic sequelae of nonorganic failure to thrive. Complete blood count, electrolytes, blood urea nitrogen, creatinine, glucose, and urinalysis are appropriate diagnostic tests for emergency department evaluation.

PRINCIPLES OF MANAGEMENT

The child who has been subjected to abuse requires medical and psychosocial management. In addition, the legal aspects of the case must be handled.

Medical Management

The physical results of abuse vary from minor contusions to major life-threatening injuries such as intracranial and intra-abdominal hemorrhages. Specific medical management varies according to the specific injury (see Chap. 4).

Psychosocial Management

During the medical management phase, the child's fears and anxieties are allayed as much as possible. Explanations to the child are frank and supportive. They should focus on the anticipated reactions of the child. It is important to confirm that the child is not guilty and did not incite the abuse. Assurance that the child will be safe and protected and that most things about his or her life will remain the same, unless he or she desires a change, is helpful. Confirmation of confidentiality is appropriate to the degree that it is feasible.

The parents need to be informed of the physician's suspicion of child abuse as well as the intention to report the case. This can be a very upsetting situation, and potential conflict can be assuaged by focusing on concern for the child rather than on accusations. A statement such as "I am required by law to report to the child protective service whenever I see a child with this kind of injury" may help to avoid a confrontation. The practical implications of the child's condition as well as those of the report itself are explained so that the parents know what to expect in the subsequent period.

Legal Implications and Reporting

Laws on reporting child abuse vary from state to state and usually specify who must report (mandated) and who may report (nonmandated) cases of suspected child abuse, as well as to whom and under what circumstances the report should be made. As stated before, the physician must know the laws of the state in which he or she practices. Physicians tend to be fearful of testifying in court and have cited this as a reason for not reporting abuse. Although the experience in court may not be pleasant, all states provide immunity from liability for the reporting person (Table 38–4). Reporting and testifying are part of a physician's duty in preserving the health and well-being of children as well as a legal mandate.

Team Approach

Due to the inherent psychosocial and legal issues involved in child abuse cases, a multidisciplinary approach is helpful in the management of abused children. These cases can result in a significant expenditure of time and emotion on the part of the emergency physician. A team approach allows each team member to compare impressions, make decisions mutually, and provide more extensive follow-up of these patients. The composition of the team will vary depending on available resources. The emergency physician and nurse, a pediatrician, and a pediatric social worker constitute an effective child abuse team.

PROBLEM 1 This child had multiple old injuries but no acute medical problems and therefore required no immediate medical intervention. The psychosocial and legal aspects of the case were more immediately important.

At 4 years of age, a child will usually be very fearful, especially at the prospect of being separated from his mother. A member of the team, usually a nurse or social worker, is charged with explaining the situation to the child, reassuring him, and maintaining close emotional and physical contact. The mother is informed of the suspicion of abuse. In this discussion, attention is centered on the child's well-being, not on the perpetrator. Nonjudgmental language is used, but the gravity of the situation is made clear. The case is immediately reported to the appropriate legal authority. The reporting and response system varies from location to location.

SPECIAL CONSIDERATIONS

Sexual Abuse

The issues involved in sexual abuse of children are similar to those in physical abuse cases in that medical and psychological trauma is encountered and evidence is collected. Sexual abuse cases can be complicated by considerations of legal statutes and by prevention of pregnancy and disease. It is advisable for physicians to become familiar with their state laws so that the history and physical evidence can be gathered properly. For example, force or a threat of force has important legal implications in Pennsylvania and other states. The National Center for Child Abuse and Neglect has defined sexual abuse as "contacts or interactions between a child and an adult when the child is being

TABLE 38–4. Child Abuse Laws in States

	Penalty Fine for Failure to Report	Immunity for Reporters of Abuse	Physician-Patient Privilege Abrogated	Photos Can Be Taken by Physicians as Evidence	Child Can Be Taken into Protective Custody by Physician
Alabama	x	x	x	–	x
Alaska	x	x	x	x	–
Arizona	x	x	x	x	–
Arkansas	x	x	x	x	x
California	x	x	x	–	x
Colorado	x	x	x	x	x[1]
Connecticut	x	x	–	–	x
Delaware	x	x	x	–	–
District of Columbia	x	x	x	x	–
Florida	x	x	x	x	–
Georgia	x	x	–	x	–
Hawaii	x	x	x	–	–
Idaho	–	x	x	–	–
Illinois	–	x	x	x	x
Indiana	x	x	–	x	–
Iowa	x	x	x	x	x
Kansas	x	x	x	–	–
Kentucky	x	x	x	x	x
Louisiana	x	x	x	–	–
Maine	x	x	x	x	–
Maryland	–	x	x	–	–
Massachusetts	x	x	–	–	–
Michigan	x	x	x	x	x[2]
Minnesota	x	x	x	–	–
Mississippi	–	x	x	–	–
Missouri	x	x	x	x	x
Montana	x	x	x	x	x
Nebraska	x	x	x	–	–
Nevada	x	x	x	–	–
New Hampshire	x	x	x	x	–
New Jersey	x	x	–	x[3]	x
New Mexico	x	x	x	–	–
New York	x	x	x	x	x
North Carolina	x	x	x	x	x
North Dakota	x	x	x	x	x
Ohio	x	x	x	x	–
Oklahoma	x	x	x	–	–
Oregon	x	x	x	–	–
Pennsylvania	x	x	x	x	x
Rhode Island	x	x	x	–	x
South Carolina	x	x	x	x	–
South Dakota	x	x	x	x	–
Tennessee	x	x	x	–	x
Texas	x	x	x	–	–
Utah	x	x	x	x	x
Vermont	x	x	–	x	–
Virginia	x	x	x	x	x
Washington	x	x	x	–	x
West Virginia	x	x	x	x	–
Wisconsin	x	x	x	–	–
Wyoming	–	x	x	x	x

x = Specified in state law, – = unspecified or not allowed by state law.
[1]With call to court.
[2]With call to hospital supervisor.
[3]With court order.
Adapted from Child Abuse Laws, National Center for Child Abuse and Neglect, Washington, DC, 1984.

used for the sexual stimulation of the perpetrator or another person. Sexual abuse may also be committed by a person under the age of 18 when that person is either significantly older than the victim or when the perpetrator is in a position of power or control over another child." Most sexual abuse is not assaultive in nature but is family related. It is uncommon for sexual abuse to be perpetrated by strangers.

The occurrence of sexual abuse may be recent or remote when it is encountered by the physician, and the presented condition may be directly or remotely related to it. Complaints may range from genital injury to bedwetting to sexually explicit behavior (Table 38–5). False accusations are rare, and detailed, explicit accounts of sexual experiences are considered firm evidence, particularly in the younger child.

A quiet, calm environment is especially important in taking the history. Optimally, a physician and a nurse interview the child together. This is imperative if a parent is not in attendance. First, the child's behavior and sexual vocabulary are ascertained. Then the child is asked to describe the events in his or her own words. Although a child under 6 years of age is often more comfortable using anatomically correct dolls to act out what happened, the use of these dolls is reserved for professionals who have had experience in such cases. Asking a younger child to draw a picture of what happened may be helpful. The child is encouraged to provide as much detail as possible. Specific points of the history, such as menstruation, occurrence of ejaculation, and the use of force or the threat of force, are elicited when appropriate. The child normally requires emotional support at what may be a time of great conflict and should be praised for the decision to discuss the situation.

In examining a suspected sexual abuse victim, the physician pays particular attention to the skin, genitalia, rectum, and oropharynx. Most prepubertal girls can be examined by simple inspection of the external genitalia and vagina using the knee-chest or frog-leg posture. In prepubertal girls active vaginal bleeding from an unidentified site or a history of penetrating vaginal injury is an indication for more detailed examination. Gynecologic consultation is necessary in these cases because exploration and repair may require general anesthesia. A routine pelvic examination is indicated for postmenarchal patients who are subject to sexual abuse. Care is taken not to traumatize the victim further. Often there will be no physical evidence of sexual abuse, and the history is sufficient. The specific details of evaluation and collection of evidence of sexual assault are discussed in Chapter 54.

PROBLEM 4 This young pregnant runaway might simply have been referred to a social service agency. A careful history revealed that the reason she ran away

TABLE 38–5. Identification of Sexual Abuse

Physical Complaints	Behavioral Complaints
Specific	*Specific*
Genital injury	Inappropriate knowledge of adult sexual behavior
Bruises	(explicit descriptions on sexual play)
Lacerations	Compulsive masturbation
Rectal laceration	Excessive sexual curiosity
Vaginal or urethral discharge	
Vaginal or rectal pain	
Pregnancy	
Nonspecific	*Nonspecific*
Anorexia	Excessive fear
Abdominal pain	Nightmares
Bedwetting	Phobias
Dysuria	Refusal to sleep alone
Encopresis	Runaways
Evidence of physical abuse	Aggression
	Suicide
	Any abrupt change in behavior

from home was that she was pregnant with her mother's lover's child. He had been forcing his sexual attentions on her for some time before she ran away.

With this additional information, it became clear that physical and laboratory examinations were indicated and that the patient needed appropriate psychological counseling as well as obstetric follow-up. The patient was also assisted in making the appropriate reports to the authorities.

Neglect

Child neglect is probably the most prevalent form of child abuse. Its effects are manifest most severely in younger children because they cannot fend for themselves. Noncompliance must be distinguished from neglect in that harm must have come to the child as a result of noncompliance to be considered neglect. Often the parents feel that they are taking care of their child appropriately, and in such cases parental education about health and child-rearing are at issue. The history should focus on the child's daily routine: Who is the child's caretaker? What is the child fed and how much? What are the child's activities?

Overt signs of neglect are the result of poor physical care. The child may be dirty, inadequately clothed, have a diaper rash or cradle cap, or be dehydrated or hungry. Manifestations of neglect, ranging from truancy to abandonment, may be present.

Nonorganic failure to thrive (FTT) (Fig. 38–7) is recognized, now widely, as a complicated manifestation of neglect. It is found almost exclusively in children less than 3 years old. It must be distinguished from organic FTT, but usually this distinction can be made on the basis of the history and physical examination. A history that is highly suggestive of nonorganic FTT includes:

1. An erratic feeding schedule,
2. An idealized feeding history, and
3. A chief complaint that is unrelated to FTT.

Emotional Abuse

Emotional abuse is a particularly insidious form of child abuse because physicians have the least developed ways of recognizing, categorizing, and managing it. But it may have the most permanently damaging effects on children. As a result of verbal abuse or excessive and unreasonable demands, the child develops a negative self-image and feels undervalued and unloved. This may result in a vicious cycle in which poor self-image and behavior problems feed on each other and make other forms of abuse more likely. Families that have an increased risk of perpetrating emotional abuse are those in which (1) the child is unwanted, (2) the child has a drug or alcohol problem, or (3) the parents are divorced or estranged

The diagnosis is made more readily if the physician has frequently witnessed family interactions. The emergency physician and the emergency department staff have only a brief opportunity in which to observe parent-child interactions, and therefore it is difficult to identify emotionally abusive patterns of interaction. Intervention by a physician is more successful when an ongoing relationship exists between the physician and the family. Although initially counseling may be provided in an emergency department setting, referral to specialized counseling or child welfare agencies is more appropriate.

DISPOSITION AND FOLLOW-UP

The primary question to be asked and answered is *"Is the child safe at home?"* If the answer is negative or uncertain, the child must be hospitalized despite the medical diagnosis or any hospital-based admission policy. The medical and moral obligation is to

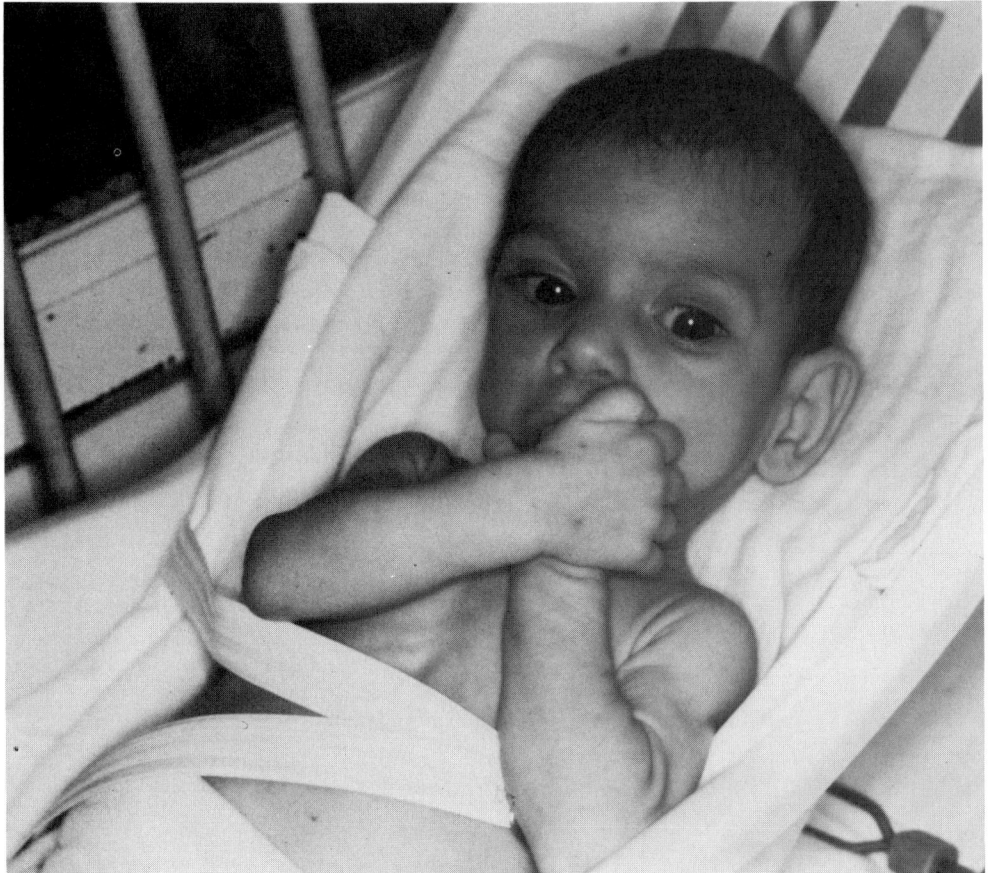

FIGURE 38–7. Nonorganic failure to thrive in a 4 month old child brought to the hospital still at birth weight. Note loose skin, protuberant abdomen, autostimulating behavior, and avoidance of eye contact.

protect the child from further abuse. In some circumstances, through the efforts of social agencies or family members, it may be possible to secure a safe place for the child, and then and only then should discharge from the emergency department take place.

Traumatized children often need referral for counseling and certainly need consistent follow-up care with a pediatrician or family physician. Some self-help groups exist (e.g., Parents Anonymous), and the family is told about this option when it is available. The physician communicates any new information that becomes available, as confidentiality permits, to the appropriate caseworker or counselor and may ask for feedback about the outcome on a case if the community service system functions appropriately. The community service system may not be as helpful as the situation demands, and the primary physician can be instrumental in coordinating the service system and an adequate long-term therapy system in his or her community. Whatever the extended service system may be, the child's progress and the family's ability to handle the stress should be monitored carefully.

PROBLEM 1 This child was admitted to the hospital, not for medical management but for protection while investigation determined the perpetrator of the abuse.

In some instances, the perpetrator can be identified, and the child can then be placed in a safe environment away from that individual rather than being admitted to the hospital. If discharge is planned, close medical and psychological follow-up should be ensured.

DOCUMENTATION

1. The events should be recorded in the child's own words whenever possible. Impressions are not as helpful as objective data.
2. Specific findings such as burns, lacerations, or contusions are noted. Photographs or detailed drawings are useful when the physical evidence is visually obvious.
3. Observations of family interactions are noted.
4. The appropriate reports are documented.
5. Provision of a safe environment is documented if the child is discharged from the hospital.

SUMMARY AND FINAL POINTS

- Child abuse is a prevalent but often unrecognized problem in our society.
- An appropriate level of suspicion of child abuse is developed after consideration of the findings obtained from the history, physical examination, radiologic studies, and observation of family interactions.
- Focusing attention on the needs of the child allows nonjudgmental but truthful communication with the parents.
- The proper management of child abuse, after diagnosis, involves medical, psychosocial, and legal interventions.
- The far-reaching needs of children in these circumstances are best met by the early involvement of a team of professionals, including emergency and pediatric physicians, nursing personnel, and specially trained social service counselors.

BIBLIOGRAPHY

Texts

1. Gil DG: Violence Against Children: Physical Child Abuse in the United States. Cambridge, Harvard University Press, 1970.
2. Kempe CH, Helfer R: The Battered Child (3rd ed). Chicago, University of Chicago Press, 1980.
3. Ludwig S: Child abuse. In Fleisher G, Ludwig S (eds): Textbook of Pediatric Emergency Medicine. Baltimore, Williams & Wilkins, 1988.
4. Sgroi S: Handbook of Clinical Intervention in Child Sexual Abuse. Lexington, MA, Lexington Books, 1982.

Journal Articles

1. American Medical Association: AMA diagnostic and treatment guidelines concerning child abuse and neglect. JAMA 254(56):796–800, 1985.
2. Barwick D: Nonorganic FTT. Pediatr Rev 1:625, 1980.
3. Fontana VJ: Child abuse reporting: The physician's responsibility. Missing/Abused 2:11, 1986.
4. Helfer R: Why most physicians don't get involved in child abuse cases and what to do about it. Children Today 4(3):28, 1975.
5. Jones J: Sexual abuse of children. Am J Dis Child 136:142, 1982.
6. Ludwig S: Shaken baby syndrome: A review of 20 cases. Ann Emerg Med 13(2):104–109, 1984.
7. Newberger EH, Bithoney WG: Pediatric understanding of child abuse and neglect. Pediatr Rev 2(7):197, 1981.
8. Rosenberg NM, Marino D: Frequency of suspected abuse/neglect in burn patients. Pediatr Emerg Care 5(4):219–221, 1989.
9. Sargent DA, et al: AMA diagnostic and treatment guidelines concerning child abuse and neglect. Chicago, AMA Advisory Panel on Child Abuse and Neglect, 1984.
10. Sills RH: Don't overlook environmental causes of FTT. Contemp Pediatr 3:25, 1986.
11. Wilson EF: Estimation of the age of cutaneous contusions in child abuse. Pediatrics 60:750, 1977.

CHAPTER 39

DEHYDRATION

JONATHAN SINGER, M.D.

PROBLEM 1 A previously healthy 18 month old boy was brought to the emergency department by his parents. His chief complaint was vomiting and diarrhea for 3 days. The illness was heralded by several episodes of vomiting followed by 10 to 15 stools per day.

PROBLEM 2 A 2 year old girl was brought by the rescue squad to the emergency department for evaluation of repeated vomiting, altered mental status, and rapid respirations.

QUESTIONS TO CONSIDER

1. How is the severity of dehydration estimated?
2. What ancillary tests are helpful in this determination?
3. When can oral methods of rehydration be considered for emergency department therapy of dehydration? What solutions are appropriate for this use?
4. When is it appropriate to choose parenteral rehydration therapy?
5. How is vascular access achieved in the severely dehydrated child?
6. Which patients require admission to the hospital for diagnosis and treatment of dehydration?

INTRODUCTION

Fluid balance is maintained if oral intake of water is sufficient to replace ongoing insensible (respiration, sweat) and urinary losses. In childhood many diseases may diminish or interrupt normal fluid intake. Burns, hyperglycemia, febrile states, illnesses associated with increased respiratory rates, and gastrointestinal derangements associated with vomiting or diarrhea cause abnormal fluid losses leading to dehydration. Gastroenteritis is by far the most common cause. Viral agents, usually a rotavirus, are the most frequent offenders. Bacteria are the second leading cause, the usual agents being *Shigella* species, *Salmonella* species, *Escherichia coli*, *Yersinia enterocolitica*, and *Campylobacter fetus*. Parasites are a rare cause.

The majority of cases of dehydration seen by the emergency physician are mild in nature and are easily managed on an outpatient basis. Moderate dehydration, which may require a holding room or inpatient care, is more commonly encountered in the United States during winter epidemics of viral gastroenteritis. Severe dehydration is a rare occurrence in the United States but is the leading cause of infant mortality worldwide, accounting for the deaths of approximately 5 million infants a year. Severely dehydrated children die as a result of diminished delivery of oxygen and energy substrate to the brain, heart, and kidneys.

The presentation of dehydration varies depending on the relative loss of water and sodium. When there is a proportionate loss of both water and sodium, the serum sodium level remains in the normal range, and the result is *isotonic dehydration*. This is the most common form of dehydration, occurring in 70% to 80% of dehydrated children. *Hypertonic dehydration* occurs when there is a greater loss of water than of sodium or when isotonic dehydration is treated with high-sodium replacement fluids such as chicken soup. This form occurs in 10% to 15% of dehydrated children and is more common in children under the age of 6 months. The hypertonic serum results in fluid shifts out of the cells. Intracellular dehydration is poorly tolerated by the brain, and lethargy, coma, or seizures frequently result. *Hypotonic dehydration* occurs when there is a greater loss of sodium than of water or when hypotonic fluids such as water are used exclusively for rehydration. Seizures and cardiovascular collapse are early and prominent features of hypotonic dehydration.

PREHOSPITAL CARE

Although most children with mild to moderate dehydration are brought to the emergency department by their parents, the severely dehydrated child who shows mental status changes or circulatory collapse will benefit from field care and rapid transport by the rescue squad.

History

1. How long has the child been sick?
2. How much vomiting or diarrhea has the child had? The number of episodes per day or per hour is useful to gauge the severity.
3. What fluids have been given by mouth?
4. When did the child last urinate or have a wet diaper?
5. Have other children at home, in school, or in day care had similar problems?
6. Are there preexisting medical problems?

Physical Examination

1. Vital signs including pulse and respiratory rate are taken.
2. The adequacy of ventilation and oxygenation is judged by observation of respiratory chest excursion, auscultation of the chest, and skin color.
3. The level of consciousness is measured against a norm, i.e., the child is alert, responsive, and interactive.
4. Signs of dehydration are actively sought. These include poor skin turgor, depressed fontanelle, lack of tears, and dry mucous membranes.

Intervention

Mild dehydration, evidenced by normal vital signs and minimal evidence of dehydration such as decreased tearing and dry mucous membranes, does not require intervention in the field.

More severely dehydrated children, who present with signs of hypovolemia (delayed capillary refill, tachycardia) or mental status changes, will benefit from immediate fluid administration.

Vascular Access. Establishment of a peripheral line is attempted. If this is unsuccessful in 3 minutes or with two attempts, an intraosseous infusion is used if the squad has been trained in its use. Otherwise, further therapy is deferred, and the patient is transported to the emergency department.

Fluid Administration. Isotonic crystalloid solution, 20 ml/kg, is appropriate for initial infusion in the hypovolemic or mentally depressed child.

PROBLEM 2 The 2 year old girl was awakened in the morning at her usual hour. She refused breakfast, vomited repeatedly, and became listless. When reawakened by her parents before noon, she had rapid respirations and felt warm. A rescue squad was called.

En route to the hospital the patient slept if she was undisturbed but responded to verbal commands of the parents. Her pulse was 140 beats/min and respirations were 44/min. She was not distressed and had good color but somewhat dry mucous membranes.

This child appears to be only mildly dehydrated, and the lethargy and tachypnea seem out of proportion to the degree of dehydration. Hypernatremic dehydration is a possibility, although the child is older than the usual victim of this type of problem. The replacement fluids given to the child, if hypertonic, could account for this result. The patient's tachypnea is consistent with dehydration, but other causes need to be evaluated. The child appears to be stable enough for transport without treatment in the field.

INITIAL APPROACH IN THE EMERGENCY DEPARTMENT

Children brought to the emergency department with complaints of vomiting, diarrhea, and poor oral intake are immediately assessed with regard to the adequacy of respiratory, circulatory, and central nervous system function. Unless other problems coexist, *airway and ventilatory status* are usually adequate. Physical assessment of the *circulatory* status is done by noting the following signs:

Skin signs
    Decreased capillary refill
    Pallor or cyanosis
    Mottling
    Decreased turgor
Head, eyes, ears, nose, and throat signs
    Depressed fontanelle
    Absence of tears
    Dry mucous membranes
    Soft, sunken eyeballs
Vital signs
    Tachycardia
    Tachypnea
    Hypotension

The *rapid neurologic assessment* includes assessment of responsiveness, which may be graded as alert and interactive, lethargic or poorly interactive, responsive only to pain, or unresponsive. Seizures may be focal or generalized.

Intervention

Patients who are severely volume depleted are given a bolus infusion as rapidly as possible of 20 ml/kg of isotonic crystalloid solution. Such an infusion may be carried out even if the pulse and blood pressure are normal for age. A second bolus is required if the patient remains in shock. If vascular access cannot be established promptly by peripheral venous line, an intraosseous infusion is initiated.

Patients who have dehydration and seizures, marked lethargy, or coma may have a hypertonic form of dehydration. Initial treatment is the same, but subsequently slow rehydration with gradual return of the serum sodium concentration to normal is undertaken. Too rapid a drop in serum sodium level can result in cerebral edema and seizures.

Seizures are treated with diazepam if they are persistent or recurrent. The airway and ventilatory status are carefully monitored, and endotracheal intubation is accomplished if the respiratory status is marginal or inadequate.

PROBLEM 1 The 18 month old infant had been in his usual state of health until 3 days prior to admission. He had been discharged from day care 48 hours prior to evaluation owing to anorexia, malaise, nonbilious vomiting, and passage of loose stools without mucus or blood. His parents had transported him by car to the emergency department on the advice of their private physician.

Like 85% of pediatric emergency department patients, this patient arrived by private conveyance. Occasionally, serious illness is not recognized by caretakers, who, sensing no urgency, leisurely transport the child. It is the responsibility of triage personnel to alert definitive caregivers of an ill child who may be deprived of the rapid attention typically given to those who arrive by rescue squad.

PROBLEM 2 Vital signs were blood pressure 80/60 mm Hg, pulse 140 beats/min, respirations 44/min, and temperature 102.2°F (39°C). The respirations were noted to be deep, and her gag reflex was intact. The child had a fruity odor on her breath and was hard to arouse. The child's mucous membranes were dry, but there were no other signs of dehydration. An intravenous (IV) line of normal saline was started, and she was given 20 ml/kg during the first 20 to 30 minutes.

The patient's altered mental status, abnormal vital signs, and breath odor represent a severe dehydration of potentially metabolic or infectious origin. Once the airway is secure, volume replacement is the first priority.

DATA GATHERING

In a patient with adequate airway, ventilation, circulatory status, and vital signs, evaluative procedures can precede therapeutic interventions.

History

The history is directed toward determining the kind and amount of fluid lost, the kind and amount of fluid replaced, the cause of the fluid loss, and the patient's usual state of health.

1. When did the child *become sick*?
2. *How much vomiting* or *diarrhea* has occurred? What do these *fluids look like*?
   Stool consistency and odor as well as the presence of mucus or blood are noted. Emesis is examined for color and content, especially blood.
3. Is the child *tolerating oral fluid*? What *oral fluids* have been *given* and in what *amounts*?
   High-solute fluids (boiled milk, soups) and low-solute fluids (Jello or water, colas) can lead to hypernatremia and hyponatremia, respectively.
4. When did the child *last urinate* or have a *wet diaper*?
5. Has the child had a *fever*?
6. Has the child been *unusually sleepy* or *poorly responsive*?
7. Are there *other children* at home, in school, or in day care with *similar problems*?
   If others are asymptomatic, did this child eat anything different from the others? Viral, bacterial, and protozoan enteric organisms can be transmitted through contaminated food, water, or direct contact with fecal material. Person-to-person

transfer is quite prevalent in day care centers. Enteric disease is commonly found in other family members.

8. Does the child have *preexisting medical problems*?
Endocrine, metabolic, and renal diseases are particularly pertinent. Recent antibiotic use arouses suspicion of pseudomembranous colitis as a cause for diarrhea. Acute or chronic use of salicylates, acetaminophen, or nonsteroidal anti-inflammatory drugs should be considered in acidotic, dehydrated patients. Inquiries about preexisting disease states should include queries on prior hospitalizations and pertinent family history.

9. *When* was the *last time* the child was *weighed* and *what was* his *weight*?
Comparing the premorbid weight with the present weight is the best way of estimating the degree of dehydration.

Previous weight − current weight = weight loss (kg)

% *Weight loss* = fraction of weight loss × 100

Current weight (kg) × fraction of weight loss = fluid deficit (liters)

An alternative calculation can be used based on the total body water (TBW):

TBW = 0.6 × weight (kg)

Fluid deficit = (premorbid weight − morbid weight) × 0.6

Physical Examination

The physical examination allows the physician to:
1. Estimate the magnitude and type of fluid and electrolyte imbalance that is present.
2. Focus on systemic toxicity associated with dehydration.
3. Confirm the history in seeking specific potential disease processes.

A complete examination is performed. Emphasis is placed on the following areas:

Vital Signs. Supine pulse and blood pressure measurements are traditionally recorded. In adults one can test the patient's cardiovascular reserve in maintaining perfusion in the face of decreased intravascular volume by repeating the pulse and blood pressure measurements in an upright position. Orthostatic depression of 20 mm Hg or elevation of the heart rate by 20 beats/min suggests volume depletion. However, since normovolemic children may have a 30 to 40 beats/minute increase on standing and variable blood pressure changes, and since orthostatic changes may also be absent in the presence of significant dehydration in the pediatric patient, this test is limited to use in older children and adolescents.

Tachycardia is consistently found in patients with significant dehydration, but hypotension is usually a late finding, occurring only after the child's marked capacity for compensation is exhausted. With hypotonic dehydration, hypotension occurs earlier and is more prominent.

An accurate measure of the respiratory rate is necessary in that substantial water loss can occur through the lungs during marked hyperventilation. Deep Kussmaul ventilations suggest metabolic acidosis.

Elevated temperature also increases the insensible loss of fluid through the skin. Water requirements increase by 7 ml/kg/24 hr for each degree of temperature elevation beyond 99°F (37.2°C) rectally.

The child's current weight is obtained. If there is a known previous weight, this is obtained in comparable clothing.

Hydration Status. The physical examination is instrumental in assessing the status of hydration regardless of the cause of dehydration. Signs and symptoms of dehydration result from extracellular volume depletion. When interstitial fluid is depleted, there may be loss of skin elasticity, with tenting and altered skin turgor (doughy or rubbery skin with hypernatremia), reduction of both retro-orbital tissue fluid, creating sunken eyeballs, and intraocular fluid, causing soft eyeballs, or reduction of cerebrospinal fluid volume, manifested by a flattened fontanelle. In dehydrated patients the physician will find depressed tear formation, thickening of saliva, and drying of mucous membranes. Intravascular volume depletion leads to reduction in urine volume and peripheral vasoconstriction with cold, mottled, and poorly perfused skin. An important indicator of hydration status is the capillary refill time. After 5 seconds of cutaneous pressure or squeezing of the nail bed, release of pressure allows the patient's capillary beds to reperfuse. The compressed tissues normally refill within 2 seconds. A capillary refill time of more than 2 seconds is indicative of dehydration. Other abnormalities seen with dehydration include decreased spontaneous motor activity, tachycardia, tachypnea, altered consciousness, and, as a late phenomenon compared to adults, depressed blood pressure.

Altered Consciousness. Infants may have poor glycogen stores and with poor oral intake may become hypoglycemic. Irritability, obtundation, and seizure may result. Similar manifestations may occur with hypernatremic dehydration due to brain desiccation.

General Physical Examination. In the pursuit of metabolic, infectious, neoplastic, or toxicologic derangement, the clinician searches for focal neurologic abnormalities, nuchal rigidity, petechiae, abdominal guarding, rebound tenderness, abdominal mass, and rectal tenderness or mass.

DECISION PRIORITIES AND PRELIMINARY DIFFERENTIAL DIAGNOSIS

Once the data are gathered, they are collated to assist in management decisions. The first question to answer: *What is the estimated degree of dehydration?*

By convention, dehydration is expressed as mild, moderate, or severe (Table 39–1). Patients with mild dehydration have lost between 1% and 5% of body weight. With the possible exception of decreased tearing or dry mucous membranes, their physical examination results are normal. Patients with moderate dehydration have lost 5% to 10% of body weight. Moderate dehydration is manifested by a sunken fontanelle, sunken eyes, dry mucous membranes, dry lips, and minimal loss of skin elasticity. The loss of

TABLE 39–1. Gauging Magnitude of Dehydration

Assessment	Mild	Moderate	Severe
Percent of loss of body weight	1–5	6–10	Over 10
Signs and symptoms	Variable	Present	Severe
Thirst	+	+	+
Absence of tears	+/−	+	+
Dry mucous membranes	+/−	+	+
Depressed anterior fontanelle	−	+	+
Sunken eyeballs	−	+	+
Soft eyeballs	−	+	+
Reduced turgor of skin	−	+/−	+
Hyperpnea	−	+/−	+
Hypotension, shock	Absent	Imminent	Usually present
Urine			
Volume	Small	Oliguria	Oliguria-anuria
Osmolality (mOsm/liter)	600	800	Maximal
Specific gravity	1.022	1.025	1.032
Blood			
Urea nitrogen	10–19 mg/dl	20–40 mg/dl	>40 mg/dl
pH	7.40 to 7.22	7.30 to 6.92	7.10 to 6.80

Adapted from Barkin RM, Rosen P (eds.): Emergency Pediatrics (3rd ed). St. Louis, CV Mosby, 1990.

skin elasticity can be demonstrated over the abdomen, where the skin tents or remains in a sharp fold when picked up. Patients with severe dehydration have lost more than 10% of their body weight. They will have intense vasoconstriction with cold, mottled, poorly perfused skin, delayed capillary refill, and definite loss of skin turgor. They have altered motor activity, altered consciousness, a rapid, thready pulse, and collapsed vessels. These events may be followed by a precipitous drop in blood pressure.

Once the degree of dehydration has been determined and the need for immediate fluid resuscitation is assessed, the second question is: *What is the probable cause of fluid loss?*

Sometimes the cause will be obvious from information obtained in the history and on physical examination. An acute onset of vomiting and diarrhea without blood or mucus, associated with fever and occurring in a setting where other children are ill with a similar problem almost certainly represents viral gastroenteritis. No laboratory testing will be needed unless the degree of dehydration or alteration in mental status is moderate to severe. In other cases the cause will not be so obvious, and diagnostic testing will be necessary to define the exact etiology (Table 39–2).

PROBLEM 1 At a well-child examination 1 week before this illness the child weighed 7.5 kg. He now weighed 7.0 kg. He was refusing solids and taking homogenized milk poorly with the current illness. The stools were characterized as loose, voluminous, brown, not particularly malodorous, and containing no mucus or blood. He had fair skin turgor but tacky mucous membranes and soft, sunken eyeballs. A diaper was still dry after 2 hours. Blood pressure was 80/60 mm Hg, pulse 150 beats/min, respiratory rate 32/min, and temperature 102.2°F (39°C).

TABLE 39–2. Causes of Dehydration by Organ System

Gastrointestinal	Renal
Infants	Renal dysplasia
Carbohydrate malabsorption	Nephrogenic diabetes insipidus
Duodenal atresia	Renal tubular acidosis
Annular pancreas	Sickle hemoglobinopathy
Pyloric stenosis*	
Necrotizing enterocolitis	**Endocrine**
Neural crest tumors	Cystic fibrosis
Short bowel syndrome	Diabetic ketoacidosis*
Intussusception	Central diabetes insipidus
Children	Adrenogenital syndrome
Viral gastroenteritis*	Adrenal hemorrhage
Bacterial gastroenteritis	Addison's disease
Pseudomembranous colitis	Hypothalamic disorders
Giardiasis	Thyrotoxicosis
Cryptosporidium	**Iatrogenic**
Entamoeba	Salicylates
Hirschsprung's disease	Ipecac
Midgut volvulus	Diuretic abuse
Peritonitis	Mannitol
Adolescents	Glycerol
Food poisoning*	High solute intake*
Pancreatitis	Nasogastric suctioning
Regional enteritis	**Mixed**
Ulcerative colitis	Hemolytic uremic syndrome
Anorexia nervosa	Reye's syndrome
Bulimia	Stomatitis
Scleroderma	Burns*
Carcinoid	Steven-Johnson's syndrome
	Hyperthermia

*Most common causes.

By clinical assessment, this child was moderately (5% to 9%) dehydrated. He had a rapid heart rate and dry mucous membranes, but skin turgor and other parameters were still normal or borderline. Because a recent weight was known, this observation could be quantified as follows:

Previous weight = 7.5 kg
Current weight = 7.0 kg
Weight loss = 0.5 kg
Percent dehydration (assuming no other reason for weight loss) = 6.6%
Fluid deficit = 6.6% of 7.0 kg (current weight) = 0.462 liters = 462 ml
Alternatively,
$TBW_1 = 0.6 \times 7.5$ kg = 4.51 liters
$TBW_2 = 0.6 \times 7.0$ kg = 4.21 liters
Fluid deficit = 0.31 liter = 310 ml

Although the numbers obtained are fairly divergent, both are reasonable estimates of the fluid lost.

PROBLEM 2 Owing to the mental status change that was out of proportion to the degree of dehydration, the hyperpnea, and the fruity breath odor, the physician suspected diabetic ketoacidosis (DKA). Bedside glucose screening by reagent strip revealed a glucose concentration of 60 to 80 mg/100 ml.

This serum glucose is inconsistent with the suspected diagnosis of DKA. Additional laboratory studies and perhaps more history are necessary. Volume replacement with isotonic crystalloid continues.

DIAGNOSTIC ADJUNCTS

Laboratory adjuncts may aid diagnostic reasoning or facilitate management decisions in those patients who have 5% dehydration or more. Maximum information will be derived from the urinalysis, blood chemistries, and hemogram. Other testing, such as radiologic imaging, is tailored to the clinical setting.

Laboratory Studies

Urinalysis

Specific Gravity. A random specific gravity of between 1.016 and 1.022 indicates clinical fluid balance, whereas 1.023 or more indicates an absolute or relative water-restricted state. Diluted urine in an apparently dehydrated child should raise the suspicion of adrenal insufficiency, aldosteronism, or chronic renal disease.

Glucose Concentration. The presence of glucose implies overload of the renal tubular reabsorptive capabilities and mandates measurement of the serum glucose level.

Protein. Proteinuria, if transient, is benign and nondiagnostic.

Ketones. Ketonuria, though commonly found in patients with uncontrolled diabetes mellitus, is more often present in pediatric nondiabetic patients with any anorectic state and with many febrile illnesses.

White Cells. Pyuria, defined as 10 or more leukocytes/mm^3 in uncentrifuged urine, may reflect a renal parenchymal reaction to the presence of bacteria or may simply be an inflammatory response to an extrarenal lesion. Sterile pyuria is common in patients with viral gastroenteritis and many febrile illnesses associated with dehydration.

Bacteria. The presence of bacteria in an uncentrifuged, high-power microscopic examination suggests a urinary tract infection, which during infancy can cause vomiting, diarrhea, and abdominal distention without micturitional complaints.

Serum Electrolytes. The infrequency of electrolyte abnormalities in patients with mild dehydration does not warrant their measurement. With moderate to severe dehydration, physiologic derangement of sodium, potassium, chloride, and bicarbonate often occurs. Serum electrolyte measurements provide information on acid-base status and are essential for calculating replacements of electrolyte deficits.

Blood Urea Nitrogen, Creatinine. Determinations of blood urea nitrogen (BUN) and serum creatinine are of value in helping to ascertain the adequacy of renal function in a clinically dehydrated patient. The two determinations are best viewed in concert, observing their absolute values as well as their relation to one another. BUN and creatinine ratios of greater than 20:1 are seen in patients with severe dehydration.

Glucose. Many infantile illnesses may be accompanied by poor oral intake, decreased gluconeogenesis, and depressed glycogen stores, leading to symptomatic hypoglycemia. In dehydrated patients with altered mental status blood glucose should be rapidly estimated by reagent strip while awaiting formal laboratory confirmation of glucose level.

Complete Blood Count

Hemoglobin/Hematocrit. Reduced intravascular fluid volume without a corresponding loss in red cell mass leads to hemoconcentration. This finding may be a useful means of confirming dehydration.

White Blood Cell Count and Differential. The peripheral leukocyte count and peripheral smear may help to bolster the subjective impression of a diarrheal illness due to either *Shigella* or *Campylobacter*. The presence of more than 10% immature neutrophils (bands), particularly when associated with a normal or low leukocyte count, suggests an infection by either of these enteric pathogens.

Blood Gas Analysis. A capillary or arterial blood gas analysis provides specific information about the respiratory, circulatory, and metabolic state of the dehydrated patient. Many laboratories report the pH and Pco_2 from the venous specimen submitted for other chemical analyses. However, in patients with severe dehydration, a conventional arterial blood gas determination should be performed because the Pao_2 should be known in such a critically ill patient.

PROBLEM 1 No laboratory adjuncts were requested in the reasonably well hydrated child with the presumptive diagnosis of gastroenteritis.

Arterial blood gas measurements revealed Pco_2 30 mm Hg, Po_2 105 mm Hg, pH 7.42, bicarbonate 18 mEq/L. These results were perplexing, because with the primary metabolic acidosis of DKA, overcorrection by respiratory compensation is not physiologic.

PROBLEM 2 Blood was submitted for determination of serum electrolytes, salicylate level, BUN, creatinine, glucose, and ketones. A prothrombin time and partial thromboplastin time were ordered. An in-dwelling Foley catheter was inserted for collection of a specimen for urinalysis and to monitor urinary output. Further history obtained from the parents revealed no family history of diabetes. The mother then volunteered that she had found the child playing with an empty baby aspirin bottle about 12 hours earlier. She thought the bottle had been empty but admitted that some tablets could have been ingested. A salicylate level was ordered.

Either hypoglycemia or hyperglycemia may occur with salicylism and may account for mental status changes. Hepatic dysfunction and coagulopathy may complicate the course of salicylate toxicity.

REFINED DIFFERENTIAL DIAGNOSIS

After laboratory evaluation, the likely origin of dehydration can be established. The history of the present illness is most likely to aid in determining whether dehydration is due to a gastrointestinal disorder, endocrine disturbance, chronic renal disease, iatrogenic disorder, or multisystemic affliction (Table 39–2). The physician interprets the historical information within the framework of an epidemiologic trend. The physical examination may confirm the clinical suspicion. Laboratory studies are helpful in establishing a metabolic derangement that may be occult on the basis of the physical examination.

Gastrointestinal diseases are the most common cause of water loss in all pediatric age groups. Acute diarrheal states far exceed any other gastrointestinal disorder in causing water and electrolyte imbalance. Recognition of the mechanism and etiologic agent responsible for excessive stool losses may be improved with characterization of stool patterns (Table 39–3).

Following gastrointestinal disease, the most common causes of total body water loss are the febrile illnesses characteristic of early childhood. These problems are predominantly viral in origin and often lead to multisystemic dysfunction, poor feeding, and low fluid intake. Hyperpnea and hyperpyrexia may exaggerate insensible water loss. Fortunately, these childhood afflictions are shortlived, and only mild to moderate states of dehydration ensue.

Acute salicylate ingestion leads to hyperpnea, hyperthermia, vomiting, and increased excretion of an excessive solute load, imposed by the accumulation of organic acids. Dehydration follows if the condition is untreated. Other dehydrating entities that may present with altered mental status, acidosis, and altered carbohydrate metabolism include sepsis, diabetes mellitus, uremia, and intoxications with ethanol, methanol, isopropyl alcohol, chloral hydrate, ethylene glycol, and isoniazid.

PRINCIPLES OF MANAGEMENT

The therapeutic principle for managing dehydration is to restore perfusion and cellular function by providing rehydrating fluids while monitoring the patient's progress. The type of fluid given, route of fluid administration, and speed of administration rest with the initial assessment of the degree and type of dehydration.

Severely dehydrated patients who are in hypovolemic shock need airway management, oxygen, ventilation, and intravenous access. Two IV lines are placed using the largest cannulae that can be inserted into the peripheral veins. Failure to cannulate immediately is an indication for intraosseous infusion, venous cutdown, or central line placement. Isotonic crystalloid solution is infused at 20 ml/kg, ideally over a period of no more than 5 minutes. After the initial fluid bolus has been given, the child is assessed for improvement by noting the sensorium, capillary refill time, pulse rate, and blood pressure. If there is no improvement, the 20 ml/kg bolus is repeated. After the second bolus, if there is still no improvement, central venous pressure measurement is required in an intensive care setting to monitor further fluid replacement.

Under less severe circumstances, management of dehydration in the emergency department is directed toward:

1. Estimating the amounts of fluid and electrolytes required to maintain the child in a healthy state.
2. Estimating the water and electrolyte content of the deficits.
3. Determining the therapeutic route.
4. Developing a therapeutic plan that provides fluid maintenance and replaces deficits and ongoing losses.

TABLE 39–3. Characteristics of Diarrhea

Stool Descriptors	Disease
Watery, without mucus or blood	*Giardia, Cryptosporidium, Escherichia coli, Aeromonas,* viral, food poisoning
Watery, with mucus or blood	*Campylobacter, Shigella, Yersinia*
Loose, slimy, with variable mucus or blood	*Salmonella*
Loose, mixed with blood, "currant jelly" appearing	Intussusception

5. Refining the estimates based on the patient's progress or analysis of laboratory results.

Establishing Maintenance Levels of Fluid and Electrolytes

The major losses of water by the body occur through insensible evaporation of water from the lungs and skin and from water lost through excretion of urine and feces. Maintenance fluids and electrolytes are best estimated using the surface area method (Fig. 39–1). Insensible water loss amounts to 500 ml/m^2/day. Hence, the obligatory water replacement for the pediatric patient ranges from 950 to 1300 ml/m^2/day.

The normal intake of sodium is between 30 and 80 mEq/m^2/day. The amount of 50 mEq/m^2/day is widely prescribed for calculating maintenance regimens. The daily intake of potassium is 40 mEq/m^2/day.

Estimating Fluid and Electrolyte Composition Under Circumstances of Loss

In general, fluid loss that occurs rapidly will resemble extracellular fluid in its composition (140 mEq sodium/liter), whereas fluid loss that occurs insidiously resembles intracellular fluid (150 mEq potassium/liter).

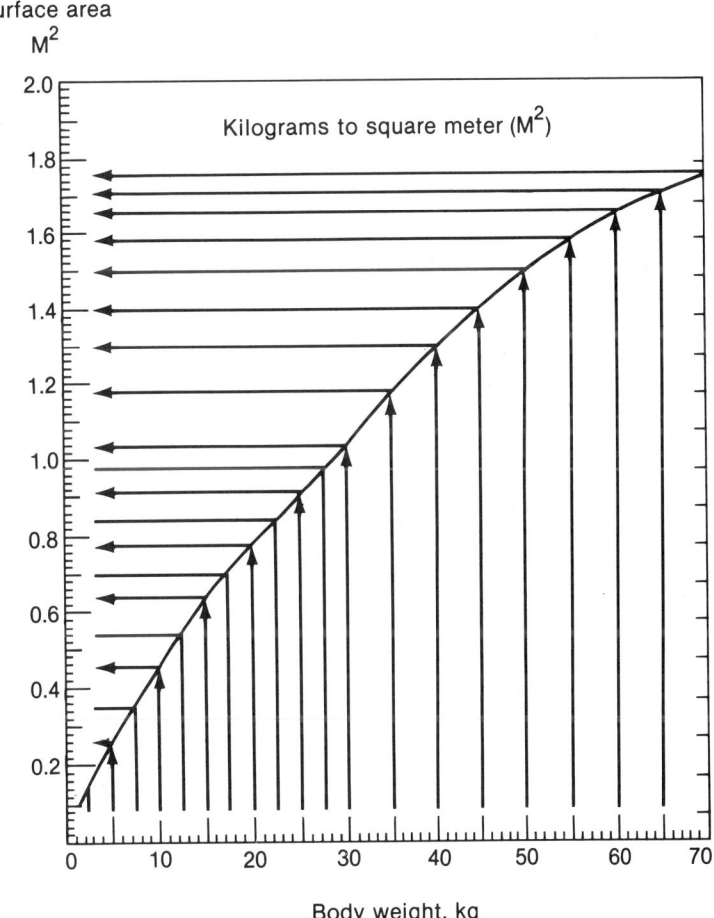

FIGURE 39–1. Body weight to surface area nomogram. (From Sinkinson CA: Simplifying the complexities of pediatric dehydration. Emerg Med Rep 10(7):53, 1989.)

If stool loss can be quantitated, it is known that a liter of diarrheal stool contains 45 to 50 mEq sodium, 10 to 80 mEq potassium, 10 to 100 mEq chloride. If one can accurately determine the volume lost by diarrheal stools, electrolyte losses can be projected based on body weight. In the usual case of acute diarrhea, 9 mEq/kg of sodium is lost and 10 mEq/kg of potassium is lost.

Gastric fluids contain 10 to 80 mEq sodium, 10 to 20 mEq potassium, and 100 to 150 mEq chloride per liter.

Therapeutics: Oral Versus Parenteral

Oral glucose-electrolyte rehydration solutions (ORS) have been shown during the past decade to be highly effective in the treatment of dehydration, especially dehydration secondary to acute diarrhea. This therapy is based on the physiologic observation that active glucose absorption in the small bowel promotes the absorption of sodium. Oral rehydration therapy has had a dramatic impact on the morbidity and mortality of diarrheal disease in the developing world. There has been less acceptance of oral rehydration therapy as a primary treatment for dehydrating diarrhea in the developed world. The reservation is not justified. The World Health Organization ORS (2% glucose, 90 mmol Na/liter, 20 mmol K/liter, 80 mmol Cl/liter, 30 mmol HCO_3/liter) has been successfully employed in patients of all ages, malnourished to well-nourished, with mild to moderate dehydration. Similarly, several marketed pharmaceutical preparations with sodium concentrations ranging from 45 to 75 mmol/liter (Pedialyte RS, Pedialyte, Lytren, Resol, Infalyte) have proved to be safe and cost-effective means of treating dehydrated children in the United States.

Intravenous fluids historically have been the main form of pediatric rehydration, even in milder cases. However, intravenous fluids can now be reserved for patients with moderate to severe dehydration who need rapid restoration of intravascular volume. Intravenous fluids are also given to those patients who do not respond to oral rehydration attempts.

Therapeutics: Maintenance, Deficits, Ongoing Losses

Regardless of the route of administration, the goals of fluid therapy are to overcome incipient circulatory disturbances, restore extracellular and intracellular fluid deficits, correct acid-base abnormalities, and modify electrolyte disturbances. The rate of replacement is linked to the underlying disease state and degree of dehydration. In general, the aim is to modify any metabolic derangement in 6 to 8 hours and provide total body repletion in 24 to 36 hours. Rehydration of children with isotonic or hypotonic dehydration can proceed along these lines, the only difference being that initial fluid resuscitation may have to be more aggressive in the hypotonic child. Rehydration of hypertonically dehydrated children is slower and is guided by the serum sodium level. Reduction of the serum sodium concentration by 15 mEq/liter/day is a safe approach that reduces the risk of precipitating cerebral edema. This gradual reduction may require 48 hours or more. The calculated amounts of fluid and electrolytes should be sufficient to replace the estimated fluid deficit, maintenance fluids, and ongoing losses. A plethora of differing guidelines exist in the literature, but a common feature of all of them is the provision of bolus fluid at the start.

Oral Bolus. A rapid rate of early repair can be provided by giving up to 40 to 90 ml/kg of a 75- or 90-mmol Na/liter solution over 4 to 6 hours.

Parenteral Bolus. Many intravenous solutions are available for bolus therapy. Plasma volume expansion can be implemented by giving 10 to 20 ml/kg of 5% dextrose one-half normal saline, 5% dextrose normal saline, normal saline, lactated Ringer's solution, or 5% dextrose–lactated Ringer's administered over 20 to 30 minutes. Dextrose-containing fluids are imperative for individuals who are symptomatic from hypoglycemia. Conversely, non–dextrose-containing solutions are indicated for individuals with hyperglycemia.

Oral Solutions Given Post Bolus. Following 4 to 6 hours of a higher solute fluid, maintenance solutions with a sodium concentration of 45 or 50 mmol/liter can be given. A total daily volume of fluid in the range of 150 to 250 ml/kg is safely administered.

Parenteral Post Bolus Solutions. Pending serum electrolyte measurements and adequate urine output, the ideal maintenance fluid beyond the emergency phase in moderate or severely dehydrated children is 5% dextrose one-half normal saline. Further decisions are based on the patient's status and the laboratory profile.

Refined Estimates Based on Patient Progress

The rate of fluid administration is largely influenced by the length of time the patient will remain under the care of the emergency physician. Suggested emergency department regimens include:

1. Therapy for 3 to 6 hours: Up to 30 ml/kg given over 30 minutes, followed by 10 ml/kg/hr.

2. Therapy for 6 to 8 hours: Bolus of 10 to 20 ml/kg given over 30 minutes, followed by 1500 to 2000 ml/m^2 given over 24 hours (maintenance rate); goal is to replace at least 50% of the projected deficit.

3. Therapy for 12 hours: Bolus, followed by maintenance rate and replacement of 75% to 100% deficit.

4. Therapy for 24 hours: Bolus, followed by replacement of half the deficit and one-third of the maintenance requirements in first 12 hours, followed by half the deficit and two-thirds of the maintenance needs in the remaining 24 hours.

Fluids are continued for at least 8 hours in the patient who presents with a serum sodium level of between 125 and 130 mEq/liter or between 145 and 150 mEq/liter, a potassium concentration of less than 3 mEq/liter, and bicarbonate less than or equal to 14 mEq/liter or acidosis (pH less than 7.10). Fluids are given until there is a urinary output of at least 1 ml/kg/hr. Vital signs are recorded at 2-hour intervals at least, and examination is repeated at 2-hour intervals if possible.

PROBLEM 1 Fluid and electrolyte calculations for this 7.0 kg (0.7 m^2) child were as follows:

Maintenance Fluid Required per 24 Hours	Losses
Water: 1500 ml × 0.7 m^2 = 1050 ml	7.5 kg × 0.6 = 4.5 liters premorbid body water
	7.0 kg × 0.6 = 4.2 liters morbid body water
Sodium: 50 mEq × 0.7 m^2 = 35 mEq	Sodium: 9 mEq × 7.5 kg = 67 mEq
Potassium: 40 mEq × 0.7 m^2 = 28 mEq	Potassium: 10 mEq × 7.5 kg = 75 mEq

Total Projected Needs

Water: 1050 ml + 300 ml = 1350 ml
Sodium: 35 mEq + 67 mEq = 102 mEq
Potassium: 28 mEq + 75 mEq = 103 mEq

This child was monitored in a holding area. He was given 20 ml/kg/hr of Pedialyte RS (75 mEq sodium and 20 mEq potassium per liter) for 6 hours. This provided 900 ml of fluid. He had an adequate urinary output, and a repeat examination showed good improvement. Parents were instructed to give an additional liter of Pedialyte (45 mEq sodium and 20 mEq potassium per liter) during the next 18 hours. The total daily intake during 24 hours would be 1.9 liters of fluid containing 112 mEq sodium chloride and 38 mEq of potassium chloride.

Excess fluid was administered, reflecting the possibility of ongoing stool losses. Hypokalemia is a rare occurrence despite the potential deficit provided by the low concentration of potassium in oral electrolyte solutions. Any of the commercial preparations are preferred over homemade salt or sugar mixtures.

PROBLEM 2 The severity of salicylate intoxication can be estimated in patients with a single ingestion by referring to the Done nomogram (Chap. 19). As predicted by the physical examination and confirmed by the salicylate level, this child showed a marked metabolic derangement including moderate dehydration.

Treatment of salicylate intoxication is directed at enhancing excretion of salicylate by the kidneys, taking advantage of the fact that excretion is more rapid at high rates of urine flow and when the urine is alkaline.

DISPOSITION AND FOLLOW-UP

Admission

The decision to admit a severely dehydrated patient to the hospital is usually made based on the history and physical examination. In cases of mild to moderate dehydration the decision to admit is delayed until the response to therapeutic endeavors has been witnessed. A decision on disposition is based on the age of the patient, the underlying disease state, past medical history, an estimate of parental compliance, and the availability of holding unit facilities.

Admission to the hospital for dehydrating illness is considered in the following circumstances:

Etiology. Hyperpyrexic (temperature of more than 104°F [40°C]) children less than 6 months of age known to have *Shigella* or *Salmonella* gastroenteritis are admitted for treatment with intravenous antibiotics.

Age of Patient. Patients less than 2 months of age with any degree of dehydration are admitted.

Degree of Dehydration. All patients with severe dehydration are admitted to the hospital.

Chemical Derangements. Admission is warranted for patients with levels of sodium less than 125 mEq/liter or more than 150 mEq/liter, potassium less than 2.5 mEq/liter or more than 6 mEq/liter, bicarbonate less than 10 mEq/liter, pH less than 7.0, BUN more than 30 mg/dl, and creatinine more than 1 mg/dl at presentation.

Past Medical History. Patients with underlying malnourishment, diabetes mellitus, chronic renal disease, or hemoglobinopathy are best rehydrated as inpatients.

Parenting. If the managing physician is not assured of parental or patient compliance with plans for continued outpatient management, rehydration is carried out on an inpatient basis.

Facilities. Attempts at outpatient rehydration in the emergency department may not be possible if there are inadequate personnel or physical facilities to address the patient's needs.

Efficacy of Prior Treatment. Patients with persistent electrolyte or acid-base imbalance, despite attempts at oral rehydration, are admitted for further therapy.

Discharge

The patient evaluated for a dehydrating illness may be discharged when the managing physician is confident of the diagnosis, degree of dehydration, adequacy of parenting skills, and availability of follow-up arrangements.

Instructions. Compliance is likely to be improved when the family is given explicit written instructions that are verbally reinforced by both the physician and the nursing staff. Such written instructions indicate both preferred and prohibited fluids. For the child with isolated diarrhea, parents are encouraged to provide one of the 45 to 50 mEq sodium/liter proprietary oral glucose solutions on an ad lib basis. For patients who have had vomiting, parents are advised to administer small volumes of fluid at frequent intervals to minimize gastric distention. Volumes may be increased and intervals between feedings can be advanced gradually. After 24 hours of clear fluid replacement, infants are returned to dilute formula and advanced slowly to full-strength formula during 2 to 3 days. Strict regimens of clear liquids are not encouraged for longer than 24 hours. Reintroduction of partial strength formula (especially nonlactose products) or bland solids such as rice, cereal, and potatoes (nonlactose carbohydrate foods) may prevent or minimize the deficit of calories and may promote the repair of the intestinal mucosa. Breast-fed infants are not discouraged from suckling in the presence of any dehydrating illness. Following a 24-hour clear liquid regimen, older children may be fed a high-carbohydrate, low-fat diet, which can be provided by bananas, rice, apple sauce, and toast or saltines (BRAT diet).

Follow-up. Parents are encouraged to seek medical attention if their child cannot tolerate the above-described dietary regimen or shows signs and symptoms of dehydration. Emergency department reassessment is recommended for unexplained fever, abdominal discomfort, irritability, seizure, neck stiffness, or nonblanching rash. When possible, an appointment with the patient's regular physician is arranged within 24 hours of emergency department discharge. If he or she is not available, the emergency department can fulfill the need for monitoring the patient's progress. The follow-up physician will adapt the graduated feeding regimen to the child's needs.

DOCUMENTATION

1. Type and amount of fluid loss.
2. Type and amount of oral replacement fluids.
3. Weight change.
4. Physical findings indicating dehydration: absence of tears, dry mucous membranes, prolonged capillary refill time, soft or sunken eyeballs, flat fontanelle.
5. An estimate, usually in percentage, of the degree of dehydration.
6. Serial determinations of vital signs and circulatory and mental status in moderate to severely dehydrated children.
7. Preliminary diagnosis including degree of severity of dehydration.
8. Detailed discharge instructions including dietary and fluid management and signs and symptoms requiring reevaluation.
9. Follow-up physician and time for appointment within 24 hours.

SUMMARY AND FINAL POINTS

- The problem-solving approach in the emergency department attempts to establish the clinical estimate of fluid loss and underlying disease process responsible for dehydrating illness.
- The clinician establishes by history and physical examination the magnitude and type of fluid and electrolyte imbalance.
- The clinical impression can be supported with laboratory data.
- Therapy is directed toward increasing plasma volume immediately, followed by giving therapeutic fluids and electrolytes that restore deficits, provide maintenance, and replace ongoing losses.
- The principles of oral rehydration therapy that have saved hundreds of thousands worldwide have broad application to emergency department practice. Oral rehydration therapy is safe and cost effective.
- Intravenous routes or intraosseous routes are used when life-threatening vascular deficits exist.
- The patient with dehydrating diarrheal illness requires explicit discharge instructions and timely follow-up examination.

BIBLIOGRAPHY

Texts

1. Barkin RM: Problems in the management of vomiting, diarrhea and dehydration. In Luten R, Harwood-Nuss A (eds): Problems in Pediatric Emergency Medicine. New York, Churchill-Livingstone, 1988, pp. 173–187.
2. Martin DL: Oral rehydration therapy. In Barken R (ed): The Emergently Ill Child. Rockville, MD, Aspen Publications, 1987, pp. 245–258.

Journal Articles

1. Barkin RM: Acute infectious diarrheal disease in children. J Emerg Med 3:1–99, 1985.
2. Bruck E: Fluid and electrolyte therapy. Pediatr Clin North Am 19:193–220, 1972.
3. Finberg L: Therapy of dehydration in infancy. Pediatr Rev 3:113–120, 1981.
4. Gottlieb RP: Dehydration and fluid therapy. Emerg Med Clin North Am 1:113–124, 1983.
5. Kumate J, Isibasi A: Pediatric diarrheal diseases: A global perspective. Pediatr Infect Dis 5(1 Suppl):S21–28, 1986.
6. Lattanzi WE: Simplifying the approach to fluid therapy. Comtemp Pediatr 6:72–88, 1989.
7. Listernick R: Simplifying the complexities of pediatric dehydration. Emerg Med Rep 10(7):49–56, 1989.
8. Listernick R, Zieserl E, Davis AT: Outpatient oral rehydration in the United States. Am J Dis Child 140:211–214, 1986.
9. Perkin RM, Levin DC: Common fluid and electrolyte problems in the pediatric intensive care unit. Pediatr Clin North Am 27:567–586, 1980.

SECTION TWELVE

MUSCULOSKELETAL DISORDERS

CHAPTER 40

THE SWOLLEN AND PAINFUL JOINT

J. STEPHAN STAPCZYNSKI, M.D.

PROBLEM 1 A 20 year old female presented with a 2-day history of aching in her left wrist and pain and swelling in her left knee associated with a low-grade fever. She had noted some new "spots" on the extensor surfaces of her distal forearms and shins.

PROBLEM 2 A 62 year old male presented with exquisite pain, redness, and swelling of his great toe.

PROBLEM 3 A 40 year old female had noted occasional stiffness in her hands with so much swelling that she could not remove her ring. She was concerned about pain and swelling in her left wrist.

QUESTIONS TO CONSIDER

1. In patients with swelling and pain of one or more joints, what aspects of the history and physical examination need to be explored?
2. How is arthritis differentiated from periarticular disorders?
3. What role do laboratory tests, radiographs, and arthrocentesis play in the initial diagnosis of the acutely swollen joint?
4. What studies are obtained for analysis of synovial fluid?
5. What are the most likely causes of an acutely swollen joint?
6. When is emergency department therapy indicated for acute arthritis?
7. How is appropriate disposition arranged for the patient with diagnosed arthritis? Undiagnosed arthritis?

INTRODUCTION

The skeletal articulations in the body are designed to facilitate movement. Their mobility ranges from immovable to freely movable. Syndesmoses, such as the tibiofibular attachment and the sutures of the skull, are immovable and rarely affected by inflammation. The cartilaginous joints include the epiphyseal plates in growing bone, the intervertebral disks, and the pubic symphysis. These have a slightly increased risk of problems. The freely movable, diarthrodial joints, which make up nearly all of the joints of the extremities, are the most prone to inflammation. These joints are composed of an articular cartilage that covers the weight- or stress-bearing surfaces and a fibrous joint capsule lined by synovium. Articular cartilage is distinguished by a low concentration of cells and a lack of blood vessels, lymphatic channels, and nerves. Nourishment is obtained from synovial fluid. The synovial lining is highly vascular and richly innervated by branches from the nerve roots that innervate muscles crossing the joint. Inflammation or irritation of the synovial lining produces pain and increased fluid. The synovium is thrown into folds at the margin of the articular cartilage but does not cover the weight-bearing surfaces. These folds allow the lining to be stretched with motion. The joint cavity contains a small amount of highly viscous fluid that lubricates the joint surfaces. Synovial fluid is composed of a transudate of plasma plus mucin, a complex macromolecule added by the type B cells in the synovial lining. Mucin is responsible for the high viscosity of this extremely effective lubricating fluid.

The articulation is additionally supported by ligaments, tendons, and muscles. Some diarthrodial joints, such as the knee, radiocarpal, and sternoclavicular joints, contain intra-articular fibrocartilaginous menisci that act as stress-reducing washers, allowing the opposing articular surfaces to glide freely past each other. The menisci are attached at their periphery to the fibrous capsule.

These complex joint structures may be affected by inflammatory processes, which usually have an immunologic, crystalline, or infectious origin. Inflammation is a pathologic process involving white blood cells, enzymes, and physiologically active substances. The end result is tissue damage, particularly to the articular cartilage. The inciting agent may be unknown, e.g., rheumatoid arthritis, or recognized, e.g., gout. Trauma is the most common cause of the swollen, painful joint. Previous injury is a predisposing factor in nontraumatic causes also.

PREHOSPITAL CARE AND THE INITIAL APPROACH IN THE EMERGENCY DEPARTMENT

Joint pain and swelling is not a life-threatening problem. Patients are triaged and evaluated in turn, based on their acuity. They belong in the "urgent" category because they may have severe pain and can suffer permanent joint damage if they are not evaluated appropriately and treated promptly. Analgesia may be given after the physician's evaluation.

DATA GATHERING

The history and physical examination provide information that will allow the physician to determine the most likely cause for the patient's problem and the need for further diagnostic testing.

History

Patients presenting with joint pain or swelling often carry the self-diagnosis of "arthritis." An effort is necessary to avoid accepting this self-diagnosis and possibly precluding a thorough assessment.

The following information is obtained:

1. *How long have the symptoms been present?*
   Arthritic symptoms of less than 6 weeks' duration are considered acute; those of over 6 weeks' duration are termed chronic.
2. *Did the problem develop gradually or suddenly?*
   Rapid onset of joint swelling or pain is typical of trauma, crystalline-induced disease, and infection. Normally, the joint space is small and the capsule is poorly compliant; therefore it takes only a small amount of increased synovial fluid to cause pain.
3. *Has it been steadily getting worse, or do the symptoms wax and wane?*
4. *Are other joints involved at any time?*
   Symptoms may be migratory (moving from joint to joint with complete resolution in the first joints) or additive, with new joints becoming involved while the first joints still hurt).
5. *Has there been any recent trauma to the area or any known injury to the joint in the past?*

6. *Is there a prior history of arthritis, joint pain, or surgery?*
7. *Does the patient take medications or a drug of abuse?*
8. *Is the patient sexually active, and, if female, what is the menstrual history?*

Physical Examination

The physical examination is important to ascertain objective criteria for arthritis, determine the pattern of joint involvement, and seek extra-articular signs of a causal process.

Joint Examination. Any involved joint is evaluated in a systemic fashion.

Inspection. Erythema of the overlying skin is commonly associated with gout and septic arthritis. Swelling may represent an effusion or edema of the surrounding tissue. In the knee, elbow, and distal joints intracapsular fluid causes a symmetrical swelling and can be palpated as a "bogginess" or "fluctuant" feeling of the capsule. Periarticular swelling is usually more localized. The two findings may be combined, complicating the differentiation. Deformity may represent chronic bony changes or acute fracture or dislocation.

Palpation. Warmth is usually noted first. It is best to begin proximally and move distally over the joint to determine the skin temperature. Tenderness is often exquisite, and a gentle examination is essential. Pain is often diffuse in the joint with intra-articular disease. Palpation will usually differentiate effusion from tissue edema.

Motion. Without inducing too much pain, it is important to determine the range of motion in all joint directions. Patients with pain and limitation of motion in all directions are likely to have intra-articular disease processes.

Other Joint Involvement. In addition to the joint initially identified by the patient, other joints may be involved. A complete joint examination, including the temporomandibular joint (TMJ) and vertebral column, is important to determine the number of joints involved and assist in narrowing the differential diagnosis.

General Examination. In addition to the joint examinations, other systems may provide valuable clues to the etiology.

Vital Signs. Fever is present in more than 50% of cases of septic arthritis and may be present in other forms of arthritis as well.

Skin

1. Petechial rash is associated with arthritis in vasculitis and systemic lupus erythematosus (SLE).
2. Pustulovesicular skin lesions on the extremities are characteristic of disseminated gonococcal infection.
3. Subcutaneous nodules are seen in rheumatoid arthritis.
4. Erythema chronicum migrans (ECM) is seen with Lyme disease.
5. Erythema marginatum is seen with acute rheumatic fever.
6. Pitting of the fingernails is associated with psoriatic arthritis.
7. Needle tracks suggest intravenous drug abuse, which can be a precipitating factor for septic arthritis.
8. Tophi (uric acid crystals in subcutaneous tissue) are associated with gout but are rarely seen today.

Eyes. Conjunctivitis and iritis in association with arthritis are part of the presentation of Reiter's syndrome.

Chest. Ausculation may reveal pleural or pericardial friction rubs due to inflammatory reactions found in rheumatic diseases such as SLE.

Abdomen. An enlarged or tender liver may indicate infectious hepatitis, which may cause arthritis.

Pelvic and Genital Area. A genital examination with a culture for gonococci is indicated when septic arthritis is a possibility.

DECISION PRIORITIES AND PRELIMINARY DIFFERENTIAL DIAGNOSIS

On completion of the history and physical examination, it is useful to make three important diagnostic decisions.

1. *Is the pain articular (from the joint) or nonarticular (from tendons, bursae, or other periarticular structures)?*
   Pain from articular and synovial surfaces worsens with both active and passive movement, whereas nonarticular pain worsens with active movement much more than with passive motion. The degree of tenderness of the periarticular tissue and pain localized to this area point to problems outside the joint capsule.
2. *Are there objective criteria for inflammation ("arthritis") or is there only subjective pain ("arthralgia")?*
   Important criteria for arthritis include (1) joint pain on passive movement, (2) swelling consistent with joint effusion, (3) limitation of motion of the joint, (4) warmth emanating from the joint, and (5) erythema over the joint. The first four criteria are the most useful in diagnosis.
3. *How many joints are involved?*
   Monoarticular (one joint) and oligoarticular (two to four joints) diseases possess a similar list of diagnostic possibilities, whereas polyarticular (more than four joints) disease usually is due to other etiologies (Table 40–1).

Once the diagnosis of acute arthritis is made, the patient's data and the number of joints involved can usually provide a "ballpark" diagnosis. Systemic disease of immunologic origin most often causes polyarticular disease. Monoarticular disease is of particular importance to the emergency physician because of the possibility of a septic joint, which can rapidly destroy the joint surface.

PROBLEM 1 This young, sexually active female without any previous history of joint problems had a fever and a red, hot, swollen left knee. The "spots" are three to four small, distal, erythematous-based ulcers.
   The findings are consistent with a monoarticular arthritis. Because of the rapidity of onset, physical findings, and age group, she was at high risk for septic arthritis, a process that can rapidly destroy a joint.

PROBLEM 2 This older man gave a history of similar episodes in the past. He recently began taking a thiazide diuretic. The toe began to ache one week earlier but "exploded" overnight. The swelling, tenderness, and erythema were quite obvious. The patient denied a history of trauma.

TABLE 40–1. Common Causes of Acute Arthritis

Monoarticular or Oligoarticular	Polyarticular
Infection	*Infection*
Bacterial	Viral
Granulomatous	*Inflammatory*
Crystal-Induced	Small joint pattern
Gout	Rheumatoid arthritis
Pseudogout	Systemic lupus erythematosus
Traumatic	Polymyositis
Hemarthrosis	Progressive systemic sclerosis
Synovitis	Large joint pattern
Nontraumatic Hemarthrosis	Rheumatoid variant
Inherited coagulopathy	Ankylosing spondylitis
Anticoagulant-induced	Reiter's syndrome
Degenerative Joint Disease	Psoriatic arthritis
	Rheumatic fever
	Lyme disease
	Degenerative Joint Disease

A monoarticular arthritis involving the great toe may involve the metatarsophalangeal joint as well as the surrounding tissue. The likelihood of monoarticular arthritis from gout is high, but definitive diagnosis depends on analysis of the joint fluid. Differentiating joint from periarticular inflammation may be very difficult.

PROBLEM 3 The patient had varying degrees of bony deformity without edema of the phalangeal joints. Her wrist was warm, with slight erythema and swelling.

The subacute onset of bilateral symptoms and signs was highly suggestive of a polyarticular process. However, this patient's specific complaints relative to the left wrist make evaluation to exclude septic arthritis important.

DIAGNOSTIC ADJUNCTS
Laboratory Studies

Laboratory tests are not usually helpful in the diagnosis of the painful joint. A leukocyte count (WBC), erythrocyte sedimentation rate (ESR), and serum uric acid level occasionally confirm the clinical impression but are not routinely recommended. In the majority of proved cases of septic arthritis, leukocyte counts are within the normal range and elevated counts may arise from a number of different causes. An elevated ESR indicates inflammation, but the test is nonspecific, and the overlap between patients with and without various inflammatory diseases is great. The serum uric acid level does not correlate with gouty attacks and can be within the normal range in up to one-third of cases of acute gouty arthritis. Tests such as serum complement, rheumatoid factor, and antinuclear antibodies have no diagnostic value in the emergency department.

Radiographic Imaging

Radiographic changes due to arthritis require weeks to develop, and therefore initial radiographs have limited diagnostic value. For most joints, standard radiographic views are adequate, but occasionally weight-bearing or stress views are necessary to gauge joint stability in patients with traumatic arthritis.

The radiographic assessment of joints includes inspection of alignment, bones, cartilage, and soft tissues. Specific abnormalities that are looked for are remembered by using the mnemonic SECONDS.

1. *Soft* tissue swelling is almost universal and nonspecific.
2. *Erosions* classically occur at the cartilage-synovial junction in patients with rheumatoid arthritis (symmetrical "punched out" erosions without bony overgrowth) and chronic gout (asymmetrical lesions with an overlying thin rim of bony overgrowth).
3. *Calcification* can be intra-articular (indicating a fracture or degenerative fragment) or periarticular (indicating tendonitis or bursitis).
4. *Osteopenia* is most pronounced near the involved joint in osteomyelitis, rheumatoid arthritis, and septic arthritis.
5. *Narrowing* of the joint space indicates loss of articular cartilage and is found early in individuals with rheumatoid arthritis.
6. *Deformity* is due to chronic destructive changes of whatever etiology.
7. *Stippling* refers to early chondrocalcinosis that produces punctate radiodensities in hyaline cartilage (Fig. 40–1). Subchrondral cysts and sclerosis are seen in people with advanced degenerative joint disease.

The most common plain film finding in acute monoarticular arthritis (AMA) is a normal joint with soft tissue swelling. At present, computed tomography, nuclear medicine techniques, and magnetic resonance imaging do not contribute significantly to the diagnosis of the swollen and painful joint.

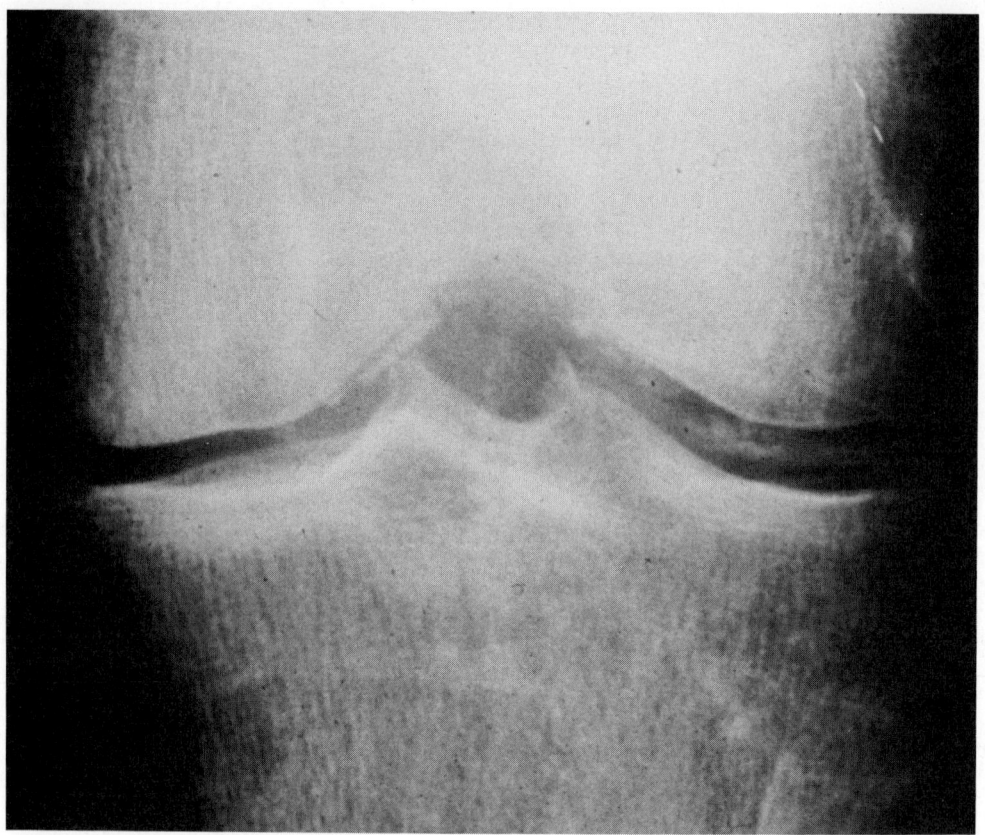

FIGURE 40–1. *The radiographic findings of chondrocalcinosis in the knee joint.*

Other Tests

Arthrocentesis

Arthrocentesis and appropriate analysis of synovial fluid are necessary to help the physician arrive at a specific diagnosis for AMA in the emergency department. Although synovial fluid can be analyzed in many ways (Table 40–2), it is diagnostic only in patients with bacterial and crystal-induced arthritis. Emergency department analysis is directed toward diagnosing these disorders.

The most important function of arthrocentesis is to exclude bacterial infection. No other technique differentiates septic arthritis from other causes of inflammatory arthritis. It is appropriate to perform arthrocentesis at the initial presentation of a patient with acute arthritis. Because different types of arthritis can coexist, it is worthwhile to obtain

TABLE 40–2. Synovial Fluid Analysis

Routine for the emergency department	Not indicated in the emergency department
General appearance	Mucin clot (acetic acid) test
String test	Spontaneous clot
Polarized light microscopic examination for crystals	Protein
Gram's stain	Acid-fast (mycobacteria) stain
Aerobic culture	Anaerobic, mycobacterial, and fungal culture
Gonococcal culture	Lactate, other organic acids
Occasionally useful in the emergency department	
Leukocyte count (WBC)	
Glucose	

synovial fluid during an exacerbation ("flare") in a patient with known arthritis, especially if the exacerbation is atypical for the patient's known disease.

Arthrocentesis is a safe procedure and has a low complication rate and few contraindications. Arthrocentesis is not performed when the joint space might be seeded by passage through infected tissue or when the results would not influence therapy. When obviously infected skin is avoided, the risk of bacterial arthritis resulting from arthrocentesis is less than 1 in 10,000. When necessary, arthrocentesis can be safely performed in a patient with bleeding disorders, although in such cases it would be prudent to treat the hemorrhagic diathesis prior to arthrocentesis.

Elements of Synovial Fluid Analysis

General Appearance. Normal joint fluid is clear and light yellow. Clouding of joint fluid is due to the presence of fibrin and leukocytes. Pink or bloody joint fluid, especially with a "fat sheen" on the surface, represents some disruption in the articular surface (intra-articular fracture), synovial lining, cartilage, or ligaments.

Viscosity. Normal joint fluid has a high viscosity owing to mucin, a complex of protein and hyaluronic acid. With inflammation, mucin is denatured, and viscosity decreases. Normal joint fluid will "string" about 1 to 2 inches when a drop is placed between the gloved thumb and forefinger and the digits are quickly separated. The mucin clot test using 3% acetic acid is the traditional test for intact mucin, but the string test done at the bedside gives immediate results and is almost as good.

Polarized Microscopic Examination. Examining a drop of fluid with a polarizing microscope is necessary to detect monosodium urate (gout) and calcium pyrophosphate dihydrate (pseudogout) crystals. Polarizers are placed above and below the specimen and then turned 90 degrees to each other so that no light can reach the examiner's eye unless it has been affected by an object between the polarizers. This specific property is called birefringence, which means that the plane of polarized light passing through such an object is rotated. Thus, light passing through a birefringent object is also able to pass through the polarizer in front of the observer's eye, causing the object to appear to glow against the black background (Fig. 40–2). The direction in which the birefringent crystal rotates the plane of polarized light is determined by use of the first-order red compensator. Urate crystals have negative birefringence, resulting in a gold-yellow color when the axis of the compensator is parallel to the crystal. Calcium pyrophosphate crystals have positive birefringence, giving a blue color when the axis of the compensator is parallel to the crystal. The use of a compensator is not mandatory because the appearance of these two crystals is very different. Urate crystals are usually needle-shaped, numerous, and strongly birefringent, glowing brightly. Calcium pyrophosphate crystals are smaller, rhomboid-shaped, fewer in number, and weakly birefringent. Other objects or crystals sometimes found in joint fluid may be birefringent, but they can be differentiated from these crystals by shape and size.

Leukocyte Count. Normal synovial fluid has a leukocyte count of less than 200 cells/mm^3, with a differential that includes 10% to 60% polymorphonuclear cells (PMNs). Inflammatory fluid has more than 5000 cells/mm^3. With increasing inflammation, the number of white cells and the percentage of PMNs increase, but the overlaps are too great for single values to be diagnostic of a specific disease (Table 40–3). Synovial fluid protein and glucose values are of little diagnostic value and are not routinely recommended.

Gram Stain. The Gram stain of synovial fluid can be diagnostic. Bacteria can be seen in 70% to 90% of culture-proven bacterial arthritides due to gram-positive bacteria, in about 50% due to gram-negative bacteria, and in 20% to 30% due to gonococci.

Cultures. Cultures for aerobic bacteria and gonococci are required. Because gonococci are fragile, the fluid is placed immediately in an appropriate carrying medium or on warmed chocolate agar. Thayer-Martin (TM) agar, which contains vancomycin, colistin, and nystatin, is not used. TM agar is used when one is attempting to culture gonococci from body areas with indigenous flora. About 10% of gonococci will be inhibited by the

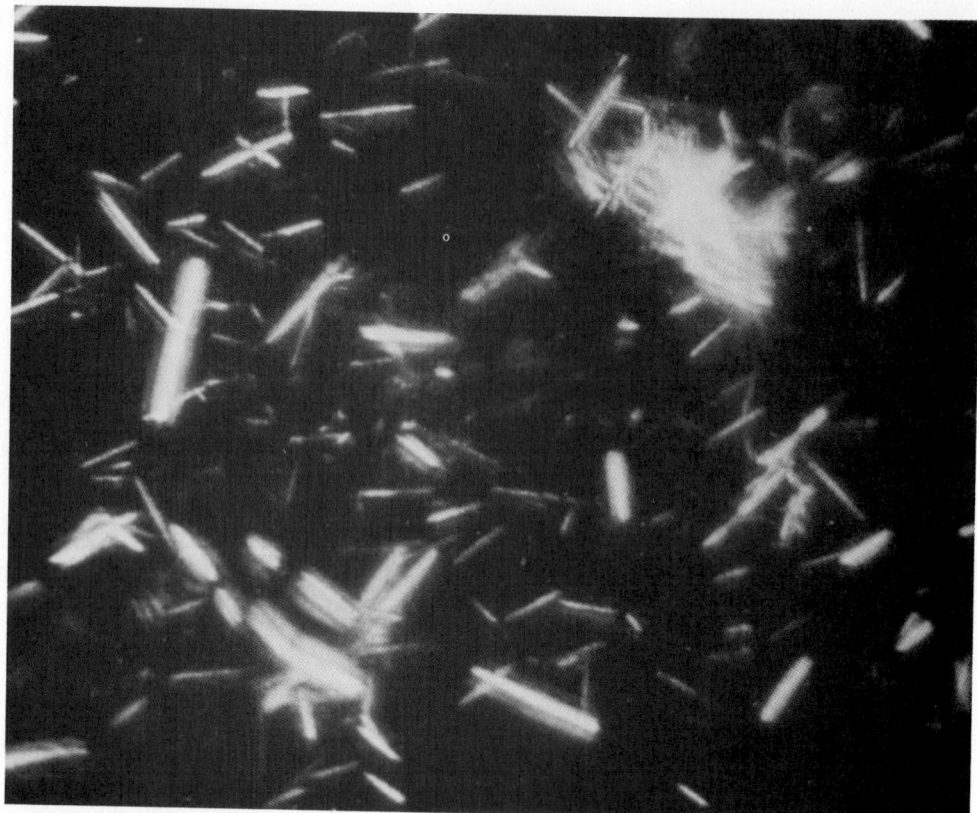

FIGURE 40-2. *Numerous urate crystals seen with the polarized microscope. Note the characteristic needlelike shape and strong birefringence.*

antibiotics in TM agar and there is no indigenous flora in joint fluid. Anaerobic, mycobacterial, and fungal cultures are not routinely indicated. Blood cultures are useful because they are positive in about half of patients with gram-positive bacterial arthritides and in 10% to 20% of those with arthritis due to gram-negative bacterial causes.

Lactate and Other Acids. Synovial fluid lactate and other organic acids have been studied for their ability to detect bacterial infection, but there is no clear benefit to their use at this time.

PROBLEM In each of these patients, the emergency physician performed an arthrocentesis. Analyses of the synovial fluid showed:

Problem	Appearance	Viscosity	Crystals	Cells	Gram Stain
1	Purulent	No string	None	70,000/mm^3 95% PMNs	Negative
2	Cloudy	Weak string	Urate	5000/mm^3 75% PMNs	Negative
3	Cloudy	Poor string	None	15,000/mm^3 60% PMNs	Negative

PROBLEM 1 Purulent synovial fluid with a high leukocyte count and an overwhelming preponderance of PMNs points to bacterial infection. The Gram stain is very helpful if it is positive, but a negative result does not exclude a septic joint, especially one due to gonococci.

PROBLEM 2 The presence of urate crystals establishes the diagnosis of acute gout. However, Gram stain and culture are still indicated because acute gout and septic arthritis can coexist.

PROBLEM 3 The cloudy synovial fluid and cell count indicate inflammation, but the values are not diagnostic of any specific process.

REFINED DIFFERENTIAL DIAGNOSIS

Based on the history, physical examination, radiographic examination, and laboratory evaluation, including joint fluid analysis, the emergency physician can establish a specific diagnosis in a significant number of cases of AMA (Table 40–3). The most important cause of AMA needing diagnosis in the emergency setting is septic arthritis. Polyarticular disease may be impossible to diagnose specifically in the emergency department, requiring extended follow-up and testing to arrive at the underlying cause.

Septic Arthritis

Acute bacterial arthritis has the potential to destroy a joint in only 3 to 4 days. No joint is immune, but the knee is the most common site (about 50% of cases), followed by the hip and shoulder. Hematogenous spread is the most common means by which bacteria infect a joint, but direct inoculation into the joint or spread from adjacent structures is also possible. The causative organisms vary with age and host factors (Table 40–4). In sexually active patients the most common infecting organism is *Neisseria gonorrhoeae*.

Disseminated gonococcal infection (DGI) complicates about 0.2% of gonococcal genitourinary infections. Arthritis is one of its most frequent manifestations. Fever is present in about 90% of such cases, and skin lesions are found in about 50%. The most commonly affected joints are the knee and ankle, although the hip and phalangeal joints are also vulnerable. Polyarticular, often migratory arthralgia is seen in about 75% of cases

TABLE 40–3. Diagnosis and Management of Major Types of Acute Monoarticular Arthritis

Diagnosis or Class	Laboratory	Radiography	Synovial Fluid	Treatment
Septic		Soft tissue swelling, osteopenia, joint space narrowing, subchondral erosions	WBC >50000 PMN >85% Glucose <50 mg/dl Gram stain positive in 65% of cases Culture positive	Admission IV antibiotics Splinting Drainage
Gout	Serum uric acid elevated 70%–90%	Soft tissue swelling, tophi	WBC 2500–50000 PMN 40%–90% Urate crystals	Oral NSAIDs Colchicine, IV or PO
Pseudogout		Soft tissue swelling, chondrocalcinosis	WBC 2500–50000 PMN 40%–90% Calcium pyrophosphate crystals	Oral NSAIDs Colchicine, IV or PO
Inflammatory joint disease	ESR elevated in 60%–80%	Soft tissue swelling, erosions	WBC 10000–50000 PMN 65%–85%	Oral NSAIDs
Degenerative joint disease		Joint space narrowing, marginal osteophytes, subchondral sclerosis	WBC <5000 PMN <25%	Oral NSAIDs
Traumatic		Soft tissue swelling	Bloody WBC <10000 Fat droplets (usually represent a fracture)	Aspiration Compression Splint

TABLE 40-4. Organisms Commonly Found in Bacterial Arthritis

Child: age 2 months to 2 years	
Hemophilus influenzae	40%
Streptococcus pneumoniae	25%
Staphylococcus aureus	25%
Child: age >2 years	
S. aureus	45%
Group A streptococci	25%
H. influenzae	10%
Adults	
Neisseria gonorrhoeae	>50%
Nongonococcal	
S. aureus	40%
Group A streptococci	25%
Enterobacteriaceae	20%

of DGI, usually preceding the arthritis. Most series report that twice as many women are affected as men.

Nongonococcal septic arthritis occurs most commonly in children and immunocompromised individuals. *Hemophilus influenzae* and other Gram-negative organisms account for about 50% of cases in children under 2 years old and for about 20% of cases in children between 2 and 6 years. In adults, staphylococci and streptococci account for more than 80% of cases of nongonococcal septic arthritis.

Crystal-Induced Arthritides

Gouty attacks have an acute onset with escalation of symptoms over 12 to 24 hours. The symptoms are monoarticular or oligoarticular and most commonly involve the metatarsophalangeal joint at the base of the first toe, the ankle, the dorsum of the foot, the wrist, or the knee. Usually there is associated soft tissue inflammation that resembles cellulitis. Gout is predominantly a disease of men. Women are affected usually only after menopause. The process is produced by an inflammatory reaction to uric acid crystals in the joint and periarticular tissues. The serum uric acid level is not necessarily elevated during an acute attack.

Pseudogout is an acute monoarticular arthritis due to calcium pyrophosphate crystals in the joint fluid. Pseudogout usually occurs in older patients and affects men and women equally. The knee is the most common site. There is little correlation between the radiographic finding of chondrocalcinosis (see Fig. 40-1) and the clinical occurrence of acute attacks of pseudogout.

Traumatic Synovitis or Hemarthrosis

Acute injury to a joint may result in immediate swelling (less than 2 hours after injury) or delayed effusion within 12 to 24 hours. Immediate swelling, with marked effusion and pain, is usually secondary to bleeding into the joint (hemarthrosis). Because of its exposed position, the knee is the joint most commonly involved with traumatic hemarthrosis, and in 90% of cases there is associated intra-articular disruption or damage. Meniscal or anterior cruciate ligament tears are the most frequent injuries. Although acute joint instability may not occur, significant long-term disability can result after this type of injury. Traumatic synovitis is a less serious injury and is infrequently associated with internal joint damage. The usual outcome is full recovery.

Nontraumatic Hemarthrosis

Bleeding into a joint is common in patients with inherited coagulopathies and occasionally occurs in patients being treated with anticoagulants (see Chap. 24).

Polyarticular Arthritides

Patients with rheumatoid arthritis, spondyloarthropathies ("rheumatoid variants"), and other collagen-vascular diseases may occasionally present to the emergency department with complaints of joint pain. Although these problems are usually polyarticular, pain in an isolated joint can be out of proportion to the others. It is important to consider the need for arthrocentesis to determine if infection is the cause of the more painful or inflamed joint. If infection is excluded to a reasonable degree, the patient is treated for the underlying disease.

Inflammatory polyarthritis has two common patterns. One is the small joint, symmetrical pattern typical of rheumatoid arthritis but also seen in systemic lupus erythematosus, polymyositis, progressive systemic sclerosis, and transiently in some viral infections such as rubella and hepatitis B. The other pattern is the asymmetrical large joint or axial skeletal involvement characteristic of anklyosing spondylitis, Reiter's syndrome, psoriatic arthritis, enteropathic arthritis, acute rheumatic fever, and Lyme disease. This latter pattern of joint involvement and group of diseases is sometimes termed the rheumatoid variant(s).

Degenerative Joint Disease

Degenerative joint disease (DJD) is a disease of age and overuse. Ninety percent of elderly patients have some degree of DJD in their hands, and 30% to 50% have involvement of their hips by age 65. Symptoms are usually mild, but acute exacerbations with swelling and evidence of inflammation may occur. Stiffness is the most common complaint, and physical examination shows bony enlargement and limitation of motion. Radiographs will demonstrate osteophytes, joint space narrowing, and bony deformity.

Periarticular Syndromes

Bursitis is inflammation of a closed space that is adjacent to but isolated from the synovial cavity. The prepatellar, olecranon, and subdeltoid bursae are most frequently affected. Idiopathic bursitis occurs in young, healthy individuals and is probably due to overuse or repetitive injury. It does not have associated systemic symptoms. Septic bursitis is more common in older individuals with predisposing disorders such as diabetes.

Tendonitis is inflammation of a tendon, usually due to repetitive injury or overuse. Common locations are the biceps tendon of the shoulder and the extensor pollicus at the thumb. There is associated tenderness and pain, especially with active movement, but little swelling and no systemic manifestations.

Osteomyelitis is bacterial infection of bone and may occur adjacent to or spread to involve a joint. Systemic manifestations of infection are usually present. Radiographic changes take up to 3 weeks to appear.

PRINCIPLES OF MANAGEMENT

The therapeutic approach to acute arthritis depends on the specific diagnosis. Available treatment modalities include
1. Aspiration of the joint fluid
2. Antibiotics
3. Anti-inflammatory medications
4. Splinting and pressure dressings
5. Intra-articular injections

The goals are joint rest, decreasing inflammation, and aggressive treatment of intra-articular infection. Specific treatments are discussed below and listed in Table 40–3.

Septic Arthritis

Antibiotics. The key to successful treatment of bacterial arthritis is initiation of appropriate antibiotic therapy as early as possible after the onset of symptoms. Therefore, early diagnosis and presumptive selection of antibiotics are essential. A relatively limited number of bacteria produce most cases of bacterial arthritis (Table 40–4). In children less than 2 years old, the major pathogens are *Hemophilus influenzae, Streptococcus pneumoniae,* and *Staphylococcus aureus.* With increasing age, *S. aureus* becomes more frequent, and in the sexually active population *Neisseria gonorrhoeae* is the most common organism. Because of this limited range of potential pathogens, antibiotics can be initiated empirically based on Gram stain interpretation, age, and host factors (Table 40–5). High-dose, intravenous antibiotics are required for patients with bacterial arthritis. The one exception is patients with disseminated gonococcal syndrome who have polyarthritis or tenosynovitis and do not have a septic joint. These patients can be treated with oral or intramuscular antibiotics, although patient compliance and reliability are concerns. Intra-articular antibiotics are not required for septic arthritis.

Joint Drainage. In most patients with septic arthritis, the joints are adequately drained by repeated arthrocentesis. Initially they may require two or three aspirations per day. Most patients require between six and nine arthrocenteses before resolution of the effusion. The process is slightly more successful if it is initiated within 3 days of the onset of symptoms. Occasionally, open drainage is required in patients in whom needle drainage cannot remove the fluid owing to the presence of intra-articular adhesions or marked thickness of the fluid. Patients with septic arthritis of the hip cannot easily undergo repeat arthrocentesis, so they are often treated by open drainage.

Splinting. Splinting of the involved extremity is important and should be done soon after the initial arthrocentesis.

Analgesia and Anti-inflammatory Agents. Septic arthritis can be very painful. Analgesia and anti-inflammatory agents are given in proportion to pain.

TABLE 40–5. Empiric Antibiotic Selection for Bacterial Arthritis

Gram's Stain	Likely Organism	Antibiotic
Gram-positive cocci	*S. aureus*	Beta-lactamase–resistant penicillin[1] *or* Vancomycin
Gram-negative cocci		
Adult or teen	Gonococci	Penicillin *or* Ampicillin *or* Ceftriaxone
Young child	*H. influenzae*	Ampicillin *and* chloramphenicol *or* Cefuroxime
Gram-negative bacilli	Enterobacteriaceae	Aminoglycoside[2] *and* Antipseudomonal penicillin[3]
None seen		
Adult or teen	Gonococci	Penicillin *or* Ampicillin *or* Ceftriaxone
Child	*H. influenzae*	Beta-lactamase resistant penicillin *and* Cefuroxime *or* Vancomycin *and* Cefuroxime
Compromised host	*S. aureus* Enterobacteriaceae	Beta-lactamase–resistant penicillin *and* aminoglycoside *or* Vancomycin and aminoglycoside

[1]Beta-lactamase–resistant penicillins: cloxicillin, dicloxacillin, methicillin, nafcillin, oxacillin.
[2]Aminoglycosides: amikacin, gentamicin, tobramycin.
[3]Antipseudomonal penicillins: azlocillin, carbenicillin, mezlocillin, piperacillin, ticarcillin.

Crystal-Induced Arthritis

Nonsteroidal Anti-inflammatory Agents. Nonsteroidal anti-inflammatory drugs (NSAIDs) are effective in hastening the resolution of acute attacks of gout and have a lower incidence of side effects than the traditional treatment with colchicine. Indomethacin has been used most often in this regard, but other NSAIDs are probably just as effective if given in high doses for short periods of time. Most attacks resolve within a few days, and therapy is rarely indicated for longer than 1 week. The typical dose of indomethacin is 50 mg three times a day for 3 days followed by 25 mg three times a day for 3 to 4 more days.

Colchicine. Colchicine is the traditional agent used for treatment of acute gout, with a response rate of about 70% within 48 hours compared to a spontaneous resolution rate of 30% to 40%. Colchicine is also effective in acute pseudogout, with a response rate of about 40%. Colchicine is administered orally or intravenously in small doses until (1) clinical improvement begins, (2) early gastrointestinal toxicity develops with nausea or diarrhea, or (3) the maximum safe dose is reached. A common protocol is an oral dose of 1 mg initially followed by 0.5 mg every 2 hours until one of the three endpoints is reached. For intravenous use, the initial dose is 1 to 2 mg with repeat doses of 1 mg every 4 to 6 hours. There are limits in dosing for elderly patients and those with impaired renal function. The therapeutic margin of colchicine is extremely narrow, and significant toxicity can occur with single doses as low as 6 mg orally or 4 mg intravenously. For this reason, NSAIDs are the drugs of choice.

Aspiration. Complete aspiration of the involved joint is occasionally followed by resolution of the inflammation. Intra-articular injection of steroids is effective in attacks of gout and pseudogout but is recommended only for physicians experienced in their use.

Analgesics. Acute gout can be exquisitely painful. Narcotic analgesics may be required for 24 hours until the anti-inflammatory medications take effect.

Traumatic Hemarthrosis

The most important point concerning the acute management of traumatic hemarthrosis is its high association with significant intra-articular damage. An acute traumatic hemarthrosis of the knee is associated in approximately 90% of cases with significant intra-articular disruption. Almost two-thirds of such injuries are ligamentous or meniscal tears. The 5- to 10-year follow-up studies of these injuries indicate that about 80% of patients will have continued problems after a single traumatic hemarthrosis of the knee.

The role of aspiration in the management of an acute traumatic hemarthrosis is unsettled. Some clinicians are advocates of always aspirating and some are proponents of never aspirating. Three reasons favor routine aspiration: (1) reducing swelling relieves the patient's pain, (2) blood in the synovial space is an irritant and may lead to further cartilage damage, and (3) the presence of fat globules in the synovial fluid is highly predictive of a significant intra-articular disruption. The argument advanced against routine aspiration is usually the risk of infection or further joint damage from arthrocentesis.

Whether aspiration is done or not, the involved joint is placed in a compression dressing, splinted, elevated, and treated with intermittent ice for at least 24 to 36 hours. Analgesics such as acetaminophen with or without narcotics are preferred, since aspirin and NSAIDs may impair platelet function.

Nontraumatic Hemarthrosis

An occasional patient may present with an acute nontraumatic hemarthrosis. Patients with an inherited coagulation factor deficiency and those using anticoagulant drugs have an obvious reason for bleeding. In rare patients bleeding into a joint may occur for no obvious reason. When investigated, some of these patients may turn out to have synovial pathology. Blood within the synovial space is irritating, and repeated joint bleeds produce chronic changes in the synovium leading to localized degenerative joint damage. It is appropriate to remove the irritating blood from the joint with arthrocentesis. This can be done safely in most patients, even those with prolonged coagulation times.

Other than rest and splinting, these patients do not require specific therapy unless it is necessary to adjust their anticoagulant dose or administer a deficient coagulation factor. The use of aspirin and NSAIDs may impair platelet function and exacerbate bleeding.

Polyarticular Arthritis

For patients presenting with inflammatory polyarticular arthritis, the emergency physician must first exclude bacterial infection. If this can be done to a reasonable degree, symptomatic treatment can begin with oral NSAIDs. Intra-articular steroids are not recommended as a treatment for the first presentation of inflammatory arthritis. Although rheumatoid arthritis and the "rheumatoid variants" are usually polyarticular, they may present initially with monoarticular involvement. The polyarticular pattern usually becomes evident within 6 months.

Degenerative Arthritis

Management of DJD is complicated by the fact that there is no specific treatment that reverses joint damage or halts further progression. The physician's role is to educate the patient, stress the avoidance of further joint abuse, and use medications and physical modalities to maximize patient function. Aspirin is often used to control painful episodes, although there is conflicting evidence about its clinical usefulness. Indomethacin and the sulindac derivatives appear to be more helpful in controlling pain and improving functional ability than aspirin or other NSAIDs.

Intra-articular Injections

Arthrocentesis and intra-articular injections may be used for a variety of arthritic problems. Simple arthrocentesis may markedly relieve symptoms, especially in the setting of a tense, tender effusion due to trauma. Instillation of local anesthetics can provide further relief, but, particularly in weight-bearing joints, continued ambulation during the anesthetic period can result in further joint injury.

PROBLEM 1 The history, clinical findings, and results of the joint fluid analysis all pointed to septic arthritis secondary to disseminated gonococcal infection. The patient's left leg was immobilized after arthrocentesis and intravenous ceftriaxone was started.

PROBLEM 2 Results of the work-up were consistent with the initial impression of gouty arthritis. The patient was started on a week-long course of indomethacin, 50 mg tid, with a planned decrease beginning on the fourth day. Additional analgesia was supplied.

PROBLEM 3 No definitive diagnosis was reached, but one of the polyarthritis syndromes was suspected. The patient was started on a NSAID and referred for appropriate follow-up. More definitive therapy will await specific diagnosis.

DISPOSITION AND FOLLOW-UP

Admission

Patients with septic joints are admitted to the hospital for intravenous antibiotic therapy and possible surgical drainage. Patients with incapacitating acute arthritis of other etiologies are admitted for medical and physical therapy to restore functional ability.

Discharge

Most other patients can be discharged with outpatient follow-up. Before patients are discharged from the emergency department, the following conditions are met: (1) the synovial fluid Gram's stain shows no bacteria, (2) the involved joint is splinted or immobilized and the patient has crutches or supports, (3) the patient has received a first dose of medication, and (4) the patient understands the diagnosis and the importance of follow-up.

Referral and Follow-Up

The patient with an inflammatory joint in whom the possibility of infection exists is checked in 24 hours. Patients with gout and other inflammatory conditions are checked within 3 to 5 days. Patients with joint injury are checked after the swelling has diminished, usually in 5 to 7 days.

Discharge instructions should stress resting the joint, avoidance of weight bearing on the large joints of the leg, use of elevation and ice to reduce edema, and recommendations to return if the pain is not improved in 24 to 48 hours.

> **PROBLEM 1** This patient was admitted for treatment with intravenous antibiotics. She had a grossly septic joint and appeared ill. Patients with disseminated gonococcal syndrome who do not have a grossly septic joint may be treated on an outpatient basis.
>
> **PROBLEM 2** Outpatient treatment with NSAIDs or colchicine is standard treatment for patients with gout, with follow-up by the primary physician. Response is rapid, often occurring within hours.
>
> **PROBLEM 3** The importance of follow-up and further evaluation by the primary care physician or rheumatologist was stressed to the patient.

DOCUMENTATION

1. Duration of joint pain and swelling.
2. History of trauma.
3. Prior history of arthritis.
4. Patient's use of medications for pain.
5. Specific examination of the joint noting erythema, warmth, swelling, joint effusion, limitation of motion, and stability.
6. A procedure note for arthrocentesis with a description of the fluid removed, what tests were ordered on the synovial fluid, and the preliminary Gram's stain report.
7. Radiographs taken and their interpretation.
8. A preliminary diagnosis.
9. Specific discharge instructions.

SUMMARY AND FINAL POINTS

- The cause of acute monoarticular arthritis can be found in many cases by careful history, physical examination, and use of diagnostic tests in the emergency department.
- The most important task for the emergency physician, when presented with a patient who has acute arthritis, is to diagnose or exclude septic (bacterial) arthritis.
- Arthrocentesis is the only definitive means of diagnosing bacterial arthritis.
- When the diagnosis is determined in the emergency department, specific therapy is initiated. If the diagnosis remains unclear, symptomatic treatment with analgesics and immobilization is used.
- In either case, appropriate follow-up is arranged for further evaluation and treatment.

BIBLIOGRAPHY

Texts

1. Kelley WN, Harris ED, Ruddy S, et al: Textbook of Rheumatology. Philadelphia, Saunders, 1985.
2. Schumacher HR: Primer on the Rheumatic Diseases (9th ed). Atlanta, Arthritis Foundation, 1988.

Journal Articles

1. Currey HLF, Vernon-Roberts B: Examination of synovial fluid. Clin Rheumatol Dis 2:149–177, 1976.
2. Eisenberg JM, Schumacher HR, Davidson PK, et al: Usefulness of synovial fluid analysis in the evaluation of joint effusion. Arch Intern Med 144:715–719, 1984.
3. Freed JF, Nies KM, Boyer RS, et al: Acute monoarticular arthritis. A diagnostic approach. JAMA 243:2314–2316, 1980.
4. Goldenberg DL, Reed JI: Bacterial arthritis. N Engl J Med 312:764–771, 1985.
5. McCarty DJ: Arthritis associated with calcium-containing crystals. Med Clin North Am 70:437–454, 1986.
6. Moskowit RW: Primary osteoarthritis. Am J Med 83(5A):5–10, 1987.
7. Nanji AA, Whitlow KJ: Clinical utility of lactic acid measurement in body fluids other than plasma. J Emerg Med 1:521–526, 1984.
8. O'Meara PM, Bartel E: Septic arthritis. Orthopedics 11:623–628, 1988.
9. Reginato AJ, Schumacher HR: Crystal-induced arthropathies. Clin Geriatr Med 4:299–322, 1988.
10. Sanford JP: Guide to Antimicrobial Therapy. West Bethesda, MD, Antimicrobial Therapy, Inc., 1989.
11. Zarins B, Adams J: Knee injuries in sports. N Engl J Med 318:950–961, 1988.

CHAPTER 41

UPPER EXTREMITY INJURY: CLOSED INJURIES

GEORGE HOSSFELD, M.D.
T. J. RITTENBERRY, M.D.

PROBLEM 1 A 17 year old high school quarterback presented with right (dominant) shoulder pain after being "sacked" while trying to get off a pass. Physical examination revealed the patient slumped forward while supporting his right forearm with his left hand. The shoulder was externally rotated and there was an abnormally sharp step-off to the shoulder contour. Pain was severe and was exacerbated with attempts at passive range of motion.

PROBLEM 2 A 10 year old girl complained of pain about the elbow after a fall from the "monkey bars." There was no obvious fracture line on radiograph, but there was impressive ecchymosis and tenderness about the child's elbow.

PROBLEM 3 The concerned parents of a 2 year old anxiously brought in their child with a "paralyzed" right arm. The senior resident briefly manipulated the crying child's arm. Within minutes the child was smiling, playing, and using the arm normally.

PROBLEM 4 A 30 year old man fell on his outstretched arm, but no fracture was found on the wrist radiograph. His wrist and hand were diffusely tender.

QUESTIONS TO CONSIDER

1. How does the mechanism of injury help to predict the specific injury that will be seen?
2. What objective findings are commonly present in patients sustaining sprains, fractures, and dislocations?
3. What examination techniques are helpful in confirming an initial suspicion that a given injury has occurred?
4. What views and specific radiographic signs are useful in confirming the diagnosis?
5. What injuries require immediate intervention? Which can be splinted and referred for orthopedic follow-up?
6. What are the techniques of reduction and immobilization used by the emergency physician?

INTRODUCTION

Emergency diagnosis of acute traumatic orthopedic injuries is facilitated by a history of the mechanism of injury, specific physical findings, and a knowledge of common syndromes. Twenty-five percent of all emergency department visits are for orthopedic complaints. Approximately half of these involve acute injuries to the upper extremity. Although these are seldom life-threatening injuries, they may have a major impact on an individual's lifestyle and livelihood.

The hand and the upper extremity are important in almost every activity of daily living, routine personal care, occupational activities, and recreational activities. This active role predisposes the hand and arm to injury whether at work, play, or rest. The protective response of the body, using the arm to ward off a blow or to brace the body during a fall, increases the risk of injury.

Failure to diagnose adequately and treat an upper extremity injury appropriately may result in major functional impairment. Because the majority of patients incurring upper extremity injury are young and otherwise healthy individuals, the functional, financial, and potential medicolegal impact is even greater. A thorough knowledge of the anatomy of the upper extremity, the potential injuries that can occur, and the mechanisms that are likely to result in specific injuries form a solid basis for the evaluation and management of these injuries.

PREHOSPITAL CARE

Extremity injuries may be obvious and impressive, but the rescue squad attends to life-threatening injuries before treating limb-threatening ones. Once the injured patient is stabilized, the search for less obvious but potentially significant extremity injuries begins. The following information is obtained by the rescue squad in preparation for discussion of the patient with the emergency department staff.

History

1. What was the nature of the accident and what were the forces applied?
2. What parts of the body were injured?
3. Exactly what happened to the injured body parts? Delineation of the mechanism of injury is not always possible, but it is important in predicting specific injuries. The chances of determining the mechanism of injury are best immediately after the accident has occurred while the patient and caregivers are still at the scene.

Physical Examination

1. Vital functions are assessed. Problems with airway, ventilation, and circulation are attended to as they are recognized.
2. Evaluation is performed for nonorthopedic trauma: neck, head, chest, abdomen.
3. Evaluation for injured extremities is performed.
    a. Neurovascular status: pulses, capillary refill time, and sensation are determined distal to all injuries.
    b. Injury site: swelling, tenderness, deformity, and any open fractures are noted.

Intervention

1. Vital functions are stabilized: intubation, assisted ventilation, oxygen, and intravenous fluids are given as indicated.
2. Nonorthopedic traumatic injuries are managed as indicated (Chap. 4).
3. Open fractures are covered with a clean, preferably sterile, dressing and splinted. The contaminated bone fragment is not replaced into the wound.
4. Distal ischemia is an indication for rapid transport. If transport time will be prolonged, in-field reduction of an angulated fracture may be indicated.
5. Immobilization may be necessary. Supplies and procedures will vary, but most

paramedics are taught to splint extremities in the position in which they are found, without manipulation. Inflatable plastic splints are commonly used.

6. Amputated parts are cleaned of gross debris, packaged in a plastic bag, and transported with the patient. If transport time is prolonged, the sealed bag is placed in ice water.

7. In patients with open injuries, hemorrhage control is achieved with direct pressure. The inflatable splint serves as both a "pressure" dressing and an immobilizer.

8. Notification of the receiving hospital, especially if there is vascular compromise or an open fracture, will allow mobilization of appropriate services prior to the arrival of the patient.

INITIAL APPROACH IN THE EMERGENCY DEPARTMENT

As in prehospital care, priority is given to resuscitation of vital functions (airway, breathing, and circulation) and to other injuries that are potentially life-threatening (Chap. 4).

Once immediate life threats have been treated or ruled out, attention can be focused on injuries of the extremities. The following sequence is performed rapidly:

1. A vascular examination to rule out any deficits requiring immediate reduction is performed. The morbidity of limb ischemia is directly proportional to time elapsed without blood flow. A cold, pale, pulseless distal extremity is an indication for immediate reduction prior to radiography.

2. Jewelry and constricting clothing are removed to avoid a tourniquet effect in conjunction with local swelling.

3. Elevation of the extremity and ice, with a carefully interposed barrier such as a hand towel to protect against thermal injury, will help to minimize edema formation.

4. Padded, preformed aluminum splints, inflatable air splints, or other "universal" devices will increase patient comfort initially. In general, these devices are suitable for temporary use only and will be replaced with a molded splint before disposition.

5. Open wounds are covered with sterile, saline-soaked gauze applied to minimize contamination and tissue loss through drying. Local application of a disinfectant such as povidone-iodine is advisable.

6. If there is an open fracture, broad-spectrum antibiotics such as first- or second-generation cephalosporins are given intravenously.

7. Application of splints, fracture or dislocation manipulation, and movement needed for radiologic assessment all cause discomfort for the patient. In most cases, providing analgesia early will result in a grateful, more comfortable, and more cooperative patient.

DATA GATHERING

History

Histories of extremity injury are brief, but the details of the events are important in assessing the likelihood of various specific injuries.

1. What kind of *activity* was the patient involved in at the *time of injury?* This information helps to assess the patient's usual level of activity and also to determine a logical sequence between the activity and the injury. It is important to consider the possibility that a different disease process caused the injury—for example, a "fall" may turn out to be syncope on more specific questioning.

2. *Exactly what happened* to the injured extremity? The mechanism of injury is very helpful in identifying the injury.

3. What *symptoms* has the patient noticed since the injury? (The occurrence of increasing pain, numbness, or tingling, and the course of the symptoms are all explored.)

4. What sort of *occupational* and *leisure activities* does the patient engage in? The significance of an upper extremity injury may be magnified many times depending on the patient's livelihood.

5. Which is the patient's *dominant hand?*

Physical Examination

Exposure. The entire extremity must be uncovered to allow adequate examination. One joint above and one joint below the suspected site of pathology are included in the examination. This allows the physician to examine the impact of forces transmitted along the bone to the joint structure.

Inspection. *Deformity* may be due to displaced or angulated fractures, dislocations, or edema. *Ecchymosis* requires time to develop, but with major disruptions it may be present on the initial examination. *Skin integrity* is important because any open wound over or adjacent to a fracture site is considered to communicate with the fracture (open fracture).

Palpation

Neurovascular status is determined by checking for the presence and strength of the brachial and radial pulses as well as for capillary refill time and skin temperature. Motor and sensory integrity of the radial, median, and ulnar nerves, which supply the hand, is evaluated as described in Chapter 42. The axillary nerve innervates the skin over the lateral shoulder, and the musculocutaneous nerve innervates the dorsum of the forearm.

Tenderness is the observation of a painful response to palpation. Although pain may be perceived over a wide area, the point of maximal tenderness is an objective sign that correlates well with the location of the pathology. Careful palpation, working from uninvolved to involved areas, is needed to determine where this is.

Swelling, like ecchymosis, is time dependent but is likely to be present to some degree at the time of initial evaluation.

Bony crepitus is perceived when bone fragments move against one another. If noted during palpation, this sign is significant, but it is not necessary for diagnosis. Since it is associated with significant pain, it is not routinely sought in the examination.

Range of motion is determined in active and passive modes. Active range of motion implies patient-originated movement. Diminished active range of motion is evidence of either loss of joint integrity or injury to the musculotendinous elements that produce the movement. Passive range of motion, in which the examiner initiates the movement, is a means of evaluating joint integrity alone. An abnormally large passive range of motion implies complete rupture of the joint capsules and supporting ligaments. Testing of range of motion may lead to severe pain, complicating interpretation of these tests.

DECISION PRIORITIES AND PRELIMINARY DIFFERENTIAL DIAGNOSIS

After completion of the history and physical examination, the following questions are asked:

1. *Is there a likelihood of a bony injury, i.e., a fracture or dislocation?*
   If there is a strong likelihood of such injury, appropriate radiographic assessment is ordered to confirm this suspicion and to delineate the exact pathology.
2. *Is the fracture or dislocation causing a complication that requires immediate reduction?*
   Although rare, neurovascular complications of injuries to the extremities must always be anticipated. If present, they can often be relieved by bony realignment. Some injuries have a high incidence of neurovascular complications, e.g., supra-

condylar fracture (vascular ischemia) and distal radioulnar ligament disruption (median nerve injury).
3. *If bone or joint disruption is not suspected because of lack of supporting physical findings, or if it has been ruled out radiographically, the next question is, What other form of soft tissue injury may be present?*
The soft tissue injuries considered after a fracture or dislocation has been clinically or radiographically ruled out are contusions, sprains, and strains.
   a. *Contusions* are usually due to direct blows. They are associated with tenderness, swelling, and, with time, ecchymosis. There is no deformity, and any reduction in range of motion of the adjacent joints is minimal and is due to the discomfort of the contusion. Occasionally, it will be necessary to rule out an underlying fracture radiographically.
   b. *Sprains* result from abnormal or excessive joint movement that is less than that necessary to result in dislocation. There is some disruption of the ligamentous structures surrounding the joint. This amount of ligament tear is clinically divided into three classes according to severity: (1) *First-degree* (minimal) *sprains* result in tenderness on stressing the joint but do not result in joint instability. (2) *Second-degree* (partial) *sprains* are significant enough tears to allow abnormal joint motion. Signs of swelling, tenderness, and ecchymosis make fracture a distinct possibility. (3) *Third-degree sprains* result in complete ligamentous disruption and a grossly unstable joint. Signs of swelling, tenderness, and ecchymosis are invariably present, and a joint effusion is frequently palpable. Associated fractures are relatively common. These injuries may heal slowly and incompletely.
   c. *Strains* are injuries to musculotendinous units due to a violent contraction or overstretching. Mild strains are diagnosed by local tenderness and pain in the muscle or tendon with contraction. Severe or complete disruptions result in severe pain and often a palpable defect in the muscle. Avulsion of bone where the tendon inserts is sometimes seen.

DIAGNOSTIC ADJUNCTS

Radiologic Imaging

Radiographs are the mainstay of diagnosis in injuries of the extremities. They do not replace the history or examination of a tender extremity. Differentiating the point of maximal tenderness from the subjective location of pain is necessary for proper selection of radiographs. A *standard radiographic series* of various anatomic locations consists of anteroposterior, lateral, and occasionally oblique views. These are applicable to most clinical situations, but special views exist to fit unusual cases. Stress views, in which the integrity of one or more ligamentous structures is indirectly evaluated, may be of tremendous benefit in some cases. If suspicion of significant bony pathology is not confirmed by the standard views, one may request a magnified "coned-down" view to enhance the image of a well-localized injury site. Frequent communication with the radiology technician can enhance tremendously the usefulness of the films obtained.

Trauma to a long bone seldom creates an isolated injury. The joint articulations at either end are often affected. Therefore, the joints on either side of the site of pathology must be adequately visualized. In the case of joint trauma, standard views generally display several centimeters of long bone on either side of the injury.

At the extremes of age or in the presence of degenerative bone disease, bony injury is more difficult to detect. With increasing familiarity with "normals," detection becomes easier. "Mirror image symmetry" can be used in questionable cases by obtaining comparison views of the presumed normal extremity. Most often, this technique is used in evaluating epiphyseal regions, such as the pediatric elbow, where considerable variation among patients exists.

Certain orthopedic injuries defy standard radiographic diagnosis because the classic radiolucent fracture line is lacking. Secondary radiographic evidence may be useful. The "fat pad" sign about the elbow, described later under Specific Injuries, is a good example. Ultimately, clinically suspected fractures should be treated with immobilization regardless of the presence or absence of radiographic signs. After a sufficient period of time, bone resorption and callous formation make radiographic diagnosis possible. Initial immobilization of any injured extremity is indicated until fracture is definitely ruled out.

Modalities used less commonly are *tomography* and *computed tomography*, in which selective "slices" of a given bone or joint are visualized. *Bone scans* are infrequently used but take advantage of the increased bone metabolism found at a fracture site to identify occult fractures. *Magnetic resonance imaging* (MRI) may play a useful role in assessing soft tissue injury and determining the presence of intramuscular or ligamentous hemorrhage.

Although there are "grading systems" to aid physicians in deciding what types of injuries are to be assessed radiographically, most bony injuries of the upper extremity are imaged. It is important not to overestimate the diagnostic powers of radiography. Subtle fractures and most soft tissue injuries are missed with present techniques.

Laboratory Studies

There are no tests to assist in the diagnosis of upper extremity injury.

PRINCIPLES OF MANAGEMENT

General Principles

The major principles of management for all orthopedic injuries are reduction to anatomic alignment, immobilization to allow healing, and rehabilitation. Pain control and measures to limit inflammation are useful adjuncts.

Reduction. Closed reduction of fractures and dislocations can, in most cases, be performed in the emergency department. Fractures and dislocations are invariably associated with spasm or contraction of the surrounding musculature. The resultant deformities can be explained with a knowledge of the involved anatomy. Reduction is much easier after spasm has been alleviated with analgesia or anesthesia. Overriding or shortening at the site of a fracture or dislocation is overcome by applying longitudinal traction to fatigue the contracting musculature. In most cases, this can be followed by appropriate manipulation of the distal bone to produce anatomic alignment. Periarticular fractures are often not amenable to closed reduction because the lever arm is too short to be manipulated. In cases of distal ischemia, reduction is attempted immediately to improve circulatory status. In less urgent circumstances, orthopedic consultation is obtained, after which the emergency physician or the orthopedist may perform the indicated reduction.

Analgesia or Anesthesia. Early administration of analgesics is indicated for patients who are stable and have purely orthopedic injuries. Major fractures and dislocations are extremely painful, and narcotic analgesics such as meperidine or morphine are appropriate. For minor reductions, such as interphalangeal dislocations, no anesthesia is needed. For major reductions, such as shoulder dislocations, intravenous analgesics and muscle relaxants such as diazepam are used. Reduction of fracture deformities is extremely painful. Anesthetic techniques that are used include hematoma blocks, nerve blocks, and intravenous regional anesthesia. Nitrous oxide-oxygen (Nitronox) by inhalation has been successfully used in the prehospital and emergency department setting.

Immobilization. Short-term immobilization is the appropriate emergent treatment for extremity injuries without complications. When there is a questionable fracture, immobilization and referral are standard procedures. Invariably, if there is significant suspicion of fracture, there is sufficient soft tissue injury alone to justify a period of rest.

Since most extremity injuries seen in the emergency department are acute and tissue edema has not yet reached maximum levels, circumferential rigid casting carries the real possibility of vascular compromise. For this reason, injuries are immobilized almost exclusively with noncircumferential plaster splints. This allows the elastic bandage to be loosened as the edema increases, and the neurovascular status can be easily monitored.

Therapeutic splinting always decreases pain by limiting bony fragment movement, inflammation, bleeding, and the risk of neurovascular compromise. As a general principle, immobilization of the joints above and below the site of the pathology is indicated. Joints not involved are not included needlessly, and, unless contraindicated, joints are immobilized in the position of function.

Commercially available prefabricated splints are available from numerous manufacturers. Although they have the advantage of speed and ease of use, they have the disadvantage of fitting less well than custom-made splints, thereby limiting the degree of immobilization while increasing the chance of "cast sores." The standard technique of splinting is making a plaster of Paris splint specifically for the patient. Prior to splinting, the extremity is padded with the joints in the desired positions. The padding is applied at least two layers thick in a circumferential manner, proceeding in a distal to proximal direction. Bony prominences and taut tendons receive a minimum of two additional layers. Padding is carried well beyond the limits of the plaster both distally and proximally. Trimming excessive padding can be done easily, but plaster must not be allowed to come into direct contact with the skin. Using a roll of padding with a small diameter and applying it with tension will avoid wrinkling. Rolls of plaster are measured on the patient; a general guideline is eight to ten layers on the upper extremity. Vigorous young people may require additional layers. The splint is molded to fit the bony contours while an assistant supports the limb in the exact position desired. Any movement at this stage creates hinging and renders the splint useless. An elastic bandage is applied from distal to proximal, and the splint is allowed to dry for approximately 30 minutes. Complications of plaster casts include cast pressure sores caused by wrinkles in the padding, inadequate padding, or finger indentations in the plaster; skin maceration resulting from skin being opposed to skin without a layer of padding between; and lack of sufficient immobilization, which occurs if the splint is "hinged" by movement at a joint during the curing (or hardening) phase of plaster splinting. Also, if there is insufficient mechanical massage to ensure interlocking of the plaster crystals between layers, a weak and easily damaged splint will be formed. If fast-setting plaster is used in combination with warm water, a thermal burn may add to the patient's injury due to exothermic heat dissipation from the formation of plaster of Paris. Increased pain in the extremity after a splint is applied necessitates immediate investigation.

With the use of customized (as opposed to preformed) plaster splints, specific individualized immobilization can be designed to fit any patient with any injury or combination of injuries. Some of the more commonly applied upper extremity splints and indications for their use are presented in Table 41–1. Because in some cases these splints may be worn for several weeks as definitive therapy, emergency department splinting is designed to provide proper fit, durability, comfort, and good immobilization.

A few comments about each major type of upper extremity splint are given below.

Long Arm Posterior Splint. Fractures and dislocations near the elbow are best treated with a long arm posterior splint. This splint is applied beginning at the ulnar aspect of the metacarpal heads, proceeding over the olecranon and up the posterior border of the arm to as proximal a position as is comfortable. Standard flexion is 90 degrees at the elbow. Usually neutral pronation-supination is appropriate and is achieved by placing the patient's thumb up.

TABLE 41–1. Immobilization of Specific Injuries

Injury	Usual Treatment
Shoulder dislocation	Reduction, sling and swath
Rotator cuff tear	Sling and swath
Acromioclavicular joint sprains	Sling (pulled tight)
Clavicular fracture	Sling or "figure of eight"
Elbow dislocation	Reduction, long arm posterior splint
Supracondylar fracture	Long arm posterior splint
Radial head fracture	Sugar tong splint
Olecranon fracture	Long arm posterior splint
Subluxation of radial head (nursemaid's elbow)	Reduction only
Midshaft ulnar (nightstick) fracture	Long arm posterior splint
Both-bone forearm fracture	Long arm posterior splint
Wrist fractures	Sugar tong splint or long arm posterior splint
Navicular fracture, thumb metacarpal fracture	Short arm thumb spica splint
Metacarpal fracture, e.g., fifth metacarpal head (boxer's fracture)	Ulnar gutter or radial gutter splint
Metacarpophalangeal joint dislocation	Short arm posterior splint
Ulnar collateral ligament tear (gamekeeper's thumb)	Short arm thumb spica splint
Phalangeal tuft fracture	Aluminum splint
Proximal phalanx fracture	Short arm posterior splint
Middle phalanx fracture	Aluminum splint
Interphalangeal joint injuries	Reduction, aluminum splint

Sugar Tong Splint. This splint is used for radial head and Colles' fractures. It is a long splint extending dorsally from the metacarpal heads around the elbow and then volarly back to the metacarpal heads. The advantage of this splint is that it gives both volar and dorsal fixation without the disadvantages of circumferential casting. Supination-pronation is eliminated at the elbow, but a moderate degree of elbow flexion and extension will remain.

Short Arm Splint. More stable wrist injuries, such as wrist extensor strains and impacted distal radius fractures, may be treated with either dorsal or volar short arm posterior molds. The elbow is left free, and iatrogenic stiffness is avoided. Volar-applied splints severely limit any functional use of the hand.

Ulnar Gutter Splint. Ulnar gutter splints are applied in the same way as the simple wrist splint. The splint is extended nearly to the end of the little finger and includes the ring and little fingers.

Radial Gutter Splint. The radial gutter splint is indicated for fractures of the second and third metacarpals and proximal phalanges of index and long fingers. Application necessitates a wide hole cutout for the thumb and thenar musculature.

Thumb Spica Splint. An effective thumb spica splint can be made by applying a dorsal wrist splint along with a 2- to 3-inch strip of plaster applied to the dorsum of the thumb. The thumb should be placed in opposition to the fingers as if a beverage can were being held in the hand.

Padded Aluminum Splint. Fractures of the middle and distal phalanges and post-reduction dislocations of the interphalangeal joints are treated with padded aluminum splints applied to the involved digit from the finger tip to the distal wrist crease. In general, all hand joints are placed in moderate flexion to avoid shortening of collateral ligaments and resultant stiffness. If there is rotatory deformity, as in spiral or long oblique fractures, an adjacent digit should be "buddy splinted" to the involved one.

Slings. Simple slings are useful in a number of situations simply to immobilize the upper extremity. For hand or wrist injuries, they should be applied so that the hand lies higher than the heart rather than with the traditional 90-degree flexion at the elbow. Slings may be used in combination with a swath, a circumferential bandage holding the arm adducted to the trunk to limit motion at the shoulder.

SPECIFIC INJURIES

Some of the more commonly encountered injuries of the upper extremity will be discussed with regard to mechanism of injury, presentation, radiologic diagnosis, and specific management.

Shoulder Injuries

Given the extensive range of motion of the shoulder joint, it is no surprise that shoulder stability is easily compromised. The shallow glenohumeral joint allows for extremes in movement. Joint stability is provided primarily by muscular and ligamentous attachments.

Anterior Shoulder Dislocation (Problem 1)

Shoulder dislocation is the most common major joint dislocation. Ninety-eight percent of cases are anterior dislocations, i.e., the head of the humerus comes to lie anterior, inferior, and medial to its normal position in relation to the glenoid.

Mechanism. The usual mechanism of injury that results in anterior dislocation is the application of leverage forces to the arm when it is in abduction and external rotation. Occasionally, direct force from behind, applied to the humeral head, can result in the same injury.

Presentation. Patients present in extreme pain, slumped forward supporting the injured arm with the well arm; extreme pain occurs with internal or external rotation. There is a characteristic "pointed" contour of the shoulder and a palpable hollow in the deltoid where the head of the humerus has vacated the glenoid cavity. Associated injuries include a usually transient nerve injury to the axillary nerve, producing hypesthesia over the deltoid, and avulsion fractures of the head of the humerus and inferior lip of the glenoid.

Radiologic Diagnosis. The standard anteroposterior and lateral views of the shoulder usually demonstrate the humeral head anterior, inferior, and medial to its normal position in the glenoid fossa. If these views are inconclusive, axillary views or scapular Y views are obtained. Axillary views are excellent for diagnosis of dislocation but are difficult to obtain owing to the requirement for abduction of the injured extremity. The scapular Y view avoids this difficulty and is the preferred view.

Management. The dislocation is reduced by reproducing the external rotation in combination with longitudinal traction. A multitude of methods have been advocated to accomplish this. The common theme is fatigue of the patient's shoulder muscles through continuous traction and intravenous muscle relaxants and *gentle* external rotation. Successful reduction is usually appreciated palpably and visually and is confirmed by the patient's ability to rotate the shoulder completely internally, as evidenced by the ability to touch the uninvolved shoulder with the index finger of the injured side.

After reduction the shoulder is held in adduction and internal rotation with a sling and swath device, and confirmatory radiographs are done. In general, a period of 3 weeks of immobilization is necessary to reduce the incidence of repeat dislocations. Patients are informed that there is a 25% chance of recurrence after one episode, a 50% chance after two, and nearly all patients who have had three dislocations require a surgical procedure to prevent chronic recurrent dislocation.

Rotator Cuff Tear

This is an injury to a group of muscles that cross the shoulder joint and give stability to it. The rotator cuff muscles are often mnemonically referred to as the SIT muscles: supraspinatus, infraspinatus, and teres minor (Fig. 41–1A).

Mechanism. A fall on the outstretched arm may tear any of these muscles without producing a fracture or dislocation.

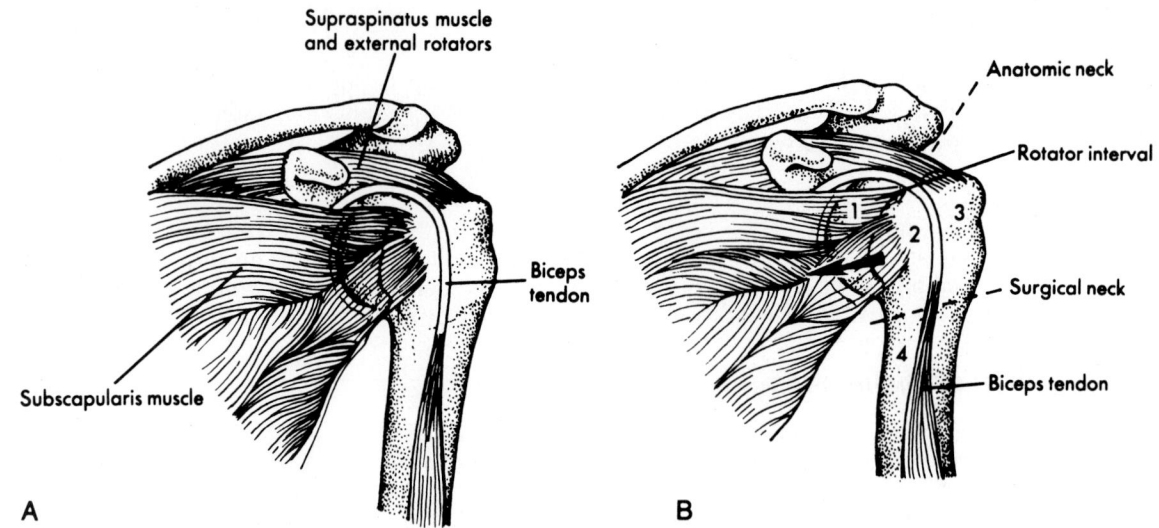

FIGURE 41–1. *Anatomy of the shoulder. (1, Head; 2, lesser tuberosity; 3, greater tuberosity; 4, shaft.) (From Orban DJ: Shoulder. In Rosen P, et al (eds): Emergency Medicine: Concepts and Clinical Practice (2nd ed), vol. 1. St. Louis, The C. V. Mosby Co., 1988.)*

Presentation. There is *relatively* painless passive range of motion. Active range of motion, notably initiation of external rotation and abduction, is very painful because the patient is asked to contract forcefully a muscle that has been partially torn.

Radiologic Diagnosis. The shoulder joint is intact and has a normal radiographic appearance.

Management. Emergency treatment consists of a short-term sling and swath and analgesics. When consultant referral may be delayed, the physician should instruct the patient in passive range of motion exercises. Pendulum motion with the olecranon describing larger and larger diameter circles is used to avoid the development of adhesive capsulitis, which can result in decreased range of motion.

Acromioclavicular Separations

The clavicle is bound to the scapula by two sets of strong ligaments, the coracoclavicular and acromioclavicular ligaments, and an acromioclavicular joint capsule.

Mechanism. When a strong force that displaces the scapula inferiorly is applied, these ligaments may tear. A common scenario is a football player carrying the ball with adducted arm who is tackled and lands on the lateral shoulder.

Presentation. A complete tear (class 3) is evidenced by a "free floating" clavicle. Physical examination displays a superiorly displaced, easily visualized lateral end of the clavicle, which is ballotable. Lesser tears may produce partial separations that result in displacement only with stress (class 2) or that result only in point tenderness at the sites of attachment, anterior and inferior to the lateral aspect of the clavicle (class 1).

Radiologic Diagnosis. Comparison x-rays of the normal side may be made, looking for relative widening. Weights can be held in the hands to confirm a suspected class 2 injury.

Management. Most partial separations are treated with a sling to elevate the scapula indirectly into apposition with the clavicle, along with analgesics. Complete separations are sometimes corrected surgically.

Clavicular Fractures

The clavicle functions as a strut that fixes the arm to the thorax.

Mechanism. A fall on the lateral aspect of the proximal arm is the usual mechanism of injury, and the middle third is the usual site of fracture.

Presentation. There is well-localized pain, swelling, and tenderness over the site of fracture. The arm is usually held against the chest to minimize movement.

Radiologic Diagnosis. Standard clavicular views demonstrate the fracture without difficulty.

Management. Realignment of fragments is difficult because the clavicle is the site of attachment of so many strong muscles both superiorly and inferiorly. Unless cosmesis is a strong concern, symptomatic treatment consists of a sling (to remove the weight of the arm from the lateral fragment) and possibly the "figure-of-eight" bandage for more anatomic alignment. No great effort need be made for anatomic alignment because it is said that "two pieces of clavicle in the same area code will heal fine." The patient is told that a visible and palpable subcutaneous callous will form as the clavicle remodels.

Humeral Fractures

Proximal Humerus. The proximal humerus is anatomically divided into four functional parts: anatomic neck, greater and lesser tuberosities, and surgical neck (Fig. 41–1B). The surgical neck is the site of most fractures.

Mechanism. Most proximal humeral fractures result from distal forces transmitted from a fall on the outstretched arm. A direct blow to the lateral shoulder may also be responsible.

Presentation. There are usually no findings except for pain and tenderness in the proximal upper arm and shoulder.

Radiologic Diagnosis. Standard shoulder views (anteroposterior and lateral) demonstrate the fracture in most cases.

Management. Rather impressive angular deformities may be tolerated in the interest of early movement. The inherent range of motion of the shoulder joint is far greater than that used by most individuals, so the shoulder is able to compensate for deformities that in other locations could not be tolerated. The issue of early motion of the shoulder joint is paramount. Even an uninjured shoulder that is immobilized for as little as 1 to 2 weeks may form an extremely debilitating adhesive capsulitis or "frozen shoulder." For this reason, proximal humerus fractures are immobilized acutely with sling and swath, and definite orthopedic referral is arranged within 48 hours.

Humeral Shaft Fractures

Mechanism. A blow to the lateral aspect of the arm is the common mechanism of injury.

Presentation. The patient complains of well-localized upper arm pain, and the extremity may be shortened or rotated. A wrist drop may be present owing to radial nerve injury. Most of the neurovascular bundle of the arm courses medial to and separated from the humerus, which affords it a certain amount of protection. The radial nerve, however, travels in the spiral groove of the humerus throughout most of its length and is frequently injured with midshaft humeral fractures.

Radiologic Diagnosis. These fractures are readily appreciated on plain radiographs of the humerus.

Management. Early management consists of sling and swath. Intramedullary rods, side plates, or passive traction may be elected later. Return to early motion is, again, of paramount importance.

Supracondylar Fractures (Problem 2)

Mechanisms. A fall on the outstretched arm with the elbow in flexion is the usual mechanism of injury.

Presentation. Supracondylar fractures are more common in children than in adults. The child usually presents while holding the arm as still as possible at 90 degrees of flexion at the elbow. There is usually marked swelling and tenderness about the elbow, and this injury can be clinically indistinguishable from an elbow dislocation.

Radiologic Diagnosis. The intra-articular hemorrhage produced by the fracture displaces the fat occupying the coronoid fossa anteriorly and the olecranon fossa posteriorly. These displacements are seen radiographically as a triangle-shaped radiolucency anterior to the distal humeral shaft (sail sign) and a more linear lucency posterior to the distal humeral shaft (Fig. 41–2). These signify joint effusion—always presumed to be blood in the context of acute trauma. To evaluate the degree of posterior angulation that is present, a straight line is traced down the anterior border of the capitellum (Fig. 41–3).

Management. Supracondylar fractures are potentially limb-threatening owing to a possible compromise of the blood supply due to shearing forces or pressure from developing hematoma and edema. Ischemia of the forearm is devastating. Close monitoring of vascular status is necessary. Long arm splinting, maintaining accessibility to both the antecubital fossa and the distal neurovascular examination sites, is recommended. Hospitalization to monitor neurovascular status closely is indicated.

Elbow Injury

Elbow Dislocation

Mechanism. Falls on the outstretched arm, usually with the elbow in some degree of flexion, are responsible for this injury.

Presentation. The patient presents with shortening of the forearm and with the olecranon tenting the skin posteriorly. This injury can be confused with a supracondylar fracture.

Radiologic Diagnosis. Anteroposterior and lateral views of the elbow reveal the coronoid process below the trochlea and displaced posterior to the humerus (Fig. 41–4). The coronoid and medial epicondyles are commonly fractured in conjunction with the dislocation.

Management. Reduction should be prompt. It is performed by reproducing the mechanism of injury with inferior traction on the proximal forearm, followed by longitu-

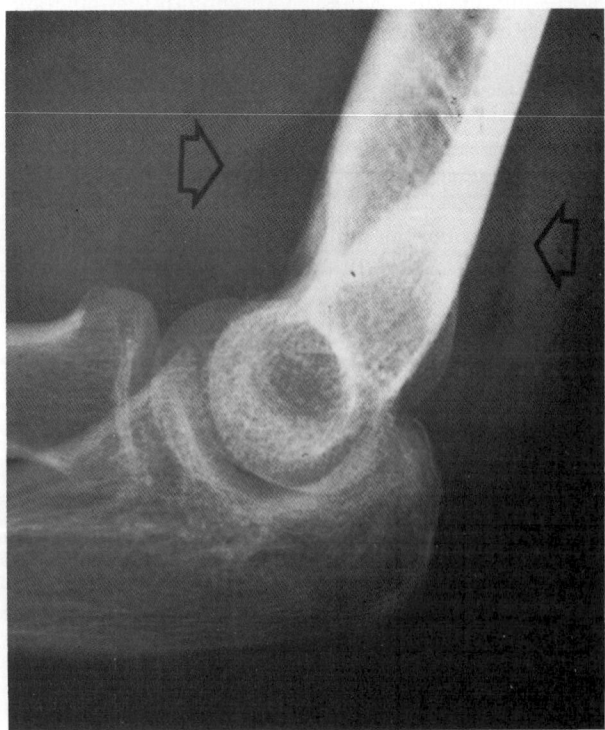

FIGURE 41–2. The typical roentgen configuration and appearance of the anterior and posterior olecranon fat pad signs (open arrows) in the lateral radiograph. (From Harris JH, Jr, Harris WH (eds): The Radiology of Emergency Medicine (2nd ed). © 1981, The Williams & Wilkins Co., Baltimore.)

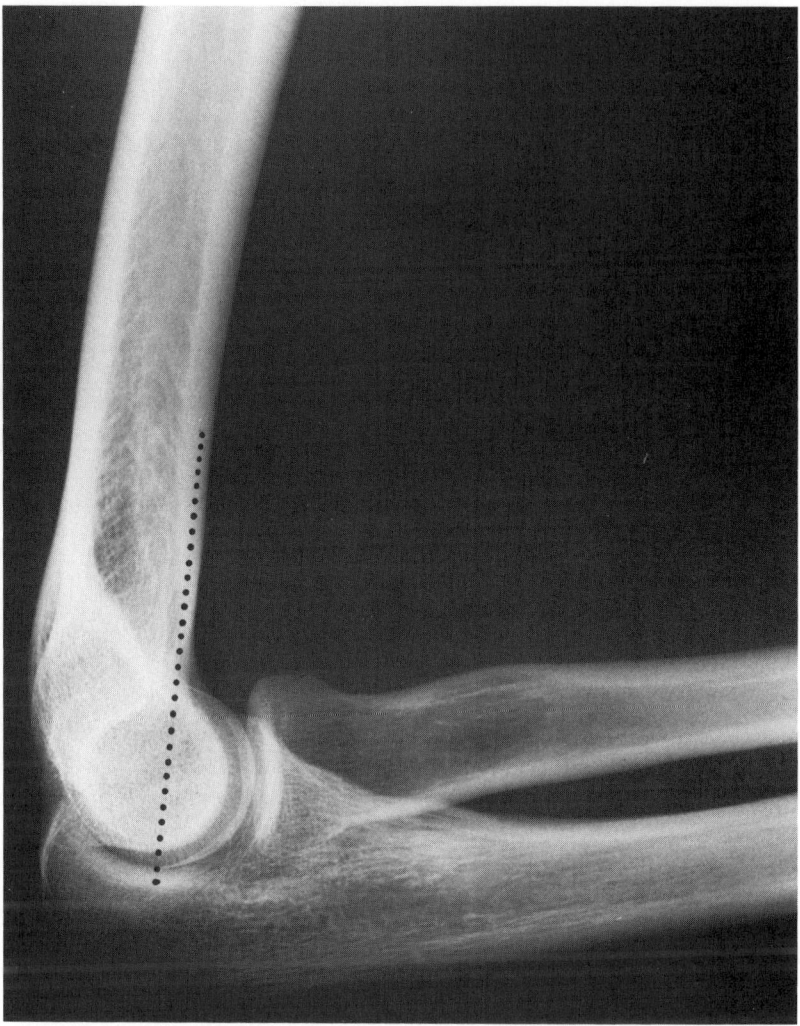

FIGURE 41–3. Supracondylar fracture: line traced down anterior border of capitellum to evaluate degree of posterior angulation.

dinal traction on the forearm and then flexion. Reduction of the radius may not occur simultaneously with that of the ulna and is confirmed with smooth supination-pronation.

Radial Head Fracture

Mechanism. Force absorbed when a person falls and lands on the outstretched arm is transmitted up the forearm, thrusting the radial head against the capitellum. Although the capitellum of the humerus may be fractured, the radial head is fractured far more commonly.

Presentation. The usual presentation is point tenderness of the radial head deep in the proximal extensor forearm muscles that is exacerbated by supination of the forearm, which the patient holds in pronation.

Radiologic Diagnosis. Often no fracture line is visible on radiologic examination. The pathologic fat pad signs discussed earlier under Supracondylar Fracture may be seen, leading to the diagnosis.

Management. Severity varies from minimal fractures with essentially no depression of the articular surface and requiring only brief immobilization to those in which a large percentage of the articular surface is depressed; these require removal and prosthetic replacement of the radial head.

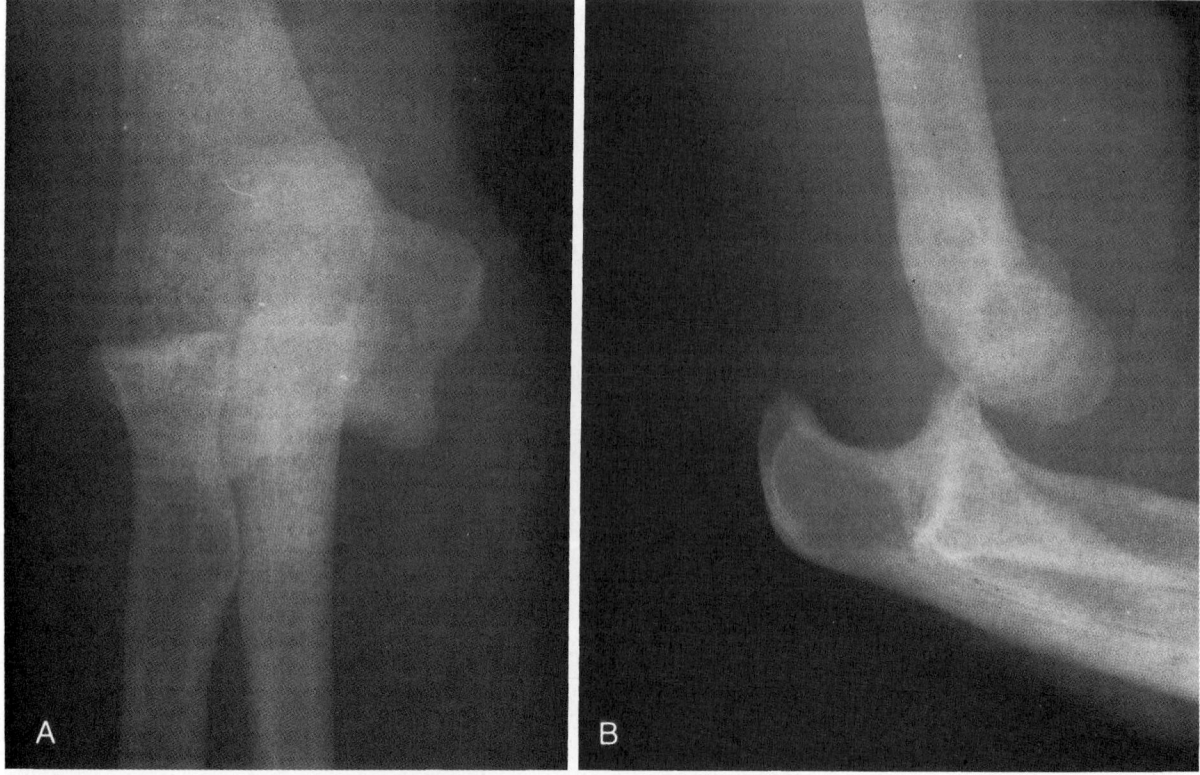

FIGURE 41–4. A and B, Complete posterior dislocation of the elbow. (From Harris JH, Jr, Harris WH (eds): The Radiology of Emergency Medicine (2nd ed). © 1981, The Williams & Wilkins Co., Baltimore.)

Olecranon Process Fractures

Mechanism. Falls directly on the elbow and forceful contraction of the triceps muscle resulting in avulsion are the mechanisms of injury.

Presentation. There is well-localized swelling and tenderness over the olecranon, and separation at the fracture site is sometimes palpable because the olecranon is covered by minimal tissue. Elbow extension will be weak or absent. Sensory and motor deficits in the hand due to ulnar nerve dysfunction are possible (Chap. 42).

Radiologic Diagnosis. The lateral view of the elbow will demonstrate the fracture nicely. Due to the distractive forces created by the triceps muscle, there is frequently proximal migration of the fragment.

Management. Long-arm splinting with the elbow held at 90 degrees is adequate emergency department management. Most of these injuries will require open reduction and internal fixation.

Radial Head Subluxation (Nursemaid's Elbow, Problem 3)

Mechanism. An unsuspected longitudinal traction applied to the hand is the cause of the injury. This usually occurs when the slowly ambulating toddler is rescued from falling or possibly "encouraged" to hurry up. This injury happens commonly in children under age 5 years and is usually caused by a well-meaning adult. It should not be construed as evidence of child abuse.

Presentation. Children display a phenomenon called "pseudoparalysis" whenever a given limb is injured anywhere along its length. Careful palpation, observation, and ingenuity in examining the extremity will elucidate the site of injury and avoid unnecessary entire limb radiographs. On careful examination, one will note that the hand itself functions normally if objects are brought to it. Similarly, shoulder motion is unlimited and is not associated with tenderness. The specific motion of supinating the pronated elbow elicits exquisite pain.

Management. The same motion, supination, followed by flexion at the elbow, reduces the injury. Within a short time (15 minutes) most children will forget that their elbow was painful and will be using the limb normally—a near miracle in the eyes of a grateful parent. No immobilization is necessary.

Forearm Fractures

The forearm, with its vulnerable position and protective function, is commonly injured. Direct blows aimed for the head are commonly absorbed or deflected by the ulnar aspect of the forearm. Falls on the outstretched arm continue to be the most common mechanism for the great majority of upper extremity injuries and account for countless forearm fractures.

An important orthopedic principle, illustrated in the forearm, is that injury to one of two bones running parallel to each other by necessity affects the other bone. This second injury may be another fracture or a dislocation at the proximal or distal end.

Ulnar Shaft Fracture (Nightstick Fracture)

Mechanism. A direct blow to the elevated ulnar shaft in a maneuver to defend the face or head is the usual scenario.

Presentation. Well-localized swelling and tenderness on the ulnar aspect of the forearm is usually the only finding.

Radiologic Diagnosis. Anteroposterior and lateral forearm views will demonstrate the fracture. This is the one exception to the previously stated principle of both-bone involvement in an injury. With neither tenderness nor radiographic evidence of radial injury at the elbow or wrist, one may presume the ulna alone to be injured.

Management. The intact radius and significant amounts of surrounding muscle bellies provide a splint. A long arm plaster splint adds to the immobilization and provides protection against further injury.

Combined Radial and Ulnar Shaft Fracture

Mechanism. A very forceful direct blow is necessary to fracture both bones. Sometimes the bones of the forearm will fracture if too much force is applied to either end.

Presentation. These patients frequently present with marked swelling and tenderness involving a large portion of the forearm. The elbow or the wrist may be involved.

Radiologic Diagnosis. With the splinting action of the intact radius lost, these fractures tend to be displaced or badly angulated. Commonly, subluxations at the wrist or elbow are associated.

Management. These injuries generally require urgent orthopedic referral for reduction under general anesthesia.

Wrist Fractures

The wrist in its role of supporting and moving the hand is prone to many injuries. By far the most common mechanism of injury is a fall on the outstretched hand. Depending on the exact vector of forces applied, distal radial and ulnar fractures, carpal fractures, or intercarpal dislocations (lunate and perilunate dislocations) can occur. The dorsally displaced radial and ulnar fracture (Colles' fracture) is by far the most common type.

Forced volar flexion of the wrist is an unusual mechanism of injury but can occur during falls or fights. A dorsal sprain of the wrist joint is possible, but if there is significant ligamentous injury, instability will again lead to intercarpal dislocation.

Smith's fracture may result from severe volarly directed forces on the distal forearm. The result is a distal radial and ulnar fracture with volar displacement.

Colles' Fracture

Mechanism. The common mechanism is a fall on the outstretched arm with the wrist in dorsiflexion.

Presentation. Swelling and tenderness at the wrist are present, and, depending on the degree of displacement, there may be significant deformity with the distal radial fragment angulating dorsally to form the "dinner fork" deformity. Median nerve dysfunction may result in numbness in the hand (Chap. 42).

Radiologic Diagnosis. Fracture of the distal radius with dorsal displacement is obvious on standard anteroposterior and lateral views of the wrist. Sixty percent of patients have an associated ulnar styloid fracture.

Management. A dorsal-volar splint such as a "sugar tong" is the preferred treatment. Orthopedic follow-up within 24 hours is recommended.

Navicular Fractures (Problem 4)

Mechanism. A fall on the outstretched arm is the cause.

Presentation. These fractures are suspected when the maximal point of tenderness is at the anatomic snuffbox with ulnar wrist deviation. The anatomic snuffbox is the depression formed at the radial aspect of the wrist when the thumb is abducted and extended, as in a hitch-hiking sign. The tendons forming the anatomic snuffbox are the abductor pollicis longus and the extensor pollicis brevis on the volar boundary and the extensor pollicis on the dorsal boundary.

Radiologic Diagnosis. The absence of radiographic visualization of an acute fracture must not dissuade the clinician from treating this injury. These fractures are notoriously difficult to visualize and may require a repeat radiograph in 2 weeks when resorption of bone along the fracture line allows visualization.

Management. Immobilization must include the forearm, wrist, and thumb to minimize an impressive 30% rate of nonunion or avascular necrosis. A tenuous blood supply, distal to proximal, combined with the absence of any muscular attachments contributing perforating arteries predisposes this bone to poor healing. A period of immobilization followed by repeat radiographs is often necessary. Even with optimal care these fractures have high complication rates (Fig. 41–5).

Hand Fractures and Joint Injuries

The hand is subject to a great array of trauma given its vulnerable position and its relationship to labor. Associated disability is also devastating economically.

Metacarpal Fractures

Mechanism. The fifth metacarpal is by far the most commonly fractured bone in the hand, usually when its owner strikes a mandible, wall, or other nonforgiving structure with a closed fist (boxer's fracture).

Presentation. The patient may be reluctant to give an honest history. Any abrasion, laceration, or puncture wound in the area should arouse the suspicion of a human bite. Even an apparently trivial skin disruption over a metacarpophalangeal joint may have been caused by a tooth entering the joint with subsequent bacterial seeding.

Radiologic Diagnosis. Anteroposterior, lateral, and oblique views of the hand are standard. Metacarpal shaft fractures are usually obvious but a minimally displaced fracture of the head of a metacarpal can be quite subtle.

Management. Immediate exploration or at least admission for elevation, intravenous antibiotics, and observation is indicated when joint penetration is a possibility. It is indeed fortunate that this most commonly fractured metacarpal is also the most mobile. This mobility allows compensation for the volar angulation of the distal fragment without loss of function.

An identical fracture of the index or long finger metacarpal needs anatomic reduction through operative means to avoid functional loss. Percutaneous k-wires are usually placed to hold the reduction in place. Fractures of the fourth metacarpal fall somewhere between these two extremes. Twenty-four-hour orthopedic referrals are recommended because many of these fractures will start to heal quickly, in whatever position the bones are in.

UPPER EXTREMITY INJURY: CLOSED INJURIES — 719

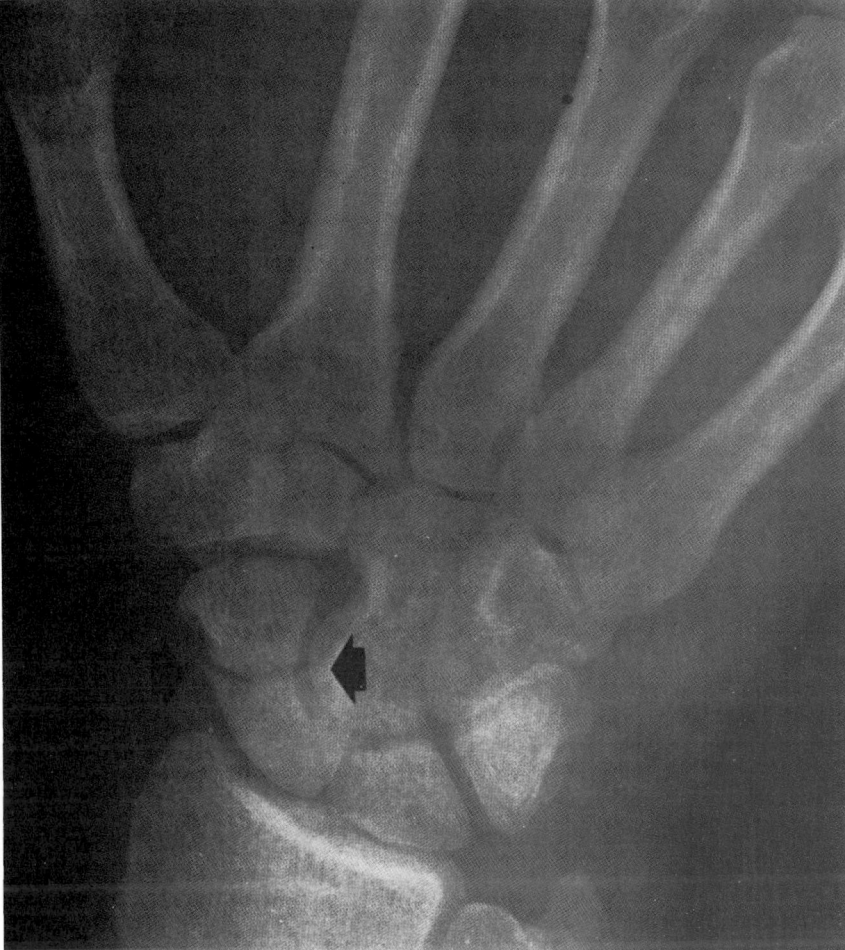

FIGURE 41-5. Navicular fracture. (From Harris JH, Jr, Harris WH (eds): *The Radiology of Emergency Medicine* (2nd ed). © 1981, The Williams & Wilkins Co., Baltimore.)

Fractures of the first metacarpal result in the thumb becoming unstable relative to the rest of the hand. The proximal fragment invariably carries with it the only strong ligamentous attachments to the carpals. Repair requires operative management, but in the acute situation the joint can be splinted with a thumb spica pending further treatment.

Metacarpophalangeal Dislocations

The fifth and index metacarpophalangeal (MCP) joints are most likely to be involved in dislocations. These injuries are termed *dorsal dislocations* because of the dorsal position of the proximal phalanx relative to the metacarpal.

Mechanism. The mechanism is a volar depression of the head of the metacarpal through the volar plate (Fig. 41-6). The metacarpal head comes to lie in a bayonet apposition with the proximal phalanx, and the finger flexors come to lie in a nooselike fashion around the neck of the metacarpal.

Presentation. There is well-localized tenderness and swelling at the base of the involved finger.

Radiologic Diagnosis. Standard hand films reveal dorsal dislocation of the MCP joint—i.e., the proximal phalanx comes to lie dorsal to the metacarpal head. The fifth and index MCP joints are most likely to be involved owing to their greater mobility.

Management. Longitudinal traction on the digit to effect a reduction results in tightening of these tendons and inability to reduce the metacarpal head through the rent in the volar plate. Operative reduction is necessary.

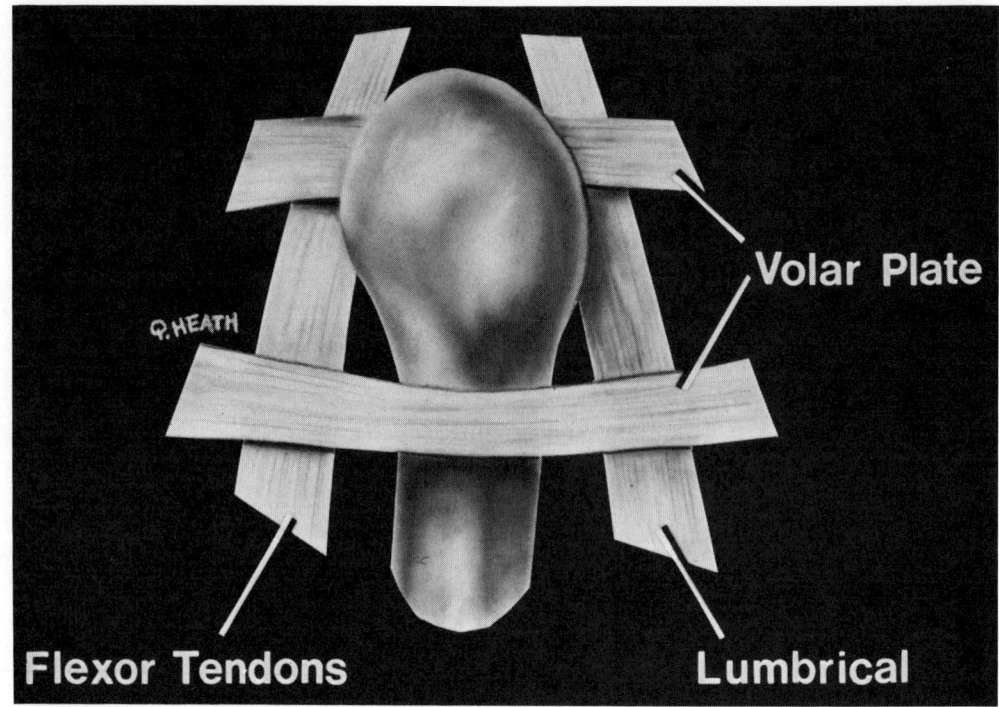

FIGURE 41–6. *Irreducible dislocation of the digital metacarpophalangeal joint, with metacarpal head rupturing through the volar plate. Arranged in a tight, sphincterlike fashion are the split-volar plate, lumbricals, and long flexor tendons. Attempts at reduction with longitudinal traction further tighten the ring by tightening the lumbricals and flexors against the thin metacarpal neck. (From Hossfeld GE: Joint injuries of the hand. Reprinted from Trauma Quarterly, vol. 1, No. 2, p. 80, with permision of Aspen Publishers, Inc., © February 1985.)*

Thumb MCP Ulnar Collateral Ligament Sprain (Gamekeeper's Thumb)

Mechanism. The mechanism of this injury is transient lateral dislocation of the thumb at the metacarpophalangeal joint that has spontaneously reduced. Strong acute or repeated lateral stresses act to deviate the mobile thumb away from the fixed elements of the hand, with subsequent rupture of the ulnar collateral ligament. Today it is seen most commonly with ski pole injuries.

Presentation. Stress testing of the ulnar collateral ligament will display more than 40 degree angulation with the MCP in extension if there is complete rupture.

Radiologic Diagnosis. Radiographic assessment of the joint will be normal.

Management. Surgical repair is necessary because in two-thirds of cases the abductor pollicis lies interposed between the two ends of the torn ligament, and no amount of immobilization will allow healing. Repair can be done electively at a later date.

Middle and Proximal Phalangeal Fractures

Mechanism. Hyperextension, torsion, and direct blows to the digit are common mechanisms.

Presentation. Deforming forces of the musculotendinous attachments may result in angulation or rotational deformity. Both abnormalities must be sought and corrected.

Radiologic Diagnosis. Standard hand or single finger views adequately demonstrate the disruption of the shaft.

Management. Many of these injuries are unstable to closed reduction and require internal wire fixation. This is true even of avulsion fractures. The insertions of the extensor and flexor tendons as well as the volar plate and collateral ligaments all may avulse their bony attachments given a strong enough deforming force. These injuries are often best treated with open wire fixation. Emergently, splinting in the position of relaxation of the involved avulsed structure with timely (within 48 hours) referral to an orthopedist is indicated to ensure rapid return to functional stability without unnecessary stiffness due to prolonged immobilization. Fractures entering the articular surfaces are also generally unstable and are best treated by prompt referral. Anatomic reopposition of the articular cartilage is mandatory to minimize joint stiffness.

Distal Phalangeal Tuft Fractures

Mechanism. These injuries usually result from a crush mechanism.

Presentation. These fractures may be open or may be associated with subungual hematoma. The patient complains of marked throbbing of the fingertip.

Radiologic Diagnosis. The specific finger in question can be visualized separately if the injury is isolated. Comminution of the tuft is common.

Management. These fractures heal satisfactorily if they are protected with a padded aluminum splint. Prophylactic antibiotics may be given if the fracture is open.

Dislocations of the Proximal Interphalangeal Joints

Mechanism. These injuries occur with or without concomitant fracture, but all involve rupture of the ligamentous structures. Hyperextension or a lateral force with the joint extended are common mechanisms.

Presentation. Due to minimal surrounding soft tissue, the dorsal displacement of the middle phalanx relative to the proximal phalanx is obvious.

Radiologic Diagnosis. A radiograph is useful in identifying concomitant fractures. It is repeated after reduction.

Management. Reduction is easily accomplished with longitudinal traction to reduce the bayonet apposition, followed by appropriate manipulation of the middle phalanx to alignment. Reduction is best done after a digital block, both for patient comfort and to enable the physician to assess the stability of the joint after reduction. If the reduced joint can be passively or actively put through a range of motion without recurrent dislocation, management is conservative. Avoidance of open repair obviates foreign body reaction with resultant stiffness.

Dislocations of the Distal Interphalangeal Joints

Mechanism. Strong hyperextension or a lateral deforming force with the joint in extension is necessary to produce these injuries. Multiple strong osteocutaneous fibers stabilize these joints.

Presentation. These injuries usually present as open dislocations. The same osteocutaneous fibers that provide stability result in shearing injuries to the overlying skin.

Radiologic Diagnosis. These dislocations are obvious. Radiographs may reveal concomitant fracture.

Management. Irrigation, debridement, reduction by longitudinal traction, and prophylactic antibiotics are indicated.

Sprains of the Finger Joints

Mechanism. Hyperextension and abduction forces applied across the proximal interphalangeal (PIP) joint are the most common mechanisms. These injuries occur most frequently in contact sports.

Presentation. The patient complains of tenderness about the PIP joint. Stress testing of the lateral collateral ligaments and joint capsule, after adequate anesthesia, may demonstrate incomplete ligamentous tears.

Radiologic Diagnosis. Standard films will be normal. Stress views will demonstrate the instability, but these are rarely done in the emergency department.

Management. Although the ligamentous disruption may be nearly complete, surgical repair is seldom indicated because the remaining intact fibers align the torn segments anatomically, where they will heal nicely with minimal fibrosis. Stiffness rather than instability is a more likely complication.

Whenever possible, immobilization should be accomplished with the joint in the flexed position and should be of brief duration. Referral is helpful to ensure proper rehabilitation.

Mallet Finger

Loss of extensor tendon attachment to the distal phalanx by disruption of the tendon or avulsion of a chip from the base of the distal phalanx results in the deformity of the fingertip described as the mallet finger.

Mechanism. Forceful flexion of the distal interphalangeal (DIP) joint, such as occurs from jamming the fingertip, is the mechanism of injury.

Presentation. Patients may present acutely with a tender DIP joint and flexion deformity. Others may present with a history of trauma that occurred days to weeks before and with a persistent deformity.

Radiologic Diagnosis. Plain films may be normal or may reveal an avulsed fragment at the base of the distal phalanx.

Management. Dorsal splinting of the DIP joint only, in slight hyperextension, is usually effective if it is maintained for 6 to 12 weeks. If there is an avulsed fragment or if splinting is ineffective, open reduction and internal fixation are indicated.

SPECIAL CONSIDERATIONS

Pediatric Patients

Although many of the principles of adult orthopedics can be applied to the pediatric population, there are many special considerations also. Accurate historical information is often unavailable, and an adequate physical examination may be difficult. Moreover, roentgenographic diagnosis is difficult owing to the radiolucency of developing bone and the variable appearance of secondary centers of ossification. Comparison radiographic views of the contralateral "normal" extremity are often essential in diagnosing abnormalities. In general, children's fractures heal more rapidly and are more likely to undergo extensive remodeling with age compared with adults, but epiphyseal (growth plate) injuries may lead to growth arrest or progressive deformity of the extremity. The pediatric patient with an extremity injury cannot be treated merely as a "little adult."

Torus and Greenstick Fractures. Torus and greenstick fractures are common and unique to children. These fractures occur when the relatively resilient bone of children allows only a localized break in the cortex. As the analogy implies, a greenstick fracture occurs when bowing of a long bone results in an incomplete fracture. A part of the cortex breaks while the cortex opposite it undergoes only a plastic deformity. The torus fracture is similar but involves a localized buckling of the cortex due to an axial load rather than bending (Fig. 41–7A and B). The torus fracture may be quite subtle and is often missed on initial review of the radiographs.

Epiphyseal Injuries. The presence of epiphyseal plates in the growing bones of children creates a whole class of injuries that are unknown in adulthood. Because their ligaments are strong relative to the areas of calcifying cartilage in the growth plate, stress near a joint is likely to cause a fracture or fracture-separation in the zone of the epiphysis. With this in mind, one cannot dismiss stress-induced pain and swelling near a joint in a child as a "sprain." Several classifications of these fractures have been proposed, but the Salter-Harris classification (Fig. 41–8) has provided the basis for discussion of these injuries for the last 30 years. Not only does classifying a pediatric fracture according to Salter-Harris criteria provide a clear picture of the fracture to the consulting orthopedist on the phone, it also provides some prognostic value.

Salter-Harris type I fractures involve only the epiphyseal plate. No fracture line is seen because the epiphyseal plate is radiolucent. Displacement of the epiphysis makes diagnosis obvious, but a nondisplaced type I fracture may appear radiographically normal. It is of paramount importance that any injury in a child sustaining trauma with tenderness over an epiphyseal plate be treated as a nondisplaced type I injury in spite of the normal appearance of the appropriate x-rays. *This is a clinical diagnosis.* Failure to immobilize and protect this injury adequately may lead to subsequent subluxation of the epiphysis, thereby causing additional injury to the growth plate and necessitating a reduction. The epiphyseal area of growing bone is delicate. Failure to treat these injuries may increase the incidence of growth disturbance and subsequent dysfunction.

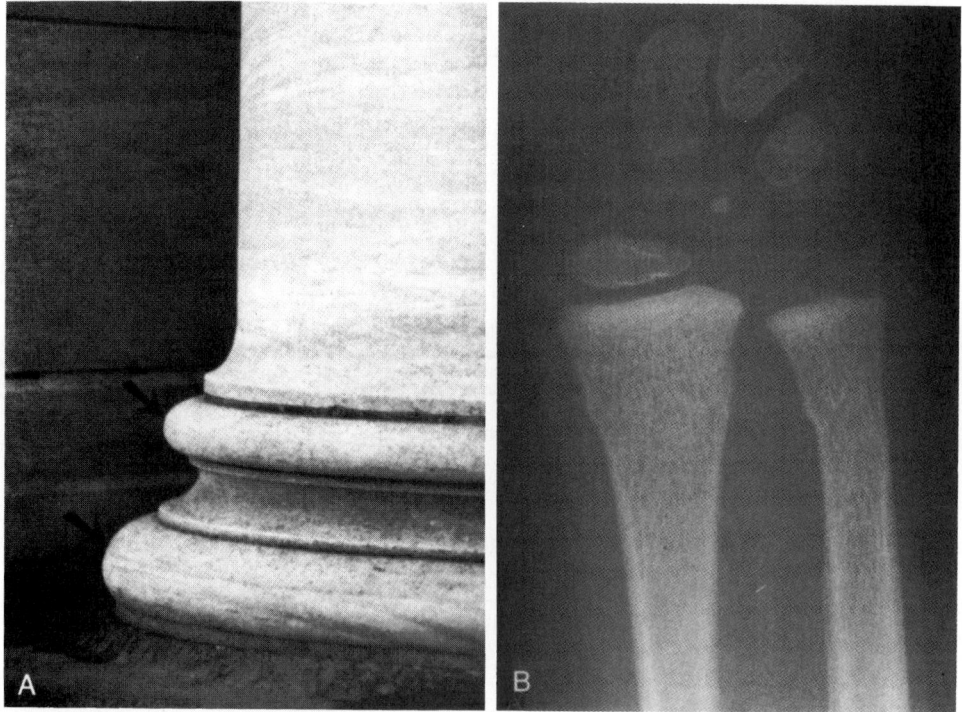

FIGURE 41-7. A, *The convex moldings at the base of a column are the origin of the term* torus fracture. *The tori are indicated by arrows.* B, *The pronounced bulging of the cortex* (arrows) *represents buckling bone, a so-called torus fracture.* (From Kirschner SG, et al (eds): Advanced Exercises in Diagnostic Radiology. Philadelphia, W. B. Saunders, 1981.)

Type II Salter-Harris injuries are similar to type I injuries in that the translucent epiphyseal plate remains contiguous and attached to the epiphyseal fragment. Type II injuries differ only in that the fracture line exits from the metaphyseal bone, creating a small radiologically visible fragment. Because the epiphyseal plate remains intact, type I and type II injuries have a lower incidence of growth disturbance and later deformity. The most common epiphyseal injury is a type II fracture-separation of the distal radius.

The type III Salter-Harris fracture describes an injury in which the fracture line exits through epiphyseal bone, revealing an epiphyseal fragment on the radiograph. The fracture is not only intra-articular but also causes injury to the epiphyseal plate. The epiphyseal plate, although radiographically invisible, always remains with the visualized epiphysis.

Salter-Harris type IV fractures have a fracture line vertical to the epiphyseal plate, which results in epiphyseal *and* metaphyseal fragments. As in type III fractures, they are intra-articular and injurious to the epiphyseal plate. Types III and IV injuries may require open reduction to restore articular and epiphyseal anatomy. Both have a poorer prognosis than type I and II fractures.

Type V injuries are potentially devastating injuries that may appear radiographically benign. An axial loading force may crush the epiphyseal plate, but only a subtle decrease in the height of the radiographically lucent space represents the area of calcifying cartilage. As in nondisplaced type I injuries, this injury must be suspected and diagnosed clinically.

All epiphyseal injuries (except presumptively diagnosed nondisplaced Salter-Harris I fractures) require prompt orthopedic consultation. The injury is immobilized in a plaster splint. Rapid follow-up is important because children undergo rapid bone repair, and extensive bony bridging may hinder reduction if it is performed late. Hospitalization may

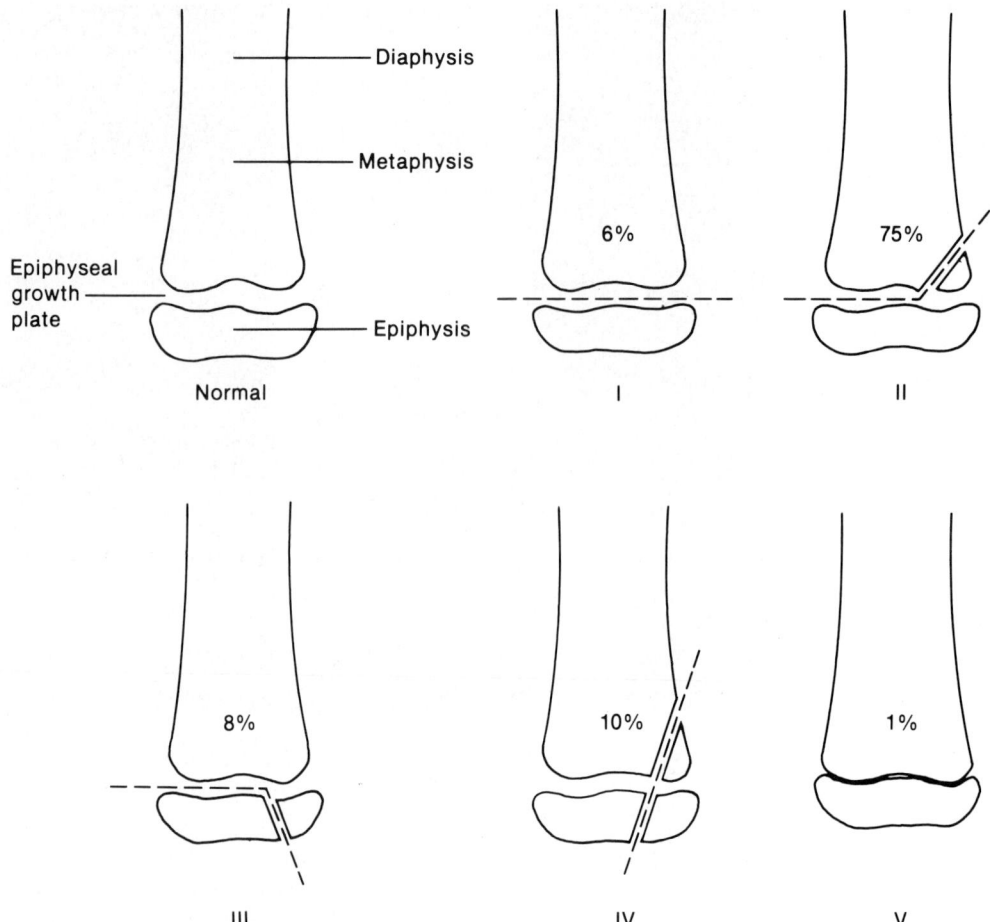

FIGURE 41–8. Salter-Harris classification of epiphyseal injury. Percentages shown represent the relative incidences. Dotted lines represent the path of fracture.

be indicated for Salter-Harris types III, IV, and V fractures. Parents are made aware immediately that epiphyseal injuries may give rise to deformity or growth arrest in the involved limb in spite of appropriate and timely care.

Geriatric Patients

The important principle in treating fractures or postreduction dislocations in the elderly is to limit the time of joint immobilization. This may be difficult because healing times may be longer, but recovery from a "frozen" joint is slow and painful.

DISPOSITION AND FOLLOW-UP

Admission or Immediate Orthopedic Consultation

Certain orthopedic injuries will require urgent operative intervention, and others are associated with complications frequent enough to warrant immediate telephone or on-site consultation. These include:
1. Open fractures or dislocations.
2. Injuries associated with real or potential neurovascular compromise.

3. Injuries known to be unstable to closed management.
4. Salter-Harris types III, IV, and V epiphyseal injuries in pediatric patients.
5. Irreducible fractures and dislocations.
6. Any injury with which the emergency physician feels uncomfortable.

Discharge and Follow-Up

Most orthopedic injuries can be effectively treated with emergency department management and timely orthopedic follow-up. Follow-up is essential, and the patient's compliance with the recommended referral is improved markedly if he is given explicit instructions as to who he is to see, the location of the doctor's office, and the specific time of the appointment.

Patient education includes instructions for
1. Keeping splints dry
2. Elevating the limb and using ice packs liberally for the first 24 hours
3. Loosening the Ace wrap if tingling or coolness of the fingers develops or if there is increased pain
4. Returning to the emergency department if these problems do not promptly resolve or if any difficulty with treatment or follow-up is encountered.

Adequate pain medication is supplied. The type and severity of injury will dictate the need for oral narcotics, nonsteroidal anti-inflammatory drugs, aspirin, or acetaminophen.

DOCUMENTATION

1. Mechanism and timing of injury.
2. Occupation and leisure activities.
3. Signs on presentation: deformity, edema, ecchymosis, crepitance, skin and neurovascular integrity, tenderness, range of motion.
4. Results of x-ray examination.
5. Procedures such as reduction of fractures or dislocations and the results of such procedures.
6. Immobilization, including the type and neurovascular status before and after application.
7. Medications and instructions for their use.
8. Therapeutic instructions, warnings, and follow-up instructions.

SUMMARY AND FINAL POINTS

- Upper extremity injuries are rarely life-threatening, and they must never take priority over threats to life.
- Injuries to the hands and arms may have significant impact on a patient's ability to hold gainful employment and enjoy leisure activities.
- The mechanism of injury is delineated when possible because it will assist in determining potential injuries.
- Physical findings on careful examination will reveal the specific site of injury in most patients and will guide the ordering of diagnostic radiographs.
- Emergency department reduction and immobilization followed by orthopedic referral are appropriate for most fractures and dislocations.
- Immediate orthopedic consultation and consideration for admission are indicated for open fractures or dislocations, neurovascular compromise, fractures that are not amenable to closed management, irreducible fractures or dislocations, and high-grade epiphyseal fractures.

BIBLIOGRAPHY

Texts
1. Eaton RG: Joint Injuries of the Hand. Springfield, Charles C Thomas, 1972.
2. Hoppenfeld S: Physical Examination of the Spine and Extremities. New York, Appleton-Century-Crofts, 1976.
3. Rockwood CA Jr, Green DP: Fractures (Vol 1). Philadelphia, Lippincott, 1975.
4. Salter RB: Textbook of Disorders and Injuries of the Musculoskeletal System (2nd ed). Baltimore, Williams & Wilkins, 1983.
5. Simon RR, Koenigsknecht SJ: Emergency Orthopedics: The Extremities. New York, Appleton-Century-Crofts, 1987.

Journal Article
1. Hossfeld GE: Joint injuries of the hand. Trauma Q 1(2):74–82, 1985.

CHAPTER 42

OPEN INJURIES TO THE HAND AND WRIST

DENNIS T. UEHARA, M.D.

PROBLEM A 24 year old man was injured at work when his hand was accidentally caught in the machine he was operating. Co-workers freed his hand, wrapped it with a towel, and brought the patient to the emergency department.

QUESTIONS TO CONSIDER

1. Which surface landmarks of the hand assist in identifying potential deep structure involvement?
2. What important nerves, tendons, and arteries may be involved in volar and dorsal lacerations of the wrist?
3. What motor functions and sensory distributions correspond to the radial, median, and ulnar nerves?
4. What techniques of physical examination are used to identify arterial, nerve, and tendon injuries in the wrist and hand?
5. Which infectious complications must be considered when treating open hand injuries?
6. When is it necessary to refer the patient to a hand surgeon?

INTRODUCTION

Most traumatic injuries to the hand are initially managed by physicians who have little or no formal training in hand surgery. The majority of these can be treated appropriately in the emergency department, but others require treatment by specialists in hand surgery. Since functional recovery is often determined by initial management, it is essential that all physicians managing injuries of the hand understand the intricacies of its evaluation and treatment. A thorough knowledge of the structural and functional anatomy of the hand is the basis for the proper care of hand injuries.

Acute injuries to the hand constitute 5% to 10% of all patient complaints evaluated in the emergency department. The male-to-female ratio is approximately 2:1. Sixty percent of patients are between the ages of 16 and 32. Lacerations are the most common injuries, accounting for over 50% of all hand-related complaints. An emergency physician working in a busy department will see approximately 400 hand injuries per year. Because many of these involve injuries to deep structures, it is imperative that all wounds be evaluated thoroughly for injuries to nerves, tendons, arteries, and bone.

PREHOSPITAL CARE

The rescue squad's responsibility is first to ensure respiratory and hemodynamic stability and then to care for the injured hand.

History

The rescue squad at the scene should determine:
1. The mechanism of injury if not obvious ("how did it happen?")
2. An estimate of the amount and kind of contamination at the scene

Physical Examination

1. Is the hand grossly intact? Are there amputated parts?
2. Is the basic grasp function intact?

Intervention

1. If bleeding is present, it is controlled by direct pressure.
2. In the presence of significant blood loss, an intravenous infusion of isotonic crystalloid solution is established.
3. The hand is then wrapped in saline-moistened sterile gauze, a splint is applied, and the hand is elevated during transport.
4. Amputated parts are placed in saline-moistened sterile gauze, sealed in a plastic bag, and placed on ice, if available.

INITIAL APPROACH IN THE EMERGENCY DEPARTMENT

Most open injuries to the hand can be managed in the minor treatment area. Exceptions include exsanguinating injuries caused by lacerations of the radial or ulnar arteries, major amputations, and injuries associated with life-threatening conditions unrelated to the hand. Evaluation of these patients includes the following steps:

Primary Assessment and Resuscitation. Mutilating injuries of the hand are impressive and seem to demand immediate evaluation and treatment. If, however, the hand injury is part of multisystemic trauma, the general principles of evaluation and resuscitation are attended to before the hand is evaluated (see Chap. 4).

Exposure. The hand is completely exposed and examined to assess the type and severity of injury.

Hemostasis. Bleeding is controlled by applying direct pressure. Since arteries are in close proximity to nerves, tendons, and muscle, blind clamping can lead to further injury and is therefore contraindicated.

Reduction of Edema. The hand is elevated, and ice is applied when significant soft tissue swelling is anticipated. Constricting jewelry, such as rings and bracelets, is removed.

Analgesia. It may be impossible to examine the hand if the patient is unable to cooperate because of pain. If severe, pain may be relieved by parenteral narcotic drugs or by local or regional anesthesia. Sensation is assessed before anesthetizing the hand.

PROBLEM The patient was brought to the hospital by private car. In the emergency department the vital signs were blood pressure 120/90 mm Hg, heart rate 90 beats/min, respiratory rate 16/min, temperature 98.6°F (37°C). Initial examination revealed moderate swelling of the hand with diffuse tenderness and bleeding from a volar wrist laceration.

Early inspection, ice, elevation, and initiation of pain management are appropriate. With the passage of time, swelling and pain increase, and evaluation becomes much more difficult. Also, based on the initial examination one may order a plain radiograph early, thus avoiding further delay in diagnosis and treatment.

DATA GATHERING

History

An organized and carefully performed history is a valuable asset in assessing the hand. When done well, it will suggest possible diagnosis as well as help the examiner anticipate specific complications. Important components of the history are:

1. *Nature of the injuring force.* Tidy injuries are clean, sharp, and recent, and do not cause extensive tissue destruction. Untidy injuries are contaminated, caused by blunt trauma, associated with significant tissue destruction, and have a tendency to become infected. A knowledge of the mechanism of injury will determine how the wound is managed, the likelihood of surgical consultation, and the need for radiography.

2. *Time since the injury.* All traumatic wounds are contaminated. As the time elapsed since injury increases, the bacterial count also increases until a point is reached when no amount of wound cleansing is sufficient to allow the laceration to be closed primarily. In general, hand wounds more than 6 hours old are subject to impaired healing and a greater incidence of infection.

3. *Contamination of the injuring force.* Grossly contaminated wounds cannot undergo primary closure regardless of appropriate wound care or time since injury. These wounds are best irrigated and left open and the patient started on antibiotics and referred for follow-up care.

4. *Associated medical illnesses.* Certain medical illnesses such as diabetes mellitus, peripheral vascular disease, and malnutrition will alter the wound healing process. Also, patients who are immunosuppressed or are taking medications such as steroids may have an altered response to wound healing.

5. *Tetanus status of the patient.*

6. Handedness of the patient and level of use, e.g., professional guitarist.

PROBLEM Further history revealed that the machine the patient was using cuts metal forms. His hand was injured when the machine was accidentally turned on while he was performing routine maintenance. Two metal bars that move across one another lacerated his hand. His hand was trapped between these bars under pressure for approximately 5 minutes. There were no rollers, and heat was not used or generated by the machine.

Injuries to the hand are quite common in industrial settings. Because it is not practical for physicians to have a working knowledge of all industrial equipment, it is essential for the patient to describe carefully the mechanism of injury. The following questions are helpful:

1. What type of machine caused the injury?
2. Were rollers used? How wide is the space between rollers?
3. What normally passes through the machine?
4. Was heat generated in the process?
5. Is there a release mechanism? If not, how was the hand released?
6. How long was the hand trapped?

Physical Examination and Functional Anatomy

The physical examination is the most important step in evaluating open injuries of the hand. A thorough examination will reveal the majority of injuries. To perform this assessment and interpret the findings, one must be familiar with the functional anatomy of the hand. The following discussion will review the physical examination in the context of functional hand anatomy. Of special significance is the concept of *topographical anticipation.* This refers to the process of anticipating a deep structural injury based on a knowledge of the surface anatomy.

Three lines on the palm accurately establish the position of the underlying structures (Fig. 42–1). The first line, the cardinal line of Kaplan, extends from the apex of the

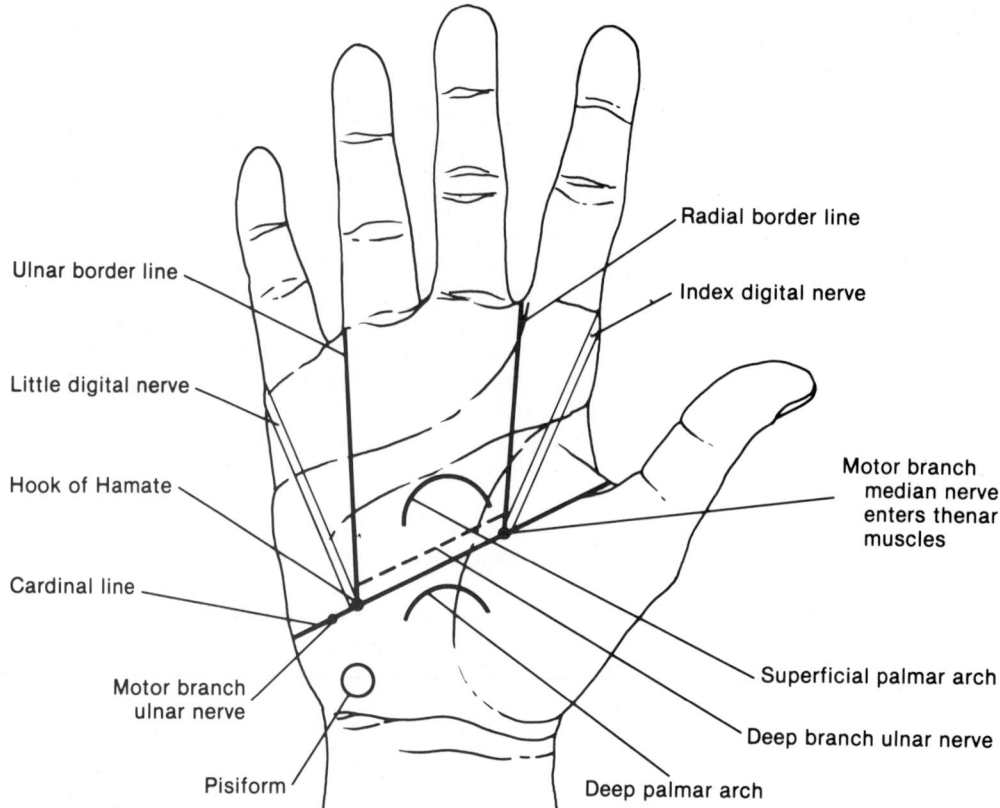

FIGURE 42-1. *Emmanual Kaplan described reference lines that accurately established the position of deep structures of the hand. (Adapted from Spinner M: Kaplan's Functional and Surgical Anatomy of the Hand (3rd ed). Philadelphia, J. B. Lippincott, 1984.)*

thumb-index interdigital fold across the palm parallel to the midpalmar crease. The radial border line is an extension of the radial border of the long finger. The point of intersection with the cardinal line represents the point where the motor branch of the median nerve enters the thenar muscles. A line drawn from this radial reference point to the radial border of the base of the index finger overlies the course of the radial digital nerve to that finger. The ulnar border line is an extension of the ulnar border of the ring finger. The place where it intersects the cardinal line closely approximates the location of the hook of the hamate. A line drawn from this point to the base of the ulnar border of the small finger overlies the course of the ulnar digital nerve to that finger. The pisiform is easily palpated at the base of the hypothenar eminence at the wrist crease.

The ulnar nerve and artery enter the palm radial to the pisiform and ulnar to the hook of the hamate (Guyon's canal). The nerve then divides, sending a deep motor branch across the palm. The course of this nerve is just distal to the cardinal line. The ulnar and radial arteries form the superficial palmar arch, which is approximately 2 to 3 cm distal to the cardinal line, and the deep palmar arch, which is just proximal.

With these surface landmarks in mind, the examination proceeds as follows:

Observation. Lacerations, puncture wounds, soft tissue swelling, deformity, and color are noted. The normal posture of the resting hand reveals increasing flexion from the index to the small finger. Deviation from this resting posture may indicate a laceration of an extensor or flexor tendon (Figs. 42-2 and 42-3).

Palpation. Gently performed palpation of the injured hand may yield valuable information. The examination is performed with the patient's hand resting comfortably

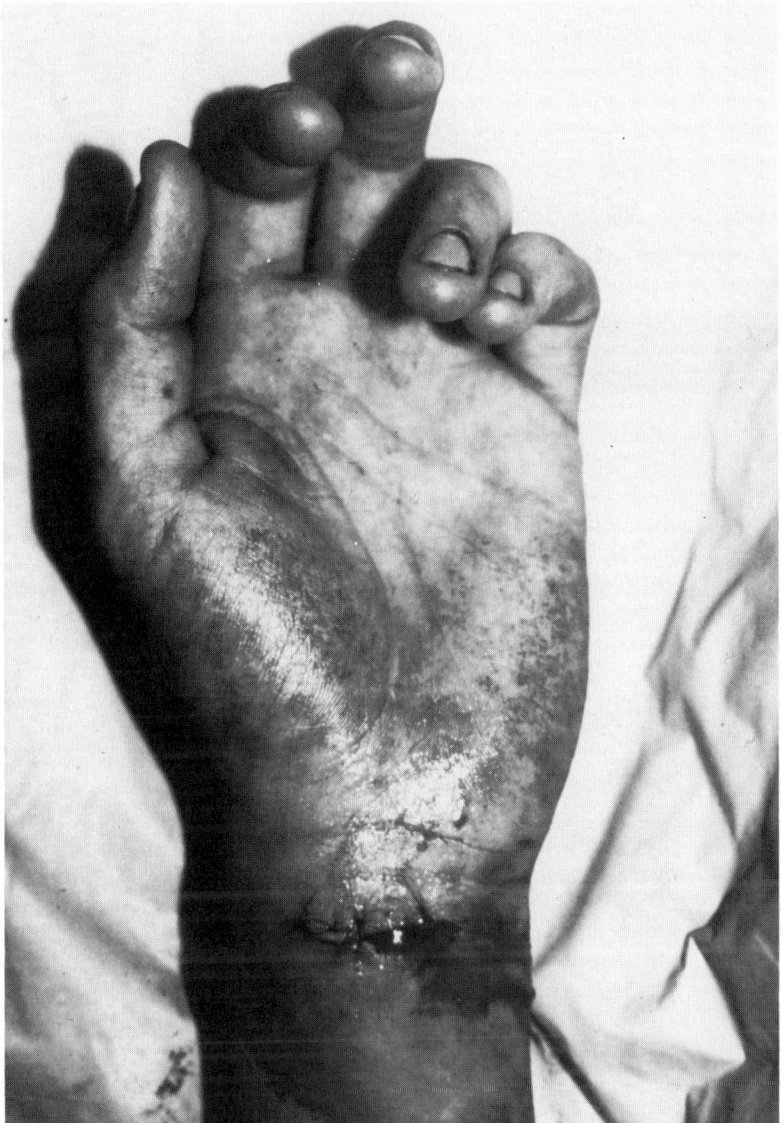

FIGURE 42-2. Laceration of the wrist with flexor tendon injuries to the middle finger. Notice the middle finger falling outside the normal resting patterns of increasing flexion from index finger to little finger.

on the table. The finger or an instrument such as the eraser end of a pencil or a cotton-tipped applicator can be used to find the exact location of maximal tenderness.

Circulation. The major blood supply to the hand is supplied by the radial and ulnar arteries. These arteries terminate by branching into deep and superficial branches, which anastomose to form the superficial and deep palmar arches (Fig. 42-4). Blood to the superficial arch is supplied mostly by the ulnar artery, and it is usually larger and more important than the deep arch.

Circulation is evaluated by observing the color, capillary filling time, and temperature of the skin. A hand that is edematous and cyanotic has venous insufficiency. A pale cool hand with poor capillary filling has arterial insufficiency.

Neurologic Examination

Sensation. Sensation to the hand is mediated by three nerves: the ulnar, median, and radial nerves (Fig. 42-5). The ulnar nerve supplies sensation to the small finger and

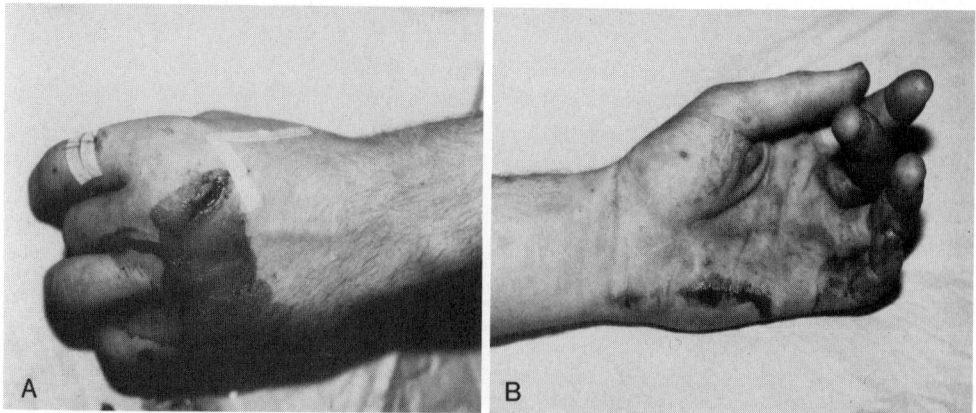

FIGURE 42–3. (A) *Glass laceration on the dorsal surface of the hand, and* (B) *complete transection of the extensor tendon to the middle finger demonstrated by altered normal alignment at rest.*

the ulnar half of the ring finger. The median nerve supplies sensation to the thumb, index, long, and radial half of the ring finger, the central palmar area, and the distal portions of the dorsum of the ring, long, and index fingers. Sensation from the radial nerve is to the dorsum of the hand not supplied by the ulnar and median nerves. Although there is sensory overlap among adjacent nerves, autonomous areas do exist. These are the tip of the small finger for the ulnar nerve, the tip of the index finger for the median nerve, and the dorsal thumb-index web space for the radial nerve. The best assessment of sensory function is obtained by checking two-point discrimination, the normal range of which is 2 to 5 mm.

Motor. The median and ulnar nerves innervate all the intrinsic muscles of the hand, and the radial nerve innervates all of the extrinsic extensors (Table 42–1). Injuries to their main trunk can be diagnosed by testing one muscle only for each nerve. The ulnar nerve is tested by placing the hand on a table on its ulnar side and having the patient elevate the index finger against resistance. The muscle belly of the first dorsal interosseus is palpated in the thumb-index web space. This muscle is reliably innervated by the ulnar nerve.

The median nerve is tested by placing the patient's hand on a flat surface palm up. The patient is then asked to raise the thumb toward the ceiling against resistance (palmar abduction). The belly of the abductor pollicis brevis, which is reliably innervated by the median nerve, can be palpated on the radial border of the thenar eminence.

The radial nerve is tested by placing the patient's forearm on a table and asking the patient to extend the wrist against resistance. The thumb is then extended and abducted; extension of the other fingers follows. A laceration of the main trunk results in paralysis of the wrist and finger extensors and reveals an obvious "wrist drop." Distal forearm lacerations, however, may result only in weak thumb and index finger extension. This is due to the more proximal innervation of the muscles to the wrist and finger extensors.

Tendons. Either flexor or extensor tendons may be involved in hand or wrist lacerations. Extensor tendons are more superficial, easier to visualize, and easier to repair and generally heal without difficulty. Flexor tendons, on the other hand, run through deep structures and are encased in a tendon sheath. They can be very difficult to visualize and repair, and complications are common.

Volar lacerations and potential flexor tendon injuries require a meticulous examination. The complex anatomy and the patient's resistance to examination due to pain can make this difficult. An appropriate nerve block or local infiltration with an anesthetic agent will facilitate this part of the examination. *Sensation is documented before instillation of anesthetic agents.*

Additionally, direct observation of the tendon through the lacerated skin may not

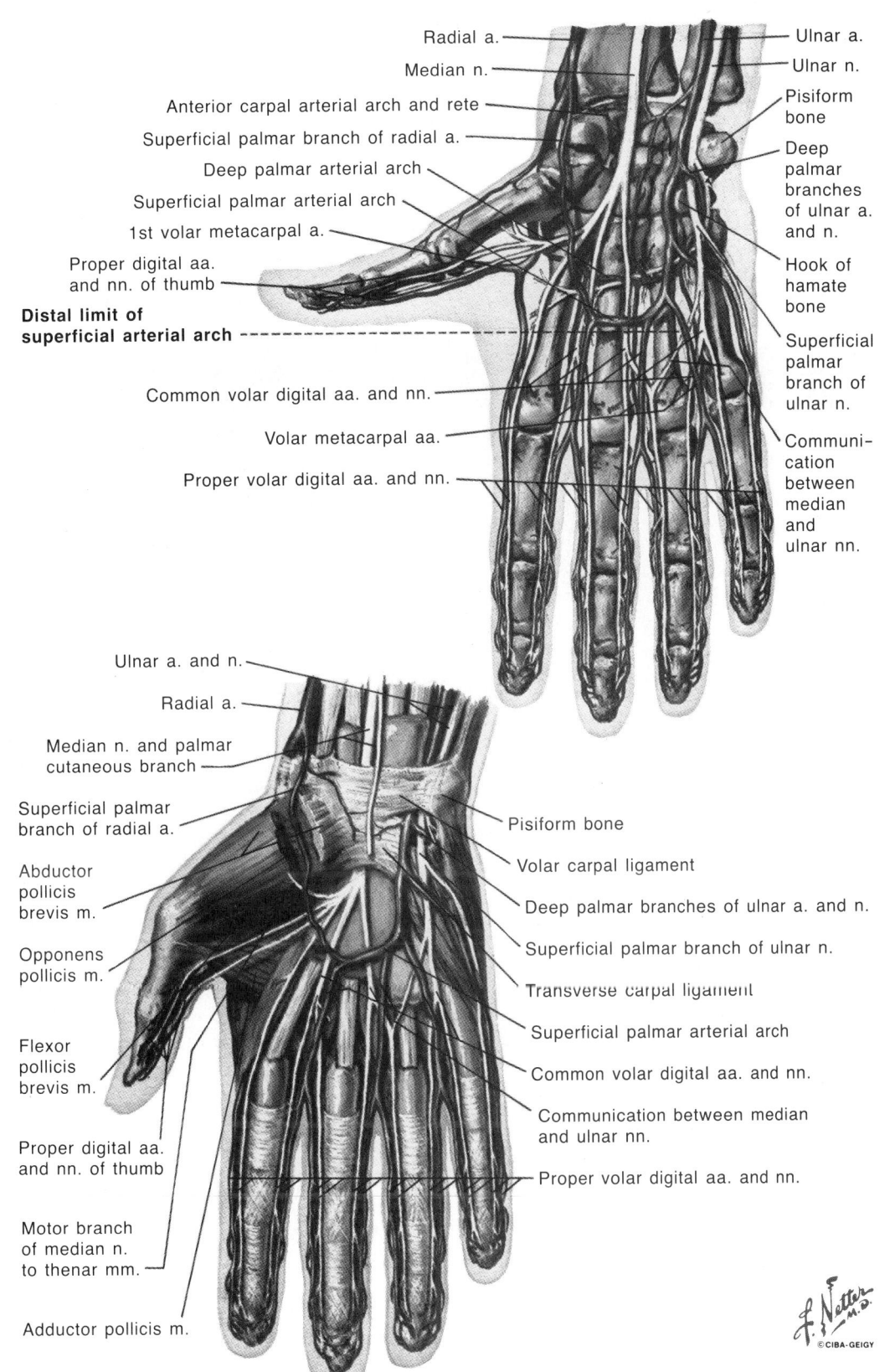

FIGURE 42–4. *Deep palmar structures. Note the superficial and deep palmar arterial arches. (Copyright 1988 CIBA-GEIGY Corporation. Reproduced with permission from the CLINICAL SYMPOSIA by Frank H. Netter, M.D.)*

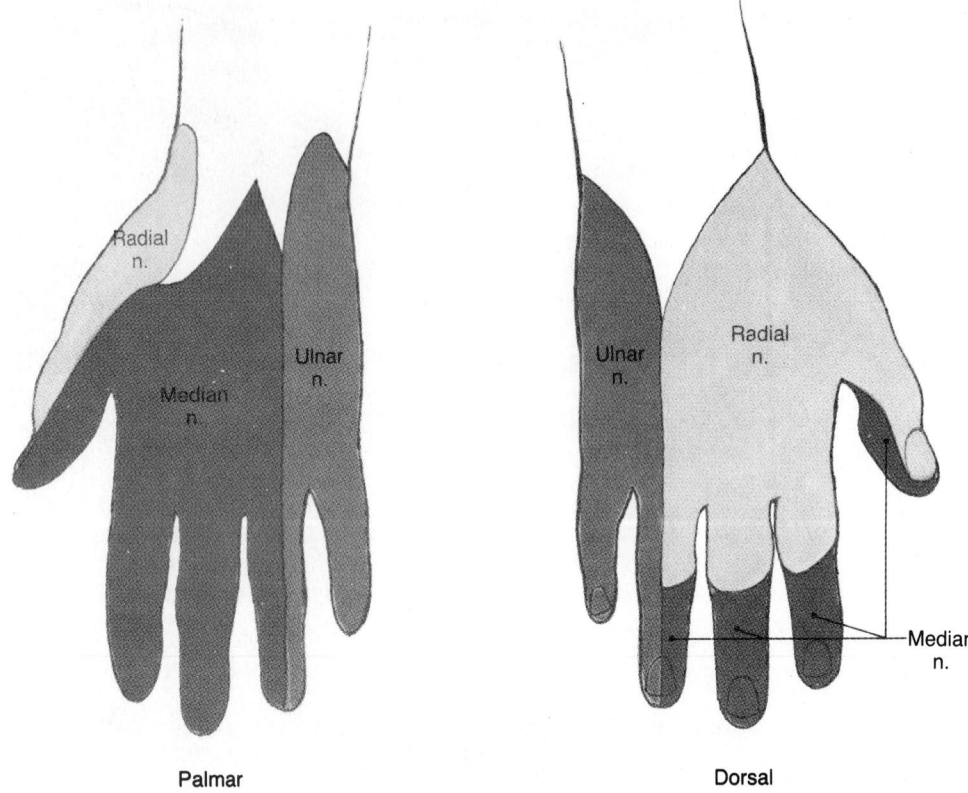

FIGURE 42-5. *Sensory distribution in the hand. (From Carter PR: Common Hand Injuries and Infections: A Practical Approach to Early Treatment. Philadelphia, W. B. Saunders, 1983.)*

reveal an injury. With potential tendon injuries an additional historical factor to consider is the position of the hand at the time of injury. Flexor tendon lacerations that occur with the fingers in flexion will not be seen through the wound when the hand is examined with the fingers in the extended position. In order to evaluate the tendon directly, the fingers must be flexed in order to reproduce its position at the time of injury. This maneuver usually brings the tendon laceration into view. If a tendon laceration is not seen but the sheath is cut, it can be assumed that the tendon is also lacerated.

The anatomy of the flexor tendons is complex (Fig. 42–6). All these tendons enter the hand through the carpal tunnel. In the palm, the flexor digitorum profundus (FDP) and the flexor digitorum superficialis (FDS) travel together to all the fingers except the

TABLE 42-1. Motor Innervation and Testing

Nerve	Innervation	Test
Ulnar	Muscles of the hypothenar eminence, two ulnar lumbricals, interossei, adductor pollicis, flexor carpi ulnaris, deep head of the flexor pollicis brevis, and flexor digitorum profundus of the ring and little fingers	Index finger abduction (first dorsal interosseus)
Median	Muscles of the thenar eminence, two radial lumbricals, palmaris longus, flexor carpi radialis, flexor pollicis longus, flexor digitorum superficialis, and flexor digitorum profundus of the index and long fingers	Thumb palmar abduction (abductor pollicis brevis)
Radial	All extrinsic muscle extensors	Wrist and finger extension

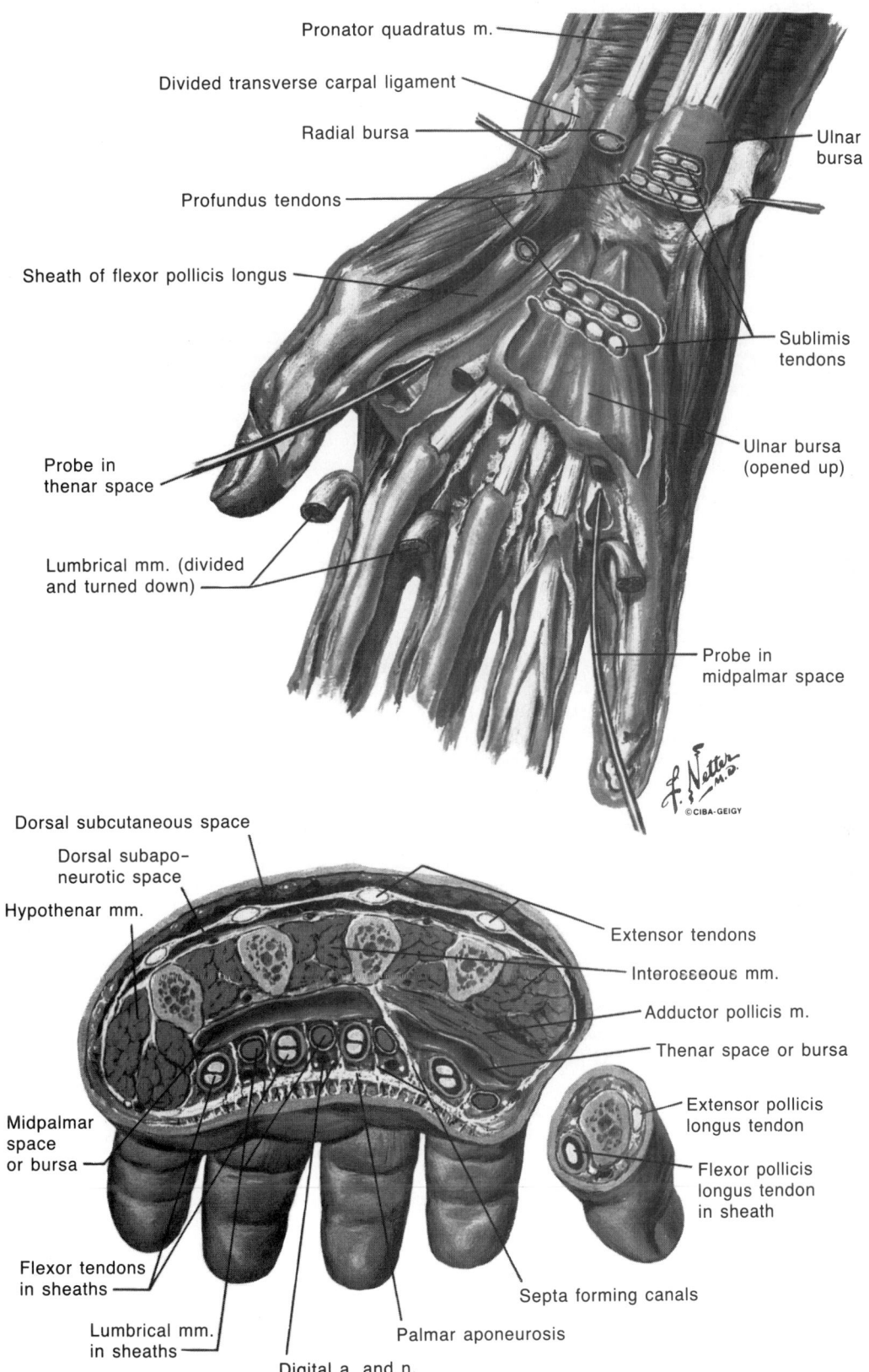

FIGURE 42–6. *Relationship of the flexor tendons to other deep structures of the hand. (Copyright 1988 CIBA-GEIGY Corporation. Reproduced with permission from the CLINICAL SYMPOSIA by Frank H. Netter, M.D.)*

thumb. At the level of the metacarpal-phalangeal (MCP) joints, they are surrounded by a fibrous canal, the flexor tendon sheath. Condensations of these sheaths form the pulley system of the fingers, which, along with the transverse carpal ligament, prevents bowstringing of the tendons and allows the flexor tendons to flex the joints fully with little dissipation of energy. At the proximal phalanx, the FDP passes through the superficialis tendon, then inserts on the proximal portion of the distal phalanges of the index, middle, ring, and small fingers. The FDP mainly flexes the distal interphalangeal (DIP) joint. It is tested by immobilizing the MCP joint and the PIP joint while the patient flexes the DIP joint against resistance.

The FDS inserts on the middle phalanx of the index, middle, ring, and small fingers. It is tested by inactivating the profundus by extending the fingers not tested and having the patient flex the PIP joint against resistance. This test is not reliable for the index finger because this finger has an independent profundus muscle belly and cannot be inactivated in this manner. The index finger is tested by having the patient flex the PIP joint while the physician feels for laxity of the distal phalanx. Another maneuver is to have the patient pinch the thumb forcefully against the index finger with the DIP joint hyperextended. Patients with superficialis tendon injuries tend to flex the DIP joint during this maneuver.

The flexor pollicis longus (FPL) inserts on the thumb distal phalanx and is tested by immobilizing the MCP joint and having the patient flex the interphalangeal (IP) joint against resistance.

Extensor tendons travel through six osseofibrous canals on the dorsal surface of the wrist (Fig. 42–7). Crosslinking of these tendons can make testing difficult. The testing of these extensor tendons is outlined in Table 42–2.

Examination in a Bloodless Field. With uncooperative patients or when occult injuries such as partial flexor tendon lacerations, open joint injuries, or retained foreign bodies are suspected, examination in a bloodless field is performed. This is accomplished by applying a layer of Webril around the patient's arm and elevating it for 2 minutes. A blood pressure cuff or a pneumatic tourniquet is inflated to 250 mm Hg. Patients can generally tolerate this procedure for 15 minutes.

PROBLEM Examination of the hand revealed moderate edema of the dorsal surface. There was a 5-cm volar laceration extending across the wrist on the distal wrist crease (Fig. 42–8A and B). Radial artery bleeding was controlled by a pressure dressing. Two-point discrimination was 4 mm, and motor function of the ulnar and median nerves was normal. The patient was unable to flex and radially deviate the wrist, nor was he able to flex either the interphalangeal joint of the thumb or the distal interphalangeal joint of the index finger. There was weak flexion of the proximal interphalangeal joint of the index and long fingers.

Observation alone is sufficient to diagnose at least four injuries. Efforts are then directed at gentle physical examination to confirm the diagnosis. Surgical consultation is obtained, and the hand and forearm are splinted, elevated, and the patient prepared for surgery.

DIAGNOSTIC ADJUNCTS

Radiologic Imaging

Radiographs are commonly used in evaluating hand injuries. The decision to use radiography depends on several factors including medical indications, patient expectations, time management, medicolegal considerations, and physician uncertainty. The medical indications for obtaining radiographs of the hand are:

1. To determine the extent of injury

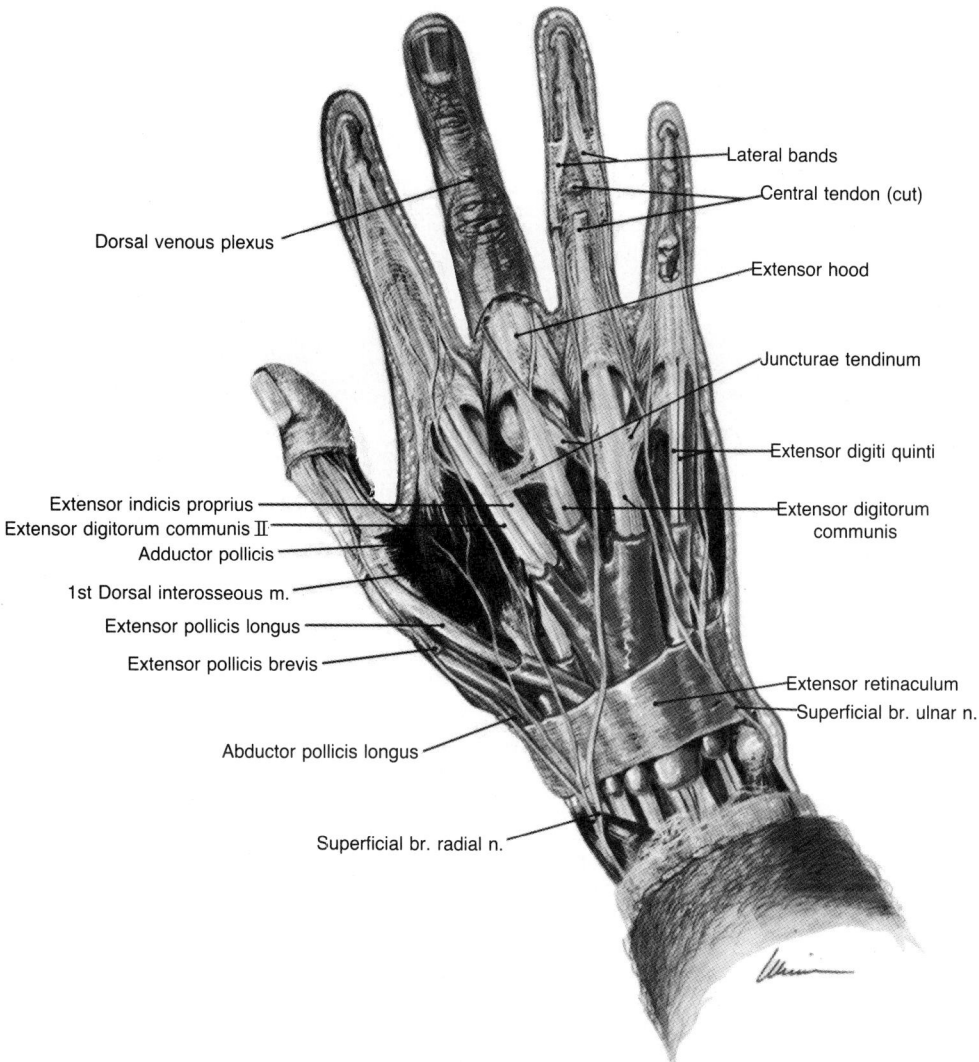

FIGURE 12-7. Extensor surface of the hand. (From Carter PR: Common Hand Injuries and Infections: A Practical Approach to Early Treatment. Philadelphia, W. B. Saunders, 1983.)

2. To diagnose an occult injury
3. To detect a foreign body
4. To document results of therapy (postreduction alignment, foreign body removal)

Routine radiographs include the anteroposterior, oblique, and lateral views. It is important that a true lateral view be obtained because any degree of obliquity may obscure a subtle but functionally significant injury. Further discussion of hand radiography is provided in Chapter 41.

PRINCIPLES OF MANAGEMENT

General Principles

Management of patients with an open injury to the hand requires attention to four factors:

TABLE 42–2. The Extensor Tendons of the Hand

Compartment	Tendons	Insertion	Test of Function
First	Abductor pollicis longus	Dorsum of the base of the thumb metacarpal	Extension and abduction of the thumb
	Extensor pollicis brevis	Dorsum of the base of the thumb proximal phalanx	Extension and abduction of the thumb
Second	Extensor carpi radialis longus	Dorsum of the base of the index metacarpal	Making fist while extending the wrist
	Extensor carpi radialis brevis	Dorsum of the base of the long metacarpal	Making fist while extending the wrist
Third	Extensor pollicis longus	Dorsum of the base of the thumb distal phalanx	Lifting the thumb off the surface of a table while the palm is flat against the table
Fourth	Extensor digitorum communis	Dorsum of the base of the proximal phalanges	Extension of the fingers at the MCP joints
	Extensor indicis proprius	Dorsum of the base of the proximal phalanx of the index finger	Extension of the index finger at the MCP joint with the other fingers in a fist
Fifth	Extensor digiti minimi	Dorsum of the extensor hood of the small finger	Extension of the small finger while making a fist
Sixth	Extensor carpi ulnaris	Dorsum of the base of the small finger metacarpal	Extension and ulnar deviation of the wrist

Hemorrhage Control. This has been discussed earlier in Initial Approach in the Emergency Department.

Wound Care. Detailed discussion of wound care is found in Chapter 15. The following elements are basic to wound care:

1. High-pressure irrigation with a 19-gauge needle, 35-ml syringe, and at least 250 ml of normal saline.

2. Skin cleansing with an agent such as povidone-iodine solution.

3. Judicious debridement of wound edges and of devitalized tissue, especially in animal and human bites.

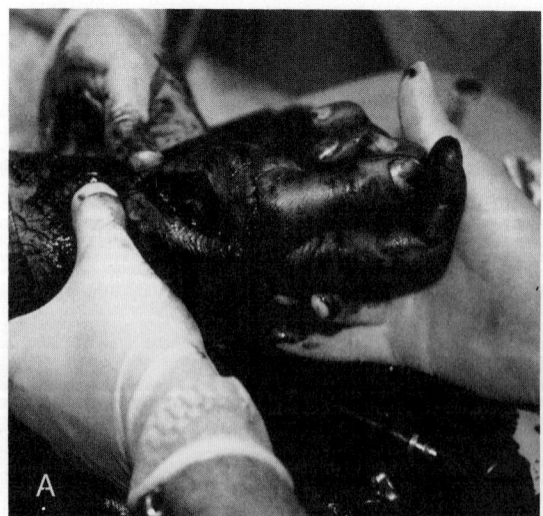
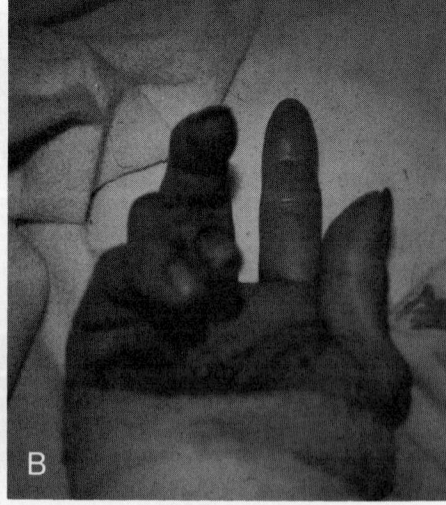

FIGURE 42–8. (A) *Photograph of the hand of a 24 year old man injured in the metal forming machine he was operating.* (B) *Suspicious positioning of index and middle fingers and thumb in the resting position.*

4. Sutures of the skin with a nonreactive monofilament material such as 5–0 nylon. Generally, a single-layer closure is sufficient.

5. Prophylactic antibiotics. Routine antibiotics for uncomplicated lacerations of the hand have not been found to be effective in preventing infections. Instead, early treatment and meticulous wound care are the more important factors.

Dressing. The dressing serves several functions: (1) absorption of drainage, (2) support and protection, (3) prevention or reduction of edema, and (4) provision of a framework for the application of antibiotic creams.

The dressing consists of three parts. The first layer is a nonadherent, fine-mesh layer that is applied directly over the wound. This layer allows seepage to occur without allowing the layer above to adhere to the wound. The second layer is the absorbent and protective layer and consists of several fluffed gauze pads. The final layer is stretchable and conforming and serves to provide even pressure without constriction.

Immobilization and Elevation. It is important to immobilize the hand in a position that will not result in functional impairment once the acute event has resolved. For most injuries this consists of placing the hand in the "safe position," with the wrist in 30 degrees of extension, the MCP joints in 60 to 90 degrees of flexion, the IP joints in 10 to 20 degrees of flexion, and the thumb in palmar abduction (Fig. 42–9). This position maximally stretches the collateral ligaments of the MCP and IP joints and reduces the danger of joint stiffness from collateral ligament shortening (Fig. 42–10). Other splinting techniques include the radial and ulnar gutter splints, the thumb spica, and the mallet finger splint. Aluminum splints as well as preformed splints may also be used (see Chap. 41).

Elevation is important when one is attempting to prevent or reduce edema. When combined with pressure and splinting, elevation markedly reduces edema and improves functional outcome.

Management of Specific Injuries

Flexor Tendon Lacerations. The anatomy of the flexor tendons is quite complex. These tendons travel through a dense osseofibrous canal and are in close proximity to bones, nerves, arteries, and other tendons. Surgery is difficult, and functional recovery

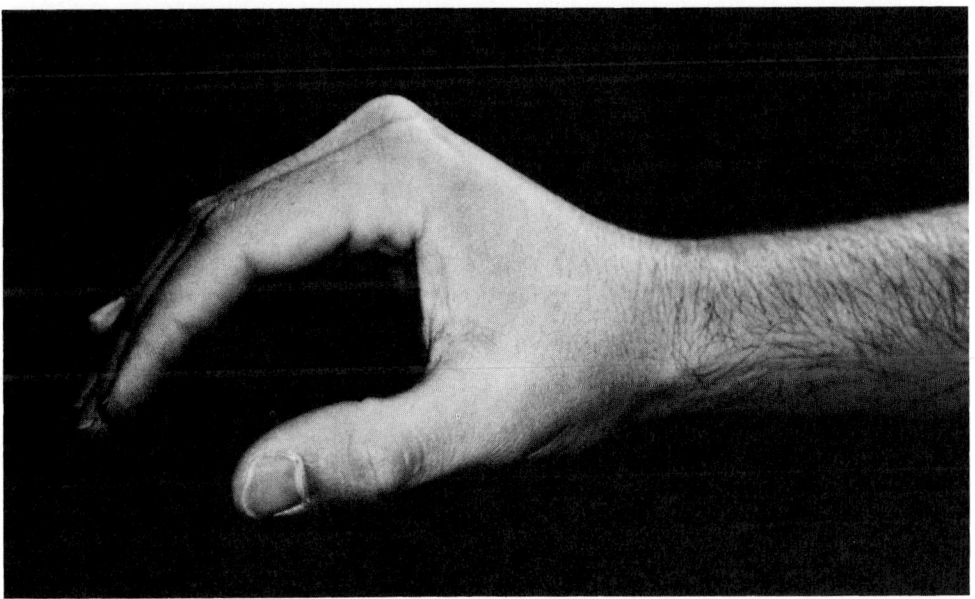

FIGURE 42–9. Position of safe immobilization.

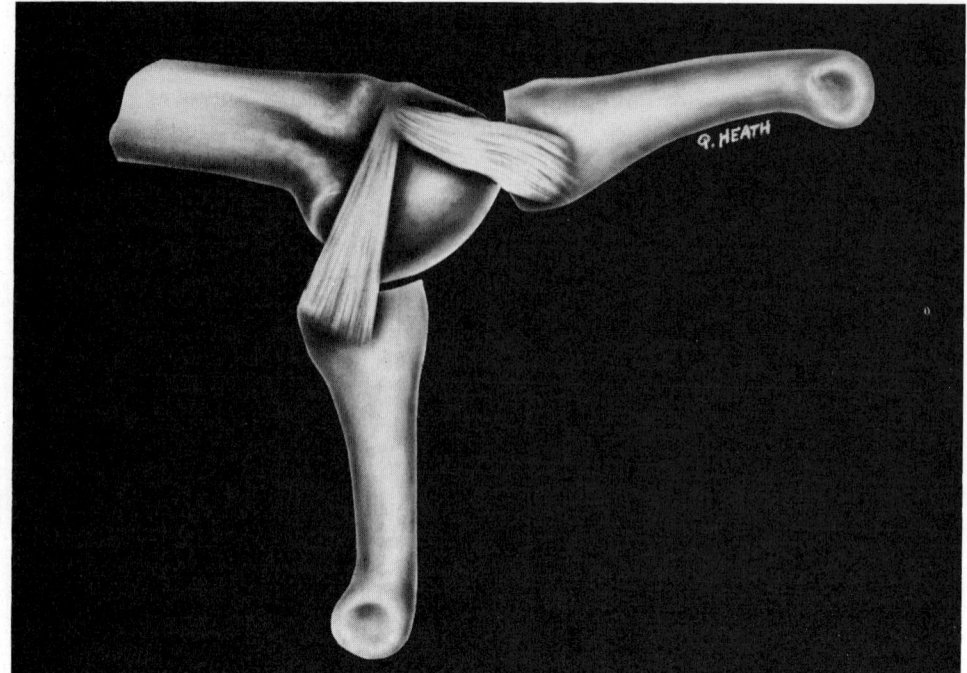

FIGURE 42–10. *Collateral ligaments at the metacarpophalangeal and interphalangeal joints are taut in flexion and lax in extension. (Adapted from Eaton RG: Joint Injuries of the Hand. Courtesy of Charles C Thomas, Publisher, Springfield, Illinois, 1971.)*

is often disappointing. Consequently, repair in the emergency department is not indicated. Instead, wound care, loosely suturing skin, prophylactic antibiotics, usually a cephalosporin, and splinting in flexion constitute the appropriate treatment. These patients should be promptly referred to a specialist in hand surgery.

Extensor Tendon Lacerations. The superficial location of extensor tendons makes them susceptible to injury and accessible to repair. Unlike flexor tendons, however, some extensor tendon lacerations may be repaired in the emergency department by experienced physicians. Although repair may take place from the distal insertion to a level proximal to the wrist, the tendons most easily repaired are those over the area of the metacarpals. If one is unfamiliar with the repair of extensor tendons, the patient is treated as above except that the hand is splinted in extension.

Nerve Injury. The diagnosis of a nerve injury is made on physical examination. Emergency treatment consists of wound care, suturing the skin, prophylactic antibiotics, and splinting. Referral to a specialist for consideration of repair is important and is preferably arranged before the patient is discharged from the emergency department.

Vascular Injury. Vascular injuries are referred to a hand surgeon.

SPECIAL CONSIDERATIONS

Infections

Infections of the hand may result from a break in the skin or, rarely, from hematogenous spread. The infections reviewed here are primary infections rather than complications of existing wounds.

Paronychia. A paronychia, or "run-around abscess," is an infection of the soft tissue surrounding the base and sides of the nail, usually caused by *Staphylococcus aureus* or *Streptococcus pyogenes* (Fig. 42–11). An abscess is drained by entering it just above the

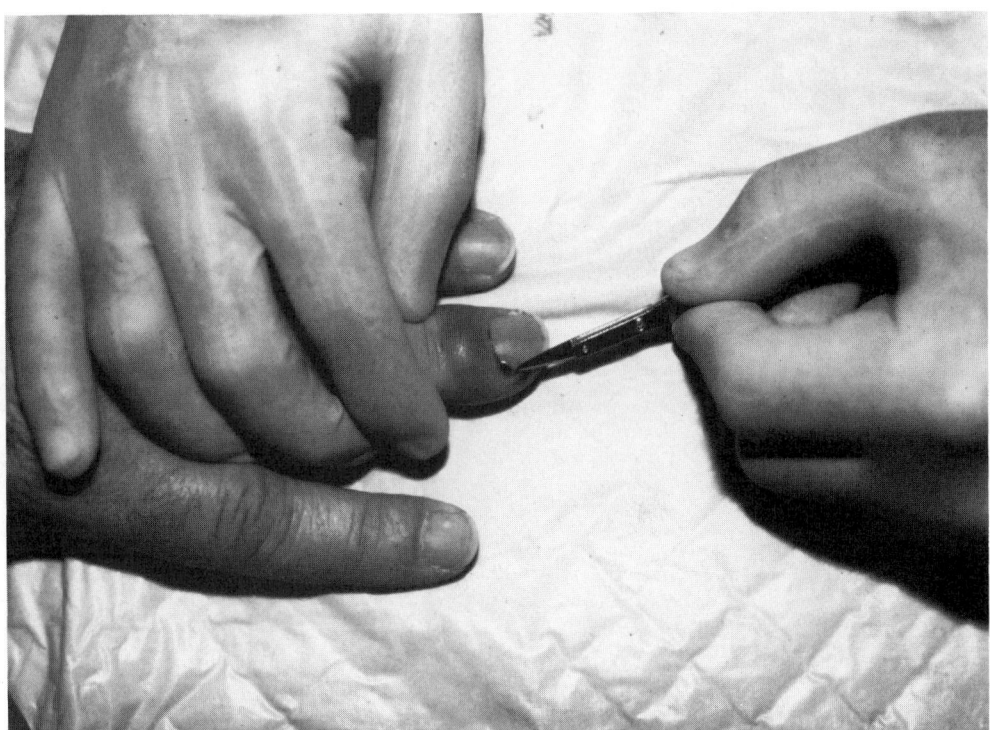

FIGURE 42–11. Incision and drainage of a paronychia.

nail with a number 11 blade. The patient is instructed to soak the finger three or four times per day.

Felon. A felon is a distal pulp space infection characterized by swelling, erythema, and pain. The causative organisms are the same as those causing paronychias. Treatment is surgical decompression. Although there are several methods of treatment, the preferred method is a longitudinal incision over the area of "pointing," which is usually over the central pad. The wound is loosely packed, and the patient is started on antibiotics such as a penicillinase-resistant penicillin or a cephalosporin such as cefadroxil. This procedure is done preferably after consultation with a hand surgeon.

Suppurative Flexor Tenosynovitis. This infection is an acute inflammation of the flexor tendon sheath characterized by Knavel's four cardinal signs of flexor tenosynovitis:

1. Finger in slight flexion.
2. Uniform swelling of the finger.
3. Tenderness along the course of the tendon sheath.
4. Pain on passive extension.

Pus forms in the closed flexor tendon sheath, which causes an increase in pressure leading to tissue ischemia, tendon necrosis, and finally tendon adhesions (Fig. 42–12). The infection may remain localized or may extend into the thenar or midpalmar bursa (Fig. 42–13). Treatment is prompt surgical decompression in the operating room.

Nailbed Injuries

The role of the fingernail is cosmetic, protective, and functional. The nail, by stabilizing the fingerpad, allows greater sensitivity and precise touch and grasp, and is therefore vitally important to the function of the hand (Fig. 42–14).

Injuries to the hand often involve the nailbed. A neglected injury may cause pain as well as splitting, ridging, and clawing of the nail. These problems are extremely

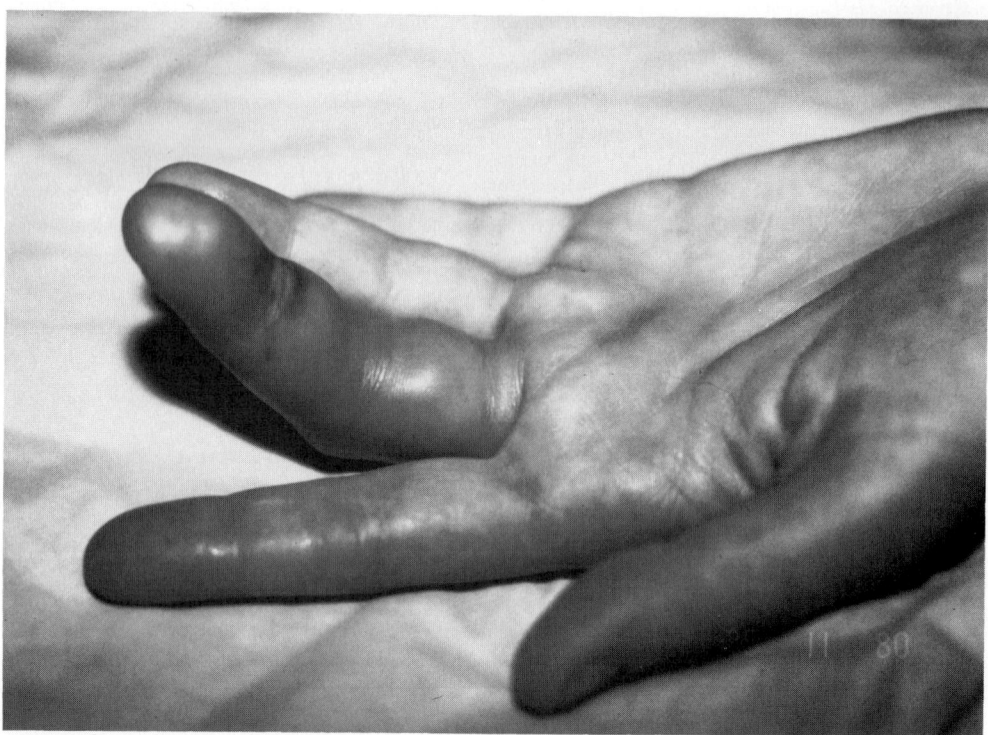

FIGURE 42-12. *Suppurative tenosynovitis of the long finger. This was caused by an untreated seemingly minor laceration at the distal interphalangeal crease. Note Knavel's signs of suppurative tenosynovitis.*

troublesome for the patient, so efforts directed at diagnosis and precise repair at the time of injury will ensure the best functional and cosmetic results.

Subungual hematomas are common injuries that often occur when a door is closed on a fingertip. The patient complains of pain, and a physical examination reveals a swollen, tender distal phalanx with a discolored nail due to the hematoma. Radiographs are taken to rule out a distal phalanx fracture. Treatment consists of nail trephination or electrocautery, which releases the blood and results in immediate relief from pain.

When a subungual hematoma is more extensive, covering more than 25% of the visible nail, or if there is an obvious nailbed injury, the nail is removed. This can be accomplished by using a mosquito hemostat while sharply dissecting the nail from the nailbed and eponychium. The nail should be thoroughly cleansed and saved. The nailbed is irrigated and minimally debrided, and lacerations are repaired using 6–0 absorbable sutures on a fine needle. The principles of repair include preservation and accurate apposition of tissue.

After the nailbed has been repaired, the nailplate is placed beneath the nailfold (eponychium). This will prevent adhesions between the nailfold and the repaired bed. If the nailplate is not available, a trimmed nonadherent material such as the aluminum wrapper of the suture may be used.

Extensive injuries such as unstable distal phalanx fractures, severe crush injuries, and nailbed avulsions are best referred to a specialist.

Amputations and Replantations

Replantation is a commonly accepted medical practice, as evidenced by the number of centers specializing in this procedure and by its popularity in the lay press. In fact, "educated consumers" expect that all amputated parts will be replanted with subsequent return to full function. Physicians responsible for the initial care of patients with

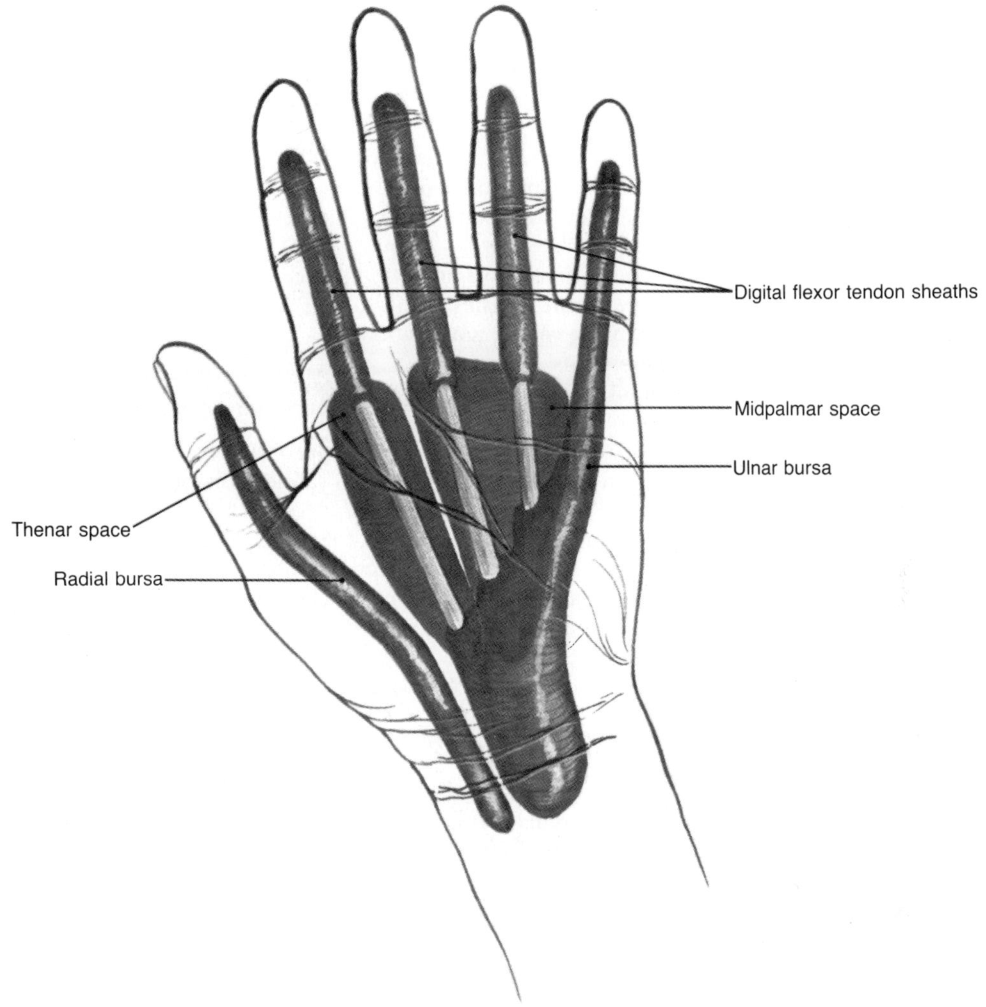

OPEN INJURIES TO THE HAND AND WRIST — **743**

FIGURE 42–13. *Relationship of flexor tendon sheaths and palmar spaces. Tendon sheath infection can spread into these spaces. (From Carter PR: Common Hand Injuries and Infections: A Practical Approach to Early Treatment. Philadelphia, W. B. Saunders, 1983.)*

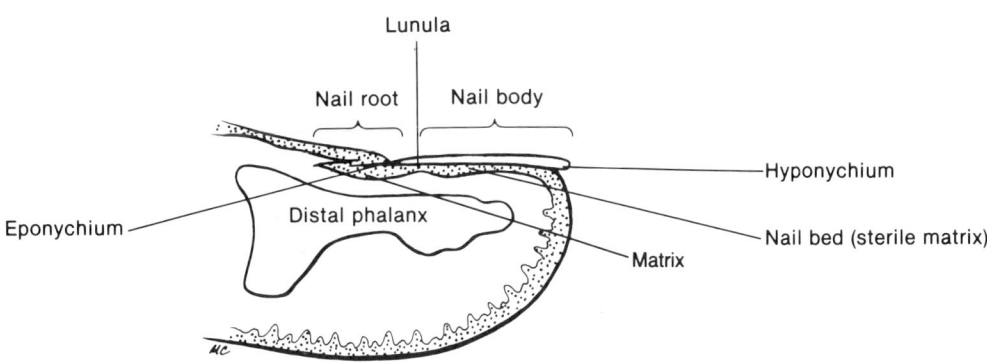

FIGURE 42–14. *Nail anatomy*

amputations need to be aware of the indications and contraindications for replantation and of the proper handling and transport of the amputated part.

Replantation is considered in the following situations:
1. Thumb amputations
2. Multiple digit amputations
3. Wrist and forearm amputations
4. Amputations in children
5. Single digit amputations in which the amputation occurs distal to the sublimis insertion.

Contraindications to replantation are generally considered to include:
1. Severe crush injuries
2. Multiple levels of amputation
3. Single digits
4. Mental instability of the patient
5. Severe medical illness

Transporting the amputated part appropriately is important if replantation is to be considered. The part is best wrapped in saline-moistened sterile gauze, sealed in a plastic bag, and placed on crushed ice.

Physicians involved in the care of patients with amputations should understand that functional recovery is never assured, prolonged morbidity is common, and multiple surgeries over years may be required. The decision to attempt replantation depends on many factors, including the age and occupation of the patient, level and condition of the amputated part, the absence of medical illness, and patient motivation. The surgeon considers these factors before a decision to reattach the amputated part is made.

High-Pressure Injection Injuries

The use of high-pressure compression equipment for the application of grease, paint, paint solvents, and hydraulic fluid is common. These devices can generate emission pressures of 1500 to 12,000 psi. Associated with the proliferation of this equipment is an increase in the number of patients who sustain high-pressure injection injuries. These injuries usually occur at work, with the index finger of the left hand the most common site.

The pathophysiology is related to two major factors. First, the amount of material injected influences the mechanical distention and hence tissue pressure. More injected material results in greater pressures, which decrease arterial inflow and reduce venous outflow. Additionally, a local physical effect results in edema, which further increases tissue pressure and ischemia. Second, the type of material injected is important. Agents such as paint and paint solvents produce an intense inflammatory reaction and are extremely damaging to tissue. These substances cause edema by direct chemical irritation, further increasing tissue ischemia. Other factors include (1) the compression pressure generated by the device, which influences the spread through tissue, (2) the anatomic areas involved, and (3) any delay in diagnosis and treatment.

The diagnosis is made by the history and observing the site of entry, which may be only 2 to 3 mm. Although the initial physical findings may be scant and the patient's complaints minimal, the injury is significant, and the likelihood of a poor outcome is great. Radiographs of the fingers and hand may demonstrate the presence of the foreign substance (Fig. 42–15). The patient is prepared for surgery, which consists of decompression, debridement, and thorough irrigation.

DISPOSITION AND FOLLOW-UP

The great majority of patients with open hand injuries and infections are managed as outpatients. A few injuries, however, demand special attention requiring hospitalization. These include:

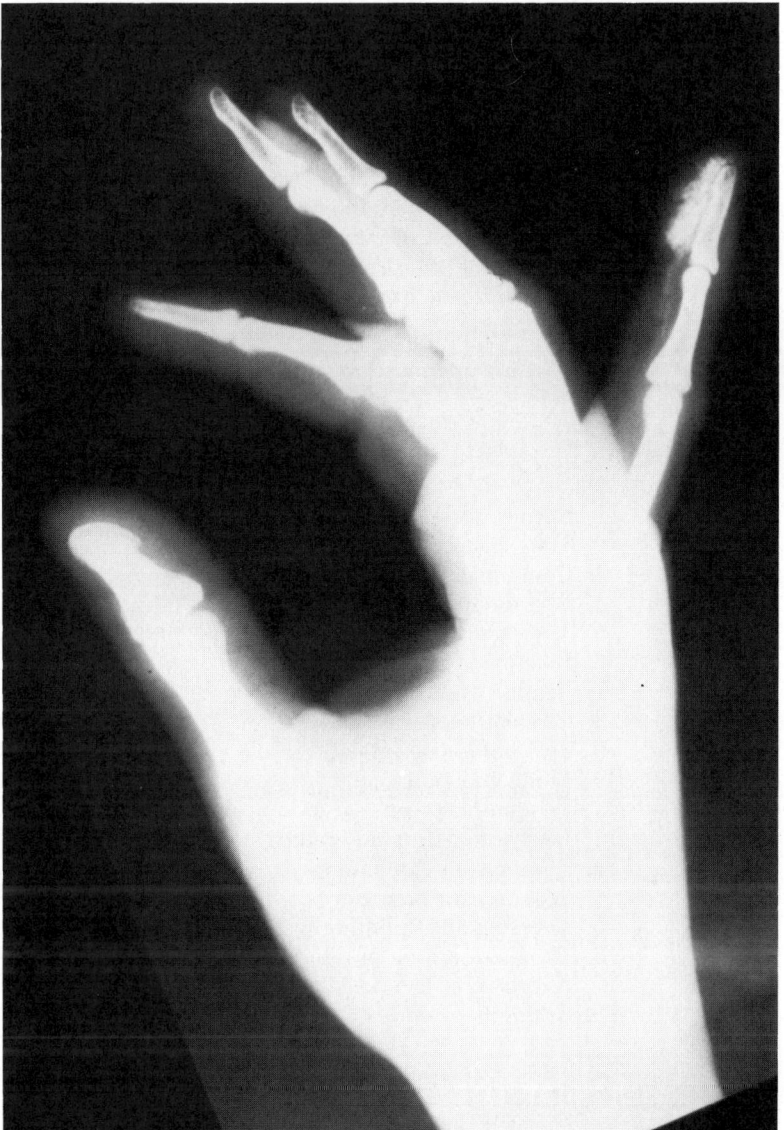

FIGURE 42–15. High-pressure paint injection to little finger. Note paint visible in soft tissue and along the course of the tendon sheath. (From Rudzinski J, Uehara D: Radiology of the hand. Reprinted from Trauma Quarterly, Vol. 2, No. 4, p. 61, with permission of Aspen Publishers, Inc., © 1986.)

1. Mutilating hand injuries.
2. Injection injuries.
3. Highly contaminated lacerations requiring operative debridement.
4. Open fractures and dislocations requiring operative intervention.
5. Complex infections such as suppurative flexor tenosynovitis, deep space infections, and septic arthritis.
6. Nerve trunk lacerations.
7. Multiple tendon or nerve lacerations.

Patients who have isolated digital nerve or tendon lacerations may have prompt surgical follow-up rather than immediate surgery. Since the type and timing of surgery are operator dependent, each surgeon will have his own preference. For tidy wounds it is appropriate to irrigate copiously, suture the skin, splint, and treat with prophylactic antibiotics. Untidy wounds are dressed and left open.

PROBLEM The patient was taken to the operating room where the following injuries were found:

- Radial artery transection
- Flexor pollicis longus laceration
- Flexor carpi radialis laceration
- Flexor digitorum profundus and sublimis laceration of the index finger
- Flexor digitorum sublimis laceration of the long finger

All injuries were repaired. One year after incident the patient is working at his previous job with nearly complete functional recovery.

DOCUMENTATION

1. Nature of the injuring force.
2. Time since injury.
3. Contamination of the injuring force.
4. Position of the hand at the time of injury.
5. Associated medical illnesses.
6. Likelihood of a foreign body.
7. Tetanus status.
8. Circulatory status.
9. Two-point discrimination.
10. Motor function.
11. Tendon function.
12. Interpretation of any radiographs.
13. Findings on exploration.
14. Wound care procedures.
15. Dressing and splinting procedures.
16. Type and timing of referral.
17. Aftercare instructions.
18. Antibiotic use.

SUMMARY AND FINAL POINTS

- Open injuries often harbor an injury to bone, nerves, tendons, and arteries. A high index of suspicion and "topographical anticipation" based on the cardinal line of Kaplan are the keys to diagnosis.
- An abnormal position of the hand at rest may indicate a tendon laceration.
- When evaluating tendon function, testing against resistance is essential.
- Sensory examination using two-point discrimination is accurate and reliable. The normal range is 2 to 5 mm.
- Examination in a bloodless field is often rewarding and is essential if the diagnosis is in doubt.
- Ice, elevation, and splinting reduce edema and shorten recovery time.
- Radiographs are used frequently to (1) determine the extent of injury, (2) diagnose occult injuries, (3) detect foreign bodies, and (4) document results of therapy.
- Principles of management of hand injuries include (1) hemorrhage control, (2) irrigation and debridement, (3) dressing, and (4) immobilization in the proper position and elevation.
- Suppurative tenosynovitis is a surgical emergency. The diagnosis can be made by

observing: (1) flexion of the finger, (2) uniform swelling of the finger, (3) tenderness along the course of the tendon sheath, and (4) pain on passive extension.
- The physical findings in patients with high-pressure injection injuries belie the catastrophic nature of this injury.
- Patients with single nerve or tendon injuries are generally referred to a hand surgeon for delayed repair.

BIBLIOGRAPHY

Texts

1. Carter P: Common Hand Injuries and Infections. A Practical Approach to Early Treatment. Philadelphia, Saunders, 1983.
2. Wolfort F: Acute Hand Injuries—A Multispecialty Approach. Boston, Little, Brown, 1980.

Journal Articles

1. Calabro J, Hoidal C, Susina L: Extensor tendon repair in the emergency department. J Emerg Med 4:217–225, 1986.
2. Canales F, Newmeyer W, Kilgore E: The treatment of felons and paronychias. Hand Clinics 5(4):515–523, 1989.
3. Frazier W, Miller M, Fox R, et al: Hand injuries: Incidence and epidemiology in an emergency service. J Am Coll Emerg Physicians 7(7):265–268, 1978.
4. Goldner R, Stevanovic M, Nunley J, et al: Digital replantation at the level of the distal interphalangeal joint and the distal phalanx. J Hand Surg 14A(2):214–220, 1989.
5. Karlbauer A, Gasperschitz F: High-pressure injection injury: A hand-threatening emergency. J Emerg Med (5):375–379, 1987.
6. Lampe E: Surgical anatomy of the hand: With special reference to infections and trauma. CIBA Symposium 40(3), 1988.
7. Mayer J, Jablon M: Tendon injuries of the hand. Trauma Q, 1(2):9–19, 1985.
8. Melone C, Jr, Grad J: Primary care of fingernail injuries. Emerg Med Clin North Am 3(2):255–261, 1985.
9. Siege D, Gelberman R: Infections of the hand. Ortho Clin North Am 19(4):779–789, 1988.
10. Urbaniak J, Roth J, Nunley J, et al: The results of replantation after amputation of a single finger. J Bone Joint Surg 67-A(4):611–619, 1985.
11. Zook E, Guy R, Russell R: A study of nail bed injuries: Causes, treatment, and prognosis. J Hand Surg 9A(2):247–252, 1984.

CHAPTER 43

LOWER EXTREMITY INJURY

T. J. RITTENBERRY, M.D.
EDWARD P. SLOAN, M.D.

PROBLEM 1 A 70 year old female was brought to the emergency department by ambulance. She complained of left hip pain and inability to walk after slipping on an icy sidewalk.

PROBLEM 2 A 23 year old male arrived on a back board after striking a sign post while riding his motorcycle. He complained only of right thigh pain. The right thigh was markedly swollen. During the work-up he became briefly hypotensive and tachycardic.

PROBLEM 3 A 17 year old male complained of a painful knee. Ambulation exacerbated the pain, and he stated that the knee felt "loose and unsteady." His symptoms began after he was "clipped" in a football game 24 hours prior to presentation.

PROBLEM 4 A 19 year old male was brought to the emergency department by his basketball coach. The patient stated that he had landed on another player's foot and had experienced immediate left ankle pain. He described an inversion stress on the ankle. Physical examination revealed swelling and tenderness at the ankle, most pronounced laterally.

PROBLEM 5 A 20 year old male, during fraternity rush activities, slid down the three-story column in front of his fraternity house and landed on both feet. He complained of severe foot and low back pain and was unable to walk owing to extreme discomfort.

QUESTIONS TO CONSIDER

1. What are the typical mechanisms of injury and findings in the patient with specific types of lower extremity injury?
2. What treatment modalities may be used in prehospital and emergency department management of common lower extremity injuries?
3. What kind of radiographic examination, if any, is necessary?
4. What common orthopedic injuries may be the cause of an acutely painful hip?
5. Which dislocations in the lower extremity are most commonly associated with neurovascular compromise?
6. What are the indications for arthrocentesis of the knee joint?
7. What differences exist in the emergency care of open fractures as opposed to closed fractures?
8. Which injuries of the lower extremity require immediate orthopedic referral, hospitalization, or surgical intervention?

INTRODUCTION

Orthopedic injuries of the lower extremity are commonly encountered in the emergency department. They usually result from trauma encountered during sports activities, falls, or vehicular accidents but may also occur with relatively normal stresses and loads. Pathologic fractures may present without apparent trauma when bone has been weakened by benign or malignant bone tumors or bone cysts. Systemic skeletal disease due to hyperparathyroidism, renal osteodystrophy, Paget's disease, osteogenesis imperfecta, and steroid-induced osteoporosis may also predispose to pathologic fractures.

Lower extremity injuries do not usually represent a threat to life, yet limb-threatening injuries do occur, mandating rapid diagnosis and management to maximize salvage. In the more likely event of injuries that are not limb-threatening, an aggressive approach aimed at pain relief, anatomic reduction, and immobilization is necessary for prompt reestablishment of lower extremity function. Failure to diagnose and treat an injury adequately may lead to cosmetic deformity, impaired function, and chronic pain. An aberration in long bone or joint architecture that results in a gait disturbance may have a "domino" effect that in time causes dysfunction and pain in other joints of the legs and back.

PREHOSPITAL CARE

Treatment ideally begins at the site of the injury. Because a physician is seldom present, bystanders, police, or emergency medical service (EMS) personnel are typically the first responders. The goals of therapy are the same as those used for managing upper extremity trauma, and immobilization aimed at reducing pain, bleeding, and further soft tissue injury is initiated prior to transport. Although rescue personnel are urged to perform an assessment of vascular status by checking for distal pulses, they are usually instructed to "splint them where they lie" and transport patients in spite of findings indicating possible limb ischemia. Manipulations aimed at reestablishing blood flow are best done in the emergency department provided that transport times are short. The risk of further injury due to incorrect though well-meaning reduction far outweighs the morbidity of transient limb ischemia.

Prehospital splinting materials are limited only by the imagination of the first responder. Umbrellas, canes, rolled newspapers, or the like may provide temporary stabilization when applied to the padded extremity. Lower extremities may be stabilized by padding and taping them to a back board or to the contralateral leg. A pillow circumferentially wrapped and taped or pinned makes an excellent splint for injuries below the knee.

The rescue squad is often equipped with preformed aluminum or inflatable splints, which are adequate for prehospital care. Femoral fractures are most effectively immobilized with a Hare traction splint. This device is composed of two telescoping rods with a proximal half-ring and a distal winding rachet mechanism. With the proximal half-ring abutting the pelvis, longitudinal traction is obtained by taking up tension with a strap placed about the ankle, and further stabilization is offered by several circumferential Velcro bands applied at the calf, knee, and thigh (Fig. 43–1).

Open fractures or open fracture-dislocations require individualized prehospital care. As in all cases of trauma, pressure is applied to the active bleeding sites. Protruding bone should not be reduced and drawn back into the wound. Hence, traction devices are contraindicated when an open injury exists. The wound should be covered as early as possible with a clean, preferably sterile, dressing.

INITIAL APPROACH IN THE EMERGENCY DEPARTMENT

Patients often present to the emergency department with isolated orthopedic injuries. The physician, however, must always suspect the presence of associated and potentially

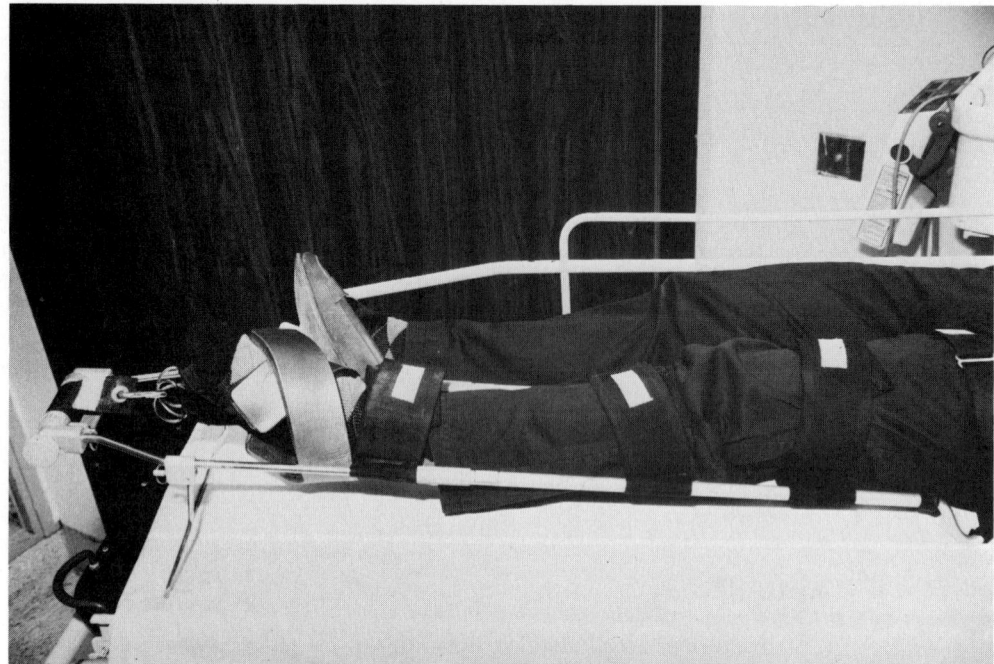

FIGURE 43-1. *The Hare traction splint provides temporary traction and stabilization of femur fractures.*

life-threatening injuries. The multiply traumatized patient who has suffered a battery, a significant fall, or a motor vehicle accident is addressed while keeping the prioritizing dictum of "life before limb" in mind. Three major problems should be looked for and addressed early: hemorrhage (internal or external), vascular compromise, and open fractures.

Hemorrhage

Victims of trauma are addressed according to the ABCs. Obvious and often impressive injuries of the extremities must not distract the physician from immediately assessing the patient's airway and breathing or establishing adequate intravenous (IV) access for aggressive volume resuscitation. Any site of external bleeding is controlled with pressure. Internal bleeding is also considered. The patient with a deformed or swollen thigh may lose up to 1500 ml of blood at the site of a femoral fracture and may present in a hypotensive state. A fractured pelvis may sequester even more blood. As with all trauma victims, concealed bleeding in the thoracic or peritoneal cavity is a major consideration.

Neurovascular Injury

All injuries are assessed for vascular compromise by palpating the femoral, popliteal, dorsalis pedis, and posterior tibial pulses. If pulses are not felt in the presence of adequate systemic blood pressure, flow can be assessed using a Doppler unit. Evaluating color, warmth, and capillary refill time in the feet and toes is also informative. Injuries commonly associated with vascular injury or compromise include anterior hip dislocations, knee dislocations (especially posterior), proximal tibial fractures, fracture-dislocations of the ankle (bimalleolar and trimalleolar fractures), and Lisfranc fracture-dislocations of the midfoot. Because major vessels are usually accompanied by nerves, associated neurologic, motor, and sensory deficits are sought on examination as well. The complete neurovascular examination is an integral part of the evaluation of the patient with *any* extremity injury.

Closed fracture-dislocations with vascular compromise are immediately reduced in an attempt to reestablish blood flow to the distal extremity. In the absence of vascular compromise, deformities usually require splinting and prompt radiologic evaluation prior to manipulation in order to obtain useful information for use in reduction as well as for medicolegal documentation.

Open Fractures

Emergency department care of open injuries differs from that of closed injuries in that manipulation is not performed. The wound should not be explored digitally. Instead, immediate cultures are obtained, and the site is first scrubbed with a povidone-iodine solution and then copiously irrigated prior to covering it with a saline or povidone-iodine-soaked dressing. This is followed by a noncompressive sterile wrap and splinting. The patient should be given intravenous antibiotics as soon as possible, most commonly a first- or second-generation cephalosporin. Fractures or dislocations with vascular compromise and all open injuries require immediate orthopedic consultation for aggressive debridement, irrigation, and reduction in the operating room.

DATA GATHERING

History

The history is an essential part of assessment in lower extremity injuries. It provides clues useful for identification of *all* the patient's injuries and may prevent iatrogenic morbidity.

1. *When did the injury occur?*
   Knowing the amount of time that has elapsed since injury is most helpful in treating open injuries or those with vascular compromise and potential vascular injury. The longer an injury is open, the greater the degree of contamination and the greater the risk of wound infection or osteomyelitis. If vascular compromise has occurred, blood flow must be reestablished in 4 to 6 hours or tissue necrosis distal to the obstruction will occur.
2. *How did the injury occur?*
   Knowledge of how an injury happened helps the physician diagnose the primary as well as associated injuries. For example, a patient who has jumped two stories to avoid a fire is a likely candidate for any combination of lower extremity injuries but is at especially high risk for calcaneal fractures. Consideration of this mechanism of injury also leads one to seek out associated injuries such as compression fractures of the lumbar spine. The mechanism of injury is also important in determining the method of repair or reduction.
3. *Has the patient had a previous injury to the same extremity?*
   A previous injury of the extremity in question will not only influence the physician's expectations during the examination but also help in interpreting the radiographs.
4. *Is there a significant past medical history?*
   Eliciting any history of past illness, current medications, or allergies is important in all cases to anticipate complications and prevent unnecessary drug interactions or reactions. All patients in need of surgery are also asked about previous surgeries, transfusions, and the time elapsed since the last meal.

Physical Examination

The physical examination will involve predominantly inspection, palpation, and a quantitative functional analysis—testing the range of motion in degrees. Auscultation is rarely used, although a Doppler blood flow detector may be necessary to confirm the distal pulses. Attention to surface structures is important and emphasizes the need to know the associated underlying bony anatomy. The uninjured opposite extremity provides the best source of what should be considered "normal" for that patient.

The Hip

The femur is the strongest bone in the human body as well as the longest. It can be divided into the head, neck, and shaft (Fig. 43–2). The hip articulation is composed of the spherical head of the femur and the acetabulum of the pelvis, forming a ball and socket joint. The capsule of this joint extends from the rim of the acetabulum to the junction of the femoral neck and the trochanters of the femoral shaft. A significant but somewhat tenuous portion of the blood supply to the head and proximal neck of the

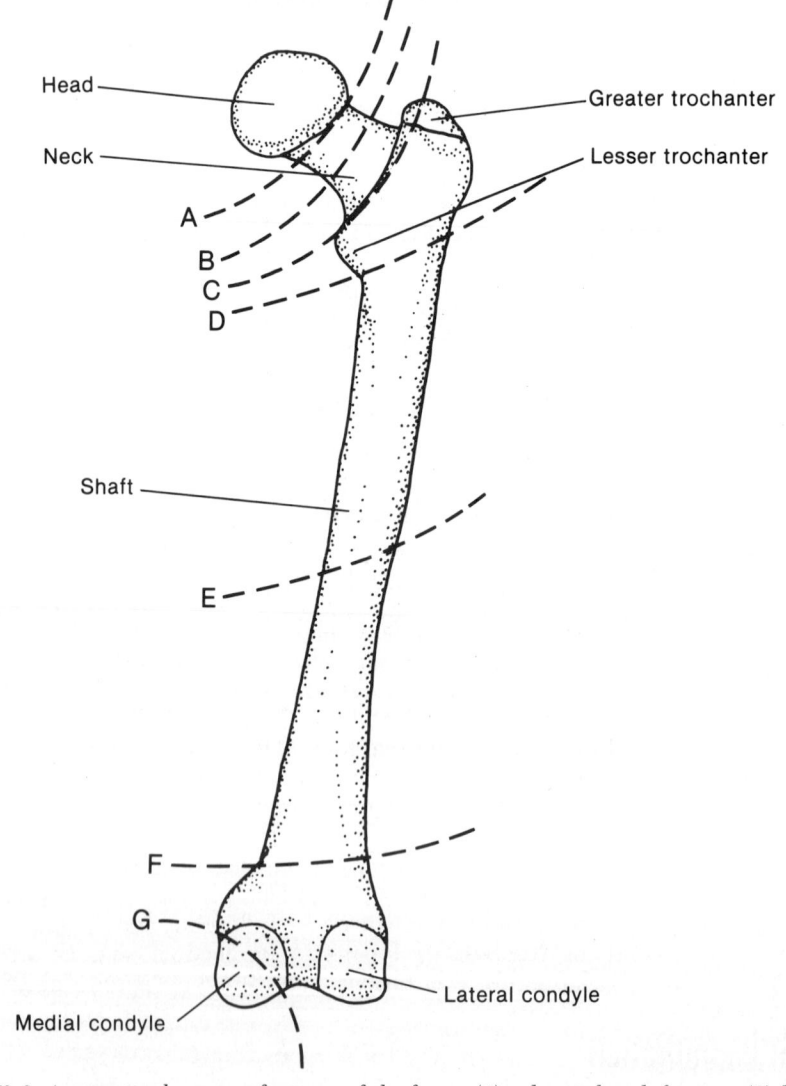

FIGURE 43–2. *Anatomy and common fractures of the femur:* (A) *subcapital neck fracture;* (B) *basilar neck fracture;* (C) *intertrochanteric fracture;* (D) *subtrochanteric fracture;* (E) *shaft fracture;* (F) *supracondylar fracture;* (G) *condylar fracture.*

femur arises from the central acetabulum through the artery of the ligamentum teres. This relationship is important in the development of nonunion or avascular necrosis after femoral neck fractures or hip dislocations.

Careful observation of the posture of the lower extremity can often lead to a strong presumptive diagnosis prior to radiographic evaluation of a hip injury. The examiner should note the presence of hip flexion as well as abduction or adduction compared to that in the uninjured leg. Comparison of the relative positions of the knees and malleoli or heels may reveal shortening of the extremity. Rotational deformity is best observed with regard to the position of the great toe and knee relative to the superior iliac crest. Range of motion of the hip in flexion, extension, abduction, adduction, and internal and external rotation is performed and quantified in terms of degrees while noting associated pain.

The Thigh

The femoral shaft and its attendant muscle groups comprise the musculoskeletal thigh. Physical examination of the thigh is as straightforward as its anatomy. Observation is often all that is necessary to make a presumptive diagnosis of a femoral shaft fracture. A swollen or deformed thigh that is tender to palpation after trauma is assumed to be a femoral shaft fracture until proved otherwise. Further evaluation and care must be undertaken on the assumption that an unstable fracture of the femur exists.

The Knee

The knee is actually a combination of three joints—the medial condylar joint, the lateral condylar joint, and the patellofemoral articulation. The articular capsule is intimately associated with the ligaments and aponeuroses of several muscle insertions as well as the knee's intrinsic ligamentous structures (Fig. 43–3A and B). The medial and lateral collateral ligaments are separate structures that provide support, especially on knee extension. Within the capsule lie the menisci and the cruciate ligaments. The anterior and posterior cruciate ligaments are strong, rounded cords arising from the anterior and posterior aspects of the tibial surface, respectively. The anterior cruciate extends posteriorly to connect to the femoral joint surface, whereas the posterior cruciate attaches to the anterior aspect of the femur. The menisci are crescent-shaped pads of fibrocartilage that extend to the outer borders of the tibial condyles; they have concave surfaces superiorly that correspond to the femoral condyles. This complex arrangement of cartilage and connective tissue gives remarkable stability to an intrinsically unstable arrangement of vertically apposed bones while simultaneously allowing weight bearing as well as free movement in the vertical plane.

During the physical examination of the knee the integrity of the supporting cartilage and ligaments is evaluated because injuries to these structures are more common than fractures of bones. The examination is approached systemically and includes the following components:

Gross Examination. Apparent swelling of the knee is often due to joint effusion rather than to local soft tissue swelling. Careful ballottement will usually help to differentiate between the two. A "patellar tap" may be noted when the patella, separated from the femoral condyles by the effusion, "taps" the femur as it is balloted. If an effusion has been present for less than 24 hours, it is presumed to be bloody; in 90% of cases it is associated with an internal injury of a cruciate ligament or meniscus.

Joint Line Palpation. If the joint line is tender, injury of the meniscus or collateral ligaments is suspected because it is here that they are attached to the bone.

Collateral Ligament Palpation. The attachments of the medial and lateral collateral ligaments to the femur, tibia, and fibula extend beyond the joint line. These attachments must be fully palpated in order to diagnose sprains about the knee. Tenderness without laxity indicates largely intact ligaments and a first-degree sprain.

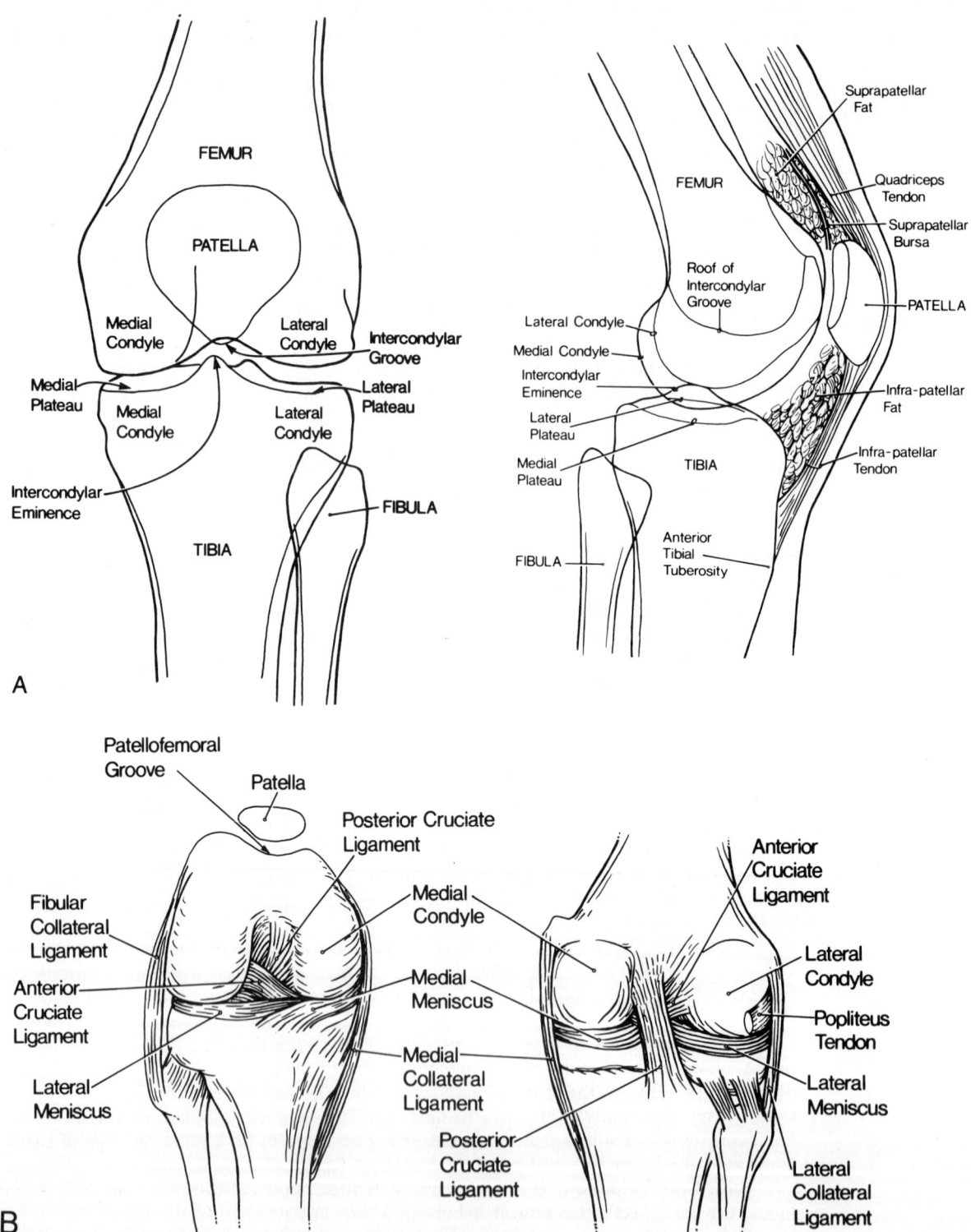

FIGURE 43–3. A, Principal anatomic structures of the knee. Anteroposterior view and lateral view. (From Rogers LF: *Radiology of Skeletal Trauma* (Vol. 2). © 1982 by Churchill Livingstone. Used by permission of the Churchill Livingstone Co.) B, Principal anatomy of the knee. Anterior view and posterior view. (Adapted from Schultz RJ: *The Language of Fractures*, Huntington, NY, Robert E. Krieger Publishing Co. © 1972 by the Williams & Wilkins Co., Baltimore. Used by permission of the Williams & Wilkins Co.,)

Ligamentous Laxity Examination. Valgus and varus stresses of the extended knee are used to evaluate the laxity of the medial and lateral collateral ligaments. With the lower leg stabilized, force applied to the lateral knee will provide a valgus stress, whereas varus stress will result from force applied to the medial knee. Anterior and posterior drawer tests of the knee in flexion are used to evaluate laxity in the anterior and posterior cruciate ligaments, respectively. For the drawer test, the patient is placed in the supine position with the hip in 45 degrees of flexion and the knee flexed to 90 degrees. While sitting on the patient's foot to stabilize it, two hands are used to push the proximal tibia posteriorly (posterior drawer test) or pull it anteriorly (anterior drawer test). There should be no movement in either of these tests in the healthy knee. The presence of laxity with stress indicates at least a second-degree ligamentous sprain. Unrestricted joint movement with stress indicates a complete ligamentous disruption.

Range of Motion. The knee joint should be evaluated for its ability to extend and flex, both actively and passively. If the injured knee cannot be fully extended, disruption of the quadriceps or patellar tendon may be present as well as a transverse patellar fracture. A "locked knee" that does not allow full range of motion suggests a meniscal cartilage tear with a loose foreign body within the joint, thus blocking movement.

Meniscal Cartilage Evaluation. Using McMurray's test, the knee is extended from the fully flexed position with the foot externally rotated. The presence of palpable crepitance, locking, or pain with full extension of the knee suggests injury to the medial meniscus.

The Leg

The anatomy of the leg is relatively simple, consisting of the parallel arrangement of the tibia and fibula, which are joined by a fibrous interosseous membrane (Fig. 43–4). On this structure are layered the various flexor and extensor muscles of the ankle divided into well-circumscribed compartments. The tibia and fibula are poorly protected by soft tissue anteriorly, increasing their vulnerability. The common peroneal nerve winds around the proximal neck of the fibula, and the anterior tibial artery penetrates the interosseous membrane in the proximal leg. Benign-appearing fractures in these two areas may be associated with unsuspected nerve or vascular injury.

The physical examination of the leg is easier than that of the knee. Fractures of the tibial and fibular shafts are often obvious owing to angular or rotational deformity and localized soft tissue injury. Palpation may elicit point tenderness. The skin is carefully examined for small wounds that can occur when bone fragments puncture the surface from within, indicating an open fracture. The compartments of the leg are also examined (as described below under Compartment Syndromes).

The Ankle and Foot

The ankle and foot consist of an intricate complex of tendons, ligaments, and bones with innumerable interdependent articulations and relationships (Fig. 43–5). The ankle is a hinge joint that has 13 tendons but no muscles that cross the joint. The weight-bearing tibia forms the plafond, or ankle ceiling, in the talocrural joint (the joint between the tibia and the talus). The support of the ankle exists circumferentially about it, with strong ligaments securing the fibula, talus, and tibia. Injuries occur either because of pulling forces along these ligaments (which cause sprains or transverse avulsion fractures) or abnormal movement of the talus within the ankle joint (which causes oblique fractures). Injuries that cause two or more disruptions in this ligament and bone ring render the ankle unstable. Fractures that occur through the malleoli above the tibial plafond are assumed to have rendered the ankle unstable.

The foot may be divided anatomically into the hindfoot, midfoot, and forefoot. The hindfoot is made up of the calcaneus and talus. It receives the majority of the weight-bearing load transferred from the tibia. The rigid midfoot is composed of the tarsal

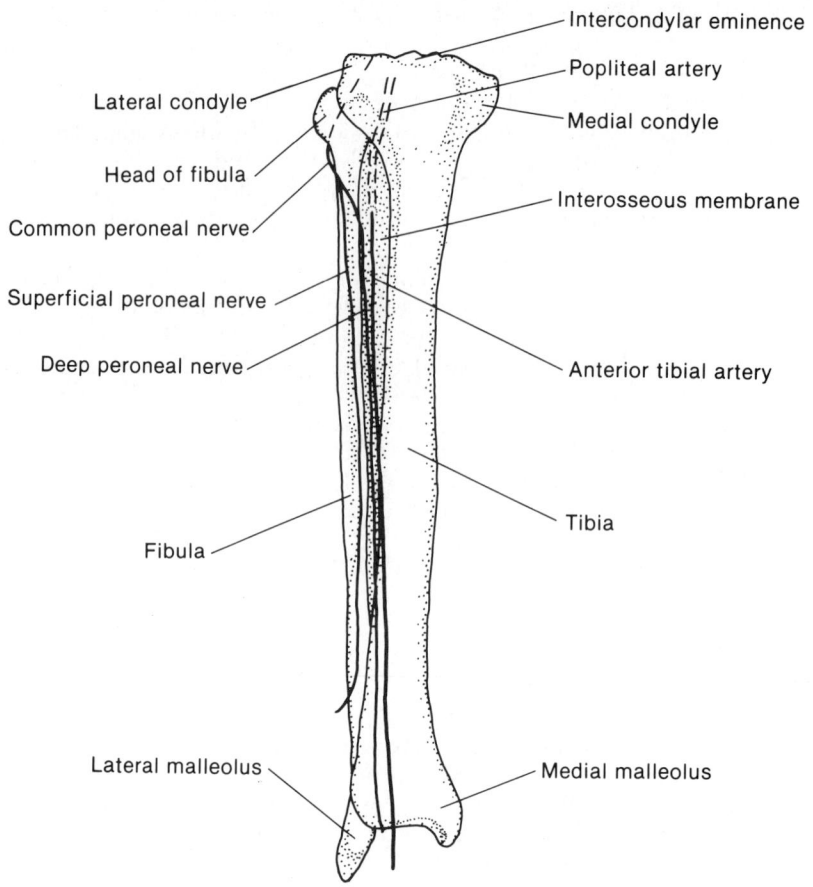

FIGURE 43–4. *Basic anatomy of the leg.*

navicular, the cuboid, and the three cuneiform bones, tightly joined by multiple ligamentous structures. The forefoot is made up of the five metatarsals and phalanges. Ligamentous connections in the forefoot decrease with increasing distance from the tarsometatarsal articulations, allowing more flexibility distally in the foot. The complex articulations and ligamentous connections in the foot help to distribute equally the loads incurred with normal gait.

Foot and ankle injuries are common and can alter this elaborate architecture, leading to dysfunctional use if they are unrecognized or untreated. A thorough examination will identify likely injuries. The examination should include the three following aspects:

Gross Examination. The presence of moderate to severe soft tissue swelling is typical in the presence of ligamentous sprains of the ankle. This is especially true of lateral ankle sprains because the lateral ankle ligaments form part of the lateral joint capsule. Ecchymosis usually occurs late after injury. Fracture-dislocations of the ankle are common and can be readily recognized by the gross deformity and extensive soft tissue swelling that accompany them. Dislocations of the tarsals, metatarsals, and phalanges are less easily diagnosed without roentgenograms owing to the diffuse pain and foot swelling that obscure bony landmarks and prevent the use of aggressive palpation to pinpoint the problem.

Palpation. Point tenderness of the ankle or midfoot ligaments suggests a common sprain. Point tenderness of the malleoli, proximal fibula, calcaneus, or base of the fifth metatarsal suggests that a fracture is more likely. All of these locations are examined in the patient with a chief complaint of an ankle "sprain."

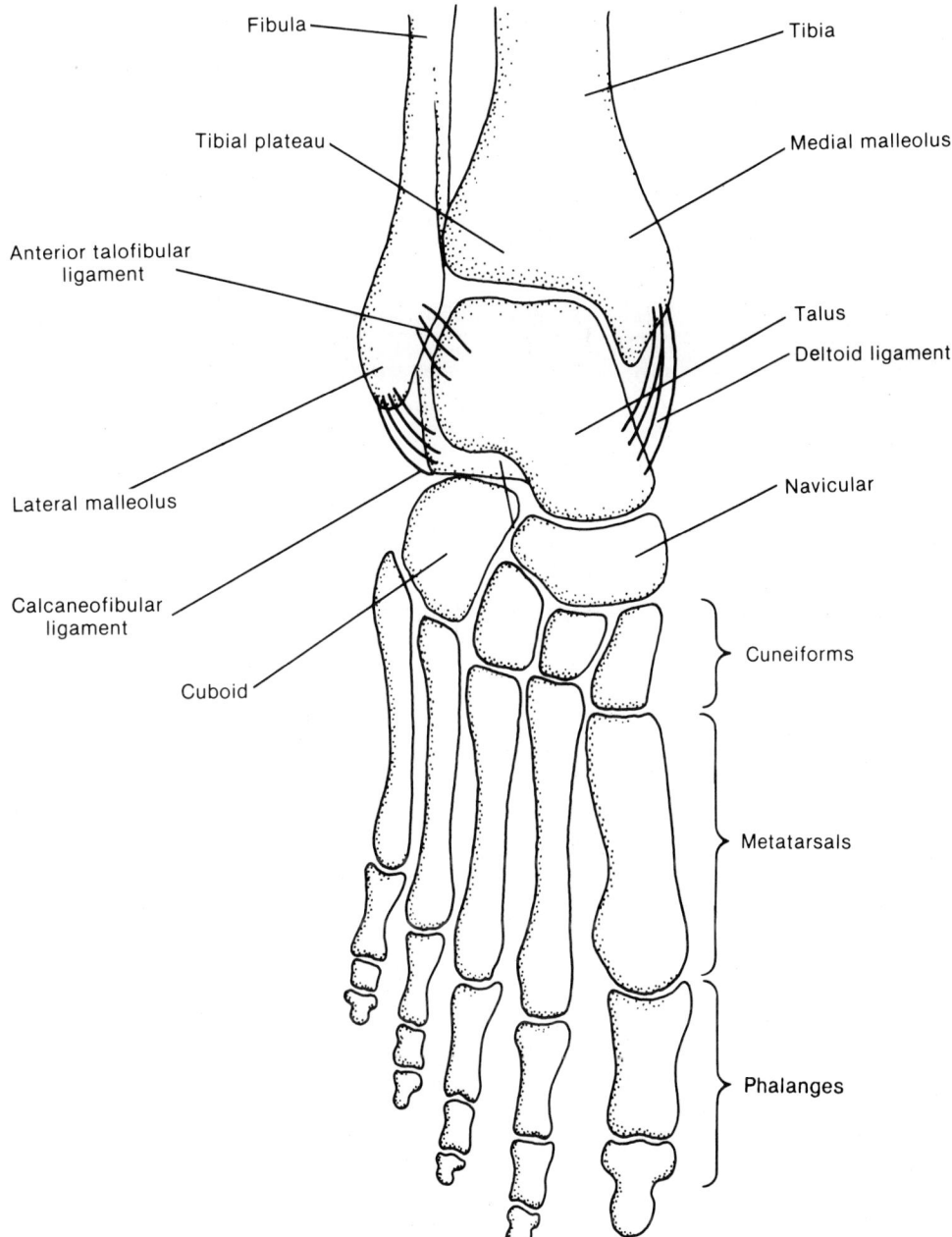

FIGURE 43–5. Basic anatomy of the ankle and foot.

Examination of Ligamentous Laxity. Laxity about the ankle is diagnosed using anterior drawer and talar tilt stress testing. The anterior drawer examination of the ankle is similar to that of the knee. It is performed by pulling the heel anteriorly while flexing the knee 45 degrees and keeping the lower leg stabilized. Movement of the foot relative to the lower leg suggests anterior talofibular ligament disruption. The talar tilt examination is performed by forcing the heel into inversion while the lower leg is stabilized. Abnormal movement of the foot reflects injury to both the anterior talofibular and calcaneofibular ligaments. These laxity tests should be performed whenever the ankle is significantly tender both medially and laterally, suggesting extensive ligamentous disruption. They are not necessary in the presence of severe ankle joint deformity, since in such cases the diagnosis of ankle instability is already made. Furthermore, the presence of severe swelling and pain may prevent adequate stressing or interpretation.

DECISION PRIORITIES AND PRELIMINARY DIFFERENTIAL DIAGNOSIS

When the data gathering is complete, the emergency physician answers three questions before moving on to diagnostic adjuncts.

1. *Is there a persistent life-threatening problem?*
   The presentation of lower extremity injury can be dramatic and can distract the physician from focusing on potentially catastrophic problems. These problems can also evolve over time. Therefore, before ordering diagnostic studies and moving on, the physician may find a brief review of the secondary survey very rewarding (see Chapter 4). This is also an appropriate time to check the volume of fluid given and the patient's tolerance to pain.
2. *Is there a persistent limb-threatening problem?*
   Limb-threatening problems from vascular, nerve, or other pressure-related damage can also evolve over time. A rapid estimate of warmth, capillary refill time, and gross neurologic status compared to these parameters on the initial examination provides valuable information.
3. *Is there a need for any further testing?*
   This is a question that applies to the more benign patient problems. Radiographs are never "routine"; it is important that there be reasonable indications for ordering them. For example, several studies have found that a careful ankle examination using specific criteria can decrease the number of ankle films ordered by almost 40% without missing significant problems. This information has not been widely accepted, however, and many films are ordered by rote rather than by reason. Each test should be thoughtfully justified before it is requested.

DIAGNOSTIC ADJUNCTS

Radiographic Imaging

Plain film radiographs are the standard measure of bone injury. As in all cases of trauma to an extremity, anteroposterior and lateral views are mandatory. A view of the full length of the long bone including both joints is necessary for optimal interpretation.

Indications for Radiographic Evaluation

Several considerations influence the need for radiographs when evaluating lower extremity trauma. Roentgenographic examination is appropriate in the following situations:

High Likelihood of Fracture. Any bone that is likely, based on the history or physical examination, to have been fractured or dislocated is radiologically examined.

High Incidence of Associated Injury. If an injury is frequently associated with a certain fracture, both areas are viewed. One example is injury to the contralateral calcaneus when a calcaneal fracture has resulted from a fall.

High Morbidity of a Missed Fracture. If the suspected fracture is known to lead to long-term complications, radiographs are used liberally. For example, failure to radiograph and diagnose a slipped capital femoral epiphysis will lead to further irreversible slippage, gait aberration, degenerative changes, and potential avascular necrosis. Therefore, any child with hip pain or a limp should undergo radiographic evaluation.

Significant Soft Tissue Injury. If there is significant soft tissue disruption of an extremity after trauma, an open fracture must be ruled out with radiographs.

High Patient Expectations. Patients or family members may be adamant in requesting radiographic evaluation of a bone that is judged clinically by the physician to be at low risk of fracture. Radiographs are strongly considered if the request is reasonable.

High Litigation Potential. Injuries that result from accidents in which one party is alleged to be at fault require radiographs to document the true extent of injury.

Poor Patient Follow-Up. If patients are thought to be poorly compliant, radiographs are obtained to document the exact injury that is present, since conservative treatment with later radiographs as appropriate is not a treatment option.

Potential Foreign Body Risk. If there is a possibility that a foreign body is present in an injured extremity, radiographs are indicated for localization and documentation.

Specific Radiographic Evaluation

Hip. Anteroposterior (AP) and lateral views of the femoral head and neck as well as an AP view of the pelvis are usually adequate for delineating hip fractures. An additional frog-leg lateral view is often obtained in children in whom a slipped capital femoral epiphysis is suspected.

Femur. AP and lateral views will reveal fractures as well as their angulation. The *entire* length of the femur should be visible in both views.

Knee. The routine knee examination includes AP and lateral views as a minimum. Most radiology departments also include an intercondylar view, which gives better visibility of the joint space and femoral condyles, as well as a patellar (or sunrise) view, which assists in identifying fractures of the patella. When an occult tibial plateau fracture is suspected, oblique views or tomograms may be indicated.

Tibia and Fibula. AP and lateral views reveal fractures as with the femur. Again, the entire length of the tibia and fibula must be visible.

Ankle. AP, lateral, and mortise views will provide information about fractures and ankle stability. The AP film will show the medial and lateral malleoli, and the lateral view reveals the talus, posterior malleolus, calcaneus, and base of the fifth metatarsal. The mortise view (an AP view with 10 degrees of internal rotation) shows the mortise en face. This view will reveal osteochondral fractures on the superior surface of the talus and will show the superior, medial, and lateral clear spaces of the talar articulation. Any variance from a constant width of 3 to 4 mm in these spaces is considered evidence of an unstable disruption of the ankle mortise.

Foot. AP, lateral, and oblique views are needed because the many bones of the foot overlap. AP and oblique views are useful in the examination of the tarsals, metatarsals, and phalanges. The lateral view reveals the calcaneus, talus, and superior portion of the tarsals.

Calcaneus. If abnormalities of the calcaneus are suggested on foot radiographs, or if tenderness and swelling are restricted to the heel, specific calcaneus films including lateral and axial views are obtained.

Specialized Techniques

Computed Tomography. Computed tomography (CT) scanning is useful in evaluating fracture-dislocations of the hip. It reveals both the fracture status of the acetabulum and the location of the femoral head. This information is particularly useful in defining central hip dislocations.

Magnetic Resonance Imaging. Magnetic resonance imaging (MRI), like CT, is useful for evaluating the femoral head and acetabulum. It also has been used for evaluating intra-articular pathology such as meniscal tears in the knee.

Radioisotope Scanning. Bone scans are rarely useful in the emergency department. Nuclear scans that reveal "hot spots" in areas of increased metabolic activity may be useful in the evaluation of systemic bone disease (Paget's disease, rheumatoid arthritis) or metastatic lesions. Bone scans may help in the diagnosis of occult fractures, stress fractures, or osteomyelitis in a patient with persistent symptoms of bone pain with unremarkable x-rays. They may also be used to evaluate local vascularity and occasionally to help define avascular necrosis of bone, as in Legg-Calvé-Perthes disease.

Arteriography. Although not useful in defining a bony injury per se, arteriography may be indicated when vascular compromise is not readily corrected by reduction of an angulated deformity. It may also be used when there is a high likelihood of arterial injury, as in posterior knee dislocations.

Laboratory Studies

Although laboratory values have little bearing on the specifics of lower extremity injuries, certain assays are important.

1. Pregnancy Test. In females of childbearing age, especially those with abnormal menstrual histories, who are about to undergo pelvic irradiation or surgery, a pregnancy test is ordered.
2. Hemoglobin and Hematocrit. These hematologic values are needed in patients with external or potential internal bleeding.
3. Type and Cross-Match. In patients with significant or potentially significant blood loss, blood type and cross-match are ordered.
4. Presurgical Testing. Presurgical testing is initiated in the emergency department for all patients whose injury will require immediate treatment in the operating room. Specific tests ordered will vary with the institution.

Other Tests
Arthrocentesis

Arthrocentesis, the needle aspiration of intra-articular fluid, is commonly used for diagnostic and therapeutic reasons in the emergency department. It is sometimes used after acute knee or elbow trauma to relieve a painful hemarthrosis and is of diagnostic value when gross blood or fat globules are aspirated from a radiographically normal joint, suggesting such intra-articular injury as a torn cruciate ligament or occult osseocartilaginous injury. In the setting of trauma, any analgesic or diagnostic value of arthrocentesis must be weighed against the risk of providing entry to the joint space for pathogenic bacteria, creating an iatrogenic septic joint. Oral analgesics and a compressive wrap may be entirely adequate treatment for a traumatic joint effusion if pain is not severe. Traumatic effusions causing more significant pain, however, require therapeutic arthrocentesis (see Chapter 40).

PRINCIPLES OF MANAGEMENT

In the emergency department management of lower extremity injuries, the physician considers all aspects of the injury: the integrity of the skin, the neurovascular status, and the severity and stability of a fracture or dislocation. Appropriate timing for surgery, if indicated, is important, as is the patient's ability to undergo and participate in the proposed treatment plan. Throughout, attention is paid to patient comfort.

Analgesia. The methods used for pain control are the same as those used with upper extremity injury (see Chapter 41).

Closed Reduction of Dislocations. Prompt closed reduction is completed if vascular compromise is confirmed. If the dislocation occurs with an open fracture in which bone is protruding from the wound, reduction should occur as soon as possible in the operating room following wound culture and irrigation. If immediate reduction is delayed and vascular compromise threatens the viability of the lower extremity, wound culture and copious irrigation are followed by reduction and immobilization in the emergency department.

Immobilization. Immobilization of lower extremity injuries minimizes pain and further soft tissue injury in prehospital as well as in hospital and outpatient settings. Emergency department splinting is a temporizing procedure until definitive casting can occur, but it can provide the long-term immobilization necessary for minor injuries. Splinting should be used *liberally* because complications of short-term immobilization are negligible, whereas failure to immobilize may indeed complicate an injury. *When in doubt, splint!*

1. *Hare Traction Splint.* As previously mentioned, the Hare traction splint (see Fig. 43–1) provides an excellent first response for suspected closed fractures below the femoral neck and above the ankle. It is especially appropriate for patients with suspected femoral fractures to reduce pain and, more importantly, to limit additional soft tissue injury and bleeding at the fracture site.

2. *Long Leg Splint.* Long leg splinting is useful with fractures of the distal femur (involving the knee joint), tibia, or tibia/fibula, and with fractures that severely disrupt the ankle mortise. The knee should be splinted in 10 to 15 degrees of flexion and the ankle in 90 degrees of dorsiflexion.

3. *Knee Immobilizer.* Knee immobilizers limit flexion and extension at the knee. Several types are available commercially. They are used most often to immobilize knees that have suspected cartilaginous or ligamentous injuries. They are ideal in this setting because they are adjustable and removable and can be placed over a bandage or clothing. Because they are adjustable, they can be used comfortably as knee swelling varies. Knee immobilizers do not, however, provide the same degree of rigidity as plaster splints, and they are easily removed by a noncompliant patient. Therefore, patients with injuries that must remain absolutely immobile, such as fractures about the knee, should receive a long leg plaster splint.

4. *Short Leg Splint.* Posterior short leg splinting, which extends from the plantar aspect of the forefoot to the proximal leg, restricts plantar and dorsiflexion of the ankle. This protects the ankle from further injury and pain in patients with ankle fractures that await definitive casting or repair. These splints also promote healing in patients with severe ankle sprains and foot fractures who are sent home. Placement of a short leg splint increases not only the likelihood that the patient will not bear weight on that extremity but also that he will seek appropriate follow-up.

5. *Sugartong (Stirrup) Splint.* Although posterior short leg splinting restricts plantar and dorsiflexion, some inversion and eversion can still occur, especially as swelling subsides and the splint loosens. Applying a strip of plaster that runs along the lateral and medial sides of the leg, encompassing the posterior plantar surface of the foot, will provide stability against eversion and inversion. Combining this stirrup splint with a posterior short leg splint provides the best ankle immobilization short of circumferential casting.

6. *Ankle Splint Alternatives.* Many minor ankle sprains can be managed without a plaster splint. Bandaging alternatives include circumferential cast padding followed by an Ace wrap, an Unna boot, or an Ace wrap alone. These bandages minimize swelling and limit motion, so that healing occurs more quickly and less painfully. As with all dressings or splints, the patient should be instructed to loosen the bandage if signs of vascular compromise occur, especially when the bandage is placed soon after the injury occurs, prior to maximal swelling.

Management of Specific Injuries

Injuries of the Hip and Thigh

The patient who complains of groin, hip, or knee pain may have one of a variety of hip injuries. In a young person who has suffered major trauma, a pelvic fracture near or at the acetabulum, an anterior or posterior dislocation of the femoral head, or a proximal femoral fracture is most likely. In an adolescent with no trauma the diagnosis of a slipped capital femoral epiphysis should be considered, whereas Legg-Calvé-Perthes disease is a possibility in preadolescent children. When the patient is elderly, a femoral neck fracture or an intertrochanteric fracture is a likely diagnosis even when a history of trauma is seemingly trivial or absent. Patients of any age who are subjected to major deforming forces may sustain any of a variety of femoral fractures (Fig. 43–2).

Femoral Neck Fractures

Mechanism. The mechanism of injury is often a trivial force applied to the greater trochanter or forced rotation of the extremity such as might occur in a simple fall. These shear forces coupled with the decreased bone density of osteoporosis may result in a fracture.

Presentation. A femoral neck fracture typically presents in an elderly patient who complains of hip pain and inability to walk. Some patients give no history of trauma. Impacted femoral neck fractures or those that are undisplaced may result in a minimum of symptoms and findings, with pain elicited only at the extremes of range of motion. Displaced fractures cause more pain and inability to walk. The hip is typically found in abduction and external rotation with associated shortening of the leg (Problem 1).

Radiologic Diagnosis. Routine anteroposterior and lateral views of the hip are usually adequate for diagnosis. With the exception of minimally displaced impacted fractures, these fractures are usually obvious. Oblique films are used when suspicion is high but routine views are nondiagnostic.

Management. All patients with femoral neck fractures (except possibly those with nondisplaced, impacted fractures that are weeks old and allow ambulation) require hospitalization to prevent further displacement until open reduction and internal fixation (ORIF) or prosthetic replacement can be performed. Due to the tenuous blood supply to the proximal femoral neck and head, failure to provide such care will increase the risk of aseptic necrosis or ultimate nonunion of the fragments.

PROBLEM 1 Shortening and external rotation of the left leg were noted in this elderly patient. Radiographs revealed a displaced femoral neck fracture. The leg was stabilized with sandbags, and the patient was hospitalized for surgical orthopedic management.

Intertrochanteric Fractures

Although femoral neck fractures occur within the joint capsule, intertrochanteric fractures occur along a line between the greater and lesser trochanters and are extracapsular. As with femoral neck fractures, they occur in older osteoporotic patients, with a higher frequency in females.

Mechanism. The mechanism of injury is almost always a fall involving both direct and indirect forces.

Presentation. The classic presentation is severe hip pain in an older patient, in whom the leg appears markedly shortened and is held in as much as 90 degrees of external rotation. Any movement of the lower limb is painful and can potentially cause further soft tissue injury or bony comminution.

Radiologic Diagnosis. These fractures are readily demonstrated on routine hip films as a lucent fracture line extending from the greater to the lesser trochanter.

Management. Patients with a possible hip fracture should have the affected limb stabilized with sandbags prior to radiographic examination. In general, more comminuted fractures are more unstable and more difficult to reduce. Immediate hospitalization and orthopedic consultation are sought. Aseptic necrosis and nonunion, however, are uncommon complications of intertrochanteric fractures owing to the generous extracapsular blood supply in this area.

Hip Dislocations

Another cause of hip pain and dysfunction is dislocation or fracture-dislocation of the hip. This was once a rare injury but has become more frequent owing to the intense forces generated in motor vehicle accidents. Less severe forces may be adequate to cause luxation of a prosthetic femoral head. Dislocations are described according to the positional relationships of the acetabulum and the femoral head and may be categorized as anterior, posterior, or central.

Posterior Hip Dislocations. Posterior hip dislocations are much more common than anterior or central dislocations.

Mechanism. The mechanism of injury is a force applied axially along the femur with the knee and hip in flexion such as may occur when a seated passenger's knee strikes the dashboard during a head-on car accident.

Presentation. The patient generally has multiple injuries. The affected hip is typically held in adduction, internal rotation, and flexion, and the leg is shortened. Ten to fifteen percent of patients with posterior hip dislocations have various degrees of sciatic nerve dysfunction because the dislocated femoral head approaches the sciatic notch, stretching or compressing the nerve. Because of the intense force necessary to produce a hip dislocation, associated damage to the femoral shaft and knee must be ruled out. As many as one-third of patients will have an associated knee injury.

Radiologic Diagnosis. Radiography will reveal the femoral head lying posterior to a coronal plane dividing the acetabulum. Additional views as well as computed tomography may be necessary to assess the femoral head's position fully as well as the integrity of the acetabulum, because an axial load applied to an abducted femur is likely to fracture the posterior acetabular lip.

Anterior Hip Dislocations. Anterior dislocations comprise less than 15% of hip dislocations.

Mechanism. The mechanism responsible for injury is similar to that causing a posterior dislocation except that the femur undergoes axial loading while in a more abducted position. An anterior dislocation may also occur if a patient is struck from behind while squatting. The femoral head may assume a superior (iliac or pubic) or inferior (obturator) position.

Presentation. A patient with an anterior-superior dislocation will present with a palpable mass in the inguinal area, with the leg held in abduction and external rotation. Because of the close proximity of this region to the femoral neurovascular bundle, direct injury to the femoral nerve, artery, or vein may result. A patient with an anterior-inferior dislocation will present with a more flexed hip.

Radiologic Diagnosis. AP, lateral, and oblique hip views will reveal the nature of the dislocation, showing the femoral head anterior to the acetabulum. Radiographs will show the femoral head overlying the obturator canal, inferior to the acetabulum, in an anterior-inferior dislocation.

Central Hip Dislocations. Central dislocations are always associated with acetabular fracture.

Mechanism. These injuries occur when an extreme axial force is transmitted to the femoral neck, shattering the acetabulum as the femoral head is driven centrally into the pelvis. The femoral head remains in contact with the comminuted acetabulum.

Presentation. The presentation is that of a pelvic fracture—severe hip and pelvic pain increase with movement. Hypotension from blood loss as well as associated intra-abdominal and genitourinary injuries are frequent accompaniments.

Radiologic Diagnosis. Plain films or CT studies will demonstrate the acetabular injury with the femoral head appearing within the confines of the pelvis.

Management. All hip dislocations are true orthopedic emergencies, and immediate orthopedic consultation is necessary. Prompt reduction will increase limb viability, decrease pressure-induced nerve ischemia, and reduce the incidence of subsequent avascular necrosis of the femoral head. Further long-term complications include myositis ossificans, post-traumatic arthritis, recurrent dislocation, and thrombosis of the femoral artery or vein. Multiple manipulations are used to reduce anterior or posterior hip dislocations; some authors advocate the immediate use of open reduction. If no fracture is present, closed reduction may be attempted in the emergency department with IV sedation and analgesia. The exception is the central dislocation, which mandates immediate surgical treatment. In the likely event that reduction is unsuccessful or cannot be maintained, general anesthesia is required for closed or open reduction in the operating room.

Fractures of the Femoral Shaft

Mechanism. Femoral shaft fractures occur commonly as a result of a direct force, torsional stress, or a high-velocity missile injury. Unless a pathologic fracture has occurred, the injury is usually the result of significant trauma.

Presentation. The patient will complain of pain exacerbated by movement or palpation of the thigh. Findings may include angulation, shortening, and rotational deformity of the lower limb. Due to the generous blood supply to the femoral diaphysis, the thigh is routinely swollen by local hemorrhage. The bleeding is significant and is often an ignored source of vascular volume loss. Up to 1.5 liters of blood may be lost at a femoral shaft fracture, leading to hypotension and tachycardia.

Radiologic Diagnosis. AP and lateral views of the entire femur are obtained to demonstrate the nature of the fracture. Depending on the mechanism of injury, the fracture may appear transverse, oblique, spiral, or comminuted, with varying degrees of angulation and shortening.

Management. Use of a Hare traction device is ideal for these fractures because it corrects angulation and shortening while preventing further soft tissue injury at the fracture site. Nerve involvement and vascular injury are rare occurrences. Patients require aggressive fluid resuscitation with large-bore intravenous catheters, admission to the hospital, and orthopedic consultation. Comminuted fractures are often treated initially with traction, whereas internal fixation with medullary nailing is often advocated in patients with simple fractures to facilitate early mobilization. The prognosis for repair of a femoral shaft fracture is generally excellent.

PROBLEM 2 This case was a typical presentation of a patient suffering a femoral shaft fracture. The high-velocity mechanism of injury associated with a swollen, tender thigh is classic. This patient's hypotension was due solely to the blood lost at the fracture site. His blood pressure responded to vigorous crystalloid fluid challenge, and his condition stabilized prior to his admission to the hospital.

Injuries of the Knee and Leg

Patellar Fractures

Mechanism. Patellar fractures occur with either direct trauma or forced flexion of the knee.

Presentation. Localized soft tissue swelling, point tenderness over the patella, and joint effusion are commonly seen. In patients with displaced transverse patellar fractures, the horizontally aligned bone defect is often palpable. The patient is usually unable to extend the knee.

Radiologic Diagnosis. Radiographs of the knee (including a "sunrise" view of the patella) facilitate diagnosis of these fractures. Since the AP view shows the patella superimposed over the knee joint, careful scrutiny is needed to discover any pathology.

Management. Nondisplaced or minimally displaced (by less than 2 mm) horizontal fractures are treated with immobilization and a compressive bandage, whereas displaced patellar fractures will require eventual surgical repair. Most patients may be discharged from the emergency department with knee immobilization and crutches after orthopedic consultation.

Distal Femoral Fractures. Fractures of the femur in or about the knee joint are infrequent. The femoral shaft is the more likely site of fracture. Fractures involving the supracondylar or intercondylar femur with intra-articular involvement are complex problems requiring immediate orthopedic referral. Such injuries are likely to require hospitalization for traction or open reduction.

Tibial Plateau Fractures

Mechanism. Patients with a history of direct knee trauma, sudden axial loading, or a violent twisting force may fracture one of the tibial condyles, disrupting the tibial plateau, which provides an articulating surface for the femur (Fig. 43–6).

Presentation. Patients are unable to bear weight without pain, and a knee effusion is typically present.

Radiologic Diagnosis. AP, lateral, and oblique views of the knee are usually adequate to define the fracture, although tomography may be necessary.

Management. Undisplaced fractures are often treated solely with immobilization, whereas displaced fractures (with greater than 5 mm of depression or widening) may require open reduction. Immediate orthopedic consultation is required to decide the disposition of the patient.

Collateral and Cruciate Ligament Injuries

Mechanism. Direct trauma to the knee can result in forced hyperextension, forced hyperflexion, valgus stress, or varus stress, any of which may be superimposed on rotational forces. These may lead to an isolated collateral ligament injury or may cause complete disruption of the collateral ligaments with injury to the cruciate ligaments.

Presentation. Marked swelling and pain (secondary to the hemarthrosis) are present as well as the patient's sensation that the knee is "giving out."

Radiologic Diagnosis. Knee radiographs will show knee effusion only.

Management. A severe traumatic effusion may require arthrocentesis. A compressive wrap, knee immobilizer, and crutches used in coordination with ice, elevation, and analgesics are prescribed until follow-up with an orthopedist can be arranged.

PROBLEM 3 The young football player suffered an injury to the anterior cruciate ligament as well as the medial meniscus when he was clipped. The opponent's force against his posterolateral knee created an acute valgus stress. On physical examination an impressive knee effusion, tenderness at the joint line, and a positive anterior drawer sign were found. Radiographs of the knee were unremarkable.

Knee Dislocation. Perhaps the most serious diagnostic consideration in acute injury of the knee is that of knee dislocation.

Mechanism. The most common type is the anterior dislocation, which is usually due to forced hyperextension. Posterior dislocation may occur when a severe force strikes the proximal tibia anteriorly—for example, when the leg strikes the dashboard in an auto

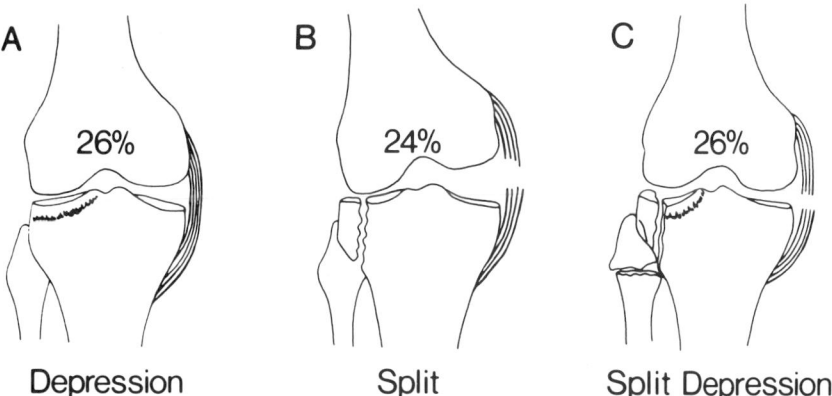

FIGURE 43–6. Classification and incidence of fractures of the tibial plateau. (Adapted from Hohl M: Tibial condylar fractures. J Bone Joint Surg (Am) 49:1455, 1967. Used by permission).

accident. This type of dislocation should be considered whenever the mechanism of injury suggests high-energy transfer to the knee.

Presentation. Massive knee swelling with deformity or complete joint instability occurs. Lack of deformity does not rule out the possibility of dislocation, since "spontaneous" reduction may occur in the prehospital setting.

Radiologic Diagnosis. If reduction has not already occurred, the lateral view of the knee will reveal the abnormal juxtaposition of the tibia and femur.

Management. Because of the high incidence of popliteal artery injury associated with knee dislocation, this injury requires immediate reduction. Placing the hip in flexion and applying longitudinal traction to the leg will facilitate the realignment of the tibia and femur. Angiography *after reduction* is indicated to rule out arterial injury. This is a true orthopedic emergency.

Patellar Dislocations

Mechanism. Patellar dislocations typically occur when there is an underlying abnormality of the patellofemoral anatomy. Direct trauma to a flexed knee may result in dislocation, but more commonly the injury occurs when the quadriceps forcibly contracts when the knee is flexed and the tibia is externally rotated, dislocating the patella laterally.

Presentation. The patient presents with a painful swollen knee, stating that the knee "went out." There is often a history of previous patellar dislocations. On examination, the knee is found to be swollen and warm due to a hemarthrosis, and the patella is palpated lateral to its normal position. If reduction has occurred prior to presentation, there will be positive results on the patellar apprehension test (Fairbands test)—on pushing the patella laterally, the patient will grasp the physician's hand because of the sensation of impending dislocation.

Radiologic Diagnosis. AP, lateral, and oblique views of the knee are required to rule out associated fracture. The patella typically appears in a lateral position, although superior, horizontal, and intercondylar patellar dislocations do occur.

Management. Lateral patellar dislocations are reduced by placing the patient in a posture of hip flexion and knee extension to achieve maximum relaxation of the knee's extensor mechanism. The patella is then gently moved medially to its normal position. After postreduction films show the patella in its normal position, orthopedic consultation is needed. Although some orthopedists elect to repair first-time dislocations surgically, others treat these injuries with a long leg cast for 6 weeks. The patient may be discharged for follow-up care with a posterior long leg splint or a knee immobilizer.

Fibular Fractures

Mechanisms. Fibular shaft fractures result from direct trauma. Isolated proximal fibular fractures are suspected in patients who are struck by a car's bumper while walking. Fibular shaft fractures tend to occur in association with tibial shaft fractures owing to their parallel positions. Ankle stress is likely to cause a distal fibular fracture but can produce a fracture throughout the length of the fibula if it is forceful enough.

Presentation. Patients with isolated fibular fractures present with local pain and swelling. Pain may not be exacerbated by weight bearing. If associated peroneal nerve injury occurs, there is weakness in ankle dorsiflexion.

Radiologic Diagnosis. AP and lateral tibia-fibula views will delineate a fracture.

Management. Because the fibula has no role in weight bearing, the rare isolated fracture of the fibular shaft usually is not problematic; it can be treated without casting when pain is minimal. Fractures of the lateral malleolus or distal fibula are more serious because the lateral support of the ankle joint is jeopardized. Depending on the severity of injury, surgical repair may be required (see section on Malleolar Fractures below).

Tibial Shaft Fractures

Mechanism. Tibial fractures occur secondary to direct trauma or torsional stress.

Presentation. Because the anterior aspect of the tibia lies immediately below the skin, fractures of this bone are often readily apparent. Examination may reveal laxity and crepitance at the site associated with pain. Nerve or vascular damage is rare except in instances of comminuted and displaced fractures of the proximal third of the tibia, near the anterior tibial artery's passage through the interosseous membrane.

Radiologic Diagnosis. AP and lateral views of the entire tibia and fibula will reveal the fracture.

Management. Emergency department treatment involves reduction of gross deformities through longitudinal traction and immobilization in a long leg posterior mold until definitive reduction and casting can be performed. Fractures of the proximal tibia may require angiographic evaluation of the popliteal and tibial arteries.

Injuries of the Ankle and Foot

Mechanisms of Ankle Injury. The ankle is a complex structure of interdependent articulations and ligamentous supports (Fig. 43–7A and B). The mechanism of injury will indicate the type of ankle pathology to be expected. The three common mechanisms of injury can be correlated with distinct constellations of findings:

Inversion Injury

1. Lateral ligamentous sprain or avulsion fracture of the lateral malleolus due to local distractive forces.

2. Oblique fracture of the medial malleolus as the talus is driven into the inferolateral tibia from below (Fig. 43–8).

Eversion Injury

1. Deltoid ligament sprain or avulsion fracture of the medial malleolus due to the local distractive force.

2. Oblique fracture of the fibula as the talus is driven into the lateral malleolus from below (Fig. 43–9A, B, and C).

External Rotation Injury

(Occurs as the foot and talus rotate externally relative to the leg)

1. Disruption of the syndesmosis between the tibia and fibula, or a fibular fracture above the plafond as the talus moves laterally.

2. Anterior or posterior tibial fracture with separation of the distal tibia and fibula.

3. Deltoid ligament sprain or tibial avulsion fracture.

These findings may occur singly, in combination, or not at all, depending on the forces involved. Keeping these patterns in mind is helpful when interpreting roentgenograms.

Ankle Sprain. Sprain is the most common diagnosis in ankle injury. An injury that appears to be a simple ankle sprain to the naïve examiner is often more complex when it is fully evaluated. The common injuries about the ankle that may simulate the pain found in simple ankle sprains are listed in Table 43–1. These must be considered and ruled out before the diagnosis of ankle sprain can be comfortably made.

Mechanism. Inversion, eversion, or rotation about the ankle lead to variable degrees of stretching and tearing of the medial deltoid ligament or lateral ligamentous complex.

Presentation. The patient presents with local swelling and pain. Lateral sprains are more common than medial sprains, due to the deltoid ligament's greater strength.

Radiologic Diagnosis. All but the most minor ankle injuries require radiographic

TABLE 43–1. Injuries Mimicking Ankle Sprain

Injury	History	Physical Findings
Calcaneal fracture	Axial load to ankle	Severe pain, swelling of heel
Proximal fibular fracture	Ankle eversion or rotation	Point tenderness along the fibula, especially near the knee
Fifth metatarsal fracture	Ankle inversion	Point tenderness at the proximal fifth metatarsal with pain on ankle inversion
Tarsal fracture midfoot	Severe foot twisting or direct trauma	Diffuse midfoot tenderness

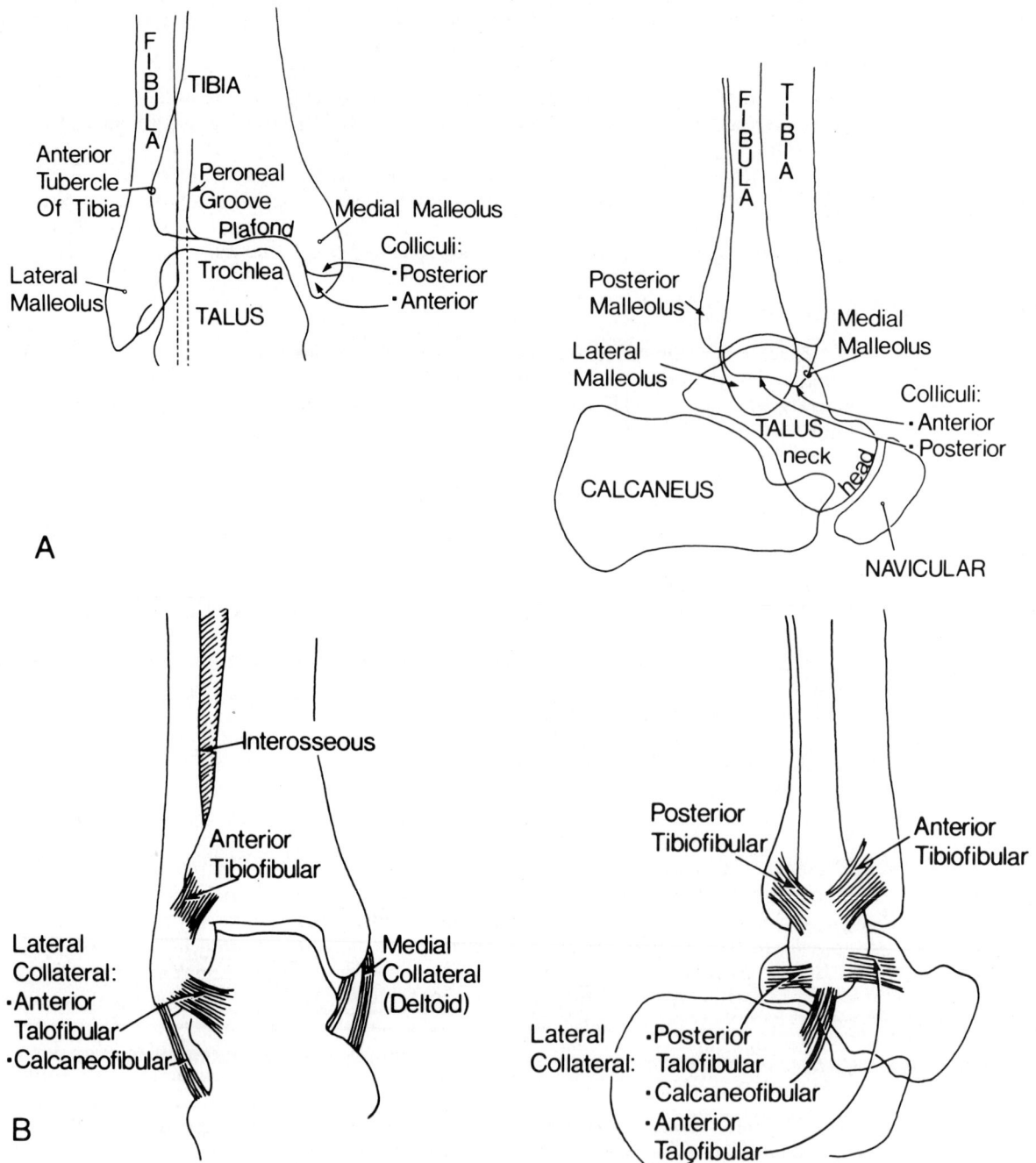

FIGURE 43-7. A, Anatomy of the ankle as seen on radiograph. (Adapted from Rogers LF: Radiology of Skeletal Trauma (Vol 2). © 1982 by Churchill Livingstone. Used by permission of the Churchill Livingstone Co.) B, Principal ligaments of the ankle. (From Rogers LF: Radiology of Skeletal Trauma (Vol. 2). © 1982 by Churchill Livingstone. Used by permission of the Churchill Livingstone Co.)

evaluation to rule out the presence of a fracture. AP, lateral, and mortise views are appropriate.

Management. Pain control, elevation, and immobilization (ranging from a bulky Ace wrap to splinting with a posterior plaster mold) are appropriate treatment regimens.

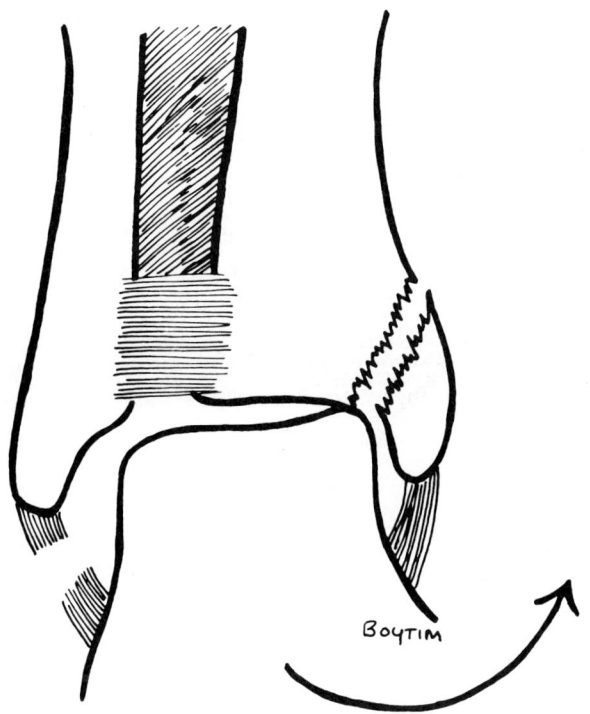

FIGURE 43–8. *Schematic representation of the type of injury caused by forced inversion of the ankle with medial displacement and rotation of the talus. The effect of the impaction force upon the medial malleolus resulting from the displacement of the talus is the vertical fracture through the base of the medial malleolus. The avulsion force may either disrupt the lateral collateral ligament (as depicted here) or, if the lateral collateral ligament remains intact, produce an avulsion fracture of the styloid process of the lateral malleolus. Note that the distal tibiofibular ligaments and the interosseous membrane remain intact. (From Harris JH, Harris WH: The Radiology of Emergency Medicine (2nd ed.) © 1981 by the Williams & Wilkins Co., Baltimore. Used by permission of the Williams & Wilkins Co.)*

Patients with all injuries are given crutches to keep them from bearing weight until they can do so without pain.

PROBLEM 4 This basketball player had suffered an ankle injury, most likely a lateral ankle sprain, based on the location of the pain and the mechanism of injury. Physical examination revealed a stable ankle joint with tenderness along the lateral ligamentous complex and associated swelling. Ankle radiographs demonstrated an intact mortise without fractures, and the diagnosis of ankle sprain was confirmed.

Malleolar Fractures

Mechanism. Transverse avulsion fractures of the medial and lateral malleoli imply pulling forces along the supporting ligaments. Oblique malleoli fractures imply injury caused by the moving talus.

Presentation. Significant ankle swelling, tenderness, and occasionally gross deformity are found in patients with malleolar fractures. Distal vascular compromise may occur with the deformity caused by a severe fracture-dislocation.

Radiologic Diagnosis. AP, lateral, and mortise views show fractures of the involved malleolus, which may appear as small avulsion injuries. The mortise view is carefully evaluated for any evidence of joint instability. A bimalleolar fracture involves the lateral and medial malleoli, whereas a trimalleolar fracture also includes the posterior malleolus (the inferoposterior lip of the distal tibia).

Management. Isolated transverse lateral malleolus fractures often can be treated much like sprains. Bimalleolar and trimalleolar fractures, however, render the ankle unstable. Gross deformity is corrected prior to immobilization in a posterior mold, and patients are usually hospitalized for open reduction and internal fixation.

Maisonneuve Fractures

Mechanism. Isolated sprains of the strong deltoid ligament are not common. Medial tenderness should raise one's index of suspicion for an associated lateral injury. This

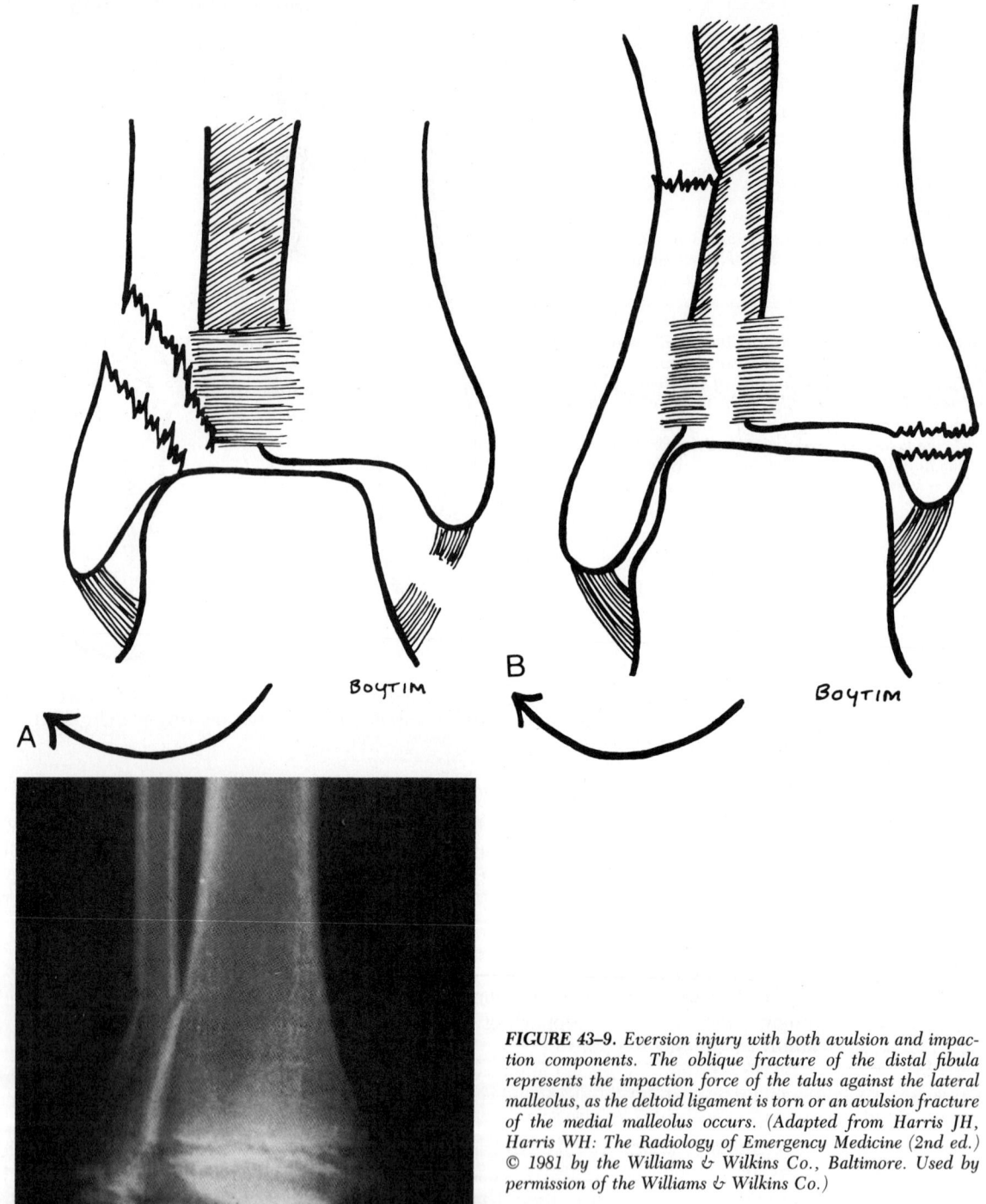

FIGURE 43–9. Eversion injury with both avulsion and impaction components. The oblique fracture of the distal fibula represents the impaction force of the talus against the lateral malleolus, as the deltoid ligament is torn or an avulsion fracture of the medial malleolus occurs. (Adapted from Harris JH, Harris WH: The Radiology of Emergency Medicine (2nd ed.) © 1981 by the Williams & Wilkins Co., Baltimore. Used by permission of the Williams & Wilkins Co.)

lateral injury could be a Maisonneuve fracture, in which the proximal fibula is fractured as forces are transferred axially and proximally along the length of the bone and interosseous membrane. This injury should be considered in an isolated fracture of either the medial or the posterior malleolus.

Presentation. In addition to pain and swelling of the medial ankle, tenderness is noted along the proximal fibula. The patient may deny any direct trauma to the area. Including palpation of the proximal fibula as a standard part of the ankle examination ensures that a Maisonneuve fracture will not be missed.

Radiologic Diagnosis. The key to this diagnosis is a high index of suspicion. Clinical examination of the area is followed by AP and lateral radiologic views of the entire tibia and fibula as well as an ankle mortise view (Fig. 43–10).

Management. Treatment principles for this injury are the same as those for ankle fractures in general. The unstable ankle, as evidenced by a disrupted mortise, is likely to require ORIF if closed reduction cannot achieve a stable, anatomic alignment. After orthopedic consultation, placement of a long leg posterior mold is appropriate, whether inpatient or outpatient treatment is chosen.

Fracture-Dislocations of the Ankle

Mechanism. The three mechanisms of ankle injury described above may lead to a fracture-dislocation. Forces strong enough to cause bimalleolar or trimalleolar fractures may force the talus out of the ankle mortise.

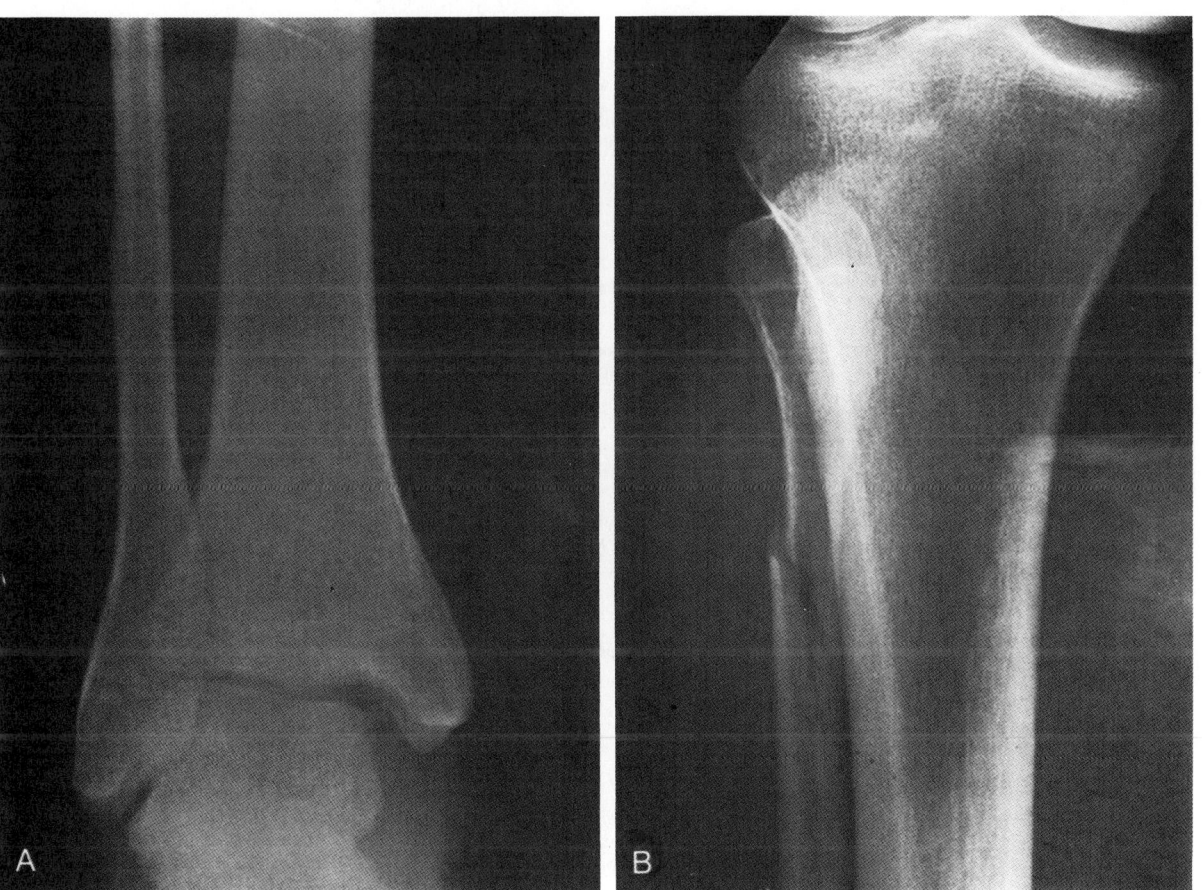

FIGURE 43–10. The Maisonneuve fracture. Note that the talus is displaced laterally indicating disruption of the distal tibiofibular ligaments while the propagation of forces proximally has caused a proximal fibular fracture. (Adapted from Harris JH, Harris WH: *The Radiology of Emergency Medicine* (2nd ed.). © 1981 by the Williams & Wilkins Co., Baltimore. Used by permission of the Williams & Wilkins Co.)

Presentation. The deformity of an ankle dislocation is readily apparent in the form of swelling and angulation. If the injury is severe, a distally cyanotic foot with an absent dorsalis pedis pulse may be noted.

Radiologic Diagnosis. The three views of the ankle will show a bimalleolar or trimalleolar fracture with disruption of the mortise.

Management. It is necessary to check immediately for the integrity of the overlying skin and distal neurovascular function. Early reduction is completed following the initial radiographs. Reduction is achieved simply by returning the talus to its position in the ankle mortise using in-line traction. Documentation of the neurovascular status following reduction and splinting is mandatory. As with other bimalleolar or trimalleolar fractures, hospitalization for ORIF is usually indicated.

Calcaneal Fractures

Mechanism. Injuries of the calcaneus result from axial loading, usually derived from a fall or jump from a significant height. Although the calcaneus is not easily fractured, it is the most commonly fractured tarsal bone. Posterior avulsion fractures due to forceful contraction of the Achilles mechanism may also occur.

Presentation. A patient may present with any constellation of lower extremity injuries after a fall. Avulsion fractures are characterized by pain, swelling, and an inability to walk owing to the impaired plantar flexion mechanism. Plantar flexion is weak or absent on examination, and the area of the avulsion is tender. Fractures of the body of the calcaneus result in severe pain and tenderness, extensive swelling and ecchymosis, and inability to bear weight.

Radiologic Diagnosis. Calcaneal fractures are often apparent on lateral views of the foot or ankle. More subtle compression fractures are diagnosed by evaluating Böhler's angle on the lateral radiograph. A decrease in the described angle (which is usually 30 to 40 degrees) indicates a fracture (Fig. 43–11A and B). Axial views of the calcaneus are also useful.

Management. Because 10% of patients have associated vertebral or contralateral calcaneal fractures, emergency department treatment is incomplete until these injuries are ruled out. It is important to institute ice, elevation, and a compressive dressing as soon as possible to prevent the extensive soft tissue swelling that follows these injuries.

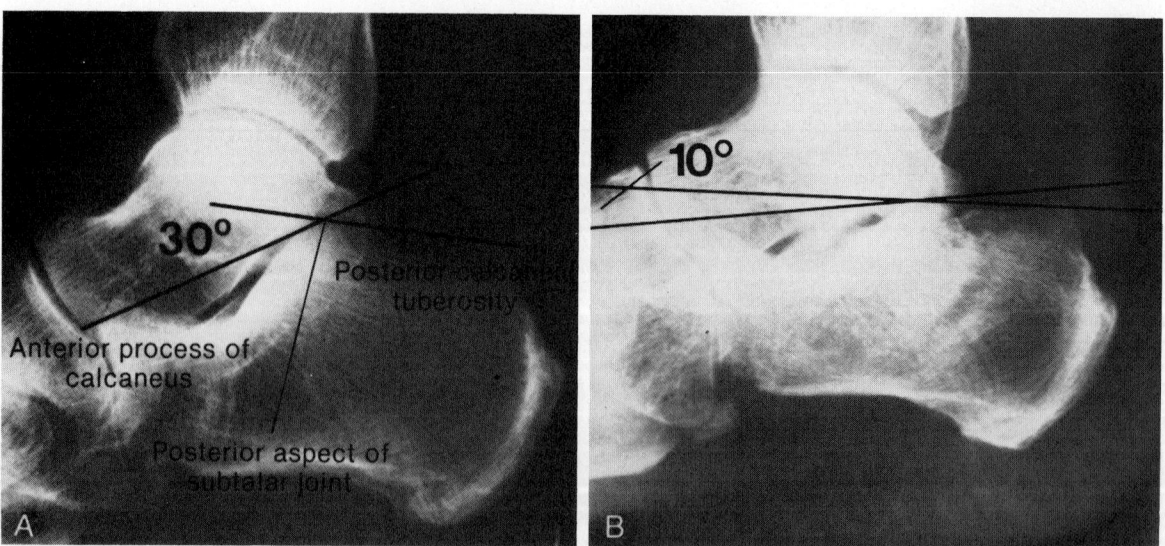

FIGURE 43–11. Bohler's angle is described by drawing a line from the posterior aspect of the subtalar joint to the anterior process of the calcaneus and another from the posterior aspect of the subtalar joint to the posterior calcaneal tuberosity. A, A normal Bohler's angle of 30 to 40 degrees; B, an abnormal Bohler's angle of 10 degrees indicates flattening of the calcaneus consistent with a fracture. (Reproduced with permission from Nance EP, et al (eds.): Advanced Exercises in Diagnostic Radiology. Philadelphia, W. B. Saunders, 1983, pp. 88, 92.)

Depending on the severity of the calcaneal pathology or the associated injuries, hospitalization may be indicated.

PROBLEM 5 Evaluation of this patient included inspection of both lower extremities and the lumbosacral spine. Many authors suggest radiographic evaluation of these areas regardless of the presence of point tenderness on palpation. A urinalysis demonstrating hematuria prompted evaluation by means of an intravenous pyelogram (computed tomography could be used also) to rule out an associated renal injury. The diagnosis in this patient was bilateral calcaneal fractures with a compression fracture of the third lumbar vertebra.

Talar Fractures

Mechanism. The talus has an anterior head, posterior body, and intermediate neck. The neck is highly vulnerable to fracture owing to its lesser diameter, relative position in bearing stress, minimal supporting cartilage, and numerous vascular foramina. These transcervical fractures are caused by forced dorsiflexion of the foot—for example, when violently forcing the foot against a car's brake pedal. The body of the talus may move posteriorly following a transcervical fracture. This results in impairment of its blood supply because the majority of the vessels of the talus enter at the neck. Avascular necrosis is a possible complication. Up to 20% of talar fractures are associated with a medial malleolar fracture. The most common fracture of the talus is an osteochondral fracture of the talar dome due to compression.

Presentation. Fracture of the talar dome has presenting signs similar to those seen with ankle sprains and is often overlooked. Clues to its presence include a click felt on ankle movement. More severe talar fractures present with intense pain and swelling and often a loss of the normal contour of the anterior ankle.

Radiologic Diagnosis. AP, lateral, and oblique views of the ankle, often with comparison views of the uninjured ankle, are needed. Small irregularities of the superior surface of the talus are seen best on the mortise view of the ankle and indicate an osteochondral fracture of the talar dome. Fractures of the head, body, or neck of the talus will cause a fracture line or an abnormal talar profile.

Management. Fracture of the neck of the talus must be reduced as soon as possible, and prompt orthopedic consultation is important. Undisplaced linear fractures of the body are less urgently addressed, needing short leg casting for 6 to 8 weeks. Displaced fractures of the talar body require prompt reduction. As with neck fractures, hospitalization for immediate surgical intervention is the rule. Osteochondral dome fractures may also require surgery to remove any fragments that may lead to locking of the ankle.

Talar Dislocations

Most ankle dislocations are examples of single talar dislocations in which only the tibiotalar joint is disrupted. More complex dislocations also involve luxation at the subtalar joint and talonavicular joint.

Mechanism. Total dislocation of the talus is rare. In this entity, the talus moves forward and laterally, losing its anatomic proximity to the tibia *and* tarsals.

Presentation. Patients have severe pain and swelling, often with severe tenting of the skin overlying the deformity.

Radiologic Diagnosis. Plain films of the ankle show complete loss of the normal position of the talus.

Management. Immediate orthopedic consultation is necessary for reduction. This injury invariably leads to avascular necrosis of the talus and a poor outcome. Failure to reduce the talus in a timely fashion can also lead to necrosis of the overlying skin.

Tarsal Fractures

Mechanism. The rigid midfoot has multiple articulations but limited joint movement. Therefore, twisting foot injuries cause only small avulsion fractures of the tarsals. Other tarsal fractures are caused by direct trauma, as when an object falls onto the foot or when violent forces twist the midfoot.

Presentation. A tarsal fracture may simulate a simple ankle sprain. However, palpation about the ankle will be unremarkable. Palpation of the painful midfoot may reveal point tenderness. A combination of tarsal fractures and dislocations may occur, causing severe soft tissue swelling and pain. Any movement of the midfoot causes discomfort.

Radiologic Diagnosis. AP, lateral, and oblique views of the foot are necessary to locate an abnormality. Because of the many articulations, multiple oblique views may be necessary to evaluate an injury fully.

Management. Orthopedic consultation is obtained. Minor injuries in inactive patients may be adequately treated with a compressive dressing, elevation, ice, and crutches. More severe injuries may necessitate a short leg walking cast once swelling subsides. Severe and complicated injuries will require ORIF and immediate hospitalization.

Tarsometatarsal Fracture-Dislocations

Mechanism. Lisfranc's joint (the tarsometatarsal joint) separates the midfoot from the forefoot. It is injured when there is severe forefoot twisting or a direct axial load on the foot with the toes hyperextended. This can occur when an equestrian falls off his horse with the foot caught in the stirrup, or when a heavy object falls on the heel while the subject is kneeling.

Presentation. Severe pain and swelling of the midfoot-forefoot complex are present, sometimes with distal vascular compromise due to involvement of the dorsalis pedis artery.

Radiologic Diagnosis. AP, lateral, and oblique views of the foot are needed. Any fracture of the base of the second metatarsal or of the cuboid is pathognomonic for disruption of the tarsometatarsal joint. The metatarsal complex is usually translocated laterally, and the dislocation is obvious on radiographs.

Management. Hospitalization for surgical reduction and stabilization is indicated. Immediate orthopedic consultation is obtained.

Metatarsal Fractures

Mechanism. Direct trauma or twisting of the forefoot is the usual cause of metatarsal fractures.

Presentation. Patients have pain on ambulation and palpable tenderness. As in other injuries of the foot, swelling and ecchymosis may be impressive if the foot has remained dependent for any length of time.

Radiologic Diagnosis. AP, lateral, and oblique views of the foot are necessary to evaluate the metatarsals fully.

Management. The soft tissue injury may become the most important focus of treatment. Patients with little or no fracture angulation and mild to moderate swelling may be managed with immobilization in a short leg splint and discharged with instructions to elevate the foot, apply ice as needed, refrain from weight bearing, and secure prompt orthopedic follow-up. Severely injured patients with poor fracture alignment and extensive swelling may require hospitalization for reduction followed by frequent skin and neurovascular checks.

March Fractures

Mechanism. Stress fractures, which occur commonly in the second and third metatarsals, result from repetitive and seemingly trivial trauma. They are so named because of their occurrence in recruits to the armed services who develop forefoot pain following extended periods of marching.

Presentation. Patients complain of foot pain that is worse with weight bearing. Localized tenderness and swelling occur at the fracture site.

Radiologic Diagnosis. These nondisplaced shaft fractures often cannot be seen on initial films. If symptoms persist, repeated radiographs or bone scans may be required to delineate the fracture.

Management. The diagnosis is presumptive when initial radiologic evaluation is unremarkable. Treatment is conservative, with splint immobilization and crutches to prevent weight bearing. Definitive treatment will require short leg casting for 3 to 4 weeks.

Fracture of the Proximal Fifth Metatarsal
Mechanism. This fracture can occur through one of three mechanisms—inversion injury with bony avulsion caused by the pull of the peroneus brevis tendon, direct trauma, or indirect stress.

Presentation. Patients with this type of fracture (Jones fracture) have history and physical findings consistent with those characteristic of an ankle sprain.

Radiologic Diagnosis. The proximal fifth metatarsal can be evaluated on either a lateral ankle or foot radiograph (Fig. 43–12).

Management. In patients with avulsion injuries in which displacement is small, a dressing that supplies some local compression followed by a posterior plaster mold is usually adequate. Patients with transverse fractures through the base of the metatarsal are treated similarly but receive a short leg cast at orthopedic follow-up.

Metatarsophalangeal Dislocations
Mechanism. Patients who "stub" their toes may dislocate the metatarsophalangeal (MTP) joint.

Presentation. The area of the MTP joint is swollen, painful, and obviously deformed.

Radiologic Diagnosis. Even though these injuries usually are not associated with phalangeal fractures, plain films are obtained prior to reduction.

Management. Reduction requires accentuation of the mechanism of injury followed by axial traction. Difficulty in reduction can be caused by entrapment of the plantar joint capsule (similar to entrapment of the volar plate in phalangeal dislocations) or entrapment of a sesamoid bone. Either taping the involved toe to its neighbor, using a metallic splint, or using a cast shoe is appropriate treatment.

Phalangeal Fractures
Mechanism. Stubbed toes that do not dislocate may fracture instead.

Presentation. Any tender, swollen foot phalanx is potentially a fractured phalanx.

Radiologic Diagnosis. A limited survey of the toes or a complete view of the foot will demonstrate a fracture.

Management. Any marked angulation can be reduced with axial traction, and the injured toe can be "buddy taped" to a neighboring toe. In the case of a fracture of the great toe, buddy taping is inadequate stabilization; plaster splinting is needed.

Phalangeal Dislocations
Mechanism. Direct trauma is usually involved in phalangeal dislocations.

Presentation. The patient with a history consistent with this mechanism of injury presents with a tender, deformed phalanx.

Radiologic Diagnosis. Views of the toes or entire foot will show loss of the normal alignment at the interphalangeal joint.

Management. Interphalangeal joint dislocations are evaluated in the same way as MTP dislocations. Similar problems with reduction occur. Great toe phalangeal dislocations are most often dorsal and are significant because of their tendency to redislocate with weight bearing. Buddy taping is usually adequate. The great toe will need stabilization with a plaster splint, however.

SPECIAL CONSIDERATIONS

Legg-Calvé-Perthes Disease

Legg-Calvé-Perthes disease, also known as *coxa plana* or *osteochondrosis of the femoral head*, results from transient ischemia and consequent avascular necrosis of the femoral head. The exact etiology of the condition is controversial, but it is presumed to be directly related to the particularly tenuous blood supply of the capital femoral epiphysis in children between the ages of 3 and 11. The typical presentation is a preadolescent

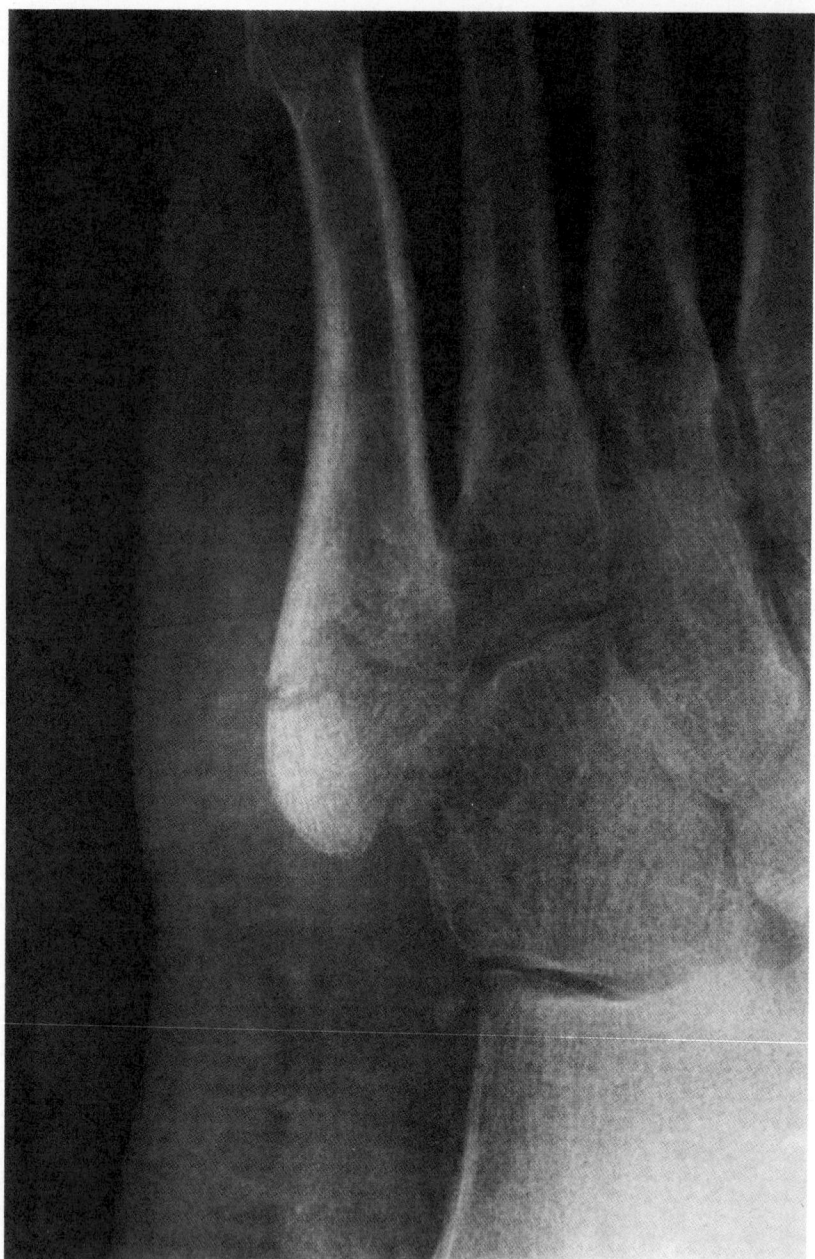

FIGURE 43–12. *The transverse lucency at the base of the fifth metatarsal represents a nondisplaced Jones fracture. (Reproduced with permission from Nance EP, et al (eds.): Advanced Exercises in Diagnostic Radiology. Philadelphia, W. B. Saunders, 1983, p. 64.)*

male complaining of hip or knee pain with an antalgic gait. Males are affected four times as often as females. Range of motion at the hip may be limited in abduction and external rotation. Clinical suspicion is confirmed by hip radiographs, including one with the patient in a frog-leg position. Early abnormalities include flattening (coxa plana) or increased bone density of the femoral capital epiphysis. Radiolucent areas below the cortical margin of the epiphysis consistent with subchondral fractures may also be seen. Radiologically, the disease progresses over 4 to 6 years, resulting in further fragmentation and flattening of the epiphysis, shortening and widening of the femoral neck, and femoral head subluxation. Later in life, this residual joint incongruity will lead to degenerative joint disease. Once the diagnosis has been made, the child should have prompt orthopedic referral. A variety of treatment regimens exist, all of which incorporate containment of the femoral head well within the acetabulum by long-term splinting of the hip in abduction and flexion. This "protects" the femoral head and minimizes further flattening of the epiphysis.

Slipped Capital Femoral Epiphysis

Another cause of hip pain and limp in children is a slipped capital femoral epiphysis. This entity is most common in older children and adolescents from 9 to 16 years of age. It occurs predominantly in obese males and is a bilateral disease in 30% of cases. Chronic shear stress encountered by the obliquely situated upper femoral epiphyseal plate coupled with other possible predisposing factors (previous radiation or chemotherapy, hypothyroidism, renal osteodystrophy) leads to separation of the growth plate and progressive posterior and medial slippage of the femoral head. The history is typically significant for an absence of direct trauma. The development of hip or knee pain and limp is generally insidious. Range of motion at the hip is painful and is limited in adduction and internal rotation. Diagnosis is made by often subtle roentgenographic findings (Fig. 43–13A and B). Radiographs may show widening and irregularity of the proximal epiphyseal plate. AP and frog-leg views of the hip will show the epiphysis projecting beyond the inferior border of the femoral neck while remaining flush or caudad to the superior edge of the neck. This abnormality is more easily seen when comparison views of the healthy hip are obtained. The overall picture is one of ice cream (the femoral head) sliding off an ice cream cone (the femoral neck). The slipping capital femoral epiphysis that remains undiscovered is likely to progress until bone maturity and fusion of the epiphyseal plate occur, decreasing hip mobility and increasing the risk of avascular necrosis or early osteoarthritis. Patients must refrain from weight bearing, usually in the hospital, until surgical pinning can be performed.

Osgood-Schlatter Disease

Another entity to be considered in the differential diagnosis of adolescent knee pain is Osgood-Schlatter disease. Repeated forceful contraction of the quadriceps mechanism causes serial partial avulsions of the tibial tubercle at the site of insertion of the patellar tendon. This apophysis is particularly prone to injury in active males between ages of 10 and 15. Repeated injuries of this growing tubercle, with subsequent avascular necrosis of the proximally avulsed portion, lead to local swelling and pain, which is exacerbated by palpation as well as extension of the knee against resistance. Radiographically, the tubercle appears elevated, irregular, and fragmented compared to the normal tibia. Treatment is usually conservative. Avoidance of kneeling, jumping, and excessive running will allow healing to occur. Some authors recommend a more aggressive approach, keeping the knee immobilized and non-weight bearing for 4 to 6 weeks and resuming normal activities after 3 months. Fusion of the apophysis with increasing bone maturity at 16 to 18 years of age makes Osgood-Schlatter disease a self-limiting problem.

Compartment Syndromes

A compartment syndrome is a condition in which the vascular supply and function of tissues within a closed space are compromised by increased pressure within that space. The fascia, skin, and bones of the lower leg form the anterior, lateral, deep posterior, and superficial posterior compartments, any of which may be involved in an acute compartment syndrome. Compartment syndromes in the thigh and gluteal regions may occur but are rare. Failure to recognize an impending compartment syndrome will lead

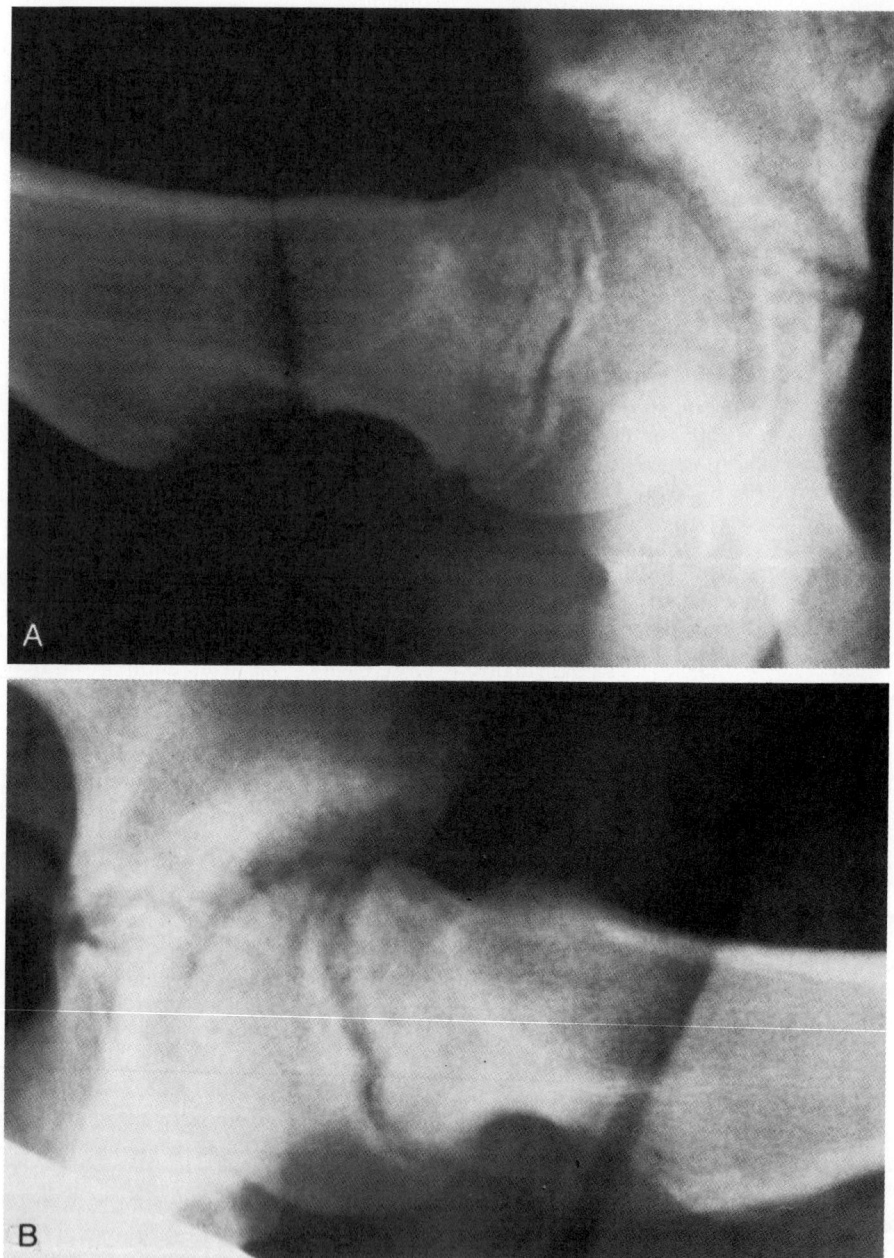

FIGURE 43-13. A, *This lateral view of the femoral head is normal.* B, *This lateral view of a slipped capital femoral epiphysis shows a loss of continuity along its superior edge where the metaphysis has moved cephalad with respect to the epiphysis. One might imagine this pathology to be similar to "the ice cream sliding off the cone." (Reproduced with permission from Nance EP, et al (eds.): Advanced Exercises in Diagnostic Radiology. Philadelphia, W. B. Saunders, 1983, p. 15.)*

to progressive ischemic necrosis of nerve and muscle, with subsequent loss of function of the extremity.

Since the development of a compartment syndrome depends on the relationship between the available enclosed space and the tissue contents within it, any decrease in compartmental size or increase in compartmental content can initiate this entity. Decreased compartmental size may result from inordinately tight dressings or casts.

Prolonged use of the military antishock trousers (MAST) has also been implicated. Compartment volume may increase owing to intercompartmental edema resulting from direct trauma such as crush injuries, or from postischemic swelling, as in cases of proximal vascular occlusion. Less common causes include burns, vigorous exercise, intracompartmental bleeding (as may occur in patients with coagulopathies), venous obstruction, muscle hypertrophy, and nephrotic syndrome.

Clinically, the most important symptom that arouses a physician's suspicion of an impending compartment syndrome is pain that is out of proportion to that expected for the degree of soft tissue or bony injury present. This ischemic pain will not be relieved by immobilization or elevation. Patients may also complain of distal paresthesias. Early findings include swelling and palpable tenseness of an entire muscular compartment, which is often hard to appreciate in the presence of extensive but more superficial soft tissue swelling. Pain with passive stretch of the muscles within the compartment is common. Paresis is difficult to appreciate because motor testing may be biased by pain. The most reliable physical finding is a deficit in soft touch and pinprick sensation in an area supplied exclusively by a nerve that travels through the compartment in question. In all compartment syndromes, a pulse deficit is an uncommon early finding. Dependence on a diminished pulse to make the diagnosis is a grave error. Among the five "Ps" characteristic of compartment syndrome—pallor, paralysis, pulselessness, paresthesias, and pain (out of proportion to injury as well as with passive muscle stretching)—the latter two are the most important early findings in making a prompt diagnosis.

Of the specific syndromes, the anterior compartment syndrome is encountered most commonly (Fig. 43–14). As intercompartmental pressure increases, passive stretching of the tibialis anterior, extensor hallucis longus, and extensor digitorum longus muscles (as in plantar flexion of the ankle or toes) will be painful. Weakening of these muscle groups may be detected on forced extension of the toes or dorsiflexion of the ankle against resistance. Impairment of anterior tibial nerve function will lead to hypesthesia in the distribution of its sensory branch, the deep peroneal nerve, which supplies the dorsum of the foot and, most exclusively, the dorsum of the web space between the great and second toes.

In deep posterior compartment syndrome, hypesthesia develops on the sole of the foot with weakness noted in the toe flexors. Passive extension of the toes will elicit pain in the calf.

The lateral compartment syndrome results in sensory loss on the lateral dorsum of the foot, weakness in foot eversion, and pain with passive inversion of the foot.

The key to diagnosing all compartment syndromes is a high index of suspicion and frequent, careful examinations of the extremity to elicit these findings.

DISPOSITION AND FOLLOW-UP

Indications for Immediate Operative Intervention

The following lower extremity injuries usually require immediate orthopedic consultation and operative intervention:
  1. Open fracture with gross bone or joint contamination
  2. Irreducible fracture-dislocation associated with neurovascular compromise
  3. Partial or complete amputation in which the limb can be salvaged or that is associated with uncontrolled hemorrhage
  4. Compartment syndrome

Indications for Admission

The following lower extremity injuries usually require orthopedic consultation and admission of the patient to the hospital:

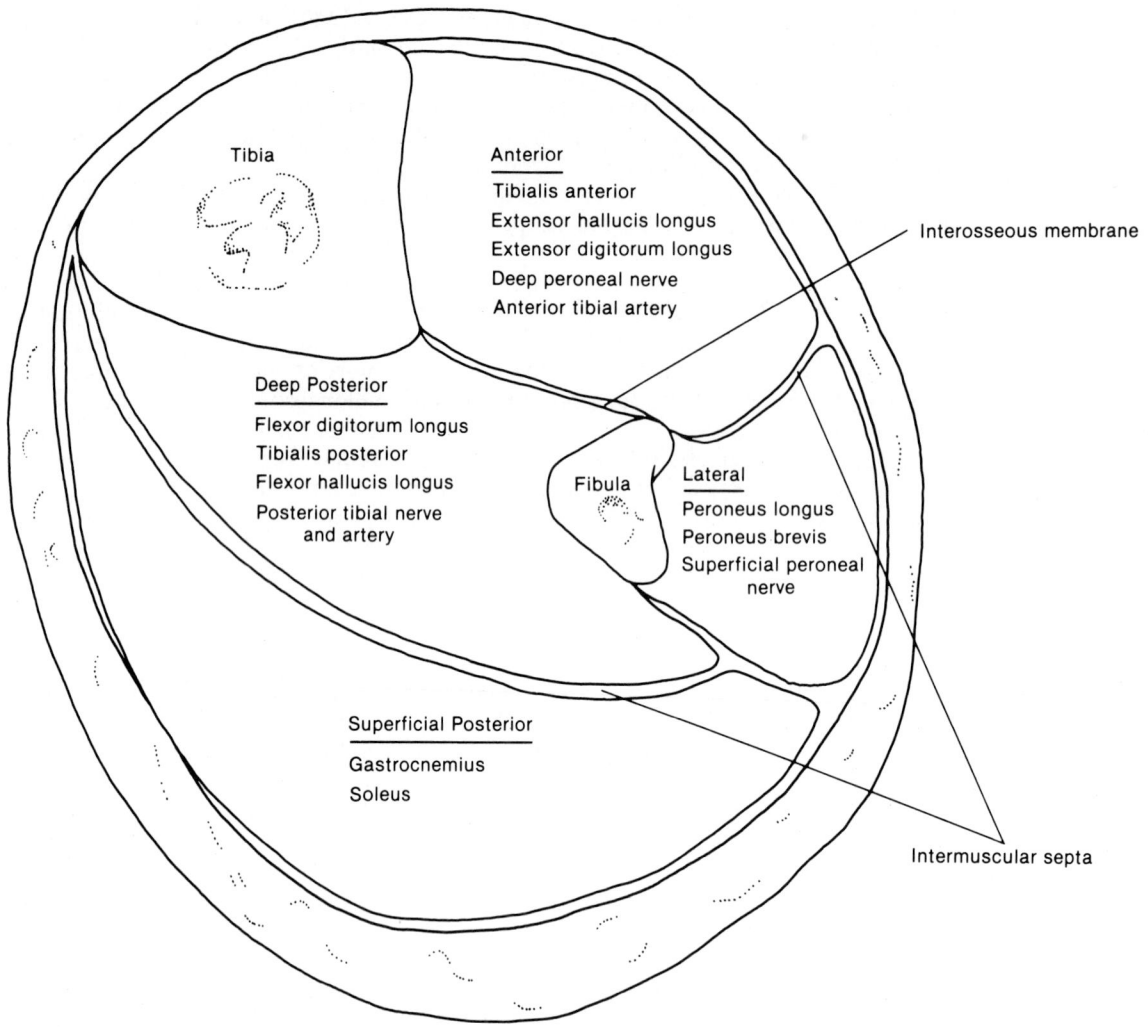

FIGURE 43–14. *Cross-sectional anatomy of the leg showing the contents of the anterior, lateral, posterior, and deep posterior compartments.*

1. Hip fracture
2. Femoral fracture, because of the severity of the trauma that caused the fracture, the potential for local hemorrhage, and the need for operative management or traction
3. Knee fracture or dislocation, because of the likelihood of increased displacement of fracture fragments with even partial weight bearing and the high probability of operative management
4. Fracture of the tibia and fibula, because of gross instability and the potential for development of vascular compromise or compartment syndrome
5. Unstable ankle fracture (bimalleolar or trimalleolar fracture)
6. Calcaneal fracture, because of the significant associated pain and swelling
7. Open fractures that require operative irrigation or intravenous antibiotics

Outpatient Management

Minor sprains, strains, and contusions are best treated with (1) RICE therapy (rest, ice, compression, elevation) for 24 to 48 hours, (2) weight bearing only when it is painless,

(3) nonsteroidal anti-inflammatory therapy for 5 to 7 days, and (4) follow-up if pain persists beyond 3 to 5 days.

Minor fractures or suspected cartilaginous or ligamentous injury of the knee may be treated with (1) RICE therapy for 24 to 48 hours with plaster immobilization or knee immobilizer, (2) absolute absence of weight bearing, (3) narcotic analgesics (acetaminophen with codeine) for 24 to 72 hours as needed, (4) nonsteroidal anti-inflammatory therapy for 5 to 7 days, and (5) follow-up with an orthopedic consultant in 2 to 3 days for splint removal, reexamination, and casting as appropriate.

Crutches

Lower extremity injuries that are initially managed with the RICE method can be expected to heal more quickly and less painfully. To improve outcome and to limit liability, patients are told to refrain from weight bearing during the first 24 to 48 hours following the injury. This can be best achieved with crutches, but a cane can be used if the patient cannot tolerate or handle crutches.

DOCUMENTATION

1. *History*
    a. Time of injury
    b. Mechanism of injury
    c. Prehospital treatment
    d. Pain with weight bearing or ambulation
    e. Past history of injury to the extremity
2. *Physical Examination*
    a. Description of presenting deformity
    b. Location of greatest point tenderness and soft tissue swelling
    c. Integrity of the skin at the site
    d. Neurovascular status
    e. Joint stability
    f. Status of the joint proximal and distal to the injury
3. *Radiologic Examination.* The body of the chart should reflect the reading of any radiographs obtained, specifically commenting on:
    a. Direct or indirect signs of fracture
    b. Position of major fracture fragments
    c. Presence of foreign bodies or subcutaneous emphysema
    d. Presence of intra-articular pathology
4. *Management*
    a. Medications given (analgesics or antibiotics)
    b. Local care given (surgical cleansing, irrigation, or debridement)
    c. Attempted or successful reductions with subsequent neurovascular examination results
    d. Splints or bandages applied
    e. Instructions given for ambulation with crutches, cane, or walker as well as notation of the patient's ability to do so
    f. Consulting orthopedist with brief account of conversation and decision to admit or discharge
5. *Follow-up.* Instructions are written in lay terms and a copy is included with the chart.
    a. RICE, instructions about weight bearing
    b. Prescriptions given
    c. Physician and time for follow-up
    d. Reasons for immediate return to the emergency department (increasing pain, swelling, or numbness in the extremity)

All of the examinations, radiographs, and management options offered should be documented, even if the patient defers treatment.

SUMMARY AND FINAL POINTS

- The emergency medicine approach to lower extremity injury begins with prehospital immobilization by first responders.
- Patient comfort should be addressed early with the use of immobilization, ice, elevation, and appropriate analgesics.
- A neurovascular examination of the leg is *always* required, *before and after* any manipulations.
- Identifying an injury prompts a search for associated injuries.
- Discharged patients need not only clear instructions about RICE therapy and medications but also readily accessible follow-up and definite guidelines for symptoms that should prompt their immediate return to the emergency department.
- When in doubt, splinting and immediate orthopedic follow-up is always appropriate.

BIBLIOGRAPHY

Texts

1. Blauve HCT, Nelson FRT: A Manual of Orthopedic Terminology (3rd ed). St. Louis, CV Mosby, 1985.
2. Murabak SJ: A practical approach to compartmental syndromes. In American Academy of Orthopedic Surgeons: Instructional Course Lectures. St. Louis, CV Mosby, 1981, pp. 91–104.
3. Nance EP, Heller RM, Kirchner SG, et al (eds): Advanced Exercises in Diagnostic Radiology: Vol 17. Emergency Radiology of the Pelvis and Lower Extremity. Philadelphia, Saunders, 1983.
4. Rockwood CA, Green DP: Fractures in Adults (Vols 1 and 2). Philadelphia, Lippincott, 1984.
5. Salter RB: Textbook of Disorders and Injuries of the Musculoskeletal System (2nd ed). Baltimore, Williams & Wilkins, 1983.
6. Simon RR, Koenigsknecht SJ: Emergency Orthopedics: The Extremities (2nd ed). New York, Appleton and Lange, 1982.

Journal Article

1. Masten FA: Compartment syndrome. An unified concept. Clin Orthop Rel Res 113:8–14, 1975.

CHAPTER 44

LOW BACK PAIN

HERBERT N. SUTHERLAND, D.O.
GARY R. STRANGE, M.D.

PROBLEM 1 A 40 year old man presented with a complaint of low back pain (LBP). The pain began as he was bending to pick up an object and was somewhat relieved with bed rest. He experienced extreme difficulty in standing and walking.

PROBLEM 2 A 56 year old fireman noted a gradual onset of low back pain. The pain was more severe in the lower back, but there was some lower abdominal pain as well. The pain was equally severe in all positions.

QUESTIONS TO CONSIDER

1. What are the common musculoskeletal causes of LBP?
2. What are the catastrophic illnesses that can present as LBP?
3. What aspects of the history and physical examination are helpful in differentiating these problems?
4. What additional tests can be helpful in differentiating primary and secondary causes of LBP?
5. What constitutes a conservative management regimen that is applicable for most patients with musculoskeletal back pain?
6. Which patients with LBP are admitted?
7. What are the appropriate follow-up arrangements for patients who are discharged home?

INTRODUCTION

It is estimated that 80% of the population will at some point in their lives develop low back pain. LBP is the number one cause of impairment of activity in individuals below the age of 45 in the United States, the most common musculoskeletal disorder for which people visit a physician, and the condition that leads most frequently to radiographic evaluation in the outpatient setting. Over 7 million radiographs of the low back, at a cost of over $500 million, are taken each year.

Considering lost productivity due to this type of pain, workmen's compensation payments, disability payments, and litigation, it is estimated that over $14 billion is spent each year on LBP. The diagnosis and treatment of LBP add another $6 billion per year.

Patients with LBP come to the emergency department for a variety of reasons in addition to the pain itself. Some have missed work and want an excuse. Some have been sent in for evaluation by their employers because of on-the-job injuries. In some cases with chronic pain, drug dependence, depression, and maladaptive personalities have resulted. The patient may also derive secondary gain from family and friends due to back problems.

Evaluation of low back pain is a difficult process. A thorough understanding of the anatomy and physiology of the lumbosacral spine and an appreciation for other structures that may cause pain referred to the lumbosacral area are essential as a foundation for accurate assessment.

The lumbosacral spine is complex in terms of anatomy and mechanical functions. It consists of the lumbar vertebrae with the interposed vertebral discs. The disc is made up of a collagenous material that surrounds the nucleus pulposus. It provides for shock absorption and smooth movement of the vertebrae above and below. Each vertebral unit is made up of a three-joint interface consisting of two articular facets that are true synovial joints as well as the disc itself. The stability of the spine is derived from its ligamentous and muscular supports. The major ligaments are the anterior longitudinal ligament and the posterior longitudinal ligament. The lumbar musculature as well as the abdominal muscles maintain the actual stability of the lumbar spine (Fig. 44–1).

Many of the anatomic elements of the lumbosacral spine have the potential to cause pain. Distinct qualities of pain are associated with specific structures in the spine. Primary LBP consists of pain originating from the spine, spinal column, or peripheral nerves. It is divided into three classes based on the source of the pain: superficial somatic, deep somatic, and radicular.

Superficial somatic pain results from processes involving the skin or subcutaneous tissues. It is usually sharp or burning in character, e.g., herpes zoster infection.

Deep somatic (spondylogenic) pain results from processes involving the vertebral column, surrounding muscles, attaching tendons, ligaments, fascia, dura, or vertebral venous plexus. Deep somatic pain is perceived as a deep, dull ache. Its most common cause is a strain with avulsion of tendinous attachments of muscles or rupture of muscle fibers or sheaths. Muscle pain may also occur without overt injury when there is persistent use of specific muscle groups or when reflex spasm develops secondary to inflammatory or degenerative processes. Other spondylogenic contributors to LBP include mechanical disruption of bones, joints, and ligaments; inflammation of joints and ligaments; neoplasms of bone; infections of bones and joints; distention of the vertebral venous plexus; and compression of the spinal dura.

Radicular pain results from stimulation of the proximal spinal nerves. It is typically lancinating, sharp, or burning in character. Mechanical disruption and degeneration are the most common processes leading to radicular pain, most commonly resulting from herniated intervertebral discs or spinal stenosis.

Although most cases of LBP are related to lumbosacral musculoskeletal disorders, a number of pelvic, retroperitoneal, and abdominal structures can be the source of pain referred to the lower back. It is important to diagnose these causes of referred or "secondary" back pain because their management differs markedly from that for primary

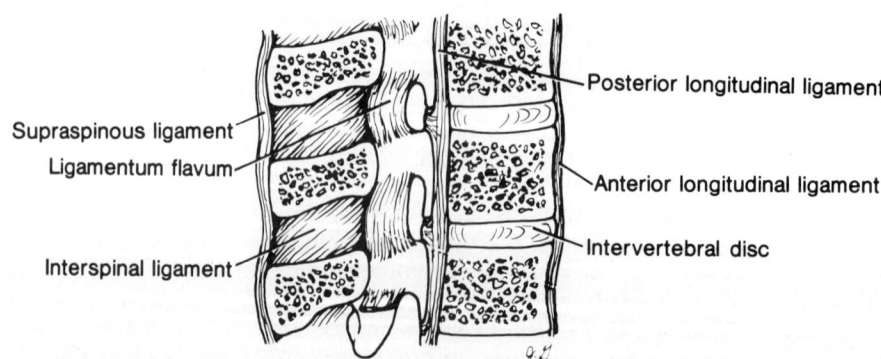

FIGURE 44–1. *Lateral view of the lumbar spine demonstrating the ligaments that support the anterior (anterior longitudinal, posterior longitudinal) and the posterior (supraspinous, intraspinous) elements of the vertebrae. Note the position of the ligamentum flavum forming a smooth posterior wall of the neural foramen. (From Borenstein DG, Wiesel SW: Low Back Pain: Medical Diagnosis and Comprehensive Management. Philadelphia, W. B. Saunders, 1989.)*

LBP. Additionally, some of these problems can be life-threatening. The goals of the emergency department evaluation are to determine the likely cause of the patient's pain, to rule out life-threatening and debilitating conditions, to initiate appropriate therapeutic interventions, and to ensure appropriate referral for further evaluation and treatment.

PREHOSPITAL CARE

Patients with LBP do not usually come to the emergency department by rescue squad. An ambulance may be necessary if the patient is completely incapacitated by pain or if there are associated serious symptoms such as syncope or severe abdominal pain. The rescue squad is expected to obtain the following information:

History

1. Where is the back pain located?
2. When did it begin?
3. Have there been previous episodes?
4. Are there associated symptoms such as weakness, lightheadedness, dizziness, syncope, or abdominal pain?
5. Has any injury occurred?
6. Is there a history of major medical problems?

Physical Examination

1. Is the patient in severe distress?
2. What are the vital signs?
3. Is the skin diaphoretic, pale, mottled, or cyanotic?
4. Is there palpable abdominal tenderness?
5. Is there palpable lumbosacral tenderness?

These few observations can be made quickly and allow the squad to determine the hemodynamic stability of the patient and the probability of primary lumbosacral back pain. These factors determine the need for intervention in the field.

Intervention

1. Patients in severe distress with a history of syncope or dizziness and those with hypotension and tachycardia require rapid transportation to the emergency department for stabilization and definitive therapy. On-scene or in-transport interventions that are initiated if they do not significantly delay transport include:

   - High-flow supplemental oxygen
   - Large-bore intravenous lines with isotonic crystalloid
   - Cardiac monitoring
   - Pneumatic antishock garment (the use of this device remains controversial, and it is considered primarily when hypotension is present and transport times are prolonged)

2. Patients with acute back trauma or those in severe distress with localized back pain, palpable lumbosacral tenderness, or spasm require careful lifting, immobilization on a back board, and transportation to the emergency department. Analgesics are generally not recommended prior to evaluation by a physician.

PROBLEM 2 This 56 year old patient had a prior history of low back pain but not like the pain of the last 2 to 3 days. He had hypertension and was taking a "medication for his heart." The pain had gradually become worse, and just before calling the rescue squad he had become sweaty, dizzy, and felt as if he were going to pass out. The rescue squad noted that the patient was in severe distress from lower back and abdominal pain; he appeared pale and had a blood pressure of 110/60 mm Hg with a pulse rate of 120 beats/min. The squad was instructed to place the patient on oxygen and a cardiac monitor and to begin transport. An intravenous line was attempted while they were en route to the hospital.

This patient, who had a history of hypertension and cardiovascular disease, is at risk for additional cardiovascular problems. In light of the history of hypertension, the blood pressure of 110/60 mm Hg can represent borderline hypotension, and the pulse is rapid. These findings combined with low back *and* abdominal pain are suggestive of various intra-abdominal pathology. Rapid transport to the emergency department is essential because deterioration can be abrupt.

INITIAL APPROACH IN THE EMERGENCY DEPARTMENT

Patients with low back pain who require immediate care on arrival are those with:
1. Hemodynamic instability
2. Significant trauma
3. Incapacitating musculoskeletal pain

The first group is the most critical. Hemorrhagic shock is invariably the cause of the instability, although the exact etiology may vary from rupture of an abdominal aortic aneurysm to rupture of an ectopic pregnancy to traumatic bleeding from pelvic, retroperitoneal, or intra-abdominal sources. Regardless of the etiology, early intervention includes:

1. Supplemental oxygen at 8 to 10 liters/min by nonrebreathing mask
2. Establishment of large-bore intravenous lines (at least two) and isotonic crystalloid administration
3. Cardiac monitoring
4. Early notification of the surgical team
5. Preoperative laboratory, radiologic, and electrocardiographic studies, including type and cross-matching for blood
6. Blood transfusion. In patients with profound or refractory shock, type-specific or type O blood may be required prior to the availability of cross-matched blood
7. Pneumatic antishock garment (PASG) may be effective in tamponading bleeding sites in the pelvis and abdomen. It may be useful while preparations are made for operative intervention.

Patients with significant trauma involving the lower back require thorough evaluation for traumatic problems as outlined in Chapter 4. Patients with severe, incapacitating musculoskeletal pain often have severely limited movement. They need reassurance, careful movement, and early examination. Analgesics (usually parenteral narcotics) may be administered if the patient has a history of onset with strain, a exertion, or unaccustomed activity, previous similar episodes, and the finding of localized lumbosacral tenderness or muscle spasm combined with normal vital signs or mild to moderate tachycardia and hypertension consistent with severe pain. A more comfortable patient will be able to cooperate better with the data gathering to follow.

PROBLEM 1 The 40 year old man stated that the acute onset of severe back pain occurred soon after he lifted a package. He appeared to be in severe distress and moved very carefully to avoid increasing his pain. The triage nurse promptly placed him on a cart and requested that he be seen expeditiously. The patient was cautiously trying to get undressed as the physician approached. There was palpable tenderness in the lumbosacral area but no obvious muscle spasm. His blood pressure was 140/90 mm Hg, pulse rate 110 beats/min.

This preliminary evaluation can be accomplished in a few minutes and virtually ensures that the pain is of musculoskeletal origin. Since the vital signs are consistent with the degree of pain observed, early use of analgesics is both safe and appropriate. With this degree of pain, narcotic analgesics such as meperidine are appropriate and will make the patient both appreciative and more cooperative for a thorough history and physical examination.

PROBLEM 2 The 56 year old man with back and abdominal pain was transported rapidly by the rescue squad. An intravenous line of normal saline was initiated while en route and was running wide open. On arrival in the emergency department the patient appeared pale, diaphoretic, and in severe pain. Blood pressure was 90/50 mm Hg, and pulse rate was 140 beats/min.

There is no time to waste in a situation like this. Hypotension, tachycardia, back pain, and abdominal pain are indicative of intra-abdominal or retroperitoneal bleeding. In an older patient with risk factors for cardiovascular disease, this scenario almost certainly represents a ruptured abdominal aortic aneurysm.

Intervention includes high-flow oxygen, additional large-bore intravenous lines and rapid fluid administration, blood replacement, and mobilization of the surgical team. If there is not a prompt response to fluid administration or if the blood pressure falls further, type O or type-specific uncross-matched blood will be used. If there will be a significant delay in moving to the operating room, the PASG may be used in an attempt to tamponade the bleeding.

DATA GATHERING

History

The history is perhaps the most essential tool in evaluating these patients. A thorough review, including social, work, and past medical histories, is needed to understand the patient's presentation fully. The key questions are as follows:

1. *When did the pain begin and what were the circumstances surrounding its onset?*
   Acute onset of pain while lifting or twisting or after a jump or fall is highly suggestive of musculoskeletal pain. An insidious onset over days to weeks suggests a degenerative, infectious, neoplastic, or inflammatory origin.
2. *What is the severity and character of the pain?*
   Severe, sharp, agonizing pain is characteristic of nerve root compression. Nagging pain of varying intensity is characteristic of muscular pain. Vague or bizarre pain descriptions suggest a psychological origin.
3. *When is the pain present? What makes it better or worse?*
   Pain that is better in the morning and gets worse with progressive activity is usually muscular in origin. Pain due to nerve root compression is aggravated by all motion, especially rotation of the trunk. Coughing or sneezing will also aggravate pain due to nerve root compression. When a herniated intervertebral disc is the cause, sitting results in more pain than standing or lying down because of the increased intradiscal pressure that occurs with sitting.
4. *Does the pain radiate?*
   Radiation of pain over the peripheral distribution of a nerve root is pathognomonic for nerve root compression. Pain is usually the earliest presenting symptom. Paresthesia, hypesthesia, weakness, and areflexia may develop later. The pain

can radiate to the groin, buttock, lateral aspect of the thigh, or posteriorly down the thigh. The nerve roots commonly involved and their pattern of radiation are shown in Table 44–1.

5. *Where is the pain located?*

Pain located diffusely across the lower back is suggestive of muscular strain. Unilateral pain is more consistent with nerve root compression, although bilateral radicular pain is possible when the nerve roots in the cauda equina are compressed. This is because they run caudally in the midline. Pain over the sacroiliac joint is common and may represent either a sprain of the tissues around the joint or inflammation within the joint. The latter is seen as part of ankylosing spondylitis. Abdominal, pelvic, or costovertebral angle pain suggests nonmusculoskeletal causes.

6. *Is there loss of bowel, bladder, or sexual function?*

LBP with unilateral or bilateral radiation, perineal anesthesia, and lower extremity weakness may progress to bowel and bladder dysfunction, usually urinary retention. This syndrome results from compression of nerve roots in the cauda equina and can result in permanent dysfunction unless surgical decompression is achieved.

7. *Are there symptoms related to other systems, particularly urinary, reproductive, cardiovascular, and gastrointestinal symptoms?*

These symptoms suggest secondary, nonmusculoskeletal causes for LBP. Endocrinopathies, malignancies, and metabolic bone disease may directly affect the lumbosacral structures. Rheumatic and connective tissue disorders may have a direct effect as well, and arthritides associated with psoriasis and colitis may involve the lower back. Prior cardiovascular disease may be important in suggesting secondary causes of LBP, such as abdominal aortic aneurysm.

8. *Is there a prior history of back problems? Are there other medical problems that may contribute to the presentation or affect the therapeutic modalities selected?*

Old, often forgotten injuries may represent the initial episode that has now led to degenerative disc disease. Though time-consuming, a detailed history of prior back problems, including treatment and response, can be very helpful in under-

TABLE 44–1. Examination for Nerve Root Compression

Site of Disc Herniation	Nerve Root Involved	Reflex Changes	Motor Changes	Pain Distribution and Sensory Changes	Comment
L3–L4	L4	Decreased knee jerk	Weakness of quadriceps	Anterolateral thigh, across knee, and down anteromedial leg	Uncommon site for disc herniation
L4–L5	L5	Usually not associated with reflex changes; occasionally knee jerk is decreased	Weakness of anterior tibial, peroneal, and extensor hallucis longus muscles (weak dorsiflexion of foot and big toe)	Posterolateral thigh, anterolateral leg, and dorsal foot and big toe. Occasionally numbness of heel and bottom of foot	Trouble with heel walking
L5–S1	S1	Decreased/absent ankle jerk	Weakness of gastrocnemius and soleus muscles (weakness of plantar flexion)	Posterior thigh, posterior leg, and lateral foot (fourth and fifth toes)	Trouble with toe walking or standing on tiptoes
Cauda equina	S2, S3, S4, S5 Possibly lower lumbar roots	Decreased rectal tone, loss of bulbocavernosus reflex and anal wink	Diffuse motor weakness in lower extremities may progress to paraplegia	Perineal or "saddle anesthesia"	Bowel and bladder problems—especially urinary retention—may present with bilateral sciatica

From Roberts JR: In focus: Sciatica and disc disease. Emerg Med Ambulatory Care News, May, 1989. Reprinted with permission.

standing the patient's perspective on this problem. This information often gives a first clue as to the patient's expectation of this visit.

Physical Examination

The physical examination of the LBP patient is conducted with the patient in four positions: standing, supine, prone, and sitting. The examination includes passive maneuvers performed with the patient remaining still and active maneuvers that require the patient's involvement and cooperation. Although the entire examination may not be possible in the severely ill or very uncomfortable patient, the initial examination is as complete as possible. Depending on the patient's presentation, the physical examination is expanded to include examination of other organ systems.

Standing

1. The patient's posture and any abnormal spinal contour are noted. Scoliosis may result from a difference in leg length. It is assessed during the supine examination. Kyphosis or excessive lumbar lordosis is also noted.
2. The lumbar paravertebral muscles are palpated for tenderness or spasm. Tenderness localized over the sacroiliac joint is noted. Trigger points may be detected during palpation.
3. Active range of motion is assessed by asking the patient to flex the spine, extend it, and bend to each side. Normal range of motion is 90 degrees of flexion, 15 degrees of extension, and 45 degrees of side bending.
4. The patient's normal gait is observed, and the ability to walk on the heels and the toes is tested. The ability to heel- and toe-walk is an indication of good lower extremity strength. It tests L4–L5 and L5–S1 (Table 44–1).
5. The stoop test is performed by having the patient go from a standing position to a squatting position. In the squatting position, intrathecal pressure is increased; the cerebrospinal fluid then reduces skeletal pressure on the spinal cord. In patients with central spinal stenosis, squatting will result in reduced pain.

Supine

1. A thorough abdominal examination is performed, paying particular attention to any organomegaly or masses that are present. A diligent search for a pulsatile mass, abdominal bruit, or abnormal femoral pulses is essential, especially in older patients who are at greater risk for development of abdominal aortic aneurysm. Rectal examination is performed, looking for evidence of masses, bleeding, or abnormal rectal tone.
2. Passive straight leg raising (PSLR) is performed. PSLR is positive if pain radiates down the posterior or lateral aspect of the thigh. Increased pain in the back is not a positive result of this test. Increased pain without radiation is most consistent with a muscular origin of the pain, whereas radiation indicates stretching of nerve roots over a herniated disc, resulting in pain along the course of the nerve root. The nerve root is not actually stretched until the angle of the raised leg reaches 30 degrees. Pain from the beginning of PSLR is suggestive of malingering.
3. Crossed straight leg raising (XSLR) is a variation of PSLR that has been found to be highly specific for lumbar disc herniation. In this test, the asymptomatic leg is raised. If pain is increased in the contralateral leg when the asymptomatic leg is raised, the result of the XSLR test is positive, a finding that has been shown to correlate with disc herniation in a high percentage of cases.
4. Leg length differences are assessed by measuring the leg from the anterior superior iliac spine to the superior aspect of the medial malleolus. Discrepancies greater than 1.5 cm are considered significant for scoliosis or other structural abnormalities.
5. Atrophy of the quadriceps and calf muscles is evaluated. Muscle weakness over a

period of weeks will result in atrophy. Lack of atrophy in the presence of long-term complaints of weakness is suggestive of malingering.

6. Motor strength is assessed by checking dorsiflexion and plantar flexion of the great toe against resistance.

7. Sensation is checked over the lower extremities by evaluating perception of light touch, pinprick, and sharp-dull discrimination. Corresponding dermatomes are compared in each leg.

8. Patellar (knee-jerk) and Achilles (ankle-jerk) reflexes are checked.

9. A palm-heel test is conducted by the examiner by placing his palms under the patient's heels. The patient is then asked to raise the leg while keeping it straight, first on one side and then on the other. When the patient is cooperating and attempting to raise one leg, the opposite heel should press firmly on the examiner's palm. If it does not, the patient is not exerting adequate effort. This suggests malingering.

Prone

(A pillow is placed beneath the abdomen to reduce lumbar lordosis and increase patient comfort.)

1. The patient is asked to localize the pain again. Localization of pain in different locations with a change in position is suggestive of malingering.

2. Palpation for tenderness is repeated. Tenderness in the costovertebral angle and spinous process is noted, as well as paravertebral muscle tenderness and spasm.

3. Reverse straight leg raising (the bow-string test) is performed by hyperextending each leg posteriorly. Pain radiating into the thigh is a positive result of this test, indicating nerve root stretching over the herniated disc.

4. The sensory examination is completed. The perineal and perianal areas are included because these areas are affected by compression of nerve roots in the cauda equina.

Sitting

1. A motor examination of the quadriceps is performed by having the patient extend the lower legs, actively and passively.

2. Hidden straight leg raising test is performed as follows: With the patient in the sitting position, the lower leg is extended at the knee, giving 90 degrees of flexion at the hip. This action gives the same result as the straight leg raising test performed with the patient in the supine position. Results are positive if the pain radiates down the sciatic nerve distribution on the affected side. A discrepancy between this test and the supine PSLR suggests malingering.

3. Deep tendon reflexes of the patellar and Achilles tendon may be rechecked.

4. Muscle strength testing by dorsiflexion and plantar flexion of the foot against resistance is completed.

PROBLEM 1 The 40 year old man was in good physical condition. He recalled a few episodes of mild back pain in the past but had had no previous severe episodes. He recalled bending over to pick up a package (weighing approximately 25 pounds); as he straightened, a popping sensation occurred, followed by the pain. He lifted packages repeatedly in his work and there was nothing unusual about this situation. The pain was severe, sharp, and aggravated by any movement; especially by rotation of the trunk. It ran down the right side of his back into the hip and posterior thigh. He had no other symptoms, specifically no numbness or tingling in the lower extremities and no bowel or bladder problems.

Examination in the standing position showed normal posture without abnormal spinal curvature. There was tenderness over the right paravertebral muscles in the lower lumbar area. With coaxing, the patient was able to bend forward about 30 degrees. He would not side-bend at all, but extension was relatively painless and he could bend backward about 15 degrees. His gait was cautious and shuffling but steady, and he was able to walk on his heels and toes. A stoop test was attempted, but he was unable to comply because of pain.

In the supine position the abdomen was scaphoid and nontender. PSLR resulted in radiation of pain into the right posterior thigh beginning at 30 degrees. When the left leg was raised, pain radiating into the right leg was again reported. Motor and sensory examination of the lower extremities revealed no deficits, and the patellar and Achilles reflexes were normal. The palm-heel test revealed good effort on the part of the patient.

In the prone position, with a pillow beneath the abdomen, the pain was again localized in the lower lumbar area on the right. Reverse straight leg raising produced radiation into the right posterior thigh. The sensory examination was completed by checking the perianal and perineal skin, where sensation was found to be intact. In the sitting position, hidden straight leg raising again resulted in radiation of pain into the right posterior thigh.

A thorough musculoskeletal back pain examination is time-consuming but essential. Cursory examination can miss important findings or may indicate positive findings that, if checked in all four recommended positions, would be negative or questionable.

PROBLEM 2 Abdominal examination revealed no masses, organomegaly, or distention. Femoral pulses were weak but palpable.

The finding of a pulsatile abdominal mass is not essential to the diagnosis of abdominal aortic aneurysm, nor are distention and loss of distal pulses. A very high index of suspicion for this problem is essential in older patients with risk factors for cardiovascular disease. Little time for further history-taking is available in this patient, and further information is not necessary to recognize the critical condition of the patient and make the proper disposition to the operating room.

DECISION PRIORITIES AND PRELIMINARY DIFFERENTIAL DIAGNOSIS

On completion of the history and physical examination, the physician is usually able to answer the following questions:

1. *Is the back pain a symptom of a life-threatening problem that requires immediate intervention?*
   Problems such as abdominal aneurysm and ectopic pregnancy that can result in hemorrhagic shock are generally identified and management is started at the time of the initial approach to the patient. However, at times the presentation is less obvious and the diagnosis is more difficult to make. Close monitoring of the patient's vital signs and clinical course during the data-gathering phase is essential because deterioration is possible at any time. If the patient remains stable, studies to confirm these diagnoses are performed, as outlined in Table 44–2. Surgical intervention may be necessary should the patient's condition deteriorate before the test results are available.
2. *Is the back pain secondary to a disease process in a system other than the musculoskeletal system or is it due to a primary musculoskeletal process?*
   The history and physical examination are usually sufficient to differentiate primary musculoskeletal from secondary back pain. Diagnostic studies in the emergency

TABLE 44–2. Secondary (Nonmusculoskeletal) Causes of Low Back Pain

System	Diagnosis	Pain Characteristics	Physical Findings	Diagnostic Tests	Therapy	Comments
Urinary	Pyelonephritis	Insidious onset; aching, dull pain; associated fever, chills, dysuria, urinary frequency	Flank tenderness, suprapubic tenderness, fever	Urinalysis, complete blood count	Antibiotics, antipyretics, urinary analgesics	Common; may be confused with LBP when presentation is vague
	Ureterolithiasis	Acute onset; severe pain, genital radiation, associated hematuria	Flank tenderness	Urinalysis, intravenous pyelogram	Analgesics, hydration	Common; may be confused with LBP when presentation is vague
Male reproductive	Prostatitis	Perineal pain, associated fever, chills, dysuria, urinary frequency	Painful, swollen, boggy prostate on rectal examination, fever	Urinalysis before and after prostatic massage	Antibiotics, antipyretics, prostatic massage	Common; may be confused with LBP when presentation is vague
	Prostatic carcinoma	Insidious onset, associated urinary retention	Enlarged, hard prostate	Acid phosphatase	Surgery, radiation therapy	Suspected mainly in men over age 50
Female reproductive	Pregnancy	Insidious onset; associated with enlarging uterus, amenorrhea	Gravid uterus	Pregnancy test	Rest, left lateral decubitus position	Due to direct pressure from the uterus as well as lumbosacral strain
	Ectopic pregnancy	Acute onset; associated vaginal bleeding, syncope, unilateral abdominal pain	Abdominal tenderness, hypotension, tender, enlarged adnexa	Pregnancy tests, pelvic ultrasound, culdocentesis	Surgery	Pelvic and back pain often precede acute rupture
	Pelvic infection	Insidious onset; bilateral abdominal pain, vaginal discharge	Abdominal tenderness, cervical motion tenderness	Cervical cultures	Antibiotics, rest, analgesics	Common, abdominal/pelvic pain usually predominant
	Uterine fibroids and tumors	Insidious onset; aching, dull	Enlarged, asymmetric uterus	Pelvic ultrasound	Surgery in some cases, radiation or chemotherapy for malignancy	Common, usually diagnosed on pelvic examination
	Endometriosis	Insidious onset; associated with menstruation	Variable, often none	Laparoscopy	Analgesics, surgery	Difficult to diagnose but may be suspected based on history
Gastrointestinal	Colitis	Associated abdominal pain, diarrhea	Abdominal and rectal tenderness, blood or mucus in stool	Stool cultures, colonoscopy, contrast radiology	Antibiotics, steroids, surgery	Variable etiologies including bacteria, protozoans, and inflammatory conditions
	Rectal or colon tumors	Insidious onset; associated weight loss, constipation, obstipation	Abdominal or rectal mass; blood in stool	Colonoscopy, contrast radiology	Surgery	

Table continued on following page

department do not often add significant information. Diagnostic tests are usually necessary to confirm secondary causes (Table 44–2).

3. *Is there an immediate risk of long-term neurologic impairment?*

The majority of the primary musculoskeletal back pain syndromes are managed conservatively. However, two problems may be encountered that require expeditious intervention to prevent permanent neurologic deficits—the cauda equina syndrome and spinal cord compression.

The cauda equina syndrome is an uncommon but very serious complication of lumbar disc disease. The patient typically presents with LBP, unilateral or

TABLE 44–2. Secondary (Nonmusculoskeletal) Causes of Low Back Pain *Continued*

System	Diagnosis	Pain Characteristics	Physical Findings	Diagnostic Tests	Therapy	Comments
Vascular	Aortic aneurysm	Insidious onset; unrelenting, associated abdominal, groin, or testicular pain; syncope, history of other cardiovascular disease	Pulsatile abdominal mass, hypotension, diaphoresis, diminished pulses	Abdominal ultrasound, CT scan	Immediate surgery, pneumatic antishock garment, fluid resuscitation, blood replacement	The most immediately life-threatening cause of LBP; must be considered in every case
Psychological	Psychosomatic, malingering	Vague or bizarre descriptions; nonanatomic distribution, nothing helps. Worse at night, at rest, or present only with specific activities	Nonanatomic distribution; inconsistent localization. Hidden straight leg raising negative. Absence of effort on palm-heel test	May require extensive testing to rule out other causes	Supportive, constructive attention; lifestyle evaluation; counseling for depression; exercise program	Difficult to diagnose and treat; key in the emergency department is constructive support and appropriate referral to rule out organic causes first and then rehabilitate

bilateral radiation, perineal anesthesia, motor weakness of the lower extremities, and bowel or bladder dysfunction (usually urinary retention). Onset may be acute or signs and symptoms of disc herniation may precede the development of the cauda equina syndrome for some time. Classically, surgical intervention within 6 hours of the onset of symptoms is considered essential to prevent permanent paralysis and bladder dysfunction.

Acute spinal cord compression, as by an expanding tumor mass, is another problem that can present as LBP with lower extremity, bowel, or bladder deficits; it requires immediate intervention to prevent permanent neurologic deficit. Spinal cord compression may also be due to central disc herniation, abscesses, hematomas, and displaced fracture fragments.

PROBLEM 1 The preliminary evaluation of this patient, which required 1 to 2 minutes of the physician's time, confirmed the presence of a localized musculoskeletal process in the lower lumbar area and vital signs consistent with the presentation of severe pain. No evidence of a life-threatening problem was found. After more extensive evaluation (10 minutes), neurologic function was found to be completely intact, including perianal-perineal sensory function.

There was no evidence of either a life-threatening problem or a neurologic deficit that might lead to permanent impairment. Findings are consistent with the initial impression of musculoskeletal origin of pain.

PROBLEM 2 From the vital signs and the history of near-syncope, it was clear from the time of the arrival of the rescue squad that this patient was unstable. Some patients with abdominal aortic aneurysm, ectopic pregnancy, or other, less common forms of retroperitoneal or intra-abdominal bleeding present with less pronounced symptoms and signs. The complaints of back pain *and* abdominal pain and the presence of risk factors for cardiovascular disease or ectopic pregnancy should prompt a thorough evaluation for these problems even when vital signs are normal.

DIAGNOSTIC ADJUNCTS

Radiologic Imaging

Many different imaging techniques are currently used for the evaluation of patients with LBP. When properly selected and appropriately timed in the course of the patient's problem, diagnostic imaging can be very helpful. However, overuse, improper selection, and inappropriate timing of tests often impair their usefulness. Table 44–3 serves as a guide to the selection of tests based on the specific problem suspected after the history and physical examination are completed.

Lumbosacral Spine Films. Lumbosacral spine films are rarely needed to diagnose the cause of LBP. They may be helpful when there is:

1. A history of or signs and symptoms suggestive of malignancy with possible metastasis to the lumbar spine.
2. Fever and localized tenderness suggesting osteomyelitis or disc infection.
3. Significant trauma to the lumbar area or a history of falls or jumps translating force to the lower back.
4. Acute, unexplained neurologic deficit.
5. A fall or similar accident while the patient was at work or in a public place, involving the possibility of legal action.
6. Inability to convince the patient of the lack of need for the study.
7. Failure to respond to a conservative regimen of treatment.

Abnormal findings on lumbosacral spine films, such as hypertrophic spurs, spina bifida occulta, spondylolysis, lumbarization of S1 and sacralization of L5, abound but may not have any relation to the patient's current symptoms. Although there is poor correlation between radiologic findings and clinical symptoms related to mechanical lower back problems, there is a closer correlation with medical problems. Fuzziness of the sacroiliac joint is an early sign of sacroiliitis and therefore of ankylosing spondylitis. Lytic lesions in the area of the facet joints, referred to as the "winking owl sign," are usually due to metastatic tumors.

Computed Tomography. Computed tomography (CT) is excellent for defining spatial relationships in the lumbosacral area and may be used as the initial study when disc herniation, spinal stenosis, tumors, or fracture-subluxations are suspected. With regard

TABLE 44–3. Radiographic Studies for the Diagnosis of Specific Causes of Low Back Pain

Disease Category	Plain Lumbosacral Films	Computed Tomography	Magnetic Resonance Imaging	Myelography	Bone Scan
Herniated nucleus pulposus		√ (many false positives)	*	√	
Spinal stenosis	√	*		√	
Ankylosing spondylitis	* (sacroiliitis)				
Osteomyelitis, disc infection	√		√		* (gallium)
Tumor	√ (winking owl sign)	* (myeloma)	* (intraspinal)	* (cord compression)	* (metastatic)
Osteoporosis	√				
Trauma	√	*		√	(occult fractures)

Key: √ = useful; * = imaging technique of choice.
Adapted from Borenstein DG, Wiesel SW: Low Back Pain. Philadelphia, W.B. Saunders, 1989.

to herniated discs, however, the usefulness of CT is reduced owing to the number of false-positive readings that occur.

Magnetic Resonance Imaging. Magnetic resonance imaging (MRI) displays small differences in tissue density with sharp contrast without exposing the patient to radiation or contrast material and is an excellent technique for visualizing the spinal cord within the spinal canal. The true correlation between symptoms and MRI findings remains to be determined, but MRI is the diagnostic procedure of choice for intramedullary tumors and may avoid many of the false-positive readings associated with herniated discs. In addition, MRI demonstrates changes resulting from disc infection very early in the infectious process. In spite of its relative unavailability and high costs, MRI is achieving a major role in the diagnostic approach to LBP.

Myelography. Myelograms are excellent confirmatory studies for evaluating pressure on neural elements when invasive procedures are being contemplated. However, myelography is the most invasive visualization technique and is associated with many more side effects than other techniques. MRI may obviate the need for myelography in patients with herniated discs, abscesses, tumors, hematomas, or vascular malformations. CT may obviate the need for myelography in patients with trauma or spinal stenosis.

Bone Scans. Radionuclide imaging with technetium-99m is an excellent technique for visualizing metastatic lesions and occult fractures. Gallium scans, in which the radionuclide binds to polymorphonuclear neutrophils, is excellent for demonstrating osteomyelitis and septic arthritis.

Other Techniques. Techniques for visualization of structures that may give rise to nonmusculoskeletal LBP include:

1. Intravenous pyelography. Intravenous pyelography (IVP) is very useful in diagnosing ureterolithiasis and renal colic.

2. Barium enema. Barium enema may be useful in diagnosing colon or rectal tumors and some forms of colitis.

3. Computed tomography of the abdomen. CT of the abdomen is an excellent study for diagnosing an aortic aneurysm in the more stable patient.

4. Ultrasonography. Abdominal ultrasound studies are useful in the diagnosis of an aortic aneurysm. Pelvic ultrasound studies are the diagnostic test of choice for pelvic masses and ectopic pregnancy.

5. Cross-table lateral radiographs of the abdomen. A lateral view of the abdomen with the patient supine will demonstrate a calcified aneurysm of the abdominal aorta in 60% of cases. Ultrasound and computed tomography are now preferred techniques for diagnosing aneurysms.

Laboratory Studies

Patients with primary mechanical LBP do not benefit from laboratory evaluation. Laboratory tests may be useful when specific problems are suspected as outlined below.

1. Complete blood count. An elevated white blood cell count is supportive of an infectious cause of LBP such as osteomyelitis or disc space infection. Its chief use, is, however, for supporting the diagnosis of secondary causes of back pain such as pyelonephritis or pelvic infection.

2. Erythrocyte sedimentation rate. An elevated erythrocyte sedimentation rate is supportive of an inflammatory cause of LBP such as ankylosing spondylitis. This test may serve as a useful screen for medical as opposed to mechanical causes of LBP.

3. HLA-B27. HLA-B27 is a histocompatibility antigen that is present in over 90% of patients with ankylosing spondylitis and in over 80% of patients with Reiter's syndrome. Eight percent of normal whites and 4% of normal blacks also have HLA-B27. The diagnosis of ankylosing spondylitis is usually made on the basis of the history, physical examination, and radiographic findings. Histocompatibility testing is rarely needed but may help when the radiographs are equivocal.

4. Rheumatoid factor. Rheumatoid factor (RF) occurs in association with a wide

variety of autoimmune and chronic infectious diseases. It is most closely associated with rheumatoid arthritis, being present in approximately 80% of these patients. RF may also support the diagnosis of subacute bacterial endocarditis in the LBP patient.

5. Serum alkaline phosphatase. Serum alkaline phosphatase (ALP) is associated with osteoblastic activity and will be elevated in patients with metastatic carcinoma, hyperparathyroidism, osteomalacia, and Paget's disease. ALP is decreased in hypophosphatasia.

6. Serum acid phosphatase. Serum acid phosphatase (ACP) is most closely associated with the prostate gland and is markedly elevated with prostatic metastases to bone.

7. Serum uric acid. Uric acid level may be elevated in patients with sacroiliac gout.

8. Serum calcium. The serum calcium level is elevated in patients with primary hyperparathyroidism and in some malignancies. It is decreased with osteomalacia.

9. Urinalysis. LBP of genitourinary origin is usually associated with an abnormal urinalysis. Hematuria may herald nephrolithiasis, infection, or neoplasia. Pyuria and bacteriuria are indications of infection.

PROBLEM 2 When a patient is in critical condition, there is no time for diagnostic imaging. However, in more stable patients, radiographic or ultrasonographic confirmation of the suspected aneurysm is indicated. The preferred imaging technique is computed tomography. Close monitoring during the study is essential because movement of the patient to the operating room may become necessary at any time. Laboratory tests to be ordered include complete blood count, hemostatic studies, type and cross-match for blood components, and renal function tests. Other tests such as measurements of electrolytes, serum glucose, and arterial blood gases are also included.

REFINED DIFFERENTIAL DIAGNOSIS

With the additional data supplied by the diagnostic test results, a specific diagnosis can usually be reached. The secondary causes of low back pain are discussed in other chapters and are briefly outlined in Table 44–2. The primary (musculoskeletal) causes of low back pain are given in Table 44–4. The most common and clinically important causes are discussed below.

Herniation of the Intervertebral Disc

The intervertebral disc is composed of a gel-like substance (nucleus pulposus) located in the posterior aspect of the disc. It is surrounded by a fibrous capsule called the annulus fibrosis. The annulus is much thinner posteriorly, making herniation of the nucleus pulposus much more likely to occur in this area. The posterior longitudinal ligament is the other posterior support, and it is thinnest at the L5–S1 interspace. The most common form of herniation is, therefore, posterior or posterior-lateral herniation at L5–S1 or L4–L5. Herniation results from gradual degeneration due to aging and repetitive stress. The final rupture leading to herniation may occur with such minor stresses as coughing or light lifting.

After herniation, the disc material may impinge on the lumbosacral nerve roots, producing pressure and irritation (Fig. 44–2). Irritation leads to pain in the distribution of the nerve root, followed by paresthesias, hypesthesia, weakness, and areflexia. Table 44–1 describes the specific findings associated with the different levels of herniation. Radiation of the pain into the lumbosacral dermatomes of the thigh and leg is termed *sciatica*. Herniated discs are the most common cause of sciatica. Other problems resulting in the same symptoms are epidural abscesses, tumors, hematomas, and direct irritation of the sciatic nerve by external pressure or by the tendon of the piriformis muscle.

TABLE 44–4. Primary Causes of Low Back Pain

Etiology	Diagnosis	History	Physical Findings	Useful Tests	Additional Aspects/Treatment
Congenital	Facet tropism (asymmetrical facets) Transitional vertebrae (sacralization of L-5, lumbarization of S-1)	History of nagging back pain, worse after exertion or sporadic activities such as gardening	May have paravertebral muscle spasm. Usually localized area of pain	Lumbosacral radiographs (Radiographs are not necessary, but these conditions may be noted when films are obtained)	Conservative treatment: heat, rest, analgesics
Tumors	Benign 1. Tumors involving nerve roots or meninges (hemangioma) 2. Tumors involving vertebrae (osteoid osteoma, Paget's disease)	Gradual onset of pain, worse at night. Often relieved with aspirin initially	Pain not usually changed significantly by position change. No associated muscle spasm. Spinal tenderness may be present. If weakness or paralysis is found, emergency evaluation is necessary	Radiographs may show a lesion. Proceed to CT or MRI if there is high suspicion and radiographs are negative. CT or MRI is used to rule out spinal cord or nerve root compression	LBP precedes radiographic changes. Thirty percent of bone density must be lost before it is visible on plain films Immediate surgical decompression or radiation therapy may be needed if there are signs of spinal compression
	Malignant 1. Primary bone tumors, multiple myeloma 2. Primary neural tumors 3. Metastatic tumors (breast, prostate, kidney, lung)	Older population, gradual onset. May have other associated symptoms relating to primary site. Poor response to analgesics or muscle relaxants		Myelogram may be necessary if surgery is contemplated	
Toxicity	Heavy metal poisoning	Gradual onset after exposure to heavy metals, usually job-related	No focal abnormality usually found	Specific levels directed by possible exposure	Rare—suspect if there is a history of exposure
Metabolic	Osteoporosis	Occurs in females over age 50. Slow onset of debilitating pain. Often associated with arthritis. If sudden exacerbation, think about compression fracture	Limited ROM. May have kyphosis. Muscle wasting of thoracic and lumbar muscles is present	Radiographs may show loss of bone density, Schmorl's nodes, loss of height, or compression fracture	A trivial amount of trauma may be required to produce a compression fracture in a patient with osteoporosis. Treatment is conservative, may require admission for pain control
Trauma or overuse	Fracture (vertebral body, transverse process)	Associated with axial loading or flexion/extension injury. Transverse process fracture usually results from direct trauma to low back	Possible bruising in the area of trauma. Examination should rule out spinal cord and associated injuries (urologic, pelvic)	Significant pain in the low back after an injury requires radiographic evaluation	
	Lumbar strain (overuse or improper use syndrome)	The history can be focused on an acute event: improper lifting, falls, athletics, minor trauma	Muscle tenderness and spasm. Radiation of pain may occur. Other tests are negative	None	Conservative treatment with bed rest, heat, analgesics, muscle relaxants
	Posterior facet syndrome	Commonly due to overuse. Pain may radiate to buttocks. Usually unilateral	Lumbar muscle spasm. Limited motion, negative results on straight leg raising	None	Conservative treatment with bed rest, heat, analgesics, muscle relaxants
	Sacroiliac joint sprain	History of flexion rotational load placed on torso, usually due to lifting a load while bending at the hip and twisting the torso	Unilateral pain at sacroiliac joint. May be reproducible by palpation. Limited ROM	None	Pain maximal over posterior, superior iliac spine but may radiate into buttocks or posterior thigh

Table continued on following page

TABLE 44-4. Primary Causes of Low Back Pain *Continued*

Etiology	Diagnosis	History	Physical Findings	Useful Tests	Additional Aspects/Treatment
Trauma or overuse *Continued*	Myofascial pain syndrome (fibrositis)	May not be a clear history of an antecedent event. Pain usually due to an activity that the patient is not used to performing	Paravertebral muscles are in spasm and have a ropey feeling. Trigger points may be found. Normal results on neurologic examination	None	This syndrome may have a radicular radiation of pain especially when pressure is put on the trigger point. Pain is increased with passive stretch while the trigger point is being stimulated. This test helps to differentiate myofascial pain from nerve root compression. Injection with anesthetic ± steroid at trigger point may benefit patient. Otherwise, treatment is conservative
Inflammation	Rheumatoid arthritis	Age 25–45. Female:male ratio 3:1. Back pain due to connective tissue degeneration. Other joints usually already involved prior to LBP	Pain with movement of spine. ROM may be limited. Usually not associated with muscle spasm. Hands and hips are usually already involved by the time of spine involvement	Rheumatoid factor	Trial of patient on aspirin or nonsteroidal anti-inflammatory medication and referral to an internist or rheumatologist is appropriate. Arthritis due to any cause may present as low back pain. The posterior facets are true synovial joints and are subject to all pathologies that affect this type of joint
	Ankylosing spondylitis	Males in early 20s. Pain in early morning, improved throughout the day	Sacroiliac joints and spine become fused causing kyphosis	HLA-B27 positive. Plain films may reveal sacroiliac sclerosis	
Degeneration	Spondylosis	Older patients, precipitated by fatigue or abnormal stress on back	Examination may reveal limited ROM and diffuse pain	Radiographs show degenerative changes. They are helpful, but not always indicated in the emergency department	Conservative treatment: Bed rest, heat, analgesics, muscle relaxants
	Degenerative arthritis (osteoarthritis)	Repeated trauma of daily living, obesity, and age. Loss of disc height may cause radiculopathy	Limited ROM, poor muscle tone, kyphosis or kyphoscoliosis common. Sciatica may be present due to nerve root entrapment from loss of disc height	Radiographs show degenerative changes	Conservative treatment: Bed rest, heat, analgesics, muscle relaxants
	Herniated disc	Pain precipitated by exertion; may begin in back and radiate down buttock to posterior or lateral thigh. Occasionally perceived in back of knee, calf, or ankle, and the patient may not have back pain as the major complaint. Patchy numbness or tingling	Pain should be reproduced by passive straight leg raising, crossed straight leg raising, and hidden straight leg raising. Chronically there is muscle wasting, loss of strength, sensory changes, and reflex changes	CT, MRI, and myelogram are usually diagnostic. They are not usually indicated in initial evaluation	Conservative treatment as above. Hospitalization may be needed if the pain does not improve. In hospital, traction is beneficial because it ensures bed rest

Spinal Stenosis

Severe degenerative arthritis resulting in marked spur formation may lead to impingement on nerve roots as they exit the neural foramina. Osteophytic formations can also impinge directly on the spinal cord, producing central stenosis. Motor and sensory deficits as well as bowel and bladder dysfunction are possible results. Increasing the intrathecal pressure by assuming the squatting position may result in improvement in symptoms, thereby

TABLE 44–4. Primary Causes of Low Back Pain *Continued*

Etiology	Diagnosis	History	Physical Findings	Useful Tests	Additional Aspects/Treatment
Degeneration *Continued*	Spinal stenosis with nerve root entrapment	Pain is worse with ambulation (symptoms similar to claudication). Pain improved with sitting and rest. Patient may have urine or stool incontinence	Central—The stoop test is usually positive. Lateral—There may be positive results on straight leg raising and a sciatic distribution of pain	Plain films reveal severe spurring or osteophytic formation. MRI, CT, or myelograms are diagnostic for central stenosis; MRI and CT are helpful for lateral stenosis	If there is bowel or bladder pathology, the patient is admitted. Conservative treatment usually results in improvement
Infectious	Acute (pyogenic disc, paraspinous or epidural abscess)	Patients usually have fever, chills, or sweats. Pulmonary, skin, and urinary infections are common sources	Fever in a patient with LBP is an important red flag. It may be the only clue to this rare cause of LBP. Percussion over spine may reveal extreme tenderness	CBC, ESR may be helpful. Plain films may show disc space fuzziness, lytic lesions of vertebral bodies, or soft tissue swelling	Look at other systems to locate source of infection. Blood cultures may be of some benefit if this cause is suspected, but source is uncertain
	Chronic, (tuberculosis, osteomyelitis, fungal infections)	Anorexia, weight loss, weakness, sweats, and fevers may be present			

ROM = range of motion; ESR = erythrocyte sedimentation rate; LBP = low back pain.

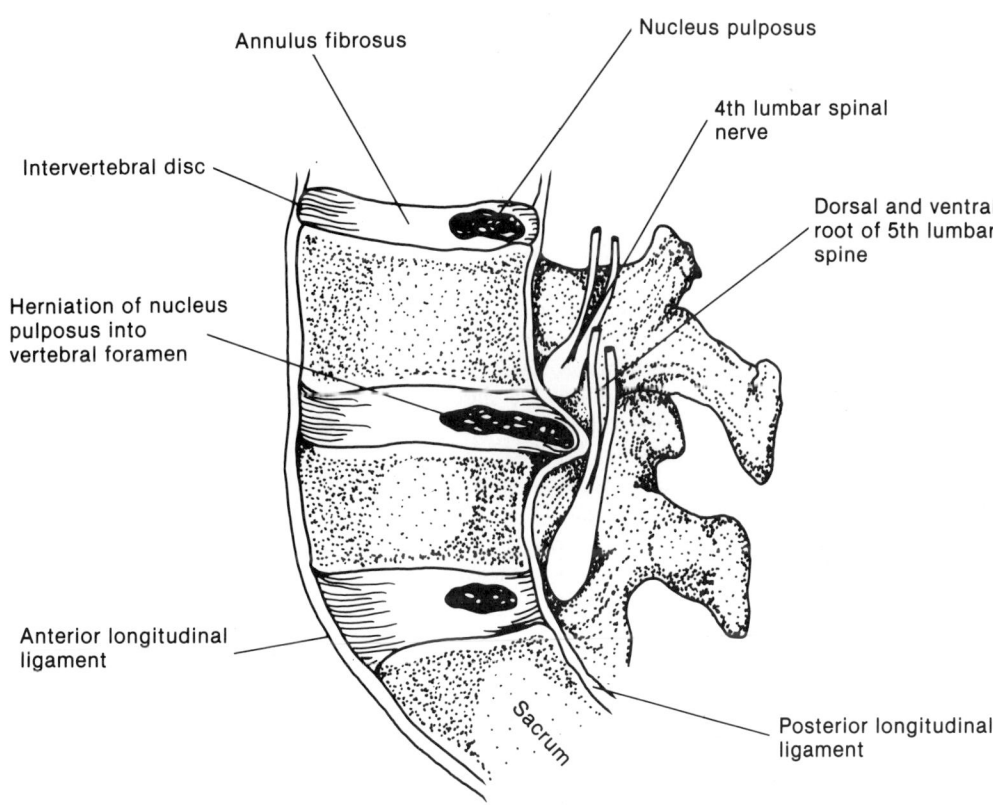

FIGURE 44–2. *Anatomy of a herniated intervertebral disc. Note that the annulus is thinner in the posterior region, predisposing the patient to posterior herniation. As noted, an L4–L5 disc causes compression of the fifth lumbar nerve root. Central or massive herniation may compress the cauda equina. (From Roberts JR: In focus: Sciatica and disc disease. Emerg Med Ambulatory Care News, May, 1989.)*

suggesting the diagnosis. Radiographic confirmation is accomplished by computed tomography, magnetic resonance imaging, or myelography. Plain films may suggest the diagnosis but are not diagnostic.

Overuse or Improper Use Syndromes

A number of low back problems may result from overexertion, especially when the patient is not in good physical condition. There is normally a balance in the support of the spinal column between the back muscles and the abdominal muscles. When one of these groups is underdeveloped, the patient is susceptible to problems that include strain of the lumbar muscles, posterior facet syndrome, sacroiliac joint sprain, and myofascial pain. In all these problems there is usually some degree of tenderness to direct palpation, and muscle spasm may be present. Tenderness over the sacroiliac joint or tenderness in that location with pelvic rocking is suggestive of sacroiliac sprain specifically. It is usually unnecessary to differentiate among these common overuse syndromes because conservative treatment is effective for all of them.

PROBLEM 1 This patient's history of repeated stress followed by acute onset of pain after a relatively trivial stress is the classic pattern of herniation of an intervertebral disc. Consistent location of the pain in the right lower lumbar area with consistent radiation into the right posterior thigh during multiple examination techniques in many patient positions is very diagnostic. Other problems, such as tumors and abscesses may result in the same physical findings, but these findings in combination with acute onset after stress virtually confirm the diagnosis of disc herniation.

This patient had no neurologic findings at the time, but the radiation of pain into the posterior thigh suggested involvement of the S1 nerve root owing to L5–S1 disc herniation. Findings that may follow are paresthesias and hypesthesia in the posterior thigh and lateral foot, weakness of plantar flexion and toe-walking, and decreased ankle jerks.

PRINCIPLES OF MANAGEMENT

The management of patients with secondary (nonmusculoskeletal) LBP varies depending on the system and specific problem diagnosed. A few of these problems—abdominal aortic aneurysm, ectopic pregnancy, and major pelvic trauma—may result in life-threatening hemorrhagic shock. These cases are managed with fluid resuscitation, blood replacement, and surgical control of bleeding.

For patients with primary musculoskeletal LBP, the major principles of management are (1) muscle relaxation, (2) relief of pain or inflammation, and (3) spinal cord or nerve root decompression.

The great majority of cases are managed with a conservative regimen of therapy, the goal of which is muscle relaxation and relief of pain or inflammation.

Muscle Relaxation

Muscle relaxation is accomplished by placing the patient on bed rest, using heat or ice, and administering muscle-relaxing medication. *Bed rest* is essential for muscle relaxation. The lower back muscles are most at rest in the semi-Fowler's position—with the shoulders elevated, the knees bent, and the feet propped up. The bed should provide firm support to the lower back. Acute-phase bed rest of 2 to 3 days with slow resumption of activity leads to improved recovery and less time lost from work. If the patient is hospitalized for severe unrelenting pain, traction may be added. The major advantage of traction is that it ensures that the patient remains at bed rest.

Either *heat* or *ice* leads to increased blood flow into the area treated, resulting in muscle relaxation. Moist heat is superior in this regard, but some patients experience good relief from ice as well. Ice provides some degree of pain relief and, after the initial cooling effect wears off, results in increased blood flow into the area and subsequent muscle relaxation.

Muscle-relaxing medications may also be added. A number of preparations such as cyclobenzaprine (Flexeril), orphenadrine (Norgesic), and methacarbamol (Robaxin) appear to be effective when used in this way. Their effectiveness may be due to analgesic or sedative properties rather than to direct muscle relaxation. Benzodiazepines such as diazepam are useful in the same way.

Relief of Pain or Inflammation

Relief of pain or inflammation is another important aspect of treatment for patients with acute musculoskeletal back pain. Aspirin and the other nonsteroidal anti-inflammatory drugs are effective for mild to moderate pain. When the patient is in severe pain, intramuscular narcotics such as meperidine are used, followed by oral administration of codeine preparations.

Spinal Cord or Nerve Root Decompression

Spinal cord or nerve root decompression may become necessary when a patient develops progressive weakness of the lower extremities or bowel or bladder dysfunction as a result of pressure on the neural tissue from a herniated disc, tumor, abscess, hematoma, osteophytic spur, or fracture fragment. The most commonly used and widely applicable method is surgical decompression. When a tumor mass is the offending agent, radiation therapy is the preferred method of decompression.

Beyond the acute phase of management, further therapy is determined by the patient's response to the conservative regimen of rest, heat, and analgesics. Once the patient begins to feel better, moderate *stretching exercises* are begun. After the problem is resolved, the patient is referred for back and abdominal muscle *strengthening exercises.*

For patients who do not respond to conservative therapy and have radiographically documented herniation of a disc, *laminectomy or microdiscectomy* is considered. Fewer than 10% of patients who present with a neurologic deficit will require surgery if 3 to 6 weeks of conservative therapy are undertaken before a decision about surgery is made. *Nonsurgical techniques* such as chemonucleosis and radiofrequency facet denervation are used in some centers.

PROBLEM 1 In this patient herniation of the L5–S1 intervertebral disc was diagnosed on clinical grounds. In such patients treatment consists of muscle relaxation and pain relief. Bed rest in the semi-Fowler's position, firm support to the lower back, moist heat applications, and adequate analgesics comprise the optimum management plan. A muscle-relaxing medication may be added and is especially helpful if it has a sedative effect that may encourage bed rest. Good choices for medications are acetaminophen given with codeine and diazepam. For patients with less severe pain, aspirin or ibuprofen with or without a muscle relaxant such as orphenidrine or methacarbamol is appropriate.

DISPOSITION AND FOLLOW-UP

Admission

Surgical treatment is required for patients with:
1. A ruptured abdominal aortic aneurysm.

2. A ruptured ectopic pregnancy.
3. Major pelvic trauma (surgery may be required).
4. The cauda equina syndrome.
5. Spinal cord compression syndromes (except when these are due to a tumor that may respond to radiation therapy).

Other patients to be admitted include the following:

1. Those with infections such as pyelonephritis, prostatitis, or pelvic infections may require admission for antibiotic therapy.
2. Those with compression fractures or transverse process fractures may be admitted for observation and evaluation for associated injuries. This decision is influenced by the severity of trauma causing the fracture and the patient's pain tolerance.
3. Those with neurologic deficits are admitted for close monitoring because immediate intervention is indicated if the deficit progresses.
4. Those with intractable pain.

Discharge

Patients to be discharged from the emergency department are given specific instructions for home care and follow-up. They are supplied with adequate pain medication, muscle relaxants, and specific instructions for activity. Generally, bed rest is recommended for a minimum of 48 to 72 hours, with slowly increasing activity guided by the patient's tolerance. Patients are instructed to return to the emergency department if the pain increases or if numbness or weakness develops in the legs. Bowel or bladder problems should also prompt immediate return. After two to three days, the patient is reevaluated, preferably in a back pain treatment center or by a physician skilled in treating low back pain.

PROBLEM 1 For patients with herniated discs without neurologic findings, outpatient management is preferred. If pain is intractable, admission is necessary. This patient received considerable relief from meperidine, and outpatient management was selected. He was instructed to make a follow-up appointment with an orthopedic surgeon in 2 to 3 days for reevaluation and to return to the emergency department if the pain increased or if he developed numbness or weakness in the legs or bowel or bladder problems.

PROBLEM 2 This patient was taken expeditiously to the operating room where a ruptured abdominal aortic aneurysm was found. Prompt surgical intervention was successful, and this patient recovered with sequelae. With an 80% mortality from this lesion, this outcome is more the exception than the rule. Delaying diagnosis or surgical intervention in patients with an abdominal aneurysm will invariably lead to a poor outcome. Approach to this problem in the urgent fashion described is essential to maximize the likelihood of a successful outcome.

DOCUMENTATION

1. Complete pain history, including precipitating factors, duration, character, severity, location, radiation, and factors that relieve or exacerbate the pain.
2. Associated symptoms related to systems other than the musculoskeletal system.
3. Results of the complete physical examination of the back in the standing, supine, prone, and sitting positions.
4. Results of the neurologic examination of the lower extremities.
5. Results of the abdominal, rectal, and perineal sensory examinations.

6. Radiographs obtained and their interpretation.
7. Treatment provided in the emergency department, response to treatment, and subsequent treatment plan.
8. Disposition and specific follow-up recommendations.

SUMMARY AND FINAL POINTS

- Patients with concomitant back and abdominal pain are at risk for serious intra-abdominal or retroperitoneal bleeding and require prompt evaluation and close monitoring.
- Patients in severe distress from musculoskeletal back pain with stable vital signs can safely and appropriately be given potent analgesics after preliminary evaluation.
- A complete musculoskeletal back pain examination is time-consuming but necessary. Examination in the standing, supine, prone, and sitting positions is essential to ensure accurate detection and interpretation of findings.
- Patients with progressive neurologic deficits or with bladder or bowel dysfunction require prompt surgical decompression. Nonprogressive neurologic deficits may resolve with conservative treatment.
- The indications for radiographic evaluation in the emergency department are few. Most musculoskeletal back pain problems are diagnosed on the basis of the history and physical examination.
- Sciatica, the radiation of back pain into the dermatomes of the legs, is commonly due to herniation of an intervertebral disc.
- Spinal stenosis due to advanced degenerative arthritic changes can result in pain and neurologic impairment. The stoop test is useful in diagnosing spinal stenosis.
- A variety of overuse-improper use syndromes exist. There is much overlap among these, and treatment is always conservative.
- Conservative treatment is the mainstay of back pain management and consists of muscle relaxation facilitated by bed rest, heat or ice, muscle-relaxing medications, and adequate analgesia. Even in the presence of neurologic deficits, 90% of patients will respond to a conservative regimen and will not require surgical intervention.
- Outpatient management is the norm, with admission usually reserved for patients with neurologic deficits or intractable pain.
- Appropriate follow-up is essential, preferably with a physician or clinic experienced in back pain care. Return to the emergency department is indicated for increased pain, onset of numbness or weakness in the legs, or onset of bowel or bladder problems.

BIBLIOGRAPHY

Texts

1. Blacklow RS: Back pain. In Macbryde's Signs and Symptoms (6th ed). Philadelphia, Lippincott, 1983.
2. Borenstein DG, Wiesel SW: Low Back Pain. Philadelphia, Saunders, 1989.
3. Cailliet R: Low Back Pain Syndrome (2nd ed). Philadelphia, F. A. Davis, 1968.
4. Mooney B (ed): Evaluation and care of lumbar spine problems. Orthoped Clin North Am 14(3), 1983.

Journal Articles

1. Abram SR, Tedeschi AA, Partain CL, et al: Differential diagnosis of severe back pain using MRI. South Med J 81(12):1487–1492, 1988.
2. Bail GR, Rothman RH: Conservative treatment of sciatica. Spine 9:54, 1984.
3. Bernard TN, Kirkaldy-Willis WH: Recognizing specific characteristics of nonspecific low back pain. Clin Orthoped Rel Res 217:266–280, 1987.
4. Deyo RA, et al: How many days of bed rest for acute low-back pain? A randomized clinical trial. N Engl J Med 315:1064–1070, 1986.
5. Hudgins WR, et al: Crossed straight leg raising test. J Occup Med 21(6):407, 1979.
6. Keim HA, Kirkaldy-Willis WH: Low back pain. Clin Sympos 32(6):2–35, 1980.
7. Kostiuk JP, et al: Cauda equina syndrome and lumbar disc herniation. J Bone Joint Surg 68A:386, 1986.
8. Lucas PR: Low back pain. Surg Clin North Am 63(3):515–528, 1983.
9. Nachemson AL: Advances in low back pain. Clin Orthoped 200:266–273, 1985.
10. Rockey PH, et al: The usefulness of x-ray examinations in the evaluation of patients with back pain. J Fam Prac 7(3):455–465, 1978.
11. Wiesel SW, et al: Study of computer-assisted tomography: The incidence of positive CAT scans in an asymptomatic group of patients. Spine 9(6):949, 1984.

SECTION THIRTEEN

NERVOUS SYSTEM DISORDERS

CHAPTER 45

ALTERED MENTAL STATUS

SIDNEY STARKMAN, M.D.

PROBLEM 1 A 50 year old man was found unconscious in a downtown park. He appeared disheveled and smelled of alcohol. The rescue squad was called to the scene by bystanders.

PROBLEM 2 A 30 year old man dressed in a business suit was found walking the streets, babbling incoherently. He was agitated and confused. The police brought him to the emergency department for "psychiatric evaluation."

QUESTIONS TO CONSIDER

1. What are the emergency conditions requiring immediate treatment in patients with altered mental status?
2. What are the most common causes of altered mental status in patients seen in the emergency department?
3. Which elements of the history and physical examination are most important in assessing patients presenting with altered mental status?
4. What ancillary tests are most helpful in diagnosing these patients?
5. How are organic causes of altered mental status differentiated from psychiatric or functional illnesses?
6. What is the role of computed tomography in the evaluation of these patients?
7. When is a lumbar puncture indicated and contraindicated in this clinical setting?
8. What are the standard initial management steps for all patients presenting with altered mental status?

INTRODUCTION

The term *altered mental status* describes a change from the "normal" mental state. The term *level of consciousness* indicates the patient's state of awareness and is only one aspect of an individual's mental status. Other manifestations of an altered mental status include disturbances in behavior, appearance, memory, mood, affect, judgment, and thought content. An abnormal mental status can be caused by an organic, functional (psychiatric), or mixed disorder. Organic illnesses are recognized as having a structural, biochemical, or pharmacologic basis—for example, brain tumors, Alzheimer's disease, or a toxic ingestion. Functional illnesses have no clearly defined pathophysiologic basis. They include disorders such as paranoid schizophrenia, manic-depressive states, and hysterical conversion reactions.

This chapter focuses on five clinical conditions characterized by an altered mental status: coma, acute confusion with depressed consciousness, delirium, amnesic states, and dementia. Sources of altered mental status often overlap in their clinical presentation, and a precise diagnosis is not always made in the emergency department. Each has distinguishing features that allow it to be categorized into one of the five broad conditions.

Coma

Coma is defined as a condition in which neither arousal nor awareness is present. *Arousal* (alertness or wakefulness) is dependent on an intact reticular activating system (RAS). This system runs through the brain stem and projects to the thalami and cortical cerebral hemispheres. *Awareness* depends on the proper functioning of the cerebral hemispheres. Coma can be induced if either the reticular activating system or *both* cerebral hemispheres are structurally damaged or chemically depressed by an endogenous or exogenous agent. A unilateral cerebral hemispheric lesion will not alter the level of consciousness unless it causes significant distortion of the brain stem and affects the reticular activating system. Identifying the brain stem and cerebral hemispheres as the foci of processes altering mental status assists in directing the physical examination and differential diagnostic pursuit. Management is often very different for causes of coma affecting the cerebral hemispheres as opposed to the brain stem.

An altered level of consciousness may indicate a primary brain disorder or systemic disease. Structural lesions of the brain most often affect the brain stem, whereas systemic disease usually exerts its influence on wakefulness through the cerebral hemispheres. Eighty percent of patients with coma have systemic or metabolic disorders. Drug ingestions are the most common cause. Structural lesions account for 10 to 15%, and functional disorders the remainder. The diagnostic principles applied in evaluating coma are useful in other patients with altered mental status.

Acute Confusion with Depressed Consciousness

Acute confusional states present in a wide variety of ways and have a large number of causes. The acute confusional state is defined clinically as a decrease in alertness and an inability to think clearly. Patients have difficulty maintaining attention to a stimulus or task. These patients are described as being stuporous or obtunded or having a clouded consciousness. The category exists on the continuum line leading to coma.

The most common causes of acute confusional states with a depressed consciousness are metabolic or drug related. They account for 70 to 80% of cases. Hypoglycemia and hypoxia are the most common metabolic causes of patients seen in the emergency department. Other causes are hyperglycemia, uremia, metabolic acidosis and alkalosis, hepatic failure, and hyper- or hyponatremia. The drugs most often causing acute confusion fall into the alcohol, opiate, sedative hypnotic, and antidepressant groups. Acute confusion also can result from structural disorders, including subdural hematoma, cerebral vascular accident, brain tumor, and brain abscess. Infection is another important cause of confusional states, e.g., meningitis and encephalitis.

The underlying anatomy and physiology involved in the acute confusional state are complex. Specific lesions to the nondominant hemisphere, parietal lobe, and nondominant side of the thalamus can cause acute confusion. Metabolic disorders tend to affect all regions of the brain. The physiologic suppression of synapse and cellular function has multiple origins, including altered action potentials, dysfunctional neurotransmission, and decreased ATP production.

Delirium

Delirium is an acute confusional state associated with an increased alertness. Patients are disoriented, show increased psychomotor activity, and often hallucinate. Classic examples of delirium are the abstinence syndromes associated with alcohol withdrawal and acute cocaine intoxication (see Chaps. 20 and 23). Other toxic ingestions causing delirium include amphetamines and atropine derivatives. Delirium also can result from a cerebral vascular accident or central nervous system infection, e.g., meningitis and encephalitis. Hypoglycemia and hypoxia can manifest as delirium, though this is far less often seen than a depressed consciousness.

Delirium is thought to result from disturbances in the temporal lobes, high midbrain, and subthalamus. These areas are responsible for hallucinatory activity and have a close relationship with the reticular activating system.

Amnesic States

The salient clinical feature in amnesic states is an impaired ability to recall events before an illness (retrograde amnesia) and to form new memories (anterograde amnesia). Patients with amnesia are usually alert and attentive. Amnesic states are characterized by varying degrees and speeds of recovery. Those causes having potential for full recovery include temporal lobe seizures, postconcussive states, and transient global amnesia from metabolic or drug-related problems. Injuries with primary tissue damage have high potential for incomplete recovery, e.g., cerebral vascular accident and severe head trauma.

Defects of memory can be traced to the medial dorsal nuclei of the thalamus and the hippocampal formation of the temporal lobe. Disorders affecting these structures can cause a memory deficit out of proportion to other cognitive functions.

Dementia

Diseases causing dementia usually appear later in adult life. Approximately 5% of the adult population over the age of 60 years can be described as having dementia. Dementia is characterized by a gradual deterioration of all intellectual functions. A failing memory is one of the most common signs of the problem. In addition to intellectual deterioration, patients undergo behavioral and personality changes. The most common identifiable cause of dementia is Alzheimer's disease. It is followed in frequency by alcoholic dementia, multi-infarct dementia, normal-pressure hydrocephalus, intracranial masses, and postinsult dementia (subarachnoid hemorrhage, encephalitis, hypoxia, or trauma). Psychiatric disorders can mimic dementia. Common causes of pseudodementia are schizophrenia, depression, and mania.

Three primary pathophysiologic processes may evolve into dementia. The first, best illustrated by Alzheimer's disease, is degeneration and loss of neurons in the association areas of the cerebral cortex. Arteriosclerotic vascular disease has a role in destroying neurons in the thalamus, basal ganglia, brain stem, and cerebrum. The second mechanism is compression of the cerebral tissue from a chronic increase in the intracranial pressure from hydrocephalus. It causes a widespread disturbance of cerebral function. The third is neuronal damage from infection, e.g., syphilis, meningitis, or encephalitis.

The emergency physician is confronted with the full range of altered mental status and its numerous etiologies. Its mystery and complexity must be unraveled in a relatively short time, while continuously protecting the patient from further insult and injury. It may not be possible to assign a clear cause in the time available, but the patient's symptoms usually will fall into one of the five major groups.

PREHOSPITAL CARE

Evaluating patients with coma or altered mental status in the prehospital setting focuses on accurately determining the severity of the problem and identifying readily reversible etiologies.

History

1. What is the basic history of this illness? Who is giving the history?
2. Is there a history of trauma, seizures, diabetes, or other medical problems? How long has the patient had altered consciousness? When was the patient last observed as "normal"?

3. Are any bottles or medication containers seen or available to be brought to the hospital?

4. Is anything notable about the environment in which the patient was found? Indoors or outdoors? Any unusual odors? Any other people in the vicinity in a similar state?

Physical Examination

1. What are the patient's vital signs? Is the airway patent and protected? Is there adequate ventilation?

2. What is the patient's level of consciousness? What is the size of the pupils and their response to light? Is there any evidence of trauma? If the patient has a depressed level of consciousness, methods of arousal are voice, touch, or noxious stimuli, such as pressure to the sternum or to the nailbed of the middle finger of each hand. The patient's response is observed and recorded. The Glasgow Coma Scale (Table 45–1) is used to quantify the patient's condition. The worst possible score is 3. The score for the motor response is based on the best response. Therefore, a hemiplegia on one side and a normal response on the other side receives a score of 6. The Glasgow Coma Scale serves as a valuable comparative standard to monitor subsequent deterioration or improvement in the patient's level of consciousness. The use of this scale in head trauma is discussed in Chapter 50, Head and Neck Trauma.

Intervention

Certain interventions are performed simultaneously while gathering information.

Airway Support and Oxygen. If respirations are adequate but the airway is impeded, a jaw-thrust or chin-lift maneuver is performed, and respirations are assisted as necessary. A nasopharyngeal airway, oropharyngeal airway, or endotracheal tube is placed, depending on the patient's airway patency and protection. High-flow oxygen supplement is routinely given to all patients with altered mental status.

Spine Stabilization. The comatose patient or patient with depressed consciousness may have a head injury and complicating cervical spine injury. The injury could be the initiating event or secondary to a fall while becoming unconscious. In these cases, a cervical spine fracture is always assumed to be present and the cervical spine immobilized.

Intravenous Access. A large-bore intravenous catheter is inserted. An isotonic

TABLE 45–1. Glasgow Coma Scale

Eye opening	
Spontaneously	4
To verbal command	3
To pain	2
No response	1
Best motor response	
Obeys commands	6
Localizes to pain	5
Withdraws to pain	4
Abnormal flexion	3
Abnormal extension	2
No response	1
Best verbal response	
Oriented, converses	5
Disoriented	4
Inappropriate words	3
Incomprehensible sounds	2
No response	1

crystalloid is the initial fluid of choice. Before infusion, a blood sample for subsequent electrolyte and glucose analysis is taken.

Cardiac Monitoring. A cardiac monitor is placed and the rhythm observed throughout transport.

Glucose. A dose of 25 to 50 ml of 50% dextrose is given intravenously. In children, 2 ml/kg of 25% dextrose is used to prevent hyperosmotic complications. Thiamine, 100 mg, is also given intravenously to adults. The patient is observed and changes in consciousness or the lack thereof are recorded.

Naloxone. A dose of 2 mg is usually given intravenously. If the patient is suspected of narcotic overdose, the first dose is decreased to 0.4 or 0.8 mg. This is repeated depending on the patient's response. Emergency department personnel must prepare for the patient with a narcotic overdose to awaken, become combative, and resist further medical evaluation.

PROBLEM 1 The paramedics arrived and found the patient comatose. His Glasgow Coma score was 7 (no eye opening = 1; unintelligible sounds = 2; nonspecific withdrawal movements = 4). His breathing was noisy but improved with a jaw-thrust maneuver. His gag reflex was intact but weak. He was placed on a backboard with spine precautions. Vital signs were blood pressure 140/90 mm Hg; pulse 90 beats/min; respiratory rate 24/min. He was given thiamine, glucose, and naloxone with no response. An empty bottle of wine was found in his jacket, along with a nearly full bottle of phenytoin capsules dated 2 weeks earlier. A companion stated that his friend had complained of headaches for about 2 weeks. The patient reeked of alcohol, and his pants were urine-stained. His right pupil was 6 mm and did not appear reactive. The left pupil was 3 mm and reactive.

Though the patient is a known alcoholic and appears to be in an alcoholic stupor or possibly in a postictal state, the history and physical point to a more urgent situation. The pupil asymmetry is particularly troublesome and suggests that the coma is due to a structural rather than metabolic condition. Rapid transport is indicated, with early hospital notification. Though the airway is patent, the gag reflex is weak, and the patient may benefit from hyperventilation (true coma, focal finding). Therefore, an orotracheal tube is put in place, with the head and neck immobilized, prior to transport and the patient hyperventilated.

INITIAL APPROACH IN THE EMERGENCY DEPARTMENT

The initial assessment of patients with altered mental status involves stabilizing basic life functions, protecting the patient from further injury, and promptly treating reversible etiologies. The following sequence is performed by the nursing staff and the physician as a team. Slight variations may exist, e.g., use of indwelling urinary catheter, depending on the degree of altered mental status and the patient's ability or willingness to cooperate.

History

1. The prehospital history is reviewed with the rescue squad or relatives, if they are available.
2. Clothes pockets are examined for identification, suicide notes, and drug bottles. A Medical Alert bracelet is sought. Telephone calls are initiated to obtain background information or history relating to the present illness.

Physical Examination and Intervention

Airway/Breathing and Oxygen. The airway is managed while maintaining cervical-spine precautions. Endotracheal intubation is performed in the patient who cannot protect the airway. Supplemental oxygen is provided for all patients.

Vital Signs. Vital signs, including rectal temperature, are obtained and compared with the field values. Hyperthermia or hypothermia necessitates instituting appropriate management.

Cardiac Monitoring. ECG monitor leads are attached and the rhythm observed. Treatment is instituted for significant dysrhythmias as necessary.

Level of Consciousness. The patient's level of consciousness is confirmed and compared with the Glasgow Coma Scale score from the field, if available.

Pupillary Responses. The pupillary responses are evaluated. Asymmetry, extremes of dilation or constriction, or poor reactivity is each a sign of a potentially serious central nervous system process.

Intravenous Access. Intravenous access is established with one or more lines, depending on the patient's hemodynamic status. An isotonic crystalloid is the fluid of choice. The rate is dependent on the patient's vital signs and the clinical estimate of adequate perfusion.

Glucose, Naloxone, and Thiamine. If glucose has not already been administered, a rapid, bedside analysis of freshly drawn blood by glucose oxidase test strip is performed. If the patient is not hypoglycemic, giving a glucose load may worsen the brain injury. For patients with hypoglycemia, 25 to 50 ml of 50% dextrose are administered. This amount should raise the glucose level 50 to 75 mg %. The test strips are more accurate in the hypoglycemic range but may underestimate high glucose levels. It is *always* necessary to confirm this bedside test with a serum glucose measurement. Two milligrams of naloxone are administered intravenously, as is thiamine, 100 mg. Thiamine is always given to suspected alcoholics or other undernourished patients because of the potential for a glucose load to aggravate an underlying thiamine deficiency.

Urine Output. An indwelling catheter is placed if necessary to monitor urine output. A urine specimen is obtained for laboratory testing.

Seizure Precautions. The patient is observed for seizure activity. A rhythmical twitching of some of the digits of either hand or a rhythmic, small-amplitude horizontal jerking of the eyes may be the only clue that the patient is in status epilepticus. If the patient is seizing and does not respond to the aforementioned treatments, the seizures are controlled with IV diazepam or lorezepam (see Chap. 48). Further assessments of mental status are obviously influenced by the addition of a sedative.

Suspected Meningitis. If meningitis is suspected, a lumbar puncture is performed early in the patient's care. Altered mental status and fever raise the possibility of meningitis in any patient. If there are signs of increased intracranial pressure or focal deficits on examination, the lumbar puncture is delayed pending results of a computed tomographic scan of the head. Appropriate antibiotics are initiated prior to lumbar puncture if there is a high suspicion of meningitis (see Chap. 47).

Elevated Intracranial Pressure. If a rapid decrease of consciousness is observed and a unilaterally dilated pupil sluggish or unresponsive to light is present, cerebral herniation is suspected. The patient is intubated and hyperventilated to a P_{CO_2} of about 25 mm Hg, intravenous mannitol, 0.5 to 1 gram/kg, is administered, and a computed tomography scan of the head is obtained. The neurosurgical consultant is notified immediately. More information is given in Chapters 49, Stroke, and 50, Head and Neck Trauma.

Initial Laboratory Data. Initial screening laboratory tests are usually sought early in the patient's care. These include complete blood count, electrolytes, glucose, blood nitrogen, creatinine, and urinalysis. Arterial blood gases are included if respiratory insufficiency is suggested by findings. Blood and urine samples are saved for other tests.

PROBLEM 1 Upon arriving at the emergency department, the rescue squad's findings were confirmed. The patient remained comatose with a Glasgow Coma score of 7 and a nonreactive, 6-mm–dilated right pupil. The vital signs were unchanged. However, the patient's respirations had become somewhat irregular. Old scars were noted on his forehead, and a more recent wound with encrusted sutures was found. In response to noxious stimuli, his left side moved much less than his right. The placement of the orotracheal tube was checked by direct visualization. Hyperventilation was continued with 100% oxygen. A ventilator was requested from respiratory therapy. A second IV line was placed. There was no response to the glucose, thiamine, and naloxone given in the field. Mannitol, 50 gm, was given intravenously. Blood for laboratory tests, including arterial blood gases, was drawn. The patient was transported for computed tomography of the head and other radiologic studies. The neurosurgeon was called and the operating room staff notified. The patient's belongings were searched for phone numbers to call. Prior medical records were requested.

The patient's physical findings are consistent with increased intracranial pressure and uncal herniation. Emergency treatment to reduce intracranial pressure by hyperventilation and osmotic agents is indicated. Preparations for urgent neurosurgical intervention are begun. The entire emergency department team is mobilized and motivated to maximize the efficiency and effectiveness of the patient's care.

DATA GATHERING

The patient in an altered state of consciousness often arrives in the emergency department without anyone available to give a medical history. The patient may not be able to give a history, certainly not a reliable one. In this situation, it is necessary to seek aggressively information from other sources. If only an address is available, the police are asked to go to the site for information. A conscientious effort can have a significant return.

History

1. *Did the patient verbalize any complaints or concerns prior to the onset in the change in mental status?*
   Patients with headache prior to their change are suspected to have an intracranial hemorrhage. Headache is also common in carbon monoxide poisoning. Patients who express feelings of depression are obviously at risk for having taken an overdose of medications.
2. *When was the patient last seen in a normal state of mental health? What is the normal state?*
   The time elapsed prior to being discovered is important because other conditions, such as dehydration, can complicate the original cause of the change in mental status.
3. *Was there a gradual or abrupt deterioration of mental status?*
   Abrupt changes are usually the result of more serious and catastrophic disorders. A patient with a significant change in status over a few hours usually has a metabolic problem. Hypoglycemia and intoxication are commonly found. Nonmetabolic causes are trauma and intracranial hemorrhage.
4. *Has the condition changed since it was initially recognized?*
   Serial monitoring of the patient's status is critical. Rapid deterioration in mental status is indicative of increasing intracranial pressure or a worsening metabolic process. Meningitis can have a rapid downhill course from both spreading infection and an increase in intracranial pressure.

5. *What is the patient's past medical history? Has the patient ever had a similar episode in the past?*
   It is necessary to know the patient's underlying medical illnesses, and whether the patient has been recently ill. Diabetes, hypertension, cerebrovascular disease, alcoholism, and depression are common concurrent disorders in patients who present with onset of a change in mental status.
6. *What are the patient's current medications?*
   Many medications, as well as drugs of abuse, can alter mental status. The most common are amphetamines, cocaine, sedative hypnotics, opiates, and antidepressants.
7. *Is the patient an alcoholic or other substance abuser?*
   In many patients in the emergency department, alcohol or substance abuse is complicating their lives. The difficulty is differentiating abuse as a primary cause of the patient's condition versus being a contributor to another process. Unfortunately, this group of patients is more susceptible to a number of disorders causing altered mental status, e.g., trauma, infection, uncontrolled hypertension, or diabetes mellitus.

Physical Examination

A thorough physical examination will (1) assess vital functions, (2) discover systemic causes of altered mental status, (3) determine whether focal neurologic signs are present, and (4) more accurately characterize the mental status changes.

Vital Signs

1. *Blood pressure.* Hypotension is rarely due to intracranial causes unless the patient is preterminal. When hypotension is present, volume loss, redistribution from venodilitation, or cardiac insufficiency is the probable cause. Cushing's triad of hypertension, bradycardia, and bradypnea is a late finding associated with increased intracranial pressure.

2. *Respirations.* Altered ventilatory patterns can provide some clues to causes. Hyperventilation may indicate acidemia and is also seen in pontine lesions. Cheyne-Stokes breathing is often associated with inadequate cerebral blood flow and diffuse cortical dysfunction. Ataxic breathing occurs when only the lowest brain stem functions are preserved.

3. *Temperature.* Fever is found primarily in infectious disorders but can occur after prolonged seizures. Environmental hyperthermia is also seen when weather conditions are appropriate. Hypothermia may be subtle and contribute to a depressed mental status.

Head, Ears, and Nasopharynx. The skull is inspected for external signs of trauma. Ecchymoses of the mastoid (Battle's sign) and hemotympanum are indicative of a basilar skull fracture. The breath odor is noted for alcohol or ketones.

Eyes. The eye examination is especially important in evaluating the patient with altered mental status. Its major value is in the comatose or consciousness-depressed patient.

1. *Pupillary size and reactivity.* Pupillary asymmetry of 1 to 2 mm with reactivity can be seen in 10% of normal people. Pupillary asymmetry or unilateral dilation of a pupil with absent reactivity can be caused by uncal herniation. Raised intracranial pressure forces the medial temporal lobe down through the tentorial membrane against the third cranial nerve. The loss of parasympathetic tone results in an ipsilateral dilated and nonreactive pupil (Fig. 45–1). Bilateral unreactive and fixed pupils are an ominous finding, indicative of significantly elevated intracranial pressure or brain death. The use of mydriatic eye drops by the patient can confound interpretation of pupillary responses.

Bilateral pupillary constriction is seen in patients with opiate overdose or in pontine lesions. The reactivity of pupils is an important differentiator between structural lesions and metabolic disorders. In most metabolic disorders, reactivity is present.

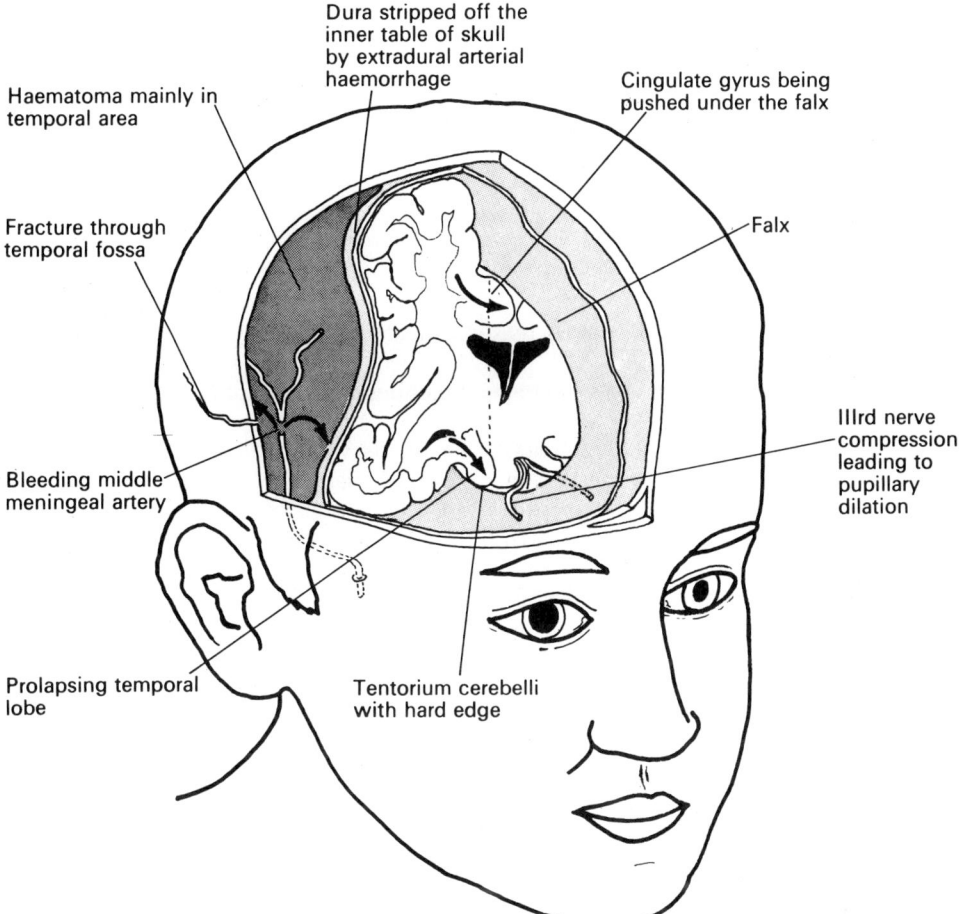

FIGURE 45–1. Uncal herniation causing compression of third cranial nerve and ipsilateral pupillary dilation in a patient with an epidural hematoma. A subdural hematoma from torn bridging veins can have the same effect. (From Patten J: Neurological Differential Diagnosis. New York, Springer-Verlag, 1977.)

2. *Corneal reflexes.* Corneal stimulation will produce a blink response if the fifth and seventh cranial nerves are intact. It is another gauge of brain stem function.

3. *Extraocular movements.* In the patient with coma or a significant depression of consciousness, brain stem function can be evaluated by testing for extraocular muscle function. Brain stem function represented by cranial nerves III through VIII is preserved if "doll's eyes" are present. When rotating the head from side to side, the patient appears to fix the eyes on the same object in spite of the head position. This is a normal oculocephalic reflex. A clearance of cervical spine status is essential before oculocephalic testing. It is suppressed in the conscious patient, present in the unconscious patient with an intact brain stem, and absent if the brain stem is dysfunctional or suppressed metabolically. If no extraocular movements are present, then the oculovestibular reflex is tested with caloric stimulation from cold water irrigation of the ears (Fig. 45–2). Before irrigating, the tympanic membranes are noted to be intact, and the head is flexed 30° from supine. If brain stem function is preserved, the eyes will deviate to the side of the stimulus. This test may be positive when oculocephalic testing is negative or equivocal. The two are usually done in sequence.

4. *Funduscopic examination.* Hemorrhages can be seen in the area of the retina when a severe subarachnoid hemorrhage has taken place. The presence of papilledema

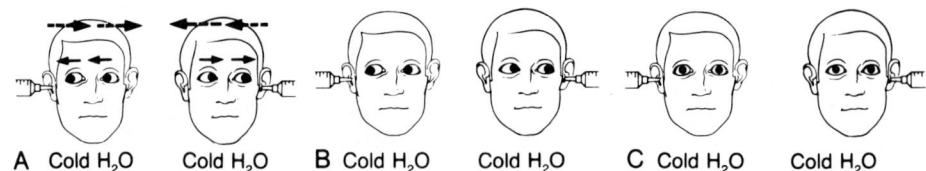

FIGURE 45–2. *Responses to caloric stimulation of the vestibular apparatus with the head placed in 30° of flexion. (A) Awake or psychogenic coma. (B) Indicates coma with brainstem intact. (C) Severe brainstem injury or deep toxic-metabolic depression. (Adapted from Plum F, Posner JB: The Diagnosis of Stupor and Coma (3rd ed). Philadelphia, F.A. Davis, 1980.)*

usually indicates increased intracranial pressure that has been present for more than 6 to 12 hours.

Neck. The presence of meningismus can indicate either meningitis or a subarachnoid hemorrhage.

Cardiopulmonary. All patients with altered mental status require a careful cardiac and lung examination. Dysrhythmias, valvular disorders, and heart failure can be responsible for, contribute to, or complicate their condition. Respiratory insufficiency, infection, or metastasis from pulmonary cancer also can cause mental changes.

Abdomen. The examination is directed toward confirmatory evidence of infection, mass lesions, and renal or hepatic insufficiency.

Neurologic Examination

1. *Level of consciousness.* The Glasgow Coma Scale is applied periodically to monitor the progress or deterioration of the patient.

2. *Cranial nerves.* Eye function is the best measure of cranial nerve integrity. If the patient's level of consciousness changes, the gag reflex is reassessed.

3. *Motor responses.* Purposeful avoidance of painful stimuli denotes an intact corticospinal tract and a nearly awake patient. Spontaneous flexion (decorticate posturing) of the arms at the elbows and wrists indicates damage at the level of the hemispheres. Arm extension with pronation (decerebrate posturing) is the result of lesions or a metabolic effect in the midbrain area. Flaccidity, despite a painful stimulus, is an ominous finding. Care must be taken in interpreting the patient without motor responsiveness because a massive overdose of the sedative/hypnotics or opiates can mimic a deathlike state.

Mental Status Examination. A mental status examination is performed to attempt to distinguish between organic and psychiatric (functional) etiologies (see Chap. 52, Behavioral Disorders). The patient must be capable of responding to questions. The elements of a complete mental status examination are listed in Table 45–2. The most important components test cognitive function. These include level of consciousness, orientation, attention, memory, and fund of information. Any impairment of cognitive function strongly suggests an organic problem causing the altered mental status.

While interacting with the patient, assessments are quickly made about appearance, behavior, mood, and affect. Note patient's speech and examine language function. Insight into a patient's judgment or thought content may not occur until specific circumstances arise or certain questions are asked. Subtle changes may be difficult to determine and must be compared with information about the patient's "usual" mental status. It is not unusual for patients with mild Alzheimer's disease to elude discovery of their marked memory deficit by being affable, displaying intact remote memory (address, telephone number, old friends and acquaintances), and giving a plausible, though totally erroneous, history of their presenting illness. Therefore, attention and memory are important measurements. Testing attentiveness is another means of assessing mental function in the alert patient. Typically, it is tested by using numbers—repeating a series of numbers presented or reciting serial 7s (serially subtracting 7 from 100). Recent memory is tested by presenting three different items, like "red tie, Hawaii, 33" and asking the patient to repeat the list of three in 5 minutes. A correct response demonstrates that attention and memory are intact. Recent memory dysfunction usually manifests itself early in organic

TABLE 45–2. Mental Status Examination

Behavior and appearance
Mood, affect
Judgment, thought content
Level of consciousness—alert, lethargic, obtunded, stupor, coma
Attention
Orientation—time, place, person
Mentation (memory)
   Registration, retention, recall
   Immediate, recent, remote
Language function (aphasia)
   Spontaneous speech
   Comprehension
   Repetition
   Naming
   Writing
   Reading
Ability to carry out purposeful movements (apraxia), including constructional ability
Recognizing ability (agnosia)

disorders. If one questions patiently and persistently, even apparently uncooperative psychiatric patients can prove they have intact recent memory.

PROBLEM 2 The 30 year old man was wearing a business suit and tie but was disheveled. He was clean shaven. He intermittently walked rapidly about the small examining room, then stopped and sat quietly. He appeared alert but was easily distracted. He correctly knew his name, the day, month, and year and recognized that he was in a hospital. In response to why he was in the hospital, he stated he didn't know, but thought he was losing his mind. He then walked away babbling. He spelled his name, Smith, but was unable to spell it backward. Similarly, he failed to recite serial 7s after the first two numbers. He appeared unable to concentrate. The remainder of the physical and neurologic examination was unremarkable. He had no medications or drugs on his person. His wife was called. She stated he had been in excellent health when he left home that day. He never had anything like this before.

This patient demonstrates problems with attentiveness and short-term memory. There are no focal neurologic signs, and the vital signs are normal. At this point, both organic and psychiatric disease are possible. The lack of a previous history, the rapid onset and findings on the mental status examination are suggestive of an organic problem.

DECISION PRIORITIES AND PRELIMINARY DIFFERENTIAL DIAGNOSIS

Following the history and physical examination, decision priorities are established, and the preliminary differential diagnosis is constructed by asking the following questions:

1. *Is the cause of the alteration in mental status life-threatening?*
   Most causes of altered mental status requiring immediate attention are cardiopulmonary. The priorities of advanced life support are instituted in these patients. Stabilizing the airway status and oxygenation comes first, then cardiac dysrhythmias and volume status. Once the cardiopulmonary systems are stabilized, the following potentially catastrophic processes are considered:
   a. Abnormalities of temperature regulation (hypo- and hyperthermia)
   b. Poisoning (carbon monoxide, cyanide)
   c. Infection (meningitis)

d. Causes of raised intracranial pressure, particularly herniation syndromes from focal lesions (mass lesions, post-traumatic brain injury). See Chapters 49, Stroke, and 50, Head and Neck Trauma.

All these can be lethal *and* are reversible.

2. *Is the altered mental status due to a primary central nervous system disease or is it the consequence of a systemic illness?*

Differentiating between primary or secondary central nervous system diseases is based primarily on the presence or absence of focal abnormalities on the neurologic examination. Focal findings strongly suggest the presence of a specific lesion in the central nervous system. Systemic problems, such as a lack of nutrients (glucose, oxygen), metabolic problems (sodium, calcium), or an accumulation of toxins (carbon dioxide, carbon monoxide, alcohol) causes diffuse central nervous system dysfunction manifesting as an altered mental status. Occasionally, hyponatremia or nonketotic hyperosmolar coma can present with focal neurologic signs. In all cases of focal neurologic signs, a search for a structural intracranial lesion is initiated. As noted in the pupillary reactivity discussions, preserved reactivity is characteristic of a systemic process. The absence of focal findings in no way rules out a primary CNS process. The search for structural lesions must continue.

3. *Is it an organic problem or a functional illness?*

The patient presenting with unusual behavior may have a functional or organic disorder. Table 45–3 is helpful in distinguishing functional from organic illness, though a mixed picture is seen in up to one-third of patients. For a patient with an organic cause, an attempt is made to categorize the causes further. Coma, confusion with depressed consciousness, and amnesia are more readily identified and have been discussed in the Introduction. The criteria for dementia are listed in Table 45–4, and the criteria for delirium in Table 45–5. Behavioral disorders are also discussed in Chapter 52.

DIAGNOSTIC ADJUNCTS

The sequence of ordering laboratory tests depends on the history and physical examination. The first three tests that follow are ordered for the majority of patients with altered mental status. The remaining tests are selected on the basis of the patient's findings.

Laboratory Studies

Complete Blood Count (CBC) and Differential. A CBC is obtained to measure the hemoglobin and hematocrit, particularly if anemia is suspected. An elevated white blood

TABLE 45–3. Distinguishing Between Functional and Organic Illnesses*

Functional	Organic
Onset under 40 years of age almost always	Onset at any age
Vital signs usually normal	Abnormal vital signs may be present
Usually oriented	Frequently disoriented
Sensorium intact	Altered sensorium usually present
Mentation usually intact	Mentation often impaired
Hallucinations usually auditory, may be persecutory or derogatory	Hallucinations usually visual
Involuntary movement disorders absent unless secondary	Involuntary movement disorders may be present
Absence of any focal neurologic signs	May have focal neurologic signs, including aphasia
Incontinence unusual	Incontinence may be present

*Initially indeterminate in about 30% of patients with altered mental status.

TABLE 45-4. Dementia

An acquired (not mental retardation), persistent impairment of intellectual function with compromise affecting at least three of the following spheres of mental activity:
1. Speech and/or language
2. Memory (not amnesia)
3. Cognition (manipulation of knowledge)
4. Visuo-spatial skills
5. Personality change

The disturbance significantly interferes with work or usual social activities or relationships with others. The sensorium usually remains intact until late in the process.

(From Diagnostic and Statistical Manual of Mental Disorders, 3rd ed, rev. Washington, DC, American Psychiatric Association, 1987, with permission.)

cell count and, in particular, a differential count with a left shift support the presence of underlying infection or inflammation.

Serum Chemistries. Serum glucose, electrolytes, calcium, blood urea nitrogen, and creatinine assess most of the metabolic causes of altered states of consciousness. Hepatic function tests are ordered if warranted by the clinical presentation.

Alcohol and Toxicologic Screen. An alcohol screen and ethanol level are indicated for any patient in whom alcohol intoxication is suspected. Screening for other toxicologic substances is necessary when a drug ingestion is suspected but cannot be accurately confirmed by other means. Drug levels are useful when specific antidotes or interventions are available and necessary, e.g., acetaminophen, salicylates.

Arterial Blood Gas Analysis (ABG). Arterial blood gas measurements are indicated when hypoxia, hypercapnia, or metabolic acidosis/alkalosis is considered. As a general rule, ABG's are obtained in all patients with coma, with significantly depressed consciousness, or those needing ventilatory support.

Carboxyhemoglobin (CO) Level. This test is obtained in all patients with a suspected exposure to CO.

Radiologic Imaging

Chest Radiographs. A chest radiograph may help elucidate pulmonary causes of an altered mental status, such as pneumonia or congestive heart failure. Rarely, a source of brain metastases may be found.

TABLE 45-5. Criteria for Delirium

A. Reduced ability to maintain attention to external stimuli, e.g., questions must be repeated because attention wanders, and to appropriately shift attention to new external stimuli, e.g., perseverates answer to a previous question
B. Disorganized thinking, as indicated by rambling, irrelevant, or incoherent speech
C. At least two of the following:
  1. Reduced level of consciousness, e.g., difficulty keeping awake during examination
  2. Perceptual disturbances: misinterpretations, illusions, or hallucinations
  3. Disturbance of sleep-wake cycle with insomnia or daytime sleepiness
  4. Increased or decreased psychomotor activity
  5. Disorientation to time, place, or person
  6. Memory impairment, e.g., inability to learn new material, such as repeating the names of several unrelated objects 5 minutes after learning them, or to remember past events, such as history of current episode of illness
D. Clinical features develop over a short period of time (usually hours to days) and tend to fluctuate over the course of a day
E. Either (1) or (2):
  (1) Evidence from the history, physical examination, or laboratory tests of a specific organic factor (or factors) judged to be etiologically related to the disturbance
  (2) In the absence of such evidence, an etiologic organic factor can be presumed if the disturbance cannot be accounted for by any nonorganic mental disorder, e.g., manic episode accounting for agitation and sleep disturbance

(From Diagnostic and Statistical Manual of Mental Disorders, 3rd ed, rev. Washington, DC, American Psychiatric Association, 1987, with permission.)

Skull Radiographs. These studies are usually not indicated in evaluating the patient with an alteration of mental status unless skull fracture is suspected clinically. If a skull fracture is suspected, computed tomography is a more useful test.

Computed Tomography (CT). A head CT is ordered under the following circumstances in the face of an altered mental status: (1) suspected trauma, (2) suspected intracranial hemorrhage, (3) presence of unexplained focal neurologic deficits, (4) papilledema, (5) other nonintracranial causes of coma ruled out, and (6) altered mental status unexplained after emergency department evaluation.

Magnetic Resonance Imaging (MRI). At present, this valuable test is not commonly used in the emergency setting. It is used after the patient is stabilized and other causes of altered mental status have not been found. It is very sensitive for revealing the common changes consistent with the various dementias. It is not yet specific enough to diagnose individual causes with precision.

Electrocardiogram

An electrocardiogram is indicated for all patients with altered mental status to evaluate for dysrhythmias, ischemia, and metabolic effects on ECG, such as a widened QRS from tricyclic antidepressants.

Lumbar Puncture

A lumbar puncture is indicated in any patient in whom meningitis is suspected. It can be done safely in patients without papilledema or other evidence of raised intracranial pressure (deepening of coma, changes in respiratory pattern, Cushing's response, decorticate or decerebrate posturing) and in whom a thorough neurologic examination reveals no focal deficits. If meningitis is suspected but a lumbar puncture is contraindicated, then appropriate antibiotics in doses appropriate to treat meningitis are administered before the patient is transported to the computed tomography department for further evaluation.

PROBLEM 1 The CT scan showed a large, right parietofrontal chronic subdural hematoma. Fresh blood within the subdural probably explained his recent deterioration. His alcohol level was only 50 mg%.

The patient's alcohol level does not account for a significant alteration in mental status, much less outright coma. When this mismatch is a low alcohol level and a high degree of mental status impairment, then other serious conditions must be aggressively sought. In this case, findings consistent with uncal herniation prompted a rapid diagnostic effort.

PROBLEM 2 The patient was noted to have a white blood cell count of 12,000 with 5% immature neutrophils (bands). Otherwise, his laboratory tests were unremarkable. Because of the clinical presentation, low-grade temperature elevation, and the elevated white blood cell count, a lumbar puncture was performed. A clinical judgment was made not to begin antibiotics. Before the LP was performed, it was reconfirmed that there were no signs of raised intracranial pressure, papilledema, or focal neurologic findings. The cerebrospinal fluid showed 200 lymphocytes and 30 red blood cells. Glucose was normal and protein elevated. A CT scan was ordered. It showed hypodense regions in both temporal lobes.

The decision to perform the LP at this point is appropriate. An infectious etiology for the altered mental status has to be ruled out. CT scanning is diagnostically supportive of the findings on lumbar puncture.

REFINED DIFFERENTIAL DIAGNOSIS

The causes of altered mental status are numerous. Table 45–6 lists the various disorders by group to facilitate classification. It is important for the practicing physician to understand clearly the treatable and reversible causes of an altered mental status. The most common treatable sources of altered mental status may be remembered by the

TABLE 45–6. Differential Diagnosis of Coma and Other Causes of an Altered Mental Status

I. **Coma**
   A. *Intracranial hemorrhage*
      Subdural hematoma
      Epidural hematoma
      Subarachnoid hemorrhage
      Intracerebral hemorrhage
   B. *Cerebrovascular ischemia*
      Large cerebral infarction
      Brain stem infarction
      Basilar artery migraine
      Pontine infarction
      Vasculitis
   C. *Metabolic*
      Hypoglycemia
      Ketoacidosis/hyperglycemia
      Uremia
      Hypercalcemia
      Hepatic failure
      Hyponatremia
      Reye's syndrome
   D. *Drug-related*
      Sedative hypnotics
      Opiates
      Tricyclic antidepressants
      Carbon monoxide
   E. *Infections*
      Meningitis
      Encephalitis
      Brain abscess
   F. *Tumor/mass*
      Malignant—primary
      Malignant—metastasis
      Benign—large
   G. *Other*
      Epilepsy
      Conversion reaction
      Thrombotic thrombocytopenic purpura
      Advanced Alzheimer's disease
      Shock

II. **Acute Confusional States with Depressed Consciousness**
   A. Essentially all the same etiologies as coma. Those listed represent more common causes
   B. *Metabolic*
      Hepatic failure
      Uremia
      Hypoxia
      Hypoglycemia
   C. *Drug/toxin-related*
      Sedative hypnotics
      Opiates
      Tricyclic antidepressants
      Carbon monoxide
   D. *Cerebrovascular*
      Abscess
      Encephalitis
      Intracranial hemorrhage, including subarachnoid hemorrhage, hematomas
      Ischemia
      Meningitis
      Tumor
   E. *Others*
      Congestive heart failure
      Dementia complicated by fever, drugs, or other acute diseases
      Postictal state

III. **Delirium**
   A. *Abstinence states*
      Alcohol
      Barbiturates
      Benzodiazepines
   B. *Drug-related*
      Cocaine
      Amphetamine
      PCP (phencyclidine)
      Atropine derivatives
      Ergotamine
   C. *Cerebrovascular*
      Ischemia to temporal lobes or upper brain stem
      Cerebral contusion
      Subarachnoid hemorrhage
      Postictal state
      Postconcussion
   D. *Infections*
      Bacterial/tubercular/viral meningitis
      Encephalitis, e.g., herpes simplex
      Typhoid fever
      Pneumonia
      Sepsis
      Rheumatic fever
   E. *Others*
      Thyrotoxicosis
      Postoperative states

Table continued on following page

TABLE 45–6. Differential Diagnosis of Coma and Other Causes of an Altered Mental Status *Continued*

IV. **Amnesic States**
   A. *Metabolic*
      Wernicke-Korsakoff syndrome (thiamine deficiency)
      Carbon monoxide
      Hypoxic insult
   B. *Craniocerebral*
      Hippocampal infarction
      Trauma to diencephalon
      Subarachnoid hemorrhage
      Temporal lobe seizures
      Postconcussive states
      Transient global amnesia
   C. *Infections*
      Encephalitis
      Meningitis
   D. *Others*
      Tumors of 3rd ventricle or temporal lobes
      Alzheimer's disease (early state only)

V. **Dementia**
   A. *Degenerative disorders*
      Alzheimer's disease
      Huntington's chorea
      Leukodystrophies
      Lipid storage diseases
      Jakob-Creutzfeldt disease
   B. *Craniocerebral*
      Cerebral arteriosclerosis
      Normal pressure hydrocephalus
      Brain tumor
      Chronic subdural hematoma
   C. *Metabolic*
      Hypothyroidism
      Cushing's disease
      Nutritional deficiencies
   D. *Others*
      Neurosyphilis
      Hepatolenticular degeneration
      Chronic drug intoxication (barbiturates)
      AIDS

mnemonic AEIOU–TIPPS. Table 45–7 illustrates how the mnemonic is used. The majority of these cases present as confusion with depressed consciousness or coma.

1. **Alcohol.** Alcohol intoxication is the most common cause of altered mental status seen in the emergency department. The odor of alcohol is usually detectable on the patient's breath. The level of intoxication depends on the patient's tolerance to alcohol. It is important to remember that patients with altered states of consciousness may have multiple processes simultaneously. The intoxicated patient can fall and hit his or her head, resulting in primary brain injury and a secondary complication such as a CNS hemorrhage. A difficult decision in clinical emergency medicine is whether to attribute the patient's clinical state to alcohol intoxication or to search for alternative causes (see Chap. 20). Some general guidelines:
   a. Is the patient's clinical status consistent with the blood alcohol level? While the individual patient's tolerance to alcohol varies, a blood alcohol level of less than 250 mg % rarely causes true coma.
   b. Is the patient's mental status improving with time? Decreased mental status due to ethanol intoxication should improve gradually as the alcohol metabolizes. A worsening condition, as observed by a changing neurologic examination, prompts the need to find other etiologies.
   c. Focal neurologic deficits are not attributable to alcohol intoxication.
   d. When in doubt, search for other sources.
2. **Epilepsy, Electrolytes, Encephalopathy.** Seizures cause an altered mental status during the ictal and postictal phases. They may be due to a known seizure disorder,

TABLE 45–7. Mnemonic for Treatable Causes of Altered Mental Status

A—alcohol	T—trauma
E—epilepsy, electrolytes, encephalopathy	I—infection
I—insulin	P—psychiatric
O—opiates	P—poison
U—urea (metabolic)	S—shock

primary CNS diseases like meningitis or intracranial hemorrhage, or a secondary systemic problem, e.g., hypoxia. The postictal phase of a seizure usually lasts minutes to hours and shows gradual clearing. The emergency department approach to seizures is discussed in Chapter 48.

Electrolytes are primarily represented by changes in sodium (see Chap. 27, Hyponatremia) and calcium (see Chap. 29, Hypercalcemia). Encephalopathy is related to hepatic disease.

3. **Insulin.** Hypoglycemia is usually secondary to diabetes and insulin treatment or to depleted lesion glycogen stores and inadequate diet. It is diagnosed by the glucose oxidase test strip measurement and the improvement in mental status following the administration of adequate intravenous dextrose (25 to 50 grams). Hyperglycemia and accompanying hyperosmolarity represent the other extreme of glucose metabolism causing altered mental status. It almost always presents as depressed consciousness. Diagnosis is confirmed by laboratory testing. See Chapter 26, Diabetes, for more information on hypo- and hyperglycemia.

4. **Opiates—exogenous toxins.** Opiates cause respiratory depression, decreased mental status, and symmetric pinpoint pupils. Patients may have needle tracks if intravenous injection is used. A prompt waking response to naloxone is diagnostic. In narcotic addicts, naloxone may trigger a withdrawal syndrome and vomiting. Other exogenous toxins can cause coma or altered mental status. A history of drug abuse, suicide attempt, or depression may help elucidate specific toxins. Laboratory studies may demonstrate a metabolic acidosis or increased anion gap. Toxicology screen usually reveals the presence of medications or drugs of abuse.

5. **Urea/metabolic.** Renal insufficiency is a relatively rare cause of altered mental status. Creatinine levels of over 7 mg % or a BUN of over 100 mg % can contribute to mental changes directly or by decreased excretion of renal metabolized substances. Other metabolic causes include endogenous toxins, such as are found in hepatic failure and bowel ischemia.

6. **Trauma.** Head trauma can result in primary brain parenchymal injury, or it can produce central nervous system hemorrhage. Focal neurologic signs are often seen and suggest increasing intracranial pressure. A computed tomographic scan of the head is usually necessary to diagnose the sites of bleeding. Chapter 50 reviews the diagnosis and management of head trauma.

7. **Infection.** Infections of the CNS can produce altered mental status or coma. Herpes simplex is a frequent cause of encephalitis, whereas *S. pneumoniae, N. meningitidis,* and *H. influenzae* most commonly cause bacterial meningitis. Viruses, fungi, and carcinoma can cause aseptic meningitis. Although antibiotics may be started empirically, a spinal fluid analysis is necessary to diagnose meningitis. Infection in other sites, e.g., lung or urinary tract, with associated bacteremia or sepsis, often results in mental status changes. This is most often seen at the extremes of age.

8. **Psychiatric.** Psychogenic coma or depressed consciousness is frequently seen in the emergency department. Usually it resolves with patience and support. Psychogenic seizures, which can sometimes be difficult to diagnose by the most astute neurologists, are probably the most common form of psychogenic altered mental status. Clues to the diagnosis of a psychogenic origin are the presence of eyelid fluttering, Bell's phenomenon (elevation of the globes when eyelid opening is resisted by the patient), and absence of a postictal phase after generalized seizures. In psychogenic amnesia, patients often forget who they are and perhaps where they are, but otherwise know the day and date and have normal memory function. This is inconsistent with the organic disease processes described earlier. The neurologic examination is otherwise normal. In hysterical coma, ice-water calorics give normal ipsilateral deviation with fast-phase nystagmus in the opposite direction. Because of the intensity of the stimulus and the associated nausea and unpleasant vertiginous sensation, the patient may be unsteady and vomit on arising. In a patient suspected of hysterical coma, caloric testing is used only as a last resort.

9. **Poisons.** These are mentioned under Opiates. Chapter 19 reviews the approach to the poisoned patient.
10. **Shock.** Inadequate cerebral perfusion is a common cause of altered mental status. The vital signs are usually sufficient for assessment, but the operative equation is cerebral perfusion pressure = mean arterial pressure − intracranial pressure. Therefore, the intracranial pressure level is also considered. It is possible to have a normal mean arterial pressure without adequate cerebral perfusion.

PRINCIPLES OF MANAGEMENT

An organized, sequential scheme of management for patients with altered mental status is presented in Figures 45–3 and 45–4. Figure 45–3 is recommended for patients with delirium or agitated confusion. Figure 45–4 is for depressed consciousness or comatose patients. The basic general principles of management include the following:

Prompt Empiric Treatment of Reversible Metabolic Etiologies. As discussed in the Initial Approach section, empiric treatment with glucose, naloxone, thiamine, and oxygen is given immediately to all patients with altered mental status.

Support of Vital Signs. Abnormalities in the vital signs are immediately addressed. Endotracheal intubation may be needed to control the airway, prevent aspiration, and support ventilation. Shock is treated with crystalloids initially. Blood replacement and pressor agents may be used once the etiology is determined. Severe hypertension (diastolic pressure greater than 130) is treated with antihypertensives (see Chap. 13, Hypertension). Hyperthermia or hypothermia is appropriately corrected (see Chap. 21, Heat Illness, or Chap. 22, Hypothermia).

Prevention of Complications or Further CNS Damage. Patients with signs of increased intracranial pressure are treated with hyperventilation and osmotic diuresis using mannitol. Active seizures can be controlled with a benzodiazepine, followed by phenytoin to prevent further seizures. The cervical spine is immobilized in all comatose patients until a cervical spine fracture can be ruled out. More information on preventing secondary complications is given in Chapter 50, Head and Neck Trauma.

Definitive Specific Therapy Based on the Determined Etiology. The history, physical examination, and diagnostic tests will give a definitive diagnosis in most patients with altered mental status. Patients with drug overdoses or toxic exposures are decontaminated and treated specifically. Central nervous system hemorrhage is evaluated for neurosurgical evacuation (see Chap. 49, Stroke). Meningitis is treated with antibiotics (see Chap. 47, Meningitis). Psychotherapy is initiated in patients in psychogenic coma (see Chap. 52, Behavioral Disorders).

PROBLEM 1 The patient was taken immediately to the operating room to have the subdural hematoma evacuated. He remained stable. After successful evacuation, he was transported to the recovery unit in stable condition.

Even in the face of cerebral herniation, early intubation and measures to reduce intracranial pressure can successfully, but temporarily, stabilize a patient so that proper resuscitation and diagnosis can be carried out prior to surgical intervention. Only rarely is it necessary to perform skull trephination ("burr holes") in the emergency department to evacuate a life-threatening hematoma.

PROBLEM 2 The findings on the LP and CT scan were suggestive of herpes simplex encephalitis. The patient was admitted to the neurosurgery service, and the diagnosis was confirmed by brain biopsy. Intravenous acyclovir was initiated for this diagnosis.

This case provides a good example of an altered mental status caused by a serious treatable condition that could have been easily mistaken for a

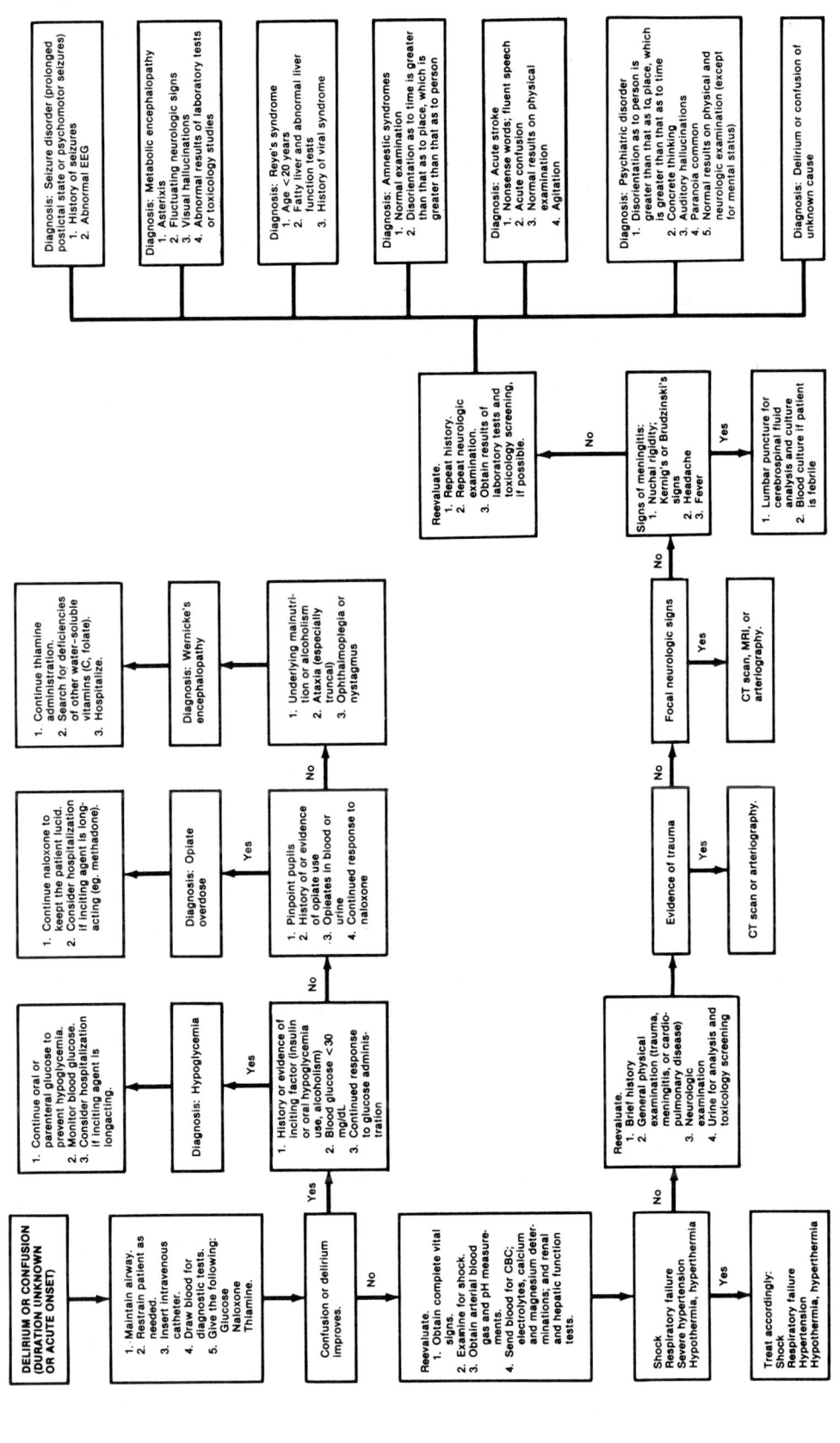

FIGURE 45–3. Suggested management steps for the patient with delirium or acute confusion. (Adapted from Mills J, Ho MT: Delirium and acute confusional states. In *Current Emergency Diagnosis and Treatment.* Los Altos, CA, Lange Medical Publications, 1990.)

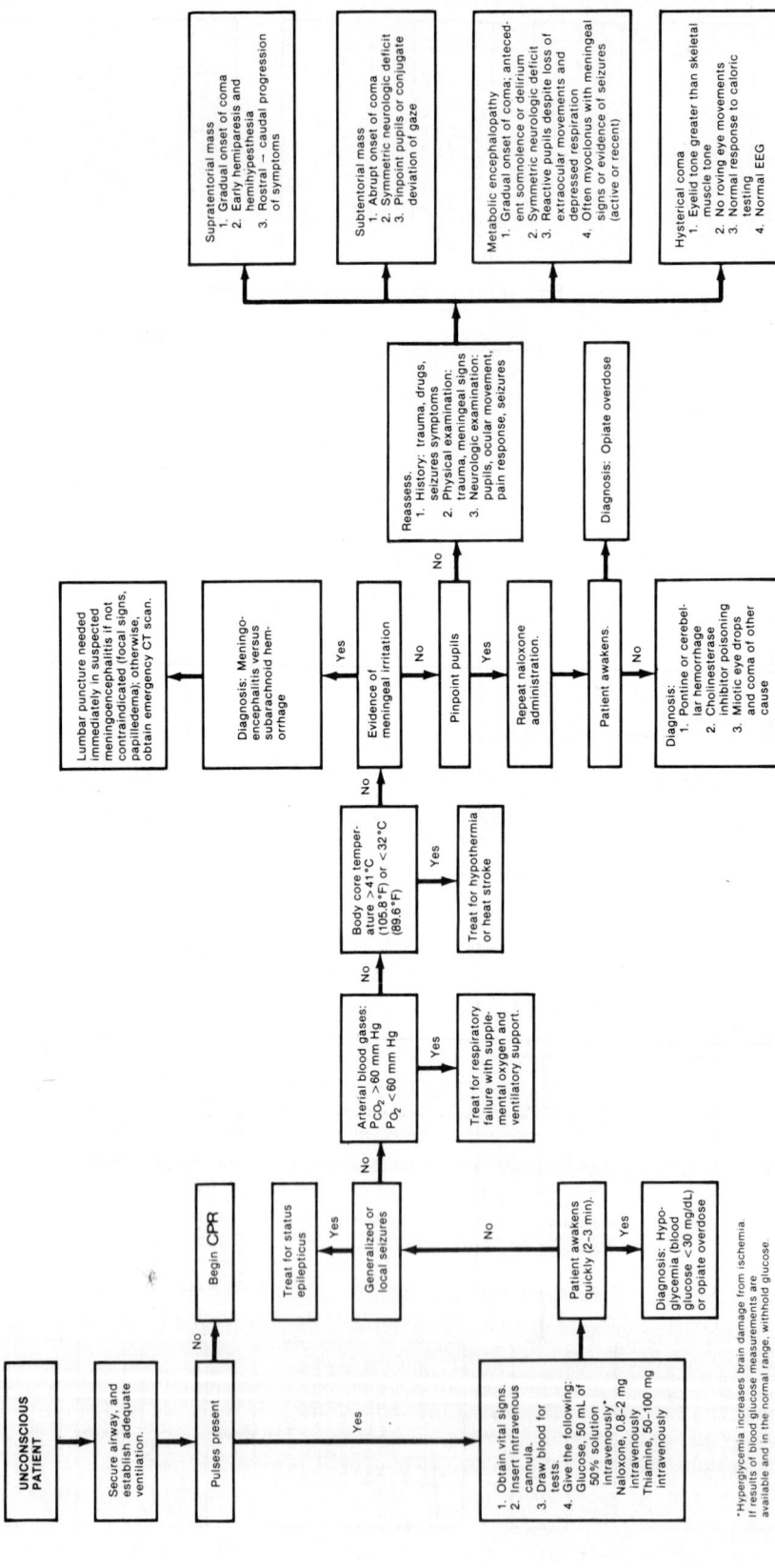

FIGURE 45–4. Suggested management steps for the patient who is comatose. Most apply to confusion with depressed consciousness. (Adapted from Mills J, Ho MT: Delirium and acute confusional states. In *Current Emergency Diagnosis and Treatment*. Los Altos, CA, Lange Medical Publications, 1990.)

psychiatric or alcohol-related problem. The history of recent normal mental health from the spouse was valuable information. Attention was paid to the changes noted on the mental status examination and related appropriately to the early signs of infection.

SPECIAL CONSIDERATIONS

Pediatric Patients

Head injuries in children differ in several ways from those in adults. Children in traumatic coma more often do not have a surgically correctable lesion, though one is always sought. A child with a relatively minor injury can have an apparent initial recovery, followed by several hours of a decreased level of consciousness with waxing and waning signs, followed by complete recovery. This condition is referred to as delayed nonhemorrhagic encephalopathy.

Following seizures, the postictal state in children occasionally can be prolonged. Reye's syndrome is a serious cause of altered mental status. This postviral illness is associated with specific entero- and influenza viruses. Taking salicylates during the infection may increase the risk of it. Patients present with gastrointestinal symptoms and a decreased level of consciousness. Elevated ammonia levels are far more common in children than adults.

Geriatric Patients

Cerebrovascular disease is primarily a disease of older individuals. An important example is giant cell (temporal) arteritis. Chronic subdural hematomas present much more commonly in the elderly. About half the time, a history of head trauma that can be very minor is obtained. Metabolic deficiencies, such as hypothyroidism and B_{12} deficiency, are also more frequent in this age group. Alzheimer's disease and other dementias are diseases occurring in the aged. Some of these are potentially reversible, such as reversible normal-pressure hydrocephalus. The elderly patient can be very sensitive to medications. Hypnotic medications, amantadine, H_2-antagonists, or quinolone antibiotics can result in an altered mental status even when taken in therapeutic dosages. Also, the elderly may accidentally or intentionally take an overdose of drugs.

DISPOSITION AND FOLLOW-UP

The disposition of patients with altered mental status depends on the broad categorization or specific diagnosis made, the clinical course in the emergency department, and the patients' support system at home.

Admission

1. All patients who remain in coma need intensive care unit monitoring and neurologic or neurosurgical consultation along with their emergency management and diagnostic regimen. Patients with other forms of continuing altered mental status are admitted for diagnosis and therapy.

2. Patients with seizures or coma due to hypoglycemia are usually admitted for observation and re-evaluation of their diabetic management. Patients with less severe altered mental status may be discharged only if they have returned to normal and fully comprehend the possible consequences of another episode. They are discharged optimally to a support system of family or friends. Follow-up with their physician is arranged. An exception to discharge in this circumstance is if they have taken long-acting oral hypoglycemics. Such patients are admitted because of the high potential for recurrence.

3. The narcotic-overdosed patient may awaken in response to naloxone, become combative, and resist further medical evaluation. Since the naloxone duration of action is 1 hour and the opiate taken (methadone or propoxyphene) may have a much longer half-life, the patients are admitted to the hospital and observed. Another reason is to evaluate possible complications that occurred during the comatose state.

4. Patients without a clear etiology for their symptoms are usually admitted for observation and diagnostic workup, even if their symptoms have cleared. The origins of altered mental status are complex, and symptoms can wax and wane. As in many medical decisions, the conservative path is the best choice in this situation.

Discharge

1. Patients in acute confusion with depressed consciousness due to alcohol intoxication are observed and monitored until they fully recover to their normal state. Psychologic or social worker intervention regarding the problem of alcoholism is addressed prior to discharge to home.

2. Patients presenting with an altered mental status due to ingestion of drugs can be discharged home if the drugs do not have delayed absorption, and after the patients are toxicologically decontaminated. Discharge should be delayed until a "normal" mental status is observed. Any patients with suicidal attempts or gestures are evaluated psychiatrically prior to discharge.

3. Patients presenting in psychogenic coma can be discharged if they have "fully recovered." If they persist in "coma" or have any residual, they require neurologic and psychiatric consultation. Similarly, if patients appear to be malingering or are diagnosed as hysterical conversion reaction, a consultation is obtained when the patient does not return to a "normal" state in a short time.

4. Upon discharge from the emergency department, all patients, their family, and friends are informed that the patient should return immediately if there is any recurrence of symptoms. It is important to arrange follow-up for these patients in 24 to 48 hours and to have a back-up plan for the people in the patient's support system should the patient refuse appropriate follow-up. Specific disposition is dependent on the underlying cause of the altered mental status.

PROBLEM 1 After evacuation of the subdural hematoma, the patient had an uneventful course and recovered completely. He swore to give up his drinking habit.

This patient was successfully treated because the life-threatening process was recognized early. The obvious distraction of this patient being alcoholic was properly interpreted as a *risk factor*, rather than a convenient means of explaining his symptoms.

PROBLEM 2 After several weeks on the neurology service and a course of acyclovir therapy for the herpes simplex encephalitis, the patient was discharged with only a subjective minimal residual of cognitive deficit.

In this case, a careful mental status examination indicated organic dysfunction even though the patient had normal vital signs and no focal neurologic deficits. Often, "something is wrong and it's not getting better" is the emergency physicians best rationale for admission.

DOCUMENTATION

1. Circumstances in which the patient was found, past history of similar problems. Sources of history.

2. Details of examining other organ systems.

3. Full neurologic examination with attention to pupils and extraocular eye movements, and mental status examination.
4. Changes in mental status or neurologic examination from onset of care.
5. Response to treatments, such as glucose, naloxone, and thiamine.
6. Results of the laboratory studies and radiologic imaging.
7. Consultation opinion of the neurologist, neurosurgeon, or psychiatrist.
8. Final assessment of probable etiology. Classifying the disorder into one of the five categories is a minimum.
9. If discharged, detailed plans for follow-up, altered medication regimen, and the name of the person responsible for the patient until next appointment. It is important to get the phone number of a contact on the chart for future recurrences.

SUMMARY AND FINAL POINTS

- Coma is at the extreme of findings manifested by depressed levels of consciousness. Delirium is an alteration of mental status with increased psychomotor activity.
- Dementia is characterized by an acquired impairment of recent memory.
- When a person loses the sense of orientation owing to an organic illness, it is usually in the sequence of time, place, and, finally, person.
- Patients with an organic cause of their alteration in mental status are usually disoriented, whereas patients with a psychogenic cause are not disoriented.
- The Glasgow Coma Scale is an important clinical tool to quantify changes in the patient's level of consciousness objectively.
- Pupillary reflexes and eye motor function are important clinical signs. They best represent the condition of the central nervous system, particularly the brain stem.
- Patients with altered mental status may have multiple etiologies at the same time. Serious life-threatening diseases are always considered and ruled out first.
- Altered mental status is empirically treated to cover reversible causes without waiting for diagnostic tests.
- The most common treatable causes of altered mental status may be remembered by the mnemonic AEIOU–TIPPS.
- Whenever meningitis is suspected, antibiotics are given immediately. A CT scan should not delay the first dose.

BIBLIOGRAPHY

Texts
1. Henry GL, Little N: Neurological Emergencies: A Symptom-Oriented Approach. New York, McGraw-Hill, 1985.
2. Plum F, Posner JB: Diagnosis of Stupor and Coma, 3rd ed. Philadelphia, F.A. Davis, 1980.

Journal Articles
1. Bates D, Caronna JJ, Cartlidge NEF, et al: A prospective study of nontraumatic coma: Methods and results in 310 patients. Ann Neurol 2:211, 1977.
2. Buettner UW, Zee DS: Vestibular testing in comatose patients. Arch Neurol 46:561, 1989.
3. Levy DE, Bates, D, Caronna JJ, et al: Prognosis in nontraumatic coma. Ann Intern Med 95:293, 1981.
4. Libowski ZJ: Delirium (acute confusional states). JAMA 258:1789, 1987.
5. McEvoy JP: Organic brain syndromes. Ann Intern Med 95:212, 1981.
6. Rabins DV, Folstein ME: Delirium and dementia. Br J Psychiat 140:149, 1982.
7. Ropper AH: Lateral displacement of the brain and level of consciousness in patients with an acute hemispheral mass. N Engl J Med 314:953, 1986.
8. Ropper AH: A preliminary MRI study of the geometry of brain displacement and level of consciousness with acute intracranial masses. Neurology 39:622, 1989.
9. Sabin TD: Coma and the acute confusional states in the emergency room. Med Clin North Am 65:15, 1981.
10. Spanos A, Harrell FE, Durack DT: The differential diagnosis of acute meningitis. JAMA 262:2700, 1989.

CHAPTER 46

HEADACHE

JUDITH C. BRILLMAN, M.D.

PROBLEM 1 A 60 year old female called the rescue squad because she was frightened. She was having the worst headache of her life and was having trouble thinking.

PROBLEM 2 A 45 year old male told the triage nurse that he had had a headache for 2 days and had come to find out why.

PROBLEM 3 A 30 year old male came to the emergency department saying that he was having a migraine headache and wanted pain relief.

QUESTIONS TO CONSIDER

1. What are the potentially catastrophic illnesses to be considered immediately in all patients with a headache?
2. What points of the history and physical examination can help in differentiating serious from less serious causes?
3. How may headaches be classified to assist the emergency physician in their management?
4. What is the role of diagnostic adjuncts in the evaluation of headaches?
5. Under what circumstances should treatment precede diagnosis?
6. What are the goals of management in most patients with headache?
7. Are there circumstances when narcotic analgesia is appropriate in the patient with headache?
8. How are disposition plans for these patients formulated?

INTRODUCTION

Headache is a patient complaint encountered daily in the emergency department. It is the ninth most common cause of visits to an ambulatory care facility. Approximately 90% of the population will experience headache at some time in their lives. It may represent a simple short-lived event, a chronic emotional difficulty, or it may herald an intracerebral catastrophe. The great majority of headaches managed in the emergency department do not represent medically serious conditions.

The term *headache* technically refers to any head pain including pain in the face, neck, and ears, but it is generally used to describe pain perceived in the scalp and cranium. Pain-sensitive structures in this area are:

1. The structures between the epidermis of the scalp and periosteum of the skull
2. The venous sinuses and their branches within the cranium
3. The structures at the base of the brain including the dura mater
4. The arteries of the dura mater
5. The cranial nerves

The parenchyma of the brain, most of the meninges, and the skull are not pain sensitive. Thus, headache is not a sensitive indicator of serious intracranial pathology.

Pain in the head results from tension and traction of pain-sensitive structures, vascular causes, and inflammation. Tension results from constriction of neck and scalp muscles due to causes such as cervical arthritis, irritating lesions, or emotional distress. Traction may result from an intracranial mass and may be felt at the base of the head prior to a rise in intracranial pressure. Vascular distention or dilation can manifest as the throbbing pain characteristic of migraine and cluster headache. Inflammation is associated with meningitis, arteritis, or sinusitis. It is usually infectious in origin but may be caused by intracerebral irritants such as blood.

PREHOSPITAL CARE

The emergency medical system is not often used by patients complaining of headache. Should this situation occur, management of the patient is similar to that described under Initial Approach in the Emergency Department.

INITIAL APPROACH IN THE EMERGENCY DEPARTMENT

The initial triage interview determines the priority by which the patient will be examined by the physician. Since headache can be a symptom associated with serious disease, the triage nurse preferentially errs on the side of the patient.

History

Severity and Onset of Pain. In patients who describe the worst headache of their lives or who have a sudden onset of pain, the pain is very likely to have a vascular origin. Intracranial bleeding, particularly a subarachnoid hemorrhage (SAH), is of paramount concern for the emergency physician in such cases.

Prior History of Headaches. The presence of a headache in a patient who does not have a prior pattern of headaches can indicate serious intracranial pathology. Unfortunately, the "headache prone" patient is also subject to serious illness. In these patients, some variation from the usual pain pattern is sought.

History of Head Trauma. Acute or subacute intracranial bleeding, e.g., subdural hematoma or subarachnoid hemorrhage, may be preceded by head trauma. A period of 3 to 4 weeks is addressed to cover the potential of a subacute process. In the elderly or patients with coagulopathies even "minor" head trauma is worthy of suspicion.

Physical Examination

Vital Signs

Blood Pressure. A diastolic pressure of greater than 130 mm Hg can indicate hypertensive encephalopathy (see Chap. 13) or cerebrovascular response to a mass lesion.

Tachypnea. Mild to moderate hypoxia can cause headaches. A particularly important cause is carbon monoxide poisoning.

Fever. Infections such as meningitis, encephalitis, or brain abscess must be considered when the patient is febrile. Headache may also be part of a "nonspecific" viral illness.

Meningismus. The presence of a stiff neck, fever, and headache alerts the physician to the risk of meningitis (see Chap. 47).

Mental Status. Is the patient oriented and responding appropriately? Altered level of consciousness generally indicates serious intracranial pathology such as stroke, intracranial hemorrhage, or meningitis.

Intervention

Tachypnea. Patients with suspected oxygenation or respiratory problems are placed on 100% oxygen. Blood samples for measurement of arterial blood gases and carbon monoxide levels are drawn.

Blood Pressure. Patients with hypertensive encephalopathy (papilledema, diastolic blood pressure of more than 130 mm Hg) need to have their blood pressure controlled with intravenous antihypertensive agents. The arterial pressure is closely monitored to reduce it by 15% to 20% within 60 minutes.

Altered Level of Consciousness. Patients are given 100 mg of thiamine, 25 to 50 gm of 50% dextrose, and 2 mg of naloxone intravenously and are then observed for changes in mentation.

Fever and Meningismus. If there are no signs of increased intracranial pressure, a lumbar puncture is performed and depending on findings, an appropriate antibiotic is given (see Chap. 47).

Seizures. Seizure activity is indicative of significant intracranial pathology. Diazepam is used to terminate an active seizure, and phenytoin will prevent further seizure activity (see Chap. 48).

Intracranial Pressure. Increased intracranial pressure secondary to hemorrhage, trauma, or tumor may be controlled with osmotic diuresis achieved with mannitol and hyperventilation (see Chap. 50).

PROBLEM 1 The 60 year old woman was in severe pain. She stated that she had had previous headaches related to severe cervical arthritis, but this pain was different. The nurse obtained a history of a transient loss of consciousness and called the emergency physician for a prompt evaluation. The physician found that the patient did not know the month or day but otherwise answered appropriately. Supplemental oxygen was given by nasal cannula; an intravenous (IV) line was started and thiamine, glucose, and naloxone were administered. No change in mentation was noted.

Severe headache is assumed to be potentially life-threatening until proved otherwise. Early in the course of care it is always best to believe the patient's assessment of pain completely. Additional data gathering may support or modify the initial impression.

DATA GATHERING

The history and physical examination are structured to corroborate the patient's description of pain and to elicit signs and symptoms of focal neurologic deficits. A search for findings of systemic disease that may cause headaches is also part of the assessment.

History

Key points in the history will distinguish an acute from a chronic process causing the headache.

Nature of Pain. Can the pain be characterized as *sharp, dull, aching,* or *throbbing*? A patient with a severe headache due to a subarachnoid hemorrhage may be unable to characterize the pain except to say that "it is the worst in his life." Vascular headaches throb, whereas muscle contraction headaches may be felt as a band or tightening around the head.

Onset. Is this a *new headache,* has it *occurred before,* or is it *chronic*? Time of onset is ascertained. Migraines begin in the early morning hours, and cluster headaches occur at night. Both may awaken the patient. Headaches of vascular origin are usually acute in onset.

Location. Is the headache *localized* or *generalized*? *Migraine* is derived from the Greek word *hemikrania*, meaning an affliction of half of the cranium. It usually occurs on the same side as previous headaches. A generalized headache may represent increased intracerebral pressure or a psychogenic disease. Occipital headaches more often originate from tension or traction.

Duration. *How long* has the headache *lasted*? Migraines may last hours to days. Cluster headaches may last minutes to hours. Progressive mass lesions cause headaches of increasing duration and intensity. A constant headache of long duration is rarely due to an urgent medical condition.

Severity/Psychologic and Physiologic Importance. Intense pain may represent a SAH or vascular headache. Tension headaches are usually dull and persistent and do not awaken the patient at night. An important part of the examination is trying to assess how the pain has affected the patient's life. Incapacitating headache is an urgent or emergent problem no matter what the underlying diagnosis.

Prodrome. Migraine may be preceded by visual or tactile auras.

Associated Symptoms. Associated symptoms may include nausea, vomiting, dizziness, loss of consciousness, weakness, eye problems, and neck stiffness. Meningeal symptoms and signs are commonly associated with SAH and meningitis. Focal motor paresis indicates a cerebrovascular accident, a subdural hemorrhage, mass lesion, or migraine. Nausea and vomiting may accompany a migraine, hypertensive, or fever-associated headache. It may also be secondary to increased intracranial or intraocular pressure.

Precipitating Factors. A history of trauma, recreational drug use, exertion, fatigue, alcohol use, or sexual activity may help elucidate the cause of the headache. Migraines may be precipitated by fatigue, stress, menstruation, and ingestion of certain foods. Emotional stress and depression are important contributors of headache. Sleep, appetite, and sexual disturbances may suggest headache secondary to psychogenic factors. Onset of headache during sexual activity is often vascular in origin.

Family History. A familial history of migraine is present in 60% of migraine sufferers. Depression may also be familial.

Medical and Medication History. Alcoholism, recent trauma, bleeding disorders, and use of anticoagulant medication are all associated with an increased risk of subdural hematoma. Acute trauma also suggests cerebral edema or focal hemorrhage.

Medical conditions such as hypertension, hypercapnia, hypoxia, hypothyroidism, metastatic malignancies, acute anemia, hypoglycemia, and steroid deficiency can all result in headache. Exposure to nitrates or ergotamines may also cause headache. Oral contraceptives may exacerbate migraine.

Medications taken in the past for head pain and their effectiveness serve as a guide to evaluation and treatment of headache. A patient who has taken ergotamine in the past and has experienced headache relief probably has migraine headaches.

Toxic Exposures. Has the patient been exposed to any toxic gases such as carbon monoxide? Do other people in a similar environment have headaches? For example, two or three family members presenting with headache should raise the suspicion of carbon monoxide in the home.

PROBLEM 1 The patient's headache was throbbing in nature and occurred suddenly. She had a transient near-syncopal episode shortly after the headache began. She now preferred to lie quietly in a darkened room. Her past medical history was noncontributory.

The suddenness of onset and severity suggested an SAH. Although her previous history of cervical arthritis supported the possibility of a flare-up, the present history was different and suggested a more catastrophic illness. A physical examination was performed expeditiously.

PROBLEM 2 The 45 year old man was from Mexico and was in the United States on business for the trucking company he owned. He had had a headache for 2 days and did not remember how or when the headache began. His head throbbed and his back ached. He had not seen a doctor in many years. His mother had migraines.

This patient was worrisome. His headache must have been troubling him significantly to force him to interrupt business and seek medical care in a foreign country. However, the headache did not fit any typical pattern.

PROBLEM 3 The 30 year old man had had migraine headaches for many years. The headache fit his typical migraine pattern. It was not preceded by an aura, was unilaterally throbbing, and was accompanied by photophobia and nausea. He had been treated with ergotamine and propranolol unsuccessfully in the past. He requested Demerol. His physician's name was obtained.

Many people label all severe headaches as migraine. Directed questioning will reveal whether the headache fits a typical migraine pattern. The history given in this case was consistent with a migraine, but other factors should raise one's suspicions about possible drug-seeking behavior. Physicians always need to be wary of patients who specifically request narcotics. If possible, the patient's history of "migraine" should be corroborated. A call is made to the primary physician before any therapy is given.

Physical Examination

The physical examination is a focused search for neurologic abnormalities or systemic signs that might explain the headache's origin.

Vital Signs. Abnormal vital signs in the patient with headache often suggest serious illness.

1. Fever without meningismus may indicate systemic illness contributing to headache.

2. Hypertension rarely causes headache unless the diastolic blood pressure is greater than 130 mm Hg.

3. Tachycardia and tachypnea may occur with a headache due to hypoxia, anemia, or carbon monoxide poisoning. More often, tachycardia reflects severe pain.

General Appearance. Is the patient in severe distress, agitated, or anxious? Conversely, is the patient resting comfortably or conversing with family or friends? Is the patient resting quietly in a darkened room? The latter is typical of a patient with migraine headache, SAH, or any other cause associated with photophobia.

Head and Neck. The head, face, and neck are inspected for evidence of trauma or other abnormalities.

1. The skull is palpated for hematoma, the sinuses and teeth for tenderness. The latter may represent a periapical abscess. A tender scalp or neck muscles may indicate a muscle contraction headache or irritation secondary to another cause. The temporal arteries are palpated for firmness or tenderness in all patients over 50 years old.

2. Auscultation for carotid bruits may reveal carotid stenosis or arteriovenous malformation (AVM).

3. Meningismus is assessed carefully. Many patients with tension headaches may have a "stiff neck." Meningismus is a reflex flexion rigidity. It may result from meningitis, encephalitis, or SAH. The patient whose neck is stiff on rotary or lateral motion is less likely to have serious disease.

4. The ears are inspected for hemotympanum or infection.

Neurologic Examination

1. Mental status. A directed mental status examination includes evaluation of orientation, memory, concentration, and speech (see Chap. 45 or 52). Marked alteration in level of consciousness indicates a true medical emergency. Delirium and dementia

may result from meningitis, cerebral anoxia, hypercarbia, or trauma. Personality changes may indicate a frontal lobe mass. Focal speech deficit may indicate a mass lesion or cerebrovascular accident (CVA).

2. The ocular examination is very important in patients with headache. A steamy cornea is usually seen in patients with acute glaucoma, whereas an irregular pupil that causes pain when reacting to direct or consensual light indicates iritis. A unilateral dilated pupil, unreactive to direct and consensual light, coupled with a decreased level of consciousness is indicative of imminent temporal lobe herniation. A visual field deficit may indicate a pituitary adenoma, brain tumor, or arteriovenous malformation. The funduscopic examination allows visual access to the small vasculature of the body and the optic nerve tract. Both have a close anatomic relationship with the meningeal coverings and the subarachnoid space. Funduscopy may show papilledema caused by increased intracranial pressure. This finding usually takes hours to days to develop. Retinal hemorrhages may be seen, suggesting intracerebral or subarachnoid hemorrhage. Vascular spasm, flame hemorrhage, and exudate consistent with malignant hypertension is also found.

3. Motor and sensory examination of both cranial and peripheral nerves is imperative. Localized weakness or abnormal sensation may result from mass lesions, hemorrhage, CVA, or migraine.

4. Cerebellar function is assessed. Dyscoordination and ataxia may be the only signs of a posterior fossa mass or hemorrhage.

5. Testing of the biceps, patella, and Achilles deep tendon reflexes as well as the Babinski reflex is standard. An asymmetric response may be the only localizing finding.

Selected Examinations. The history, vital signs, and general appearance can indicate the presence of systemic disease. A rapid screening physical examination including cardiovascular, pulmonary, and abdominal examinations is recommended. Potential high-yield sources of infection (e.g., the ears, nose, and throat area, the lungs, and the genitourinary tract) are explored in the patient with a fever.

PROBLEM 1 The patient's vital signs were normal except for a heart rate of 110 beats/min. She appeared uncomfortable and was lying in a darkened room. She spoke with her eyes closed. The head and neck examination was positive only for photophobia and mild resistance to neck flexion. The patient was lethargic but answered questions appropriately. The remainder of the neurologic examination showed normal results.

The patient's altered level of consciousness indicated serious intracranial pathology even though no focal findings were present. Her resistance to neck flexion was highly suggestive of SAH or meningitis.

PROBLEM 2 The patient's vital signs were normal. He was in mild to moderate distress and was waiting patiently for the examination to be concluded. He was alert and oriented. The results of the physical examination, including the neurologic examination, were completely normal.

This case continued to be troublesome, and more information was necessary. A second, more detailed history revealed that the patient was under a great deal of stress. He had recently acquired another trucking company and did not have enough drivers to staff this company.

DECISION PRIORITIES AND PRELIMINARY DIFFERENTIAL DIAGNOSIS

Following the history and physical examination, a distinction is made between emergent, urgent, and nonurgent cases of headache. These categories are defined by considering how quickly the diagnosis must be made or treatment begun to prevent loss of life or functional capacity. A number of pathologic processes are classified in this manner in

Table 46–1. A prioritized differential diagnosis is constructed by considering three questions.

1. *Is a potentially catastrophic disease process occurring?*
   The signs and symptoms reviewed in the sections on Initial Approach in the Emergency Department and Data Gathering may indicate the presence of catastrophic illness (Table 46–2). Since emergent causes of headache are often dynamic, these signs and symptoms may develop at any time during the evaluation.
2. *If emergent processes can be ruled out, what urgent processes must be considered (Table 46–3)?*
   Migraine and cluster headaches are often diagnosed by their characteristic histories. The history of giant cell arteritis is less specific, but a tender temporal artery and elevated erythrocyte sedimentation rate (ESR) mandate treatment. Cerebral vascular accidents or "stroke" (see Chap. 49) usually result in objective neurologic abnormalities. The history and stigmata of head trauma (Chap. 50) will cause the physician to investigate this possibility. An intracerebral mass without abnormal neurologic findings is difficult to diagnose. Here the progressive nature of the headache or evolving neurologic findings are the most significant points. Remember, if the pain has interrupted the patient's ability for leading a normal life, it is at least an urgent problem. Therefore, both the underlying pathology and the severity of symptoms have a role in the categorization.
3. *Is a less urgent process occurring?*
   Characteristics of these conditions are given in Table 46–4.
   There is considerable overlap between migraine-like symptoms and underlying tension/traction headaches. Nausea, throbbing unilateral pain, and scalp muscle tenderness occur frequently in tension headache, and migraine headaches do not always fit the classic pattern. In this context, the emergency physician can only treat the headache relative to its severity and strive to differentiate the true emergent and urgent causes from the less urgent ones.

PROBLEM 2 It did not appear that this gentleman's headache was emergent or urgent. The headache did not fit well into any typical headache pattern. He had none of the typical symptoms of migraine or cluster headache. He was relatively young for giant cell arteritis. The short duration (2 days) argued

TABLE 46–1. Common Causes of Headache Presenting in the Emergency Department

I. Emergent causes
   A. Intracranial hemorrhage—subarachnoid hemorrhage, subdural, epidural, or intracerebral hematoma
   B. Meningitis or encephalitis
   C. Severe hypertension with encephalopathy
   D. Disorder of oxygenation or respiration: hypoxia, hypercarbia, carbon monoxide poisoning
II. Urgent causes
   A. Vascular—migraine, cluster, cerebrovascular accident, arteriovenous malformation, altitude sickness, giant cell arteritis
   B. Mass—brain tumor, abscess, arteriovenous malformation
   C. Potential head trauma or chronic subdural hematoma
   D. Secondary to systemic disorder, hypoglycemia, fever, hypothyroid, anemia
   E. Miscellaneous—glaucoma, benign intracranial hypertension
III. Less urgent causes
   A. Muscle contraction (tension)
   B. Secondary to diet or medications
   C. Fatigue, postexertion, postcoital
   D. Post trauma
   E. Post lumbar puncture
   F. Sinusitis without complications
   G. Myofascial pain syndrome

TABLE 46–2. Characteristics of Emergent Causes of Headache

Cause	Affected Population	History	Associated Symptoms	Physical Examination	Diagnostic Adjuncts	Management Principles
Subarachnoid hemorrhage	Adults aged 20–50 years old. May be post-traumatic. May occur during strenuous activity, e.g., sexual intercourse. Account for 1% of headaches seen in emergency department	Pain is abrupt in onset, throbbing in nature, and often described as "the worst headache in my life." The pain may radiate to the neck or back. Patient may have history of headache or blood dyscrasia	Commonly nausea, photophobia, neck and back pain. May have diplopia, transient loss of consciousness, or seizure. Increased pain with straining	Nuchal rigidity commonly present. May see seizure (10%), focal neurologic deficit, or depressed level of consciousness	Head CT is definitive in over 90%. Lumbar puncture will show either RBCs or xanthochromia in 99%	These patients are kept quiet, admitted to intensive care. A neurosurgeon is consulted early in their care
Bacterial meningitis	Most often seen in infants and elderly. Causes 1% of headaches seen in emergency department	The prodrome is highly variable. Usually onset of severe diffuse pain over hours. Seldom precipitating factors, though there may be another site of infection, e.g., otitis media	Almost always occurs with complaint of neck pain, malaise, photophobia. More severely affected patients are confused and have vomiting	Patients have fever (90%), nuchal rigidity. Often depressed or heightened level of consciousness. Skin may show hemorrhagic or petechial rash	Lumbar puncture definitive, characteristically elevated WBC >50, elevated protein, normal or decreased glucose. Immunologic studies of CSF may be helpful	All patients are taken to intensive care. Treatment with antibiotic coverage is top priority
Hypertensive with encephalopathy	Primarily patients with long-standing hypertension	Onset of pain is usually rapid and may awaken patient from sleep. It is severe, global, and throbbing. May have headache history or problem with poorly controlled hypertension, often poor compliance	Patients are often confused. May have chest pain or shortness of breath. Can present with seizure activity	Blood pressure usually (>80% of patients) above 130 mm Hg diastolic. Funduscopic changes including vasospasm, hemorrhage, and papilledema. Patients often have depressed level of consciousness but are rarely comatose unless there is intracerebral hemorrhage	Renal insufficiency is common. Elevated protein level in urine. Other organ to evaluate is heart (ECG, enzymes)	Parenteral blood pressure control is essential

against an intracerebral mass. He reported no head trauma and had no signs of systemic disease. A muscle contraction headache from tension was considered possible.

PROBLEM 3 The patient's vital signs were normal. He did not appear to be in much discomfort. His affect was flat, although it was thought that this was due to the pain. Results of the physical examination were otherwise normal. This man's physician returned the call, stating that the patient was under treatment for schizophrenia and substance abuse. He did not have a history of migraine.

Patients may easily learn the correct symptoms and vocabulary for a specific disease. All efforts must be made to obtain a complete and consistent history. This includes calling other physicians, talking to family, and reviewing old medical records. Other area emergency departments may be contacted to determine if the patient has visited there.

DIAGNOSTIC ADJUNCTS

There are no routine laboratory tests for the patient with headache. Results of the history and physical examination dictate the appropriate diagnostic tests.

TABLE 46–3. Characteristics of Urgent Causes of Headache

Cause	Affected Population	History	Associated Symptoms	Physical Examination	Diagnostic Adjuncts	Management Principles
Migraine	Sixty percent of patients are female. May begin in childhood, usually before age 40	Pain is dull ache evolves to a severe throbbing over minutes to hours. Usually affects the same hemicranium. Onset occurs in the morning, has a recurrent pattern lasting hours to days. In some patients (35%), scotomas, flashing lights, paresthesias, hallucinations occur as prodrome; more often there is no prodrome. Precipitated by stress, fatigue, diet, hormonal changes. Family history in 60%	Photophobia, nausea, vomiting	Patient usually resting in dark with eyes closed. Uncomfortable with pain. Affected hemicranium may be tender. Rare to find neurologic or funduscopic abnormalities	No useful tests. May respond to parenteral phenothiazines	Usually outpatient treatment unless intractable vomiting. Pain relief given because prophylactic medications (e.g., beta-blockers, ergotamine) do not work by time patient appears in emergency department
Cluster	Eighty percent of patients are male. Appears between 20 and 40 years of age. Not commonly seen in emergency department. Patients often aware of the pattern	No prodrome. Pain is a burning, often severe sensation. Commonly periorbital. Occurs at night and in clusters lasting weeks to months. Usual duration is 15 min to 4 hr. Often occurs after ethanol ingestion or use of vasodilators. Family history rare, but patients are often heavy smokers	Nasal congestion, rhinorrhea, tearing, conjunctival flush	Patients are uncomfortable from pain. Face may be flushed or blanched. Increased secretions from eye and nose. Horner's syndrome sometimes seen	None	Once diagnosed, management is prophylactic. Pain can be decreased occasionally with oxygen or ergotamine. Primary treatment is analgesia

Table continued on following page

Laboratory Studies

Erythrocyte sedimentation rate (ESR) is indicated in patients over 50 years of age who have pain in the region of the temporal artery. Almost all patients with temporal arteritis have an elevated sedimentation rate. A normal sedimentation rate virtually rules out arteritis. Each laboratory establishes the normal values based on the type of test used.

Complete blood count with differential is indicated in patients with fever, meningismus, or suspected anemia. Both the white cell count and the differential may be nonspecific indicators of infection or inflammation.

Carboxyhemoglobin level is indicated in patients who were confined in a closed environment and exposed to smoke or a faulty heater, or when several people from the same house complain of headache.

Arterial blood gas measurements are ordered in any patient with signs, symptoms, or situations suggestive of risk for hypoxia or acidosis.

Radiologic Imaging

Computed tomograms (CT) of the head are indicated in patients with abnormal neurologic signs, sudden onset of a severe headache, or associated head trauma. It is a

TABLE 46-3. Characteristics of Urgent Causes of Headache *Continued*

Cause	Affected Population	History	Associated Symptoms	Physical Examination	Diagnostic Adjuncts	Management Principles
Giant cell (temporal) arteritis	Almost always over 55 years. Females comprise 60% of patients	No prodrome. Pain is a deep, aching, throbbing, and burning. Can be moderate to severe. May be very slow to rapid in onset. Usually located over temples, often unilateral. Seldom has precipitating factors. Family history positive on occasion	Pain may also be in ear, teeth, or temporal area with mastication. Visual scintillating or fleeting loss of vision (amaurosis fugax) noted in up to 10% of patients. This is a serious complication	Tenderness over temporal artery most common finding. Visual changes are usually gone by time of examination, but careful testing is important. Some patients experience relief with pressure on the carotid artery	Almost always elevated ESR. Anemia is common	Early corticosteroid use in high doses (at least 60 mg prednisone)
Space-occupying lesion (tumor, abscess, hemorrhage)	Only 30%–50% of patients with mass lesion have pain. It usually occurs after ICP has increased	Pain is without prodrome and is deep, dull, and aching. Intensity ranges from moderate to severe. Location is typically bifrontal or occipital. It is worse in early morning, but rarely awakens patient from sleep. Increased by straining, exertion. Pain may last weeks to years and often steadily progresses in severity. Abscess may be preceded by ear or sinus infection. History may point to source of metastasis	Aching in neck muscles. Nausea and vomiting. Seizures	Up to 50% of patients have neurologic abnormalities, most often focal findings or changes in funduscopic examination, e.g., papilledema. Altered mental status is diagnostic	Radiologic imaging with CT and MRI is diagnostic	Must always be suspected in patients with recurrent headache. Early referral and ICP control is limited goal in emergency department

useful tool for the patient with a severe headache who does not have a "headache prone" history. The widespread availability of head CT has had a significant and positive impact on the emergency department evaluation of headache. A head CT with contrast will delineate a tumor, bleed, abscess, or AVM. A head CT for the stable patient with a suspected brain tumor is not always required emergently. The normal head CT is just as important as an abnormal one demonstrating intracranial pathology because it can go far to allay the concerns of both physician and patient. A normal head CT may direct the physician to consider nonstructural causes of headache, although early CVAs are not seen on head CT, and it is falsely negative in 6% to 8% of patients with subarachnoid hemorrhages.

Sinus radiographs are indicated for patients with tenderness over their sinuses, congestion, and other signs of sinusitis. A screening view for maxillary sinusitis is a Waters' view in a skull series.

Skull radiographs are rarely indicated to assess patients with headache.

Special Tests

Lumbar Puncture. A lumbar puncture (LP) for cerebrospinal fluid (CSF) analysis is performed early in a patient with fever and meningismus to diagnose bacterial meningitis. The fluid is analyzed for white blood cell count and differential, red blood cell count,

TABLE 46–4. Characteristics of Less Urgent Causes of Headache

Cause	Affected Population	History	Associated Symptoms	Physical Examination	Diagnostic Adjuncts	Management Principles
Muscle contraction (tension)	Patients aged 20–60. Females affected more than males	Pain begins without prodrome. Mild to moderately severe, steady ache, constricting "band" or "vice" around head. May appear in forehead or temple but most often in neck and occiput. Onset insidious at varying times of day. Lasts for hours to years. Precipitated by fatigue and stress. Patient may have history of depression, or "headache-prone" family member	Anxiety, sadness, depression, insomnia	Normal neurologic examination. Muscles tender over area of pain, particularly neck and occiput	No specific test	A frustrating problem for both patient and physician. Oral analgesia and nonsteroidal anti-inflammatory medication are mainstays of treatment. Majority of care is given by primary physician. Important to avoid complacency and monitor for changing symptoms
Post-traumatic	Seen in up to one-third of patients who have been hospitalized for head trauma. Can follow "minor" head injury	No prodrome. Pain is dull, mild to moderate in severity. Onset occurs hours to days after injury. May last for years. Prior history of trauma	Sense of disequilibrium, fatigue, memory and attention deficits. Mood swings can occur	Normal	Head CT considered to rule out subacute or chronic subdural hematoma or contusion	May be difficult to treat. Oral analgesia is best choice. Early referral to neurologist or neurosurgeon important
Sinusitis	Any age	No prodrome. Pain is due to pressure and fullness in frontal area. Pressure increases with leaning forward. Pain can be mild to severe and is constant; can last for years. Often initiated by URI, dental infections. Patient may have history of allergies, rarely some element of immunosuppression (e.g., diabetes mellitus)	Nasal congestion, postnasal drip. May have nasal obstruction	Low-grade fever, tenderness over involved sinus	Sinus films may show air-fluid levels or mucosal thickening	Broad-spectrum, gram-positive oriented antibiotic and decongestant therapy initiated in emergency department. ENT referral is given if persistent. May be a subtle cause of headache

ICP = intracranial pressure, ESR = erythrocyte sedimentation rate, CT = computed tomography, MRI = magnetic resonance imaging, URI = upper respiratory infection, ENT = ear, nose, and throat.

glucose, protein, and Gram stain; a culture is made for bacteria, virus, or fungus. Turbid CSF, elevated opening pressure, high lactate and protein levels, and a low glucose level are consistent with bacterial meningitis (see Chap. 47). CSF analysis is also performed in patients suspected of subarachnoid hemorrhage if the head CT is negative. The diagnosis is confirmed by finding blood in the CSF or by the presence of xanthochromia, the latter representing hemorrhage of more than 6 to 12 hours old. If intracranial hypertension is a possibility, a CT of the head is obtained prior to lumbar puncture to give a diagnosis or to lend support to this concern. The LP is performed after the CT is interpreted as normal. If the CT is abnormal, a discussion with the radiologist and neurosurgical consultant is held before proceeding.

REFINED DIFFERENTIAL DIAGNOSIS

Following the data-gathering process, a diagnosis will be evident in most patients with headache. A brief summary of the major diagnostic considerations is given below. Additional information on the emergent, urgent, and less urgent causes of headache are given in Tables 46–2, 46–3, and 46–4.

Emergent Causes

Subarachnoid hemorrhage is a true medical emergency and accounts for approximately 1% of persons with headache seen in the emergency department. Most bleeding occurs from rupture of a saccular aneurysm, although AV malformations are a common source of subarachnoid bleeds in patients under 20 years of age. Approximately 35% to 40% of patients die before reaching the hospital. The clinical picture of patients with subarachnoid bleed varies from patients who are asymptomatic to those who are comatose. Most patients experience a sudden onset of a severe diffuse headache, although occasionally the lesion may present in a less acute manner. It is not a cause of chronic head pain but may cause a worsening of a previous headache pattern. It is usually associated with nausea, vomiting, dizziness, stiff neck, photophobia, diplopia, confusion, or depressed mental status. Subhyloid or preretinal hemorrhages with blood layered between the retina and vitreous sac may be seen on funduscopic examination. A head CT scan will demonstrate a subarachnoid bleed in about 92% to 94% of patients.

Meningitis is the cause of headache in approximately 1% of patients. The most common causative organisms in adults are *Streptococcus pneumoniae* and *Neisseria meningitidis*. Clinical signs include fever, nuchal rigidity, nausea, and vomiting. Diagnosis is made by cerebrospinal fluid analysis. Meningitis is reviewed in Chapter 47.

Severe hypertension is the cause of headache in approximately 4% of emergency department patients. The pain is diffuse and throbbing, worse in the morning, and may awaken the patient from sleep. If the headache is associated with diastolic pressures greater than 130 mm Hg, altered mental status, and papilledema, hypertensive encephalopathy may be diagnosed (see Chap. 13).

Urgent Causes

Migraines are diagnosed in approximately 20% of patients who complain of headache. Although the precise cause is unknown, they are associated with decreased cerebral blood flow and extracerebral vasodilatation. Classically, migraines are associated with premonitory sensory, motor, or visual symptoms, followed by a throbbing unilateral headache with associated nausea, vomiting, and photophobia. Some patients have focal neurologic signs as part of the migraine. Migraines may be precipitated by a number of factors including stress, menstruation, oral contraceptives, physical exertion, certain foods, and lack of sleep. Common or atypical migraine has similar symptoms, although a prodrome does not occur and the location of head pain is often unilateral.

Cluster headaches are less common than migraines. They usually occur in men between the ages of 20 and 50 years. Cluster headaches are characterized by an abrupt onset of intense unilateral periorbital pain. The pain peaks in a few minutes and lasts for about 45 minutes. Attacks tend to come at the same hour each day for several weeks and then disappear for months. There are often associated symptoms of lacrimation, conjunctival injection, ptosis, nasal stuffiness, rhinorrhea, and Horner's syndrome. During the active period, ethanol can precipitate attacks.

Cerebrovascular accidents can cause headaches. Almost invariably, however, there are associated focal symptoms with CVAs, usually weakness. The history, physical examination, and CT scan usually give the diagnosis. Stroke is discussed in Chapter 49.

Giant cell arteritis is an uncommon disease of the elderly characterized by painful inflammation of the temporal and other arteries. It is highly associated with polymyalgia rheumatica and occurs primarily in patients 55 years of age or older. Systemic symptoms such as fever, malaise, and weakness occur in addition to localized tenderness over the superficial temporal artery. The erythrocyte sedimentation rate is invariably elevated. The diagnosis is supported by a temporal artery biopsy.

Intracranial mass lesions from tumors, hematomas, or abscesses account for approximately 3% of people with headaches seen in the emergency department. The headaches usually recur with increasing frequency and intensity. The pain is more intense in the morning and may wake the patient from sleep. Personality or mental status changes are frequently seen. A head CT scan is usually necessary to make the diagnosis.

Acute angle closure glaucoma can cause intense periorbital pain, nausea, and vomiting from increased intraocular pressure. Physical examination reveals a cloudy cornea, a mid-dilated and poorly reactive pupil, and a firm, tense globe due to marked elevation of the intraocular pressure (see Chap. 34).

Less Urgent Causes

Muscle contraction or tension headaches account for one-third of all patients with headache coming to the emergency department. The headache is usually bilateral and is described as dull, pressing, or bandlike. It varies with intensity during the day and decreases with sleep. There is clinical overlap with migraine headaches, and some patients have nausea, vomiting, photophobia, and lightheadedness. The patient will generally give a history of similar headaches in the past.

Acute sinusitis accounts for less than 1% of complaints of headache in the emergency department. The pain is localized over the involved sinus and is described as a constant ache or pressure. This sensation can be accentuated by bending forward. The headache is more intense in the morning and may be associated with rhinorrhea, fever, chills, and postnasal drip. The involved sinuses are tender to percussion. Radiographs show air-fluid levels in acute sinusitis and cloudiness with chronic inflammation.

PROBLEM 2 There was still no clear diagnosis in this patient, although he was believed to be in significant pain. An ESR was ordered to rule out giant cell arteritis and a CBC to screen for anemia or infection. These test results were normal. The physician considered obtaining a head CT. However, the patient did not have abnormal neurologic signs, a sudden onset of a severe headache, or associated head trauma. A lumbar puncture was considered, but there was no fever or meningismus.

Patients with headache often present diagnostic dilemmas. The emergency physician must do everything reasonably possible to rule out serious illness. An extra effort in obtaining additional data, serial observations of the patient, and consultation with other physicians is often necessary.

PRINCIPLES OF MANAGEMENT

The principles of management include (1) prompt attention to life-threatening signs and symptoms, (2) pain control, (3) volume replacement if anorexia and vomiting are significant symptoms associated with the headache, and (4) treatment of specific diseases. Prompt attention to life-threatening signs and symptoms includes airway and blood pressure control and observation for increased intracranial pressure and seizures. Immediate management was discussed earlier in the Initial Approach in the Emergency Department section.

Analgesia for headache usually depends on the specific diagnosis. Patients with structural lesions such as tumors, abscesses, or bleeding may be given parenteral narcotics such as meperidine (Demerol) or morphine. These are often given in combination with antiemetics (Phenergan, Vistaril) for relief of the acute headache (e.g., meperidine 50 mg and Phenergan 25 mg intramuscularly). These medications have the unfortunate side effect of depressing the patient's level of consciousness. Recent studies have demonstrated that patients with severe headaches, especially migraines, can often be treated successfully in the emergency department with intravenous phenothiazines. Chlorpromazine is given at 5 to 10 mg over 3 minutes and can be repeated up to 30 mg. Prochlorperazine, 10 mg IV over 3 minutes, is given as a single dose. Side effects include postural hypertension and extrapyramidal signs. The latter, should they appear, are treated with an antihistamine (diphenhydramine). Relief is noted in up to 75% of patients.

Caution is advised regarding outpatient use of narcotics for patients with recurrent or chronic headaches. In selected circumstances, and preferably after a call to the primary physician, a limited number of oral codeine-containing compounds such as Tylenol No. 3, Vicodin, or Percodan may be prescribed. Non-narcotic medications are the most commonly prescribed agents. They may include the physician's nonsteroidal anti-inflammatory drug of choice, e.g., Fiorinal, and may be combined with a mild sedative such as diazepam.

Specific Treatment
Emergent Causes

Subarachnoid hemorrhage is associated with significant morbidity and mortality. The prognosis for patients with subarachnoid hemorrhage depends on the initial presentation and has not significantly changed during the past 30 years. Morbidity and mortality are caused by the initial bleed, rebleeds at 24 hours to 1 month, and cerebral vasospasm. Approximately 40% to 70% of patients with a subarachnoid bleed will survive only 1 month despite treatment. Medical management includes bed rest and hypertension control. The head of the bed is raised slightly (about 30°). Anticonvulsant treatment, antifibrinolytic therapy, and volume control are controversial and may be instituted after discussion with, and agreement by, a consultant. Prompt neurosurgical consultation is indicated to assess the need for emergency surgery.

Bacterial meningitis and *hypertensive encephalopathy* are treated as described in Chapters 47 and 13, respectively.

Urgent Causes

Migraine headaches may be treated with ergotamine derivatives when the initial symptoms begin. Patients seen in the emergency department usually have had symptoms lasting for hours, and ergotamines will not be effective. Recent studies have shown that parenteral phenothiazines, such as prochlorperazine 10 mg IV, are effective in relieving headache symptoms in most patients. For those headaches not relieved by phenothiazines, parenteral narcotics are required. Preventative therapy with beta-blockers, tricyclic antidepressants, and other medications may be started in consultation with the patient's primary physician.

Cluster headaches are treated with 100% oxygen, which may produce cerebrovasoconstriction and some relief. Parenteral narcotics are needed if oxygen does not abort the acute attack. Prophylaxis with ergotamines, prednisone, and other treatment is appropriate as part of the patient's chronic care.

Giant cell arteritis is treated with oral steroids. The major morbidity is blindness associated with extension of the arteritis to involve the ophthalmic artery. Steroids result in an initial improvement in 80% to 90% of cases.

A mass lesion such as a tumor or abscess is treated symptomatically. If there are signs of elevated intracranial pressure, initial measures including hyperventilation, osmotherapy, and steroids are begun after consultation with a neurosurgeon.

Acute glaucoma is treated with miotics (pilocarpine), topical beta-blocking agents (timolol), carbonic anhydrase inhibitors (acetazolamide), and osmotic diuretics (mannitol or sorbitol). Ophthalmologic consultation is obtained in the emergency department.

Less Urgent Causes

Muscle contraction and post-traumatic headaches can generally be managed with non-narcotic analgesics such as acetaminophen, aspirin, or ibuprofen. A short course of muscle relaxants is sometimes useful. Chronic symptoms may be treated by tricyclic antidepressants, relaxation training, or biofeedback. Persistent post-traumatic headache requires full assessment, including CT of the head.

Acute sinus headache is treated with topical vasoconstrictors, antibiotics, and analgesics. Consultation with an otolaryngologist is appropriate if the frontal sinuses are involved or the infection does not resolve quickly.

PROBLEM 1 The head CT scan showed an SAH. A neurosurgeon was consulted, and plans were made to admit the patient. The patient was kept in a quiet room, at bed rest with her head elevated. Narcotic analgesics were administered.

The patient's fluctuating level of consciousness was a worrisome sign. She was at risk for rebleeding and cerebral vasospasm. Consultation was important to consider the benefits and risks of medical versus surgical treatment.

SPECIAL CONSIDERATIONS

Pediatric Patients

Headache is a common presenting complaint in children. It is estimated that 40% of children aged 7 and 75% of 15 year olds will have experienced headache. Any headache accompanied by fever, lethargy, meningeal signs, or other neurologic abnormality must be considered meningitis until proved otherwise. Most of the causes of headache listed in Table 46–1, except giant cell arteritis, can also cause headache in children. Muscle contraction, migraine, and sinusitis are the common localized causes of acute headache. Muscle contraction is the most common cause of chronic headache in the pediatric population. Migraine variants are more common in children than in adults. Sinusitis should be suspected in children with respiratory symptoms and an acute or chronic headache. Systemic illness, e.g., viral upper respiratory tract infection, may also cause a headache. Resolution of the headache should parallel improvement in the systemic illness.

Geriatric Patients

Headache is less common in older people than in other adults. This statement applies particularly to the frequency and severity of muscle contraction and tension headaches. Although all causes of headache listed in Table 46–1 can result in headache in the elderly, some entities are relatively more important. Cerebrovascular accidents are common in the elderly. In patients with cerebral infarction the headache rarely predominates, whereas in those with hemorrhage it may be a prominent symptom. Approximately 8% to 18% of patients with cerebral emboli have headache as a presenting symptom. Giant cell arteritis is considered in any patient who is 50 years old or more. Primary CNS tumor or metastasis often results in a persistent and progressive headache that increases with activities that increase intracranial pressure, e.g., cough or straining at stool.

DISPOSITION AND FOLLOW-UP

In addition to the acuity of the condition, the patient's disposition is influenced by his support structure, the emergency physician's level of comfort in considering discharge, and the pain status at the time of discharge.

Admission

All patients with emergent causes of headache are admitted for definitive care, and consultation with a neurologist or neurosurgeon is arranged (see Table 46–1). Among those with urgent causes of headache, patients with CVA, AVM, altitude sickness, giant cell arteritis, mass lesion, head trauma, and glaucoma are admitted. Admission is considered in patients with frontal sinusitis.

Discharge

Patients with muscle contraction, mild to moderate post-traumatic headache, sinusitis, and vascular origin headaches may be discharged to home. The majority of patients with migraine-type headaches are treated and discharged by their primary physician or a neurologist prior to complete resolution of the pain. All patients leaving the emergency department are given comprehensive discharge instructions including when, where, and why to follow up. Patients must understand their diagnosis and the dose, indications, and side effects of the prescribed medication. If narcotic analgesia is given, the patient is advised not to drive, and transportation is arranged.

Patients are asked to return to the emergency department if their headache:
1. Becomes significantly worse
2. Changes in character
3. Results in a change in mental status
4. Results in multiple episodes of vomiting
5. Results in neurologic deficit

In approximately 30% of patients who present to an ambulatory care setting with headache, no definitive diagnosis can be made. Often the headache corresponds to features found in several types of headache. At a particular stage in development, a headache caused by a mass lesion or trauma might easily be confused with a muscle contraction headache. A headache may have the combined features of a viral meningitis, migraine, and muscle contraction headache. Diagnostic testing such as head CT scanning or lumbar puncture may help solve some of these dilemmas but will be unable to resolve all of them. The emergency physician has several options in this situation. It is less important to make a specific diagnosis than to formulate a rational plan that anticipates catastrophic illness and protects the patient from its consequences. This includes:

1. Clear identification and treatment of life-threatening symptoms and conditions.

2. Serial observation of the patient for complications and identification of relevant signs and symptoms. These observations may be made during a several-hour stay in the emergency department or during follow-up in 24 to 48 hours at the primary physician's office.

3. Depending on the level of physician concern, careful instructions are given as to what potential problems to anticipate, signs and symptoms that should prompt return, and when and where to follow up. If the data point to less serious causes of headache, the patient is given non-narcotic analgesics and is asked to keep a headache diary.

4. If the patient is discharged, he should understand that a definitive diagnosis has not been made. The differentiation between headache types may be made several weeks later after follow-up.

PROBLEM 2 This patient was discharged with a nonsteroidal anti-inflammatory analgesic. He was asked to return in 1 to 2 days for a reevaluation. He returned 2 days later. His headache was worse, and he had neck and back stiffness. A male physician obtained a history of onset of the headache during sexual intercourse; the patient had not felt comfortable giving this information to the female physician who had previously examined him. A head CT demonstrated an SAH.

Since the same process may present with different levels of progression or severity, reevaluation is a valuable tool when a diagnosis or condition is uncertain. One needs to be aware of cultural, sexual, and religious factors. Although most patients with SAH present with obvious neurologic symptoms, up to 10% have minimal signs and symptoms. A high index of suspicion is necessary if the headache does not fit a typical pattern.

PROBLEM 3 The patient was informed of the discussion with his primary physician. He was told that narcotics would not be dispensed to him on this or future emergency department visits for his complaint of "migraine." He was asked to continue his care with his primary physician. A notice was written informing other doctors in the emergency department about this patient's presentation and care.

The symptom of headache can be used by patients to abuse narcotics. A careful review of a patient's past history and medical records will often reveal this problem. Although parenteral narcotics are given to relieve the pain of the acute attack, oral narcotics are rarely given from the emergency department.

DOCUMENTATION

1. History: nature of pain, severity, prodrome, and associated symptoms.
2. Physical examination: vital signs, general appearance, level of consciousness, results of neurologic examination.
3. Ancillary test findings including head CT and LP.
4. Interventions and response to therapy.
5. Consultants contacted and recommendations.
6. Repeat neurologic and mental status examinations.
7. Symptoms prior to discharge: resolving or progressing.
8. Reasons for reaching a final diagnosis and disposition.
9. If patient not admitted, discharge instructions and follow-up.

SUMMARY AND FINAL POINTS

- Headache may represent a catastrophic illness or a minor problem.
- A meticulous history and neurologic examination are important to distinguish serious from less serious causes of headache.
- The sudden onset of a headache in a patient who does not normally have headaches may indicate serious intracranial pathology.
- Up to 8% of patients with subarachnoid hemorrhage will have normal head CT scans. A lumbar puncture is necessary in this group.
- Migraine and muscle tension headaches are the most common causes of headaches in the emergency department.
- Management often coexists with and response influences the diagnosis. The patient's condition may change at any time.
- Although a definitive diagnosis cannot always be made, serious pathology should be ruled out and the patient given clear follow-up instructions.
- In up to 30% of patients there may not be a clear diagnosis of the headache after their evaluation in the emergency department.

BIBLIOGRAPHY

Texts
1. Diamond S, Dalessio DJ: The Practicing Physician's Approach to Headache (4th ed). Baltimore, Williams & Wilkins, 1986.
2. Peatfield R: Headache. New York, Springer-Verlag, 1986.
3. Water ME: Headache. Littleton, MA, PSG Publishing, 1986.

Journal Articles
1. Diehr P, Wood RW, Barr V, et al: Acute headaches: Presenting symptoms and diagnostic rules to identify patients with tension and migraine headache. J Chron Dis 34:147–158, 1981.
2. Fenichel GM: Migraine in children. Neurol Clin 3:77–94, 1985.
3. Jones J, Sklar D, Dougherty J, et al: Randomized double-blind trial of intravenous prochlorperazine for the treatment of acute headache. JAMA 261:1174–1176, 1989.
4. O'Hare TH: Subarachnoid hemorrhage—a review. J Emerg Med 5:135–148, 1987.
5. Scheife RT, Hills JR: Migraine headaches: Signs and symptoms, biochemistry and current therapy. Am J Hosp Pharm 37:365–374, 1980.
6. Shinnar S, D'Souza BJ: The diagnosis and management of headaches in childhood. Pediatr Clin North Am 29:79–94, 1981.

CHAPTER 47

SUSPECTED MENINGITIS

MYRON L. MILLS, M.D.

PROBLEM 1 A 3 month old infant was brought to the emergency department by his mother. She stated that he had not been eating well since the night prior to admission. He had vomited once or twice and had been irritable and crying. On examination the physician found a low-grade fever, irritability, and a supple neck. The patient was not consolable.

PROBLEM 2 An 8 year old child was rushed to the hospital by her parents after she collapsed following a brief febrile illness. The child was febrile, pale, and in shock; she had meningismus and diffuse petechiae.

PROBLEM 3 A 20 year old college student returned to the emergency department a second time complaining of a fever, severe headache, and myalgias. He stated that he had noticed a faint rash followed by some vomiting and diarrhea 2 days before the headache had begun.

QUESTIONS TO CONSIDER

1. What are the common causes of meningitis in pediatric, adult, and immunocompromised patients?
2. Are the classic symptoms and signs of meningitis reliable for diagnosis in the emergency department?
3. When is a lumbar puncture indicated in the patient suspected of having meningitis?
4. Why is cerebrospinal fluid (CSF) analysis valuable in selecting the diagnostic probabilities in patients with meningitis?
5. Can the distinction between viral and bacterial meningitis be made by CSF analysis?
6. Can meningitis be present in spite of normal results on lumbar puncture?
7. What is the role of computed tomography (CT) of the head in evaluating the patient with suspected meningitis?
8. What is the appropriate timing of antibiotic treatment for the patient with suspected bacterial meningitis?

INTRODUCTION

About 50,000 patients a year are treated for meningitis in the United States. Meningitis is one of the most serious infectious emergencies, and yet it can present with only nonspecific findings, especially in very young, elderly, and immunocompromised patients. Many of these patients first seek medical attention in the emergency department. Bacterial meningitis accounts for almost one-half of the reported cases. Seventy percent of bacterial meningitis occurs in children less than 5 years old. Viral meningitis comprises most of the other cases. It is also most often seen in young children.

The blood-brain barrier provides good protection from bacterial invasion. However, once organisms have gained access to the subarachnoid space, host defenses are very limited. Bactericidal levels of the appropriate antibiotic must be achieved quickly for effective treatment. In meningitis, the infectious process extends throughout the subarachnoid space, usually including the outer brain, spinal cord, and ventricles. Both bacterial and viral pathogens reach the subarachnoid space most often by hematogenous spread. Bacterial infections also enter this space by direct invasion, e.g., after an open head injury, commonly a basilar skull fracture, or by extension of a contiguous infection, such as from the middle ear, paranasal sinuses, orbits, or oral cavity.

The most common pathogens causing bacterial meningitis are *Hemophilus influenzae* (50%), *Neisseria meningitidis* (30%), and *Streptococcus pneumoniae* (10%). One of these three organisms is found in more than 90% of all cases of bacterial meningitis. Many other strains of bacteria can cause meningitis including group B *Streptococcus*, gram-negative coliforms, enterococci, *Listeria monocytogenes*, and *Mycobacteria*. The gram-negative infections have almost doubled in frequency in the last two decades. Specific strains of bacteria are found more often in different age groups. During the newborn period (under 1 month of age), group B *Streptococcus*, *Escherichia coli*, enterococci, *H. influenzae*, and *Listeria* are the most common pathogens. During infancy and early childhood, *H. influenzae* is the most common organism, with a peak incidence between 3 months and 6 years of age. In older children and young adults, *N. meningitidis* is the most common organism. Elderly patients have a higher proportion of *S. pneumoniae* infections than any other age group. Many viruses can cause meningitis. The most common are the enteroviruses (over 80%), such as echovirus and coxsackievirus. Arbovirus, mumps, herpes, varicella, and measles virus are all known pathogens.

In spite of the advent of antibiotic therapy, the mortality from bacterial meningitis remains high, with death rates ranging from 5% to 10% in patients with *Hemophilus influenzae* and up to 20% to 40% in patients infected with *S. pneumoniae*. Patients who survive have a high rate of mental retardation, seizure disorders, speech disorders, and hearing deficits. Most viral meningitides are benign and self-limiting. They rarely have long-term sequelae. These disorders must be differentiated from viral encephalitis with its contrasting high mortality and serious long-term deficits.

The most important aspect in the management of meningitis is rapid recognition and treatment. Each hour of delay can significantly affect the outcome. Delays often occur when parents or physicians do not recognize that a child is seriously ill. Partial treatment of meningitis by administration of antibiotics prior to the onset of the infection can mask some of the clinical findings associated with meningitis, thus causing delay in recognition and consequently treatment.

INITIAL APPROACH IN THE EMERGENCY DEPARTMENT

Meningitis is considered in the differential diagnosis of any patient presenting with any combination of the following symptoms: fever, headache, photophobia, stiff neck, alteration in mental status (level of arousal and/or cognitive function), or vomiting. Decreased feeding, jaundice, or respiratory distress may also be present in newborns. Often, many of these symptoms are not present in an individual patient. Newborns with meningitis may present with only decreased feeding and irritability. Elderly patients may show only a change in mental status or have a fever without a known source. Immunocompromised patients may have only a fever because their inflammatory response is often impaired.

The same priorities apply in the management of suspected meningitis as in any other medical emergency. A rapid primary survey is conducted and simultaneous treatment is given for any airway, ventilatory, or circulatory problem found. In patients with altered mental status or hypotension the following interventions are performed:

   1. Airway and breathing are managed as necessary. Supplemental oxygen is provided.

   2. An intravenous line with isotonic crystalloid is started. Hypotension is treated

by conservative volume resuscitation. The amount of fluid given and the rate are carefully monitored because potentiating cerebral edema is a concern in these patients.

3. Continuous cardiac monitoring is established.

4. Blood specimens are taken for a complete blood count (CBC), electrolytes, glucose, blood urea nitrogen (BUN), creatinine, and culture.

5. Patients with decreased mental status or seizures are given thiamine 100 mg IV, 50% dextrose 25 to 50 gm (1 gm/kg of 25% dextrose in children), and naloxone 2 mg IV (0.01 mg/kg in children).

6. Hyperthermic patients (temperature over 105°F or 40.5°C) are treated with cooling measures: a cooling blanket, damp wash cloths, and a fan to maximize convection heat loss.

7. Patients with seizures are given diazepam 5 to 10 mg IV slow push for initial control. In adults a loading dose of phenytoin is administered at 15 mg/kg if the patient is not already taking phenytoin. In children phenobarbital 15 mg/kg is given slowly, intravenously. *If the child has already received diazepam, there is a high likelihood that respiratory depression or apnea will follow the administration of phenobarbital. The respiratory status must be closely monitored, and assisted bag-valve-mask ventilation or endotracheal intubation and ventilation is carried out at once if necessary.*

8. In most patients with suspected meningitis the traditional sequence of diagnosis followed by treatment can be followed. About 10% of patients are seriously ill, with obtundation, coma, seizures, delirium, or shock. In these circumstances, if the diagnosis of meningitis is likely, antibiotic therapy is started prior to any procedures (Table 47–1). The goal is to minimize any unnecessary delays.

9. A lumbar puncture is performed as soon as possible in patients with suspected meningitis. If intracranial hypertension or an expanding mass lesion is suspected from the findings on the physical examination, e.g., papilledema, anisocoria, bradycardia, hypertension, or focal neurologic deficit, a head CT scan is done before proceeding with a lumbar puncture. If no contraindication exists, the lumbar puncture is performed. An extra tube of spinal fluid is collected for a Gram's stain to be performed immediately after the tap, and, if the tap was traumatic, for centrifugation while the CSF is sent to the laboratory for analysis.

10. After the lumbar puncture, the patient is treated with a broad-spectrum antibiotic

TABLE 47–1. Common Pathogens and Antibiotic Treatment of Meningitis*

Age	Usual Organism	Antibiotic
Neonate	Group B streptococci Gram-negative bacilli Enterococci *Hemophilus influenzae* *Listeria*	Penicillin 75,000 units/kg/day Ampicillin 100–200 mg/kg/day and Gentamicin 5.0–10 mg/kg/day or Cefotaxime 200 mg/kg/day
Infants and children	*H. influenzae* *Neisseria meningitidis* *Streptococcus pneumoniae*	Ampicillin 300 mg/kg/day and Chloramphenicol 100 mg/kg/day or Cefotaxime 200 mg/kg/day or Ceftriaxone 100 mg/kg/day
Adults	*N. meningitidis* *S. pneumoniae*	Penicillin 12–24,000,000 μ/day or Ampicillin 12 gm/day or Cefotaxime 12 gm/day or Ceftriaxone 4 gm/day

*These are guidelines. Precise dosing is determined at the time of need.

regimen appropriate for age and immune status until the CSF culture results reveal the specific causative agent (Table 47–1).

PROBLEM 2 The 8 year old girl was poorly responsive and hyperventilating and had a blood pressure of 60/40 mm Hg. Her temperature was 102.2°F (39°C). She had no allergies to medication. Her airway was open with an intact gag reflex, and she was ventilating well. Venous access was established, and the patient was given a fluid challenge of 20 ml/kg of isotonic crystalloid solution. A blood sample was drawn for culture while the IV was started. A rapid assessment of the patient revealed meningismus in addition to the petechial rash in the axillae, flanks, and wrists. She was given ampicillin, chloramphenicol, and a corticosteroid intravenously.

The clinical appearance of a fulminant onset of fever, meningismus, petechiae, and shock is consistent with a presumptive diagnosis of meningococcal meningitis complicated by meningococcemia and possible Waterhouse-Friderichsen syndrome (adrenal insufficiency due to intracortical adrenal hemorrhage). *Hemophilus influenzae* and *Streptococcus pneumoniae* infection can also present with a petechial rash and shock; therefore, broad-spectrum antibiotics are begun even before the diagnosis is made. Although there is still much to learn about this child, this case illustrates the need for early action in critically ill patients.

DATA GATHERING

History

A history exploring the patient's current illness, possible predisposing factors for meningitis, and any recent treatment with antibiotics is obtained. Antibiotic treatment can mask the early clinical findings and prevent the appearance of organisms on Gram's stain or culture.
1. Are *symptoms present that are consistent with a diagnosis of meningitis?*
    a. *Headache.* Most alert patients with meningitis have a headache, but the quality of the pain may not be very helpful; most of the time the pain is severe, diffuse, and often throbbing. It is usually increased by cough or straining.
    b. *Photophobia.* Many patients complain of photophobia, a symptom related to meningeal irritation.
    c. *Stiff neck.* Patients with meningitis will complain of a stiff neck. This complaint is evaluated as part of the physical examination.
    d. *Change in mental status.* Most patients with bacterial meningitis have some change in mental status: a history of changes in level of arousal (lethargy, obtundation, irritability, or delirium), and/or changes in cognitive function, behavior, or personality. Viral meningitis rarely alters mental status. This finding points to a more serious involvement of the brain parenchyma—encephalitis.
    e. *Nausea and vomiting.* These are nonspecific symptoms that can be caused by meningeal irritation. A history of projectile vomiting raises the possibility of increased intracranial pressure.
    f. *Decreased feeding.* Decreased feeding may be an early symptom of meningitis in newborns and infants.
2. *Onset.* How *rapidly* did the *symptoms develop?* Patients tend to fall into one of two groups in regard to onset of infection: there is either a sudden, explosive onset with rapid progression of symptoms (occurs in about 10% of patients) or a more gradual progression from a mild preceding febrile illness (occurs in 90% of patients). The former history is more common with meningococcal meningitis.

3. *Systemic symptoms*
   a. Myalgias and backache are common, particularly in patients with meningococcal disease.
   b. There may be upper airway or facial infections, which may have been treated recently.
   c. Malaise is commonly noted.
4. Are there *predisposing factors?* These may include:
   a. Recent infection of the head or neck—paranasal sinusitis, otitis media, orbital cellulitis, periodontal abscess, pharyngitis. These upper airway and head infections are factors leading to pyogenic meningitis.
   b. Septic arthritis, which may be a predisposing factor or may cause all three most common bacterial infections.
   c. An immunocompromised state—e.g., newborn, diabetes, alcoholism, cirrhosis, sickle cell anemia, splenectomy, cancer, chemotherapy, AIDS. Pneumococcal and *Hemophilus* meningitis are most often associated with these conditions.
   d. Recent exposure to someone with meningitis—this is typical of meningococcemia.
   e. Recent head trauma, which is associated with increased frequency of pneumococcal and gram-negative bacillary meningitis.

Physical Examination

The physical examination is directed toward detecting signs supporting the diagnosis of meningitis and assessing the patient's tolerance to the disease.

1. Vital signs
   a. Temperature. Most patients with bacterial meningitis have a fever. It may not be present in newborns (60%), young infants, or the elderly.
   b. Pulse rate. The pulse rate may be high owing to fever and hypovolemic or septic shock. A slow pulse rate or bradycardia can be caused by increased intracranial pressure.
   c. Blood pressure. Blood pressure may be elevated owing to increased intracranial pressure, or low owing to hypovolemia or septic shock.
   d. Respiratory rate. Respiratory rate may be elevated in infants who present in respiratory distress, a finding associated with meningitis in the newborn period.
2. Mental status. The patient's orientation, cognitive functions, ability to concentrate, and awareness of the environment need to be assessed. Infants are evaluated for tracking, curiosity (reaching out for objects), irritability, and consolability. Any infant or child showing lethargy, decreased awareness of the environment, or inconsolability must be suspected of having meningitis. On the other hand, a smiling infant who maintains eye contact is less likely to have meningitis.
3. Head. A bulging anterior fontanelle is suggestive of meningitis in children whose anterior fontanelle is still open (usually 6 to 9 months of age). Still, this sign is found in only 30% of cases.
4. Face. Tenderness over the sinuses or mastoid bone or opacity on transillumination may suggest sinusitis as a possible source of the infection.
5. Eyes
   Pupils. A unilateral, large, unreactive pupil suggests third cranial nerve involvement, uncal herniation, local trauma, or medication to the eye. Up to 10% of the population have pupils that are unequal in size, but they react to light and accommodation.
   Papilledema. Papilledema is seen more often with a cerebral abscess than with meningitis and suggests increased intracranial pressure. Up to 50% of patients with a cerebral abscess have papilledema. This finding usually indicates the need to do a head CT scan before proceeding with a lumbar puncture.
6. Ears. An erythematous, bulging tympanic membrane suggests otitis media as a possible source.

7. Neck. With meningismus, one finds resistance to flexion only, whereas other neck disorders cause pain and resistance to movement in the lateral and rotational planes also. Meningismus is the most helpful and specific finding for meningitis, but it is often absent in children less than 18 months of age (in whom it is seen in only 15% of cases). It can also be difficult to evaluate in the elderly because of neck stiffness due to degenerative arthritis of the cervical spine. Meningismus may be present with parameningeal inflammations, e.g., cervical adenopathy, sinusitis. It can be differentiated from other causes of a stiff neck by checking the cervical spine range of motion.
8. Brudzinski's sign. Involuntary flexion of the hips and knees with flexion of the neck is a sign of meningeal irritation.
9. Kernig's sign. An inability to fully extend the leg (passively) with the hip flexed at 90 degrees is a sign of nerve root irritation caused by inflammation of the meninges.
10. Neurologic examination

    Cranial nerves. Deficits in the cranial nerves are more common with cerebral abscess and encephalitis, less common in bacterial meningitis. Still, up to 20% of patients will have a dysfunction of the third, fourth, sixth, or seventh cranial nerve. Such deficits are rarely seen in viral meningitis.

    Motor examination

    Tone. The patient may have flaccid muscle tone or opisthotonos, a posturing with rigid hyperextension of the neck and back, in which the whole body appears arched. This is a sign of diffuse meningeal irritation.

    Strength. Hemiparesis or hemiplegia is more common with cerebral abscess or encephalitis. It is seen in less than 15% of patients with bacterial meningitis.

    Movement disorders. Athetosis, choreoathetosis, and hemiballismus have been reported in patients with bacterial meningitis.

    Reflexes. Deep tendon reflexes may be hyperactive and the Babinski reflex often shows upgoing toes in patients with bacterial meningitis, cerebral abscess, and encephalitis. No changes are noted in those with viral meningitis.

    Cerebellar signs. Ataxia may be present with meningitis, but a cerebellar hemorrhage or abscess is more common and must be ruled out.
11. Skin

    Jaundice. Jaundice may be associated with meningitis in the newborn.

    Petechiae, purpuric, or ecchymotic rash. A rash is classically seen with meningococcemia but also appears with *Hemophilus* and streptococcal bacteremia. It is assumed to be meningococcal in origin, and prompt treatment is indicated.

PROBLEM 1 The 3 month old child had a history of otitis media 2 weeks prior to admission. The mother gave the child the amoxicillin prescribed for 3 days, and then, since he seemed to feel better at the time, she stopped giving him the medication. The mother stated that since the night before admission, the infant had lost his appetite, was not playful as usual, and seemed to cry a lot. On examination, the rectal temperature was found to be 102°F (38.9°C). The child was constantly crying, seemed unaware of his environment, and had a slightly bulging fontanelle.

The history of previous infection, inappropriate antibiotic dosing, unconsolable state, and slightly bulging fontanelle in a child this age all point to a very high probability of meningitis. It is important to generate a preliminary differential diagnosis. Still, a lumbar puncture is required in this infant.

PROBLEM 2 Other than the fact that she had recently been at camp, there was little more information to be gathered from the child's very distraught parents. The child's vital signs responded to therapy, and a lumbar puncture set-up was ordered.

An early call to the child's pediatrician is very important. In many cities with children's hospitals, such a patient may be considered for transfer prior to the lumbar puncture. Infectious disease precautions to protect the emergency physician and staff are necessary.

PROBLEM 3 On the first visit the student had been told that he had an upper respiratory infection, and he was treated symptomatically. No antibiotics were given. Since then his major symptoms had become a throbbing, frontal headache, neck and back ache, and some photophobia. Physical findings included a temperature of 101°F (38.3°C), a preference for a darkened room, slight resistance on flexion, and an inability to touch chin to chest. A faint macular rash was noted over the trunk and face.

This patient is typical of an evolving process that did not declare itself initially. The suspicion of meningitis exists, but pursuit of the diagnosis is highly dependent on the experience of the physician and just "how ill" the patient seems to be. This second visit is best considered as very significant.

DECISION PRIORITIES AND PRELIMINARY DIFFERENTIAL DIAGNOSIS

Following the history and physical examination, the emergency physician suspecting meningitis seeks answers to these questions:
1. *Does the patient have meningitis?* Meningitis must be differentiated from other diseases that present with fever, headache, altered mental status, vomiting, malaise, and meningismus.
    a. *Encephalitis* is often accompanied by clinical findings related to cerebral, cerebellar, or brain stem involvement: hemiparesis, gustatory or olfactory hallucinations, temporal lobe seizures, aphasia, cranial nerve deficits, ataxia, or movement disorders. These findings are unusual in the early course of meningitis. The CSF profile for encephalitis is usually similar to that for a viral meningitis.
    b. *Subarachnoid hemorrhage* may cause a fever, headache, photophobia, and meningismus, but the features that differentiate it from bacterial meningitis are a sudden onset of severe headache, low-grade fever, and blood in the CSF.
    c. *Cerebral abscess* often presents with fever, headache, and altered mental status and can be difficult to differentiate from bacterial meningitis. The onset of the illness usually occurs more gradually compared with meningitis. Patients with a cerebral abscess are often afebrile, especially if the abscess is encapsulated. If a fever is present, it is usually lower than in meningitis. Intracranial hypertension and signs of a mass lesion are much more common with cerebral abscess than with meningitis. Up to half of patients with cerebral abscess have papilledema and focal neurologic deficits. These findings are dependent on the duration and location of the abscess. Early cerebral abscesses located in "silent" areas such as the frontal or occipital lobes may cause minimal symptoms. If an abscess is suspected, the patient is treated with broad-spectrum antibiotics and evaluated with a head CT scan before a lumbar puncture is performed.
    d. *Subdural hematoma* usually causes some alteration in mental status and may be associated with a fever secondary to posterior hypothalamus injury. Usually a known history of head trauma is present, and differentiating it from meningitis is not a problem. If the patient is "found down," and nothing is known about the onset of the illness, head trauma is always a consideration. In this circumstance, evidence of external head trauma should be sought, the cervical spine cleared, and the neck checked for meningismus. If doubt about possible trauma remains, the patient may be treated expectantly with broad-spectrum antibiotics and a head CT scan before proceeding with a lumbar puncture.

e. *Reye's syndrome* has some of the features of meningitis: altered mental status and vomiting in a child. Usually a fever is not present, the child may not complain of a headache if he or she is conscious, and meningismus is absent. The hypoglycemia and liver function abnormalities that accompany Reye's syndrome are usually not features of bacterial meningitis.
f. *Retropharyngeal abscess* may cause a severe headache and resistance to anterior flexion of the neck, but it is usually associated with a severe sore throat and sometimes airway obstruction, suggested by a muffled voice, drooling, and stridor.

2. If the preliminary diagnosis remains meningitis, then the question is, *What type of meningitis is it?* Although most meningitis is infectious, an oncologic process can cause similar symptoms. The infectious causes can be bacterial, viral, fungal, or parasitic. This chapter will emphasize the common bacterial and viral causes of meningitis because they are most often seen in the emergency department. An educated guess can be made on the basis of age, risk factors, and clinical presentation (Table 47–2). Still, the assessment of suspected meningitis is not complete without a lumbar puncture.

DIAGNOSTIC ADJUNCTS

The only way to diagnose meningitis is to analyze the cerebrospinal fluid. Because of the severe morbidity and mortality associated with bacterial meningitis, a lumbar puncture is done for any patient with signs or symptoms of meningitis, particularly the combination of altered mental status, fever, headache, meningismus, and irritability. Because of the lack of many symptoms or signs in neonates and infants, lumbar puncture is performed more liberally in those with lethargy, poor feeding, or irritability whether or not fever is present.

Lumbar Puncture and Cerebrospinal Fluid Analysis

CSF is sent to the laboratory for a cell count, differential, Gram's stain, culture, and measurements of glucose, protein, and cryptococcal antigen (if the patient is immunocompromised). An extra tube is kept for a Gram's stain and centrifugation if the fluid is grossly bloody. Table 47–3 summarizes the CSF analysis results in patients with viral and bacterial meningitis and in different age groups.

Opening Pressure. The normal opening pressure with the patient in the lateral decubitus position is up to 20 cm (200 mm) of water. The top of the fluid column should fluctuate with respiration after it has equilibrated. The pressure may be falsely elevated if the patient is straining (Valsalva maneuver). It is necessary for the abdominal muscles to be relaxed to obtain a reliable measurement of pressure. Elevated pressures are typical but not diagnostic of meningitis.

TABLE 47–2. Frequency of Clinical Findings in Bacterial versus Viral Meningitis

	Bacterial	Viral
Acute presentation (symptoms <24 hr)	25%	5%
Headache	Prominent	Prominent
Meningeal signs	80%	60%–70%
Fever	Common: 80% >38.9°C*	Common: 30%–40% >38.9°C*
Alteration in mental status	80%–90%	25%–50%
Seizures	30%	5%
Focal neurologic deficits	50%	<10%

*38.9°C = 102°F

(From Rennie C: Meningitis. In Tintinalli JE, Krome RL, Ruiz F (eds): Emergency Medicine: A Comprehensive Study Guide (2nd ed). New York, McGraw-Hill, 1988.)

TABLE 47–3. Cerebrospinal Fluid Findings in Different Age Groups

	Open Pressure (mm H$_2$O)	Cell Count (cells/mm^3)	Glucose (mg/dl)	Protein (mg/dl)
Normal neonate	Up to 200	Up to 30 (60% polys)	1:1 with serum	Up to 150
Infant (>1 mo)	Up to 200	Up to 10 (monos)	1:1 with serum	Up to 150[a]
Normal adult	Up to 200	Up to 5[b] (monos)	>/= 1:2 serum	Up to 45
Bacterial meningitis	May be >200	>5 usually[c] (polys—depends on time)	<1:2 serum	May be >45
Viral meningitis	May be >200	>5 usually[d] (monos)	>/= 1:2 serum	Usually <150

polys = polymorphonuclear cells; monos = mononuclear cells.
[a]Does not drop to adult levels until 1 year of age.
[b]More than one poly is suspicious for early bacterial meningitis.
[c]Usually hundreds to thousands but may be less depending on time from onset of infection lumbar puncture was done.
[d]May be predominantly polys during first 24 hours.

Cell Count. Normal CSF in an adult is clear and contains fewer than 5 mononuclear cells. Cloudy fluid contains more than 200 white blood cells (WBC)/mm^3 or more than 400 red blood cells (RBC)/mm^3. The presence of more than one polymorphonuclear cell (PMN)/mm^3 in an adult is suspicious for early meningitis. In neonates, normal CSF may contain up to 30 WBC/mm^3 with 60% PMNs. After 1 month of age there should be no more than 10 WBC/mm^3.

Traumatic Tap. Problems in interpretation arise when the spinal tap is traumatic, i.e., contains a large amount of blood. When this happens, the fluid is immediately centrifuged to determine whether xanthochromia is present. If it is, a subarachnoid bleed is suspected in the absence of jaundice, hypercarotenemia, or a markedly elevated CSF protein level. In addition, the first and last specimens collected are sent to the laboratory for an RBC count. In a traumatic tap, the count decreases between the first and last tubes collected. Various methods have been devised to "estimate" mathematically the WBC count in a traumatic tap. In one formula the CSF RBC count is divided by 500 and 1000 to derive a range for the "expected" WBC count. The calculated "expected" WBC count is then compared with the actual WBC count in the bloody fluid. In another method, the CSF RBC count is multiplied by the ratio of WBC to RBC in the peripheral CBC to derive the "expected" CSF WBC count. This figure is then compared with the actual CSF WBC count to determine whether there is a higher WBC count than expected. Studies to date have shown that mathematical methods tend to "overcorrect" the WBC count. The presence of blood in the CSF does not change the results of glucose measurements, Gram stain, or other tests. If serious doubt remains, the best course of action is to treat the patient expectantly with the appropriate antibiotic regimen.

CSF Glucose. In adults the normal CSF glucose concentration is usually at least 50% that of a concomitant blood glucose level, whereas in children it is usually the same as the blood glucose concentration. Bacterial but not viral meningitis alters the normal ratio.

CSF Protein. In adults the normal CSF protein level varies from 15 to 45 mg/dl, but in neonates it may be as much as 150 mg/dl. CSF protein levels do not drop to adult levels until 1 year of age. Most patients with bacterial meningitis have an increased CSF protein concentration.

CSF Lactate. CSF lactate levels of more than 35 mg/dl are consistent with a diagnosis of bacterial meningitis.

CSF Serology

C-Reactive Protein. A positive CSF C-reactive protein level strongly suggests bacterial meningitis in children. In cases in which there is a high probability of this diagnosis, the predictive value exceeds 95%.

Counterimmune Electrophoresis. Counterimmune electrophoresis (CIE) can be used to detect bacterial antigen in the CSF; it is particularly helpful when WBCs are present in the CSF but no organisms are seen on the Gram's stain, a condition seen in patients with early or partially treated meningitis. This test is also very helpful if the culture is sterile owing to previous antibiotics. The advantage of this test is that results are available in 45 to 60 minutes, whereas cultures take at least 24 hours. CIE is 90% sensitive for detecting *H. influenzae*, 80% for *S. pneumoniae*, but less than 50% for *N. meningitidis*.

Latex Particle Agglutination. Latex particle agglutination has the same uses and advantages as CIE. It is technically easier to perform (5 to 15 minutes), and it is reported to be significantly more sensitive than CIE. For these reasons, it is becoming more popular than CIE for the rapid detection of bacterial organisms. Unfortunately, it also has a low sensitivity for detecting *N. meningitidis*.

CSF with Prior Treatment. Another problem arises in partially treated patients who have received antibiotics for some other illness. The use of antibiotics prior to infection may result in a negative Gram's stain and sterile culture, but they do not significantly change the cellular or chemical elements of the CSF. There may be a slight increase in the proportion of lymphocytes. Again, CSF lactate, C-reactive protein, counterimmune electrophoresis, or latex particle agglutination may help establish a definitive diagnosis.

Other Laboratory Studies

Serum Electrolytes. Serum electrolyte measurements are ordered, and particular attention is paid to the serum sodium level. A number of patients with meningitis develop the syndrome of inappropriate secretion of antidiuretic hormone (SIADH), and hyponatremia is a known complication with few specific symptoms (see Chap. 27).

Serum Glucose. Knowledge of the blood glucose concentration is important so that one can properly determine if the CSF glucose is low. The CSF glucose level should be at least 50% that of the blood level. If the blood glucose level is low, one cannot infer that an associated hypoglycorrhachia is due to bacterial meningitis.

Cultures. Blood and urine cultures may help to identify the organism causing meningitis, although urine cultures usually are not helpful in infants and children.

Radiologic Imaging

Head CT. If the patient has clinical findings consistent with a diagnosis of bacterial meningitis, a CT scan is not indicated. One proceeds directly to an LP or immediate antibiotic treatment. If a patient has findings that suggest a possible intracranial abscess or other mass lesion, especially if papilledema or focal neurologic signs are present, then a CT scan is obtained before an LP is performed. If the patient is very ill, treatment with antibiotics is started first, and then a CT scan and LP follow. If a cerebral abscess is suspected, CT scan with contrast is included, since a mature abscess will demonstrate a "ring" lesion due to the vasculature in the abscess wall.

Magnetic Resonance Imaging. Magnetic resonance imaging is more sensitive than CT scanning in detecting a cerebral abscess, subdural emphysema, and other mass lesions, but it has no utility in making the diagnosis of meningitis itself.

PROBLEM 1 On LP grossly purulent CSF was found with a WBC count of more than 50,000/mm^3, a low glucose level, and a high protein level. No organisms were seen on Gram's stain.

This case is all too typical of meningitis in infants. The adage about meningitis in this age group—"if you are thinking about it, do the LP"—usually holds true. The emergency physician's next step is rapid, appropriate antibiotic use and referral.

REFINED DIFFERENTIAL DIAGNOSIS

The results of the CSF analysis will answer the question of whether the patient has meningitis. The refined differential diagnosis addresses the question: *Is it bacterial or nonbacterial meningitis?* The distinction between bacterial and viral meningitis is the most common and important. Table 47–2 lists the clinical differences, and Table 47–3 lists the CSF analysis in these two groups.

Nonbacterial Meningitis. "Aseptic meningitis" is most commonly caused by a viral infection. Fungal infections, leukemia, lymphoma, and chemicals may also cause aseptic meningitis. Patients with aseptic meningitis may have all the features of bacterial meningitis: fever, headache, meningismus, and sometimes altered mental status, but usually the clinical course is milder. In addition to the patient's presenting signs and symptoms, CSF analysis is the most useful differential aid. Usually, there are less than 100 WBCs/mm^3—most of them are mononuclear cells, although a preponderance of PMNs may exist during the first day of the infection. The CSF glucose level is normal, and the Gram stain is negative. *This same CSF profile may be present in patients with partially treated bacterial meningitis.* Therefore, it is essential to determine whether prior antibiotic therapy has been given. A predominantly lymphocytic pleocytosis with a *low* CSF glucose level suggests a fungal, tubercular, or carcinomatous meningitis.

Bacterial Meningitis. In order, the most common bacterial causes of meningitis are *H. influenzae, N. meningitidis,* and *S. pneumoniae. Hemophilus influenzae* type B meningitis is most common in children between 4 months and 2 years of age. Newborns are usually protected by the presence of maternal antibodies. *Hemophilus influenzae* is an encapsulated gram-negative rod that frequently inhabits the respiratory tract. Patients frequently have an antecedent infection such as otitis media, pharyngitis, sinusitis, epiglottitis, mastoiditis, or pneumonia. These infections may obscure or delay the diagnosis of meningitis. A transient unilateral sixth nerve palsy occurs in 20% of patients with meningitis. An autoimmune related anemia is more often seen with this infectant.

Meningococcal meningitis is a severe, often lethal disease caused by a gram-negative diplococcus. Infections are most common in children and young adults and frequently occur in winter and early spring. Infections are spread by aerosol means and by direct contact. Asymptomatic nasopharyngeal infections can last for weeks. A minority of infected patients will develop a rapidly progressive disease with sore throat, fever, and headache. A skin rash progresses from a morbilliform to petechial to purpuric form. Cultures from the purpuric lesions may grow meningococcus. Some patients develop focal neurologic signs such as sixth, seventh, or eighth cranial nerve defects. The Waterhouse-Friderichsen syndrome with adrenal hemorrhage, massive purpura, hypotension, and disseminated intravascular coagulation (DIC) is associated with a poor prognosis. Specific treatment for meningococcal meningitis is high-dose penicillin. Since other pathogens can cause a purpuric meningitis, broad-spectrum rather than specific antibiotic coverage is indicated until culture results confirm the diagnosis. Meningococcemia exists in 20% of patients without meningitis. It may also recur after an episode of meningitis, and such patients require close follow-up.

Pneumococcal meningitis is the most common bacterial cause of meningitis in adults. Frequently pneumococcal infections of the sinuses, mastoid, middle ear, or lung precede the meningeal symptoms. Patients with skull fractures, alcoholism, sickle cell disease, and multiple myeloma are particularly susceptible to pneumococcal infections. Petechial lesions, adrenal hemorrhage, and DIC are not common but may occur in patients with overwhelming infection.

PROBLEM 3 The emergency physician decided to do an LP. The opening pressure was 190 mm H_2O, and the fluid was clear. The cell count showed 65 cells, 90% lymphocytes. The CSF glucose level was 60 mg/dl, and the protein concentration was 40 mg/dl. Gram's stain showed no organisms.

The CSF was consistent with a diagnosis of viral meningitis. The CSF analysis and the rash and diarrhea pointed to an enterovirus infection. Echovirus or coxsackievirus are the most common viruses. Although the patient's symptoms were mild, an echovirus meningitis can present with confusion, delirium, and papilledema.

PRINCIPLES OF MANAGEMENT

General Principles

Overall management of the patient with meningitis involves control of the airway, circulation, fever, seizure, and early use of antibiotics. Guidelines for the first four were reviewed in the section Initial Approach in the Emergency Department.

Antibiotics

Antibiotics are the cornerstone of specific management. Antibiotic selection is done on an empiric basis in at least 25% of patients with bacterial meningitis. In this situation, treatment can be guided by the patient's age and immune status because particular organisms tend to predominate in different age groups (Table 47–1). The traditional antibiotics of choice during the neonatal period have been ampicillin and gentamicin. In the past, gentamicin has been given intrathecally, but recent studies suggest that there is no advantage to the intrathecal route compared with systemic administration. In children, ampicillin and chloramphenicol have been the drugs of choice, but the resistance of *H. influenzae* to ampicillin has increased to 25% since 1974! Recently, there have been reports of a low rate of resistance to chloramphenicol also. In adults, penicillin has been the drug of choice, but *S. pneumoniae* resistance to penicillin (up to 7%) has been reported. To date, there have been no reports of resistance of *N. meningitidis* to penicillin.

Because the sensitivities of the major pathogens to traditional antibiotic regimens are changing, new agents are being investigated for the treatment of bacterial meningitis. So far, the third-generation cephalosporin antibiotics hold the most promise. The first-generation cephalosporins do not penetrate the blood-brain barrier; except for cefuroxime, the second-generation cephalosporins have not been effective in the treatment of meningitis even though some reach adequate CSF levels. Among the third generation cephalosporins, cefotaxime and ceftriaxone are the most effective. These antibiotics, used as single agents, have cure rates that are at least equal to those of the multidrug regimens that have been used traditionally to treat the three major pathogens. Nonetheless, morbidity and mortality have not significantly changed with use of these newer agents. Finally, cephalosporins are ineffective for the treatment of *Listeria* infections, which are still treated with ampicillin.

The point that antibiotic therapy must be started as soon as possible cannot be overemphasized because morbidity and mortality from meningitis are often directly related to the promptness of treatment. Every attempt is made to start antibiotic treatment within one hour of admission to the emergency department.

PROBLEM 2 After the IV fluid and antibiotics were administered and the patient was improving hemodynamically, an LP was performed. The CSF was purulent, and a Gram's stain showed gram-negative cocci consistent with a diagnosis of meningococcal meningitis. The patient was switched to penicillin therapy for the remainder of the treatment period.

SPECIAL CONSIDERATIONS

Immunocompromised Patients

Meningitis presents special problems in patients who are immunocompromised. The incidence of AIDS and organ transplantation has increased considerably, as has the longevity of patients with cancer, renal failure, and other terminal diseases. Diabetes, alcoholism, cirrhosis, sickle cell anemia, and splenectomy are other common causes of the immunocompromised state that must be taken into consideration in the diagnosis and treatment of meningitis. Elderly patients, particularly those with chronic debilitating diseases, also fit into this category. These patients are very susceptible to the three major bacterial infectants, and most of the time their illness is caused by one of these three. Occasionally they may be infected by a more unusual organism. The emergency physician must consider a wide range of infectious possibilities in these patients. This difficult process optimally cannot delay the initiation of therapy. *Listeria* or *Pseudomonas* infections may be associated with some of the above disorders. In addition, these patients may develop an infection from fungi or protozoa, organisms rarely seen in the normal population. Such organisms may include *Cryptococcus, Aspergillus, Mucor, Nocardia,* or *Toxoplasma*. Patients with AIDS seem to be predisposed to *Mycobacterium avium*. Most of these organisms cause meningitis that has a subacute to gradual onset, but the patient may present with an acute illness. Assessment of the immunocompromised patient must include a cryptococcal antigen titer and fungal and mycobacterial cultures. Ampicillin is added to the antibiotic regimen to cover possible *Listeria* infection. Amphotericin B remains the drug of choice for fungal infections. In the particular case of *Cryptococcus*, amphotericin B and 5-flucytosine are synergistic.

DISPOSITION AND FOLLOW-UP

Most of these patients are admitted to the intensive care unit. They can be divided into two groups according to whether they have bacterial or nonbacterial meningitis.

Bacterial Meningitis

Patients with bacterial meningitis are admitted. Those with altered mental status or seizures or who are in shock need to be placed in an intensive care unit. Patients and family may ask about the potential for residual damage. It is important not to underplay this issue because 10% to 20% of patients who recover will have some problems. These may include hearing loss, seizures, mental retardation, and emotional lability. In infants, significant sequelae occur in 30% to 50% of patients.

Nonbacterial Meningitis

The question often arises about the disposition of patients who have viral meningitis. Some of these patients may be sent home if the following conditions are met:
 1. The presence of an early or partially treated bacterial meningitis has been ruled out.
 2. The CSF is completely consistent with an aseptic meningitis (lymphocytic pleocytosis, no organisms on Gram's stain, normal CSF glucose level).
 3. The patient is not lethargic or obtunded.
 4. The patient has no vomiting or diarrhea (sometimes associated with the enteroviruses causing the meningitis).
 5. The headache is tolerable (sometimes the headache associated with a viral meningitis may be severe enough to require narcotic analgesia for relief).
 6. The patient and his or her family are reliable.

7. The patient will not be alone but under close observation (by family or a friend).
8. Follow-up care is readily available.

The issue of possible exposure to an infecting agent, particularly *N. meningitidis*, must be discussed with the family and emergency department staff. Information pertinent to this discussion is available in Chapter 18.

DOCUMENTATION

1. Symptoms and onset: headache, fever, stiff neck, nausea, or vomiting
2. Any changes in mental status noticed by family or friends, such as lethargy, confusion, or behavioral or personality changes
3. Recent infections (especially of the head or neck)
4. Any prior use of antibiotics
5. Any contact with others with a diagnosis of meningitis
6. Vital signs including temperature
7. Physical examination results including mental status, pupils, and funduscopic examination results, presence or absence of meningismus, general status
8. Neurologic examination results including mental status, cranial motor status, sensory nerve status, and reflexes
9. Assessment of the need for LP or CT and also reasons against performing these tests
10. Lumbar puncture—time of procedure, consent, opening pressure, gross appearance of fluid, results of Gram's stain and centrifuge if a traumatic tap is present, requested CSF studies sent to the laboratory, and results. How well the patient tolerated the procedure is also noted.
11. Date and time antibiotics were given, and type, dose, and route of administration
12. Disposition plans and instructions, including transfer or referral arrangements

SUMMARY AND FINAL POINTS

- Detection of early meningitis requires consideration of this diagnosis in any patient presenting with a fever, headache, alteration in mental status, or flu-like syndrome.
- Bulging fontanelles and meningismus are not always present in the very young, and meningismus can be difficult to evaluate in the very old.
- If you think about a lumbar puncture, you should probably do it!
- The results of the LP guide therapy. Prompt treatment is the key to a good outcome. If there will be a significant delay for any reason, the patient should be given broad-spectrum antibiotic(s) appropriate for age and immune system.
- If results of the initial LP are normal but a high suspicion of meningitis remains, it is repeated in 8 to 12 hours. It is far better to do one LP too many than to miss the diagnosis.

REFERENCES

1. Schlech WF, Ward JI, Band, JD, et al: Bacterial meningitis in the United States, 1978–1981: The National Bacterial Meningitis Surveillance Study. JAMA 253:1749, 1985.

Suggested Reading

1. Benson CA, Harris AA: Acute neurologic infection. Med Clin North Am 70:987–1011, 1986.
2. Bolan G, Barza M: Acute bacterial meningitis in children and adults. Med Clin North Am 69:231–241, 1985.
3. Dagbjartsson A, Ludvigsson P: Bacterial meningitis: Diagnosis and initial antibiotic therapy. Pediatr Clin North Am 34:219–229, 1987.
4. Dougherty JM, Roth RM: Cerebrospinal fluid. Emerg Clin North Am 4:281–297, 1986.
5. Henry K, Crossley K: Meningitis—principles of diagnosis, advances in treatment. Postgrad Med 80:59–71, 1986.
6. Task Force on Diagnosis and Management of Meningitis: Diagnosis and management of meningitis. Pediatrics Suppl 78:959–982, 1986.
7. Weinstein L: Bacterial meningitis. Med Clin North Am 69:219–223, 1985.

# CHAPTER 48

SEIZURES

MARC S. NELSON, M.D.

PROBLEM 1 The rescue squad radioed the emergency department that they were at the scene where a 50 year old man was observed to have a grand mal seizure while waiting in line to purchase a bottle of wine at the local liquor store. They reported that he was a well-known chronic alcoholic.

PROBLEM 2 An 18 month old girl was brought in by her parents after she "stopped breathing and began to shake all over." The child had no prior seizure history. The parents did note that she was febrile to a temperature of 104.2°F (40.1°C) earlier in the day.

PROBLEM 3 A 17 year old boy was brought in by the rescue squad after having a 2- to 3-minute grand mal seizure at school. There was a note from the school nurse stating that he had a long-standing seizure disorder.

QUESTIONS TO CONSIDER

1. What are the life-threatening concerns when caring for a patient who has seizures?
2. What aspects of the history and physical examination are important for patients presenting with seizures?
3. What are the common causes of seizures in patients presenting to the emergency department?
4. How can true seizures be differentiated from conditions that mimic them?
5. What ancillary tests are important in the management of seizures?
6. When is consultation with a neurologist appropriate?
7. Which patients are admitted to the hospital?
8. Which patients with seizures who are being discharged need to be started on an anticonvulsant regimen?

INTRODUCTION

A seizure is the physical manifestation of a sudden, disorderly discharge of cerebral neurons. This neuronal discharge may appear as tonic-clonic (convulsive) movements, loss of consciousness, sensory deficits, repetitive behavior (automatisms), or some combination of these phenomena. *Epilepsy,* a Greek word meaning "to seize upon" or "to take hold of," is often used interchangeably with *seizure.* It is preferably used to describe the clinical condition associated with repetitive seizure activity caused by a discernible focus of abnormal electrical activity in the brain. It is not completely understood why neurons in or near a focal lesion discharge spontaneously. Some studies suggest that the membranes of these cells have an increased permeability and hypersensitivity that make them more susceptible to stimuli such as hypoxia or hypoglycemia.

The convulsive movements may be generalized or partial (focal) in appearance. Focal seizures are the result of a lesion in a specific part of the cerebral cortex. Depending on the location, different patterns may be seen. For example, lesions of the superior temporal cortex give rise to auditory and vertiginous sensations, whereas lesions from the mesial temporal cortex cause olfactory sensations. Patients who have seizures so frequently that they do not regain consciousness between seizures are in "status epilepticus." Such activity can produce neuronal damage, cerebral edema, and the development of new irritable foci.

Seizures have always been a significant cause of morbidity. It is estimated that more than 1 million Americans have epilepsy. The incidence of seizures is estimated to be 30 to 50 per 100,000 population per year with even higher rates if febrile and isolated seizures are included. Approximately 35% to 40% of seizures are of undetermined origin (idiopathic). Many of these patients have diffuse developmental abnormalities that are demonstrated only on postmortem histologic studies. Complex partial seizures have been correlated with changes in nerve cell density and the glial supporting tissue in the temporal lobe called mesial temporal sclerosis. These changes may be due to an ischemic insult. Abnormal nerve cell migration or orientation is seen in other patients with seizures. All these mechanisms result in an abnormal focus of electrical stimulus within the brain. Idiopathic or primary seizures may be precipitated by stress, fatigue, loss of sleep, hyperventilation, menstruation, photic stimulation, or alcohol. About 60% of seizures are secondary to other disease processes. These include metabolic, traumatic, toxic, infectious, vascular, degenerative, and endocrine pathologies.

PREHOSPITAL CARE

The rescue squad plays an important role during active seizures by preventing complications and injury to the patient. In the postseizure state they also must protect the patient from injury. The information supplied by the prehospital personnel should include the following data.

History

1. What happened during the event (preferably information obtained from on-scene observers). What activity immediately preceded the event?
2. What was the patient's condition at the time of arrival of the rescue squad and at the present time?
3. Does the patient have a known seizure disorder? If so, what medications are being taken?
4. Is the seizure related to trauma, drugs, or alcohol?

Physical Examination

1. Is the airway clear and breathing spontaneous? During active seizures patients are at high risk for aspiration. If the seizure is prolonged, they may become severely hypoxic and acidotic.
2. Does the patient have a pulse and blood pressure? Taking a blood pressure on a patient who is actively seizing is difficult. However, assessment of the pulse is necessary to rule out severe hypotension or cardiac arrest as a cause of the seizure.
3. Does the patient respond to voice or painful stimuli? Following the active seizure phase, or ictus, most patients experience a postictal phase. The nature of the postictal period can be a diagnostic clue to the type of seizure that occurred. The postictal phase in generalized seizures is characterized by decreased responsiveness, gradually abating over minutes to hours. In partial seizures there may be no ictal or postictal altered level of consciousness.

Interventions

1. Airway control. Patients who are actively seizing and do not have signs of trauma are placed in the lateral decubitus position to prevent aspiration. A nasopharyngeal airway is placed and supplemental oxygen provided by nasal cannula. If available, a padded bite protector may be placed between the teeth to prevent injury to the tongue.

2. Cervical spine. If the seizure is secondary to trauma, and the cervical spine is potentially at risk, an attempt is made to maintain alignment. This is extremely difficult during a seizure, and definitive immobilization efforts are applied in the postictal state. Fortunately, a seizure associated with trauma is short-lived and seldom recurs. Of course, the trauma may have been caused by seizure activity.

3. Intravenous catheter. An intravenous (IV) line with 5% dextrose in water as the fluid of choice is started to administer glucose and anticonvulsants or other medications as needed. Starting an intravenous line in an actively seizing patient is almost impossible. It is best accomplished in the postictal phase.

4. Cardiac monitor. Patients are monitored for cardiac dysrhythmias. These may be the cause of the seizure or secondary to the metabolic abnormalities producing the seizure.

5. Hypoglycemia prophylaxis. A blood sample is drawn and placed in a red top tube. The serum glucose level is measured by a test strip, or thiamine (100 mg) and 50% glucose (12.5 to 25 gm) are administered intravenously.

6. Anticonvulsant therapy is administered to patients who have recurrent seizures without regaining consciousness or a single seizure lasting more than 5 minutes. Diazepam may be administered intravenously in 2- to 5-mg boluses up to a maximum of 20 mg to terminate the seizure. The patient is closely monitored for respiratory depression and hypotension.

PROBLEM 1 The patient was having a generalized seizure when the rescue squad arrived at the scene. From bystander reports it was determined that the seizure had lasted about 8 minutes. The patient had a pulse, but blood pressure could not be measured. He was placed on oxygen and a cardiac monitor, and an intravenous line was started with difficulty. Thiamine and glucose were administered intravenously without producing any change in condition. The paramedics requested permission to use an anticonvulsant drug. The emergency physician ordered 5 mg of intravenous diazepam, which terminated the seizure in 2 to 3 minutes. Transport time to the hospital was estimated to be 5 to 10 minutes.

Alcohol withdrawal seizures generally terminate spontaneously and do not need anticonvulsant therapy. Even before the patient arrives, the emergency physician should be thinking of other causes for this patient's seizures.

INITIAL APPROACH IN THE EMERGENCY DEPARTMENT

The initial approach in the emergency department is directed toward (1) supporting the patient's vital signs, (2) treating life-threatening causes of seizures, and (3) controlling active seizures.

The prehospital history and physical examination results are confirmed, paying special attention to a history of previous seizures and circumstantial evidence of drug use or trauma.

The patient's vital signs are supported, as noted previously, with (1) airway control—use of nasal airway, supplemental oxygen, and positioning the patient to prevent aspiration; (2) IV line, to administer drugs as needed; and (3) cardiac monitoring, to diagnose cardiac dysrhythmias.

Life-threatening causes of seizures can be immediately addressed.

Hypoglycemia. Serum glucose concentration is immediately determined using a test strip bedside technique. If the patient is diabetic or taking hypoglycemic agents, or if the blood glucose level is not immediately available, empiric treatment with 12.5 to 25 gm of 50% glucose is indicated.

Hypoxia. Supplemental oxygen is administered, and the potential causes of hypoxia are reviewed. If the patient is cyanotic or has abnormal findings on pulmonary examination, a chest radiograph and an arterial blood gas determination are obtained immediately. In appropriate circumstances (e.g., fire, suicide attempt), a carbon monoxide (CO) level is obtained. Definitive airway management may be necessary to deliver a higher percentage of oxygen.

Cardiac Dysrhythmias. Ventricular fibrillation can present as a seizure. The vital signs and cardiac monitor help to assess the presence and nature of dysrhythmias.

Intracranial Hemorrhage. Patients with a history or signs of head trauma, or with focal or progressive neurologic signs may have central nervous system hemorrhage. Immediate computed tomography (CT) of the head is indicated. Patients with progressive signs of an expanding mass lesion are treated with hyperventilation, furosemide (Lasix), and mannitol to decrease intracranial pressure. Prompt neurosurgical consultation is obtained.

Drug or Poison Ingestion. Ingestion of any of a wide variety of toxins may present as a seizure. Although supportive therapy alone is the mainstay of treatment for many of these agents, those with specific antidotes must be considered: cyanide, tricyclic antidepressants, methanol, ethylene glycol, and heavy metal poisoning.

Meningitis. It may be difficult to evaluate a patient who has recently seized for signs and symptoms of meningitis. Seizures can cause a fever, and meningismus may be difficult to evaluate. A prior history of fever, headache, vomiting, stiff neck, and new-onset seizures should arouse a high suspicion for meningitis and should prompt an immediate diagnostic lumbar puncture (see Chap. 47).

Eclampsia. Eclampsia is suspected in patients who are in their third trimester of pregnancy. Blood pressure, reflexes, proteinuria, and prior history can help in diagnosing this condition. Magnesium sulfate is the drug of choice for treating seizures associated with eclampsia.

Patients who are actively seizing may be given diazepam in 2- to 5-mg boluses up to a maximum of 20 mg. Blood pressure and respirations must be closely monitored when diazepam is given.

PROBLEM 1 The patient arrived in the emergency department lethargic and purposefully responsive to painful stimuli only. The rescue squad had no other history. They believed that the patient was improving and repeated the history of chronic alcohol abuse. The patient was breathing spontaneously and had an intact gag reflex. A serum glucose test strip showed a glucose concentration of 140 mg/dl. Supplemental oxygen was continued at 4 liters/min. The cardiac monitor showed a sinus tachycardia, rate 120 beats/min. The patient was afebrile and without meningeal signs.

Many major catastrophic problems had been ruled out in this patient. Intracranial hemorrhage remained a significant possibility, as did drug or poison ingestion. Assessment of meningeal signs before clearing the cervical spine in a patient without a history of significant trauma is appropriate.

DATA GATHERING

The history and physical examination allow the physician (1) to determine whether the event was a true seizure or something that mimics seizures, and (2) to look for clues indicating whether the seizure was primary or secondary to another disease process.

History

Obtaining an accurate history from a patient with a seizure disorder often requires a number of sources. These include the patient himself, his friends and family, the paramedics, and an old chart if available. Several key points need to be elicited.

1. A *detailed description* of exactly what happened *prior*, *during*, and *after* the *event* is important. Was there an *aura*, onset in *specific muscles, loss of consciousness, tongue biting,* or *incontinence?* Was there a *postictal* state? What was the *time course* of these events? Were there any *precipitating events*, such as stress, fatigue, or lack of sleep?

2. What *type* of *seizure* was it? Seizures may be classified by distinguishing generalized seizures (bilaterally symmetric and without local onset) from partial (focal) seizures (seizures that begin locally). Knowledge of the type of seizure allows one to localize the part of the brain that is responsible.

3. Does the patient have a history of a *prior seizure disorder?* If so, how *frequently* does the patient have seizures? How *compliant* is the patient in taking his or her medications? One of the most common reasons patients with seizures come to the emergency department is a subtherapeutic level of an anticonvulsant drug.

4. A complete *list* of the *medications* being taken by the patient is necessary. Seizures can represent toxic effects of drugs listed in Table 48–1.

5. Is the seizure secondary to a *traumatic event?* Although the approach to a seizure secondary to head trauma is similar to that used for a nontraumatic seizure, some additional precautions must be taken (see Chap. 50).

6. Does the patient have a history of *drug* or *alcohol abuse?* Grand mal seizures are common when people addicted to alcohol, barbiturates, or sedative-hypnotics suddenly abstain or go through withdrawal.

7. Has the patient been in his usual *state of health* or has he been *recently ill*, e.g., complaining of fever, headache, stiff neck, lethargy, or vomiting?

8. Past medical history/review of pertinent systems.

Cardiac Disease. Is there a history of coronary or valvular heart disease? Are there known cardiac dysrhythmias? Is the patient taking cardiac medications such as quinidine?

Pulmonary Disease. Does the patient have chest pain or shortness of breath? Any disease that causes significant hypoxia may lead to seizures.

Endocrine Diseases. Does the patient have diabetes, thyroid disease, or parathyroid disease? Is he taking hypoglycemics? Hypoglycemia and hyperglycemia, hypocalcemia, hyponatremia, and thyrotoxic storm may all present as a seizure.

Renal Disease. Does the patient have a history of kidney disease? Is the patient being dialyzed? Uremia can lead to seizures.

TABLE 48–1. Etiologies of Seizures

Primary (idiopathic)	
Secondary	
Toxic	Intoxication with cocaine, tricyclics, theophyllines, penicillin, lidocaine, physostigmine, oral hypoglycemics, isoniazid, phenothiazines, pentazocine, lithium, lead
	Withdrawal from alcohol, barbiturates, hypnotics
Traumatic	Concussion, contusion, bleed
Neoplastic	Primary or metastatic
Infections	Meningitis, encephalitis, brain abscess, neurosyphilis, parasites
Vascular	Cerebral hypoxia or bleed, arteriovenous malformation, vasospasm, hypertensive encephalopathy
Metabolic	Hyponatremia, hypoglycemia, uremia, hepatic failure, hypercarbia, hypoxia, hypocalcemia, hypomagnesemia, hyperosmolar states
Endocrine	Addison's disease, hypothyroidism, hyperthyroidism
Obstetric	Eclampsia

Oncologic Diseases. Is there any history of cancer? Metastasis to the brain is common, the most frequent sites of origin being the lung, breast, skin (melanoma), and gastrointestinal tract. Tumors may also affect electrolyte balance through paraneoplastic syndromes and inappropriate secretion of antidiuretic hormone (SIADH).

Immunocompromised Patient. Patients who are immunocompromised, such as those with AIDS, may have a variety of parasitic, fungal, viral, and bacterial infections as well as neoplastic diseases that cause seizures.

9. Family history. Although it is most significant in patients with classic petit mal seizures, heredity plays an important role in many types of seizure disorders.

Physical Examination

The physical examination allows the physician to determine the presence of systemic diseases that may cause or imitate seizures.

Vital Signs. Vital signs are reassessed during the physical examination. An elevated body temperature is not attributed to seizure activity but should prompt a search for a source of infection.

Head, Eyes, Ears, Nose, Throat. Even in the absence of a history of trauma the head is carefully palpated. The tympanic membranes are examined for hemotympanum. The size and shape of the pupils and how they react, extraocular movements, and the optic disc margins and venous pulsations are carefully noted. Evidence of oral injuries such as tongue lacerations is sought as well as gingival hypertrophy secondary to phenytoin (Dilantin).

Neck. The neck is examined for stiffness, which may indicate meningeal irritation, and bruits, which indicate cerebrovascular disease.

Chest. Examination for rales, rhonchi, rubs, or tachypnea is carried out. Pulmonary disease may be the cause of seizures. In addition, aspiration pneumonia may be a complication of seizures.

Cardiac Disease. Heart murmurs, gallops, and irregular rhythms may be indicative of heart disease.

Extremities. A search is made for traumatic injuries that may have occurred as a complication of the seizure such as a shoulder dislocation. Seizures are the most common cause of posterior dislocations of the shoulder.

Neurologic Examination. Attention is directed toward finding focal deficits and locating a specific area in the brain as the source if possible. The neurologic examination is usually repeated because the recovery from a seizure is a dynamic process. Occasionally patients have a transitory focal deficit after a seizure termed *Todd's* or *postictal paralysis*. The paralysis gradually improves during minutes to hours.

1. Mental status examination. Is the patient alert and oriented? Does he remember what happened? An accurate account of the postictal period can help to characterize the seizure. Patients with generalized tonic-clonic seizures have postictal lethargy and confusion lasting minutes to several hours. There is no postictal period in patients with generalized absence seizures. The postictal period of complex partial seizures is characterized by disorientation and inattention and lasts for 2 to 10 minutes.

2. Cranial nerve function.

3. Motor function. The focus is on symmetry of motor function and specific muscle groups.

4. Sensory examination.

5. Reflexes

6. Testing of gait and stance. This examination is delayed until the patient is fully able to cooperate.

PROBLEM 2 The baby had been sick with a cold for 2 days. She had no prior history of seizures. This episode lasted about 2 minutes. One hour later the baby was still lethargic and irritable. Her temperature was 104°F (40°C). Physical examination showed an erythematous, immobile right tympanic membrane. There was no meningismus. The rest of the examination showed normal findings.

Otitis media was certainly a source of infection. The question was whether a more serious infection was present. The emergency physician was concerned about the infant's continuing lethargy and irritability. Possible explanations included fever, postictal state, sepsis, and meningitis. Acetaminophen was given in an attempt to lower the temperature and observe the child's activity after defervesence. In retrospect, this should have been done on admission.

PROBLEM 3 The old chart and a call to the school nurse supplied information that the patient was known to be noncompliant with his medication. There was no suspicion of drug abuse or suicide attempt. On examination the patient was found to be postictal without focal findings. Bedside glucose level was 130 mg/dl.

There was little reason to doubt the history as presented. Significant pathology was not apparent. Therefore, the care for this patient began with watchful waiting for resolution of the postictal state and assessment of therapeutic drug levels.

DECISION PRIORITIES AND PRELIMINARY DIFFERENTIAL DIAGNOSIS

The first question to be answered in any patient who presents with a "seizure" is: *Did the patient in fact have a true seizure?*

In an event unwitnessed by the physician, this determination must be based largely on the accuracy of the history.

Factors that tend to support a diagnosis of seizures include:
1. A previous history of similar events.
2. A precipitating cause, such as sleep deprivation, stress, or fatigue.
3. The presence of an aura just prior to the event.
4. The description of tonic-clonic movement and loss of consciousness.
5. A postictal state.
6. Tongue biting.
7. Incontinence of bowels or bladder.

The information obtained from data gathering is compared to the characteristics of other conditions that may mimic seizure activity.

Cerebrovascular Insufficiency. Patients with transient ischemic attacks may have episodes that mimic seizures. Vertebrobasilar insufficiency results in decreased blood flow to the brain stem. Patients may complain of cranial nerve symptoms, such as diplopia, slurred speech, and vertigo followed by syncope. There is generally no tonic-clonic movement or postictal state.

Syncope. Patients with syncope experience a sudden, transient loss of consciousness and collapse. Some degree of muscle twitching or tonic contractions may accompany the syncope, but there is no tonic-clonic movement, tongue biting, or postictal phase. The etiology of syncope includes dysrhythmias, hypovolemia, vasovagal abnormalities, metabolic abnormalities, and primary neurologic diseases (see Chap. 12).

Cataplexy. Following stress or excitement, some patients with narcolepsy develop a sudden loss of muscle tone resulting in a fall. These episodes may resemble myoclonic seizures. Physicians should be concerned about cataplexy in patients with a history of narcolepsy.

Hyperventilation. In response to stress, patients may hyperventilate, causing a respiratory alkalosis. These metabolic changes can result in carpopedal spasm, muscle twitching, and circumoral paresthesias.

Dissociative States. Patients with severe psychiatric disturbances may present in trancelike states that may resemble petit mal absence or temporal lobe seizures. Patients with dissociative states usually are able to function mentally. Electroencephalography may assist in the diagnosis.

Pseudoseizures or Factitious Seizures. These are behavioral episodes in which patients purposely or unconsciously display seizurelike activity with no organic basis. It is estimated that between 5% and 10% of patients treated for seizure disorders have pseudoseizures. Some patients who have an organic basis for seizures have pseudoseizures as well on occasion. Factitious seizures can be difficult to diagnose even by an experienced observer. Most patients exhibit abnormal limb or trunk movements, but the orderly tonic-clonic sequence is not usually present. Attacks generally occur in the presence of a crowd to gain attention. The patient is unhurt by falling, tongue biting and incontinence are rare, and there is frequently no postictal period. The patient may respond to direct questioning or diversion tactics, or may purposefully move an ammonia capsule away from the nose while maintaining seizure activity.

Once it has been decided that the patient has had a true seizure, the second question is: *What is the cause? Primary or secondary?*

Approximately 35% to 40% of seizures have no clear source and are thus termed idiopathic. Table 48-1 lists the major causes of seizures. One important cause of seizures, alcohol, deserves special mention. Alcohol withdrawal seizures account for approximately 15% of the seizures seen in the emergency department. They are sometimes called "rum fits" and occur when total or relative abstinence from alcohol occurs after a long period of inebriation. More than 90% of alcohol withdrawal seizures occur within 8 to 48 hours after the last drink, usually peaking at 12 to 24 hours. The seizures are usually generalized motor in nature. They are usually single but may recur in patients with severe withdrawal. Status epilepticus due to ethanol is rare without some underlying disorder. Focal seizures should prompt a further work-up. It is important to remember that in patients with a preexisting seizure disorder, alcohol, even in small amounts, may precipitate a seizure. Because of the high risk of underlying organic disease, patients over 50 years old with seizures attributed to ethanol use are considered candidates for further evaluation.

The differential diagnosis of seizures also depends on the age group of the patient. Table 48-2 lists the most common causes in each age group. Many of these diseases require laboratory studies to help make the diagnosis.

DIAGNOSTIC ADJUNCTS

Diagnostic tests are performed to help determine the specific etiology of secondary seizures. There are few areas of medicine in which more unnecessary tests are ordered

TABLE 48-2. Causes of Seizures in Different Age Groups

Age of Onset	Probable Cause
Neonatal	Congenital maldevelopment, birth injury, anoxia, metabolic disorders
Infancy (3 mo–1 yr)	As above; infantile spasms
Early childhood (1 yr–3 yr)	Infantile spasms, febrile convulsions, birth injury and anoxia, infections, trauma
Childhood (3–10 yr)	Perinatal anoxia, injury at birth or later, infections, thrombosis of cerebral arteries or veins, idiopathic
Adolescence (10–18 yr)	Idiopathic, trauma
Early adulthood (18–25 yr)	Idiopathic, trauma, neoplasm, drug or alcohol withdrawal
Middle age (35–60 yr)	Trauma, neoplasm, vascular disease, alcohol or drug withdrawal
Later life (over 60 yr)	Vascular disease, tumor, degenerative disease, trauma

Adapted from Adams RD, Victor M: Principles of Neurology (3rd ed). New York, McGraw-Hill, 1985.

than in the work-up of a seizure patient. It is neither cost-effective nor practical to order every test for every patient. The patient's medical history and physical examination findings dictate the selection of laboratory tests.

Laboratory Studies

Complete Blood Count with Differential. The white blood cell count with differential is indicated if an infectious etiology is suspected. The hemoglobin level will indirectly reflect the oxygen-carrying capacity of the blood.

Serum Electrolytes. Hyponatremia can cause seizures. Recent studies have shown that electrolyte abnormalities are rarely found, and electrolyte measurements are not cost-effective as a screening device. Electrolytes are obtained in patients taking diuretics and in those who present with signs or symptoms of neoplastic disease, renal failure, or endocrine abnormalities, e.g., hypoadrenalism, hypothyroidism, or hyperthyroidism. Electrolyte measurements are also ordered in patients with new-onset seizures in whom the etiology is unclear.

Serum Glucose. A glucose level is indicated in all patients who suffer seizures. A finger stick bedside determination can be used as a screening device for hypoglycemia as a cause of seizures.

Calcium and Magnesium. Calcium and magnesium levels are obtained in patients with muscle spasms, twitching, or a positive Chvostek's or Trousseau's sign.

Toxicology Screen. This test is indicated in patients who are suspected of having taken an overdose of medications or who are known drug abusers with seizures.

Anticonvulsant Drug Levels. Anticonvulsant levels are indicated in all patients who have been prescribed or who state that they are taking anticonvulsant medications. These test results are reasonably accurate and are available in most laboratories for phenytoin, phenobarbital, and carbamazepine.

Arterial Blood Gases. Profound alterations in acid-base equilibrium occur immediately following a single grand mal seizure. The pH may go as low as 7.05. The significant lactic acidosis that occurs after a single grand mal seizure usually resolves spontaneously within 40 to 60 minutes after the seizure has stopped. Serum potassium elevation does not accompany the lactic acidosis. If arterial blood gas levels are significantly abnormal after a seizure, a repeat test is recommended in 40 to 60 minutes to uncover persistent acid-base disorders that may have caused the seizure, e.g., methanol intoxication.

Radiologic Imaging

Computed Tomography of the Head. Computed tomography (CT) has evolved into the most important imaging tool used in the diagnosis of seizures. It is indicated for patients with focal neurologic findings, first-time seizures, or suspected head trauma or CNS tumors. About 7% of patients with subarachnoid hemorrhage have normal findings on CT scan. If a subarachnoid bleed is suspected despite a negative CT of the head, a lumbar tap should be performed, looking for red blood cells or xanthochromia. Most acute cerebrovascular infarctions are not detected by the initial CT scan.

Skull Films. These films are of limited value. Much more information is obtained from a CT scan.

Magnetic Resonance Imaging. Magnetic resonance imaging (MRI) may be useful as part of the neurologic work-up, but this test is not usually available in the emergency department.

Electrocardiography. A 12-lead electrocardiogram is useful in patients suspected of seizure or seizure-like activity from hypotension dysrhythmia.

Other Tests

Lumbar Puncture. Lumbar puncture is critical for patients with a fever, headache, and nuchal rigidity. Cerebrospinal fluid analysis can identify meningitis or subarachnoid bleed.

Electroencephalography. This is a useful test in the work-up of a patient with a seizure disorder but is seldom ordered in the emergency department. It may help in differentiating true seizures from pseudoseizures.

PROBLEM 1 The alcoholic patient was gradually waking up. He complained of a bad headache and stated that he had been on a drinking binge for the past several days to relieve the headache pain. He had had rum fits several years ago when he was jailed following a brawl and drinking binge. The physical examination revealed no focal findings, although the patient remained slightly lethargic. The patient's alcohol level was 285 mg/dl. A CT was done, revealing a small subdural hematoma.

Even though this patient had no focal findings, several aspects of his course were sufficiently worrisome to warrant the CT of the head: (1) he required anticonvulsant medication to stop his prolonged seizures, (2) he had had a bad headache *prior* to his seizure, (3) his alcohol level was very high when he had the seizure. Alcohol withdrawal seizures occur when there is an abrupt fall in ethanol level. They *may last* more than 5 minutes and may require short-term anticonvulsant treatment. Alcoholics, however, often fall and hit their heads and may not have obvious signs and symptoms of trauma.

PROBLEM 3 The patient gradually awakened after 30 minutes. He said that he did have a seizure disorder and took phenytoin regularly. Physical examination was unremarkable. With normal findings on examination, the physician decided to order only a serum phenytoin level and observe the patient.

Patients with known seizure disorders who recover completely often have subtherapeutic anticonvulsant drug levels.

REFINED DIFFERENTIAL DIAGNOSIS

Once the history, physical examination, and ancillary tests are completed, the emergency physician is generally able to limit the differential diagnosis to one or two major categories (Table 48–1). If the ancillary tests do not reveal a specific etiology of the seizures, the patient is considered to have idiopathic epilepsy.

A simplified classification of seizures is presented in Table 48–3. Seizures can be either generalized or partial. Generalized seizures involve the whole body and occur in 20% to 40% of patients with epilepsy. Generalized absence or petit mal seizures can be difficult to diagnose. There is no aura, loss of posture, incontinence, or postictal confusion. The attack rarely lasts more than 20 seconds. Absence seizures invariably start in childhood, and patients are rarely brought to the emergency department for this problem. Tonic-clonic or grand mal generalized seizures occur in both children and adults. There may be a brief aura followed by loss of consciousness and rhythmic tonic-clonic movements lasting 1 to 5 minutes. There may be tongue biting, cyanosis, and bowel or bladder incontinence. Postictal confusion lasts for minutes to hours.

Partial seizures occur primarily in adults and represent abnormal electrical activity

TABLE 48–3. Seizure Classification

Partial	Generalized
Simple	Simple absence (petit mal)
Motor	Tonic-clonic (grand mal)
Sensory	
Autonomic	
Complex	
Psychomotor (temporal lobe)	

in one area of the brain, causing motor, sensory, or autonomic dysfunction. Partial seizures are considered complex if the focal discharge spreads and causes altered consciousness or combinations of motor, sensory, and autonomic dysfunction. Psychomotor or temporal lobe seizures are a type of complex partial seizure. Presentations are constant for an individual but extremely variable overall.

Status epilepticus is a life-threatening emergency. It is defined as repeated seizures without regaining consciousness. It usually occurs as three seizures or more during a 30-minute period or continuous seizure activity for more than 10 minutes. This seizure disorder is frequently secondary to withdrawal of anticonvulsant medication, CNS infection, hemorrhage, tumor, or metabolic abnormalities. The short-term mortality is under 10%, but complications can raise the mortality to more than 20%.

PRINCIPLES OF MANAGEMENT

The management of patients with seizures depends on the following basic principles:

General Supportive Measures

All seizure patients immediately receive three general supportive measures.
1. Airway protection and supplemental oxygen. A nasal or oral airway may be placed to ensure airway patency.
2. Intravenous line. A "lifeline" is established to give anticonvulsant medications as needed.
3. Seizure precautions. Many emergency departments have protocols specifying protective measures to be used for patients who may seize. Bed rails are placed up, and hard surfaces are padded. Clothing and dentures are removed. During an active seizure the patient is placed in the left lateral decubitis position to avoid aspiration. A soft object, such as a padded tongue blade, may be placed in the patient's mouth. These patients, especially in the postictal phase, may be difficult to manage, but preferably they are not restrained.

Eliminate Causal Factors of Seizure

Prompt attention is given to eliminate life-threatening causes of seizures. These include hypoxia, cardiac dysrhythmias, hypoglycemia, meningitis, eclampsia, hyponatremia, intracranial hemorrhage, and specific toxins. Specific therapies are listed in the earlier section, Initial Approach in the Emergency Department.

Pharmacologic Control of Active Seizures

Anticonvulsants are indicated if the patient has had more than one seizure or is having a single seizure that has lasted more than 5 minutes. The drug of choice is diazepam given intravenously. The patient may be given a bolus of 1 to 5 mg over 1 to 2 minutes. Peak concentrations are achieved in 1 to 2 minutes. If seizure activity does not terminate, repeat boluses may be given to a maximum of 20 to 30 mg of diazepam. Diazepam may cause respiratory depression and vasodilatation, leading to hypotension. The emergency physician must be prepared to intubate the patient and support the blood pressure with intravenous crystalloid if needed. The treatment protocol for status epilepticus is presented in Table 48–4.

Prevention of Further Seizures

Prevention of further seizures depends on correctly identifying the cause of the present or recent one. Reversible causes such as hypoglycemia, hyponatremia, and hypoxia are

TABLE 48–4. Treatment of Status Epilepticus

Time (minutes)	Procedure
0	ABCs
	Check pulse
	Place oral/nasopharyngeal airway
	Establish IV
	Obtain laboratory evaluation
	Check anticonvulsant levels
	Electrolytes
	BUN
	Glucose
	Arterial blood gases
	Place patient on cardiac monitor
	Place patient on oxygen saturation monitor, if available
	Check blood pressure
5	Thiamine, 100 mg IV
	Dextrose in water 50%, 50 ml IV push
10	Diazepam IV, 5 mg/min, repeat q 4–5 min, to 20 mg
	Phenytoin IV, 50 mg/min, to 18 mg/kg; IVP (or in 100 ml normal saline)
	Monitor BP, cardiac rhythm
30	Endotracheal intubation (may require Pavulon, 0.1 mg/kg)
	Phenobarbital,* 100 mg/min, to 20 mg/kg
60	General anesthesia with halothane and neuromuscular blockade
	or
	Paraldehyde, 0.1 mg/kg over 1 hr
	or
	Lidocaine, IV

*Phenobarbital may be used before phenytoin if
  (1) previous control with phenobarbital has been used
  (2) there are severe cardiac conduction problems
  (3) patient is allergic to phenytoin, or
  (4) patient is less than 6 years old

Adapted from Delgado-Escueta AV, Wasterlain C, et al: Current concepts in neurology: Management of status epilepticus. With permission from *The New England Journal of Medicine*, 306(22):1337, 1982.

promptly treated. Children with febrile seizures do not need anticonvulsant therapy. Patients with idiopathic seizures or seizures secondary to an intracranial hemorrhage, tumor, infection, or other discernible lesions usually need anticonvulsant therapy to prevent further treatment. The drug of choice for tonic-clonic seizures is phenytoin in adults and phenobarbital in children.

Phenytoin has multiple effects on the central nervous system including stabilization of excitable membranes, which prevents propagation of local neuronal firing. The physiologic effects of phenytoin result from changes in sodium and calcium transport across cell membranes. Most patients can be orally loaded with 400 mg of phenytoin initially, with additional doses of 300 mg at 2 and 4 hours. A therapeutic phenytoin level is 10 to 20 µg/ml. If the phenytoin level is subtherapeutic, additional doses of phenytoin may be given. Approximately 1 mg/kg of phenytoin will raise the drug level 1 µg/ml.

Phenobarbital is the drug of choice for children with grand mal seizures. The mechanism of action of barbiturates as an anticonvulsant drug is uncertain. Phenobarbital can be given in maintenance doses of 3 to 6 mg/kg/day in children and 1 to 2 mg/kg/day in adolescents. Patients can be loaded with double doses for 2 to 3 days.

Attention to Complications of Seizures

Complications of seizures include aspiration, acidosis, and fractures. Aspiration pneumonia may not be obvious on the initial radiograph, but arterial blood gas determination usually shows hypoxia. Occasionally, loose teeth are aspirated and cause bronchial obstruction. Patients who aspirate are treated with antibiotics such as penicillin that cover oral anaerobes. If bronchial obstruction is present, bronchoscopy must be considered.

The lactic acidosis accompanying seizures can be severe; however, it usually corrects itself once the seizure is resolved. Therefore, bicarbonate treatment is generally not indicated unless the arterial pH is less than 7.0.

Patients with seizures may incur musculoskeletal injuries such as fractures or lacerations. Posterior dislocations of the shoulder can occur from intense muscular contractions during tonic-clonic seizures, and these need prompt reduction (see Chap. 41). Musculoskeletal injuries and lacerations are addressed and treated specifically.

PROBLEM 3 This patient had no lacerations or bone tenderness. The phenytoin level was less than 2 μg/ml. The patient received 1 gm of phenytoin slowly over 30 minutes and was observed for another hour.

Most subtherapeutic anticonvulsant levels are due to poor patient compliance. The patient's ability to pay for the medication may be a factor.

SPECIAL CONSIDERATIONS

Pediatric Patients

Approximately 3% to 5% of children have febrile convulsions. These usually occur after 6 months of age, most commonly between 9 and 24 months. This condition is a benign disease, often familial, and usually appears as a brief grand mal seizure. The children recover completely, and there are no long-term sequelae. No further treatment is usually necessary, although the parents are asked to be aggressive in the future about monitoring and lowering the child's temperature during illness.

Seizures in this age group are not always benign. If any of the following features are present, a thorough work-up is required:

1. Seizure lasting more than 3 minutes. (The exact duration is often difficult for a ic parent to discern.)
2. Focal seizure.
3. Recurrent seizures.
4. Lethargy or anything but complete alertness after the seizure.

In both the very young and the very old, occult trauma secondary to child abuse or elder abuse is always considered.

PROBLEM 2 Lethargy persisted 30 minutes later on reexamination. Temperature was now 103.5°F (39°C). A lumbar puncture was performed in the emergency department. The cerebrospinal fluid was cloudy with gram-negative rods. Antibiotics were administered immediately, and consultation was obtained.

Because the risk of meningitis is high and the time elapsed prior to antibiotic administration is directly correlated with morbidity and mortality, the emergency physician must approach the child with a febrile seizure in an attentive and time-conscious manner. The decision to perform further evaluation, particularly lumbar puncture, is optimally made within 30 minutes of the patient's first being seen.

DISPOSITION AND FOLLOW-UP

The disposition of patients with seizures depends on making a reasonable diagnosis of the etiology and ruling out serious disease processes.

Admission

Patients with the following types of seizures are admitted to the hospital:
1. Status epilepticus

2. Seizures secondary to infectious etiology
3. New-onset seizures in patients over 50 years old
4. Eclampsia
5. Seizures due to intracranial hemorrhage or tumor
6. Seizures due to hypoxia, hyponatremia, hypoglycemia, cardiac dysrhythmias, or drug toxicity

Patients who have not regained full consciousness or who have metabolic or hemodynamic abnormalities that need close monitoring are admitted to an intensive care unit. Hospital admission is also considered in (1) patients who have alcohol or drug withdrawal seizures who are observed to be stable, (2) children with febrile seizures, and (3) young patients with new-onset seizures. Admission depends on the reliability and support system of the patient to follow up and return as needed.

Neurology Consultation

Consultation with a neurologist is indicated under the following circumstances: (1) all patients admitted as above, (2) patients with new-onset seizures, and (3) breakthrough seizures in a patient with therapeutic anticonvulsant drug levels.

Discharge

Patients with a known seizure disorder and subtherapeutic drug levels may be sent home after anticonvulsant supplementation. All patients who are sent home are given clear discharge instructions and instructions to follow up with their primary physician or in a clinic. Levels of anticonvulsants are rechecked in 1 to 2 weeks by their primary physician.

DOCUMENTATION

1. History of trauma, both recent and remote. Occult trauma in an alcoholic who may not remember having fallen is always considered.
2. Prior seizure history.
3. Detailed neurologic examination, especially the presence or absence of focal deficits.
4. Laboratory studies and results.
5. Consideration of life-threatening conditions. It should be clear that potentially life-threatening conditions (Table 48–2) have been addressed and either treated or ruled out.
6. Disposition, including details of discharge instructions and follow-up.

PROBLEM 1 The 50 year old man was taken to surgery for evacuation of the subdural hematoma. The emergency physician must always have a high index of suspicion for intracranial hemorrhage in alcoholic patients. Symptoms of altered mental status cannot be attributed solely to acute alcoholism or withdrawal.

PROBLEM 3 The 17 year old boy was sent home. His primary physician was called, and arrangements were made to have the patient's phenytoin level rechecked in 2 weeks.

The patient's regular dose of anticonvulsants is not adjusted unless the emergency physician is certain of compliance. Consultation with the patient's family and primary physician is necessary to assess compliance and meaningful follow-up.

SUMMARY AND FINAL POINTS

The work-up of a seizure patient is as easy or as difficult as one makes it. By obtaining a careful history and ordering laboratory tests judiciously, most patients are managed without difficulty.

- Any potentially life-threatening diseases, specifically cardiac dysrhythmias, hypoglycemia, hyponatremia, toxic ingestions, and meningitis, are assessed and ruled out or treated.
- The best observer account of what actually took place prior to, during, and just after the event is obtained and documented.
- Other conditions such as syncope, factitious seizures, and cataplexy can mimic seizures.
- Precautions are taken to prevent further seizures.
- Status epilepticus is associated with significant morbidity. It is treated in a rational stepwise manner.
- The history and physical examination dictate the need for ancillary tests.
- Complications of seizures include aspiration, acidosis, lacerations, fractures, and dislocations.

REFERENCES

Texts

1. Adams RD, Victor M: Principles of Neurology (3rd ed). New York, McGraw Hill, 1985.
2. Lechtenberg R: The Diagnosis and Treatment of Epilepsy. New York, Macmillan, 1985.
3. Luders H, Lesser RP (eds): Epilepsy. New York, Springer-Verlag, 1987.
4. Niedermeyer E: Epilepsy Guide. Baltimore, Urban and Schwarzenberg, 1983.

Journal Articles

1. Delgado-Escueta AV, Wasterlain C, et al: Current concepts in neurology: Management of status epilepticus. N Engl J Med 306(22):1337–1340, 1982.
2. Earnest MP, Marx JA, Drury LR: Complications of intravenous phenytoin for acute treatment of seizures. JAMA 249(6):762–765, 1983.
3. Eisner RF, Turnbull TL, Howes DS, et al: Efficacy of a "standard" seizure workup in the emergency department. Ann Emerg Med 15:33–39, 1986.
4. Orringer CE, Eustace JC, Wunsch CD, et al: Natural history of lactic acidosis after grand mal seizures: A model for the study of an anion-gap acidosis not associated with hyperkalemia. N Engl J Med 297:796–799, 1977.
5. Walsh-Kelly CM, Berens RJ, et al: Intraosseous infusion of phenytoin. Am J Emerg Med 4:523–524, 1986.

CHAPTER 49

STROKE

LOUIS S. BINDER, M.D.

PROBLEM 1 A 55 year old male smoker presented with a 1-hour history of sudden vision loss to the left eye, "like a curtain coming down over my eye." His symptoms were totally resolved by the time he arrived in the emergency department.

PROBLEM 2 A 66 year old male was brought to the emergency department by the rescue squad with sudden onset of right arm and leg weakness and inability to speak.

QUESTIONS TO CONSIDER

1. What is a "stroke?"
2. How are the following terms defined: transient ischemic attack (TIA), stroke in evolution, completed stroke?
3. What are the important elements of the history and physical examination to be obtained in patients presenting with symptoms of stroke?
4. What are the common causes of stroke?
5. What ancillary tests are considered in patients with stroke?
6. Which therapies are available in the emergency department for managing patients with symptoms of stroke?
7. What common complications are seen in patients with stroke?
8. What criteria are used in making disposition decisions in patients with stroke?

INTRODUCTION

The blood supply to the brain comes from four vessels arising off the aortic arch: two carotid and two vertebral arteries. Figure 49-1 illustrates the pertinent anatomy of the cerebral blood supply. The common carotid artery bifurcates into internal and external carotid arteries at the level of the hyoid bone. Only the internal carotid artery enters the skull through the carotid canal. At the cavernous sinus the internal carotid artery gives rise to the ophthalmic arteries and then trifurcates into the anterior and middle cerebral arteries and posterior communicating artery. The vertebral artery ascends through the foramina in the cervical vertebral transverse processes and enters the skull at the foramen magnum. They join at the level of the upper medulla to form the basilar artery, which divides at the midbrain to form the two posterior cerebral arteries. Anastomosis between the anterior and posterior cerebral vessels by means of the anterior and posterior communicating arteries creates the circle of Willis. This circular arterial linkage lies at the base of the brain surrounding the optic chiasm and pituitary stalk.

A stroke is defined as a sudden neurologic deficit, usually due to cerebral vascular rupture or occlusion. Common clinical manifestations include:

1. *Transient ischemic attack (TIA)*—a transient episode of neurologic deficit of acute onset. It is usually lateralized and lasts a few minutes. It can persist for up to 24 hours.

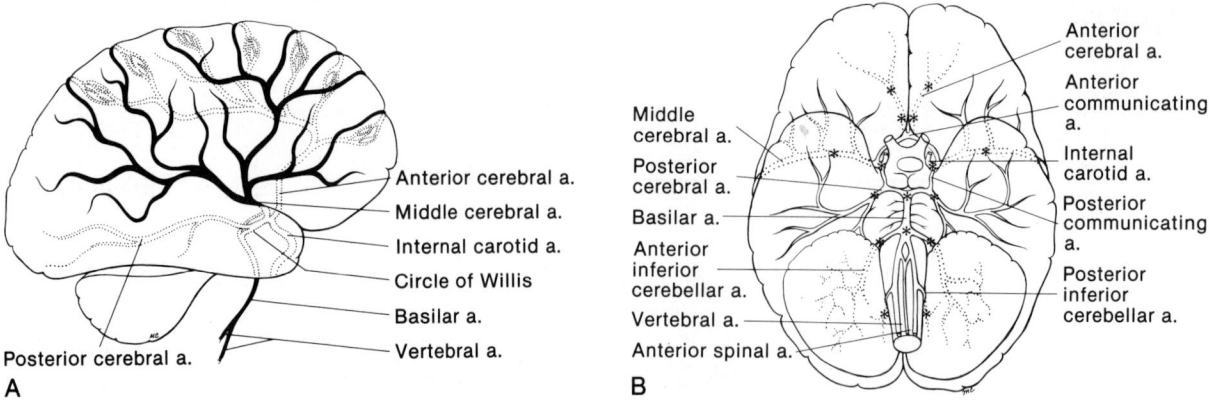

FIGURE 49-1. *Anatomy of cerebral blood supply.* A, Lateral view. B, Basal view. Asterisks denote common areas for atheroma.

2. *Complete stroke*—a stable and permanent neurologic deficit, usually consisting of weakness or paralysis. It may be sudden in onset or evolve to completion. It is usually lateralized.

3. *Stroke in evolution*—the sudden onset of a neurologic deficit with progression over hours to days. It implies a dynamic process of neuronal ischemia and infarction resulting from the initial insult or its complications.

Strokes most commonly result from an atherosclerotic process that causes localized narrowing and thrombus formation in cerebral vessels. The disease is silent until a critical narrowing occurs in one or more vessels, resulting in neuronal ischemia and dysfunction in the distribution of that vessel. Alternatively, strokes may result from atheromatous emboli, most often from the bifurcation of the carotid arteries. Emboli also can be of cardiac origin, e.g., left ventricular mural thrombus, atrial mural thrombus, valvular heart disease, or septal defects. Hemorrhagic strokes usually result from cerebral emboli, which first cause ischemic damage to blood vessels. The emboli then become friable and allow reperfusion of the damaged vessel, resulting in hemorrhagic infarction. Infrequently, other pathologic processes may cause a stroke syndrome, such as developmental malformations, tumor, aortic or carotid dissection, intracerebral inflammation, or infection. Lastly, other noncerebrovascular entities may mimic an acute stroke, e.g., tumor, subdural hematoma.

Stroke is the third leading cause of death in the United States after heart disease and cancer. It is the most lethal and disabling of the neurologic diseases. It is estimated almost 5% of the U.S. population over 65 years of age has had a stroke at one time in their lives. More than 400,000 patients are discharged from the hospital with a diagnosis of stroke. From an economic and functional standpoint, it is one of the most devastating problems in medicine. Timely and appropriate medical intervention in its early stages may minimize the patient's neurologic injury and improve the eventual functional outcome.

PREHOSPITAL CARE

Most patients brought to the emergency department by rescue squad have completed strokes. The information gathered is primarily directed toward possible causes and potential complications. Acquisition of this information should follow a standardized format to be applied quickly and professionally.

History

1. What are the symptoms? When did they begin, and how long have they lasted?
2. Is there a significant history of known diseases predisposing to stroke, e.g., diabetes or hypertension?

3. What medications is the patient taking?
4. What is the estimated time of arrival at the emergency department?

Physical Examination

1. The airway status and adequacy of ventilation are assessed.
2. The vital signs and general appearance of the patient are noted.
3. Level of consciousness is either described or measured according to the Glasgow Coma Scale.
4. Pupil size, equality, and reaction to light are noted.
5. A description of the weakness present is given, including any abnormal responses to stimulation, e.g., posturing.

Intervention

Oxygen. Supplemental oxygen is given by either nasal cannula or mask as tolerated, 4 to 6 liters per minute; 1 to 2 liters per minute are given initially if obstructive pulmonary disease is present.

Intravenous Access. An intravenous (IV) catheter is started; the infusate is usually 5% dextrose in water, but isotonic crystalloid is used if the patient is hemodynamically unstable. Vascular access is necessary to administer medication and restore volume as necessary.

Cardiac Monitor. A cardiac monitor allows the prehospital personnel to describe the cardiac rhythm and observe it in transit. Up to 30% of patients with a new neurologic insult will have an abnormal cardiac rhythm.

Dysrhythmia Management. If ventricular ectopy or other significant dysrhythmia is detected, treatment by protocol or physician order is necessary.

PROBLEM 2 The rescue squad reported that the patient had experienced sudden right-sided weakness and inability to speak 3 hours ago. He was taking hydrochlorthiazide for hypertension and had a history of several similar transient episodes of weakness on the right side. He was alert and awake. Vital signs were blood pressure 200/120 mm Hg, pulse 65/min with irregular rhythm, respirations 18/min and adequate. There was a right facial, right arm, and right leg weakness. Oxygen by nasal cannula at 4 liters/min was started, and an IV line of dextrose in water 5% was placed at a keep-open rate. The cardiac monitor showed one to two unifocal premature ventricular contractions (PVCs) per minute. The squad reported a 5-minute estimated time of arrival to the hospital.

This patient's age, sex, previous history of transient neurologic deficit, hypertension history, and current symptoms all point to the probability of cerebrovascular disease. No dysrhythmic prophylaxis is indicated at this time. Optimally, a family member who knows the patient and his medical history well should accompany the patient. Other information, such as lists of medications, physician's name, hospital card, and any lists of diagnoses or medical records in the family's possession can be of help to the emergency physician.

INITIAL APPROACH IN THE EMERGENCY DEPARTMENT

All patients in whom acute cerebrovascular disease is suspected are brought immediately to a monitored bed in the emergency department. The following activities are performed by the nursing staff in advance of, or simultaneously with, the physician's examination:

1. The ABCs—airway, breathing, and circulation—are assessed rapidly. The level of consciousness, color and general appearance, patency of the airway and adequacy of ventilation, blood pressure, and adequacy of peripheral perfusion are assessed next.
2. The basic history is confirmed from either the rescue squad or family members.
3. The patient is undressed, allowing full exposure for assessment.
4. Cardiac monitoring and supplemental oxygen are reestablished and placement or assessment of the IV line is carried out.
5. The complications of acute cerebrovascular disease are anticipated. The emergency physician should be prepared to treat emergent complications including:
   a. *Airway Compromise.* If the stroke victim is having respiratory difficulties or cannot protect the airway, he should be nasotracheally or endotracheally intubated.
   b. *Dysrhythmias.* Ventricular dysrhythmias are to be anticipated. Treatment with defibrillation is appropriate in an unstable patient with ventricular tachycardia or fibrillation. Lidocaine may be given if the patient is hemodynamically stable.
   c. *Hypertension.* Hypertension is often seen in patients presenting with acute cerebrovascular disease. In acute situations hypertension may be physiologic, allowing adequate cerebral perfusion if intracranial pressure is elevated. An acute lowering in pressure may result in failure of perfusion of a stenotic or thrombosed cerebral vessel, leading to neuronal ischemia in the tissue supplied by that vessel. Therefore, mild to moderate hypertension in stroke does not require treatment. Severe hypertension, greater than 180 to 200 mm Hg systolic or 130 to 140 mm Hg diastolic, or hypertensive encephalopathy is treated with agents that relax smooth muscle in peripheral arterioles and reduce peripheral vascular resistance—agents such as diazoxide, hydralazine, and nitroprusside. The diastolic pressure is gradually reduced to 110 mm Hg while the patient is closely monitored (see Chap. 13).
   d. *Cerebral Edema or Herniation Syndrome.* Acute herniation is uncommon in the early hours of a cerebrovascular accident. It is due to brain edema, mass effect, and uncal herniation through the tentorial notch. The goal of management is to reduce intracranial pressure, and intervention includes intubation and hyperventilation, elevation of the head of the bed, fluid restriction, and use of diuretics (see Chap. 50).

DATA GATHERING

The history and physical examination can differentiate a cerebrovascular occlusion from other causes of stroke, establish the initial extent of the neurologic deficit, and identify complications. It is important to repeat the initial examination serially to detect changing neurologic signs and symptoms.

History

1. How did the symptoms evolve? The patient or family is asked to describe the *exact onset, duration, and progression* of the symptoms.
2. What is the *nature* of the symptoms? The type of weakness, speech impediment, vision impairment, gait change, and changes in level of consciousness are identified. What can't the patient do now that he could do before?
3. Are there *associated symptoms?* Is there numbness, tingling, vertigo, syncope, nausea or vomiting, chest pain, or palpitations? Cardiac symptoms, significant weight loss, or fever may point to pathologic processes causative for stroke.
4. Has the patient had *similar symptoms before?* Prior reversible presentations of cerebrovascular disease consistent with a diagnosis of TIA are harbingers of impending stroke.
5. In evaluating patients with chronic medical problems and impairments (i.e., a

nursing home patient who may have had a stroke), an attempt is made *first to establish a "functional baseline"* from information given by the caretaker. What were the patient's capabilities before the acute event, i.e., dressing, eating, bathing, transferring independently? Changes or deviations from that baseline are explored next.

6. Does the patient have any *risk factors* for stroke (Table 49-1)?
7. *Current medications* and any *known* allergies are noted.
8. *Past medical history*, including hospitalizations, surgical procedures, and chronic illnesses are noted. The cardiac history, valvular disease, and any prior neurologic presentations are emphasized.

PROBLEM 2 The patient stated that he had experienced an acute onset of right-sided weakness about 3 hours earlier while watching television. His family noted that he had been unable to speak more than one to two words, and this required great effort. There were no other associated symptoms. He had had previous occurrences of "slight weakness" resolving in 3 to 5 minutes during the last 3 months but had not sought medical attention. He took hydrochlorthiazide for hypertension but was noncompliant. He had no known allergies.

A review of risk factors is positive for age, male sex, hypertension, cigarette smoking, and history of TIAs. The patient's previous medical records are ordered early. They can be of immense help in clarifying a confusing history, supplying a comparison electrocardiogram (ECG), developing a problem list and medical regimen, and providing a functional baseline for comparison. The medical records confirm the problem list and medication regimen in this aphasic patient and mention a grade 2 to 3/6 systolic murmur that "needs evaluation and possible anticoagulation therapy."

Physical Examination

In the physical examination the physician seeks evidence of cardiac or atherosclerotic vascular disease, increased intracranial pressure, or herniation syndrome and establishes a neurologic and functional baseline for future comparisons. Table 49-2 lists the pertinent elements of the physical examination in the patient with suspected stroke.

PROBLEM 1 The patient described an acute painless loss of vision in the left eye. It was preceded by a "flickering" sensation. After an hour, he decided to drive to the hospital and noticed return of his vision while in transit. He was asymptomatic in the emergency department. Physical examination results, including funduscopy, and neurologic assessment were essentially within normal limits, with the exception of a blood pressure of 160/100 mm Hg and a left carotid bruit. He was unaware of any risk factors for stroke but did smoke two packs of cigarettes per day.

The fleeting nature of neurologic findings in patients with stroke syndromes is often frustrating. The physical examination is used not only to establish the extent of the deficit but also to seek possible causes of the signs or symptoms. The physician should not be dissuaded by the patient

TABLE 49–1. Risk Factors for Cerebrovascular Disease

Age >50 years	History of TIAs
Male sex	Atherosclerotic cardiovascular disease
Hypertension	Other cardiovascular disease, e.g., atrial fibrillation, congestive heart failure, aortic
Diabetes mellitus	valvular disease
Cigarette smoking	Hypercoagulable state, usually associated with hematologic or gastrointestinal cancer
Hyperlipidemia	

TABLE 49–2. Important Components of the Physical Examination in the Patient with Stroke

Area of Examination	Important Components	Comments
Vital signs	Blood pressure	May be elevated, often in response to need for increased cerebral perfusion pressure
	Heart rate	Usually normal or bradycardic. The latter is due to a parasympathetic mediated baroreceptor response. Extrasystolic beats are common and usually ventricular in origin
	Respirations	Variable. If they slow suddenly, consider impending herniation
	Temperature	Patient usually afebrile. Elevated temperature points to an infectious process that may be a cause or complication
General appearance	Position, movement, color, diaphoresis	Rough gauge of how the patient is tolerating the event
Eye	Conjugate deviation	May indicate frontal or brain stem lesion or visual field cut
	Pupils—asymmetry and reaction	If abnormal, consider herniation and midbrain dysfunction
	Fundi	Nicking, hemorrhage, "cotton wool" spots indicate hypertension or diabetes. Degree of capillary thickening ("silver or copper wiring") is indicative of chronic hypertension. Papilledema indicates increased intracranial pressure. Subhyaloid or preretinal hemorrhage may be seen in patients with subarachnoid or intracranial hemorrhage
Neck	Carotid bruits	Direct evidence of cerebrovascular disease
Lungs	Auscultation	Signs of consolidation, rales, wheezes often due to aspiration as a complication
Cardiac	Auscultation	Irregular rhythm may indicate atrial fibrillation or extrasystoles. Murmurs suggest valvular disease (aortic stenosis is the most important lesion)
Neurologic	Level of consciousness	Progression to coma may signal impending herniation
	Speech	Poor fluency and one- to two-word phrases indicate an expressive (Broca's area) aphasia. Comprehension of commands is intact in expressive aphasia, lost in receptive aphasia (Wernicke's)
	Cranial nerves	Dilated and unreactive pupil may indicate uncal herniation. Central seventh nerve palsy ipsilateral to hemiparesis is consistent with hemispheric infarct. Peripheral seventh nerve palsy or other cranial nerve palsy contralateral to hemiparesis is consistent with brain stem infarct
	Motor	Assess for focal weakness. If leg is weakest, suspect anterior cerebral artery infarct. Middle cerebral artery lesions manifest as hemiplegia or face and arm weakness exceeding leg weakness. Subtle weakness of arms may be assessed by "drift" test. Have patient hold arms at 90-degree angle in front with eyes closed and watch for downward drifting of affected arm
	Sensory	Check response to pain, touch, and proprioception in all extremities
	Reflexes, at biceps, knee, ankle, and foot	Reflexes are usually decreased in distribution of weakness in acute stages. Inequality of reflexes and Babinski sign (upgoing great toe) are lateralizing signs
	Coordination, station, and gait	Gait, heel, and toe walking (if able), finger/nose and heel/knee/shin for cerebellar testing

who states that the neurologic symptoms that caused him or her to come to the emergency department are now resolved. A careful examination is still necessary to avoid missing subtle findings.

PROBLEM 2 On physical examination the patient was found to be alert and in acute distress. Blood pressure was 200/100 mm Hg, pulse 60/min and irregular, respirations 18/min, and temperature 98.4°F.

HEENT (head, eyes, ears, nose, throat): Mild arteriovenous nicking and early "copper-wiring" changes in the fundi, otherwise negative.
Neck: No bruits or JVD distention.
Lungs: Clear.
Cardiac: Grade 3 to 4/6 holosystolic murmur with palpable thrill at the base of the heart. One to two extrasystoles/min. No gallops.

Abdomen: Unremarkable.
Extremities: Unremarkable.
Neurologic: Obvious expressive aphasia, comprehends commands.
> Cranial nerves II to XII intact except for mild right central seventh nerve palsy.
> Motor: Right hemiparesis, greater in the upper extremity.
> Sensory: Decreased on right side to pain.
> Reflexes: Decreased on right side. Babinski reflexes positive on right.
> Cerebellar examination: Impaired on right side due to weakness, intact on left.

The findings were consistent with acute cerebrovascular disease. Before pursuing this pathway, other nonvascular disorders need to be considered, e.g., tumor, metabolic problem, subdural hematoma.

DECISION PRIORITIES AND PRELIMINARY DIFFERENTIAL DIAGNOSIS

Following data gathering, the emergency physician focuses on three questions.

1. *Are the findings due to a noncerebrovascular cause that may mimic a stroke syndrome?* Noncerebrovascular diseases to consider include:
   a. *Subdural and epidural hematoma.* Both forms may manifest with lateralizing signs. Subdural hematoma is more likely to be confused with stroke (see Chap. 50).
   b. *Postictal state with Todd's paralysis.* This condition is preceded by a history or physical findings consistent with seizure; it usually lasts 2 to 3 hours and has a rapidly improving neurologic pattern.
   c. *Occult neoplasm.* Rarely the onset is acute if a hemorrhage occurs within the tumor. More often there is an insidious onset associated with systemic symptoms, e.g., anorexia, weight loss.
   d. *Drug toxicity.* Although lateralizing deficits are rare, stroke can be caused by abuse of narcotics or sedative-hypnotics. This diagnosis is usually supported by a characteristic toxidrome (see Chap. 19). It can also be a complication of abuse because intravenous drug use increases the potential for brain abscess, septic emboli, and thrombotic stroke.
   e. *Metabolic encephalopathy.* Stroke syndromes rarely occur in patients with hypoxia, hypoglycemia, hyperthermia, or nonketotic hyperosmolar coma. Data gathering usually gives clues to these systemic diseases.
   f. *CNS infections.* Meningitis, encephalitis, and brain abscess rarely present as a stroke. Other signs of infection such as fever, elevated white blood cell count, immunosuppression, meningismus, headache, or a prodromal history may be present.
   g. *TIAs* have their own differential, including focal seizures, migraine aura, syncope, and dysrhythmias.
2. *What type of stroke is present?* Table 49-3 lists the major categories of stroke, along with a description of the typical presentation, associated symptoms and risk factors, and examination findings. The emergency physician considers which time course, progression, and overall pattern best fits the clinical picture. Choosing a specific stroke syndrome helps in selecting which patients will be benefited by computed tomography (CT) of the head and influences management. Questions that can help make this choice include:
   a. Are the neurologic examination results normal or abnormal at this time? If the examination results have returned to normal, the diagnosis is most consistent with a transient ischemic attack.
   b. Is the clinical course progressive, constant, or fluctuating?

TABLE 49-3. Stroke Symptoms—Differential Diagnosis

	Presentation	Associated Symptoms	Risk Factors	Physical Examination	Useful Tests	Additional Aspects
TIA	Sudden onset of symptoms (vision or speech change, focal weakness) Short duration—minutes to hours (maximum 24 hr)	Numbness/sensory loss Vertigo (basilar TIA) Speech change (dysarthria, aphasia) Gait change—ataxia Vision change (diplopia, field cut, monocular or bilateral vision loss)	Age Male sex Smoking ASCVD Hyperlipidemia Heart disease Hypercoagulable states	Usually normal unless attack still in progress Funduscopic changes Cardiac examination (murmur) Carotid bruits	Good HX/PE Noninvasive carotid evaluation Carotid arteriogram	20% to 60% of TIA patients have a stroke within 2–5 years
Stroke in evolution (progressive stroke)	Sudden onset of symptoms Duration >24 hr Progressive neurologic signs and symptoms	Same as above Nausea and vomiting on occasion	Same as above	Hypertension/bradycardia typical Possible dysrhythmia Neurologic examination findings are referable to involved area Funduscopic, carotid, and cardiac changes as above	Baseline laboratory studies CT scan of head Cerebral angiography (?)	Seen in approximately 15%–25% of stroke patients
Completed stroke	Sudden onset of symptoms Duration—permanent No progression or regression of symptoms	Same as above	Same as above	Same as above	Same as above	If thrombotic, may commonly develop during sleep with symptoms perceived on awakening in the morning (resulting from low flow through a stenotic area)

Embolic stroke	Sudden onset of symptoms Duration >24 hr	Same as above	Same, especially heart disease, e.g., atrial fibrillation and cardiac mural thrombus	Same—emphasis on cardiac examination	Same as above	May occur at any time; often follows exertion Often responsible for hemorrhagic infarction; friable clot dissolves with perfusion through ischemic vessels May be acutely associated with seizures in up to 20% of patients
Subarachnoid hemorrhage	Sudden onset of symptoms Severe headache, syncope and nuchal pain Focal neurologic signs, including cranial nerves	Nausea and vomiting Obtundation, sometimes comatose	None (aneurysms are congenital)	Hypertension/bradycardia Nuchal tenderness and rigidity to movement Fundi-subhyaloid hemorrhage or papilledema Dilated pupil if posterior communicating artery aneurysm Neurologic examination is nonfocal	Same as above LP considered if CT scan negative and if diagnosis still suspected	One-third from anterior communicating artery aneurysms One-fourth from middle carotid artery aneurysms One-fifth from posterior communicating artery aneurysm
Intracerebral hemorrhage	Sudden onset of symptoms (dense hemiplegia, hemianesthesia, field cut, obtundation) Duration >24 hr usually permanent	Usually comatose Rapid progression to loss of consciousness Reticular activating system impairment	Hypertension (brain-stem and basal ganglia) Anticoagulant therapy (frontal, parietal, temporal, and occipital lobes)	Usually comatose Cranial nerve findings, e.g., cranial nerve III palsy Hemiparesis/hemisensory loss, pinpoint pupils (pontine or cerebellar) Posturing Ataxia, vertigo, vomiting (cerebellar) Upgoing Babinski sign	Same as above, except LP not done	Occurs in approximately 10%–20% of stroke patients

ASCVD = atherosclerotic cerebrovascular disease
HX/PE = history and physical examination

c. Are there potential sources of cerebral emboli? Most of these sources are cardiac in nature. These patients require investigation for mural thrombus, atrial fibrillation, or valvular heart disease.
d. Most important, the possibility of intracranial hemorrhage must always be considered. Factors supporting this diagnosis are hypertension, anticoagulation therapy, headache, altered mental status, nuchal rigidity, and subhyaloid hemorrhage.

3. *Are any complications of stroke present or evolving?* The patient must be reassessed and treated for the major early complications noted in the initial approach:
   a. Airway compromise
   b. Dysrhythmias
   c. Hypertension
   d. Cerebral edema or herniation syndrome.

PROBLEM 1 There were no findings consistent with noncerebrovascular disease in the 55 year old white male who presented with fleeting loss of vision. The carotid bruit was very supportive of vascular disease. The resolution of symptoms pointed to a TIA, most likely embolic in origin. There was no reason to suspect intracranial hemorrhage. No complications were present.

PROBLEM 2 Two possibilities were entertained for this patient. The presentation was consistent with a completed stroke, and the patient's risk factors strongly support this diagnosis. However, the unexpected presence of a cardiac murmur and the reference to it in the patient's chart suggested the possibility of an embolic stroke. No complications were present, but the patient was at high risk and required repeated evaluation.

DIAGNOSTIC ADJUNCTS

The questions asked in the preliminary differential diagnosis allow the physician to select ancillary testing to either evaluate conditions that mimic stroke syndromes or determine whether an intracranial hemorrhage has occurred.

Laboratory Studies

In the patient with stroke-in-evolution or completed stroke, the first three sets of tests are usually ordered, with the exception of liver function tests.

1. Measurement of electrolytes and glucose and renal and liver function tests are ordered for patients suspected of having metabolic encephalopathy.

2. Complete blood count and clotting studies (prothrombin time [PT] and partial thromboplastin time [PTT], and platelets) are indicated in all patients in whom anticoagulation is being considered.

3. Measurement of arterial blood gases helps to evaluate patients for hypoxia and acidosis.

4. Drug screening is indicated if there is a history of drug ingestion or signs of a specific toxidrome.

Radiologic Imaging

Computed Tomography of the Head. CT is the most important diagnostic adjunct for diagnosing stroke syndromes. It has excellent sensitivity (greater than 90%) in detecting hemorrhagic or ischemic stroke. It can also differentiate between different disease processes that result in stroke symptoms (Fig. 49–2). Its advantages include its availability, simplicity, noninvasiveness, and relatively low cost. Indications for performing emergent CT imaging in stroke are (1) persistent, nonreversing, or progressive focal neurologic

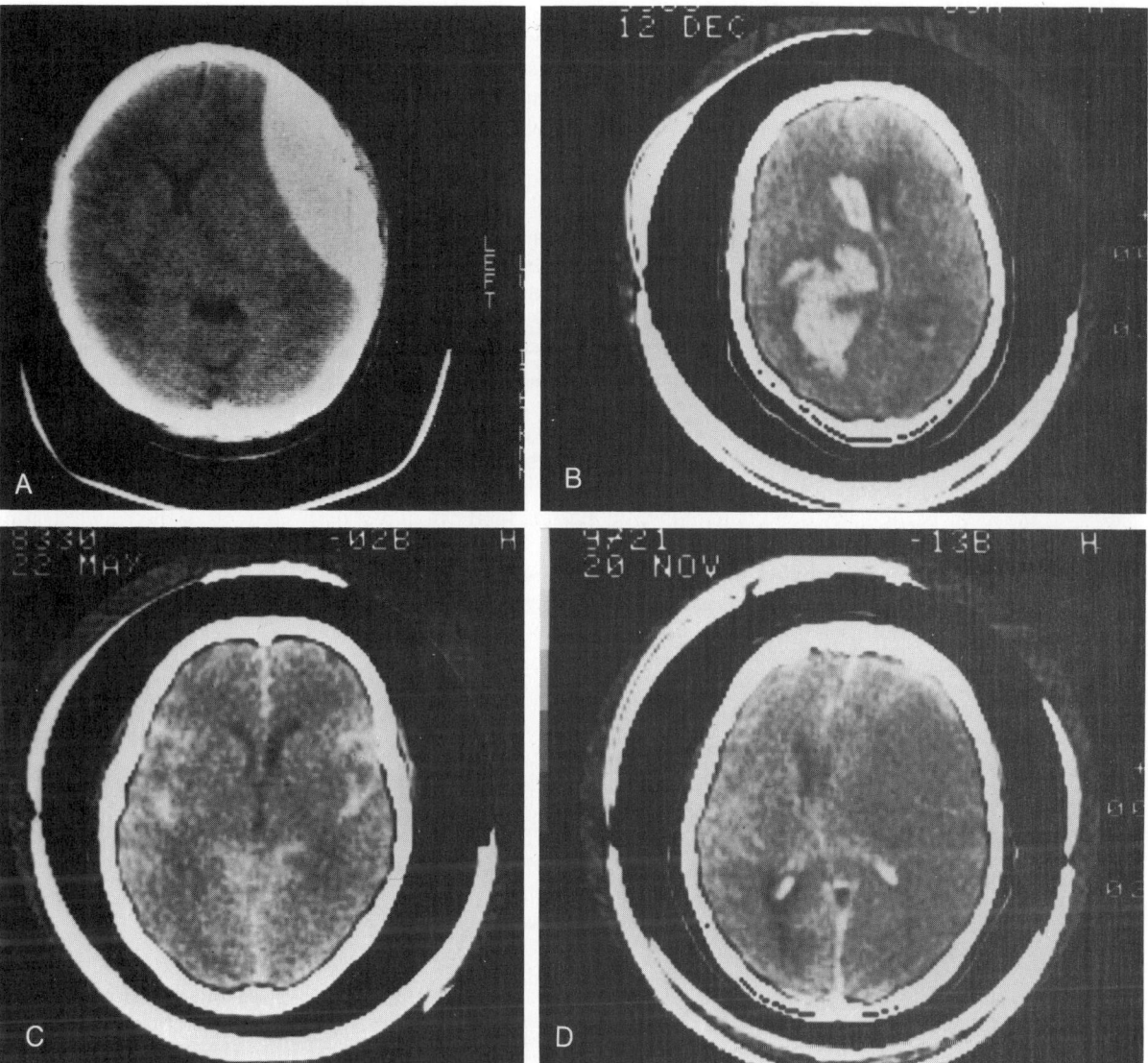

FIGURE 49–2. CT of head. Examples of discernible lesions that may manifest as an acute neurologic deficit. A, Acute epidural hematoma with midline shift secondary to mass effect and edema. B, Right thalamic intracerebral hemorrhage with surrounding edema. C, Subarachnoid hemorrhage with blood visible in the sylvian fissures and intracerebral sulci. D, Acute left hemispheric completed stroke with edema and midline shift.

findings on examination, (2) history or examination findings consistent with a diagnosis of subarachnoid hemorrhage, or (3) possibility that a structural brain lesion (e.g., hemorrhage, intracranial hematoma, aneurysm, tumor) is causing a depressed level of consciousness.

Caution is exercised in interpreting CT scans obtained within the first few hours of a completed stroke. Generally, an acute cerebral infarction is isodense radiographically. Acute changes may not be seen in the first 12 to 24 hours following an ischemic insult. An early "negative" CT scan does not rule out the possibility that cerebral infarction has occurred. A consistent sign found more than 24 hours after infarction is hypodensity in the affected area. Intracerebral hemorrhage, hemorrhagic infarctions, and up to 95% of subarachnoid hemorrhages are readily apparent on early CT scans.

Chest Radiographs. Standard posteroanterior and lateral chest films are ordered for patients with complete stroke, stroke-in-evolution, and those for whom admission is anticipated. A search is made for signs of aspiration, pneumonia, or tumor.

Cerebral Angiography. Angiography of the four cerebral arteries is performed by trans-femoral catheterization. It is used to visualize vascular abnormalities of the brain (arteriovenous malformations, tumors, or aneurysms), demonstrate displacement of cerebral vessels by mass effect, or, therapeutically, to occlude arteries with emboli or induced thrombi.

Carotid Angiography. Carotid angiography is a two-vessel, contrast-enhanced imaging procedure that reveals the common, internal, and external carotids. It is indicated in patients with symptomatic bruits of carotid origin or occasionally in patients without bruits who are symptomatic for TIA. It can delineate the nature of the lesion and the extent of arterial stenosis as well as the presence of other extracranial or intracranial vascular lesions. Arteriography is generally contraindicated during the acute stages of a stroke because the rate of complications and mortality is unacceptably high.

Magnetic Resonance Imaging. Magnetic resonance imaging (MRI) has the advantage of avoiding exposure to ionizing radiation and contrast media. It can visualize structures at the brain-bone interface and images some lesions that are not well visualized on CT, particularly demyelinated white matter. MRI can detect early changes in the concentration of brain water that occur in the first hours after an ischemic insult. In animal studies, brain ischemia of more than 6 hours' duration is routinely demonstrated by this means. Although it is too early to be definitive, MRI has the potential to become the imaging tool of choice in stroke patients in the emergency department.

Electrocardiogram

Electrocardiograms (ECG) are ordered in acute stroke to identify dysrhythmias diagnosed on the cardiac monitor. Some ischemic strokes have concomitant coronary ischemia. Atrial fibrillation suggests embolic stroke.

Special Procedures

Lumbar Puncture. Examining a sample of the cerebrospinal fluid (CSF) may allow detection of blood or xanthochromia indicative of an intracranial or subarachnoid hemorrhage that is not evident on the CT scan (occurring in approximately 5% to 10% of patients). This is the principle indication and benefit of lumbar puncture in patients with acute cerebrovascular disease. Rarely, it has been used to distinguish between hemorrhagic and nonhemorrhagic infarction when a CT scan is not available. It has many false negatives in this role, and a decision to anticoagulate a patient based on this test is not recommended. It is also done if there is a possibility of meningitis.

The procedure carries a risk of transtentorial herniation if increased intracranial pressure or a mass lesion exists. Therefore, unless meningitis is suspected, a CT scan is obtained first. The risk of herniation is relatively small in the absence of the signs and symptoms of increased intracranial pressure (e.g., headache, papilledema, decreased level of consciousness, unilateral dilated pupil, or other evidence of herniation).

Noninvasive Carotid Evaluation: Ultrasound Imaging and Oculoplethysmography. Asymptomatic carotid bruits are initially evaluated by noninvasive means. Though expert opinions vary, most do not require carotid angiography. These imaging techniques can differentiate external carotid and subclavian bruits from those of common and internal carotid origin. The latter are of greater clinical concern and may require carotid arteriographic evaluation. Noninvasive carotid tests are generally not available in the emergency department.

PROBLEM 1 This patient needed a noninvasive evaluation of his carotid bruits. The question in the emergency department concerned the urgency of consultation and the need for admission.

PROBLEM 2 Laboratory tests to rule out other possible causes of the patient's stroke were ordered. The values for the complete blood count, electrolytes, glucose, BUN, creatinine, arterial blood gases, and clotting studies were normal. There was no indication for a lumbar puncture in this patient. A CT scan was ordered and was interpreted as showing no mass effect, no hemorrhage, and no lucency.

REFINED DIFFERENTIAL DIAGNOSIS

The preliminary differential diagnosis emphasizes the cause of the patient's stroke, identifying the type of stroke and anticipating complications. Once it is found to be cerebrovascular in origin, the refined differential diagnosis is directed toward localizing its site in the central nervous system and determining the underlying cause. Findings on physical examination frequently help to localize the site of brain injury in a stroke. Although it is preferable to analyze the findings in the context of neuroanatomy, common findings are associated with specific vascular syndromes. The syndromes most commonly seen in the emergency department are listed below.

1. *Internal Carotid Syndrome.* This is a combination of hemiparesis, hemisensory deficit, aphasia, and hemianopsia.

2. *Middle Cerebral Artery Syndrome.* Contralateral hemiparesis or hemiplegia, contralateral impairment of sensation, dysarthria, and expressive or receptive aphasia comprise this syndrome. The face and arm are usually affected more than the leg.

3. *Anterior Cerebral Artery Syndrome.* Contralateral lower extremity paresis or paralysis, contralateral lower extremity sensory defect, urinary incontinence, and abnormalities in behavior are the main features of this syndrome.

4. *Vertebral Basilar Syndrome.* This is a combination of hemi- or quadriparesis, dysarthria, dysphagia, impaired sensation, vertigo, nausea, vomiting, nystagmus, diplopia, and internuclear ophthalmoplegia.

5. *Lateral Medullary (Wallenberg Syndrome).* The Wallenberg syndrome comprises vertigo, nausea, vomiting, nystagmus, dysphagia, ataxia, ipsilateral Horner's syndrome, and impaired sensation to face ipsilaterally and contralaterally in body.

6. *Lacunar Infarct Syndrome.* This entity involves thrombosis of the small penetrating end arteries. Patients are usually hypertensive and manifest isolated neurologic deficits. Lesions in the internal capsule produce pure motor hemiparesis, thalamic lesions cause contralateral sensory loss, and pontine infarcts produce ataxic hemiparesis.

PRINCIPLES OF MANAGEMENT

In patients with stroke most of the physician's effort is directed toward data gathering and differential diagnostic decisions. Beyond basic stabilization and anticipation and treatment of complications, most management decisions revolve around the use of antiplatelet drugs and anticoagulants.

General Management

1. Assessment and support of airway and breathing are used as indicated. Supplemental oxygen is given to improve oxygenation to the brain.

2. Circulation is assessed and supported as well. Intravenous access for IV fluid

therapy is established, and medications administered in all patients. ECG monitoring is maintained to assess cardiac rhythm abnormalities, and treatment is instituted if indicated.

3. Complications are anticipated. These include airway compromise, dysrhythmias, hypertension, and cerebral edema. Emergent management has been reviewed in the section on Initial Approach in the Emergency Department.

Treatment of Specific Syndromes

Transient Ischemic Attacks. No acute intervention is needed. Acute anticoagulation therapy with either heparin or sodium warfarin is controversial but is generally not recommended by most authorities. Both medications have unfavorable risk-benefit ratios. Aspirin is often started.

Stroke in Evolution. Intravenous heparin therapy is instituted following CT scanning if there is no evidence of bleeding. Heparin inhibits the propagation of thromboemboli and is instituted in the presence of a fluctuating neurologic picture or progressive stroke.

Complete Thrombotic Stroke. Blood pressure is monitored, and the patient is observed for signs of developing cerebral edema. Because the deficit is complete, there is no need for anticoagulation.

Embolic Stroke. Heparinization is indicated to promote mural thrombus resolution, prevent recurrences, and inhibit propagation of cerebral thromboemboli. A CT scan is done to rule out hemorrhagic infarct before anticoagulation therapy is given. This therapy may be deferred if the stroke is massive.

Subarachnoid Hemorrhage. Priorities include placing the patient in a dark and quiet room to reduce cerebral stimulation and vasospasm, maintaining adequate arterial blood pressure, and treating cerebral edema appropriately. Early neurosurgical consultation is necessary. Intracranial pressure monitoring may be indicated.

Intracerebral Hemorrhage. The mass effect caused by the intracerebral hematoma and associated cerebral edema are treated with selected use of hyperventilation, diuretics, and positional maneuvers. Acute neurosurgical intervention for evacuation of the hematoma is controversial.

Anticoagulation Therapy

Heparinization. Specific indications for acute heparinization include progressive stroke (stroke in evolution) and embolic stroke in the absence of cerebral hemorrhage on the initial CT scan.

Thrombolytic Therapy (Streptokinase, Urokinase, Tissue Plasminogen Activator [tPA]). These therapies are still undefined for the treatment of cerebrovascular disease, and there are no clear guidelines for their use.

Antiplatelet Agents. Antiplatelet agents such as aspirin, dipyridamole, and sulfinpyrazone have been advocated for patients with transient ischemic attacks. There is no evidence that the last two drugs are more effective than aspirin. Studies have found that antiplatelet agents have some beneficial effect on subsequent TIAs, cerebral infarction, and death. The sex of the patient, the degree of vascular stenosis, and the dose of the antiplatelet agent may influence these results. The decision about whether to use antiplatelet agents is generally made in consultation with the neurologist or primary care physician who will follow the patient.

PROBLEM 2 In the absence of hemorrhagic changes on the CT scan and because of concern about a potential embolic etiology of the stroke, heparinization is begun acutely. Plans are made to evaluate the murmur echocardiographically on an inpatient basis.

SPECIAL CONSIDERATIONS

Pediatric Patients

Pediatric patients presenting with a stroke usually have either an intracranial hemorrhage or a vascular occlusion. The pathophysiology of both disease processes differs from that seen in adults. Intracranial hemorrhage in children most often occurs after rupture of an arteriovenous malformation or congenital (berry) aneurysm. Less commonly, a hemostatic deficit (thrombocytopenia, hemophilia, leukemia) or occult head trauma with subdural or epidural hematoma may be seen. The clinical picture is similar to that characteristic of adults with the exception of children under 2 years of age. Any significant decrease in the level of consciousness in these patients warrants early CT evaluation. Therapy is usually supportive, with embolization of arteriovenous malformations and surgical drainage of intracranial hematomas performed at the discretion of the neurosurgeon.

Acute vascular occlusion is less common and may occur secondary to arterial embolization or thrombosis (e.g., acute infantile hemiplegia) or secondary to venous thrombosis of the cerebral sinuses. Acute infantile hemiplegia occurs most commonly in children between 1 and 3 years of age, but similar presentations may occur in older children. Most commonly, the disease is idiopathic, but it can be caused by other diseases such as sickle cell anemia, lupus erythematosus, congenital heart disease with embolization, polycythemia, or acute arteritis (polyarteritis nodosa, Takayasu's disease). The clinical presentation mimics that of an acute stroke. Treatment is supportive with concomitant treatment of the underlying or pathogenic condition. There is usually residual hemiparesis, spasticity, and mild intellectual or behavioral impairment following the illness, but the degree of functional recovery is usually greater than that seen in adults with stroke. Cerebral venous thrombosis usually occurs secondary to local sinus infection or dehydration. Secondary cerebral edema results in increased intracranial pressure, obtundation, a bulging fontanelle, and seizures. The diagnosis is primarily clinical and therapy is supportive, with concomitant treatment of cerebral edema and underlying conditions. Rarely, either traumatic or nontraumatic carotid artery dissection can be the etiology of stroke in the younger patient.

Geriatric Patients

To understand the special problems of stroke in the elderly, one must understand the pathophysiology of aging. Decreased functional reserve in most organ systems, decreased sensitivity to the perception of painful stimuli, decreased resistance to the pathophysiologic processes of infection and malignancy, increased likelihood of drug interactions and intolerances, and survival into the peak age range for many serious diseases all place the geriatric patient at significant risk. Misdiagnosis of a treatable entity mimicking acute stroke, a less obvious clinical presentation of stroke when the medical and functional baseline is previously impaired, and a more complicated clinical course due to the above factors are all commonly encountered in the treatment of elderly patients. Decisions about immediate anticoagulation in management may be extremely complex because the etiology of stroke may be unclear and relative contraindications to anticoagulation may exist.

Previously Impaired Patients

In a patient with a previous history of chronic medical diseases (e.g., the nursing home patient), the diagnosis of stroke can be exceedingly difficult. If the patient is normally obtunded, demented, has had a previous stroke, or has extreme functional impairment, the appearance of neurologic findings with acute stroke may be extremely subtle. A large number of other disease presentations may mimic that of acute stroke, may contribute to its etiology, or may complicate its clinical course. They must be considered in these patients. For example, in a patient with controlled congestive heart failure and ischemic heart disease, a routine urinary tract infection may increase demands on cardiac output, resulting in worsening heart failure, silent infarction, and development of a mural thrombus with embolic stroke. Without pain, the clinical presentation would likely be mild dyspnea, refusal to eat or ambulate, obtundation, or other functional impairment. For these reasons, evaluation of the previously impaired patient must be complete, and attention must be paid to subtle changes from the baseline level of functioning. A thorough search for other mimicking or complicating conditions is necessary. These patients are difficult to diagnose and treat.

Due to decreased physiologic reserve, specific treatment may create a complicated clinical course. For example, tube feedings may result in hyperosmolar complications; fluid therapy can cause dehydration, overhydration, or electrolyte imbalance; catheterization for incontinence may lead to urosepsis; and prolonged bed rest may lead to bedsores, thrombophlebitis, and pulmonary embolism. These considerations are more germane during the later phases of hospital management but may be contributing factors in the patient coming to the emergency department from an extended care or convalescent center.

DISPOSITION AND FOLLOW-UP

The status of the neurologic deficit and its potential source are the primary factors in disposition decisions.

Admission

Patients presenting with an acute completed or evolving stroke require admission to a monitored bed. Serial monitoring of the deficit, anticipation and treatment of complications, and patient comfort are all appropriate reasons for admission. Admission to the intensive care unit is required to manage subarachnoid and intracerebral hemorrhage, obtunded patients, and those with complications.

Discharge

The only subset of stroke patients who are considered for discharge are those presenting with transient ischemic attacks (TIAs). The preferred course of action is to admit these patients for expedited noninvasive assessment and then carotid arteriography and possible endarterectomy as necessary. However, outpatient evaluation is acceptable if the patient has completely recovered, is expected to be compliant, and arrangements for close follow-up can be made. Neurologic consultation is generally obtained over the telephone in the emergency department to discuss the case and establish clear follow-up instructions. Any early recurrence of symptoms should prompt emergent admission and expedited work-up.

PROBLEM 1 The 55 year old man with fleeting change of vision (amaurosis fugax) was seen by the neurologic consultant in the emergency department. A CT scan was obtained and was normal. Arrangements were made for noninvasive carotid studies to be done within 48 hours, and follow-up was planned with the neurologist.

Some patients, even with neurologic signs and symptoms that have completely resolved, may still have a cerebral infarction. This patient's symptoms were most consistent with an ophthalmic artery embolus causing a transient ischemic attack. Because these emboli most commonly arise from the carotid artery, diagnostic evaluation of the carotids is indicated.

DOCUMENTATION

1. Nature of symptoms, their onset, duration, and progression.
2. Functional baseline of the patient (especially if there has been previous disease or debilitation), and recent changes from that baseline.
3. Associated symptoms and pertinent absence of symptoms based on the neurologic review of symptoms.
4. Prior occurrences of neurologic symptoms (e.g., previous TIAs).
5. Risk factors for cerebrovascular disease.
6. Medications, allergies, and past medical history.
7. Vital signs, general appearance, examination findings (particularly bruits, heart, lungs, and detailed neurologic examination).
8. Ancillary test results including CT scan if available.
9. Diagnosis and disposition.

SUMMARY AND FINAL POINTS

- Initial patient care efforts are focused on basic stabilization and assessment of the extent of the deficit and its possible cause.
- A high index of suspicion and mental preparation is maintained for complications including airway compromise, dysrhythmias, high or low blood pressure, cerebral edema, or herniation syndrome.
- The history and physical examination help differentiate patients with cerebrovascular disease from patients with other diseases that produce stroke symptoms.
- Identification of candidates for CT head scanning, for anticoagulation therapy, and for emergent neurosurgical consultation early in the course of care is an important goal of management.
- Admission is usually the appropriate disposition for patients with symptoms of cerebrovascular origin. Patients with new onset of obtundation, progressive neurologic findings, or complications are candidates for admission to the intensive care unit.

BIBLIOGRAPHY

Books

1. Brant-Zawadzki M: Ischemia. In Stark DD, Bradley WG: Magnetic Resonance Imaging. St. Louis, Mosby, 1988.
2. Henry GL, Little N: Neurologic emergencies—a symptom oriented approach. New York, McGraw-Hill, 1985.
3. Issacs B: The central nervous system—stroke. In Brocklehurst JC: Textbook of Geriatric Medicine and Gerontology (3rd ed). New York, Churchill Livingston, 1985.
4. Tootle JF: Cerebrovascular Disorders (3rd ed). New York, Raven Press, 1984.

Journal Articles

1. Bosker G: Diagnostic challenges and therapeutic strategies in focal neurologic lesions. Emerg Med Rep, 9:65–72, 1988.
2. Fayle RW, Van Horn G, Grotta K: Cerebrovascular disease: Differential features and diagnostic tests. Texas Med 77:59–62, 1981.
3. Grotta JC: Current medical and surgical therapy for cerebrovascular disease. N Engl J Med, 317:1505–1516, 1987.
4. Hogan EL, Graham D: Instituting early intervention in subarachnoid hemorrhage. Emerg Med Rep 7:25–32, 1986.
5. Jordan S: Emergency department care of the stroke patient (Parts I and II). Dig Emerg Med Care 4: Vol. 6 (pp. 1–8); Vol. 7 (pp. 1–8), 1984.
6. LeBlanc R: The minor leak preceding subarachnoid hemorrhage. J Neurosurg 66:35–39, 1987.
7. Nakano KK: An overview of stroke: Epidemiology, classification, risk factors, and clinical aspects. Postgrad Med 80:82–99, 1986.
8. Stroke Prevention in Atrial Fibrillation Study Group Investigators: Preliminary report of the Stroke Prevention in Atrial Fibrillation Study. N Engl J Med 322:863–868, 1990.
9. Timerding BL, Barsan WG: Stroke patient evaluation in the emergency department before pharmacologic therapy. AJEM, 7:11–15, 1989.
10. Vollman PW: Eldrup-Jorgensen J, Hoffman MA: The role of cranial computed tomography in carotid surgery. Surg Clin North Am 66:255–268, 1986.
11. Werdelin L, Juhler M: The course of transient ischemic attacks. Neurology 38:677–680, 1988.

CHAPTER 50

HEAD AND NECK TRAUMA

KILBOURN GORDON III, M.D.

PROBLEM 1 A 24 year old man was assessed by paramedics at the scene of a motor vehicle accident. He had sustained massive facial injuries and lay semiconscious on the driver's seat. His respirations were impeded by blood accumulating in the oropharynx.

PROBLEM 2 A 21 year old man was brought to the emergency department in the back of a pick-up truck after sustaining an accident in an all-terrain vehicle. He was lying on his back complaining of neck pain and paresthesias going down both arms. He had no visible signs of trauma.

PROBLEM 3 A 45 year old alcoholic was found unconscious on the street. The paramedics suspected a head injury. His street friends said he had been in a fight 5 days earlier.

QUESTIONS TO CONSIDER

1. What is the appropriate initial management of the potentially unstable cervical spine?
2. What are the different types of injuries involving the head or neck? Which have catastrophic potential?
3. What key factors in the history and physical examination help in the diagnosis of specific head and neck injuries?
4. What are the indications for plain radiographs of the head and neck?
5. When is emergency computed tomography of the head indicated?
6. What is the appropriate emergency management of serious head and neck injuries?
7. When is consultation with a neurosurgeon important?
8. Which patients with head and neck injuries can appropriately be discharged with follow-up by their primary physician?

INTRODUCTION

Trauma to the head and neck is commonly seen in the emergency department. Motor vehicle trauma accounts for the majority of the 400,000 patients with head injuries admitted to hospitals each year in the United States. Head trauma is responsible for 1% to 3% of all deaths and 26% of trauma-related deaths each year in the United States. In 30% to 40% of this latter group, acute alcohol intoxication is a complicating factor.

Spinal cord injury is estimated to occur annually in 50 persons per 1 million population. It is often found concomitantly with head trauma. As with head trauma, spinal injury is often associated with motor vehicle accidents in which the patient is intoxicated. Other, less common causes include falls or falling objects, gunshot wounds, and water sports.

Anatomy of the Head and Neck

Knowledge of the normal anatomy of the head and neck is necessary to understand the significance of abnormal findings on physical examination or radiologic films. Figure 50–1 illustrates the normal cervical vertebrae. Their important components are the vertebral body, the pedicle, the articular process (also known as the facet), the laminae, and the spinous process. The spinal cord is enclosed in the space bordered by the vertebral body anteriorly and the laminae laterally. These basic anatomic structures are present through the entire vertebral column, although the shape varies in the cervical, thoracic, lumbar, and sacral regions. Figure 50–2 illustrates the lateral view of the cervical spine. The first cervical vertebra (C1), the atlas, has a ring structure with an absent vertebral body. The second cervical vertebra (C2), the axis, has a vertically enlarged vertebral body called the *dens axis* or *odontoid process*. The dens projects superiorly through the ring of C1 and is attached by the dentate ligament. The arrangement allows for a 180-degree plus rotation of the skull on the cervical spine. The nonbony ligamentous supporting elements of the cervical spine are important in maintaining bony alignment and are composed of the anterior longitudinal ligament, the posterior longitudinal ligament, the ligamentum flavum, and the ligamentum nuchae.

The scalp consists of five layers, the most important of which are the galea aponeurotica and the dermis. The galea is a fibrous, nonelastic covering that lies directly adjacent to the skull. The skull consists of three layers, the middle layer consisting of cancellous bone and the outer and inner aspects consisting of the outer and inner tables, respectively. The brain is enveloped by three layers of coverings—the dura mater, the arachnoid, and the pia mater. The dura is the dense, fibrous, nonelastic outermost layer and is part of the protective structure for the brain. The arachnoid is a thin, vascular middle layer. It has a role in brain nutrition and produces cerebrospinal fluid (CSF). The innermost layer, the pia, closely envelopes the brain matter throughout its sulci and gyri and has a role in nutrition.

Pathophysiology
Spinal Injuries

Causes of cervical spine injuries can be categorized into discrete mechanisms of injury according to the direction of force causing the injury. These are (1) flexion injuries, (2)

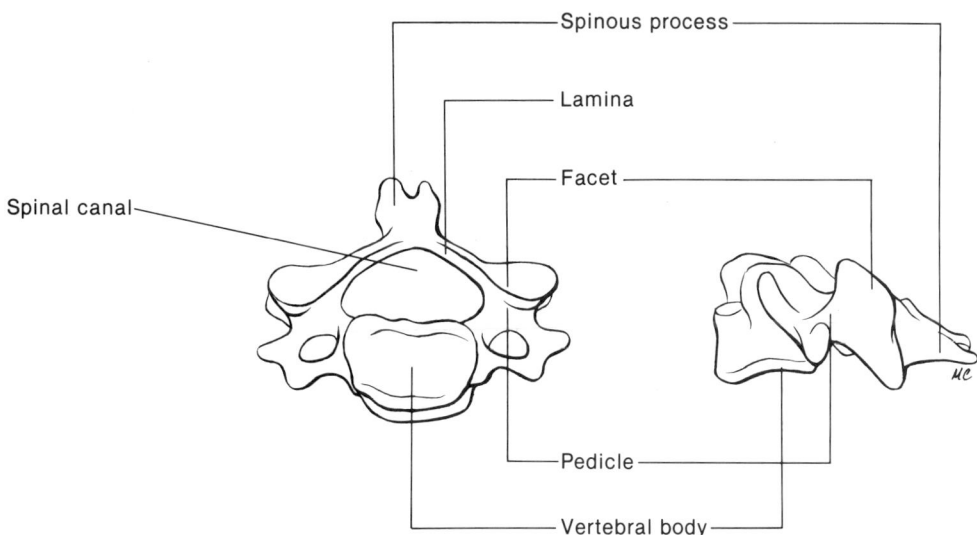

FIGURE 50–1. *Cervical vertebrae C3 through C7, superior and lateral aspects. (Redrawn from Gerlock AJ: Advanced Exercises in Diagnostic Radiology: The Cervical Spine in Trauma. Philadelphia, Saunders, 1978.)*

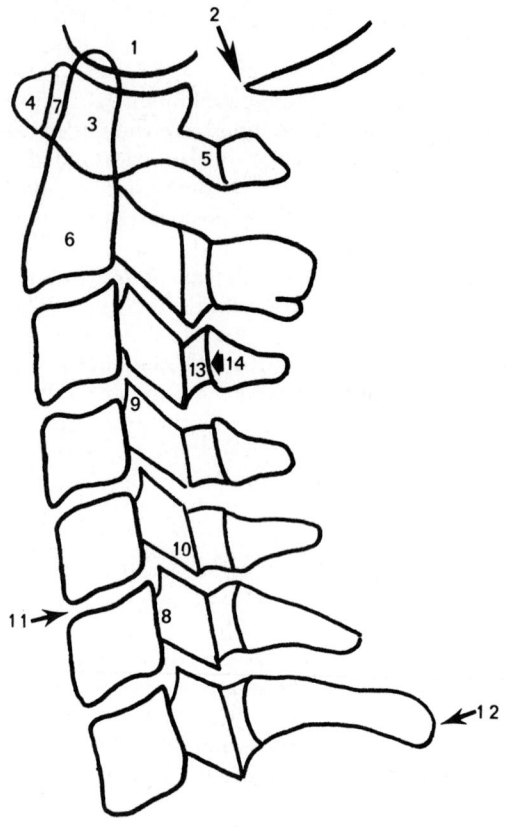

FIGURE 50–2. Cervical vertebrae C1 through C7, lateral aspects. (1) Occipital condyle of skull, (2) posterior margin of foramen magnum, (3) odontoid process or dens of C2, (4) anterior arch of C1, (5) posterior arch of C1, (6) C2 vertebral body, (7) space between the posterior surface of the anterior arch of C1 and the anterior surface of the odontoid process, (8) pedicle of C6, (9) superior articular process of C4, (10) inferior articular process of C5, (11) intervertebral disc space between C5 and C6, (12) tip of spinous process of C7, (13) lamina of C3, and (14) spinolaminar junction of C3. (From Gerlock AJ: Advanced Exercises in Diagnostic Radiology: The Cervical Spine in Trauma. Philadelphia, Saunders, 1978.)

extension injuries, (3) rotational injuries, and (4) vertical compression injuries. Flexion injuries are the most common and cause five times the morbidity and mortality compared with the other mechanisms. A spinal cord injury can be the result of a bony injury such as a fracture, dislocation, or fracture-dislocation, or a nonbony injury such as a ruptured or buckled ligament, extrusion of the disc, or vascular compromise. It is important to remember that interpretation of a cervical spine radiographic series as "normal" does not rule out significant cord pathology in the acute setting.

Head Injuries

Head trauma consists of skull injury and brain tissue injury (Table 50–1). The first category, skull injury, is divided into (1) fractures of the cerebral vault, in which the location and depth of the fracture are most important clinically, and (2) fractures of the skull base, in which the fracture may not be seen radiographically but is diagnosed by

TABLE 50–1. Classification of Traumatic Head Injuries

Skull Injuries	Focal Injuries	Diffuse Brain Injuries
Vault fracture	Epidural hematoma	Mild concussion
Linear	Subdural hematoma	Classic cerebral concussion
Depressed	Contusion	Prolonged coma
Basilar fracture	Intracerebral hematoma	Mild diffuse Axonal injury
		Moderate diffuse axonal injury
		Severe diffuse axonal injury

From Gennarelli TA: Emergency department management of head injuries. Emerg Med Clin North Am 2:750, 1984.

the clinical findings such as CSF rhinorrhea or otorrhea, periorbital ecchymosis (raccoon eyes), or a late-appearing ecchymosis located in the mastoid area behind the ear (Battle's sign).

Brain tissue injury may be divided into focal injury and diffuse brain injury. *Focal injuries* include

1. Cerebral contusion, resulting in multiple small isolated hemorrhages in the brain parenchyma.
2. Epidural hematoma, caused by arterial bleeding that produces a hematoma external to the dura. It often results from a skull fracture lying adjacent to the middle meningeal artery.
3. Subdural hematoma, caused by venous bleeding between the dura and the subarachnoid membrane following blunt trauma.
4. Intracerebral hematoma, resulting from intracerebral bleeding after severe brain parenchymal disruption or subsequent tissue ischemia and necrosis.

Diffuse brain injuries include

1. Mild concussion, manifested as rapidly resolving temporary neurologic dysfunction or short-term loss of consciousness.
2. Classic cerebral concussion, manifested as slowly resolving temporary neurologic dysfunction, typically memory loss, often accompanied by a significant loss of consciousness (more than 5 minutes to hours).
3. Diffuse axonal injury, resulting in a prolonged comatose state. Mild and moderate forms of diffuse axonal injury rarely result in coma lasting more than 24 hours. The severe form of diffuse axonal injury is associated with brain stem dysfunction and is due to the involvement of the reticular activating system; the coma may last for months.

All forms of brain injury, whether resulting from penetrating or closed head trauma, result in swelling of the cerebral tissue. Vasogenic and cytogenic pathophysiologic processes active at the cellular level result in cerebral edema and increased intracranial pressure (ICP). The cranial vault, being a closed space, can accommodate only a limited amount of brain swelling before rising ICP compromises cerebral perfusion pressure. Another complication of brain edema and increased intracranial pressure is the creation of pressure gradients across the relatively fixed membranes within the skull. Pressure across these membranes may shift tissue and result in a *brain herniation syndrome*. These herniations exist in at least four patterns:

1. Uncal herniation, in which unilateral cerebral swelling or mass lesions force the ipsilateral medial portion of the temporal lobe into the tentorial hiatus, compressing the oculomotor nerve and becoming manifest as an ipsilateral fixed, dilated pupil. The cerebral peduncle is also compressed, causing a contralateral hemiparesis and a depressed level of consciousness.
2. Central herniation, in which bilateral uncal herniation occurs owing to downward displacement of both hemispheres from diffuse swelling or bilateral lesions. This leads to coma, Cheyne-Stokes respirations, decorticate posturing, and death.
3. Cingulate herniation, in which the cingulate gyrus moves laterally underneath the falx cerebri leading to cerebral ischemia. Although interesting anatomically, it is rarely diagnosed clinically.
4. Cerebellar tonsil herniation is a relatively rare complication of blunt head trauma. It results in medullary compression with respiratory arrest and death.

Figure 50–3 illustrates the normal intracranial relationships and the first three herniation syndromes.

PREHOSPITAL CARE

Prehospital care of the head- or neck-injured victim begins with the primary survey, attention to cervical spine immobilization, and careful extrication. The following infor-

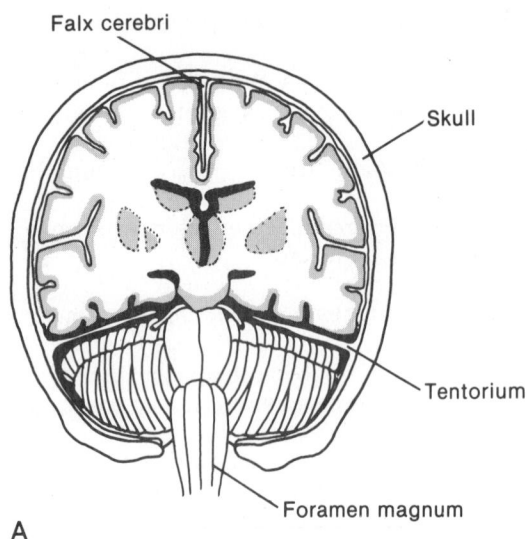
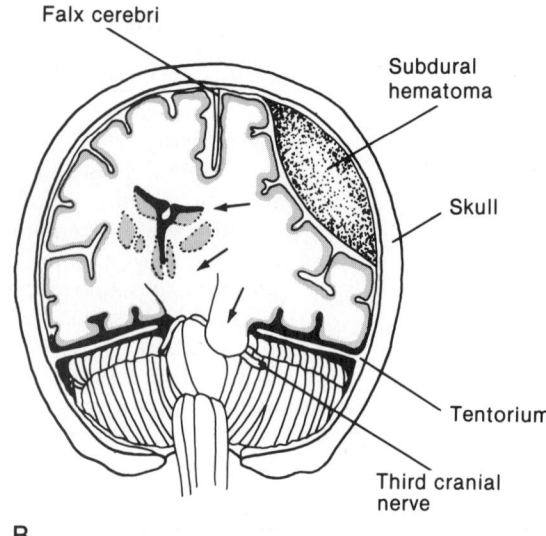
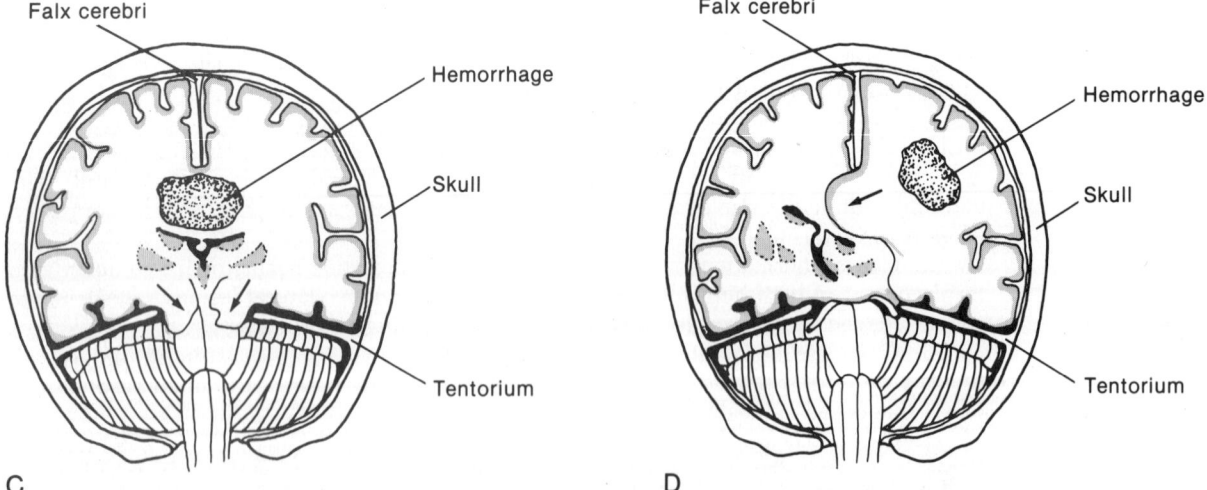

FIGURE 50–3. Herniation syndromes. A, Normal relationship of intracranial structures. B, Uncal transtentorial herniation syndrome. C, Central herniation syndrome. D, Cingulate herniation. (From Rosen P: *Emergency Medicine: Concepts and Clinical Practice.* St. Louis, Mosby, 1988.)

mation is obtained by the rescue squad and transmitted by radio, or given on arrival in the emergency department.

History

1. Mechanism of injury
   a. Motor vehicle accident—vehicle type, speed, and impact specifics are obtained. Use or nonuse of seat belt and condition of windshield and steering wheel are noted. The goal is to give early information on the forces involved.
   b. Gunshot wound—type of weapon (high- or low-velocity), caliber, and range are noted.
2. Time elapsed since injury.
3. Major medical problems.
4. Possible use of drugs or alcohol complicating the clinical presentation.

Physical Examination

1. Airway status: patency and protection of the airway (gag reflex).
2. Breathing status: spontaneous breathing, respiratory effort required (use of accessory muscles).
3. Cardiovascular status: blood pressure, pulse rate, and capillary refill time.
4. Level of consciousness: The Glasgow Coma Scale is used to measure the level of consciousness, including eye opening, verbal response, and motor response (see Table 50–2). A score of less than 8 is defined as coma.
5. Presence of neck pain.
6. Location and extent of other injuries.

Prehospital Intervention

Airway and Cervical Spine. Cervical spine immobilization is initiated in concert with airway assessment. Management of the airway can be a difficult problem for ambulance personnel. All trauma patients are placed in a supine, immobilized position. Consequently the tongue or debris may occlude the airway and attentive suctioning is often necessary. The patient who is able to protect his airway and is breathing satisfactorily is provided

TABLE 50–2. Glasgow Coma Scale

Eyes open	
Never	1
To pain	2
To verbal stimuli	3
Spontaneously	4
Best verbal response	
No response	1
Incomprehensible sounds	2
Inappropriate words	3
Disoriented and converses	4
Oriented and converses	5
Best motor response	
No response	1
Extension (decerebrate rigidity)	2
Flexion abnormal (decorticate rigidity)	3
Flexion withdrawal	4
Localizes pain	5
Obeys	6
Total	3–15

From Jennett B, Teasdale G: Aspects of coma after severe head injury. Lancet 1:878–881, 1977.

with supplemental oxygen. Patients who are unable to protect their airway or who have acute respiratory failure are treated with orotracheal intubation or an esophageal obturator airway. In both techniques, strict in-line immobilization of the cervical spine is imperative. Flexion or extension may exacerbate an obvious or occult injury. The rescue squad immobilizes the cervical spine using a firm cervical collar, e.g., a Philadelphia-type collar (Fig. 50–4). Additional support is provided by placing sandbags adjoining the base of the collar and by taping of the head to the backboard. On rare occasions, when an obvious neurologic deficit exists, personnel may immobilize the spine in the exact position in which the patient's head is oriented to the body.

Although rarely needed in the field, needle or surgical cricothyroidotomy is performed when massive facial trauma precludes the use of oropharyngeal intubation or an esophageal obturator airway. These procedures are reviewed in Chapter 2.

Intravenous Access. At least one large-bore intravenous (IV) line (16-gauge or larger) is placed. The initial flow rate is low to minimize cerebral edema. It is increased as necessary in response to hemodynamic instability. The initial fluid of choice is isotonic crystalloid.

Oxygen. All patients receive supplemental oxygen. Hypoxemia has been documented in up to 40% of patients with head injury.

Naloxone and Glucose. Patients with a depressed level of consciousness are given thiamine 100 mg, 50% dextrose 25 to 50 g, and naloxone 2 mg intravenously. The patient is observed for improvement, and changes are recorded. Optimally, blood is obtained for serum glucose determination prior to administration of 50% dextrose.

Increased Intracranial Pressure. In a patient with a severe head injury and a Glasgow Coma Scale score of less than 8, increased intracranial pressure is assumed. Moderate hyperventilation is initiated in the prehospital setting. This usually necessitates endotracheal intubation.

PROBLEM 1 The 24 year old male victim of the motor vehicle accident required multiple attempts at suctioning the blood from his oropharynx. Attempts to control

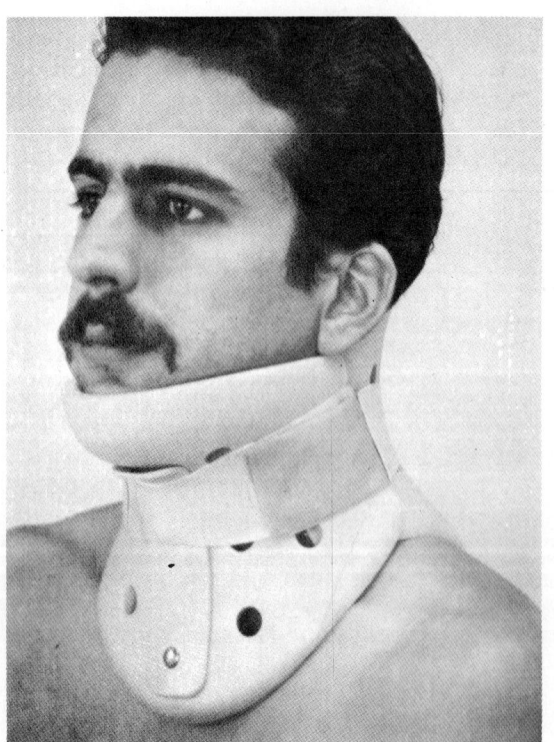

FIGURE 50–4. Philadelphia-type collar. Two-piece collar supports occiput, chin, and sides when two halves are joined by Velcro straps. (From Dick T, Land R: Spinal immobilization devices. Part I: Cervical extrication collars. J Emerg Med Services 7:29, 1982.)

hemorrhage from his nose by direct pressure were unsuccessful, and orotracheal intubation with in-line immobilization was performed. The patient showed decorticate posturing, produced only moaning sounds, and did not open his eyes on command. An IV line was started, and the "coma cocktail" was given en route to the hospital.

There are at least five reasons for active airway management in the field in this patient: questionable patency of the airway due to hemorrhage, questionable ability to protect the airway, problems with secretions, assumed need for oxygen supplementation, and a head injury with a Glasgow Coma Scale score of 6 that strongly suggested the need for hyperventilation. This patient requires transport to a qualified trauma center as fast as possible.

PROBLEM 3 The 45 year old alcoholic who was found unconscious on the street was placed in a hard cervical collar during the initial evaluation. The patient had a gag reflex and was breathing spontaneously; supplemental oxygen was given. He had spontaneous eye opening and made gutteral noises. The combination of naloxone 2 mg, thiamine 100 mg, and 50% dextrose 50 ml (25 g) was administered intravenously during transport to the hospital. No improvement in mental status was observed during the subsequent 10 minutes. He grimaced and withdrew his arm during intravenous line placement.

The most important sign in an isolated head trauma patient is the level of consciousness. The Glasgow Coma Scale is the single best approach to providing a "universal vocabulary" and provides an *objective* method for prehospital personnel to use to measure the baseline level of consciousness and assess changes during transport. The patient's Glasgow Coma Scale score as described is 10.

INITIAL APPROACH IN THE EMERGENCY DEPARTMENT

Patients with significant head or neck trauma are brought immediately into the major resuscitation room. Principles of the initial management include (1) stabilizing the cardiovascular status, (2) assessing and monitoring the level of consciousness, and (3) protecting the patient from further injury. The following activities are performed:

1. Oxygen is given at 4 to 8 liters/min flow. Adjust according to response or results of laboratory tests.
2. Vital signs, including temperature, are checked and compared with vital signs taken by prehospital personnel.
3. Intravenous access is confirmed or established. The goal is to use the least amount of fluid needed to stabilize the patient because of the presence of cerebral edema. The fluid is chosen in the context of hemodynamic stability. A frequent tally of the amount given is useful.
4. A cardiac monitor is placed, and the initial rhythm is observed.
5. The clothing is removed without disrupting head-body alignment.
6. The level of consciousness is determined and documented in descriptive terms, e.g., "response to pain is slight withdrawal of extremities," or "speech is absent spontaneously." The Glasgow Coma Scale is recalculated based on the initial examination in the emergency department.
7. Extensive hemorrhage from head or neck wounds is immediately controlled with direct pressure.
8. A screening neurologic examination is performed to assess pupillary size and reactivity, position and movement of the eyes, symmetry of motor movement and reflexes of extremities, and gross respiratory pattern.

9. The history is confirmed while prehospital personnel are still present.

10. If it was not done in the field, the neck is immobilized with a Philadelphia-type collar and sandbags. This is done while maintaining the in-line position of the head and neck. If the patient is responsive, the physician's concerns about possible neck injury are conveyed, and the patient is asked to cooperate by not moving the head.

The primary survey may reveal other trauma-related injuries. These injuries may have higher priorities for treatment than the head or neck injury (see Chap. 4). Once the airway is secured and the neck is immobilized, attention is focused on the condition of the heart, lungs, and abdomen.

PROBLEM 1 The patient's vital signs were blood pressure 140/100 mm Hg, heart rate 110 beats/min, respiratory rate 20/min and controlled. Proper endotracheal tube placement was confirmed by auscultation. A second IV line was placed. The patient continued to exhibit a Glasgow Coma Scale score of 6. Laboratory tests included arterial blood gas measurements to measure the level of oxygenation and the effect of hyperventilation, a complete blood count, and blood type and cross-match for 4 units of blood. Massive facial trauma precluded nasogastric tube placement. CT scan personnel and the neurosurgeon were notified of the patient's arrival and condition.

PROBLEM 2 This patient was alert, opened his eyes, spoke spontaneously, and followed simple commands. Vital signs were within normal limits. The Glasgow Coma Scale score was 15. He described neck pain and paresthesias of his hands. A hard collar was placed, and the patient was told about the physician's concern about spinal cord injury. He was very cooperative. A screening examination, including a neurologic examination, found only symmetric upper extremity weakness of extension at the elbow and wrist flexion.

PROBLEM 3 The condition of this patient had deteriorated. On examination, he did not open his eyes, made no noise, and had no motor response to pain. This was a Glasgow Coma Scale score of 3. His right pupil was dilated 6 mm in diameter and nonreactive. The left pupil was 3 mm and was found to be nonreactive in the primary survey. The emergency physician confirmed the prehospital Glasgow Coma Scale score of 10 with the medics and was concerned about brain herniation. The patient was endotracheally intubated, and hyperventilation was started. An immediate CT scan of the head was ordered, and a call was placed to the neurosurgeon. Other stabilizing measures were instituted.

Head trauma, neck trauma, and a potentially vulnerable airway are *always* assumed to be interconnected. Problems are anticipated in all of them, even if the initial data show only one at risk.

DATA GATHERING

The history and physical examination are important means of determining signs or symptoms of neurologic dysfunction following head or neck trauma. Serial examinations are necessary to demonstrate an evolving neurologic injury.

History

1. *Trauma event*. The history, although previously discussed with ambulance personnel, is now sought directly from the patient. The patient is asked: What *events* preceded the *trauma*? What is *remembered* of the trauma? Was there *loss* of *consciousness*? Were any *drugs* or *alcohol* involved?

a. If a motor vehicle accident: Was the seat belt worn? Was the patient a passenger or the driver? Where was the site of impact to the vehicle? Was the steering wheel crushed? Was the windshield shattered?
b. If a penetrating injury: What were the size, shape, and force of the penetrating object?

2. *Systemic symptoms*
   a. *Pain.* Is pain or discomfort present? If so, where is it located? What is its character and intensity? Where did it begin? Does it radiate?
   b. *Nausea, vomiting.* Is nausea or vomiting present? Nausea and vomiting may be indicative of increased intracranial pressure. Vomiting may predispose the patient to aspiration. If the patient is actively vomiting, he may be log-rolled on to his side, keeping his neck aligned. Consideration is given to performing endotracheal intubation for airway protection.
   c. *Numbness or weakness.* Does the patient have any area of unusual sensation or perceive a decreased strength?
   d. *Bowel and bladder function.* Does the patient sense loss of control over the anal sphincter and bladder?
3. *Medications.* What medication is the patient taking? When was the last dose taken? These medications may indicate significant underlying medical disorders or may have contributed to decreased consciousness.
4. *Past medical history.* The patient is asked about conditions that could predispose to syncope, such as prior cardiac dysrhythmia or infarction, known seizure disorder, diabetes mellitus, bleeding, hypovolemia, or dehydration.

Information about the patient's usual mental status is sought from old charts, wallet or purse, family, and primary physician. What appears to be altered mental status may actually be the patient's baseline condition.

Physical Examination

The patient with head and neck trauma receives a full primary and secondary survey (see Chap. 4). The survey's emphasis is on gauging the patient's level of consciousness, discovering neurologic deficits, and monitoring the changing nature of the findings.

Vital Signs. Blood pressure, pulse, and respirations are reevaluated. Bradycardia and hypotension are a late finding of increased intracranial pressure and impending herniation. Hypotension is usually due to bleeding elsewhere in the body, although scalp wounds may result in serious loss of blood. Hypertension is often seen with intracranial hemorrhage. The pulse has no characteristic pattern in patients with head trauma. It is usually increased secondary to pain in the conscious patient. Respirations have different patterns reflecting the level of the cortex and brain stem that is involved. These patterns are often not established in the emergency department and are of little value in predicting the patient's course. The diagnosis of "central hyperventilation" is reserved until the patency of the airway (particularly endotracheal tube patency), acid-base status, toxicologic status, and circulatory condition are evaluated.

Head. The head is carefully palpated for pain and tenderness. Special attention is given to possible entrance or exit wounds and to the presence of foreign bodies or lacerations. A sterile glove is used to examine open wounds, enabling the examiner to palpate the skull carefully for fractures.

Ears. The ears are examined for blood behind the tympanic membrane (hemotympanum), which indicates a basilar skull fracture. Serous fluid draining from the ear is presumed to be cerebrospinal fluid, and this is confirmed by the "double halo" test. In this test a small amount of the leaking fluid is placed on filter paper and allowed to separate into various constituents by its rate of diffusion across the paper. CSF reveals a layering of two circles or a "double halo" appearance. Analysis of the glucose level in the fluid to identify CSF is unreliable.

Eyes. Pupillary size, equality, and reflexes are noted. Most structural lesions influencing the pupil will affect both size and reflex reactivity, "the dilated and fixed" pupil. Extraocular movements and reflexes are important; they are discussed in Chapter 45. Examination of the fundus may reveal papilledema with absence of venous pulsations, or retinal hemorrhage. A subhyoid or preretinal hemorrhage may be seen, especially in children with head trauma; this indicates an underlying intracerebral hemorrhage.

Nose. The presence of a clear discharge may indicate a CSF leak. Testing with filter paper will help distinguish CSF from other fluid. Tenderness of the nose may indicate an underlying nasal fracture.

Face. The face is palpated for tenderness, deformity, or instability with gentle movement of the maxilla. The mandible is examined for loss of teeth, tooth approximation, tenderness of the jaw, and soundness of the temporomandibular joint.

Mouth and Throat. The mouth and throat are examined for lacerations, bleeding, foreign bodies, patency of the upper airway, and presence of a gag reflex.

Neck. In the alert and cooperative patient, the cervical spine collar may be removed while in-line immobilization is maintained. If the patient is pain-free and without deformity on palpation, he is asked to lift his head slightly. If there is no pain on limited movement, the patient is asked to raise the head more, and turn it slowly from side to side. If he remains pain-free, the posterior section of the collar is removed. If neck pain or limited movement occurs at any time, the collar is replaced. In the uncooperative or unconscious patient, the collar is not removed. The examination is postponed until the condition of the cervical spine is clearer radiologically and optimally when the patient is alert, calm, and cooperative. All patients are examined for subcutaneous emphysema, lacerations, deformity, or tracheal deviation of the anterior neck. In patients with penetrating trauma, attention is given to whether the platysma muscle is violated. If so, surgical consultation is necessary.

Neurologic Examination. The level of consciousness is the single most important indication of underlying pathology. Level of consciousness can be most objectively categorized by use of the Glasgow Coma Scale (see Table 50–2). This scale is useful to (1) standardize the degree of brain stem and cerebral function, (2) document objectively changes in the level of consciousness, and (3) predict on a preliminary basis the morbidity associated with head trauma. Patients with a score of 8 or less usually have significant morbidity. Hypothermia, ethanol, or drugs of abuse (e.g., barbiturates) can confuse the interpretation of the Glasgow Coma Scale.

Rectal Examination. A rectal examination is performed to assess sphincter tone. Absence of sphincter tone may indicate significant spinal injury.

The remainder of the initial examination includes examination of the sensory, motor, and cranial nerves. In cooperative patients, simple observations of extremity movements, symmetry of reflexes, smile, or grimace, and response to pain or touch are sufficient. Any abnormal findings prompt a detailed examination. In patients with suspected cervical spine injury, each segment of the cervical cord is examined. Motor deficit findings for each segment are listed in Table 50–3. An illustration of the sensory dermatomes is often useful in localizing findings to a particular level (Fig. 50–5).

PROBLEM 1 On arrival in the emergency department, the patient with massive facial injury continued to respond with decorticate posturing and moaning. Vital signs were blood pressure 130/90 mm Hg, pulse 110 beats/min, respiration 18/min controlled by bag-valve-mask, and temperature 37°C (98.6°F). No additional history was available. A home telephone number was found in the patient's wallet and a call was placed. On physical examination the extent of visible injuries was found to be limited to the face. The patient had a nasal fracture, a possible fractured mandible, and a large horizontal laceration at the hairline. His eyes roved conjointly, and the pupils were 4 to 5 mm in diameter, equal and reactive. Tympanic membranes were normal. During posturing and with stimulation, the patient moved all

TABLE 50–3. Motor Deficits and Corresponding Cervical Cord Segments

Motor Deficit	Cervical Cord Segment Injured
Respiratory failure	C4 and above
Quadriparesis with sole preservation of shoulder elevation and diaphragmatic breathing	C5
Wrist extension and elbow flexion. Biceps reflex may be absent	C6
Elbow extension, partial paralysis of finger and wrist flexons: result in *preachers hand*	C7
Complete paralysis of finger flexors	C8
Partial paralysis of hand muscles (interossei and lumbricals) and abductor pollicis	T1

extremities. Reflexes were symmetric and brisk. The Babinski reflex was "up-going" bilaterally. Rectal tone was normal. The remainder of the physical examination was unremarkable.

For the moment, most of the patient's injury seems to be centered in the head and neck. The physical findings are consistent with a diagnosis of significant trauma causing intracranial damage of undetermined extent. The absence of spinal cord-related deficiencies does not mean that the supporting bony or ligamentous structures are intact or stable. Considerable ancillary testing is necessary while the patient is hyperventilated and serially reevaluated.

PROBLEM 2 On direct questioning, the patient who hit his head after overturning an all-terrain vehicle stated that he felt the aura of a seizure just before he lost consciousness. He had been drinking prior to the accident. He had "epilepsy" and had run out of his medication 2 weeks earlier. The patient remembered only the ambulance ride. He was awake, alert, and complained of paresthesias along the ulnar aspects of both arms. No muscle weakness was detected. Reflexes were normal. Vital signs were within normal limits, as were the rest of the findings on physical examination.

Sensory complaints can be difficult to explain immediately. Any neurologic complaint indicates a serious problem until proved otherwise. Continued protection of the patient's cervical spine is absolutely necessary. Driving with a known seizure disorder after ethanol use, combined with "running out" of medication, suggests a noncompliant patient who has not yet accepted the reality of his disease. This psychosocial issue needs to be considered during disposition.

PROBLEM 3 The patient was unchanged, with a Glasgow Coma Scale score of 3. In addition to hyperventilation, the osmotic diuretic mannitol was given. Vital signs were blood pressure 160/100 mm Hg, pulse 100 beats/min, respiratory rate 16 and controlled by bag-valve-mask, and temperature 95°F (35°C). The patient responded weakly to stimuli on the left. Reflexes were symmetrically decreased with the exception of an "up-going" Babinski sign on the left side. The remaining findings on the physical examination were unremarkable. A number of blood studies were ordered. The neurosurgeon arrived and worked with the emergency department personnel to transfer the patient to the radiology department for a CT scan. The operating room staff was notified.

This patient has not deteriorated further and seems to be responding

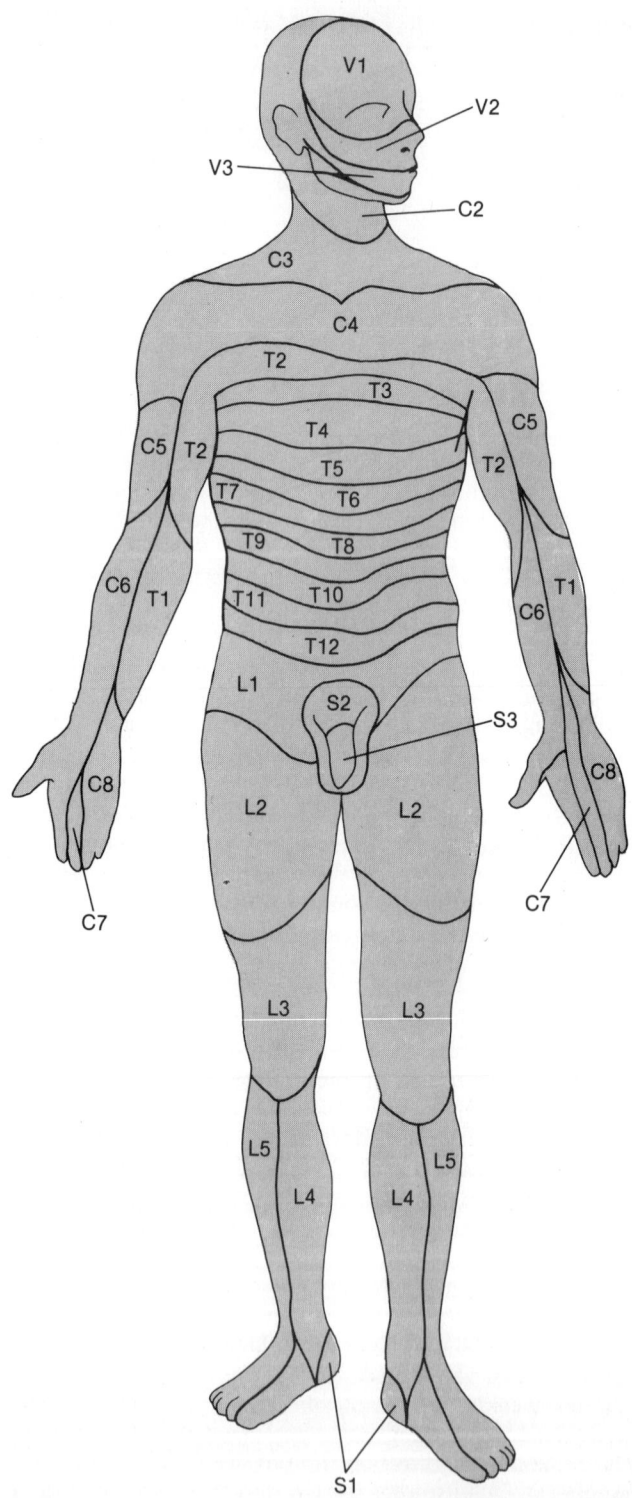

FIGURE 50–5. Distribution of spinal nerves and branches of the trigeminal nerve to segments of the body surfaces. Each segment is named for the principal spinal nerve that serves it. C = cervical segments; T = thoracic segments; L = lumbar segments; S = sacral segments; V = trigeminal segments. (From Solomon EP, Davis PW (eds): Human Anatomy and Physiology. Philadelphia, Saunders, 1983.)

to hyperventilation. Therefore, emergency "burrholes" by the emergency physician or preferably the neurosurgeon are not necessary. In this patient, the emergency physician can facilitate diagnostic studies, complete the physical examination, and anticipate metabolic problems, e.g., hypoglycemia, that may complicate the patient's course. Close cooperation with the neurosurgeon is absolutely necessary.

DECISION PRIORITIES AND PRELIMINARY DIFFERENTIAL DIAGNOSIS

Most traumatic injuries are assessed by trying to understand the nature and extent of the underlying pathologic processes by interpreting the clinical manifestations of these processes, since the physician cannot "get inside and look around." The decision priorities and preliminary differential diagnosis are derived from answering three questions.

1. *Are there obvious or suspected life-threatening injuries after data gathering? That is, are there findings indicative of problems requiring immediate management?*

   Management in this case may comprise further evaluation and consultation rather than a specific intervention. In head trauma, these findings include (1) unilateral or bilateral dilatation of pupils, (2) Glasgow Coma Scale score of 8 or less, (3) focal neurologic deficits, (4) brain stem respiratory pattern, (5) abnormal Babinski reflex, (6) decorticate or decerebrate posturing, and (7) changing or deteriorating findings on neurologic examination. Early management of head trauma is described under Question 3 below.

2. *Are there signs of acute spinal cord injury?*

   Patients with acute spinal cord injury who are treated with large doses of steroids within 8 hours of their injury have better motor and sensory outcomes than patients not treated with high-dose steroids. Therefore, patients who demonstrate signs of acute spinal cord injury should be treated initially with 30 mg/kg of methylprednisolone followed by 5.4 mg/kg/hour for the next 23 hours. High doses of steroids are thought to suppress the breakdown of membranes by inhibiting lipid peroxidation at the injury site.

3. *Are there treatable pathologic processes that could worsen the original injury?*

   The major concern in regard to head and neck trauma is its effect on the brain and spinal cord. Primary injuries comprise actual structural damage to neuronal tissue inflicted by the traumatic forces. These injuries heal with scar tissue, and recovery from them is very limited. A common set of "secondary" processes exists that can worsen the degree and extent of injury to neuronal tissue. Some of these processes are initiated as the tissue responds to injury, some may result from trauma to other organs, and others may exist at the time of the injury and contribute to its cause. To prevent the damaging effects of these secondary processes, they must always be considered early in the care of any brain-injured patient.

   Metabolic substrate replacement. Oxygen, glucose, and thiamine are important metabolic substrates in brain and spinal cord tissue. Low levels or absence of these substrates can have a damaging effect on neurons. Oxygen and thiamine are usually supplied before they are measured. Glucose is optimally measured and then supplied in the amount deemed necessary. Hyperglycemia in injured tissues is a potentially harmful effect of superfluous glucose administration.

   Toxins. The presence of endogenous (renal, hepatic) or exogenous (poisons, intoxicants) toxins is assessed in head-injured patients. Such toxins may cause or result from the injury, but in either case they can complicate the patient's presentation and clinical course and further injure damaged cells. Appropriate laboratory testing and administration of a narcotic antagonist, naloxone, are part of the management protocol.

   Mass lesions. Mass lesions result from either intracranial or intraspinal hemorrhage or edema. In the skull, they can cause pressure shifts, resulting in herniation, and may increase ischemia to tissues at and near the area of primary damage. CT scanning has dramatically changed the diagnosis and management of mass lesions. Skull trephination (burrholes) in the emergency department is reserved for only the most extreme situations.

   Metabolic rate. The metabolic rate of the brain determines its oxygen demand. Increased rates increase oxygen demand when there may not be sufficient supply; therefore, at a minimum a "normal" rate is desirable. Two controllable factors that have the potential to increase this rate are fever and seizure activity. Both are to be anticipated and suppressed.

Ischemia. Neuronal tissue does not tolerate vascular ischemia well. Cerebral vessels have the ability to autoregulate their resistance to maintain a relatively constant flow in the presence of a fluctuating blood pressure. Their lower effective operating range is about 60 to 70 mm Hg mean arterial pressure. This self-regulating ability may also be lost in severe injury. It is recommended that the mean arterial pressure be maintained between 90 and 110 mm Hg. Isotonic crystalloid and blood are the fluids of choice *up to* this level. Above this level the fluid is changed to 0.25% to 0.50% normal saline and flow is reduced to decrease cerebral edema. It is important to remember that an adequate mean arterial pressure (MAP) does not guarantee blood flow to the brain. Cerebral perfusion pressure is equal to MAP minus ICP. Therefore, the intracranial pressure is a major determinant of flow.

Tissue edema. Primary injury and secondary processes can promote tissue swelling. This can cause direct intracellular injury and ischemic injury from increased intracranial pressure. In the emergency department, tissue edema is treated, though not always successfully, with controlled hyperventilation and judicious use of diuretics. Hyperventilation reduces arterial P_{CO_2} and causes cerebral vessel constriction. Diuretics, both osmotic and loop, are thought to reduce water content in normal and injured brain tissue.

By attending to these problems, the emergency physician can exert a significant and often favorable influence on the outcome.

4. *Are any of the causes of death associated with the neuronal injury present or evolving in this patient?*

Unless neuronal injury is massive, most patients do not die from neuronal injury directly. Two results of this injury, however, are the most common causes of death—respiratory failure and hypotension. Either can be caused by brain or cervical cord injury. The patient is closely monitored to check for these problems. Since both are common sequelae of a number of other injuries, the role of central nervous system (CNS) deficits in causing them is usually considered after other sources are ruled out.

PROBLEM 1 This patient continued to exhibit a Glasgow Coma Scale score of 6 and was at risk for herniation from a mass lesion and cerebral edema. The problems of substrate, toxins, metabolism, and ischemia had been treated or were being assessed. The definitive diagnosis awaited the results of CT scanning. The neurosurgeon was notified of the severity of the preliminary differential diagnosis.

PROBLEM 2 This patient was alert and resting comfortably. There was no evidence of hypoventilation or neurogenic shock. The patient's complaint of paresthesias was sufficient to justify full protection of the cervical spine, even though the results of the examination did not clearly fit a cervical nerve distribution. As noted earlier, sensory patterns are often difficult to diagnose.

PROBLEM 3 Findings in this patient pointed to a likelihood of a mass lesion. While waiting for the CT scan, each of the other concerns were addressed. Glucose and oxygen were given. Thiamine was administered. The patient was slightly hypothermic, and the MAP was 120 mm Hg. Because of increased intracranial pressure, the real cerebral perfusion was unknown.

DIAGNOSTIC ADJUNCTS

Following the history and physical examination, radiographic studies are helpful in making a definitive diagnosis. However, serious head or neck injury can exist in the presence of apparently normal radiologic studies.

Radiologic Imaging

Computed Tomography of the Head. A CT scan of the head is the most important diagnostic test to be performed in patients with neurologic findings after head trauma. It determines structural rather than functional changes in the brain and surrounding tissue. Examples of CT head scans are given later in this chapter (Fig. 50–8) and Chapter 49. In patients with head trauma, the CT scan can define an intracranial hemorrhage and image the effects of increased intracranial pressure. This information will determine the need for emergent neurosurgical intervention. A normal CT scan, however, does not rule out a CNS bleed.

Indications for ordering CT scans in the setting of head trauma have recently been addressed by a Food and Drug Administration (FDA)-sponsored Skull X-ray Referral Criteria Panel. Based on the history and physical examination results, the panel recommends dividing patients into high-, moderate-, and low-risk groups for CNS pathology, especially intracranial hemorrhage (Table 50–4). In patients meeting high-risk criteria a CT scan is ordered.

Patients classified as having a moderate risk of brain injury often pose a dilemma for the emergency physician. A CT scan of the head is not mandatory for these patients, but each case is viewed individually. In-hospital serial neurologic monitoring for 24 hours is the best choice for these patients. A CT scan of the head is not indicated for patients meeting low-risk criteria.

CT scans may be ordered *without* intravenous contrast if the inciting trauma has occurred within 4 to 5 days prior to patient evaluation. Hemorrhage within this time period is easily noted on a noncontrast CT scan. By 7 days after injury the hemorrhage more closely matches the normal surrounding cerebral tissue. In the patient in whom trauma occurred 5 or more days prior to evaluation, a CT scan of the head is first performed without contrast. If no intracranial bleed is seen, the scan is repeated with contrast to detect an old hemorrhage.

Skull Radiographs. Skull radiographs are seldom necessary when a CT scan of the head is available in a timely fashion. In hospitals without CT scanning, skull films may demonstrate a skull fracture, allow an estimate of its depression, and reveal a shift of a calcified pineal gland in the patient with significant mass effect. Skull radiographs are not indicated for patients with mild head trauma who meet the criteria for low risk of CNS injury as detailed in Table 50–4.

Skull radiographs can be useful in the following instances:

1. In the child in whom abuse is suspected radiographs and a bone survey should be part of the workup (see Chap. 38). The presence of old fractures is documented for medicolegal purposes.

2. Anteroposterior (AP) and lateral skull films may be helpful in deciding whether a foreign body lies within the *intracranial* or *extracranial* space. The extra cost of a head CT scan may not be necessary if there is a good chance that the foreign body is extracranial and no fracture exists.

3. The location of a skull fracture over the middle meningeal artery may be of great prognostic value, since such a patient is at significant risk for an epidural bleed.

Cervical Spine Series. A complete cervical spine (C-spine) series includes the lateral, anteroposterior, and odontoid (open mouth) views. These studies can be completed with a cervical collar in place.

Indications for C-spine radiographs are liberal. They include (1) a mechanism compatible with C-spine injury, e.g., trauma to the head or neck, or flexion, extension,

TABLE 50–4. Management Strategy for Radiographic Imaging in Patients with Head Trauma[a]

Low-Risk Group	Moderate-Risk Group	High-Risk Group

Possible findings
  Asymptomatic
  Headache
  Dizziness
  Scalp hematoma
  Scalp contusion or abrasion
  Absence of moderate-risk or high-risk criteria
	Possible findings
	  History of change of consciousness at the time of injury or subsequently
	  History of progressive headache
	  Alcohol or drug intoxication
	  Unreliable or inadequate history
	  Age less than 2 year (unless injury very trivial)
	  Post-traumatic seizure
	  Vomiting
	  Post-traumatic amnesia
	  Multiple trauma
	  Serious facial injury
	  Signs of basilar fracture[b]
	  Possible skull penetration or depressed fracture[c]
	  Suspected physical child abuse
		Possible findings
		  Depressed level of consciousness not clearly due to alcohol, drugs, or other causes (e.g., metabolic and seizure disorders)
		  Focal neurologic signs
		  Decreasing level of consciousness
		  Penetrating skull injury or palpable depressed fracture

Recommendations Observation alone: Discharge patients with head-injury information sheet (listing subdural precautions) and a second person to observe them	*Recommendations* Extended close observation (watch for signs of high-risk group) Consider CT examination and neurosurgical consultation Skull series may (rarely) be helpful, if positive, but do not exclude intracranial injury if normal	*Recommendations* Patient is a candidate for neurosurgical consultation or emergency CT examination or both

[a]Physician assessment of the severity of injury may warrant reassignment to a higher-risk group. Any single criterion from a higher-risk group warrants assignment of the patient to the highest risk group applicable.
[b]Signs of basilar fracture include drainage from ear, drainage of cerebrospinal fluid from nose, hemotympanum, Battle's sign, and "raccoon eyes."
[c]Factors associated with open and depressed fracture include gunshot, missile, or shrapnel wounds; scalp injury from firm, pointed object (including animal teeth); penetrating injury of eyelid or globe; object stuck in the head; assault (definite or suspected) with any object; leakage of cerebrospinal fluid; and sign of basilar fracture.
From Masters SJ, McClean PM, Arcarese JS, et al: Skull x-ray examinations after head trauma. Reprinted with permission from *The New England Journal of Medicine*, Vol. 316, pages 84 to 91, 1987.

or axial loading of the head; (2) altered mental status with suspected head or neck trauma; (3) cervical spine pain following trauma; and (4) focal or bilateral neurologic deficits that may be consistent with cervical spine injury.

In obtaining and interpreting these films, several aspects must be clear to the emergency physician.

1. There is *no* urgency to remove the cervical collar. The patient's head must remain fixed relative to the body until the cervical spine films *and* repeat neurologic screening examination are normal. This priority is communicated to the radiology staff. In high-risk situations, a portable lateral film is obtained first, or the patient is accompanied to the radiology department by a physician.

2. The lateral cervical spine film is taken first, and absence of pathology is confirmed before the AP and odontoid views are completed. These subsequent views require some movement of the patient and may be avoided if an unstable fracture is seen on the lateral radiograph.

3. All seven cervical vertebrae should be seen on the lateral cervical spine film including the C7–T1 interspace. This may require the use of traction on the arms or special radiographic techniques such as the transthoracic view.

4. Significant injuries to the spine and cord may be present despite "normal" radiographs.

5. Patients who continue to have severe neck pain or neurologic findings despite normal C-spine radiographs are studied more definitively by CT scan or magnetic resonance imaging of the cervical spine.

A critical skill of the emergency physician is the ability to differentiate abnormal from normal cervical spine radiographs. The lateral view is most important in this regard, although the other views contribute valuable information. In the normal lateral view four contour lines must be aligned (Fig. 50–6). They are as follows: (1) the anterior vertebral line, (2) the posterior vertebral line, (3) the spinolaminar line, and (4) the line connecting the tips of the spinous processes. These four lines delineate the normal lordotic curve of the cervical spine and establish the relationship between the "anterior" vertebral body and the "posterior" structures around the spinal cord, the pedicle, lamina, facets, and spinous process.

Interpreting this view requires experience, and a few points may be helpful:

1. The absence of the normal lordotic curve may indicate a ligamentous injury or may be the result of severe cervical muscle strain.

2. Each vertebral body is identified on the lateral radiograph. If one vertebral body is "out of alignment," it is said to be "subluxed" with respect to its next lower vertebral segment. Such a subluxation is considered a serious injury until proved otherwise.

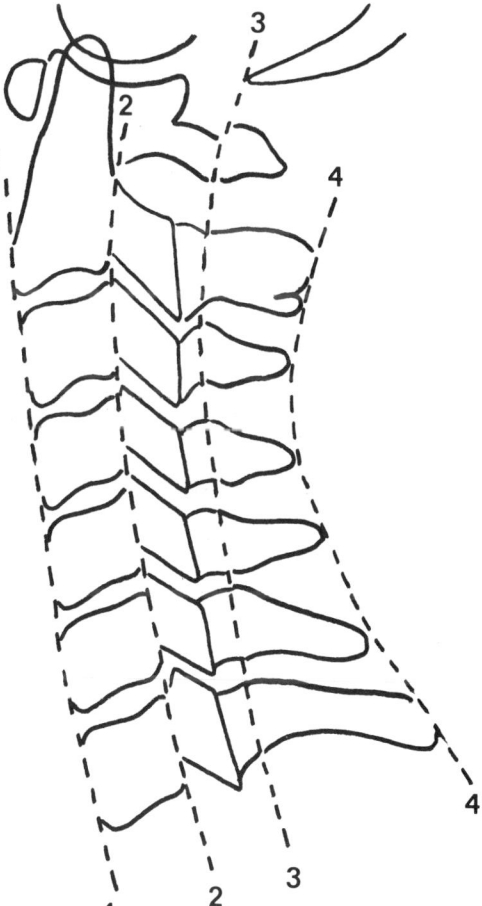

FIGURE 50–6. *The four contour lines of the cervical spine, normal anatomy. (1) The anterior vertebral line, (2) posterior vertebral line, (3) spinolaminar line, (4) line connecting the tips of the spinous processes. (From Gerlock AJ: Advanced Exercises in Diagnostic Radiology: The Cervical Spine in Trauma. Philadelphia, Saunders, 1978.)*

3. The "parallel" alignment of lines 3 and 4 to lines 1 and 2 on Figure 50–6 establish the relationship of the "anterior" and "posterior" elements.

4. The soft tissue areas ventral to the spinal column (along line 1) are important. The prevertebral soft tissue width at C3 should be less than half the width of the adjacent vertebral body (or less than 7 mm), and the width at C6 should be less than 22 mm. Any increased size of the prevertebral soft tissue may indicate a bony fracture or ligamentous disruption.

5. The normal anatomy of the spinal vertebrae and the "posterior" anatomy are recognizable and are duplicated for each cervical vertebra C2 through C7.

6. The next most important view is the odontoid (open mouth) view. This may be difficult to obtain in an uncooperative patient. The normal odontoid relationships are illustrated in Figure 50–7; the odontoid view most closely resembles the schematic depicted in Figure 50–7B. The key elements are (1) absence of a fracture of the dens itself and (2) alignment of the inferior articular facet of C1 directly over the superior articular facet of C2. Additionally, the gap between the anterior ring of C1 and the dens (predens space) should be less than 3 mm in adult patients.

Any observations inconsistent with these guidelines are brought to the attention of an experienced emergency physician and, optimally, a radiologist. Cautious interpretation is in the best interest of the patient.

Arteriography. Carotid arteriography is considered for neck wounds that penetrate the platysma muscle and may cause occult vascular injury.

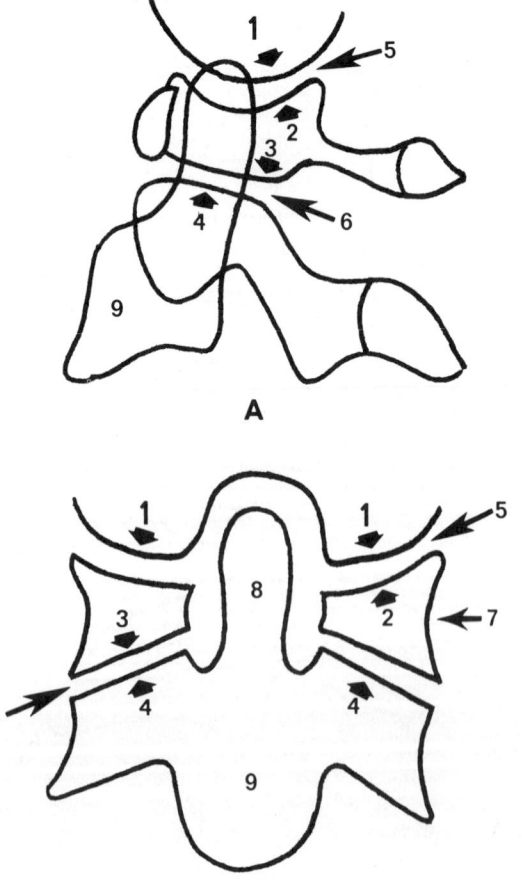

FIGURE 50–7. *Lateral and odontoid views of the occipito-atlantoaxial joints. A, Lateral view. B, Dens or odontoid view. (1) Articular surface of occipital condyles, (2) superior articular facet of C1, (3) inferior articular facet of C1, (4) superior articular facet of C2, (5) occipito-atlanto joint, (6) atlantoaxial joint, (7) lateral mass of C1, (8) odontoid process, (9) body of C2. (From Gerlock AJ: Advanced Exercises in Diagnostic Radiology: The Cervical Spine in Trauma. Philadelphia, Saunders, 1978.)*

Laboratory Studies

Laboratory testing is necessary to establish the level of metabolic substrates (oxygen, glucose) present, determine the presence of endogenous and exogenous toxins, indirectly measure the oxygen-carrying capacity of blood (hemoglobin), and assess any underlying metabolic conditions possibly complicating the clinical picture. The following tests are routinely ordered in all patients with serious head and neck injury.

Arterial Blood Gas Analysis. This test is indicated in patients with serious head trauma to ensure that the patient is adequately oxygenated (PaO_2 more than 60 mm Hg) and to confirm that hyperventilation is present in patients with cerebral edema. Hyperventilation should optimally lower PCO_2 to 25 to 30 mm Hg. In the future, the use of a pulse oximeter and end-tidal CO_2 monitor may provide continuous data on oxygen and carbon dioxide levels in seriously ill patients.

Hematology. Complete blood count and differential, platelet estimate, and coagulation studies are done. Blood type and screen or cross-match is ordered as necessary.

Chemistry. Electrolytes, blood urea nitrogen (BUN), creatinine, and glucose levels are determined. Liver function tests, if clinically indicated, are ordered.

Toxicology. A toxicology screen, preferably directed by data gathering, is ordered. Determination of ethanol level is often routine in any patient with altered mental status. Whether the result is negative or positive, the search for other sources continues. Ethanol ingestion is considered a contributing problem but is rarely the only problem.

PROBLEM 1 Arterial blood gas determinations demonstrated that the patient was not hypoxic and had a PCO_2 of 25 mm Hg. The remainder of the laboratory values were normal. The patient's lateral C-spine radiograph was read as normal. However, the odontoid views revealed that the lateral masses of C1 were displaced laterally compared to the masses of C2. The patient had a C1 ring or Jefferson's fracture. Cervical immobilization was maintained.

This type of C_1 fracture is often caused by severe axial loading on the top of the head. Cervical spine stability now is of prime importance. The CT scan revealed diffuse cerebral edema without intracranial bleed. Since there was no mass lesion, treatment for the head injury shifted more to monitoring and medical management than to surgical intervention.

PROBLEM 2 The patient's cervical spine radiographs were normal. Because of the paresthesias and severe neck pain, the emergency physician remained concerned about a cord lesion, and a CT scan of the cervical spine was ordered. The patient's serum phenytoin level was undetectable. He was given a loading dose of phenytoin to prevent further seizures.

PROBLEM 3 The alcoholic patient with a Glasgow Coma Scale score of 3 had an alcohol level of only 55 mg/100 ml. His lateral, AP, and odontoid C-spine films were found to be normal. However, the hard cervical collar was not removed before he was sent to CT scan because he remained comatose, thereby preventing the performance of a complete neurologic examination. His dilated pupil had decreased in response to the hyperventilation.

REFINED DIFFERENTIAL DIAGNOSIS

Initial data gathering and serial observations combined with proper use and interpretation of laboratory values, radiographs, and CT scan often allow the differential diagnosis to be further refined.

Head Injuries
Blunt Head Trauma

Blunt head trauma can result in epidural, subdural, intracerebral, or subarachnoid hemorrhage. An epidural hematoma is characterized clinically by transient loss of consciousness immediately after injury, followed by a lucid period. This period of consciousness may deteriorate rapidly and is often associated with signs of uncal herniation. The patient may exhibit an ipsilateral dilated pupil and contralateral hemiparesis relative to the side of the hematoma. Epidural hemorrhage is usually due to arterial bleeding and may be associated with a skull fracture over the middle meningeal artery. The bleed is distinctly seen as a biconvex density on the CT scan (Fig. 50–8A).

Subdural hematoma is the result of venous bleeding beneath the dura. Geriatric patients, alcoholics, patients with cerebral atrophy, and those with hemostatic disorders are susceptible to subdural hemorrhage. Symptoms result from direct pressure to the cortex under the bleed. Subdural hemorrhage may be classified as acute, subacute, or chronic based on the time course of the development of symptoms. Acute symptoms develop within 24 hours; subacute symptoms take 1 day to 2 weeks to develop, and chronic hematomas become symptomatic after 2 weeks. A chronic subdural hemorrhage is often difficult to diagnose because a history of head trauma days or weeks ago may not be available, and the appearance symptoms can be insidious, e.g., slightly increased

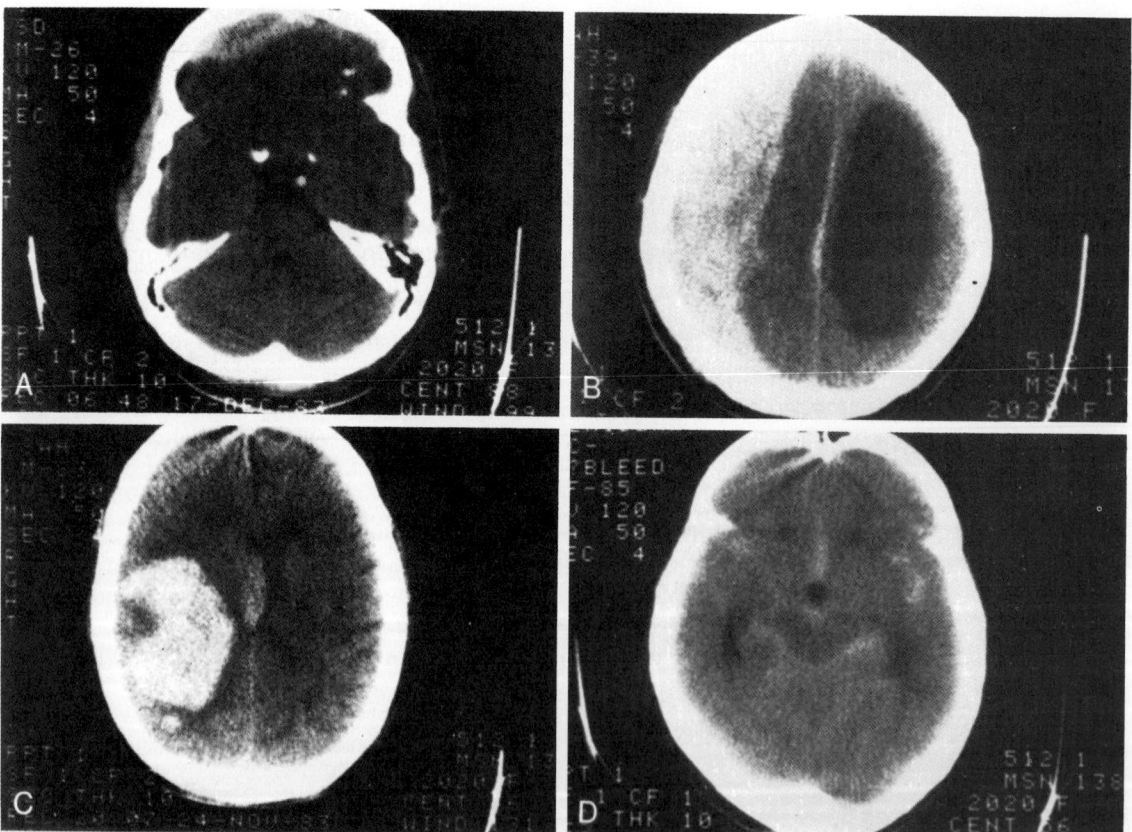

FIGURE 50–8. *A*, Frontal epidural hematoma. *The localized lenticular-shaped blood density in the frontal region is the common configuration of an epidural hematoma.* *B*, Subdural hematoma. *This massive, panhemispheric collection of blood assumes a typical shape as it outlines the cortex. There is also ventricular enlargement.* *C*, Intracerebral hematoma. *The localized blood density mass in the parietal region has associated edema surrounding it, seen as a darker band.* *D*, Subarachnoid hemorrhage. *Blood in the subarachnoid spaces appears as faint white lines in the major fissures.* (From Tintinalli JE: Emergency Medicine: A Comprehensive Study Guide. New York, McGraw Hill, 1985.)

irritability, or a chronic headache without focal neurologic findings. The CT scan of the head often shows a crescent-shaped deficit (Fig. 50–8B).

Intracerebral hemorrhage is bleeding within the parenchyma of the cerebral hemispheres. It may occur at the time of trauma or may appear a few days later. Symptoms are usually dramatic and include acutely depressed level of consciousness and signs of increased intracranial pressure (Fig. 50–8C). Subarachnoid hemorrhage may occur spontaneously as the result of an aneurysmal bleed, or it may be caused by head trauma (Fig. 50–8D).

Skull fractures are considered in all patients with head trauma and may be classified as linear, depressed, or basilar. Linear fractures are important because they may be the precursor of subsequent intracranial events such as epidural hemorrhage. Depressed skull fractures are indications of severe traumatic force and are often associated with cerebral contusion, a bruising of the cerebral cortex. If the fracture is depressed more than 5 mm, it requires elevation neurosurgically. Basilar skull fractures are usually *inferred* from the characteristic clinical signs including Battle's sign, raccoon eyes (periorbital ecchymoses), and CSF rhinorrhea or otorrhea. They are not usually well identified by radiologic imaging.

Temporary loss of consciousness (longer than 5 min) or temporary neurologic deficits that resolve in less than 24 hours may be categorized as cerebral concussion or cerebral contusion. In the patient with cerebral concussion, the CT scan is normal, whereas in the cerebral contusion patient CT shows microhemorrhages of the cerebral cortex. Patients with cerebral contusion are at high risk for subsequent intracranial bleeding.

In both cases the most common deficit is memory loss. Memory loss may be retrograde—loss of memory a time period before the injury—or antegrade—loss of current memory. In the latter situation the patient may ask the same question repeatedly, since he does not remember asking it. This can be very annoying to staff and family, and the underlying problem must be explained to them.

Penetrating Wounds of the Head

Gunshot wounds to the head are the most common cause of penetrating injury to the skull and have an extremely high mortality. Documentation of the path of the bullet is important because bullets that traverse the cerebral hemispheres almost always result in mortality. Two-view radiographs of the patient with an entrance wound are helpful in delineating the presence of the bullet or fragments. CT scanning may be difficult to interpret because of interference from the metallic projectile.

Neck Injuries
Common Fractures

A "hangman's" fracture is suspected when the spinolaminar line reveals that the spinous process of C2 is posteriorly subluxed. The anterior and posterior vertebral lines often remain in alignment. Thus, a hangman's fracture is a fracture through the pedicle of C2 (Fig. 50–9). This is a highly unstable fracture involving the posterior elements.

Another fracture best seen on lateral C-spine radiographs is the teardrop fracture, a small anterior-inferior chip fracture of the vertebral body. This is a flexion-type injury and has a high incidence of ligamentous disruption and cord compression (Fig. 50–10).

The clay shoveler's fracture is a fracture of the spinous process of C6 or C7. It may be unstable if the nuchal ligament is fully avulsed.

The dens or odontoid view may reveal a fracture in one or more areas of the atlas, the ring comprising C1. This is called a Jefferson's fracture. The odontoid view shows one or both lateral masses of C1 located lateral to their usual positions (Fig. 50–11). This very unstable fracture is usually the result of axial loading. It can result from falling from a significant height, diving into shallow water, or being thrown against the car roof in an abrupt deceleration.

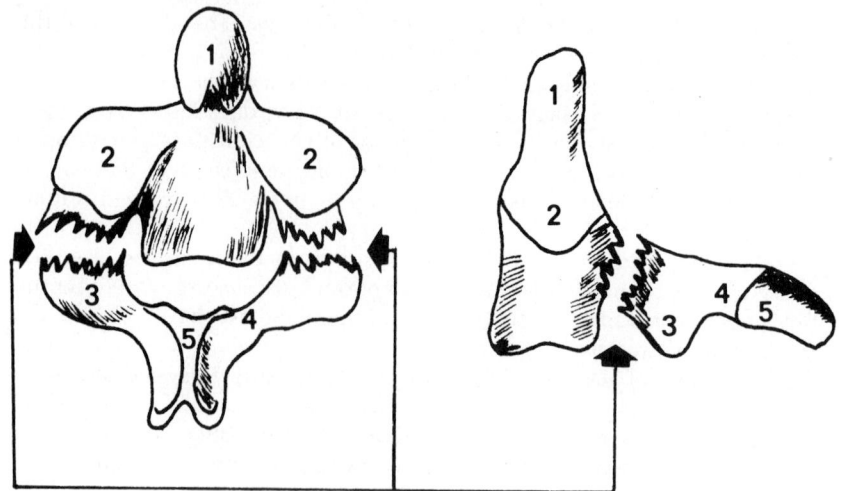

FIGURE 50-9. Hangman's fracture. The arrows point to the fractures through the pedicles anterior to the inferior articular facets and posterior to the superior articular facets. (1) Odontoid process, (2) superior articular facets, (3) inferior articular facets, (4) laminae, (5) spinous process. (From Gerlock AJ: Advanced Exercises in Diagnostic Radiology: The Cervical Spine in Trauma. Philadelphia, Saunders, 1978.)

Ligament and Muscle Strain

Abrupt deceleration in a motor vehicle accident causes a flexion-extension injury. It often damages, to varying degrees, the muscular and ligamentous supporting tissue of the cervical spine. The extent of injury depends on the prior condition of the cervical spine, the degree and direction of the force, and the patient's opportunity and ability to protect himself. Although pain usually appears during the first few hours, the full intensity and range of symptoms may be delayed for 2 to 3 days. These symptoms include stiffness, radicular pain, paresthesias, paresia, headache, and dizziness or a sense of instability. These symptoms can occur in the presence of normal alignment on the cervical spine series. All patients who have neck pain or have sustained a mechanism of injury with the potential to produce this injury are warned of these possible complications. Under controlled situations, lateral view radiographs of the neck in flexion and extension may identify instability in the cervical spine.

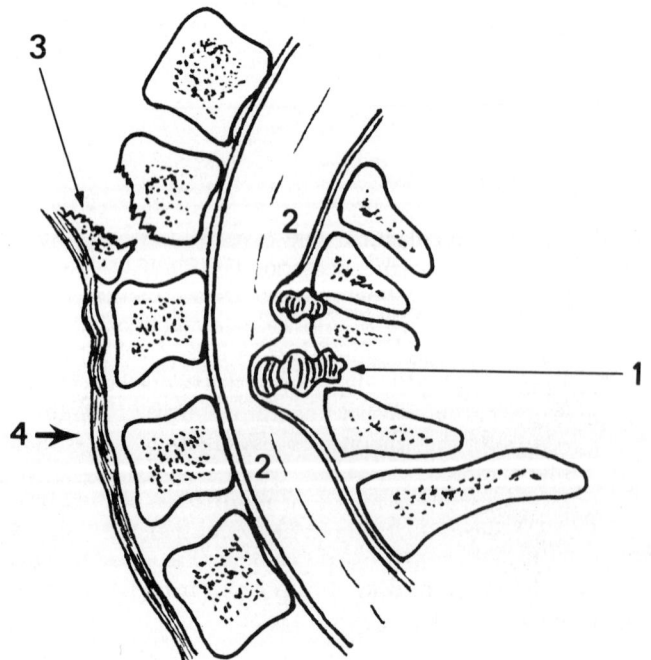

FIGURE 50-10. Teardrop fracture and contusion of the spinal cord. (1), Buckled ligamenta flava compressing the spinal cord, (2) spinal cord, (3) the teardrop—an avulsed fracture fragment from the anterior margin of a vertebral body, (4) anterior longitudinal ligament. (From Gerlock AJ: Advanced Exercises in Diagnostic Radiology: The Cervical Spine in Trauma. Philadelphia, Saunders, 1978.)

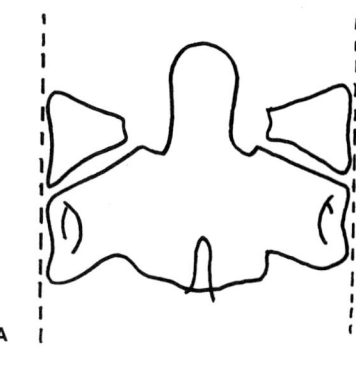

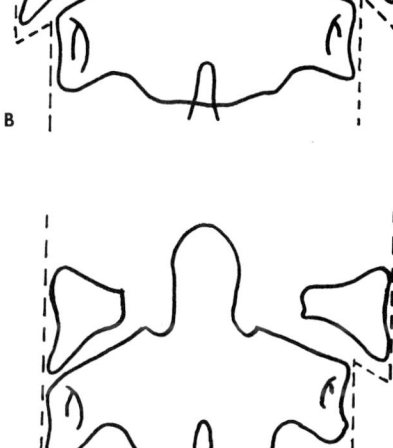

FIGURE 50–11. *Jefferson's fracture, showing relationship of C1 to C2. A, Normal atlantoaxial anatomy as seen from the odontoid view. B, Bilateral displacement of the lateral masses of C1. C, Unilateral displacement of the lateral masses of C1. (From Gerlock AJ: Advanced Exercises in Diagnostic Radiology: The Cervical Spine in Trauma. Philadelphia, Saunders, 1978.)*

Penetrating Wounds of the Neck

Penetrating neck wounds result in four types of injuries.
1. Laryngotracheal
2. Visceral (pharynx and esophagus)
3. Vascular (carotid artery and jugular veins)
4. Neurologic (spinal cord and cerebral infarction secondary to vascular injury)

Laryngotracheal injuries are suggested by dyspnea with stridor, hoarseness, or odynophagia. The neck is palpated for crepitus, loss of the normal contour, and tenderness.

Visceral injury is a life-threatening condition and is often not discovered until late in the course of care. Its presentation may include subtle degrees of odynophagia, dysphagia, hematemesis, or crepitus. Patients in whom visceral injury is suspected should undergo esophagoscopy to confirm the diagnosis. Radiographic studies may be attempted in the conscious patient but have disadvantages. Contrast esophagrams with water-soluble contrast give poor anatomic definition but have few sequelae if the contrast medium is aspirated. Barium esophagrams offer better anatomic definition but have substantial risks if the agent is aspirated.

Vascular injuries may be evident as hematoma formation or frank hemorrhage. The latter should be controlled with direct pressure, since clamps may worsen preexisting vascular or nerve injury. Because of the stellate ganglion's anatomic proximity to the carotid artery, the presence of Horner's syndrome (miosis, ptosis, anhidrosis) after a penetrating injury is assumed to represent vascular involvement.

Neurologic injuries may result from gunshot wounds involving the cervical spine or a cerebral infarction caused by a carotid artery transection, a dissection of the arterial intima layer, or a projectile embolus. Cervical spine radiographs, CT scan of the spine, and angiography are usually necessary to diagnose the problem.

Cord Syndromes

Injury to the spinal cord can occur with or without bony injury. Patients with neurologic deficits and normal radiographic studies may have a cord syndrome. A complete cord syndrome is a loss of motor and sensory function below the level of injury. It can be initiated by a concussive injury to the cord, causing "spinal shock." This usually resolves within 24 hours and is the basis for differentiating it from more permanent neuronal damage. In either case, careful testing may reveal sacral sparing on the sensory examination and an intact bulbocavernous reflex, or perceptible rectal tone. These findings point to an incomplete cord lesion. The three common incomplete cord syndromes are central, anterior, and Brown-Séquard.

The central cord syndrome is usually caused by hyperextension of the neck that contuses the central area of the spinal column. This injures the central fibers of the corticospinal tract. It is characterized by a disproportionately greater weakness in the upper extremity. Sensory deficits are variable. Resolution of the neurologic deficits is unpredictable, although a speedy recovery and preservation of bowel and bladder function are positive prognostic signs.

The anterior cord syndrome is usually caused by hyperflexion injuries. The anterior spinal artery is injured or the anterior cord contused by vertebral fragments or a herniated intervertebral disc. The syndrome is characterized by complete paralysis and loss of sensation to pain and temperature bilaterally below the lesion. Dorsal column function such as light touch, proprioception, and vibratory sensation are generally intact. Most patients show some neurologic improvement but do not completely recover.

The Brown-Séquard syndrome, a hemisection of the cord, is more commonly seen with a penetrating injury. This syndrome evolves to ipsilateral motor and contralateral sensory dysfunction. Bowel and bladder function is retained.

A mild cord contusion presents as transient neurologic signs following a traumatic injury that resolves in minutes to hours. Mild paresthesias or weakness of the upper extremities are most common. The symptoms may completely resolve during the emergency department visit. The prognosis for full recovery is excellent.

PROBLEM 1 The patient had an unstable C1 ring fracture (Jefferson's fracture).

PROBLEM 2 The cervical spine CT scan appeared normal. The patient's paresthesias had improved. The emergency physician diagnosed the problem as a cord contusion at the C7 level (see Table 50–3).

PROBLEM 3 The patient remained lethargic. A CT scan of the head revealed an acute epidural hemorrhage of the right parietal area, and bone windows showed a linear, nondepressed skull fracture over the right parietal skull area.

PRINCIPLES OF MANAGEMENT

General Principles

The general principles of head and neck trauma management are (1) to support the patient's cardiovascular status, and (2) to prevent further injury. Most of this information was given earlier in the sections on Decision Priorities and Preliminary Differential Diagnosis. A few additional points are listed below:

Measures to Decrease Intracranial Pressure. Hyperventilation is the most immediate and effective method of reducing intracranial pressure. In addition to hyperventilation, elevation of the head of the bed and osmotic or loop diuresis may be used. Mannitol is given as a 20% solution, 0.25 to 1 g/kg intravenously. Furosemide (0.5 to 1 mg/kg) is given in addition to mannitol in some patients. Intracranial pressure monitoring is useful to help guide treatment. The use of steroids in patients with head trauma remains controversial, although some recent studies support its efficacy.

Immobilization. All patients who exhibit a decreased level of consciousness following trauma are presumed to have a cervical spine injury until proved otherwise. Spinal immobilization is continued until a cervical spine fracture is ruled out. Patients with simple neck muscle strain may be treated with analgesics and muscle relaxants.

High Dose Steroids. Patients with acute spinal cord injuries should be treated with large doses of steroids. An initial loading dose of 30 mg/kg of methylprednisolone is followed by an infusion of 5.4 mg/kg/hour for 23 hours.

Nasogastric Tube. Because of the likelihood of vomiting and subsequent aspiration, nasogastric tube placement is considered in all head-injured patients. If a cribriform plate fracture or nasal fracture is a possibility, the nasogastric tube is inserted orally. Its placement is checked by listening for the sound of air at the epigastrium while instilling air through the tube.

Foley Catheter. A Foley catheter is placed if (1) a pelvic examination reveals no instability, (2) a rectal examination shows absence of a high-riding prostate, and (3) the external meatus has no blood on examination. The Foley catheter will help in monitoring the patient's fluid status.

Scalp Lacerations. Copious bleeding from scalp lacerations is treated with closure. If necessary, local anesthesia with lidocaine and epinephrine will decrease pain and bleeding. Scalp wounds involving the galea are closed in two layers, the galea separately, with absorbable suture, to avoid subgaleal hematoma formation. Most scalp wounds are closed by a one-layered nonabsorbable suture. This closes the dermis and the subcutaneous tissue simultaneously.

SPECIAL CONSIDERATIONS

Children

Neck Injury

Pediatric patients rarely suffer cervical spine injury. Children under 15 years of age represent only 1% to 3% of all patients with spinal injuries. However, children who suffer significant cervical trauma most often have pathology in the upper cervical region. These injuries are more likely to result in a catastrophic neurologic loss such as quadriplegia.

The findings on lateral cervical spine films of pediatric patients are different from those in their adult counterparts. The space between the anterior ring of C1 and the anterior aspect of the dens (predens space) normally measures up to 5 mm. (In adults, the normal measurement is up to 3 mm.) In children there is often a relationship of the C2–C3 vertebrae called *pseudosubluxation*. Apparent subluxation of the C2–C3 vertebral body alignment is a normal finding in up to 40% of children under 8 (Fig. 50–12). A true subluxation exists when the spinolaminar line at C2 is abnormal. This abnormality is seen in Figure 50–13, which depicts a C3–C4 subluxation in a 15 year old boy. Prevertebral soft tissue swelling may be an additional clue that true subluxation has occurred.

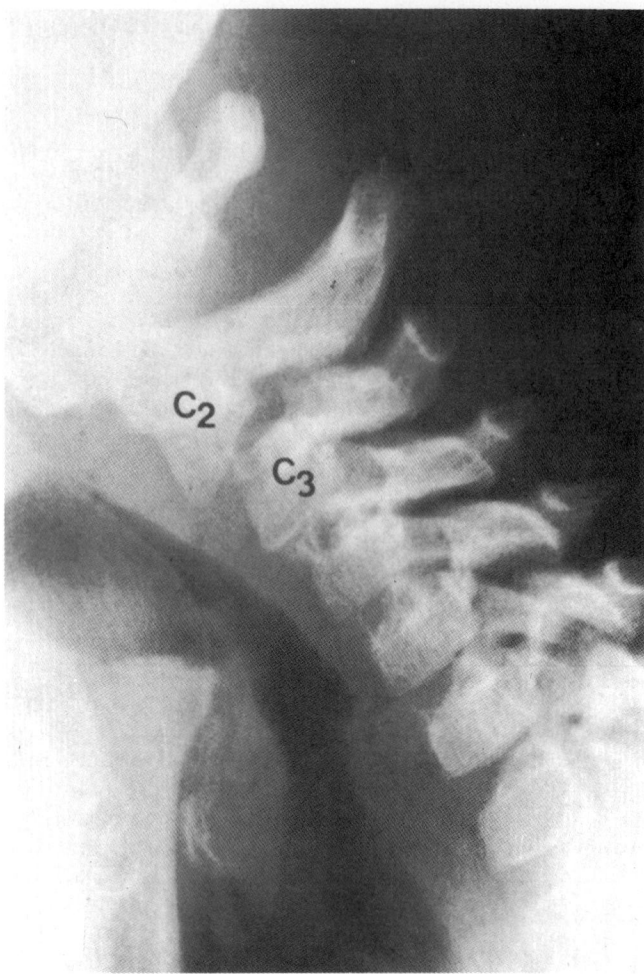

FIGURE 50-12. Pseudosubluxation of C2–C3 in a 7-year-old girl. (From Wilberger JE (ed): Spinal Cord Injuries in Children. Mt. Kisco, NY, Futura Publishing, 1986.)

Head Injury

Blunt head injury in children is very common. It may occur as isolated head trauma or in conjunction with other injuries. Head trauma in children always arouses suspicion of child abuse. A careful history may identify this problem. Children having a high potential for abuse are admitted to the hospital for a full evaluation (Chap. 38).

Children who have one to three episodes of vomiting or slight sleepiness without neurologic deficit are watched in the emergency department for several hours. Should their vomiting progress or symptoms increase, an emergency CT scan is done and they are admitted. If the child has reliable, competent parents and the vomiting ceases, he may be safely sent home providing the parents can comply with strict "head" instructions.

DISPOSITION AND FOLLOW-UP

All patients with head and neck trauma are observed for late sequelae manifested by deteriorating neurologic signs. Decisions about discharge often depend on whether the patient can be adequately observed outside the hospital.

Admission

Patients requiring admission are those with:
1. An intracranial hemorrhage of any kind.

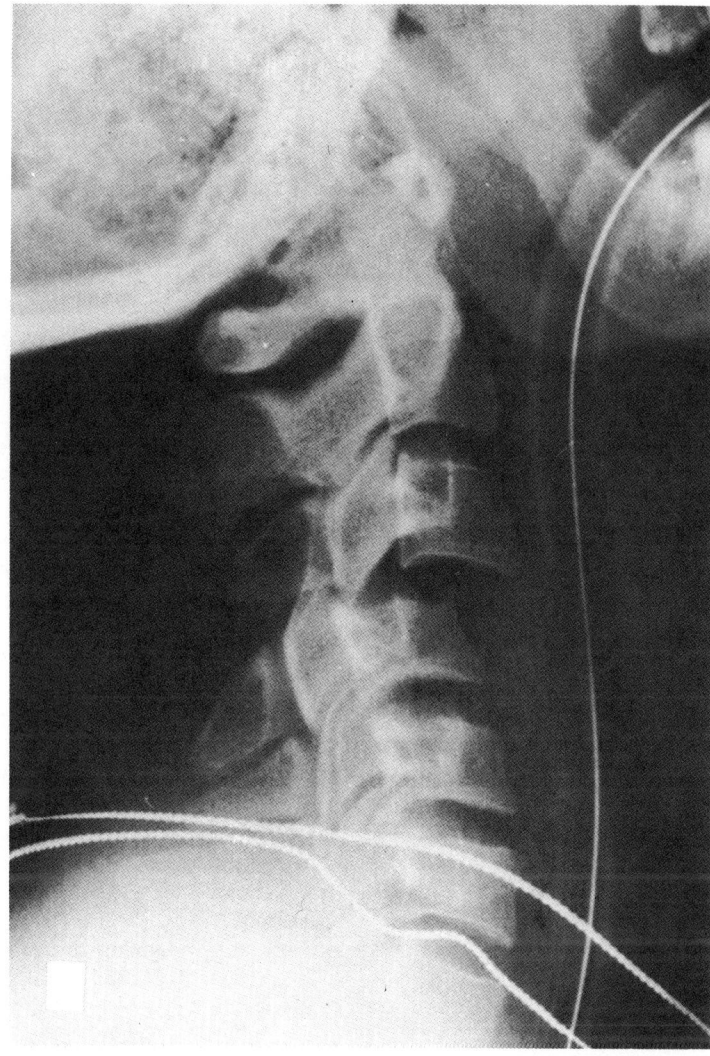

FIGURE 50–13. *Severe dislocation and subluxation at the C3–C4 level associated with quadriplegia in a 15-year-old boy involved in an automobile accident. (From Wilberger JE (ed): Spinal Cord Injuries in Children. Mt. Kisco, NY, Futura Publishing, 1986.)*

2. A skull fracture or cervical spine injury of any kind.
3. A persistent neurologic deficit.
4. Cerebral contusions confirmed on CT scan. This group can have a morbidity of up to 90%.
5. A temporary (over 5 minutes) neurologic deficit and negative results on CT scan. These patients are diagnosed as having "cerebral concussion" and observed for 24 hours.
6. Complicated clinical presentations resulting from intoxication or other injuries.
7. Persistent cervical spine pain and equivocal interpretation of the cervical spine radiographic series.
8. Bilateral or focal neurologic deficits and normal C-spine radiographs.
9. Head trauma patients who do not have family or friends to watch them overnight. These patients need to be admitted to be observed for late sequelae and neurologic deterioration.

Discharge

Patients who have sustained mild head trauma and have no evidence of neurologic deficit may be discharged from the hospital. The following factors are addressed before the patient is sent home:

1. The patient must be supervised by a responsible person. The role of this person is to wake the patient every few hours through the night and monitor the patient's responsiveness and behavior during a full 24-hour period.

2. The supervising person understands that he or she is observing the patient for lethargy, confusion, vomiting, ataxia, or increasing pain. The patient needs to return immediately to the emergency department if any of these conditions become evident.

Studies show that patients with mild head injuries may indeed suffer from subsequent deficiencies in learning, memory, or visual motor speed. Therefore, careful physician follow-up of the patient is necessary.

Patients with mild to moderate neck pain, normal neurologic findings, and normal radiologic studies may be discharged and treated for a neck muscle strain with analgesics and muscle relaxants. Follow-up is arranged with the primary care physician.

PROBLEM 1 The neurosurgeons recommended IV mannitol and intensive care monitoring. They planned to place the patient in a halo cervical immobilization device to treat the C1 fracture.

PROBLEM 2 The neurosurgical consultant evaluated the patient and agreed with the diagnosis of a cord contusion. He was admitted for observation. The patient's noncompliance and seizure while driving were noted on the chart and communicated to the admitting physician.

PROBLEM 3 The patient was taken to surgery, where a large right-sided epidural hematoma was evacuated, the middle meningeal artery reanastomosed, and the depressed fracture elevated. He was released from the hospital with residual left-sided hemiparesis. One week later, he returned to the emergency room by rescue squad. His Glasgow Coma Scale score was 8, and he was combative. A left-sided paresis was noted. The emergency physician carefully read the discharge summary from his medical chart and was aware that the hemiparesis was the result of this previous injury. Assessment of the patient for mental status change revealed a blood alcohol level of 350 mg/dl. With the concurrence of the neurosurgeon, the patient was observed. During the first 2 hours the patient's condition improved. The emergency physician did not obtain an emergent CT scan. Cervical spine radiographs were taken and cleared. The patient was carefully observed with frequent neurologic checks in the emergency department and was discharged to a shelter for the homeless the following day.

DOCUMENTATION

1. History of the traumatic event with respect to the mechanism of injury and the forces involved. Did the patient lose consciousness or have any other neurologic deficits? If so, for how long?
2. Mental status, described and measured by the Glasgow Coma Scale.
3. Past medical history, e.g., alcoholism, seizures, diabetes.
4. Medications taken.
5. Physical examination results including
    a. Vital signs
    b. Head and neck findings with specific reference to extent of injuries, bleeding, crepitus, and pain.
    c. Ears—hemotympanum or CSF drainage.
    d. Eyes—pupils, oculomotor reflexes, extraocular muscles, funduscopic findings.
    e. Neurologic status—screening neurologic examination including mental status, motor, sensory, cerebellum, and reflexes.

6. Course of care. The chart reflects serial neurologic evaluations.
7. Interventions and patient's response to them.
8. Consultants' recommendations.
9. Diagnosis.
10. Disposition plans. It is not enough to write "Head instructions" as a discharge instruction. Each patient needs to have a *written* statement of the *specific* head instructions so that he or she can reread the instructions on returning home. Discharge to the care of a responsible adult is required.

SUMMARY AND FINAL POINTS

- Head and neck trauma can be concomitant injuries.
- Careful cervical spine immobilization is essential during prehospital as well as hospital care.
- Mental status changes are the most important indicator of underlying cerebral injury.
- A normal head CT scan does not rule out a CNS bleed.
- Normal cervical spine radiographs do not rule out serious spinal cord injury. The lateral view must include all seven cervical vertebrae.
- Frequent neurologic examinations are necessary to monitor a possibly evolving injury.
- Metabolic causes of altered mental status may coexist with significant cerebral injury.
- All patients suffering head or neck trauma with associated neurologic deficits are admitted for further management.

BIBLIOGRAPHY

Texts

1. Bloch RF, Babbauar M: Management of Spinal Cord Injuries. Baltimore Williams & Wilkins, 1986.
2. Galli RL, Spaite DW, Simon RR: Emergency Orthopedics—The Spine. Norwalk, CT, Appleton & Lange, 1989.
3. Harris JH, Edeiken-Monroe B: The Radiology of Acute Cervical Spine Trauma (2nd ed). Baltimore, Williams & Wilkins, 1987.
4. Wilberger JE: Spinal Cord Injuries in Children. Mount Kisco, NY, Futura Publishing, 1986.

Journal Articles

1. Bracken MB, Shepard MJ, Collins WF, et al: A randomized, controlled trial of methylprednisolone or naloxone in the treatment of acute spinal-cord injury. N Engl J Med 322:1405–1411, 1990.
2. Gennarelli TA: Emergency department management of head injuries. Emerg Med Clin North Am 2:749–760, 1984.
3. Masters SJ, McClean PM, Arcarese JS, et al: Skull x-ray examinations after head trauma. N Engl J Med 316:84–91, 1987.
4. Mills ML, Ruisso LS, Vines FS: High yield criteria for urgent cranial computer tomography scans. Ann Emerg Med 15:1167–1172, 1986.
5. Saunders CE, Cota R, Barton C: Reliability of home observation for victims of mild closed head injury. Ann Emerg Med 15:160–163, 1986.

CHAPTER 51

DIZZINESS

ARTHUR B. SANDERS, M.D.

PROBLEM 1 A 20 year old female college student complained that she had been dizzy for 1 day.

PROBLEM 2 An 80 year old man presented to the emergency department complaining of weakness and dizziness gradually worsening over 1 week.

QUESTIONS TO CONSIDER

1. What are the common causes of dizziness in patients presenting to the emergency department?
2. How does one distinguish between vertigo and lightheadedness?
3. How does one distinguish between central and peripheral vertigo?
4. What history and physical examination are appropriate for patients complaining of dizziness?
5. What are the appropriate ancillary tests to consider for patients complaining of dizziness?
6. What is the emergency department management and disposition of patients complaining of vertigo and lightheadedness?

INTRODUCTION

Dizziness is a common complaint of patients seen in the emergency department. By 65 years of age more than 30% of people have suffered from dizziness; by age 80, 67% of women and 33% of men have reported episodes of dizziness. Dizziness occurs in all age groups; however, in patients more than 50 years of age dizziness is more likely to be caused by a serious underlying disorder.

Unfortunately, the term *dizziness* is imprecise and has multiple meanings, both to the lay public and to health care professionals. The complaint of dizziness may mean lightheadedness, disequilibrium, imbalance, weakness, unsteadiness, a sensation of movement or rotation, or the feeling that one is about to lose consciousness.

In most patients, the findings from the history and physical examination can be used to classify the complaint of dizziness into the categories of vertigo and lightheadedness. *Vertigo* is defined as the "hallucination of movement." Patients with vertigo complain of the sensation of spinning or rotation of patients or their surroundings. This hallucination of movement is often accompanied by systemic symptoms such as nausea, vomiting, and diaphoresis. Some patients, in fact, may complain of nausea and vomiting as their primary symptom. Vertigo is indicative of vestibular dysfunction, which may be peripheral or central in origin (Table 51–1).

Clinical studies have demonstrated that 23% to 38% of patients presenting to the emergency department with a complaint of dizziness will have true vertigo. The remainder have lightheadedness. *Lightheadedness* can be defined as the sensation of impending loss

TABLE 51-1. Classification of Vertigo-Nystagmus

	Central	Peripheral
Onset, type	Insidious, continuous	Sudden, intermittent
Nausea and vomiting	Minor symptom	Often severe
Head motion	Little aggravation of symptoms	Aggravation of symptoms
Tinnitus	Uncommon	Characteristic
Hearing loss	Uncommon	Characteristic
Cranial nerve examination	Abnormal	Normal
Positional nystagmus	Immediate onset, no fatigue, no adaptation	Latent periods (2–20 sec), fatigue, adaptation occurs
Spontaneous nystagmus	Multidirectional, conjugate movement, not suppressed by visual fixation	Unidirectional dissociated or disconjugate movement, no vertical nystagmus, suppressed by visual fixation
Differential diagnosis	Vertebrobasilar insufficiency Brainstem infarct Tumor (acoustic neuroma) Hemorrhage (cerebellar) Multiple sclerosis	Vestibular neuronitis Benign positional vertigo Ménière's disease Middle ear infection Cholesteatoma Perilymphatic fistula

of consciousness and is generally caused by a temporary decrease in blood flow to the brain. It may be accompanied by dimming of vision, diaphoresis, nausea, and loss of balance. Although lightheadedness has similar causes, it should be distinguished from true syncope (Chap. 12), which involves loss of consciousness and heralds a worse prognosis.

INITIAL APPROACH IN THE EMERGENCY DEPARTMENT

A small percentage of patients presenting to the emergency department with dizziness have serious life-threatening diseases. It is prudent to evaluate all patients with dizziness initially for evidence of life-threatening illness. This initial evaluation can be done by reviewing the patient's vital signs and briefly observing and communicating with the patient.

Blood Pressure. Hypotension is not an uncommon cause of dizziness, especially in elderly patients. Patients presenting with hypotension should have an intravenous line started immediately with an infusion of isotonic crystalloid. Patients presenting with poorly controlled hypertension or hypertensive urgency may also have dizziness. If the patient is significantly hypertensive (blood pressure over 190/130), he is closely evaluated for signs of the renal, cardiopulmonary, and central nervous system effects of hypertension (Chap. 13). Hypertension and bradycardia may indicate increased intracranial pressure and a primary central nervous system problem.

Pulse Rate. Dysrhythmias are a serious and treatable cause of lightheadedness and are of prime concern, especially in elderly patients. The pulse is evaluated for irregularity, tachycardia, or bradycardia. Elderly patients or patients with abnormal heart rates are immediately placed on an electrocardiographic (ECG) monitor.

Respirations. The patient's respirations are observed for any signs of respiratory distress. If the patient is tachypneic or complains of shortness of breath, one must consider hypoxia as a cause of the dizziness. Causes of hypoxia include pulmonary embolus, pneumonia, congestive heart failure, carbon monoxide poisoning, and so on.

Temperature. The patient's temperature is noted. A fever may indicate sepsis, and hyperthermia or hypothermia may be present as dizziness.

General Appearance. One determines whether the patient is alert, oriented, and responding appropriately. These initial observations may reveal a gross neurologic deficit or a problem in mental status that needs immediate evaluation.

After consideration of the vital signs and general appearance, the patient's problem can be prioritized in relation to the problems of other patients in the emergency department, and the physician can return later for a more complete history and physical examination.

PROBLEM 2 The 80 year old man was alert and oriented but sluggish in his responses. Vital signs were blood pressure 130/95 mm Hg, pulse 100 beats/min, respirations 16/min, temperature 37°C (98.6°F).

Cardiovascular disease should be of initial concern in this 80 year old patient. His vital signs showed mild diastolic hypertension and borderline tachycardia. The patient is placed on an ECG monitor to be observed for dysrhythmias and an intravenous (IV) line of dextrose in water 5% is started and kept open in case medications are needed emergently.

DATA GATHERING

History

The history is very important in evaluating patients with dizziness. The patient should be informed that there are multiple interpretations for the word *dizziness* and that it is important to describe the sensation as precisely as possible. If necessary, the emergency physician can offer a choice of terms to use, such as lightheadedness, spinning sensation, imbalance, weakness, unsteadiness, feeling about to faint, and so on. The physician can specifically inquire, *"Does the room spin?"* or *"Do you feel yourself spinning?"* From the initial history one can get a sense of whether the patient is experiencing vertigo or lightheadedness. Key historical points include the following:

Time Course. Is the dizziness *episodic* or *continuous*? How *long* have the *symptoms* been *present*? Has the patient ever had *similar symptoms* in the *past*?

Predisposing Conditions. What was the patient doing *immediately prior* to the *initial episode* of dizziness? Is there a *particular position* or *activity* that *brings on* the dizziness?

Associated Symptoms. Is there associated *nausea, vomiting,* or *diaphoresis*? Do *palpitations* accompany the dizziness? Are there any *otic symptoms* such as hearing loss, tinnitus, fullness, or pressure or pain in the ear? Are there associated headaches, weakness, numbness, or other *neurologic symptoms*? Has there been any *recent head trauma*? Are there any *symptoms* of *dehydration* such as thirst or poor oral intake?

Review of Symptoms. It is important to *review* the *symptoms* related to the cardiac, pulmonary, neurologic, and otic systems.

Medications. In almost 10% of patients presenting to an emergency department with dizziness this symptom is due to medications they are taking. Approximately 300 medications have been associated with dizziness. Some are directly ototoxic. Table 51–2 provides a list of some of the more common drugs associated with dizziness.

TABLE 51–2. Medications Associated with Dizziness

Alcohol	Antimalarials*
Antibiotics*	Chloroquine
Aminoglycosides	Quinine
Antiarrhythmics	Diuretics*
Anticonvulsants*	Ethacrynic acid
Phenytoin	Furosemide
Antidepressants	Hypnotics
Antihistamines	Hypoglycemics
Antihypertensives	Phenothiazines
Anti-inflammatory agents*	
Salicylates	
Antiparkinson agents	

*Directly ototoxic

PROBLEM 1 The college student said that she had been experiencing a "spinning" sensation all day. She had vomited three times and had not eaten since yesterday. The attacks of dizziness were episodic and were worse when she moved her head. She "almost passed out" when she got up from bed.

The patient's description of her dizziness is most consistent with a diagnosis of vertigo. However, she may also be dehydrated and orthostatic. It would be important to look for signs of nystagmus and perform orthostatic vital signs as part of the physical examination.

Physical Examination

The physical examination is often helpful in distinguishing the cause of dizziness. The emergency physician should concentrate on performing thorough cardiovascular, neurologic, and otic examinations. Specifics of the directed examination are as follows:

General Appearance. Once again, it is important to take a few minutes to observe the patient before proceeding to a full history and physical examination. Does the patient seem uncomfortable? How is he lying or sitting? Does he move cautiously because certain positions provoke the symptoms? Has he vomited since being admitted to the emergency department? Is he anxious and hyperventilating?

Vital Signs. Any abnormal vital signs are measured again by the examining physician. Have any interventions performed initially been effective? Has the patient responded to fluids? Does the ECG monitor reveal dysrhythmias?

Eyes. The patient's eyes are examined to determine any abnormality in range and pattern of motion, visual fields, pupillary reactions, corneal reflex, or funduscopic appearance. Abnormalities may indicate a primary neurologic disease such as multiple sclerosis or brain stem pathology. The eyes are examined for nystagmus in four directions. The patient is asked to follow the physician's finger with his eyes to both lateral positions as well as up and down. Be careful not to elicit end-position nystagmus by asking the patient to look to the extreme right or left. Rhythmic jerks of the eye in extreme lateral positions may occur in normal patients as a result of tired muscles rather than vestibular pathology. If nystagmus is not elicited and vertigo is suspected by this history, the special tests described later in this chapter may be used.

Ears. The patient should undergo a complete ear examination, inspecting the ear canal and tympanic membrane and performing the Weber and Rinne tests. Any indication of hearing loss or a discrepancy of hearing between the two ears can be followed with audiometric examination.

Pulmonary. The chest is examined for any signs of active disease, including rales, ronchi, wheezes, or rubs.

Cardiovascular. A complete cardiac examination is done noting heart sounds, murmurs, rubs, and gallops and including an evaluation for congestive heart failure. The carotid arteries are auscultated for bruits.

Abdomen. An abdominal examination is performed to rule out any evidence of sepsis or bleeding. A young woman presenting with dizziness should have a pelvic examination to determine whether there are signs of an intrauterine or ectopic pregnancy. A rectal examination, including a stool guaiac test for blood, is necessary to evaluate the patient for possible sites of blood loss.

Neurologic Examination. A complete neurologic examination is performed including cranial nerves, motor function, reflexes, sensation, and cerebellar tests. The Romberg or Quix test may detect body sway. In the Quix test the patient stands with the feet together, arms outstretched and chin up. He closes his eyes and is observed for body sway for approximately 1 minute. Cerebellar testing should include finger to nose and heel to shin testing as well as the ability to walk. Patients who have an imbalance in the legs generally have a cerebellar or proprioceptive disorder. True muscular weakness may indicate a primary neuromuscular disease such as myasthenia gravis, botulism, or Guillain-Barré syndrome.

Bedside Tests. Several bedside tests can be performed to help in the evaluation of the patient with dizziness.

Bárány's Test for Positional Nystagmus. The physician places the patient in the supine position and quickly rotates the head to 45 degrees in each direction (Fig. 51–1). The eyes are observed for nystagmus in each direction, and the patient is queried about symptoms of dizziness and nausea.

Hyperventilation. The patient is instructed to hyperventilate for 3 minutes to determine whether the symptoms of dizziness are reproduced.

Tilt Test for Orthostatic Hypotension. The patient's blood pressure and pulse are taken while supine and standing. An increase in the pulse rate of 20 to 30/min, fall in blood pressure of 20 mm Hg or greater, or the development of clinical symptoms indicates orthostasis.

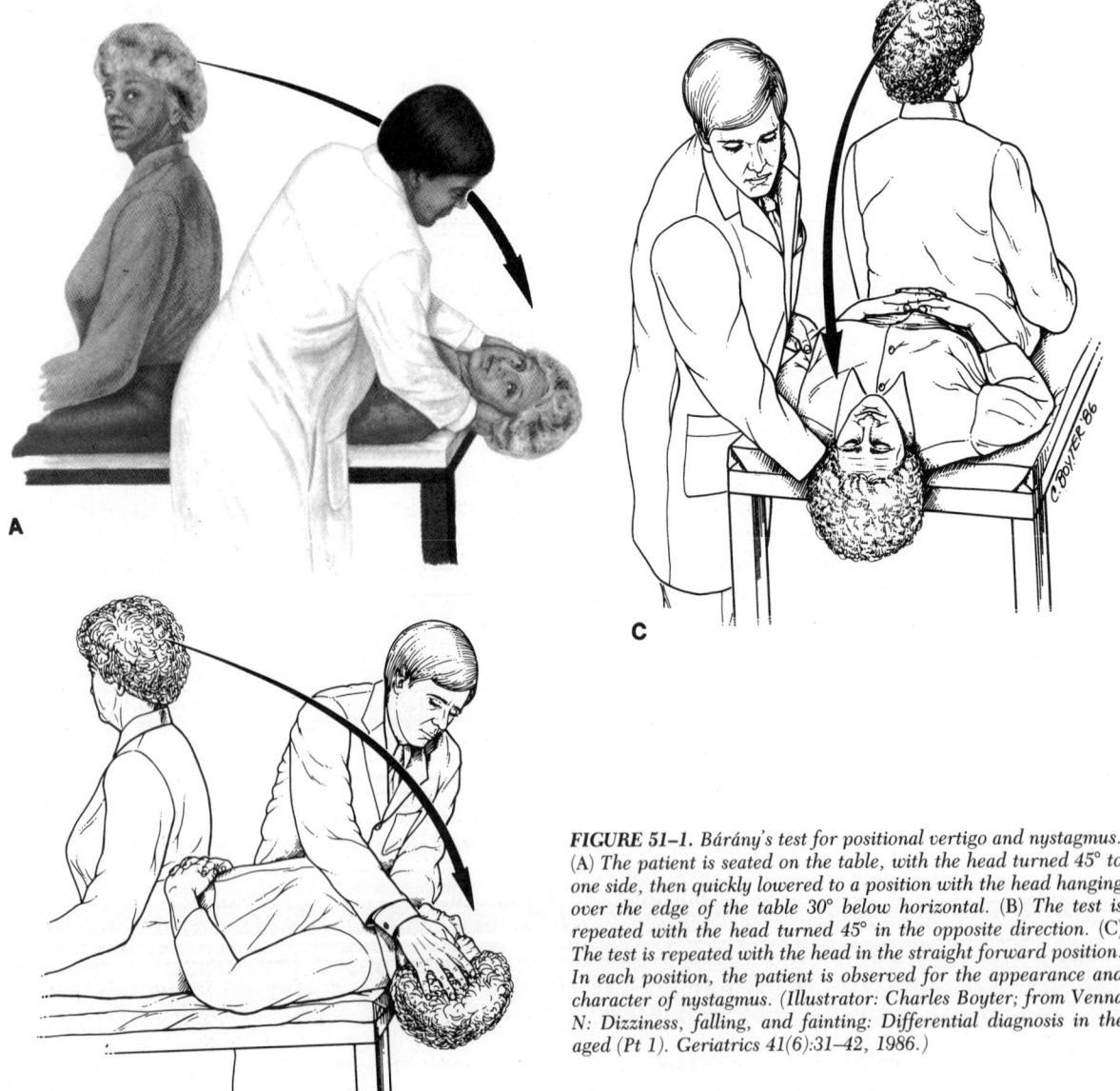

FIGURE 51–1. Bárány's test for positional vertigo and nystagmus. (A) The patient is seated on the table, with the head turned 45° to one side, then quickly lowered to a position with the head hanging over the edge of the table 30° below horizontal. (B) The test is repeated with the head turned 45° in the opposite direction. (C) The test is repeated with the head in the straight forward position. In each position, the patient is observed for the appearance and character of nystagmus. (Illustrator: Charles Boyter; from Venna N: Dizziness, falling, and fainting: Differential diagnosis in the aged (Pt 1). Geriatrics 41(6):31–42, 1986.)

Valsalva Maneuver. The patient is instructed to hold his breath in forced expiration for 15 seconds to determine whether symptoms are reproduced.

Neck Hyperextension. This test is designed to compress the vertebral arteries and test brain stem perfusion. The neck is hyperextended over the examining table and then brought back to a sitting position to determine whether symptoms are reproduced.

PROBLEM 1 The patient showed nystagmus on lateral gaze with her head back. She also had positive results on the tilt test for orthostatic hypotension. The rest of the physical examination was unremarkable. An intravenous infusion with normal saline was started to hydrate the patient.

PROBLEM 2 In the 80 year old male there were no abnormalities on the ECG monitor. He had a history of hypertension, congestive heart failure, and osteoarthritis. His drug prescriptions included digoxin and hydrochlorothiazide. He described the dizziness as a persistent "cloud." There was no nausea, vomiting, or chest pain. Physical examination revealed spontaneous nystagmus and signs of mild hypertension and congestive heart failure that seem unchanged from data recorded on previous examinations in the clinic.

The patient's description of his symptoms was vague, defying easy classification. He was taking several medications and had underlying disease processes that could cause dizziness.

DECISION PRIORITIES AND PRELIMINARY DIFFERENTIAL DIAGNOSIS

1. *Is this true vertigo or lightheadedness?*
   Based on the directed history and physical examination, the complaint of dizziness in most patients can be categorized as either vertigo or lightheadedness. Patients with vertigo describe the sensation of spinning or rotation. They often have accompanying nausea, vomiting, and diaphoresis. The physical examination generally demonstrates nystagmus, which may be spontaneous or positional on movement of the head as described. Patients with lightheadedness do not meet these criteria for vertigo. They describe symptoms consistent with decreased cerebral blood flow without true syncope.
2. *If vertigo, is it central or peripheral?*
   Vertigo can be classified as peripheral or central, as listed in Table 51–1. Peripheral vertigo is often aggravated by movement of the head and is more likely to be associated with nausea, vomiting, tinnitus, and hearing loss. The nystagmus is unidirectional (but never vertical) and is suppressed by visual fixation. Central vertigo is usually insidious in onset over weeks or months and can be associated with other neurologic signs or symptoms such as cranial nerve deficits, diplopia, or dysarthria. In general, central vertigo is associated with an older population and more serious disease processes.
3. *If lightheadedness, how are the many different causes organized?*
   The etiology of lightheadedness is not so straightforward. Multiple systems must be investigated.

   Neurovascular Causes. Multiple neurovascular diseases may be the cause of dizziness. These include vertebrobasilar insufficiency, multiple sclerosis, brain stem or cerebellar-pontine infarct or tumor, or Parkinson's disease. Further work-up will depend on the accompanying neurologic abnormalities.

   Cardiac Causes. Cardiovascular causes of dizziness include dysrhythmias, valvular heart disease, congestive heart failure, or any condition that decreases cardiac output and blood flow to the central nervous system.

   Metabolic Causes. Metabolic causes that must be considered include hypoxia, hypoglycemia, hyperventilation, toxins, drugs, uremia, hepatic failure, and hypokalemia. Specific metabolic diseases should be worked up as dictated by the history and physical examination findings.

Hematologic Causes. Anemia, hyperviscosity syndromes, and myeloproliferative disorders should be considered in patients presenting with dizziness.

Psychogenic Causes. Stress, anxiety, and hysteria may be associated with dizziness or hyperventilation syndromes.

Miscellaneous Causes. Other conditions such as sepsis, shock, autoimmune diseases, and orthostatic hypotension from multiple causes must be evaluated in these patients.

Idiopathic Causes. In approximately 20% to 30% of patients who present with a complaint of dizziness there will be no clear etiology of the complaint even after a thorough evaluation.

DIAGNOSTIC ADJUNCTS

Laboratory Studies

Laboratory studies are dictated by the clinical history and physical examination. Specific tests to consider for patients presenting with dizziness include the following:

Complete Blood Count with White Cell Differential. The CBC is used to investigate the possibility of anemia or myeloproliferative diseases.

Serum Glucose. Serum glucose is used to rule out hypoglycemia.

Serum Electrolytes. Hypokalemia can produce vague symptoms such as weakness and dizziness.

Arterial Blood Gases. These measurements may be useful in patients in whom hypoxia or hypercarbia due to pulmonary embolus, congestive heart failure, or pneumonia is suspected.

Pregnancy Tests. Pregnancy tests should be considered for women of childbearing age who present with dizziness or orthostatic hypotension.

Toxicology Tests. Tests for specific drugs such as salicylates, phenytoin, alcohol, or carbon monoxide may be useful in some patients in whom the clinical history is unclear or drug toxicity is suspected.

Selected Tests for Specific Cases. Protein electrophoresis, thyroid function tests, VDRL, sedimentation rate, coagulation tests, or immunologic tests may be appropriate to make the diagnosis of specific diseases.

Radiologic Imaging

Computer tomography (CT) and *magnetic resonance imaging* (MRI) are the most useful tests for detecting central nervous system pathology in patients in whom a central cause of vertigo or dizziness is suspected. Hemorrhage, acoustic neuromas, and other neoplasms will generally be visible on the CT scan. Small ischemic strokes may not be detected by initial CT scanning, and follow-up scans in a few days are necessary (see Chap. 49).

Electrocardiography

A 12-lead electrocardiogram is ordered in any patient with dizziness who has suspected cardiovascular disease. If the patient does not have cardiac symptoms at the time of the emergency department visit, further ECG monitoring may be necessary with either admission to an inpatient monitored bed or by means of an outpatient Holter monitor. Patients who show signs and symptoms of cerebrovascular disease should be considered for noninvasive vascular studies of the central nervous system circulation.

Other Tests
Otolaryngologic Testing

Electronystagmography. Electronystagmography (ENG) is performed in otolaryngology laboratories. In this test, electrodes detect the rate, direction, and amplitude of eye movements. This test may be used to detect nystagmus that has not been evident clinically. The character of the nystagmus may aid in differentiating between central and peripheral causes of vertigo (see Table 51–1).

Audiometry. Formal audiometric testing in an otologic laboratory will document any hearing deficit and help localize specific lesions. Hearing deficits accompany specific disease entities such as Ménière's disease and acoustic neuroma.

Brain Stem Auditory Evoked Responses (BAER). This physiologic test of auditory pathways may be done in selected patients in whom central neurologic lesions are suspected. It is particularly helpful in diagnosing patients with acoustic neuromas.

Caloric Testing. The vestibulo-ocular reflex is tested by irrigating the ear canal with cold water, which produces nystagmus in the opposite direction. Characteristics of the nystagmus produced may help to distinguish between peripheral and central lesions that cause vertigo. Caloric tests may be most beneficial when they are combined with electronystagmography and are generally done in the otolaryngology laboratory.

PROBLEM 2 The emergency physician felt that it was important to evaluate the patient's congestive heart failure and medications as possible etiologic factors for his dizziness. An ECG, chest radiograph, serum electrolytes, digoxin level, and arterial blood gas measurements were ordered.

REFINED DIFFERENTIAL DIAGNOSIS

After completing the history, physical examination, and ancillary tests, the emergency physician is usually able to classify the patient with dizziness and evaluate the likelihood of disease processes in the differential diagnosis. Table 51–3 lists the characteristics of the more common and serious diagnostic considerations. The most common diseases are benign positional vertigo and vestibular neuritis. Patients with these diseases have true vertigo by history and nystagmus on physical examination. These diseases are usually self-limiting. Acoustic neuroma is a more serious disease presenting as vertigo. There are often accompanying neurologic findings and an abnormal CT scan or MRI. Elderly patients with lightheadedness may have serious dysrhythmias or metabolic abnormalities. Cardiac examination and electrocardiogram usually allow the emergency physician to make a decision regarding the likelihood of a cardiovascular cause for the dizziness. Orthostatic hypotension may indicate dehydration or acute blood loss. A clear etiology for a patient's orthostasis must be sought during the emergency department visit.

PRINCIPLES OF MANAGEMENT

The management of patients with dizziness is geared to the specific disease process suspected. Patients with peripheral vertigo may be treated symptomatically. Intravenous diazepam can abate an acute attack, whereas oral antihistamines such as meclizine can be used to prevent further symptoms. Intravenous saline is administered if there is evidence of dehydration.

Patients with central vertigo may also be treated symptomatically. However, prompt work-up for serious disease processes such as tumor and infarction is initiated.

Treatment for lightheadedness is directed toward a specific cause or causes.

PROBLEM 1 After 2 liters of intravenous normal saline had been administered, the

TABLE 51–3. Differential Diagnosis for Dizziness

	History	Physical Examination	Ancillary Tests	Emergency Department Management
Benign positional vertigo	Spinning sensation Nausea and vomiting Worse on head movement	Positional nystagmus Normal findings on neurologic examination	Positive Bárány's test	Symptomatic treatment (antihistamines)
Vestibular neuritis (acute labyrinthitis)	Spinning sensation Nausea and vomiting Acute onset	Spontaneous nystagmus Normal findings on neurologic examination		Symptomatic treatment (antihistamines)
Acoustic neuroma	Spinning sensation Facial weakness Tinnitus	Neural hearing loss Diminished corneal reflex Abnormal BAER Ataxia	Abnormal CT scan	Surgical treatment
Ménière's disease	Spinning sensation Tinnitus Hearing loss	Spontaneous nystagmus Progressive decrease in auditory acuity Normal findings on neurologic examination	Abnormal audiometric findings Abnormal ENG	Symptomatic treatment Surgical options Referral to otolaryngologist
Hyperventilation	Lightheadedness Numbness Tingling in extremities Stress related	Within normal limits	Hyperventilation reproduces symptoms	Symptomatic treatment
Dysrhythmias	Lightheadedness Palpitations	Cardiac examination findings may be abnormal	24-hour Holter monitor	Admission to monitored bed Antiarrhythmics
Orthostatic hypotension	Lightheadedness Worse on standing up	Within normal limits	Positive tilt test results	Rule out acute blood loss Replace fluids Admit if necessary for diagnostic tests

patient was not orthostatic; however, the spinning sensation continued. The emergency physician felt that the most likely diagnosis was acute labyrinthitis with dehydration secondary to vomiting.

This patient had vertigo caused by acute labyrinthitis and lightheadedness due to dehydration. Patients with dizziness may have both vertigo and lightheadedness at the same time.

PROBLEM 2 Ancillary test results on the 80 year old man were returned. The ECG and chest radiograph were unchanged from previous studies. The digoxin level was within the therapeutic range. Electrolytes were as follows: sodium, 140 mEq/liter; potassium, 3.5 mEq/liter; chloride, 96 mEq/liter; carbon dioxide 10 mEq/liter. Arterial blood gases were pH 7.24; Po_2, 80; Pco_2, 30.

The exact cause of this patient's dizziness remains unclear. The laboratory findings point to the need for more history from this patient.

SPECIAL CONSIDERATIONS

Pediatric Patients

It is often difficult to evaluate the symptom of dizziness in children. Vertigo occurs in children and may be documented by nystagmus or special tests such as ENG. Benign positional vertigo is most common between the ages of 1 and 3 years. Vertiginous seizures, migraines, and otologic infection can be considered in children. Teen-agers may be more prone to drug abuse and hyperventilation syndromes.

Geriatric Patients

In the geriatric population arteriosclerotic cardiovascular disease or medication problems are more likely to be causes of dizziness.

DISPOSITION AND FOLLOW-UP

The definitive diagnosis of patients presenting with dizziness is frequently not made in the emergency department. Further diagnostic tests and observation over time are often necessary to be certain of the diagnosis. The challenge in the emergency department is to separate those patients who have evidence of serious or life-threatening illnesses from those who can be managed symptomatically and followed in the clinic.

Admission

Patients with evidence of central vertigo or central nervous system abnormalities need to be seen by a neurologic or ENT consultant. Most often these patients are admitted to the hospital for diagnostic tests and definitive treatment.

Patients presenting with lightheadedness are appropriately evaluated in the emergency department, and cardiovascular, neurologic, and metabolic causes are ruled out. If there is a suspicion of a cardiac dysrhythmia, the patient is admitted to a monitored bed. Patients with orthostatic hypotension may be appropriately evaluated and treated according to etiology. Admission may be necessary if blood loss is suspected.

Discharge

Patients with peripheral vertigo who are well hydrated and are able to care for themselves generally can be sent home on symptomatic treatment. The patient is cautioned about changing position, operating a motor vehicle, or assuming a position in which vertigo may cause serious harm. Follow-up by an appropriate primary care or ENT physician is appropriate to determine whether the onset of dizziness arises from a chronic or more serious condition.

Patients with negative results on metabolic, neurologic, and cardiovascular work-up can be sent home and asked to return if symptoms become worse. These patients are followed in a few days by their primary care physician. Medications that are implicated in causing dizziness need to be reevaluated and the use of alternative medications considered in consultation with the patient's primary care physician.

PROBLEM 2 The laboratory tests showed a metabolic acidosis. The emergency physician reviewed the history with the patient and his family. When asked specifically about aspirin ingestion, the patient said he often took aspirin for his arthritis and recently heard that it will also prevent heart attacks. His salicylate level was 80 mg/dl (therapeutic level is less than 30 mg/dl). He was admitted to the hospital for observation.

Medications are frequently a cause of dizziness, especially in the elderly. Some elderly patients experience toxic reactions to salicylates after inadvertently taking multiple doses for arthritis pain and then forgetting when and how much they took. This situation can lead to dizziness, nystagmus, metabolic acidosis, and other signs of chronic salicylate poisoning.

DOCUMENTATION

1. Patient's description of dizziness in his own words.
2. Associated symptoms such as positional changes and inciting events.

3. Any medications taken.
4. Past medical history of otologic, neurologic, and cardiovascular disease.
5. Physical examination results with careful attention paid to otologic, neurologic, and cardiovascular findings.
6. Response to special tests such as hyperventilation and positional changes.
7. Ancillary test results including ECG monitoring in the emergency department for evidence of dysrhythmia.
8. Response to therapy given in the emergency department such as fluids or antihistamines.
9. Consideration given to ruling out serious life-threatening diseases.
10. Clear patient instructions including cautions not to engage in any activities in which the dizziness may be harmful.

SUMMARY AND FINAL POINTS

- Dizziness is an imprecise term; careful history and physical examination can help distinguish between lightheadedness and vertigo.
- Approximately 23% to 38% of patients presenting to the emergency department with a complaint of dizziness will have true vertigo.
- The neurologic and otologic examinations can help distinguish between peripheral and central vertigo.
- Central vertigo is usually indicative of serious disease processes.
- Patients may have both vertigo and lightheadedness at the same time.
- Medications are the cause of dizziness in about 10% of patients. Over 300 medications have been associated with dizziness.
- Cardiovascular etiologies must be seriously considered in all elderly patients with lightheadedness.

BIBLIOGRAPHY

Texts

1. Dix MR, Hood JD (eds): Vertigo. Chichester, John Wiley and Sons, 1984.
2. Packer RJ, Berman PH: Dizziness/vertigo. In Fleisher GR, Ludwig S (eds): Textbook of Pediatric Emergency Medicine (2nd ed). Baltimore, Williams & Wilkins, 1988, pp. 146–149.

Journal Articles

1. Bonikowski FP: Differential diagnosis of dizziness in the elderly. Geriatrics 38:89–104, 1983.
2. Drachman DA, Hart CW: An approach to the dizzy patient. Neurology 22:323–334, 1972.
3. Lehrer JF, Poole DC: Diagnosis and management of vertigo. Comprehensive Therapy 13:31–40, 1987.
4. Luxon LM: A bit dizzy. Br J Hosp Med 32:315–321, 1974.
5. Madlon-Kay DJ: Evaluation and outcome of the dizzy patient. J Family Pract 21:109–113, 1985.
6. Nedzelski JM, Barber HO, McIlmoyl L: Diagnosis in a dizziness unit. J Otolaryngol 15:101–104, 1986.
7. Skiendzieleiwski JJ, Martyak G: The weak and dizzy patient. Ann Emerg Med 9:353–356, 1980.
8. Towler AM: Dizziness and vertigo. Br Med J 288:1739–1743, 1984.
9. Trobe JD: Dizziness. Emergency Decisions 2:41–47, 1986.
10. Venna N: Dizziness, falling, and fainting: Differential diagnosis in the aged (Part I). Geriatrics 41:30–42, 1986.
11. Venna N: Dizziness, falling and fainting: Differential diagnosis in the aged (Part II). Geriatrics 41:31–45, 1986.

SECTION FOURTEEN

PSYCHO-BEHAVIORAL DISORDERS

CHAPTER 52

BEHAVIORAL DISORDERS

MICHAEL G. MANSKE, M.D.
GLENN C. HAMILTON, M.D.

PROBLEM 1 A 34 year old male was brought to the emergency department by ambulance after apparently falling in his shower. He was awake, slightly agitated, and occasionally spoke unintelligible words.

PROBLEM 2 A 66 year old bedridden woman was transferred from a nursing home for evaluation. The staff had noted increasing confusion; the patient related visits from her husband, who had died 2 years ago.

PROBLEM 3 A 40 year old man was brought in by ambulance after police had found him acting strangely on a downtown street corner. The man was agitated and shouting, "God has instructed me to save the world . . . the final judgment will come Tuesday."

QUESTIONS TO CONSIDER

1. What are the emergency physician's responsibilities in managing patients with behavioral disorders?
2. What is a mental status examination?
3. How can a mental status examination help differentiate between organic and functional illness?
4. What are the relevant classes of functional illness?
5. When is it necessary to consult a psychiatrist? What information is important to convey during such a telephone consultation?
6. How is the issue of involuntary consent involved in the care of patients with an emotional disorder?
7. How is disposition managed for the patient who has elements of both organic and functional disorders?

INTRODUCTION

Five to fifteen percent of patients presenting to the emergency department have a psychiatric problem. If alcohol-related (7%) and drug-related (5%) problems are included, psychobehavioral problems account for almost 30% of emergency department visits. Over 10 million man hours and $12 billion are spent annually in the treatment of emergency behavioral problems. A number of factors make treatment of psychiatric problems in the emergency department difficult. The physician and staff have time constraints that reduce the opportunity for prolonged interaction. Psychiatric care requires an average of two to three times longer than most medically oriented encounters. A disproportionate number of psychobehavioral complaints occur during the night hours, when resources are limited and disposition is difficult. The bias of staff against repeat visitors or patients with psychobehavioral complaints may limit the quality of care such patients receive. Lastly, the emergency department is often the "court of last resort" for patients and families who are not satisfied with their care, have been denied access to care, or have decided care is necessary. All expect something to be done, whether it is warranted or not. To add to the difficulty, 30% to 60% of psychobehavioral problems may be partially or completely due to underlying medical illness. Some of these medical illnesses are potentially life-threatening if they are not diagnosed and treated. These circumstances place considerable strain and risk on the emergency department staff. The only way to manage the difficult setting and demands while caring for patients with psychobehavioral problems is to set realistic goals. These goals are:

1. To anticipate and manage violence.
2. To perform a basic evaluation including psychiatric history, physical examination, mental status examination, and selected laboratory tests.
3. To differentiate organic from psychiatric disease.
4. To pay attention to potentially life-threatening organic diseases.
5. If the disease is psychiatric, to classify it correctly and arrange appropriate disposition.
6. To maintain a perspective for patient advocacy.

PREHOSPITAL CARE

Many patients who present with psychobehavioral problems will arrive accompanied by a rescue squad, police, family, or friends, or they may arrive alone. The information to be obtained from any accompanying individuals includes the following items:

History

1. Description of the scene where the patient was found; were there any signs of violence or drug abuse?
2. Eyewitness accounts of patient's behavior.
3. The patient's key past medical history, e.g., diabetic, and psychiatric history from family, friends, or medical alert badge.

Physical Examination

1. General description of patient's appearance, including level of consciousness.
2. Vital signs.
3. Findings on a brief mental status examination.
4. Findings on a gross neurologic examination.

Intervention

Field intervention may range from simple reassurance to active restraint. The psychiatric training and experience of rescue squads vary greatly. A primary concern is that prehospital personnel are not placed in potentially hazardous situations. If there is any potential for violence, the police are asked to become involved.

PROBLEM 3 The patient was found on a downtown street corner. The paramedics witnessed him speaking structured sentences containing bizarre religious content while in an agitated state. No past medical history was available. The patient was well-dressed and very neat in appearance. Although he was occasionally slightly lethargic, he quickly began another outburst. He only allowed the paramedics to take his pulse. It was strong and regular with a rate of 100. Respirations were 18/min and normal. Because the neurologic findings were grossly normal, they did not perform any medical interventions but planned to transport the patient. They radioed the emergency department to request further orders.

The paramedics are advised to offer reassurance and explain the need for transport to the patient. This patient should definitely be evaluated in the emergency department. If he didn't respond to reassurance and did not agree to be transported, physical restraint might have been necessary.

INITIAL APPROACH IN THE EMERGENCY DEPARTMENT

Patients in the emergency department may be identified as "known schizophrenic," "mental health patient," or just "acting strangely." Each receives an initial screening evaluation consisting of general observation and recording of vital signs to exclude any gross abnormality.

Other specific considerations in the initial approach to the behaviorally disturbed patient include the following:

1. Unless immediate medical care is required, the patient is placed in a comfortable, reasonably private room with minimal outside intrusions.

2. Interviews with the family, friends, or witnesses of the current behavioral episode are initiated. These people are asked to remain in the emergency department, or their names and telephone numbers are obtained to permit further information gathering later.

3. Old medical records of patient are requested; these may be the only clue that the patient does in fact have a counselor, therapist, or place of residence.

4. If any suicidal or violent behavior is suspected, the patient is not left unattended.

5. Security personnel are notified as indicated and are given explicit restraint orders.

6. If the patient is threatening violence or is actively violent, restraint is necessary. Full leather restraints are preferred. A team approach works best in subduing the patient. Optimally, four people work together to immobilize each limb. After restraint, a weapons check should be done, and the patient is closely monitored.

The initial approach assumes that an organic problem is causing or contributing to the psychobehavioral problem of the patient. Both the level and content of consciousness can offer clues supporting an organic etiology.

PROBLEM 2 On admission the patient was an ill-appearing, elderly woman who was looking about the room moaning and was disoriented. Vital signs on triage were: pulse 104 beats/min, blood pressure 106/67 mm Hg, respiration 30/min, and temperature 100.3°F (37.9°C).

An abnormality in any of the vital signs forces one to consider an organic cause for a patient's altered behavior. Certainly, with the slight abnormalities in all vital signs in this patient, an organic illness must be considered. Her age and disorientation also support an organic cause. This patient's condition should be assumed to be medical in origin until proved otherwise.

DATA GATHERING

History

The general goal of the history obtained from a patient with a behavioral disorder is to determine why the disorder is an emergency at this point in time, to obtain information about the patient's previous psychiatric history, and to understand the make-up and capabilities of his or her personal support system.

The quality of the history obtained from a patient with a psychobehavioral disorder depends on the mindset of the physician, the setting, and the structure of the interview. The attitude and preconceptions of the physician greatly influence the exchange of information in the interview. The best attitude is one of detached concern in which empathy and understanding are given the patient without judgment. Most judgments are based on the physician's value system, which may not have any useful correlation with the needs and values of the patient. The setting should be quiet, reasonably private, and nonthreatening. The structure of the interview is focused on gathering information but builds to establish trust. The physician determines specifically

1. A *description of the current episode* of the emotional disorder including the *acuity of its onset* and its *duration*
2. A description of *behavior leading up to the current episode* and *any previous episodes*
3. *Suicidal or homicidal ideation*
4. *Associated symptoms.* For example,
   a. Disorientation
   b. Agitation, insomnia, anorexia
   c. Memory or thought problems
   d. Hallucinations
   e. Delusions, phobias
   f. Others
5. *Drug* and *alcohol* history
6. Place of *residence* and *employment*
7. Names of family, friends, or other members of *patient's support system*
8. History of *previous therapy programs, counselors,* or *mental health contacts*
9. *Past medical or surgical history:* medications, allergies

PROBLEM 1 The patient was described by the rescue squad as a "known schizophrenic." They were called by the patient's mother, who lived with him. He was "taking a shower" when she heard a loud "thud" in the bathroom, and found the patient slumped over in the bathtub. The paramedics noted that the patient was awake but "tired" when found. They mentioned that the patient's mother was an invalid and was remaining at home. A call to her provided the information that the patient had been completely compliant in taking his chlorpromazine. She thought he had been becoming gradually more "emotional" during the week prior to his apparent fall in the shower.

The gradual onset of confusion directs the investigation toward an organic cause. Trauma is certainly a potential secondary organic factor causing this patient's behavior.

Mental Status Examination

After obtaining the history and performing an initial screening examination (general observation, vital signs), the physician should perform a detailed mental status examination in every patient with an emotional disorder. The mental status examination consists of six components:

Appearance and Behavior. The patient's *dress* and state of *hygiene* are assessed. Is he *alert*, and what is the level of *interaction with the environment*? How does he *respond to people*? What current *activities* is he engaged in?

Orientation. Orientation to *person* (name and address), *place* (name and function of hospital), and *time* (day of week, month, year) is checked.

Affect and Mood. The patient is asked to *describe his mood*. The type of *affect* is noted, as well as its fluctuations and range. Anxiety, anger, fear, depression, and *euphoria* are considered.

Thought. The patient's *thought content* is considered next. The presence of *delusions, obsessions,* and *phobias* is noted. The patient's *thought processes* also need to be considered, i.e., his "train of thought." Is it *appropriate, logical,* and *chronological*?

Perceptions. The presence of any *hallucinations, illusions* or *unusual feelings* is assessed.

Cognitive. The patient's immediate, recent, and remote *memory* is specifically assessed. His *communication skills* are assessed, by noting vocabulary and language comprehension. *Insight* is determined: minimal—patient acknowledges that a problem exists; moderate—patient understands the nature of the problem; significant—patient understands why he has a problem. The patient's ability to use insight to function in society is considered his *level of judgment*. The person's thought content is reassessed by considering whether he has *concrete* or *abstract thought* and by estimating his level of intelligence.

Mental Status Examination Summary

An efficient way to perform a mental status examination is to:

- Introduce oneself to the patient while assessing his appearance and behavior.
- Assess orientation by asking his name, address, where he is, and the exact date.
- Ask the patient to describe his mood and observe his affect; the physician may have to provide examples such as, "Are you happy? Are you angry?"
- Ask the patient to describe what he is thinking while you assess his thought processes.
- Specifically ask whether he has hallucinations, illusions, or other disorders of perception.
- Start the cognitive assessment by checking the patient's memory: Ask if he remembers your name, what he had to eat for the previous meal, and who was president prior to the current president.
- Assess communication and thinking by asking him to perform some simple arithmetic and to explain a common proverb.
- Assess insight and judgment by asking him how he views his problem and how it affects his role in society.

General Physical Examination

A general physical examination follows the mental status examination. The patient is told simply and exactly what is going to be done. Undressing is left until the end of the examination. Rectal and pelvic examinations are deferred unless they are specifically indicated.

PROBLEM 1 The paramedics reported that the patient was awake but "tired." The physical examination showed that he was fluctuating in and out of consciousness; while awake, he was lethargic and spoke garbled words. His pupils were equal and reactive, and all four extremities moved purposefully. A large abrasion with ecchymosis was noted on his forehead.

The physical findings in this patient are significant in that they provide clues to the possibility of an organic cause for the abnormal behavior. These findings remove the bias that this patient is "just another schizophrenic."

PROBLEM 2 The mental status of the patient had been normal for her age, but during the past 3 to 4 days she had become disoriented and confused. Her husband died 2 years ago, yet she stated that he visited her yesterday. Physical examination revealed that the patient had a slight fever, tachycardia, tachypnea, and hypotension. She was ill-appearing and very lethargic. She had no neck stiffness, decubitus ulcers, or abdominal pain. The lung examination revealed bibasilar rales. The patient refused to cooperate to cough. She had signs of dehydration, respiratory compromise, and an indwelling urinary catheter that drained foul-smelling cloudy urine.

The initial screening examination supplies clues that this patient's abnormal behavior might have an organic basis. The mental status examination supports the physician's suspicions. After the physical examination, the physician has a working diagnosis of sepsis secondary to a genitourinary or pulmonary source.

DECISION PRIORITIES AND PRELIMINARY DIFFERENTIAL DIAGNOSIS

The preliminary differential diagnosis for a patient with an emotional disorder answers the broad question: *Are these findings due to an organic* or *functional (psychiatric) etiology?*

As mentioned, it is useful to assume that a patient's behavior is organic in nature. The emergency physician first considers the potentially life-threatening organic conditions that can explain the patient's abnormal behavior. Table 52–1 lists components obtained from the history, mental status examination, and physical examination that support an organic as opposed to a functional disorder.

A useful mnemonic for remembering whether changes in key components of the mental status examination suggest an organic or a functional cause is OMI HAT:

Organic	**Functional**
*O*rientation	*H*allucinations—auditory
*M*emory—recent	*A*ffect—mood
*I*ntelligence—cognitive	*T*hinking—delusions, illusions

In many patients the findings will not fit into a simple dichotomy of organic or functional etiology. Up to 30% of patients with a behavioral problem have elements of both organic and functional causes. These patients are not easily separated into either class but belong in a gray zone in which the cause of the disorder is considered ambiguous.

PROBLEM 1 It was known that the "known schizophrenic" who was found lying down in the shower had had changing behavior during the past week. The onset of the incident was relatively acute. The mental status examination showed that he was lethargic and had no memory of how he fell. He did not manifest hallucinations or delusions. The physical examination, as already mentioned, showed signs of recent head trauma.

Note that several historical and physical findings point to an organic

TABLE 52–1. Clues Gathered from Data that Differentiate Between Organic and Functional Causes of Behavioral Problems

Organic	Functional
History	**History**
Acute onset	Onset over weeks to months
Any age	Onset from age 12 to 40 years
Mental Status Examination	**Mental Status Examination**
Fluctuating level of consciousness	Alert
Disoriented	Oriented
Attention disturbances	Agitated, anxious
Poor recent memory	Poor immediate memory
Hallucinations: visual, tactile, auditory	Hallucinations: most commonly auditory
Cognitive changes	Delusions, illusions
Physical Examination	**Physical Examination**
Abnormal vital signs	Normal vital signs
Nystagmus	No nystagmus
Focal neurologic signs	Purposeful movement
Signs of trauma	No signs of trauma

cause for the recent change in this patient's behavior. Although this patient is a "known schizophrenic," to ignore these findings and to assume that he is presenting with a functional disorder is a serious error. With a past history of functional illness but current findings pointing to an organic cause, this patient is in the gray zone, with emphasis on an organic cause. Further tests are indicated.

PROBLEM 3 This patient was brought in because of bizarre behavior and periodic lethargy. On mental status examination he appeared well dressed, but his clothing was dirty. He was oriented to person and place but had a flat affect and bizarre thought processes. He admitted to auditory hallucinations, "the voice of God," and showed abnormal results on cognitive testing. Contact with family confirmed that his behavior had been more unusual during the last 2 weeks. They had had no knowledge of his whereabouts for the previous 48 hours. He had normal vital signs and normal results on neurologic examination with no signs of trauma.

Because the initial screening assessment is normal and the patient had normal vital signs, there is little indication of an organic cause of abnormal behavior in this patient. The mental status examination supports a functional cause of the behavioral problem. A general physical examination is all that was needed to confirm that no organic pathology existed.

DIAGNOSTIC ADJUNCTS

Ancillary tests are useful in two contexts. They can confirm or exclude a preliminary working diagnosis regarding organic or functional etiology. Many patients' behavior is obviously functional in origin, and no ancillary tests are necessary. More often, ancillary tests are used to clarify the origin of the behavioral disturbance of a patient with an indeterminate etiology. The following tests are considered for the patient with a suspected organic cause or for one with an equivocal cause.

Laboratory Studies

Complete Blood Count with Differential. Hemoglobin levels indirectly reflect the oxygen-carrying capacity of the blood. The white blood cell count may point to an infectious or inflammatory cause.

Serum Electrolytes (Na, K, HCO_3, Cl). The most useful value is the serum sodium level because sodium abnormalities may present as altered mental status. Bicarbonate levels are helpful in diagnosing acid-base disorders.

Glucose Concentration. Glucose measurements are often done by test strip as a screening test. Both hypoglycemia and hyperglycemia can cause bizarre behavior.

Arterial Blood Gas Measurements. pH and $Paco_2$ are necessary for acid-base calculations. Increased Pco_2 can depress the level of consciousness. Pao_2 is essential because hypoxemia commonly presents as abnormal behavior.

Blood Urea Nitrogen. The BUN is a useful screening test for renal function status.

Toxicology Screen. Toxicology screening tests are very dependent on the capability of the laboratory. With increasing drug use, they are useful tools for assessing unusual behavior, particularly if the patient is less than 40 years old (see Chaps. 19 and 23).

The following tests are ordered according to specific indications for the initial work-up of a patient with a known organic cause or to clarify the cause in a patient in the "gray zone."

- Creatinine
- Calcium

- Ammonia
- Thyroid and liver function tests
- Specific drug levels—e.g., alcohol, anticonvulsants, lithium

Radiologic Imaging

Computed Tomography of the Head. Head CT scans are the only test to be routinely included in evaluating patients presenting with an ambiguous finding, particularly if the change in behavior was acute in onset, associated with trauma, or unexplained by the other screening laboratory tests.

Other Tests

An *electrocardiogram* (ECG) may assist the diagnosis in the elderly patient, in whom myocardial infarction can present as a change in mental status. *Lumbar puncture* and other invasive procedures are performed when they are clinically indicated.

PROBLEM 1 An organic cause of abnormal behavior was likely in the patient who had apparently fallen in the shower. The working diagnosis was intracranial trauma. After the patient's cervical spine radiograph was cleared, a head CT was ordered and was reported as normal. Because the organic cause was still unexplained, the work-up continued to exclude metabolic, toxicologic, or other neurologic abnormalities. A complete blood count, serum electrolytes, BUN, creatinine, glucose, arterial blood gases, and toxicologic screen were ordered. The electrolyte values were sodium, 108 mEq/liter and chloride, 85 mEq/liter. Acute severe hyponatremia could explain the patient's presentation, and serious treatable neurotrauma was excluded.

Further work-up by the physician places the patient in the category of euvolemic hyponatremia, and other tests (urine osmolarity 8 mOsm/liter and serum osmolarity 230 mOsm/liter) exclude inappropriate secretion of antidiuretic hormone (SIADH) as the cause. Thus, the final diagnosis is polydipsia. The physician again called the patient's mother, who on direct questioning revealed that indeed the patient had been gulping huge volumes of water for the past week. He had, in fact, been in the shower drinking water from the shower nozzle when he fell.

REFINED DIFFERENTIAL DIAGNOSIS

A detailed differential diagnosis is not the goal of assessment in the emergency department. Rather, the patient is classified in order to choose between a medical evaluation for an organic disorder or a consultation with a psychiatrist or other mental health worker for a functional disorder. The final diagnosis may take days to reach. The classes of organic disease that may present as psychobehavioral problems are listed in Table 52–2. Table 52–3 describes the characteristics of the five major psychiatric categories presenting to the emergency department as functional psychobehavioral disorders.

PROBLEM 3 The behavior of this patient was most likely functional in nature. The general screening physical examination was grossly normal and reasonably excluded an organic etiology. The most obvious findings on the mental status examination were bizarre thought process with grandiosity and auditory hallucinations. The blunted affect and unusual sense of self are also classic findings in a patient with a schizophreniform disorder. After extended observation, it seemed that the patient's periods of "lethargy" were actually malingering.

TABLE 52-2. Classes of Organic Disease that may Present as Psychobehavioral Disorders

Medical (in order of frequency)
  Neurologic, e.g., hypoxia, ischemia, mass lesions, degenerative lesions
  Infectious, e.g., sepsis (pneumonia, urinary tract infection), meningitis, endocarditis
  Endocrine, e.g., diabetes, thyroid, adrenal, pituitary
  Electrolyte, e.g., sodium, acid-base, calcium, BUN/creatinine
  Nutrition, e.g., thiamine, vitamin B_{12}
  Collagen vascular, e.g., systemic lupus erythematosus, polyarteritis nodosa

Pharmaceutical Use (prescription or "borrowed")

Benzodiazepines	Corticosteroids
Propranolol	Digitalis
Cimetidine	NSAIDs
Tricyclic antidepressants	Anticonvulsants

Drug Abuse or Withdrawal

Alcohol	Amphetamines
Cocaine	Barbiturates
Opiates	Phencyclidine (PCP)

TABLE 52-3. General Classes of Functional Disorders Presenting as Psychobehavioral Problems in the Emergency Department

Affective—Depression
1. Background: Very common; about 20% of female and 10% of male adults have had at least one episode.
2. History: Anhedonia, depressed, sad, hopeless, irritable, anorexia, insomnia, fatigue.
3. Mental status examination: Patient feels worthless or sad; has poor concentration; depressed affect; thoughts of suicide.
4. Physical appearance: Poor hygiene, tired-appearing.
5. If the physician feels sad or fatigued after evaluating this patient, the diagnosis is considered.

Affective-Mania
1. Background: Uncommon, may be difficult to diagnose because of "mask" or episodic nature.
2. History: Increased activity, restlessness, talkativeness, insomnia, euphoria; unusual or risky behavior.
3. Mental status examination: Talkative, hyperactive; flight of ideas; grandiosity; short attention span; irritable; lack of judgment; impulsive; mood lability; hallucinations or delusions.
4. Physical appearance: hyperactive; tired-appearing but still pushing.

Schizophrenia
1. Background: Prodromal, active and residual phases; lifetime prevalence is around 1%.
2. History: Decreased level of performance in some activity; unusual thinking; deteriorating personal relationships; poor volition; withdrawal; psychomotor or bizarre behavior.
3. Mental status examination: Disturbance of thought content and form; hallucinations or delusions; inappropriate and blunted affect; disturbed sense of self; unusual relation to environment.
4. Physical appearance: Disheveled; repetitive psychomotor behavior.

Personality Disorder—Borderline Personality
1. Background: Personality traits that are inflexible, maladaptive, and impair functioning. Borderline personality is common, especially in women.
2. History: Instability in interpersonal behavior, mood, and self-image.
3. Mental status examination: Unpredictable behavior; dysphoric mood or feelings of anger or emptiness; affective instability; identity disturbance.
4. Physical appearance: Signs of self-damaging acts such as suicidal gestures, self-mutilation, recurrent accidents or fights.
5. If the physician feels manipulated, "pushed into a corner," or in a "lose-lose" situation, consider this diagnosis. These patients can make physicians work very hard to meet their unrealistic expectations.

Anxiety
1. Background: Common response to stressful situations.
2. History: Panic attacks, fear, apprehension; dyspnea, palpitations, dizziness.
3. Mental status examination: Apprehensive, anxious, jittery; worries, ruminates; hypervigilant; poor concentration.
4. Physical appearance: Autonomic hyperactivity, trembling, restlessness.

This patient's behavior is not consistent with an organic etiology. Furthermore, the diagnosis of a functional illness is refined to the point at which a consultation with a psychiatrist or mental health worker could provide useful information with which to initiate management and disposition of this patient.

PRINCIPLES OF MANAGEMENT

The management principles for treating psychobehaviorally disturbed patients are:
1. Establish rapport.
2. Maintain control of the situation.
3. Use medications judiciously.
4. Understand the patient's support system.
5. Maintain a positive, realistic perspective on what can be accomplished in the emergency department.

Establishing Rapport and Maintaining Control

The patient's problem is seldom cured during a brief stay in the emergency department, but a respectful approach based on genuine concern and interest will lessen the patient's (or his family's) anguish and minimize confrontation and disturbance in the department. In most acute psychiatric situations, the patient is seeking to gain control of painful emotions. Because the hospital environment is a controlling one, sometimes just being inside a hospital will help. The physician escalates the control mechanism to match the patient's response. These methods range from simple use of voice and touching ("I'm sorry you can't get out of bed" while at the same time "assisting" the patient back into bed), to a show of force ("These three guards and I will have to help you back into bed"), to actual physical restraint ("I'm sorry you wouldn't cooperate, we must place you back in bed and secure you for your own safety"). Establishing control includes judicious use of ancillary personnel including security, patient representatives, social workers, mental health workers, and psychologists or psychiatrists. These workers are often the key to controlling the situation while the patient is in the department and facilitating efficient disposition of the patient for definitive care.

Use of Medication

The emergency physician may use "chemical restraints" in dealing with patients with acute behavioral disorders. The two general classes of such drugs are the butyrophenones and the benzodiazepines, and the emergency physician must have a working knowledge of the pharmacologic principles involved in using these drugs. These drugs are used only in limited circumstances because (1) they will relieve psychotic symptoms due to organic or functional illness and they may obscure organic causes, (2) they may delay diagnosis of a psychological illness, (3) they may retard psychological growth of the patient, and (4) they may reinforce abuse of the emergency department by drug seekers.

Haloperidol is the butyrophenone antipsychotic of choice. It is indicated for
1. Control of psychotic behavior in patients with a known organic disorder that is being treated.
2. Control of a disruptive patient who is unresponsive to psychotherapy or physical restraints.
3. Initiation of antipsychotic treatment for a patient who has follow-up arranged.
4. Control of a patient who is being transferred.

The patient is always told that the medicine is being given to help him feel better, and oral medicine is offered before intramuscular injection. The initial oral dose of haloperidol is 5 to 10 mg (1 to 2 mg for elderly patients). The onset of action occurs in

30 minutes, and the duration varies from 2 to 4 hours. The initial intramuscular dose is also 5 to 10 mg; onset occurs in less than 30 minutes, and the duration varies. A repeat dose may be given every 30 minutes until symptoms are controlled. The average total dose is 4 to 20 mg. It is necessary to monitor the patient's "target" symptoms at least every 30 minutes. These include level of cooperation, organization of thinking, and lessening of anxiety. The best target symptom is sedation; if the patient becomes drowsy, enough medication has been given. The side effects of haloperidol are sedation, hypotension, and extrapyramidal effects (dystonia, akathisia, Parkinsonism, and tardive dyskinesia). The last symptom may be seen in 20% to 30% of patients in whom the drug is administered acutely. It treated with either an anticholinergic (Cogentin 1 to 2 mg intramuscularly) or antihistaminic agent (Benadryl 25 to 50 mg intramuscularly).

Diazepam is the benzodiazepine of choice, although recently midazolam has been recommended because of its shorter onset of action. Either is recommended to (1) provide muscle relaxation or patient cooperation for uncomfortable procedures, or (2) relieve situational adjustment reactions when a patient has a well-defined need. When prescribing a benzodiazepine, the patient is told that the prescription is intended to last for a very short time period. The initial oral dose of diazepam is 5 to 10 mg (1 to 5 mg for elderly patients). The onset of action is 30 minutes; the duration varies. The initial intravenous dose is also 5 to 10 mg (1 to 2 mg for elderly), the onset is immediate, and the duration varies. The patient's target symptoms are monitored at least every 15 minutes. A repeat dose may be given every 15 minutes until symptoms are controlled. Again, the best target symptom is sedation. The side effects of diazepam are sedation, respiratory depression, and hypotension.

SPECIAL CONSIDERATIONS

Pediatric Patients

The same principles that apply to adults apply to children and adolescents who present to the emergency department with psychobehavioral disorders. Functional disorders such as situational crisis, affective disorders, and schizophreniform illness are common in children. Still, organic factors, e.g., drug toxicity or overdose, metabolic disorders, and trauma are considered.

Geriatric Patients

Geriatric patients comprise a large percentage of patients presenting to the emergency department with psychobehavioral disorders. Although the prevalence of affective and schizophreniform illness is high in these patients, organic pathology is the most common cause of altered mentation in the elderly. Up to 30% of elderly patients presenting with obvious cognitive impairment have a treatable underlying physical or psychological disorder that has caused their behavior. All patients who show significant cognitive impairment should have a thorough work-up with a complete medical history including a drug inventory, physical examination, psychologic testing, laboratory assessment, and radiographic analysis.

DISPOSITION AND FOLLOW-UP

The disposition of patients with behavioral disorders is often difficult owing to the chronicity of the disorder, the uncooperative nature of the patients, and the arrival of patients at times when disposition resources are limited. This difficulty is somewhat lessened by the knowledge that the emergency physician is not alone in caring for these patients. It is essential to know the support services, mental health resources, and community programs available to the emergency department. It is useful to maintain contact with mental health caregivers, acknowledge the professional skill and effort they put into the care of emotionally disturbed patients, and follow up on the effectiveness of referrals.

Admission

Many patients can be treated in the emergency department and referred to more definitive ongoing care facilities. "Gray zone" patients with a mixed organic-functional cause or an uncertain diagnosis are usually admitted for continued evaluation. Other specific indications for admission include:

1. Initial acute psychosis
2. Acute psychosis without remission
3. Mania
4. Suicidal or homicidal ideation
5. Demented patient unable to care for self
6. Stuporously depressed patient
7. Catatonic patient
8. Acute anxiety unrelieved by medication

Psychiatric Consultation

When hospitalization or close follow-up is necessary, a formal consultation with a psychiatrist is recommended, and this usually occurs by phone. The two components of a telephone consultation are first, what to tell the psychiatrist, and second, what to expect from this specialist.

What to tell the psychiatrist:
a. Patient's name, vital information
b. How patient came to the emergency department
c. Brief history of the episode and psychiatric background
d. Mental status examination results
e. Diagnostic impression of the illness. One should try to fit the condition into one of the five groups listed in Table 52–3. If unable to do so, descriptive information may be given
f. Resources of the patient, the patient's family, and the emergency department

What to expect from the psychiatrist:
a. Clarification until it is mutually agreed that a functional problem exists
b. Focus on the patient's discomfort and the means needed to resolve it
c. Clear communication and agreement on a sensible management plan

Involuntary Commitment

Many patients with psychobehavioral disorders will not agree to be admitted to the hospital, and the emergency physician along with a consulting psychiatrist will need to intervene to commit the patient involuntarily. Involuntary commitment forms a difficult balance between the medical need to expedite treatment and the legal right to personal freedom. The emergency physician should know the state laws. A typical (Ohio) law states that (1) commitment requires two signatures (one is usually that of a physician), (2) the patient is held for 48 hours, during which time he or she must receive psychiatric evaluation, and (3) the patient must be either a threat to himself or others or must be unable to care for himself. A complete history, results of the mental status examination, physical examination results, psychiatric consultation, the indications for commitment, and the signatures of witnesses are part of the legal commitment procedure.

Discharge

The most important factor for discharging the patient is a clearly arranged follow-up appointment. This information is given to the person most responsible for the patient, and a plan is developed in case the patient does not keep the follow-up appointment. This plan usually involves the support person calling the patient's primary physician or returning with the patient to the emergency department.

PROBLEM 1 The patient had been diagnosed as hyponatremic secondary to polydipsia. He was admitted by an internist. An inpatient psychiatric consultation was arranged.

This case demonstrates the mixed organic-functional disorder seen in some patients. This patient's schizophrenia led to behavior that resulted in an organic disorder, and this organic disorder presented as a psychobehavioral problem. Indeed, the irony here is apparent only to the physician who does a full assessment of this patient!

PROBLEM 2 The problem was diagnosed as sepsis secondary to urinary or pulmonary source. The patient's internist agreed to admit her.

PROBLEM 3 The patient's problem was diagnosed as acute psychosis, and all organic factors were reasonably excluded. Because this was the initial presentation for this patient, hospitalization was required. The psychiatrist on call was telephoned and agreed to admit the patient. The emergency physician and psychiatric unit nurse both signed the involuntary commitment paper.

Not all patients with psychiatric problems will be admitted this easily. Often a final disposition or resolution of the patient's problem cannot be accomplished in the middle of the night. In the latter situation, the patient may have to be held in the emergency department until resources are more available during daytime hours.

DOCUMENTATION

1. Key historical information
   a. Suicidal or homicidal ideation
   b. Support systems available
2. Key physical findings
   a. Complete mental status examination
   b. General physical examination
3. Emergency department therapy
   a. Psychotherapy given and patient's response to it
   b. Indications for chemical or physical restraint
4. Psychiatric consultation
5. Disposition and follow-up, including back-up plan should follow-up be resisted

SUMMARY AND FINAL POINTS

The three cases described in this chapter represent the variety of medical and psychiatric problems that present as "emotional disorders." Each case provides a basic lesson in the care of patients with psychobehavioral disorders in emergency medicine.

PROBLEM 1 Known psychiatric patients may have concurrent medical conditions.

PROBLEM 2 Pure medical problems may present as emotional disorders. Differentiating functional from organic illness may be difficult.

PROBLEM 3 The major classes of functional illness must be recognized and therapy begun when indicated.

- The cause of behavioral disorders may be functional or organic, yet in up to 30% of patients the cause is mixed or uncertain etiology.
- Although the emergency physician's role is limited, his or her most important function is to exclude organic causes.
- These patients take time and resources, and usually care extends beyond the emergency department.
- Many of these patients are admitted, some involuntarily, and this requires special communication skills and an understanding of the law.

BIBLIOGRAPHY

Texts

1. Bassuk EL, Birk AW: Emergency Psychiatry. New York, Plenum Press, 1984.
2. Hyman SE: Manual of Psychiatric Emergencies. Boston, Little, Brown, 1984.
3. Soreff SM: Emergency Psychiatry. Psychiatr Clin North Am 6(2), 1983.
4. Walker JI: Psychiatric Emergencies. Philadelphia, Lippincott, 1983.

Journal Articles

1. Dubin WR, Weiss KJ, Dorn JM: Pharmacotherapy of psychiatric emergencies. J Clin Psychopharmacol 6:210–216, 1986.
2. Ellison JM, Hughes DH, White KA: An emergency psychiatry update. Hosp Commun Psychiatry 40(3):250–260, 1989.
3. Fauman MA, Fauman BJ: The differential diagnosis of organic based psychiatric disturbance in the emergency department. J Am Coll Emerg Physicians 6:315–319, 1977.
4. Gerson E, Bassuk E: Psychiatric emergencies: An overview. Am J Psychiat 137:1–9, 1980.
5. Goldberg RJ, Dubin WR, Fogel BS: Behavioral emergencies: Assessment and psychopharmacologic management. Clin Neuropharmacol 12(4):233–248, 1989.
6. Gross DA: Medical origins of psychiatric emergencies: The systems approach. Int J Psychiat Med 11:1, 1981–1982.
7. Khan MH, Johnson FC: Clinical guide to emergency room evaluation and management of the violent patient. SDJ Med 40:10–14, 1987.
8. Marson DC, McGovern MP, Pomp HL: Psychiatric decision making in the emergency room: A research overview. Am J Psychiatry 195(8):918–925, 1988.
9. Wise TN: What to expect from a psychiatric consultant. Primary Care 4:4–8, 1977.

CHAPTER 53

THE POTENTIALLY SUICIDAL PATIENT

MARK A. EILERS, M.D.

PROBLEM 1 A 48 year old man was brought to the emergency department by his family. He stated, "I am depressed." The family wanted the patient to see a psychiatrist.

PROBLEM 2 An 18 year old girl was brought to the emergency department by a rescue squad because of a suspected overdose. At the scene she was screaming and violently refusing to allow transport to the hospital.

QUESTIONS TO CONSIDER

1. How often is the potentially suicidal patient evaluated in the emergency department?
2. What presenting circumstances elicit a high suspicion of suicide?
3. How is the potential risk for suicide assessed?
4. What level of suicide risk requires that the patient be admitted?
5. When is physical restraint necessary for a patient with a potential for suicide?
6. What legal guidelines assist in managing a patient at risk for suicide?

INTRODUCTION

In 1984, more than 29,000 Americans reportedly committed suicide. Suicide was the tenth leading cause of death in the United States. There may be twice as many suicides as reported, and 15 to 20 "attempts" for every reported case. These numbers continue to increase. During the past 10 years the suicide rate among adolescents has more than doubled and is now the third leading cause of death in this group. A second growing population of potential suicidal patients is the elderly. Individuals 45 years and older have a threefold greater number of attempts and completed suicides than the general population. The likelihood of suicide reaches a plateau at the age of 60 in women but rises with increasing age in men. Potentially suicidal patients are a large and expanding group who most often present to the emergency department for evaluation. To anticipate and identify these important high-risk patients, additional demographics on suicide are necessary.

The age group at highest risk for a suicide attempt is the group aged 15 to 34 years. Men complete suicide almost four times more often than women, although women make a suicide "gesture" ten times more often than men. Men tend to use violent means more frequently than women, using firearms 50% more frequently than women. Self-poisoning is used in 7% of suicide gestures by men and 33% in women. All other methods are equally divided between the sexes.

Fifty percent of patients completing suicide have seen one or more physicians within the month prior to their death. Their chief complaints often suggest an underlying depression or an emotional cry for help. Vague somatic complaints such as persistent headache or chronic fatigue are typical. These are "acceptable" reasons to seek medical care when the underlying motive is a hope for discovery of suicidal thoughts. When depressive symptoms or emotional cries for help are treated without recognition of suicide potential, the physician may become an unwitting accomplice by providing the means. For example, a physician may prescribe a hypnotic-sedative for a patient presenting with a chief complaint of insomnia without fully exploring the underlying causes of the insomnia. This provides an avenue for a suicide attempt by overdose.

Maintaining a high index of suspicion for self-destructive intent prepares the emergency physician to recognize the potentially suicidal patient within a variety of clinical presentations. There are many clues in the patient's present and past history that should raise the physician's suspicions (Table 53–1).

PREHOSPITAL CARE

Prehospital radio communication emphasizes the suicidal patient's medical status rather than the underlying psychopathology. Discussion with prehospital personnel after the patient arrives in the emergency department is important and reveals helpful information.

History

1. If the suicidal attempt is obvious, what was the setting and the chronology of the events preceding the attempt? Did the patient leave a note? Was there any sign of the patient's affairs being put in order? This information can be useful in assessing the degree of premeditation.

2. Who called the paramedics for help and where are those individuals now? Did the patient have a secondary gain motive in mind by involving the individual who called for help?

3. If the attempt is not obvious, are there factors that might indicate that attempted suicide may have played a role in the event, for example, evidence of excessive risk taking, e.g., walking on the freeway (Table 53–1)?

Physical Examination

1. Vital signs are recorded at the scene plus any alterations during transport.
2. A general primary assessment (airway, breathing, circulation, gross neurologic status) is completed.
3. Specific information relating to altered level of consciousness or complicating injuries or illnesses is recorded.

TABLE 53–1. Clues Prompting Consideration of a Patient's Suicide Potential

Single-vehicle, single-driver accident
Accidental ingestion
Risk-taking behavior (walking on freeway, dangerous activities)
Unclear reasons for seeking medical care
Stationary object accidents, e.g., striking a bridge abutment
No evidence of avoidance attempt in accident, usually motor vehicle accident
No safety equipment used, e.g., seat belts
Previous history of multiple injuries
Major psychiatric disease (schizophrenia)
Chronic, painful, or debilitating medical illness
Victims of violence, e.g., domestic or sexual assault
Marked personality changes
Suicidal threats
Social disorder

Intervention

Prehospital care intervention involves basic and advanced life support, as necessary. Police or security forces may be required to subdue a combative patient. If patients appear to be psychotic, intoxicated, or acting in a threatening manner to themselves or others, additional personnel such as police, fire, or security officers are necessary to restrain and transport them safely. State laws provide for immunity from prosecution for false imprisonment when official or medical personnel act in a sincere belief that the patient represents a threat to themselves or others at the time of presentation and evaluation.

PROBLEM 2 The rescue squad enlisted the help of the patient's father to bring her into the ambulance. She was secured on the stretcher and accompanied throughout transport. She continued to curse the rescue personnel and threaten them with legal action.

This patient's case was managed with major difficulty. The rescue squad wisely recruited a family member to assist in the "restraint." The "legal action" threat is not uncommon. It is important for prehospital providers to be familiar with state statutes.

INITIAL APPROACH IN THE EMERGENCY DEPARTMENT

The suicidal patient may present as a critically ill individual or one of the "walking worried." Any patient with an underlying medical or surgical emergency is stabilized prior to suicide evaluation. Beyond emergency stabilization, four principles guide the initial approach to the suicidal patient. They are applied as dictated by the seriousness of the attempt. They are (1) the patient is never left alone, (2) physical restraint of the patient is applied as necessary for his or her own protection, (3) medical personnel take what measures are necessary for self-protection, and (4) rapport with the patient is the goal.

1. No matter how "ineffectual" the gesture may be, suicide attempts are always taken seriously. The patient is brought urgently to the attention of the emergency physician, nursing, and support personnel. These patients are placed in an area where they can be observed until they are evaluated. Hospital security staff may assist in observing the patient.

2. Anticipating a patient's loss of control or violent behavior allows one to institute physical restraint prior to the act. State laws allow patients to be restrained against their will if the physician suspects suicidal intent or anticipates violent behavior. The hospital environment often has its own psychological "restraining" influence, but its influence is unpredictable. Enlistment of visible security personnel can be an effective deterrent to violence and attempts to leave the department. Depending on the patient's activity, one warning may precede restraint. In maintaining the difficult balance between restraint and rapport with the patient, one should err on the side of protecting the patient (see Chap. 52).

3. If the situation is physically threatening, the interview is begun with the patient restrained or in the presence of security personnel. Self-protection during the interview process must be foremost in the care provider's mind. Sitting between an agitated patient and the only route of escape simply invites injury.

4. The manner in which a patient is received in the emergency department is critical in establishing rapport. The "tone" of the setting has a direct and important impact on the patient's trust in the care provided. Offhand comments or a lack of concern or respect from nursing, support, or medical staff can strongly influence the patient's experience. A nonjudgmental, empathetic, and respectful approach to the patient is the best way to

begin a dialogue. Insulting questions or comments from a patient, no matter how provocative, do not require an answer.

PROBLEM 1 The 48 year old man stated that he was "depressed." He was placed in the interview room, and the emergency physician was notified. The family was asked to remain with him. The triage nurse determined that his vital signs were normal.

Because of his statement about his depression, the potential for suicide is clear. Restraint is not necessary in this case. The physician must maintain a constant awareness of the emotional state of the patient and the family. Opening the history taking by asking nonjudgmental, empathetic questions will yield the most important information. Because they came together, this interview is best initiated in the presence of the patient's family. Eventually the patient's immediate and past history is explored separately with the patient and with family members.

PROBLEM 2 The 18 year old girl with an "overdose" was alert, awake, and in no apparent distress. She was unhappy at being in the hospital but was not attempting to leave. She was unaware that any of her family were coming to the emergency department. The rescue squad was aided by the patient's father, and they reported that he was coming shortly. The patient was much calmer and less abusive than when the squad responded initially at her home. Vital signs were blood pressure 110/70 mm Hg, heart rate 90 beats/min and regular, respiratory rate 14/min, temperature 98.4°F (37°C).

The patient's airway, breathing, and circulation were normal, as were the vital signs. The nurses were instructed to observe the patient continually. Restraint was unnecessary as long as the patient's behavior remained appropriate and relatively cooperative. Self-protection is probably not an issue at this time. Rapport was established by explaining each step in the assessment process to the patient as part of initiating the interview process. The patient's father will be questioned for corroborating information when he arrives.

DATA GATHERING

Once the patient is medically stable, one begins to assess suicidal potential through the interview process. Although the patient's presenting condition may establish a high suicide potential, more often the patient's status is typified by the cases illustrated. The interview is held in a location in the emergency department chosen to maintain the patient's privacy. Whether the physician speaks with the patient or family first or meets them together is decided by personal preference and the particular situation. Eventually, it is important to seek family members, friends, prehospital care personnel, police, primary physicians, and other relevant individuals to provide detail and confirm the events preceding the patient's arrival. The history is often the only guide to the establishment of suicidal intent. Because the quality of the information and the motives for offering it vary greatly, corroborating evidence is essential.

History

The interview begins by questions about less emotionally charged issues, e.g., demographic information. It quickly moves on to more specific facts surrounding the event(s) precipitating the emergency department visit.

Demographic Data. Age, sex, race, religion, marital status, work, and education are noted. The physician matches this information against the profile of the "suicide prone" individual.

Chief Complaint. The triage quote from the patient or responsible party identifies the initial subject area to be rephrased to the patient as a question. For example, the direct patient quote "Wants to see mental health," could be rephrased as, "The chart says you would like to see a mental health worker; can you tell me more? (or what would you like to discuss?)"

History of Present Event. Another approach is the open-ended question. "Why did you decide to come (or why were you brought) to the emergency department this evening?" This query may trigger a complete recitation of the event. Follow-up questions of greater specificity are usually necessary to clarify the patient's situation.

A chronology of events is constructed leading up to the emergency department presentation. This is the most time-consuming component of the history, but it is also the most important. Structuring the patient's story as a sequence of events over a period of time organizes the often confusing and conflicting versions told by both the patient and family members. The questions progress from acquiring simple background information to a direct inquiry about suicidal intent.

Past Medical History

Previous Psychiatric History. The answer to this question often requires confirmation by contacting the patient's psychiatrist. Psychiatric records are notoriously difficult to obtain, although it is important to make an attempt. Helpful information is often available on the medical record.

Family History. Any family-related disorders, previous suicide attempts, or psychiatric diagnoses are reviewed.

Marital History. Divorce itself places the patient at risk. Information about recent marital discord may be an important factor in determining risk.

Medical or Surgical History. A past history of medical or surgical illnesses may supply clues to the possibility that an underlying organic illness may be exacerbating this patient's suicidal behavior or may emphasize the role that physical symptoms play in this patient's psychiatric environment.

Medications. If a patient is taking antipsychotic and antidepressant medications from various physicians the concern about compliance, quality of care, and risk is heightened.

Direct Questions about Suicide. These questions are asked near the end of the interview. Slightly modified, they serve also as a framework for questioning the patient's friends or family.

Affective Elements

1. Have things been so bad that you have been considering hurting yourself?
2. How badly have you felt? Are you still able to function in your life? How long have you felt bad, and how hard is it for you to shake these feelings?

Somatic Elements.

1. Do you have any other troubles such as loss of interest in eating, sex, life, or sleeping?
2. Do you have any physical complaints such as headache, backache, or insomnia?

Suicidal Plan

1. Have you ever tried to commit suicide? Are you now thinking about suicide?
2. Do you have a plan for committing suicide? If so, what is it and what steps have you taken toward implementing it? Patients who have a definite plan and have taken steps toward completion of that plan are demonstrating significant intent.
3. What is stopping you now? The presence or absence of a significant person or event is taken as a sign of premeditation. If present, this individual or event can be built on during supportive psychotherapy.
4. If an attempt has been made, does the patient have any regret or insight about the experience? Lack of regret or a superficial "cover-up" response increases the patient's risk for completing the act.

Physical Examination

A physical examination is part of the assessment in all patients suspected of suicidal intent. The completeness of the examination is altered according to the clinical condition of the patient, but the basic components are as follows.

Vital Signs. Any instability requires immediate corrective action.

Skin. Signs of repeated trauma are sought, particularly razor blade cuts at the wrist or antecubital fossa. Signs of substance abuse or of being a victim of violence are sought.

Head, Eyes, Ears, Nose, Throat. Are there any obvious signs of head or facial trauma? The eyes are examined for pupil size and reflexes. Equality of light reactivity is critical in differentiating coma secondary to toxins arising from a central nervous system lesion. Are the eye movements normal? Is there nystagmus? Rotational or vertical nystagmus is highly suggestive of the influence of a CNS lesion or centrally acting drug, e.g., phencyclidine. Are there signs of trauma to the ears, e.g., hemotympanum? Is there septal perforation in the nose due to cocaine abuse? Inspection of the throat for lesions related to ingestion of caustics or foreign bodies is done.

Thorax or Lungs. Are there any signs of injury or underlying pathology? Pulmonary edema may be related to substance abuse, particularly intravenous heroin.

Cardiac. Inspection, palpation, and auscultation are part of the standard examination. Are there signs of irregular heart rate or rhythm, possibly related to drug intoxication?

Abdomen. Are visceral or somatic signs present? These may support a complication of a suicide attempt, e.g., signs of perforation in a caustic ingestion, decreased bowel sounds with a tricyclic antidepressant overdose.

Neurologic Examination. What is the patient's level of awareness and orientation? Is there spontaneous movement? Are verbal commands obeyed? What is the response to noxious stimuli? Is there purposeful movement or posturing? If there is a possible noxious ingestion, serial examination and tracking of changes are necessary.

Mental Status Examination (see Chap. 52). Evaluation of mental status is a critical aspect in determining a patient's suicidal intent and risk. A rapid examination has five components:

1. A description of the general appearance and behavior of the patient.
2. Observing the stream of conversation, both in structure and content.
3. Intellectual function: Is the patient oriented to person, place, and time? What is the patient's short-term memory? Can the patient make reasonable judgments?
4. The patient's mood, i.e., the way the patient feels.
5. Mental content: What is the patient thinking? How are the patient's thoughts organized?

PROBLEM 1 The patient's history was taken in the presence of his family. He was recently divorced and had moved back with his family after losing his job. During the interview he repeatedly referred to his situation as "just hopeless." He stated that he had lost his appetite and had not slept well in at least 3 months. He also reported, and this was confirmed by the family, that he had attempted suicide by an overdose in the last year during a period of depression. When questioned directly, the patient reported that he had a plan to take pills. He wanted to end his pain and relieve his family of the burden. He stated the necessary pills were at home. The family was unsure about the pills, but this kind of talk at home prompted them to seek medical attention. Physical examination showed normal vital signs and normal findings except for "accidental" scars on the volar aspect of both wrists. The patient was slow to respond to questions and appeared sad and depressed.

This patient's history is painfully sad and consists of a series of major losses. His somatic complaints support concerns about a serious degree of depression.

PROBLEM 2 A brief screening physical evaluation for other injuries or concomitant disorders was normal. The patient was interviewed alone. She stated that she took a few of her mother's nerve pills when she was "turned down for a date" by her new boyfriend. She stated that she was angry and embarrassed by all this attention, felt fine, and wanted to go home. She gave no prior history of suicidal attempts or psychiatric history. She hoped she never saw her boyfriend again. Physical examination revealed a well-developed, well-nourished female who was alert but demonstrated slight slurring in her speech. The results of the remainder of a more detailed physical examination were normal.

This patient was in an age group known for impulsive behavior. She could have been acting just as impulsively to get out of the emergency department. The history of ingestion and slurred speech warrant more data gathering and observation.

DECISION PRIORITIES AND PRELIMINARY DIFFERENTIAL DIAGNOSIS

The decision priorities and preliminary differential diagnosis are established in response to two questions:

1. *Are there medical diseases requiring immediate management in this patient?*
   This question includes the relatively rare possibility of organic disease masquerading as a psychiatric illness and causing a suicide attempt. More common is the medical management of intoxication or poisoning as a result of the attempt. The response is tailored to the nature of intoxicant and the patient's condition. Recognition and therapy of acute poisoning is discussed in Chapter 19. Ethanol and cocaine intoxication are addressed in Chapters 20 and 23.

2. *If a suicide attempt or gesture has been made, and the medical concerns are resolved, what risk does the patient pose to himself or others in the near future?*
   Differentiating between a suicidal "gesture" and a serious attempt at self-destruction has obvious clinical ramifications. Major environmental or clinical factors correlated with serious or lethal intent include:
   a. A general sense conveyed to the physician of overwhelming hopelessness, helplessness, depression, or despair.
   b. Age greater than 45 years.
   c. Alcoholism or drug abuse.
   d. Aloneness or poor social support.
   e. A family history of suicide or close association with someone completing suicide.
   f. Psychosis, especially psychoses associated with hallucinations, delusions, or unreal thoughts. Command hallucinations, those suggesting that the patient is evil or should commit self-destructive activities, are the most ominous.
   g. Major depressive illness, especially illnesses with somatic complaints.
   h. Victims and perpetrators of societal violence, domestic violence, incest, or child abuse.
   i. Patients with a predominance of somatic complaints such as headaches, anorexia, insomnia, anxiety, or stomach problems.

These factors are integrated with information specific to the suicide attempt obtained from the interview. The following factors indicate a high risk for completing suicide:

1. A violent or near-lethal preplanned attempt. Most of these are readily apparent, but a more subtle example is the patient who is unwilling to discuss his or her single car accident.
2. Continued suicidal intent with feasible plans.
3. Patients in possession of the means to execute their plan.
4. Secondary gain anticipated from the act. Some patients may expect self-destructive acts to elicit sympathy and sorrow from individuals that they believe are "uncaring."

5. Lack of remorse or insight regarding the recent attempt.

As the number of these factors increases, more suspicion about the true lethal intent of the patient's behavior is warranted. As the potential for lethality rises, so does the need for psychiatric consultation and admission.

"Sad Persons" Scale

In an attempt to better quantify the "risk rating" of this varied information, a risk assessment scale has been created by summating weighted factors. The utility and validity of this weighted suicide risk scale by nonpsychiatrists in assessing the need for psychiatric intervention has been demonstrated. The mnemonic SAD PERSONS is used to represent a list of significant risk factors for suicide (Table 53–2).

Ten categories are scored according to the interview and tallied. If a category is not represented, it is scored zero. In several studies, patients scoring 9 or greater correlated well with a psychiatrist's perception of the need for admission. They were considered to be at high risk for a repeat suicide attempt. Patients scoring 6 to 8 were almost equally divided between those recommended for admission and those recommended for discharge. This group had sufficient risk to justify emergent psychiatric consultation. Patients scoring 5 or less were considered in a lower risk category. They were considered appropriate for discharge and close follow-up. Two sources for error were noted: (1) failure to account for the influence of drugs or alcohol on the patient's responses, (2) failure to corroborate the patient history with a secondary source such as family, friends, or other health care professionals.

No risk assessment system is infallible. A patient may have only a single risk factor and therefore will score only one or two points on a risk assessment scale, but that factor alone may be so overwhelmingly dangerous that psychiatric intervention is justified. For example, a patient with no additional risk factors other than the possession of a quantity of cyanide and suicidal intent would score only two points on the Sad Person's scale. These, however, are of such significance that admission is mandated. Assessment of suicide risk is made very cautiously. Consultation is necessary if any doubt of the accuracy of the risk assessment exists.

PROBLEM 1 Through the interview the physician determined that the patient had no insight into the origins and potential resolution of his situation. He was at

TABLE 53–2. Modified Sad Person's Scale

Category	Points	Description
S = Sex	1	Male
A = Age	1	<19 or >45 years
D = Depression or hopelessness	2	Admits to depression or decreased concentration, appetite, sleep, libido
P = Previous attempts or psychiatric care	1	Previous inpatient or outpatient psychiatric care
E = Excessive alcohol or drug use	1	Stigmata of chronic addiction or recent frequent use
R = Rational thinking loss	2	Organic brain syndrome or psychosis
S = Separated, divorced, or widowed	1	
O = Organized or serious attempt	2	Well thought out plan or "life-threatening" presentation
N = No social supports	1	No close family, friends, job, or active religious affiliation
S = Stated future intent	2	Determined to repeat attempt or ambivalent about repeat attempt

Reprinted with permission from Hockberger RS, Rothstein RJ: Assessment of suicide potential by nonpsychiatrists using the SAD PERSON's Score. J Emerg Med 6:99–107, 1988.

high risk for a repeat attempt. He was in the right age group, was "alone" and recently divorced, had a past history of psychiatric disturbances, had somatic complaints, evoked feelings of hopelessness and helplessness, had feasible plans, and was in possession of the means. Using the Sad Person's Scale, he was male, over age 45, depressed, had made previous suicide attempts and had had psychiatric care, used alcohol, was separated, had an organized attempt in mind, had little social support, and had stated future intent. His total score was 12.

PROBLEM 2 The 18 year old female with a suspected overdose had an unremarkable past medical, surgical, and psychiatric history. The patient showed insight into her behavior appropriate for her age. Her father was strongly supportive. Using the Sad Person's Scale, she was young, not abusing alcohol or drugs, had good social support, had no family or personal history of psychosis or suicidal ideations, had no depressive illnesses, was not a victim of violence, had essentially no somatic complaints, did not use a violent means and had no workable plan, did not expect any secondary gain, and did not feel hopeless or helpless. Her total score was 1.

DIAGNOSTIC ADJUNCTS

Few ancillary tests assist specifically in managing the potentially suicidal patient. The toxicology screen is worthy of mention. Frequently patients are under the influence of intoxicating substances or are intentionally attempting to conceal the use of these agents. Selective use of the toxicology screen may be helpful in identifying unsuspected or unreported ingested substances. This test is discussed in more detail in Chapter 19.

PRINCIPLES OF MANAGEMENT

Protecting a patient from self-harm is the guiding principle in emergency intervention. Two guiding principles that will help to protect self-destructive patients from themselves are

1. A physician's high index of suspicion. When approaching a patient the physician should keep constantly in mind the possible role of suicidal intent in the patient's presentation. With this approach, several clues may be detected and their importance acknowledged (Table 53–1).

2. Appropriate restraints are applied early in the course of care if there is uncertainty or suspicion about the violent potential of a patient's behavior. Restraining the patient may require a simple show of force with a contingent of security guards. If additional control is required, a team approach is indicated, optimally with four staff members, one to control each limb at the elbow or knee. Leather restraints are applied to each limb. If a search for drugs or weapons has not been completed, it is done immediately after restraint (see Chap 52). The physician is protected by law in using restraint to protect a patient against himself or others based on his professional assessment of the patient's behavior at that time.

If pharmacologic restraint is required, the drug of choice is haloperidol. An initial dose of 5 to 10 mg given parenterally is the usual amount in most patients. One to two milligrams is the initial dose in elderly patients. Patient sedation is monitored as a target symptom. Drowsiness denotes sufficient dosage. In the suicidal population, pharmacologic restraint is used cautiously and preferably after discussion with the patient, family, or psychiatric consultant. It is not used if an unknown poison is complicating the patient's condition.

Patients who demonstrate insight into the etiology of their distress may be candidates for brief, supportive psychotherapy. This first session may be given by health care providers in the emergency department. Long-term psychotherapy and other forms of psychiatric intervention are part of an extended therapeutic relationship.

Rarely are patients sent home with medication. If so, only single doses of a medication administered in the emergency department are dispensed for home use pending immediate follow-up with a psychiatrist the following day. Major psychotropic medications, e.g., antidepressants, are administered only after consultation with a psychiatrist.

SPECIAL CONSIDERATIONS

Children and Adolescents

A recent report by the American Academy of Pediatrics Committee on Adolescents describes a disturbing increase in the suicide rate among adolescents. Adolescents share many of the same risk factors as the rest of the population. There is also an "impulsive" element in their behavior that cannot be discounted. Younger children may demonstrate other manifestations such as difficult relationships, difficulties at school, sleep disorders, social isolation, and hypochondriacal behavior. A difficult problem in identifying children and adolescents at risk for suicide is that their early symptoms often become manifest in an atypical or indirect fashion. Examples include: progressively declining school work and social activities, multiple physical complaints, and a disintegrating relationship with the family. These may be too easily explained as characteristic of the "teen-age years" instead of early symptoms predictive of suicide. Only an open mind, empathy, and a clinical suspicion will detect these subtle signals. Once detected, a detailed review of the patient's family and social support systems is necessary. The patient's living conditions and the possibility of sexual or physical abuse or drug dependency are important considerations.

The child who is seen for psychological complaints may be suffering from suicidal ideation. The physician should not hesitate to ask a child about suicidal intent. Frequently the child will be relieved to know that someone is concerned about him or her. Involving family members, loved ones, and friends is necessary to begin and sustain the counseling process.

Older Patients

There is a marked increase in the lethality of suicide attempt by patients over 45 years of age. One source suggests that for every completed suicide in the early adult years there are 50 to 200 attempts, but in the over-45 age group the ratio of completions to attempts is 1:3. Vigilance is necessary when friends or family report despondency following the death of a loved one, an anniversary, or changes in personal stature, e.g., retirement. Older patients as a rule have a higher number of risk factors when they are questioned after a suicide attempt. Discharge from the emergency department must be weighed against risk potential carefully and follow-up plans specifically arranged.

DISPOSITION AND FOLLOW-UP

One of the most difficult problems in emergency medicine is the disposition of the suicidal patient. The information gathered during the evaluation is formulated into a suicide risk assessment. Three patient categories are constructed after behavior caused by major medical problems is eliminated. They are handled in the following manner:

1. Patients at *high risk* for suicide almost always meet one or more of the following criteria: active psychosis, threatening or directing hallucinations, preplanned attempts of high lethality, continued suicidal intent with feasible plans, Sad Person's Scale scores of 9 or greater, and social isolation. They are emergently hospitalized, against their will if necessary, for psychiatric evaluation.

2. Patients at *moderate risk* will benefit from emergent psychiatric evaluation but may not require emergency hospitalization. These patients' criteria usually include major depressive illnesses, male gender, age greater than 45 years, high-risk activities, alcohol or drug abuse, feelings of hopelessness, helplessness, exhaustion, or despair, possession of a means to complete the act, patients with secondary gain, or patients with Sad Person's Scale scores of 6 to 8.

3. Patients at *low risk* may be discharged home without hospitalization or formal psychiatric evaluation. These patients have very low Sad Person's Scale scores and manifest very few of the above-listed risk factors. They usually have adequate social support, good insight into their behavior, and can express their feelings about the attempt. They have no "complicating" factors in their cases. These patients optimally have acute psychiatric follow-up arranged within 24 hours. The psychiatric follow-up arrangements are discussed with a responsible party accompanying the patient. The arrangements should include specific details of location, time, and place and contingency plans of action for the responsible party if the patient avoids the appointment.

Psychiatric Consultation

In presenting the case of a suicidal patient to a psychiatrist, certain key points of information will facilitate the quality of the evaluation. These include:

1. The patient's demographic data, chief complaint, and present physical condition.
2. A brief but complete recitation of the events leading up to the emergency evaluation.
3. The risk factors present or absent. (See the earlier section, Decision Priorities and Preliminary Differential Diagnosis.)
4. The existence of intoxication, depression, significant medical problems, or character disorder.
5. The adequacy of the patient's social support system.
6. The emergency physician's own summary assessment of suicide risk.

Consulting with a psychiatrist on the telephone or his representative (mental health worker) after he has evaluated the patient should result in resolved concerns about disposition. A written statement of the degree of risk and what factors the consultant discovered or confirmed are critical aspects of the assessment.

Prior to speaking with the patient and the family, the emergency physician assembles and clarifies the details of disposition. Voluntary admission is straightforward. Involuntary admission usually requires considerable discussion with the patient and family and thorough documentation. Security personnel may need to be involved. If plans are made for outpatient treatment, specific instructions are given to the patient *and* a support person. These instructions include time, date, and place of appointment as well as contingency plans if the patient does not keep the appointment. A "social contract" is established with the patient to follow up with the appointment.

Patients' compliance with disposition instructions after suicide evaluation in the emergency department is notoriously poor. Every effort must be made to establish a follow-up appointment and to share those details with a responsible person accompanying the patient. The details are documented on the chart and on a written form given to the patient and the accompanying support person.

PROBLEM 1 This patient had a high-risk suicide profile and was voluntarily admitted to the inpatient psychiatry service. The patient underwent 2 weeks of intensive inpatient therapy and is currently functioning reasonably well in a new job; he is taking a low dose of an antidepressant.

The physician has the option of effecting involuntary admission in such a case. It is necessary to know the state laws regarding this important responsibility.

PROBLEM 2 The facts in the case of the 18 year old girl were corroborated by her father and boyfriend. She recognized that this was an impulsive act and agreed to be discharged home in the care of her family. Specific detailed written instructions were given for an outpatient counseling appointment the next morning.

DOCUMENTATION

1. The chief complaint and the source of other historical information obtained.
2. Specific risk factors, both positive and negative, as listed in the section Decision Priorities and Preliminary Differential Diagnosis.
3. If restraint of the patient was necessary, a statement justifying the actions taken.
4. A list of precautions taken against suicide, if any.
5. A brief summary of suicide risk, including any consultations.
6. The precise details of discharge
   a. To whom instructions for discharge, follow-up, and contingency planning were given and explained.
   b. The time, date, place, directions, person, and follow-up details.
   c. Complete details of the contingency action to be taken should the patient decline follow-up.

SUMMARY AND FINAL POINTS

- The potential for suicidal intent is considered in certain clinical situations, e.g., patients in single car accidents, patients who engage in high-risk behavior, and patients with unclear reasons for seeking medical care.
- Do not leave a potentially suicidal patient alone in the emergency department.
- A series of questions probing more directly into the issue of suicidal intent may reveal the patient's motives and plans.
- Corroborating information is necessary from other sources.
- Medical, surgical, and major psychiatric diseases may masquerade as suicidal intent. This finding is still less common than are other psychobehavioral disorders seen in the emergency department.
- Differentiating a suicidal gesture from a serious lethal intent is a critical responsibility of the emergency physician. It may be facilitated by using high-risk criteria or the Sad Person's Scale.
- In questionable cases, liberal use of consultants and erring to protect the patient are recommended.
- On discharge, the support person accompanying the patient is provided with specific, detailed written instructions for follow-up as well as a contingency plan to be followed should the patient decline care later.
- Documentation must include justification for any restraint used.

■ Involuntary commitment is available to the physician if the patient is potentially harmful to himself or others or cannot take care of himself.

BIBLIOGRAPHY

Texts

1. Howton K: Attempted Suicide (2nd ed). New York, Oxford Medical Publishers, 1987.
2. Maltsberger JT: Suicide Risk: The Formulation of Clinical Judgment. New York, New York University Press, 1986.
3. Victoroff VM: The Suicidal Patient: Recognition, Intervention, Management. Oradell, NJ, Medical Economics Books, 1983.
4. Weissberg MP: Dangerous Secrets: Maladaptive Responses to Stress. New York, Norton, 1983.

Journal Articles

1. Committee on Adolescence, American Academy of Pediatrics: Suicide and suicide attempts in adolescents and young adults. Pediatrics 81:322–324, 1988.
2. Hockberger RS, Rothstein RJ: Assessment of suicide potential by nonpsychiatrists using the SAD PERSONS Score. J Emerg Med 6:99–107, 1988.
3. Murphy GE: The physician's responsibility for suicide. I. An error of commission. Ann Intern Med 82:301–304, 1975.
4. Murphy GE: The physician's responsibility for suicide. II. Errors of omission. Ann Intern Med 82:305–309, 1975.
5. Pfeffer CR: Clinical aspects of childhood suicidal behavior. Pediatr Ann 13:56–61, 1984.
6. Rosenthal PA, Rosenthal S: Suicidal behavior by preschool children. Am J Psychiatry 141:520–525, 1984.
7. Weissberg MD, Suskauer SH: The suicide crisis: Preventing the final act. Emerg Med Rep 105–112, 1986.

CHAPTER 54

SEXUAL ASSAULT

JOELLEN LINDER, M.D.

PROBLEM A 53 year old woman, on returning home from church, was grabbed and thrown to the ground just inside the driveway entrance to her home. The assailant was described as a young man, approximately 18 to 20 years old, who asked the victim to pray for him as he raped her.

QUESTIONS TO CONSIDER

1. What are the evaluation and treatment priorities in the care of the sexual assault victim?
2. How is the examination process explained to a person who may recently have been sexually violated? Is consent necessary for collection of evidence?
3. Are there protocols or standard forms for gathering evidence and recording information? What is a sexual assault kit?
4. What historical points must be documented?
5. What is involved in the physical examination? Are there specific elements to be sought in the physical examination? For example, is the location of bruises or bite marks important? When should photographs be obtained?
6. What does "chain of evidence" mean? Why is it important?
7. What precautions to preserve evidence must be addressed? When should they be mentioned?
8. What happens after the examination in the emergency department? What common reactions are seen in sexual assault victims?
9. How is law enforcement involved? What is the examining physician's role if the case comes to trial?

INTRODUCTION

Sexual conduct or act is defined as vaginal intercourse between a male and a female, and anal intercourse, fellatio, and cunnilingus between persons regardless of sex. *Sexual contact* means touching of an erogenous zone of another person for the purpose of sexually arousing or gratifying either person. *Statutory rape* is intercourse with a female below a certain age, usually 14 to 18, with or without her consent. The rationale is that the victim is not mature enough to understand the full implications of the act and to give valid consent.

Rape is defined in legal terms that vary depending on the state in which the crime occurred. In most state penal codes, rape involves penetration of the orifices of a nonconsenting victim with the use of force or coercion through physical violence or the threat of same to accomplish the acts.

Sexual assault is a crime of violence. Based on annual victimization rates for violent crimes from 1975 through 1984, an estimated five out of six of today's 12 year olds will be victims of rape, either completed or attempted, at least once during their lives. In 1986 there was one forcible rape every 6 minutes. The age range of victims is 6 months to 93 years. Half the victims know the rapist. Most rapes occur in poverty areas. Injuries occur in 8% to 45% of victims, and 1% require hospitalization. In 1977 less than 20% of reported rapes resulted in conviction. This is one of the lowest conviction rates for any violent crime.

The alleged crime usually occurs unobserved, and therefore testimony by the victim and the assailant and physical evidence found at the scene or through a methodical physical examination becomes essential for the legal process. Sixty percent of rape victims experience post-traumatic stress disorders for years following a rape, and 16% still suffered these emotional problems 15 years following this crime.

PREHOSPITAL CARE

In many instances victims of sexual assault present to the emergency department without making prior contact with anyone. Persons who render assistance to the victim of rape during the acute phase play an important role in recovery. When a call is made to 911 by a victim of sexual assault, the rescue squad should respond as a priority. Emergency medical services (EMS) personnel will be confronted with the acute phase symptoms. The care giver should maintain objectivity, give appropriate treatment, and avoid asking "why" questions. The patient should be transported in a position of comfort if EMS transportation is used.

1. Attention to the victim's physical condition is always the first priority.

2. The victim is encouraged to report the alleged crime. All victims should be examined by a physician regardless of whether or not they want to involve the law enforcement process.

3. To preserve evidence, victims are advised not to bathe, wipe their genital area, douche, insert or remove a tampon, brush their teeth, or change clothing if they are still wearing the clothing worn during the attack. Usually the clothing worn will be kept for evidence, so the victim is asked to bring an extra set of clothes.

PROBLEM This woman, having no family living in the immediate area and too embarrassed to call her fellow church members, called the local rape hotline. She decided to report the attack and was accompanied to the emergency department by a volunteer from the local rape crisis center and a law enforcement officer.

INITIAL APPROACH IN THE EMERGENCY DEPARTMENT

Three specific areas of need of the sexual assault survivor include medical needs, psychosocial needs, and legal needs. On arrival in the emergency department an initial assessment of the victim's physical needs must be made at triage to determine whether immediate medical intervention is needed. If the patient is stable, privacy is respected as much as possible, and a quiet area is found for the patient. Family and friends are allowed to stay with the victim if desired. If no one accompanies the victim to the emergency department, every effort is made to find someone to stay with the patient throughout her or his stay.

An informed consent to an examination for evidence collection is obtained as early as possible. This consent is mandatory. The local law enforcement agency is contacted if the victim is willing to report the incident. The nursing staff member who will be assisting in the collection of evidence should prepare the examination room and have the sexual assault kit ready.

PROBLEM This woman was initially triaged to a quiet area in the emergency department that was set up especially for victims of sexual assault. The rape crisis volunteer remained with her while information was obtained by registration personnel, and the nurse checked an initial set of vital signs. Informed consent regarding the examination for evidence was obtained. The emergency physician was informed of the patient's arrival in the department. The physician would see her as a priority once any patients in critical medical condition were stabilized.

Emergency care of the victim of sexual assault requires coordination of services that usually are provided outside the emergency department. The survivor of sexual assault has often been through a life-threatening experience. Many of the steps subsequently taken to gather evidence in the examination of sexual assault victims are invasive and often unpleasant reminders of the trauma of rape. One of the most important things the emergency health care personnel can provide for the victim is reassurance and a return to control. This is sometimes difficult to achieve in a busy, crowded emergency department.

DATA GATHERING

Information about the events of the alleged crime is gathered systematically under an established protocol. The State of California in 1987 established a Medical Protocol for Examination of Sexual Assault and Child Sexual Abuse Victims to meet minimum standards for evidential examinations. The protocol contains step-by-step procedures for conducting examinations of the adult female, adult male, pediatric patient, and suspect. Other states and local jurisdictions have similar protocols for evidence collection and preservation. When the victim agrees to report the alleged crime and consents to an examination for evidence, the local protocol should always be followed. The physician should avoid any judgment; his or her role is not to decide whether rape has occurred but to give medical care and collect medicolegal evidence. Information about relationships and motives are seldom available to the physician.

History

Specific information to be obtained from the adult female victim such as the one in this case includes the following (Fig. 54–1):
1. Name of person providing history, relationship to patient
2. Date and time of assault
3. Location and physical surroundings of assault
4. Name(s), number, and race of assailant(s)
5. Acts described by patient. Note: any penetration, however slight, of the labia or rectum by the penis or any penetration of a genital or anal opening by a foreign object or body part constitutes the act. Oral copulation and masturbation require only contact.
6. Physical injuries or pain described by patient
7. Methods employed by perpetrator (i.e., weapons, physical blows, restraints, threats)
8. Postassault hygiene or activity
9. Pertinent medical history
   a. Last menstrual period
   b. Any recent anal or genital injuries, surgeries, diagnostic procedures, or medical treatment that may affect physical findings?
   c. Consenting intercourse within past 72 hours?
10. DO NOT RECORD ANY OTHER INFORMATION REGARDING SEXUAL HISTORY

Text continued on page 972

State of California   Office of Criminal Justice Planning (OCJP) 923

MEDICAL REPORT—SUSPECTED SEXUAL ASSAULT

<u>Patients requesting examination, treatment and evidence collection:</u> Penal Code § 13823.5 requires every physician who conducts a medical examination for evidence of a sexual assault to use this form to record findings. Complete each part of the form and if an item is inapplicable, write N/A.

<u>Patients requesting examination and treatment only:</u> Penal Code § 11160–11161 requires physicians and hospitals to notify a law enforcement agency by telephone and in writing if treatment is sought for injuries inflicted in violation of any state penal law. If the patient consents to treatment only, complete Part A # 1 and 2, Part B # 1, and Part E # 1–10 to the extent it is relevant to treatment, and mail this form to the local law enforcement agency.

<u>Minors:</u> Civil Code § 34.9 permits minors, 12 years of age or older, to consent to medical examination, treatment, and evidence collection related to a sexual assault without parental consent. Physicians are required, however, to attempt to contact the parent or legal guardian and note in the treatment record the date and time the attempted contact was made including whether the attempt was successful or unsuccessful. This provision is not applicable if the physician reasonably believes the parent or guardian committed the sexual assault on the minor. If applicable, check here ( ) and note the date and time the attempt to contact parents was made in the treatment record.

<u>Liability and release of information:</u> No civil or criminal liability attaches to filling out this form. Confidentiality is not breached by releasing it to law enforcement agencies.

A. GENERAL INFORMATION
(print or type)   Name of Hospital:

1. Name of patient					Patient ID number		
2. Address			City		County	State	Phone (W) (H)
3. Age	DOB	Sex	Race	Date/time of arrival	Date/time of exam	Date/time of discharge	Mode of transportation
4. Phone report made to law enforcement agency: Name of officer				Agency		ID number	Phone
5. Responding officer				Agency		ID number	Phone

B. PATIENT CONSENT

1. I understand that hospitals and physicians are required by Penal Code § 11160–11161 to report to law enforcement authorities cases in which medical care is sought when injuries have been inflicted upon any person in violation of any state penal law. The report must state the name of the injured person, current whereabouts, and the type and extent of injuries.

   _____
   Patient/Parent/Guardian (circle)

2. I understand that a separate medical examination for evidence of sexual assault at public expense can, with my consent, be conducted by a physician to discover and preserve evidence of the assault. If conducted, the report of the examination and any evidence obtained will be released to law enforcement authorities. I understand that the examination may include the collection of reference specimens at the time of the examination or at a later date. Knowing this, I consent to a medical examination for evidence of sexual assault. I understand that I may withdraw consent at any time for any portion of the evidential examination.

   _____
   Patient/Parent/Guardian (circle)

3. I understand that collection of evidence may include photographing injuries and that these photographs may include the genital area. Knowing this, I consent to having photographs taken.

   _____
   Patient/Parent/Guardian (circle)

4. I have been informed that victims of crime are eligible to submit crime victim compensation claims to the State Board of Control for out-of-pocket medical expenses, loss of wages, and job retraining and rehabilitation. I further understand that counseling is also a reimbursable expense.

   _____
   Patient/Parent/Guardian (circle)

C. AUTHORIZATION FOR EVIDENTIAL EXAM

I request a medical examination and collection of evidence for suspected sexual assault of the patient at public expense.

_____
Law Enforcement Officer

Agency	ID Number	Date

DISTRIBUTION OF OCJP 923 FOR EVIDENTIAL EXAMS ONLY	HOSPITAL IDENTIFICATION INFORMATION
ORIGINAL TO LAW ENFORCEMENT; PINK COPY TO CRIME LAB (SUBMIT WITH EVIDENCE); YELLOW COPY TO HOSPITAL RECORDS	

OCJP 923

FIGURE 54–1 Example of a medical report form used in cases of suspected sexual assault. (From State of California Medical Protocol for Examination of Sexual Assault and Child Sexual Abuse Victims. Used with permission.)

Illustration continued on following page

D. OBTAIN PATIENT HISTORY. RECORDER SHOULD ALLOW PATIENT OR OTHER PERSON PROVIDING HISTORY TO DESCRIBE INCIDENT(S) TO THE EXTENT POSSIBLE AND RECORD THE ACTS DESCRIBED BELOW. DETERMINE AND USE TERMS FAMILIAR TO THE PATIENT. FOLLOW-UP QUESTIONS MAY BE NECESSARY TO ENSURE THAT ALL ITEMS ARE COVERED.

1. Name of person providing history	Relationship to patient	Date/time of assault(s)

2. Location and physical surroundings of assault (bed, field, car, rug, floor, etc.)

3. Name(s), number and race of assailant(s)

4. Acts described by patient
(Any penetration, however slight, of the labia or rectum by the penis or any penetration of a genital or anal opening by a foreign object or body part constitutes the act. Oral copulation and masturbation only require contact.)

	Yes	No	Attempted	Unsure	If more than one assailant, identify person.
Penetration of vagina by					
Penis					
Finger					
Foreign object					
Describe the object					
Penetration of rectum by					
Penis					
Finger					
Foreign object					
Describe the object					
Oral copulation of genitals					
of victim by assailant					
of assailant by victim					
Oral copulation of anus					
of victim by assailant					
of assailant by victim					
Masturbation					
of victim by assailant					
of assailant by victim					
other					
Did ejaculation occur outside a body orifice?					
if yes, describe the location on the body.					
Foam, jelly, or condom used (circle)					
Lubricant used					
Fondling, licking or kissing (circle)					
If yes, describe the location on the body.					
Other acts					

5. Physical injuries and/or pain described by patient

	Yes	No
Lapse of consciousness:		
Vomited:		
Pre-existing physical injuries:		

If yes, describe: _____

6. Methods employed by perpetrator

	Yes	No	Area of body
Weapon inflicted injuries			
Type of weapon(s)			
Physical blows by hands or feet (circle)			
Grabbing/grasping/holding (circle)			
Physical restraints Type(s) used			
Bites			
Choking			
Burns (including chemical/toxic)			
Threat(s) of harm			
To whom:			
Type of threat(s)			
Other method(s) used			
Describe:			

7. Post-assault hygiene/activity
( ) Not applicable if over 72 hours

	Yes	No
Urinated		
Defecated		
Genital wipe/wash		
Bath/shower		
Douche		
Removed/inserted tampon, sponge, diaphragm (circle)		
Brushed teeth		
Oral gargle/swish		
Changed clothing		

8. Pertinent medical history

Last menstrual period:

Any recent (60 days) anal-genital injuries, surgeries, diagnostic procedures, or medical treatment which may affect physical findings? ( ) Yes ( ) No

If yes, record information in separate medical chart.

Consenting intercourse within past 72 hours? ( ) Yes ( ) No

Approximate date/time:

DO NOT RECORD ANY OTHER INFORMATION REGARDING SEXUAL HISTORY ON THIS FORM.

HOSPITAL IDENTIFICATION INFORMATION

OCJP 923

FIGURE 54–1 Continued

E. CONDUCT A GENERAL PHYSICAL EXAM AND RECORD FINDINGS. COLLECT AND PRESERVE EVIDENCE FOR EVIDENTIAL EXAM.

1. Blood pressure	Pulse	Temperature	Respiration	2. Height	Weight	Eye color	Hair color

3. Note condition of clothing upon arrival (rips, tears, presence of foreign materials)

4. Collect outer and underclothing worn during or immediately after assault.
5. Collect fingernail scrapings, if indicated.
6. Record general physical appearance:

- Record injuries and findings on diagrams: erythema, abrasions, bruises (detail shape), contusions, induration, lacerations, fractures, bites, burns, and stains/foreign materials on the body.
- Record size and appearance of injuries. Note swelling and areas of tenderness.
- Collect dried and moist secretions, stains, and foreign materials from the body including the head, hair, and scalp. Identify location on diagrams.
- Scan the entire body with a Wood's Lamp. Swab each suspicious substance or fluorescent area with a separate swab. Label Wood's Lamp findings "W.L."
- Collect the following reference samples at the time of the exam if required by crime lab: saliva, head, hair, and body/facial hair from males.
- Record specimens collected on Section 11.

7. Examine the oral cavity for injury and the area around the mouth for seminal fluid. Note frenulum trauma.
   - If indicated by history: Swab the area around the mouth. Collect 2 swabs from the oral cavity up to 6 hours post-assault for seminal fluid. Prepare two dry mount slides.
   - If indicated by history, take a GC culture from the oropharynx and offer prophylaxis. Take other STD cultures as indicated.
   - Record specimens collected on Section 11.

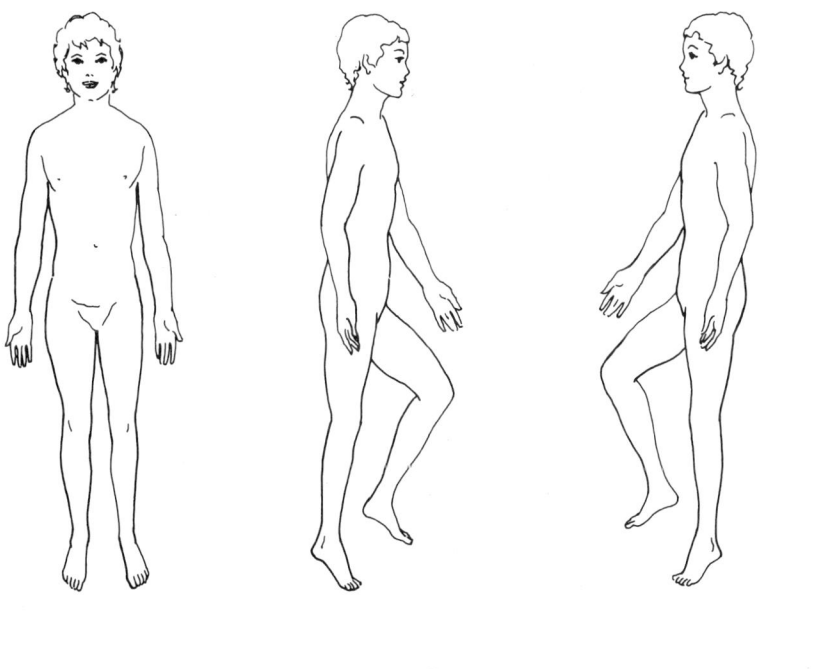
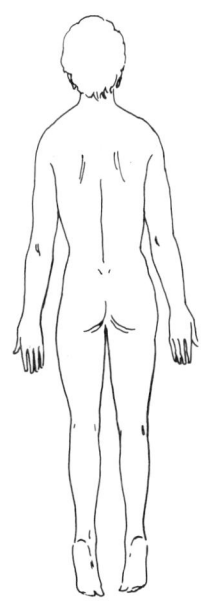
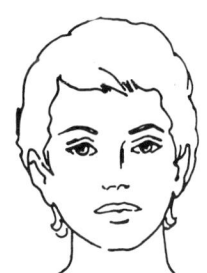

OCJP 923

HOSPITAL IDENTIFICATION INFORMATION

FIGURE 54–1 Continued

Illustration continued on following page

8. External genitalia
- Examine the external genitalia and perianal area including the inner thighs for injury and foreign materials.
- Collect dried and moist secretions and foreign materials. Identify location on diagrams.
- Cut matted pubic hair. Comb pubic hair to collect foreign materials.
- Scan area with Wood's Lamp. Swab each suspicious substance or fluorescent area. Label Wood's Lamp findings "W.L."
- Collect pubic hair reference samples at time of exam if required by crime lab.
- For males, collect 2 penile swabs if indicated. Collect one swab from the urethral meatus and one swab from the glans and shaft. If indicated by history, take a GC culture from the urethra and offer prophylaxis. Take other STD cultures as indicated.
- Record specimens collected on Section 11.

9. Vagina and cervix
- Examine for injury and foreign materials.
- Collect 3 swabs from vaginal pool. Prepare 1 wet mount and 2 dry mount slides. Examine wet mount for sperm. Take a GC culture from the endocervix and offer prophylaxis. Take other STD cultures as indicated.
- If the assault occurred more than 24 hours prior to the exam, collection of cervical swabs may be indicated up to 2 weeks post-assault if no possibility exists of contaminating the specimen with semen from previous coitus. Label cervical swabs and slides to distinguish them from the vaginal swabs and slides.
- Aspirate/washings to detect sperm are optional.
- Record specimens collected on Section 11.
- Obtain pregnancy test (blood or urine).

10. Anus and rectum
- Examine the buttocks, perianal skin, and anal folds for injury.
- Collect dried and moist secretions and foreign materials. Foreign materials may include lubricants and fecal matter.
- If indicated by history and/or findings: Collect 2 rectal swabs and prepare 2 dry mount slides. Avoid contaminating rectal swabs by cleaning the perianal area and dilating the anus using an anal speculum.
- Conduct an anoscopic or proctoscopic exam if rectal injury is suspected.
- If indicated by history, take a GC culture from the rectum and offer prophylaxis. Take other STD cultures as indicated.
- Record specimens collected on Section 11.
- Take blood for syphilis serology. Offer prophylaxis.

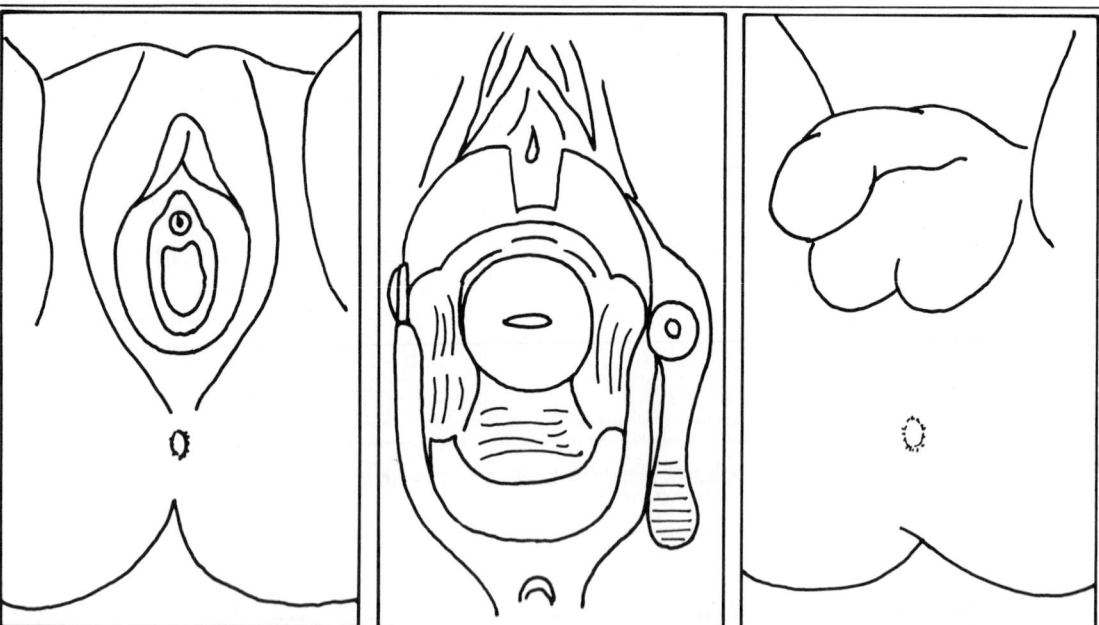

HOSPITAL IDENTIFICATION INFORMATION

FIGURE 54-1 Continued

11. Record evidence and specimens collected.

ALL SWABS AND SLIDES MUST BE AIR DRIED PRIOR TO PACKAGING (PENAL CODE § 13823.11). AIR DRY UNDER A STREAM OF COOL AIR FOR 60 MINUTES. Swabs and slides must be individually labeled, coded to show which slides were prepared from which swabs, and time taken. All containers (tubes, bindles, envelopes) for individual items must be labeled with the name of the patient, contents, location of the body where taken, and name of hospital. Package small containers in a large envelope and record chain of custody. See the State of California Medical Protocol for Examination of Sexual Assault and Child Sexual Abuse Victims published by the state Office of Criminal Justice Planning, 1130 K Street, Sacramento, CA 95814 (916) 324-9100 for additional information.

SPECIMENS FOR PRESENCE OF SEMEN, SPERM MOTILITY, AND TYPING TO CRIME LAB

	Swabs	Dry mount slides	Yes	No	N/A	Taken by	Time
Oral							
Vaginal							
Rectal							
Penile							
Aspirate/washings (optional)							

Vaginal wet mount slide examined for spermatozoa, dried, and submitted to crime lab
Motile sperm observed
Non-motile sperm observed

OTHER EVIDENCE TO CRIME LAB

	Yes	No	N/A	Taken by
Clothing				
Fingernail Scrapings				
Foreign materials on body				
Blood				
Dried secretions				
Fiber/loose hair				
Vegetation				
Dirt/gravel/glass				
Matted pubic hair cuttings				
Pubic hair combings				
Comb				
Swabs of bite marks				
Control swabs				
Photographs				
Area of the body _____				
Type of camera _____				
Other _____				

REFERENCE SAMPLES AND TOXICOLOGY SCREENS TO CRIME LAB

Reference samples and toxicology screens can only be collected with the consent of the patient. Reference samples can be collected at the time of the exam or at a later date according to crime lab policies. Toxicology screens should be collected at the time of the exam upon the recommendation of the physical examiner or law enforcement officer.

Reference samples

	Yes	No	N/A	Taken by
Blood typing (yellow top tube)				
Saliva				
Head hair				
Pubic hair				
Facial/body hair				

Toxicology screens

| Blood/alcohol toxicology (grey top tube) | | | | |
| Urine toxicology | | | | |

EXAM INFORMATION (print)

Anoscopic exam				
Proctoscopic exam				
Genital exam done with:				
Direct visualization				
Colposcope				
Hand held magnifier				

PERSONNEL INVOLVED (print) — PHONE

History taken by:
Physical examination performed by:
Specimens labeled and sealed by:
Assisting nurse:

FINDINGS

Report of sexual assault, exam reveals:
☐ PHYSICAL FINDINGS
    ☐ Exam consistent with history
    ☐ Exam inconsistent with history
☐ NO PHYSICAL FINDINGS
    ☐ Exam consistent with history
    ☐ Exam inconsistent with history

SUMMARY OF FINDINGS

PHYSICAL EXAMINER

Print name of physical examiner

Signature of physical examiner

License number of physical examiner

LAW ENFORCEMENT OFFICER

I have received the indicated items as evidence and the original of this report.

Law enforcement officer

Law enforcement agency   ID number   Date

HOSPITAL IDENTIFICATION INFORMATION

ARRANGE FOLLOW-UP FOR STD, PREGNANCY, INJURIES, AND PROVIDE REFERRALS FOR PSYCHOLOGICAL CARE.

OCJP 923

FIGURE 54–1 Continued

PROBLEM The woman provided her own history, stating that the assault occurred about noon on the lawn just adjacent to the drivegate entrance to her home. There was only one assailant, who she thought lived in the neighborhood, but she did not know his name. He penetrated her vagina with his penis; she did not know whether he had ejaculated. He had grabbed her wrists and choked her about the neck and threatened to kill her if she screamed. She still complained of some burning in her throat and perineum. She had immediately called the hotline; had not changed clothes nor used the facilities. Her last menstrual period was 8 years ago; she had not had intercourse within the previous 72 hours. She had no major medical illnesses or prior hospitalizations, no known allergies, and a hormone pill was her only medication. She had no other complaints at this time but wanted a cup of coffee if possible.

Physical Examination

In addition to collection of evidence, which is a legal requirement, the patient is simultaneously evaluated for physical and emotional trauma. The physical examination should be complete and directed by the history. It is important to document any marks, bruises, or other signs of trauma. Many medical forms include diagrams for this documentation (see Figure 54–1). Photographs should be taken before the patient leaves the emergency room if they are warranted, i.e., if there are obvious bruises, lacerations, bite marks, or burns. In performing the steps in the evidential examination one should begin with the least invasive step and proceed as outlined:

1. Note condition of clothing. Collect outer and underclothing worn during or immediately after the assault.

2. Collect fingernail scrapings if there is any dirt, debris, or other evidence from scratching the assailant under the fingernails.

3. Conduct general physical examination. Document any marks. Scan entire body with Wood's lamp. Collect dried and moist secretions and foreign materials from body including head, hair, and scalp. Document findings on diagrams.

4. Examine oral cavity for injury. Document findings. If indicated by history, swab area around mouth. For example, if the victim describes forced oral copulation or trauma, evidence is collected from the oral cavity. Collect two oral swabs up to 6 hours postassault and prepare two dry mount slides. Take specimen for Thayer-Martin culture.

5. Examine external genitalia for injury. Scan with Wood's lamp, and collect dried and moist secretions and foreign materials. Document findings. Cut matted pubic hair. Comb pubic hair to collect foreign materials and loose hair.

6. Examine vagina and cervix for injury and foreign materials. Collect three swabs from vaginal pool. Prepare one wet mount for sperm. Document findings. Avoid swabbing the cervical area unless assault occurred more than 24 hours prior to the examination and no possibility exists of contaminating specimen from previous coitus. Sperm may survive more than 72 hours in the cervical mucus. Therefore, it is best to obtain specimens for evidence from the vaginal pool in order to avoid confusion. Take specimen for Thayer-Martin culture.

7. Examine buttocks, perianal skin, and anal folds for injury. Collect dried and moist secretions and foreign materials. Document findings. If indicated by history or findings collect two rectal swabs and prepare two dry mount slides. Take specimen for Thayer-Martin culture. Conduct an anoscopic or proctoscopic examination if rectal injury is suspected.

8. Other evidence to be collected at the discretion of the physician and law enforcement officer include blood alcohol and toxicology screens. The patient has the right to refuse these tests.

9. Reference samples can be collected at the time of the examination or at a later date according to local crime laboratory procedures. These samples include blood for blood typing, saliva, 15 to 20 head hairs, and 15 to 20 pubic hairs.

10. Examination of the male victim should follow the same protocol where it applies.

PROBLEM On examination the patient appeared to be a well-kempt, neatly dressed woman who was 5 feet 3 inches tall, weighed 165 pounds, and had normal blood pressure, pulse, and respirations. As she undressed, her clothing was placed in a properly labeled paper bag. There were three parallel erythematous nonblanching marks on the right side of her neck and a slightly tender, blanching erythematous mark on the palmar surface of her right wrist. There were no oral or facial injuries. Results of chest, back, and abdominal examinations were unremarkable. The Wood's lamp scan revealed no evidence of secretions. Small periurethral tears were noted on examination of the perineum. Swabs were obtained from the vaginal pool of secretions. Under the microscope there was no evidence of spermatozoa or vaginal infection.

Contusions that are tender or slightly erythematous on initial examination are noted now. They may actually show up better a few days later in a photograph.

DIAGNOSTIC ADJUNCTS

Laboratory Studies

The collected specimens undergo a number of enzymatic and genetic tests at the "crime" or forensic laboratory. The reader is referred to reference 9 for further details.

Optional clinical tests to be considered include evaluation for pregnancy, *Chlamydia*, HIV antibody, and syphilis.

DIFFERENTIAL DIAGNOSIS

Sexual assault is a legal term that is defined by the legal system. Physicians are not required to "diagnose" legal issues. Involvement in the legal process by health care providers is necessary to gather evidence and report findings. Still, it is important to be empathetic and to provide medical care as indicated. Formulating differential diagnoses in the case of victims of sexual assault should be limited to the medical problems that may be involved. Restoring a sense of control to the victim throughout the process will help.

PRINCIPLES OF MANAGEMENT

The three areas of need noted previously under Prehospital Care guide the management of the sexual assault victim throughout the emergency department evaluation: medical, legal, and psychosocial.

Once the initial medical needs related to the assault are assessed and stabilized, two potential problems must be addressed: pregnancy and sexually transmitted disease. The risk of pregnancy from unprotected intercourse is about 1% from a single episode. Recent studies recommend the use of estrogens as postcoital therapy if treatment is started within 72 hours of unprotected intercourse: (1) A combination of norgestrel 1.0 mg and ethinyl estradiol 0.1 mg may be given orally in two doses, immediately and 12 hours later, or (2) ethinyl estradiol 5 mg/day may be given for 5 consecutive days.

Treatment to prevent sexually transmitted diseases is offered to all victims of sexual assault. The risk of contracting gonorrhea is approximately 13%, and the risk of syphilis is less than 1%. Between 5% and 10% of sexually abused children are infected with

Neisseria gonorrhoeae, Chlamydia trachomatis, or *Gardnerella vaginalis.* Prophylactic therapy should follow current Centers for Disease Control (CDC) guidelines for treatment of gonorrhea and *Chlamydia* infection at a minimum (see Table 54–1). If *Trichomonas,* candidiasis, or bacterial vaginosis is noted on microscopic examination of the vaginal secretions, appropriate treatment is given (see Chapter 61).

To satisfy legal requirements, the collection and preservation of evidence must follow procedures that will maintain the chain of custody or "chain of evidence." General guidelines are described below:

1. If the incident occurred within 72 hours prior to presentation of the victim in the Emergency Department, the patient is examined without delay. Each item of evidence is clearly marked with the patient name, identification number, date and time of collection, location where it was collected (e.g., vaginal swab), and name of the person collecting the evidence. The items are placed in individual envelopes, all of which are then placed in a box or larger envelope (the sexual assault kit) to be sealed and signed by the person collecting the evidence. All swabs and slides must be thoroughly air dried before they are packaged to allow maximum preservation of the specimens. Subsequent handling and transfer is documented to show that no breaks in the chain of custody have occurred. Proper documentation ensures that evidence has not been altered or lost prior to trial.

2. If the incident occurred more than 72 hours prior to presentation, laboratory evidence is not likely to be present, e.g., secretions or pubic hair combings. A complete physical examination should still be performed to detect any physical trauma or genital injuries or infection.

Psychosocial needs are anticipated by maintaining a kind, direct, efficient, and organized approach to the patient. Judgmental statements are avoided, and the elements of the entire procedure are explained in advance. The physical examination is mentioned, including a pelvic examination to evaluate for injury and to seek or collect evidence. The patient is informed that the potential for pregnancy and sexually transmitted disease will be discussed, and decisions will be made together.

PROBLEM In this case the victim was postmenopausal; therefore pregnancy prophylaxis was not offered. However, prevention of sexually transmitted diseases according to current recommendations by the CDC was offered. The woman accepted oral therapeutics.

Diethylstilbestrol (DES) should not be used as a postcoital contraceptive because of the risk of exposure of potential offspring to carcinoma of the vagina and congenital heart disease. If the victim is already using a reliable method of birth control or is postmenopausal, prophylaxis is not necessary.

TABLE 54–1. Centers for Disease Control Guidelines for Sexually Transmitted Diseases Prophylaxis

1. Culture for *Neisseria gonorrhoeae* and *Chlamydia trachomatis* from any potentially infected sites.
2. Examine vaginal specimens for *Trichomona vaginalis* by wet mount and, if available, culture.
3. Obtain a serologic test for syphilis.
4. Provide prophylactic treatment as follows:
    Tetracycline 500 mg PO qid for 7 days, *or*
    Doxycycline 100 mg PO bid for 7 days.
    If the patient is pregnant or allergic to tetracycline treat with:
    Amoxicillin 3.0 gm or ampicillin 3.5 gm with probenecid 1.0 gm as a single oral dose.
5. Medical follow-up with private physician, gynecologist, or STD clinic should occur in 7 days for repeat of cultures except for the syphilis serologic test, which should be done in 6 weeks.
6. Every effort should be made to determine whether STD infection is present in the assailant.

Centers for Disease Control: STD Treatment Guidelines. Atlanta, Center for Disease Control, 1985, p. 33.

SPECIAL CONSIDERATIONS

Special consideration is given to children who are victims of sexual abuse, elderly victims, male victims, and victims with special ethnic and cultural concerns. Sexual assault of these individuals may be reported by immediate family or close friends. Often the victims do not tell anyone unless they are severely injured.

Child Sexual Abuse

Sexually abused children often present with symptoms of sexually transmitted disease, psychosomatic complaints, or behavior problems of acting out or poor performance in school. Care of these victims must be carefully coordinated to effectively utilize personnel from child protective service agencies, social support agencies, and law enforcement and legal justice systems as well as health and mental health care agencies. Many communities have developed interdisciplinary teams composed of specialists with training in the evaluation and treatment of sexually abused children.

The emergency care of sexually abused children includes but is not limited to the following:

1. Symptoms and signs that identify the sexually abused child must be recognized. Some children will talk openly about sexual acts. Others may exhibit aberrant behaviors, complain of vague physical ailments, or have physical findings consistent with sexual trauma.

2. The acute medical problems of the child are managed, including physical injury, sexually transmitted disease, and pregnancy.

3. An accurate history of the assault is obtained and recorded, including who, when, what, where, and how. It may be helpful to use anatomically correct dolls in obtaining the history in toddlers and preadolescent children to demonstrate details of events that are often difficult to describe.

4. Collection of evidence, documentation, and reporting must follow local legal requirements. Issues may arise about consent, e.g., the child wants the examination and the parents do not. A court order may be necessary.

5. Protection of the child against further abuse must be ensured prior to disposition. Determination of the risk to this child and others in the home can be made by child protective service agency personnel and other agency personnel.

6. Follow-up plans should address the medical and emotional needs of the child and family members. Consultants with specialized skills in the area of child sexual abuse are included whenever possible.

Male Victims

The actual incidence of male victims of sexual assault is unknown. One source estimates that about 10% of all rape victims but less than 1% of rape reports are males. These victims often sustain trauma to the anal and oral areas as well as extragenital trauma. In addition to following the systematic protocol for collection of evidence from victims, the examiner should pay close attention to the anus and rectum. Rectal lacerations and perforation of the sigmoid colon is more commonly associated with foreign body penetration or "fisting."

Other Special Victims

At least 5% of sexual assault victims are women over the age of 50. Severe physical trauma and overwhelming feelings of vulnerability are common aftereffects in these individuals. Follow-up support is essential for the survival of victims who live alone or have sensory or motor deficits. If a victim does not speak English, every effort must be made to find a sensitive interpreter.

DISPOSITION AND FOLLOW-UP

Disposition information and instructions for the victim of sexual assault should include
1. The names of the health care providers who were involved in the emergency visit.
2. Name and identification of the law enforcement investigator handling the case and the case number.
3. Phone numbers of the rape crisis center and name and phone number of the follow-up physician.
4. The medications given and their possible side effects.

It might also be helpful to provide information about reactions the victim may expect to experience during recovery from this incident. The patient may wish to be evaluated for HIV infection resulting from the assault; this test should be performed as soon as possible after exposure and repeated at 6 months.

Several models have been developed to describe the reactions of survivors of sexual offenses. The most notable among these models, the rape trauma syndrome, describes two phases of recovery. The first stage is the acute "disorganization" phase. It occurs in the immediate hours after the event and lasts through several weeks following it. The patient may exhibit a wide range of emotions and may complain of physical trauma, skeletal muscle pain, and gastrointestinal and genitourinary symptoms. The second phase is the "long-term process: reorganization," during which the victim experiences initial disorganization of lifestyle followed by a long-term recovery process. The exact process varies with the coping behavior and support system of the individual. Most responses by the victim are felt to be normal responses to an abnormal life event. Effective crisis intervention can help to restore victims to their former lifestyles and can help to improve their skills in handling future crises.

PROBLEM The patient wanted to return to her home with a law enforcement officer. A member of her church was eventually contacted at her request and agreed to stay with her that evening. Instructions were given to the patient with recommendations for follow-up counseling through the local rape crisis center. She was scheduled to return to see her private physician in 6 weeks for a repeat examination and further serologic tests.

When a victim has sustained severe physical trauma or when other acute medical illness is involved, one must consider admission to the hospital for further treatment. The majority of survivors of sexual assault are discharged from the emergency department and will return for appropriate follow-up care as needed.

DOCUMENTATION

Accurate and complete documentation is a critical component of the sexual assault evidential examination. Documentation of all findings should be recorded on appropriate forms determined by local jurisdictions or the emergency medical record. Specific information to be included in the medical record has been described earlier in this chapter (see Figure 54–1).

Confidentiality of patient records is essential in cases of sexual assault. Many victims are afraid that the assailant may return, and they move to another home or another city.

Establishing a functional confidential file is best accomplished through a system of cross-indexing. The notation, "Medical-Legal Examination: Refer to confidential files" is included on the emergency medical record. All records pertaining to the actual examination for evidence should be placed in the hospital confidential files. Written reports required by child abuse reporting law are included in the confidential files and released only to child protective agencies. Should the case go to court, several agencies may request access to the confidential files. Consultation among the local district attorney's office, the hospital attorney, and the hospital administration is important to ensure the confidentiality for the patient.

SUMMARY AND FINAL POINTS

- Current legislation is based on the Criminal Sexual Conduct Act, sometimes referred to as the Michigan Comprehensive Reform Law, which was passed in 1974. This law redefined criminal sexual conduct and extends protection regardless of gender.
- Statutes vary from state to state, but most laws declare that rape is a sexual act, the victim did not consent to the act, and threats or force were used by the assailant.
- The crime of sexual assault is being recognized as an aberrant act by psychologically disordered individuals who overpower their victims through sexual acts. In the past 20 years, studies of both victims and perpetrators of this devastating crime have helped to promote appropriate sentencing and rehabilitation programs based on the violence of the acts.
- Understanding the patient's medical, legal, and psychosocial needs will allow the emergency physician to attend to *all* important aspects of care.
- A review of local laws and procedures and an apprentice relationship with an experienced physician is necessary before any physician enters into this difficult situation alone.

PROBLEM The assailant was arrested 1 week later based on the description given by the woman. He was released on bail the same day. After several delays in scheduling the trial, the case went to court 10 months following the initial assault. Testimony was taken from the victim, the examining physician, the crime lab technologist, and the investigating officer. In addition, testimony was heard from three other female victims ranging in age from 17 to 49 who were assaulted by the assailant during a period of time 6 months prior to this woman's assault. The assailant was found guilty and sentenced to 5 years in jail. He was released on probation 3 years later. Rehabilitation included psychological counseling as well as group therapy with other sex offenders that was to continue as part of his 2-year probation.

The woman received counseling through the local rape crisis center for a period of 1 year. She has recovered well and is currently working as a hotline volunteer at the rape crisis center in her community.

This case ends with a positive overall picture for this victim. Of 3126 offenders convicted of rape during 1985 in 28 large court systems, 65% were sentenced to state or federal prison, 1% were sentenced to jail, 17% were given a combination of jail and probation, and 16% were sentenced to straight probation.

Many victims of sexual assault continue to be haunted by physical and emotional scars for the rest of their lives. The road to recovery begins at the initial point of contact with anyone who can help to restore a sense of control to the victim. This begins in the emergency department.

BIBLIOGRAPHY

Text

1. Office of Criminal Justice Planning, Informational Guide: California Medical Protocol for Examination of Sexual Assault and Child Sexual Abuse Victims. Sacramento, 1987.

Journal Articles

1. Burgess AW, Holmstrom LL: Rape trauma syndrome. Am J Psychiatry 131(9):981–986, 1974
2. Centers for Disease Control: Publicly funded HIV counseling and testing—United States, 1985–1989. MMNR 39(9):137–140, 1990.
3. Dixon GW, et al: Ethinyl estradiol and conjugated estrogens as postcoital contraceptives. JAMA 244(12):1336–1339, 1980.
4. Dwyer BJ, Hicks DJ, Weissberg MP: Sensitive emergency management of rape victims. Emerg Med Rep 9(15):113–120, 1988.
5. Jenny C, Hooton TM, Bowers A, et al: Sexually transmitted diseases in victims of rape. N Engl J Med 322(11):713–716, 1990.
6. Kobernick ME, Seifert S, Sanders AB: Emergency department management of the sexual assault victim. J Emerg Med 2:205–214, 1985.
7. Martin CA, Warfield MC, Braen GR: Physician's management of the psychological aspects of rape. JAMA 249(4):501–503, 1983.
8. Resick PA: The trauma of rape and the criminal justice system. Justice System Journal 9(1):52–61, 1984.
9. Sensabaugh GF, Bashinske J, Blake ET: The laboratory's role in investigating rape. Diagn Med 45–53, 1985.
10. Sharma A, Cheatham HE: A women's center support group for sexual assault victims. J Counsel Dev 64:525–527, 1986.
11. Talbert S, et al: Improving emergency department care of the sexual assault victim. Ann Emerg Med 9(6):293–297, 1980.

SECTION FIFTEEN

THORACO-RESPIRATORY DISORDERS

CHAPTER 55

ACUTE DYSPNEA

SETH W. WRIGHT, M.D.

PROBLEM 1 The rescue squad responded to the house of a 57 year old man with a history of emphysema who was complaining of 3 days of increasing shortness of breath. He was well known to the rescue squad personnel and had required ventilatory support on several previous occasions.

PROBLEM 2 A 19 year old man presented with a sudden onset of left-sided chest pain and difficulty in breathing while playing basketball. He denied previous episodes of shortness of breath or trauma. On arrival he appeared uncomfortable but was in no distress.

PROBLEM 3 A 73 year old woman with no significant past medical history presented with a complaint of shortness of breath. She stated that she had had an episode of chest pain 2 days ago that had now resolved. She had spent the past two nights sleeping in a recliner chair.

QUESTIONS TO CONSIDER

1. What are the common causes of dyspnea that cause patients to seek emergency care?
2. What prehospital therapy is available for these patients?
3. Which aspects of the history and physical examination will help to differentiate between dyspnea of cardiac origin and that of pulmonary origin?
4. What are the signs of impending respiratory failure?
5. What ancillary tests are useful in evaluating the acutely dyspneic patient?
6. How are arterial blood gas values analyzed for the maximum benefit of the patient?
7. What are the essentials of treatment for the common causes of dyspnea?
8. Which patients with dyspnea are admitted to the hospital?

INTRODUCTION

Breathing is an automatic function that takes place without conscious effort or discomfort in the normal individual. A variety of disease states may interfere with normal breathing and lead to the symptom of dyspnea. Dyspnea is difficult to define accurately but is best described as an unpleasant sensation of increased effort in breathing or "air hunger" accompanied by objective evidence of difficult or uncomfortable breathing. As with pain, dyspnea has a subjective component and is perceived and expressed differently by different people. Acute dyspnea is the rapid onset of the sensation or a worsening of a baseline respiratory insufficiency that often causes the patient to seek medical care.

The pathophysiology of dyspnea is complex and poorly understood. Sensory input from the lungs, ventilatory muscles, and chemical receptors are transmitted to the central nervous system, where the conscious perception of dyspnea is generated in the higher brain centers. Contributing factors include the effort involved in breathing, respiratory muscle fatigue, the blood pH, and the arterial levels of oxygen and carbon dioxide. In general, there is good correlation between the severity of dyspnea and the cardiac or pulmonary dysfunction responsible for it.

The following terms are used in the assessment of the dyspneic patient. They need defining because they are often misused.

Tachypnea. A respiratory rate greater than normal. Normal rates range from 44 cycles/min in a newborn to 14 to 18 cycles/min in adults.

Hyperpnea. Greater than normal minute ventilation that just meets metabolic requirements.

Hyperventilation. A minute ventilation (determined by respiratory rate and tidal volume) that exceeds metabolic demand. Arterial blood gases characteristically show a normal Po_2 with an uncompensated respiratory alkalosis (low Pco_2 and elevated pH).

Dyspnea on exertion (DOE). Dyspnea provoked by physical effort or exertion. Often quantified in simple terms, such as the number of stairs or number of blocks the patient can manage before the onset of dyspnea.

Orthopnea. Dyspnea in a recumbent position. Usually measured in number of pillows (i.e., two pillow orthopnea).

Paroxysmal nocturnal dyspnea (PND). Sudden onset of dyspnea occurring while reclining at night, usually related to the presence of congestive heart failure.

PREHOSPITAL CARE

Complaints relating to shortness of breath generate almost one-quarter of telemetry calls in some emergency medical systems. The history and physical examination results relayed by the rescue squad will direct preparations for the arrival of the patient.

History

1. What is the time course of the shortness of breath? Has it been progressive gradually over several days or has there been a sudden onset?
2. Are there any associated symptoms such as chest pain?
3. Is the patient taking any medications—theophylline, diuretics, nitroglycerin?
4. Is there a known or suspected cause, such as recent chest trauma, aspiration, or underlying pulmonary disease?
5. Most important, does the patient have a history of a similar problem in the past (asthma, emphysema, congestive heart failure [CHF])?

Physical Examination

1. General examination. What are the vital signs, general appearance, and mental status? Is the patient able to talk?
2. Specific examination. The presence of cyanosis, jugular venous distention (JVD), breath sounds, wheezing, use of accessory muscles, and peripheral edema is noted. Is the airway patent and protected? What is the patient's perceived ventilatory status?

Intervention

All patients with significant shortness of breath are transported as rapidly as possible to the hospital. Prehospital treatment of all patients includes the following:

Airway. Airway patency, protection of the airway, and ventilatory status are assessed. The need for endotracheal intubation is difficult to ascertain over the radio. If they have not already done so, the rescue squad is directed to intubate any patient who has difficulty in maintaining or protecting the airway or is obviously unable to ventilate effectively. Patients who cannot be intubated can be ventilated with a bag-valve-mask apparatus. If the status of the patient is in doubt, the physician can ask, "Do you feel that the patient needs to be intubated at this time?" The treating personnel will generally state "Yes, we should intubate now" or "No, we feel comfortable with the patient's respiratory effort at this time."

Supplemental Oxygen. Oxygen is supplied to all patients with dyspnea regardless of etiology. The rate is usually 2 to 4 liters/min, delivering a fraction of inspired oxygen (FIO_2) of 24% to 28%. Higher flow rates are given as necessary. Prehospital personnel may be wary of giving oxygen to patients with chronic obstructive lung disease (COPD) because of the risk of depressing ventilation and the resultant hypercarbia. Although there is a definite risk of producing significant hypercarbia, this occurs in only a small subset of patients. Close observation will identify the depressed mental status that evolves as the hypercarbia develops. Rates of 1 to 2 liters/min are usually satisfactory for this patient group but may be increased as necessary. Administration of oxygen is essential in maintaining tissue oxygenation, even if ventilatory support is required.

Intravenous Access. An intravenous line is started in all patients if possible. The choice of solution depends on the suspected cause of the dyspnea. Dextrose in water 5% (D/W 5%) at a keep-open rate is appropriate in most situations.

Cardiac Monitor. Monitoring is essential for following the heart rate and cardiac rhythm. Patients with hypoxia are at risk for a variety of dysrhythmias.

Medical Therapy. If the cause of the dyspnea is known or strongly suspected, medical treatment can begin in the prehospital setting.

Bronchodilators. When available, an inhaled nebulizer treatment with beta-adrenergic agonists such as metaproterenol is the treatment of choice for patients with bronchospasm. Subcutaneous epinephrine remains useful in children and young adults but is contraindicated in older patients and in those with heart disease. The use of aminophylline in the prehospital setting is discouraged. It has been shown to be of little value in the patient with acute-onset bronchospasm.

Nitrates. Nitroglycerin (NTG) may be useful if myocardial ischemia or pulmonary edema is suspected as the cause of the dyspnea. The blood pressure should be carefully monitored during and after administration of NTG. The usual dose is 0.3 to 0.4 mg sublingually every 5 minutes for three doses as long as the blood pressure remains stable.

Morphine. Intravenous morphine will benefit the patient with CHF due to its preload reduction and anxiolytic effects. Blood pressure and respiratory rate are closely monitored after it is given. This drug may not be carried by the rescue squad.

Diuretics. The prehospital use of furosemide is limited to the patient with extreme respiratory distress secondary to CHF. The preload reducing action is rapid, but the diuretic effect is delayed.

Needle Decompression. Relief of a tension pneumothorax can be lifesaving but is rarely necessary for patients with a spontaneous pneumothorax. The technique is described later in this chapter.

PROBLEM 1 The rescue squad stated that the 57 year old man had a long history of emphysema and ran out of his medications 4 days ago. He had a blood pressure of 170/95 mm Hg and a pulse of 135 beats/min. Examination of the lungs revealed a respiratory rate of 36/min with bilateral wheezes and use of accessory muscles. At this point he was given oxygen by nasal cannula at 2 liters/min, and an IV of D/W 5% had been started. The squad reported that he was extremely short of breath but was still awake and alert and did not require intubation. The estimated time of arrival at the hospital is 10 to 15 minutes.

This patient will probably benefit from the use of a bronchodilator for treatment of his bronchospasm. Instructions are given to the life squad to administer a hand-held nebulizer treatment of metaproterenol and accomplish transport to the hospital as rapidly as possible. If he does not improve, increasing the oxygen to 4 liters/min with close observation may be helpful.

INITIAL APPROACH IN THE EMERGENCY DEPARTMENT

The emergency physician is usually able to determine the cause of dyspnea after a brief history, physical examination, and a chest radiograph. Treatment is directed toward the underlying disorder rather than toward the symptom of dyspnea. Patients with moderate to severe shortness of breath may deteriorate rapidly and are triaged to an area of the emergency department where facilities for airway management are available. These patients are seen immediately by the physician. Patients with less urgent conditions, such as mild asthma, are promptly triaged to an appropriate area and seen as soon as possible. The following activities are performed in the first few minutes after arrival in the emergency department:

1. Rapid assessment of the airway and ventilatory effort. Experienced emergency physicians develop a "sixth sense" about the need for intubation. Clues that the dyspneic patient may require intubation and mechanical ventilation include (1) altered mental status, (2) impending patient exhaustion, e.g., inability to answer questions, (3) patient position, particularly sitting up and leaning forward with associated diaphoresis.
2. Vital signs are obtained and compared to the prehospital values.
3. The patient's history and prehospital course are briefly discussed with the patient and rescue squad. Prolonged questioning at this time is often counterproductive. After the patient's symptoms are improved, a more detailed history is taken.
4. The patient is placed on a cardiac monitor and given supplemental oxygen. There are numerous methods of administering oxygen therapy.
    a. *Nasal Cannulas*. Nasal cannulas are simple, comfortable, inexpensive, and provide 24% to 50% oxygen with flow rates of up to 10 liters/min. They are useful for the patient with suspected acute myocardial infarction, mild dyspnea, and COPD.
    b. *Simple Oxygen Mask*. Simple masks delivery oxygen at rates of approximately 30% to 50%, but precise percentages are difficult to control. Because a flow rate of at least 5 liters/min is recommended to prevent carbon dioxide rebreathing, they are not suitable for delivering a low FIO_2.
    c. *Nonrebreather Mask*. The application of a reservoir bag that remains inflated throughout inspiration will provide up to 90% oxygen. These masks are of value in patients with CHF and in others who require a high FIO_2 (greater than 50% oxygen).
    d. *Venturi Mask*. The Venturi mask allows a set percentage of oxygen at the trachea. These masks are most effective in delivering 24% to 28% oxygen with minimum flow rates of at least 4 liters/min and 6 liters/min, respectively. At rates of more than 30% oxygen they frequently do not provide constant or predictable FIO_2. These masks are excellent for patients with COPD in whom a known and relatively constant percentage of oxygen is desired.
5. An intravenous line with D/W 5% at a keep-open rate is started if it is not already in place. Isotonic crystalloid is given if the patient is clinically dehydrated or hemodynamically unstable.
6. A rapid physical examination is performed, paying attention to the breath and heart sounds, use of accessory respiratory muscles, and the presence or absence of JVD.
7. A blood sample for arterial blood gas (ABG) analysis is often obtained during the initial assessment. Supplemental oxygen need not be withheld prior to obtaining the arterial sample. Arterial blood gas measurements are indicated for patients with severe respiratory distress, cyanosis, mental status changes, or failure to respond to therapy. Definitive airway management is not withheld pending ABG results.

PROBLEM 1 The patient arrived in the emergency department. Because of his obvious respiratory distress, he was immediately triaged to the major resuscitation area. The rescue squad personnel stated that he had momentary improvement on the metaproterenol but now seemed worse. His vital signs were unchanged; however, he was now confused and able to give only one-word answers. Auscultation of his lungs revealed decreased breath sounds bilaterally with only a few wheezes.

The information in the radio call raised concern about this patient's ventilatory status, and equipment for intubation (endotracheal tube, bag-valve-mask, suction) was set up prior to his arrival. Because of his obvious respiratory distress and confusion, he was intubated at this point. He was preoxygenated and then nasotracheally intubated. A portable chest radiograph was obtained. It showed good position of the tube and a right lower lobe infiltrate. He was placed on a ventilator. Therapy was begun with metaproterenol nebulizer treatments, aminophylline, and corticosteroids. His pulmonologist was contacted, and he was admitted to the intensive care unit for further evaluation and care. Samples for basic blood work were drawn, including ABG samples while he was on the ventilator. The patient was transferred to the intensive care unit before the results returned.

DATA GATHERING

History

The severely dyspneic patient often has difficulty giving an adequate history. Other sources, including family, the rescue squad, the patient's previous medical record, and the primary physician, are often necessary. In obtaining a history from the patient with dyspnea, several questions are asked.

1. Has there been a *similar problem in the past?* This is likely to be the single most important question the physician can ask. The majority of patients presenting to the emergency department with shortness of breath have a known underlying disorder causing the dyspnea.

2. *How long has dyspnea been present?* Was the *onset sudden or gradual?* Does anything make it *worse or better?* The longer the evolution of the symptoms, the less likely the problem can be reversed in the emergency department. Sudden onset usually reflects a structural, infectious, or acute ischemic cause.

3. *Are there associated symptoms?* Specifically, the physician should inquire about the presence of chest pain, cough, fever, sputum, hemoptysis, orthopnea, PND, and DOE. Each may point to a different etiology or a combined disorder.

4. *What medications are taken?* Knowing what medications a patient takes will often tell almost as much about his medical history as reading the old chart.

5. *What therapy has worked in the past?* Many patients know how they have responded to treatment given during previous exacerbations of their illness.

6. What is the *past medical history?* As with any other presenting complaint, it is essential that a complete past medical history be obtained.

Physical Examination

A more detailed examination is performed after initial treatment and stabilization are completed.

Vital Signs

Blood Pressure. The blood pressure is frequently elevated in patients with bronchospasm and CHF. Treatment usually reduces the blood pressure to a normal level. The presence of hypotension leads the physician to the most serious diagnoses of tension pneumothorax, cardiogenic shock, or volume depletion.

Pulse. Virtually all patients with significant dyspnea are tachycardic unless they are taking a beta-blocking agent. The slowing of the pulse to the 80 to 100 beats/min range can be followed as a *rough* gauge of the response to therapy, even when sympathomimetic agents are used.

Respiratory Rate and Pattern. The respiratory rate is a useful measure of the patient's distress and response to treatment. The normal adult should have a respiratory rate of between 14 and 18 breaths per minute or less at rest, although the accurate rate may be difficult to measure. Preferably the respirations are measured for at least 1 minute. Patients with a rate of more than 40 are likely to require mechanical ventilation. A rate of less than 14 in the dyspneic patient may be a sign of respiratory fatigue. (Further discussion and the indications for intubation and mechanical ventilatory support for the dyspneic patient in respiratory distress are contained in Chapter 56.) The respiratory pattern is occasionally useful. Deep inspiratory–expiratory respirations, usually with "air hunger," are consistent with a diagnosis of metabolic acidosis. Patients with upper airway obstruction have difficulty with inspiration, and those with lower airway obstruction complain of expiratory problems. The patient with COPD may minimize the work of breathing by maintaining a slow steady pattern of respirations with a deep tidal volume. If compliance of the lung is decreased or chest wall movement is restricted, the patient may take rapid, short respirations. Gasping respirations following recurring spells of apnea (Cheyne-Stokes respirations) occur in patients with a low cardiac output or a cerebral insult.

Fever. The presence of fever usually points to an infectious process as the cause of the dyspnea. Patients with pulmonary embolism can have a low-grade fever. A rectal temperature is obtained because oral temperatures are unreliable in the tachypneic patient.

Pulsus Paradoxus. The pulsus paradoxus is an exaggeration of the normal physiologic fall in systolic blood pressure during inspiration. It is measured by inflating the blood pressure cuff above the systolic blood pressure and slowly deflating it until systolic sounds are heard during expiration. The cuff is further deflated until sounds are heard throughout the ventilatory cycle. The difference between the sounds first heard with expiration and those heard with inspiration is usually less than 10 mm Hg. The pulsus paradoxus is classically elevated to 20 to 30 mm Hg or greater in patients with severe asthma or cardiac tamponade. Unfortunately, the test is time-consuming, not particularly sensitive, and occurs in many patients with other cardiopulmonary disorders. It has limited usefulness in the emergency department.

General Appearance

Ability to Speak. The patient's ability to speak and the length of the sentences he uses is helpful in assessing the severity of dyspnea. Patients who complain loud and long of being "short of breath" are usually less worrisome than those who give breathless one-word answers.

Mental Status. Is the patient agitated, disoriented, or showing signs of depressed mental status? All are indicators of potential hypoxia.

Positioning. The severely dyspneic patient usually sits upright and leaning slightly forward regardless of the cause of the dyspnea. A supine position is less consistent with serious illness.

Cyanosis. There is often confusion between central and peripheral cyanosis. Peripheral cyanosis (or acrocyanosis) results from increased oxygen extraction in the peripheral capillary beds in patients with circulatory failure and vasoconstriction. This leads to the typical mottled cyanotic extremities. Central cyanosis is more apparent around the mouth and face and requires the desaturation of at least 5 gm of hemoglobin. Thus, a patient with a normal hemoglobin concentration of 15 gm/dl will develop central cyanosis at an oxygen saturation of 67%, whereas the anemic patient with a hemoglobin concentration of 10 gm/dl will not develop cyanosis until the oxygen saturation decreases to 50% or less. Both peripheral and central cyanosis are likely to be present simultaneously in the critically ill patient.

Ear, Nose, and Throat. The face is palpated for signs of sinusitis because patients with asthma can have concurrent sinus infections. The mucous membranes are examined to assess hydration. The oral cavity is inspected for dentures and other foreign bodies. The neck is inspected for the presence of JVD or tracheal deviation.

Pulmonary Examination. The patient is examined to detect use of the accessory respiratory muscles, splinting, and paradoxical chest movement. Percussion is often omitted from the examination but should be done on all patients. Hyperresonance suggests a pneumothorax, especially a tension pneumothorax. The chest is auscultated for audible stridor, inspiratory-to-expiratory ratio, wheezes, rales, rhonchi, rubs, and evidence of consolidation. Each has its own significance and may be overlooked if not sought specifically.

Cardiovascular System. The neck veins are examined for evidence of elevated central venous pressure. This finding may be unreliable in severely dyspneic patients because of wide variations in intrathoracic pressure. Patients are examined for the presence of gallops, murmurs, and rubs.

Extremities. The extremities are inspected for the presence of edema, quality of pulses, and appearance of peripheral cyanosis. The fingernails are examined for signs of clubbing.

PROBLEM 2 The physical examination of the young man with the chest pain and shortness of breath showed a blood pressure of 125/85 mm Hg, pulse 105 beats/min, and respiratory rate 32/min. Decreased breath sounds and hyperresonance on the left side were significant findings. An oxygen mask was placed and adjusted to give 4 liters/min, and an intravenous (IV) line was started with D/W 5% at a keep-open rate.

The history and physical examination are very suggestive of a spontaneous pneumothorax. However, in many patients with a simple spontaneous pneumothorax the physical findings are subtle and may be overlooked in the loud and busy emergency department. Moving the patient to a quiet room where careful percussion and auscultation can be better interpreted is often the best course in the stable patient.

DECISION PRIORITIES AND PRELIMINARY DIFFERENTIAL DIAGNOSIS

The differential diagnosis of dyspnea is extensive. Fortunately, the information gathered during the history and physical examination, combined with the patient's response to initial stabilization, can help the physician establish a preliminary differential diagnosis and a prioritized approach to management. This process is aided by answering the following questions:

1. *Is it true dyspnea? What is its precise nature?*
   The definition of "an unpleasant sensation of increased effort to breathe or 'air hunger' accompanied by objective evidence of difficult or uncomfortable breathing" must be matched to the patient's presentation. This definition helps differentiate dyspnea from hyperventilation, sighing respirations, and other forms of "breathlessness." It also helps distinguish true dyspnea from limited respirations due to thoracic pain, e.g., pleurisy or rib fracture. The nature of the unpleasant sensation is important. The feeling of being unable to move air in and out is characteristic of obstructive disease of the upper or lower airway. Dyspnea on exertion is more typical of increased lung stiffness, such as that caused by pulmonary fibrosis or infiltrate. A sense of "suffocation" is often noted by patients with congestive heart failure or weakened respiratory muscles.

2. *Is it pulmonary or nonpulmonary in origin?*
   Pulmonary causes are the most common, and true "shortness of breath" with or without exercise is often the first symptom of such causes. A history of thoracic trauma may be given. Other respiratory signs and symptoms of cough, sputum production, peripheral chest pain often accentuated by respiration, wheezing, lung consolidation, effusion, pleuristic rub, and dry rales or crackles may be noted. Signs and symptoms pointing to primary pulmonary causes of dyspnea direct the physician to a differential diagnosis based on the major anatomic elements of the respiratory tract: upper airway, bronchi and alveoli, interstitium including vasculature, thoracic cage–lung interface, and respiratory musculoskeletal structure. Table 55–1 lists the common causes of pulmonary origin dyspnea based on this anatomic approach.

   Nonpulmonary causes are primarily cardiac or miscellaneous in origin. Distinguishing between dyspnea of pulmonary and cardiac origin can be difficult in some patients. Dyspnea of cardiac origin occurs when left atrial pressure is elevated, leading to accumulation of fluid in the interstitial spaces of the lung. This pulmonary congestion leads to decreased lung compliance, increased work of breathing, reflex bronchospasm, and poor gas exchange. These patients usually have a history of cardiac disease, chest pain or discomfort, orthopnea, and paroxysmal nocturnal dyspnea. Physical examination often demonstrates signs of circulatory impairment, e.g., moist or crepitant rales, wheezes, or jugular venous distention. Patients with myocadial ischemia or infarction are frequently short of breath even if clinically evident congestive failure is not present. The mechanism for this type of dyspnea is poorly understood. The miscellaneous causes relate to central nervous system stimulation of respiration, compensatory response to acid-base disorders, decreased oxygen-carrying capacity of the blood, endocrine disorders, and a few others. The major cardiac and miscellaneous causes of dyspnea seen in the emergency department are listed in Table 55–2.

   Dyspnea of mixed origin can be a difficult diagnosis without additional testing. Most cases of dyspnea in the emergency department are approached by addressing the next question.
3. *What are the common and catastrophic causes of dyspnea to be considered in each patient?*
   Table 55–3 lists the six most important pulmonary causes with their pertinent characteristics. Table 55–4 gives the nonpulmonary causes. Prior to extensive laboratory testing, the patient's findings are divided into "most probably" pulmonary or nonpulmonary and then compared to these two tables.

TABLE 55–1. Pulmonary Causes of Dyspnea: An Anatomic Approach*

Upper airway	Interstitium, including vasculature
Foreign body	Pneumoconiosis
Epiglottitis	Pulmonary embolus
Laryngospasm, angioedema	Pulmonary fibrosis (restrictive disease)
Trauma	Thoracic cage-lung interface
Bronchi (large and small airways)	Pneumothorax
Asthma	Hemothorax
Bronchitis	Effusion
Bronchiolitis	Respiratory musculoskeletal structure
Bronchogenic carcinoma	Rib fracture
Alveoli	Flail chest
Pneumonia	Guillain-Barré syndrome
Pulmonary tuberculosis	Myasthenia gravis
Emphysema	Other muscular disorders, botulism, tetanus
Toxic inhalation, e.g., paraquat	
Pulmonary contusion	
Adult respiratory distress syndrome	

*Some processes may occur in more than one site.

TABLE 55–2. Nonpulmonary Causes of Dyspnea

Cardiac
    Acute ischemia or infarction
    Cardiac valve dysfunction
    Cardiac dysrhythmia
    Congestive heart failure
    Cardiac tamponade
Miscellaneous
    CNS stimulation—head trauma, mass lesion, cerebrovascular accident, aspirin, sepsis
    Acid-base disorder—metabolic acidosis
    Decreased O_2-carrying capacity—anemia, carbon monoxide, methemoglobinemia
    Endocrine—hyperthyroidism, pregnancy
    Psychogenic—hyperventilation syndrome

PROBLEM 1 The 57 year old man had a history consistent with an exacerbation of his pulmonary problem. Another pulmonary disorder, i.e., superimposed infection, was the likely cause. At the time of admission, a nonpulmonary, and particularly a cardiac cause, could not be ruled out. The diagnosis of cardiac disease contributing to the decompensation of pulmonary disease can be very difficult. The evaluation proceeded with the diagnosis of "probably pulmonary sources, but possible mixed picture."

PROBLEM 2 The patient's complaint was rapidly localized to a pulmonary disorder occurring anatomically at the thoracic cage–lung interface, i.e., a pneumothorax. Until it was definitively diagnosed, other possibilities were not discarded.

PROBLEM 3 A rapid assessment of the 73 year old woman revealed vital signs of 190/110 mm Hg, pulse 118 beats/min, respiratory rate 36/min. She was afebrile. She had JVD, an S_3 gallop, and bilateral wheezes and rales. She had been placed on a cardiac monitor, and a nonrebreathing mask giving 100% oxygen was applied. An intravenous line of D/W 5% was started to deliver medications. Arterial blood gas measurements, chest radiograph, and electrocardiogram were ordered.

The patient's history and physical examination are very suggestive of a nonpulmonary, probably cardiac cause. Treatment may be started with this in mind, but other pulmonary causes such as pulmonary embolus or pneumonia are not ruled out.

DIAGNOSTIC ADJUNCTS

The history and physical examination will reveal the etiology of the dyspnea in the great majority of cases. Nevertheless, diagnostic tests are frequently indicated to make or confirm the diagnosis, screen for unexpected findings, or measure the response to therapy.

Laboratory Studies

Arterial Blood Gases. Arterial blood gas analysis is performed on all severely ill patients to evaluate the adequacy of oxygenation and ventilation. The arterial blood gas measurement can be used to calculate the *alveolar-arterial (A-a) gradient*. This is a moderately useful measurement for determining the efficiency of gas exchange. It measures the difference between the P_{O_2} in the alveolus and the artery and is calculated as:

$$\text{A-a gradient} = [713 \text{ mm Hg } O_2 \times F_{IO_2}] - P_{O_2} - (1.2 \times P_{CO_2})$$

TABLE 55–3. Characteristics of Common Pulmonary Causes of Dyspnea

Specific Condition	Epidemiology	Etiology	History	Physical Findings	Useful Tests
Asthma	Common in children and young adults with decreasing incidence with advancing age. Patients with adult onset usually have a worse prognosis. Frequently there is a family history of asthma	Caused by a reduction in small airway diameter. Edema, mucosal inflammation, and mucous secretion. May be related to allergic, infectious, occupational, emotional, or exercise-related causes	Most patients have a history of previous attacks. Precipitating factors usually present. The onset of wheezing is variable. Chest pain, sputum production, or fever may be present	Usually tachycardia and tachypnea. Wheezing usually present but may be absent in severe asthma. I:E ratio may be increased. Cyanosis and marked retractions are signs of severe pain	Spirometry useful for assessing severity and response to therapy. Chest radiograph and blood gas measurement may be helpful
Emphysema	Significant disease is almost always associated with tobacco use; rarely alpha-l-antitrypsin deficiency exists. Increasing incidence with advancing age. More common in men	Defined on a pathologic basis as an abnormal, permanent enlargement of the air spaces distal to the terminal bronchioles, accompanied by destruction of their walls. This is present to some extent in most people over 50 years but is much more common and severe in tobacco users	History of previous episodes of dyspnea. Most patients have smoking history	Barrel chest. Wheezes or decreased breath sounds may be present	Blood gas measurement, chest radiograph. Blood gas: Low Po_2, Normal or high Pco_2
Chronic bronchitis	Defined as daily productive cough for >3 months of the year. Seen almost exclusively in smokers, although occupational and environmental factors may play a role. More common with advancing age. Men outnumber women	Defined clinically as a chronic condition of excess mucus secretion in the bronchial tree from hyperplasia and hypertrophy of the mucus-secreting goblet cells in the large airways. Chronic hypoxemia and hypercapnia from poor ventilation lead to polycythemia, pulmonary hypertension, and cor pulmonale. Many patients have underlying viral or bacterial infections. Many have concomitant emphysema	History of dyspnea and smoking. Copious sputum production	Often cyanotic and cachectic. Wheezes, rales, and decreased breath sounds are present	Blood gas measurements, chest radiograph, sputum Gram stain. Blood gas: low Po_2, high Pco_2, low pH in acute phase

TABLE 55–3. Characteristics of Common Pulmonary Causes of Dyspnea *Continued*

Specific Condition	Epidemiology	Etiology	History	Physical Findings	Useful Tests
Pneumonia	Seen in all age groups but more dangerous in the very young and very old. Seen more frequently in alcoholics, diabetics, and patients with immunodeficiency syndromes	Causative organism varies with age and underlying medical condition. Enteric organisms and *Listeria* are more common in neonates. Viral and mycoplasma pneumonias are more commonly found in children and young adults. *Pneumococcus* is the most common cause of community-acquired bacterial pneumonia. Enteric organisms, *Hemophilus influenzae*, *Klebsiella*, and staphylococci cause pneumonia in alcoholics and debilitated patients. *Pneumocystis carinii* is common in AIDS patients	Fever, variable degree of toxicity. Cough, sputum production or hemoptysis	Fever, variable degree of toxicity. Tachypnea and tachycardia	Blood gas analysis, chest radiograph, sputum Gram stain, complete blood count
Pneumothorax	Typically occurs in patients with underlying lung disease such as asthma, chronic obstructive pulmonary disease, or malignancies. May occur in otherwise healthy people, particularly thin young males	Results from the spontaneous rupture of a pulmonary or subpleural bleb into the pleural space	Sudden onset of dyspnea and sharp pleuritic chest pain. May have history of trauma, heavy exertion or previous pneumothorax	Unilateral decreased breath sounds. Tracheal deviation, JVD, and hypotension occur with tension	Upright chest radiograph; may need expiratory view if pneumothorax is small
Pulmonary embolus	Probably occurs much more commonly than suspected, particularly in hospitalized patients. Incidence increases with advancing age, recent surgery, malignancies, prolonged immobilization, and pregnancy	Greater than ninety-five percent of emboli arise from the deep veins of the pelvis and legs. Large emboli lodge in proximal pulmonary artery and cause hypotension and shock. Smaller emboli lodge more distally and lead to dyspnea, pleuritic pain, and hypoxia	Usually sudden onset of dyspnea (85%) with sharp pleuritic chest pain (75% of patients). Hemoptysis (30%), cough (50%), and anxiety (60%) are common. Risk factors are usually present. Syncope is a rare but important presentation (10%)	Tachycardia (40%), tachypnea (90% have >16/min), cyanosis (20%), increased pulmonic valve closure (50%), increased temperature (40%)	Chest radiograph, blood gas analysis (85–90% with P_{O_2} <80 mm Hg), ventilation-perfusion scan, pulmonary angiograph

I:E ratio = inspiratory-expiratory ratio; JVD = jugular venous distention.

TABLE 55–4. Characteristics of Common Nonpulmonary Causes of Dyspnea

Specific Condition	Epidemiology	Etiology	History	Physical Findings	Useful Tests
Congestive heart failure	Incidence increases dramatically with advancing age. Most patients have a known history of cardiac disease or significant risk factors	Left ventricular dysfunction leads to elevated venous pressure and resultant fluid collection in the lung parenchyma. Common causes of heart failure include myocardial ischemia, tachydysrhythmias, increased sodium intake, and noncompliance with diuretic therapy	Variable onset of symptoms. Cough orthopnea, PND, and chest pain are common. Risk factors for heart disease	Rales, wheezes, JVD, gallop rhythm, peripheral edema. Often extremely diaphoretic	Chest radiograph, blood gas, ECG
Myocardial ischemia/infarction	The leading cause of death in most industrialized countries. Occurs at a younger age in men, but the difference evens out with advancing age. Risk factors include tobacco use, hypertension, diabetes, unfavorable lipid profile, and a positive family history	Usually caused by the gradual development of fixed atherosclerotic lesions in the coronary circulation leading to an imbalance between myocardial oxygen supply and demand. Arterial spasm may play a role in some patients	May have chest or epigastric pain, nausea, emesis, diaphoresis. Risk factors include diabetes, hypertension, tobacco, hyperlipidemia, family history	Usually normal; may be diaphoretic and have apprehensive appearance. May have gallop rhythm, new murmur, or signs of CHF	ECG, cardiac enzymes, chest radiograph
Decreased oxygen-carrying capacity	Any age, trauma victim, severe anemia, toxic exposure	Either absolute loss of hemoglobin from blood loss, or functional loss from binding with toxins, e.g., carbon monoxide, or changing structure, e.g., methemoglobinemia	Patients may have source of blood loss or other exposure. Dyspnea may be presenting complaint with toxin such as carbon monoxide. Associated weakness, fatigue	Pallor, cyanosis, source of blood loss	Complete blood count, clotting studies, carboxyhemoglobin, direct viewing of "brown blood" in methemoglobinemia. Arterial blood gas measurements are less useful since they measure dissolved O_2 in serum
Acid-base disorders	Any age at particular risk, diabetics, alcoholics	Some diseases, e.g., diabetic ketoacidosis, lactic acidosis, seem more common than others	Patient aware of "deep" breaths, not always "air hunger." Associated disorder, e.g., diabetes, aspirin ingestion, methanol ingestion	May have findings of underlying disease. Nonspecific for dyspnea	Arterial blood gas, serum bicarbonate, serum potassium
Hyperventilation syndrome	Most common in adolescent and young adults. Patients frequently have history of anxiety-related disorders in past	Often provoked by environmental or personal factors, but these are frequently not obvious to the patient or physician	History of previous stress-related attacks. Frequently complaints or circumoral and extremity paresthesias	Normal except for tachypnea and frequent sighing	Blood gas: high P_{O_2}, low P_{CO_2}, high pH

PND = paroxysmal nocturnal dyspnea; JVD = jugular venous distention.

The normal range of the A-a gradient in persons without lung disease is 5 to 20 mm Hg. Hypoxemia due to any cause except alveolar hypoventilation (narcotic overdose, neurogenic apnea, etc.) will increase this gradient.

Complete Blood Count and Differential. In the majority of patients the CBC is measured to assess the level of hemoglobin and the white blood cell count and differential to suggest or support the diagnosis of infection or inflammation.

Serum Bicarbonate Concentration. Serum bicarbonate is included as part of the electrolyte measurements if the acid-base status of the patient is suspected to be abnormal.

Gram Stain of Sputum. The sputum Gram stain is the most useful diagnostic modality for determining the presumptive etiology of a pneumonia. Acceptable specimens have 25 or more leukocytes per low-power field ($100\times$) with few squamous cells. Acceptable specimens are sent for culture.

Radiologic Imaging

Chest Radiographs. Posteroanterior and lateral views of the chest are the most important tests in the evaluation of the acutely dyspneic patient. Table 55–5 describes the radiographic findings of common causes of dyspnea. A portable anteroposterior view is obtained in any patient who is too uncomfortable or clinically unstable to be transported to the Radiology Department.

Ventilation/Perfusion (V/Q) Scanning. This minimally invasive procedure is considered when a pulmonary embolus is suspected. It involves three steps. The perfusion scan is first performed after the injection of radiolabeled albumin. A completely normal scan will rule out a diagnosis of pulmonary embolus. If the perfusion scan is abnormal, the next step is to review the patient's chest radiograph. If the perfusion defect corresponds with an abnormality on the chest film, the scan is considered indeterminate. Third, if a perfusion defect corresponds with an area of the lung that is normal on the chest radiograph, a ventilation scan is performed. The patient inhales a radioactive inert gas, and areas of decreased ventilation are then noted. The V/Q scan is considered high probability for a pulmonary embolus when perfusion defects correspond with areas of normal ventilation. A normal V/Q scan has a sensitivity of 99% and essentially rules out a pulmonary embolism.

Pulmonary Arteriography. Although V/Q scanning is often helpful in diagnosing or excluding pulmonary embolus, the "gold standard" for the diagnosis remains pulmonary arteriography. Ideally, it is performed within 24 to 48 hours of the embolic episode. Arteriography should be performed in patients when doubt exists about the diagnosis, particularly in patients with risk factors for anticoagulation.

TABLE 55–5. Radiographic Findings in Common Causes of Dyspnea

Condition	Chest Radiograph Findings
Asthma/emphysema	Usually normal, may show hyperinflation, fibrotic changes, peribroncheolar cuffing, or bullous disease
Pneumonia	Lobar or alveolar infiltrates
Pulmonary embolism	Nonspecific, may be normal. Atelectasis, infiltrates, effusion, Hampton's hump
Pneumothorax	Lung collapse, mediastinal shift, subcutaneous emphysema. Inspiratory-expiratory films may benefit the diagnosis
Noncardiogenic pulmonary edema (adult respiratory distress syndrome)	May be normal early. Later cardiogenic pulmonary edema pattern may be present without cardiomegaly
Cardiogenic pulmonary edema	Venous engorgement and redistribution, bilateral alveolar edema, Kerley's B lines. May see left ventricular enlargement

Electrocardiography

An electrocardiogram (ECG) is obtained in all critically ill patients and in any patient in whom there is a possibility of primary cardiac disease or arrhythmia.

Other Tests

Pulse Oximetry. Newer techniques involving continuous noninvasive monitoring of oxygen saturation are beginning to play an increasing role in patients with respiratory disorders. Pulse oximetry has been found to be particularly useful for following the oxygen saturation of blood in critically ill patients. The sensing unit is applied to the finger, and measurements are made by light-activated sensors. This technique correlates well with arterial blood gas measurements. It is less useful if there is significant vasoconstriction of the extremity, such as occurs in patients in shock.

Pulmonary Function Testing. Simple bedside spirometry (PEFR, FEV_1) can be used to assess the severity of dyspnea and to follow the patient's response to therapy. These tests are most used in asthmatics but can be part of the assessment of patients with any pulmonary disorder.

PROBLEM 2 The chest radiograph revealed a 50% pneumothorax on the left side. The mediastinal structures were in their normal position, indicating that tension was not present.

Occasionally there is a high suspicion of pneumothorax, but the routine inspiratory film does not reveal any collapse. An expiratory view, by reducing the chest cavity-to-lung volume ratio and the contrast between the lung parenchyma and air, may uncover the presence of a small pneumothorax.

PROBLEM 3 An electrocardiogram (ECG) was obtained, revealing an ST-depression in the precordial leads suggestive of myocardial ischemia. The chest radiograph was consistent with a diagnosis of congestive heart failure. Myocardial ischemia or infarction is a frequent cause of acute congestive heart failure.

The presence of tachydysrhythmias (atrial fibrillation, supraventricular tachycardia [SVT], ventricular tachycardia) may also lead to CHF owing to increased myocardial oxygen demand combined with impaired ventricular and coronary artery filling.

PRINCIPLES OF MANAGEMENT

The key to managing the patient with dyspnea of any cause is delivery of adequate oxygenation. Other principles include the relief of bronchospasm, elimination of edema, and treatment of infection. Each is applied as appropriate in managing the most common causes of dyspnea, listed below.

Asthma or COPD

Oxygen. Carbon dioxide retention is a concern in COPD. A venti-mask is used preferably with a controlled oxygen percentage. If this is not available, oxygen administration is begun with 1 to 2 liters/min, monitoring response. Patients become lethargic as PCO_2 rises from loss of hypoxia drive. This is rarely a problem in asthmatics.

Beta-Adrenergic Sympathomimetic Agents. Sympathomimetics, preferably in the inhaled form, have become the mainstay of therapy for patients with acute asthma (see Chap. 56).

Theophylline. The use of theophylline is not felt to be useful in acutely ill asthmatics, but it continues to be given nevertheless (see Chap. 56). It is a commonly used treatment in patients with decompensated COPD. Patients who are not taking an oral form are given a loading dose of 5 to 6 mg/kg and started on a maintenance infusion of 0.5 mg/kg/hr based on the ideal body weight. Young patients and smokers usually require a higher maintenance dose, whereas the presence of CHF or liver disease necessitates a reduction in the dose.

Corticosteroids. The early use of corticosteroids often aids the responsiveness of asthmatics and COPD patients to other medications. They are given to patients already taking them who have respiratory decompensation as well as to patients who are not responding to beta-adrenergic and aminophylline therapy. The initial dose is usually given as methylprednisolone, 40 to 60 mg, for the average adult.

Pneumonia

Oxygen. Oxygen is given directed by blood gas analysis results.

Antimicrobial Therapy. Antimicrobial therapy is directed by Gram stain analysis and the clinical setting. Penicillin, ampicillin, and erythromycin are all reasonable choices for outpatient management of community-acquired pneumonia in otherwise healthy individuals. Patients with underlying disorders (diabetes, alcoholism, emphysema, etc.) are admitted to the hospital for intravenous antibiotics. Though their efficacy is not well documented, antibiotics are often prescribed for exacerbations of COPD.

Bronchospasm Therapy. Bronchospasm, if present, is treated as listed under Asthma or COPD.

Spontaneous Pneumothorax

Patients with a tension pneumothorax require a tube thoracostomy as described below. Needle decompression can be done as a temporizing measure while the necessary equipment is being set up. A 14- or 16-gauge needle is inserted at the second intercostal space at the midclavicular line for temporary relief. Patients with a simple pneumothorax can be treated in a variety of ways depending on the experience of the treating physician.

Observation Alone. Small pneumothoraces (less than 20%) in healthy, minimally symptomatic patients can be treated in the hospital with close observation and frequent chest x-rays.

Needle or Catheter Aspiration. Aspiration of air with a needle or 16-gauge catheter connected to a three-way stopcock has been successfully used in patients with spontaneous and traumatic pneumothoraces. Patients with no air leak at 6 hours are discharged from the emergency department, and a follow-up visit is scheduled for the next day.

Tube Thoracostomy. Placement of a chest tube has remained the standard of care for patients with a large (over 20%) pneumothorax or tension pneumothorax. A 22- to 28-French tube is placed in the fifth intercostal space at the mid to anterior axillary line under local anesthesia. This procedure is supplemented with an intravenous narcotic. The tube is connected to suction at 20 cm of water. A chest radiograph is obtained to confirm reexpansion and placement.

Pulmonary Embolus

Oxygen. Oxygen is given according to the results of blood gas analysis.

Anticoagulation. Heparin is started if there is no contraindication with a bolus of 5000 to 10,000 units intravenously followed by an infusion of 1000 units/hr. The rate of the infusion is adjusted according to the partial thromboplastin time.

Thrombolytic Therapy. Thrombolytic therapy with streptokinase, urokinase, or tissue plasminogen activator may be considered in patients with massive pulmonary embolus. This is usually reserved for patients with hemodynamic instability and severe hypoxia.

Vena Cava Interruption. Patients with contraindications to anticoagulation and those with recurrent emboli despite adequate anticoagulation are candidates for vena cava interruption with a Greenfield filter.

Congestive Heart Failure

Oxygen. High-flow oxygen is given to all patients.

Diuretics. Diuretics such as furosemide have a dual action in patients with CHF. Within minutes there is a preload reduction due to an increase in venous capacitance. Second, the renal diuretic effect begins within 20 minutes. The usual starting dose is 20 to 40 mg intravenously. Patients with renal insufficiency and those on chronic diuretic therapy may need higher doses.

Nitrates. Preload and some afterload reduction with nitrates will often lead to prompt improvement in the patient's clinical status. Sublingual nitroglycerin 0.4 mg has an onset of action within 30 seconds and is usually well tolerated. This dose is repeated every 5 minutes for a total of three doses. An intravenous infusion is also useful, particularly in hypertensive patients and those with myocardial ischemia.

Morphine Sulfate. Intravenous morphine sulfate 2 to 4 mg IV reduces venous return (preload) and also acts as an analgesic and anxiolytic. It may be repeated every 5 to 10 minutes as necessary and as tolerated. Its atropinelike action may cause first- or second-degree heart block in susceptible patients.

Bronchodilators. Patients with reflex bronchospasm will benefit from inhaled beta agonists and intravenous aminophylline.

Inotropic Agents. Inotropic agents are occasionally required as second level agents in patients not responding to other agents. Dobutamine, a beta-1 agonist, is considered the drug of choice for treatment of CHF in normotensive patients. Dobutamine has a potent inotropic effect without causing peripheral vasoconstriction and is usually well tolerated. Dopamine is preferred in the presence of shock because of its constricting effect on the peripheral vasculature. Amrinone, an agent with inotropic and vasodilatory effects, has been shown to improve the hemodynamic status in patients with cardiogenic pulmonary edema.

Blood Pressure Control. Many patients with pulmonary edema have a severely elevated blood pressure. Control of pressure is important to reduce the myocardial oxygen demand. Many will experience a rapid reduction in pressure with nitrates, furosemide, and morphine therapy. Patients with refractory hypertension (diastolic pressure of more than 120 mm Hg) should be started on a nitroprusside drip to reduce the blood pressure. Recent reports suggest that sublingual nifedipine may also be effective in reducing blood pressure rapidly in this setting.

Hyperventilation Syndrome

Diagnosis. Though it may be readily apparent, it is important to consider other causes of dyspnea, particularly pulmonary embolus and myocardial ischemia. An arterial blood gas analysis will confirm the presence of a significant respiratory alkalosis and normal oxygenation.

Rebreather. The use of a paper bag "rebreather" is to be discouraged because it may lead to significant hypoxia.

Reassurance. Reassurance is of the utmost importance. These events are common, and patients should never be led to think that they are crazy or wasting the physician's time.

Medication. Discharge with a mild anxiolytic, e.g., Vistaril 25 mg up to four times a day for 1 to 2 days, is often reassuring and beneficial to the patient.

Dyspnea of Unknown Cause

If the diagnosis, or even division into pulmonary versus nonpulmonary cause remains unclear, the extent of the assessment depends on the general condition of the patient. The respiratory rate, breath sounds, and presence of underlying medical problems are reviewed in a second round of data gathering. The minimum laboratory tests include an arterial blood gas analysis and a chest radiograph to exclude hypoxemia and significant pulmonary pathology. Other studies are performed as indicated by the clinical situation.

PROBLEM 2 Because of the size of this pneumothorax the decision was made to place a chest tube. Informed consent was obtained, and the patient was prepared and draped under strict sterile technique (gown, gloves, mask). A small-bore chest tube was placed through the fifth intercostal space at the midaxillary line by means of blunt dissection. Prior to the procedure the patient was given adequate amounts of a narcotic and benzodiazepine for sedation. A portable chest film confirmed tube placement and reexpansion of the lung.

PROBLEM 3 With the diagnosis of congestive heart failure secure, specific therapy was started. Because of her cardiac ischemia and hypertension the patient was placed on a nitroglycerin drip for preload reduction. She was also given morphine sulfate 2 mg while the IV nitroglycerine infusion was being prepared. A Foley catheter was inserted, and furosemide 40 mg IV was administered. Within 20 minutes she felt considerably better.

SPECIAL CONSIDERATIONS

Pediatric Patients

A wide variety of disorders cause dyspnea in the pediatric population including most of those affecting adults and some that are unique to children (see Chap. 37). Common causes of shortness of breath in children include

Upper Airway
Foreign body aspiration
Epiglottitis
Croup
Retropharyngeal abscess

Lower Airway
Foreign body aspiration
Asthma
Cystic fibrosis
Bronchopulmonary dysplasia
Pneumonia
Bronchiolitis
Anaphylaxis

Dyspnea in children seldom resembles its manifestations in adults. It is usually brought to medical attention because of fever, cough, or generalized illness. An accurate respiratory rate is essential. The normal range in children varies with age.

Pregnancy

Compensatory changes in respiratory physiology (increased oxygen consumption, decreased functional residual capacity, increased minute ventilation) frequently lead to the complaint of dyspnea in the latter stages of pregnancy. In addition, the pregnant patient has an increased risk of pulmonary complications. The most commonly seen problems are pulmonary embolus, dyspnea in asthmatics, and pulmonary edema.

Pulmonary embolus. There is an increased incidence of pulmonary embolism during pregnancy related to compression of the vena cava by the uterus. Treatment is with heparin until the time of delivery because warfarin (Coumadin) is contraindicated during pregnancy.

Asthma. Asthma becomes worse in about one-third of patients during pregnancy, one-third improve, and one-third have no change in symptoms. Treatment is essentially the same as for the nonpregnant patient. (See Chap. 56.)

Pulmonary Edema. Pulmonary edema, related to either preeclampsia or cardiomyopathy, occasionally occurs in the peripartum period.

DISPOSITION AND FOLLOW-UP

The disposition of the dyspneic patient will depend on the cause of the dyspnea and the response to therapy in the emergency department. Suggestions for admission and follow-up for patients with common causes of dyspnea are described below.

Asthma and COPD. Most patients with a bronchospastic component to their disease improve with treatment and can be discharged home with close follow-up with their personal physician. General criteria for admission include:
1. Presence of pneumonia or pneumothorax.
2. Mental status change.
3. Failure of hypercarbia or acidosis to resolve with treatment.
4. Minimal improvement in PEFR or FEV_1 after treatment.
5. No subjective improvement after 4 to 6 hours of treatment.

Pneumonia. "Nontoxic" appearing patients who are otherwise healthy can be discharged on oral antibiotics with follow-up in 24 to 48 hours. Patients with risk factors such as age (very young and very old), significant tachypnea, multilobar involvement, preexisting lung disease, Po_2 less than 60 mm Hg, diabetes, alcoholism, sickle cell anemia, and those with emesis are admitted for intravenous therapy.

Pulmonary Embolus. All patients with confirmed or suspected pulmonary emboli are admitted. Most can be placed in a regular ward if they are hemodynamically stable.

Pneumothorax. A select group may be discharged if there is no reaccumulation of air after catheter aspiration. Otherwise, these patients are admitted.

Pulmonary Edema. Most of these patients are admitted to the intensive care unit. Many will require invasive monitoring, complicated pharmacologic therapy, and a "rule out myocardial infarction" protocol.

Myocardial Infarction. All are admitted to an intensive care unit for cardiac monitoring, serial ECGs, and cardiac enzyme analysis. These patients are at high risk for dysrhythmias, valvular complications, CHF, and hypotension.

Hyperventilation Syndrome. Symptoms usually resolve after a short period of observation in the emergency department and after appropriate reassurance has been given. These patients are then discharged home if other causes of dyspnea have been adequately ruled out. Patients are referred to a primary care physician for a follow-up visit.

Dyspnea of Unknown Cause. Patients with complaints of dyspnea and no identifiable reason for the complaint pose a challenge for the physician. These patients often have underlying pulmonary pathology but appear to be at baseline at presentation to the emergency department. If the patient appears well, has a normal or baseline Po_2, has a normal chest radiograph, and does not have significant medical problems (diabetes, cardiac disease, and so on), they can be discharged home with a follow-up appointment scheduled for the next day. Other patients are admitted to the hospital.

PROBLEM 2 The patient with the pneumothorax was admitted, and the chest tube was placed on water seal. No air leak was noted, and the chest tube was removed in 24 hours. Follow-up radiographs were normal. He was discharged with a warning that he was at high risk for a recurrent pneumothorax.

PROBLEM 3 The woman with congestive heart failure was admitted to a critical care unit for further stabilization and monitoring for a possible myocardial infarction.

DOCUMENTATION

1. Onset and severity of dyspnea.
2. Associated symptoms and past medical history.
3. List of medications being taken and any allergies present.
4. Vital signs before and after intervention.
5. Chest and cardiac examination results.
6. Interpretation of chest radiograph, ECGs, and arterial blood gas measurements.
7. Response to therapy.
8. Diagnosis and reason for reaching that diagnosis.

SUMMARY AND FINAL POINTS

- Dyspnea is one of the most common complaints in people presenting to the emergency department.
- Although the sensation of dyspnea is poorly understood, the amount of dyspnea usually correlates with the severity of the causative illness.
- The complaint of dyspnea represents a high potential for significant morbidity and should never be taken lightly by the physician.
- The respiratory rate is one of the most sensitive indicators of respiratory distress.
- The chest radiograph is the most important diagnostic test for evaluating the dyspneic patient.
- The diagnosis of dyspnea can be divided into pulmonary and nonpulmonary causes. Pulmonary causes may be explored anatomically. Nonpulmonary causes include primary cardiac disorders, acid-base disorders, central nervous system problems, and deficiencies in oxygen-carrying capacity of hemoglobin.
- Although the treatment of dyspnea should be directed at the specific cause, oxygen remains the mainstay of management in the acute phase.

BIBLIOGRAPHY

Texts

1. Murphy C: Acute dyspnea. In Callaham ML (ed): Current Therapy in Emergency Medicine. Philadelphia, BC Decker, 1987, pp. 337–342.
2. Smith PL, Bleecker ER: Common pulmonary problems: Cough hemoptysis, dyspnea, and chest pain. In Barker LR, BurtonJR, Zieve PD (eds): Principles of Ambulatory Medicine (2nd ed). Baltimore, Williams & Wilkins, 1986, pp. 617–628.

Journal Articles

1. Bennett DA, Bleck TP: Recognizing impending respiratory failure from neuromuscular causes. J. Crit Illness 3:46–60, 1988.
2. Burki NK: Dyspnea. Lung 165:269–277, 1987.
3. Cherniack NS, Altose MD: Mechanisms of dyspnea. Clin Chest Med, 8:207–214, 1987.
4. Fulmer JD, Snider GL: American College of Chest Physicians—National Heart, Lung, and Blood Institute Conference on oxygen therapy. Arch Intern Med, 144:1645–1655, 1984.
5. Littenberg B, Gluck EH: A controlled trial of methylprednisolone in the emergency treatment of acute asthma. N. Engl J Med 314:150–152, 1986.
6. Mahler DA: Dyspnea: Diagnosis and management. Clin Chest Med 8:215–230, 1987.
7. McDonald AJ: Adult respiratory emergencies. Emerg Med Clin North Am 7(2):187–430, 1989.
8. Nowak RM, Tomlanovich MC, Sarkar DD, et al: Arterial blood gases and pulmonary function testing in acute bronchial asthma: Predicting patient outcomes. JAMA 249:2043–2046, 1983.
9. Valenzuela TD: Pulmonary embolism. Ann Emerg Med 17:209–213, 1988.

CHAPTER 56

WHEEZING

ROBERT L. NORRIS, M.D.

PROBLEM The mother of an 18-year-old girl called 911 because her daughter was "wheezing and can't catch her breath." The mother was very agitated, begged for immediate help, and could give no more information to the dispatcher.

QUESTIONS TO CONSIDER

1. Which diseases other than asthma can present with the sign of wheezing?
2. Which historical points and physical findings are useful in differentiating the causes of wheezing?
3. How is the diagnosis of asthma made in the emergency department?
4. What physical findings best assess the severity of lower airway obstruction?
5. What roles do arterial blood gas measurements and pulmonary function tests serve in evaluating the patient with wheezing?
6. What therapies are available for the patient with wheezing from lower airway obstruction?
7. When is endotracheal intubation necessary in the wheezing patient?
8. What criteria are appropriate for considering discharge in the patient who presents with wheezing?

INTRODUCTION

A wheeze (sibilant rhoncus) is a continuous, musical sound produced by vibration as air moves past a resistance or partial obstruction in the lower respiratory tract. It is a common finding in patients presenting to the emergency department with shortness of breath or cough. There are numerous causes of wheezing that are important to consider in patients with no prior history of obstructive airway disease (Table 56–1). Many of these causes are discussed in other chapters (Chapters 37 and 55). Wheezing is most frequently associated with asthma and chronic obstructive pulmonary disease (COPD). These diseases are the primary focus of this chapter.

Asthma is defined by the American Thoracic Society as a disease characterized by an increased responsiveness of the trachea and bronchi to various stimuli. It is manifest by widespread airway narrowing that changes in severity either spontaneously or as a result of therapy. It affects almost 5% of the U. S. population and is responsible for more than 1 million emergency department visits annually. There are more than 130,000 hospital admissions and 2000 to 6000 deaths due to asthma in the United States each year.

The pathophysiology of asthma involves many body systems. The autonomic nervous system is important in determining bronchomuscular tone. Stimulation of beta-2 sympathetic receptors by circulating catecholamines activates adenylate cyclase, leading to an increase in intracellular cyclic adenosine monophosphate (cAMP) and bronchodilatation. Stimulating alpha-1 sympathetic receptors results in bronchoconstriction. The parasym-

TABLE 56–1. Differential Diagnosis of the Wheezing Patient (ASTHMATIC)

A—Asthma
    Asthma (extrinsic, intrinsic)
S—Stasis
    Pulmonary embolism
T—Toxins
    Toxic gases
    Smoke inhalation
    Insecticides
    Cholinergic poisonings
    Chemical irritants
H—Heart
    Congestive heart failure, pulmonary edema ("cardiac asthma")
    Noncardiogenic pulmonary edema
    Adult respiratory distress syndrome (any cause)
M—Mechanical
    Foreign body (upper airway, lower airway)
    Foreign body embolism (IV drug abuse)
A—Allergy, aspiration
    Anaphylaxis
    Laryngeal edema
    Organic particle exposure
    Extrinsic allergic alveolitis
    Aspiration of gastric contents
    Near drowning
T—Trauma, tumor
    Upper airway trauma
    Pneumothorax, tension pneumothorax
    Endobronchial tumor
I—Infection
    Bronchitis
    Pneumonia
    Bronchiolitis
    Croup, epiglottitis
    Pertussis
    Fungal diseases
C—Chronic lung disease, congenital lung disease
    Chronic obstructive pulmonary disease (emphysema, bronchitis)
    Alpha-1 antitrypsin deficiency
    Cystic fibrosis
    Congenital abnormalities of the respiratory, cardiovascular, or gastrointestinal systems
    Bronchopulmonary dysplasia

pathetic system has subepithelial irritant receptors located in the larynx and lower airways; they comprise the afferent limb of a vagus nerve reflex arc. When stimulated, these receptors cause an increase in intracellular cyclic cAMP, which causes bronchial smooth muscle constriction and increased glandular secretions. Recent theories about the pathogenesis of asthma suggest that there is both a hyporesponsiveness of beta-2 airway receptors, allowing alpha-bronchoconstrictive effects to predominate, and an increase in the number of alpha-1 receptors in asthmatic airways. There appears to be a lower firing threshold for the cholinergic irritant receptors in asthmatic airways, adding to the relative hypersensitivity ("twitchiness") of bronchial smooth muscle.

The other major pathogenetic system in asthma involves the release of various chemical mediators that act to increase airway resistance. In "extrinsic" asthma, specific extracorporeal allergens bind with IgE on mast cells lining the tracheobronchial tree, stimulating the release of various preformed mediators (e.g., eosinophilic chemotactic factor, neutrophilic chemotactic factor, and histamine), and the synthesis of others (e.g., leukotrienes, platelet-activating factors, and prostaglandins). These mediators stimulate bronchial smooth muscle constriction, mucus secretion, bronchial wall edema due to vasodilation, and interstitial influx of eosinophils and neutrophils. A similar release of chemical mediators occurs in patients with intrinsic asthma in response to intracorporeal stimuli.

These pathologic changes result in increased airway resistance, air trapping, and ventilation-perfusion mismatch. They become manifest as dyspnea and cough, and, on physical examination, as decreased air exchange and wheezing.

Chronic obstructive pulmonary disease (COPD) is a term that encompasses a spectrum of respiratory disease. Emphysema and chronic bronchitis are identifiable points on this continuum. The American Thoracic Society defines *emphysema* as an anatomic alteration characterized by an abnormal enlargement of the air spaces distal to the terminal, nonrespiratory bronchioles accompanied by destructive changes of the alveolar walls. *Chronic bronchitis* is a clinical disorder associated with excessive mucus secretion in the bronchial tree. It is characterized by a chronic or recurrent productive cough during most days of the month for a minimum of 3 months a year for not less than 2 successive years. The major predisposing factor for COPD is cigarette smoking. Other processes can lead to its development, including exposure to industrial or vegetable dusts, cystic fibrosis, and alpha-1 antitrypsin disease. Most patients with COPD have features of both emphysema and chronic bronchitis. COPD has tremendous morbidity and is responsible for almost 30,000 deaths annually in the United States. Patients with decompensated COPD are commonly seen in the emergency department.

The pathologic changes characteristic of COPD include hypertrophy and hypersecretion of mucus-secreting glands, bronchial smooth muscle hypertrophy, mucosal inflammation, and destruction and enlargement of alveoli. The end result of these changes is variably reversible airway obstruction and diminished oxygen diffusion capacity. Over time, the COPD patient usually develops carbon dioxide retention and hypoxemia. As chronic carbon dioxide retention progresses, the patient's stimulus to breathing becomes more reliant on hypoxia ("hypoxic drive") and less responsive to hypercarbia. Pulmonary hypertension and cor pulmonale are problems in patients with severe or long-standing chronic bronchitis.

PREHOSPITAL CARE

A large percentage of wheezing patients are first assessed by prehospital care personnel. The patient's condition dictates the information the physician obtains.

History

If the patient is in severe distress, the following questions are asked:

1. What is the severity of the patient's respiratory distress? Particular attention is paid to vital signs, respiratory effort, chest sounds, and level of consciousness.

2. What is the transport time from the patient's location to the emergency department? Knowledge of this time allows preparation for receiving the patient while the rescue personnel stabilize the patient during transit.

If the patient is in less distress or if transport time will be prolonged, the following additional information is obtained by the rescue squad:

1. Does the patient have a history of respiratory disease? How long has the patient been ill?

2. Are there any inciting factors discernible in the events surrounding the onset of the illness (e.g., exposure to toxic gases)?

3. Is the patient experiencing chest pain? Pneumothorax is always a consideration in patients with wheezing of acute onset.

4. What self-treatment has the patient used? Prescribed or over-the-counter medications, and inhalers are especially important.

Physical Examination

1. The level of respiratory distress is noted, e.g., skin color, level of consciousness, and ability to utter complete sentences.
2. Blood pressure and heart rate are measured.
3. Respiratory rate and use of accessory muscles are noted.
4. Breath sounds are noted, particularly if they are decreased or asymmetric.
5. Evidence of peripheral edema is sought.

Interventions

1. Oxygen is supplied at a high-flow rate, 6 to 10 liters/min by nasal cannula, for the patient in severe distress from whatever cause. Low flow oxygen is given at 2 to 4 liters/min if the patient has a history of COPD and is not in severe distress. Oxygen at 1 to 2 liters/min is reserved for the COPD patient with a known history of carbon dioxide retention.
2. Cardiac monitoring is instituted, and the patient is watched for dysrhythmias.
3. If time permits, intravenous access is established with dextrose in water 5% (D/W 5%) at a keep-open rate.
4. If the history is compatible with a diagnosis of congestive heart failure and the patient is not hypotensive, diuretics or nitroglycerin may be given after discussion with the base hospital physician.
5. If the patient is younger, subcutaneous epinephrine (0.01 mg/kg, up to 0.4 mg) can be given for bronchodilation. Older patients or those with cardiac risk factors can be safely treated with an inhaled beta-2 agonist such as metaproterenol. Intravenous theophylline is not recommended. Its efficacy during an acute attack of asthma or COPD is questionable, and it has significant risks if given intravenously in the field.

PROBLEM On arrival at the home, the rescue squad found the patient sitting upright in a chair and unable to talk owing to shortness of breath. Her mother said she was an "asthmatic" who was taking theophylline, but she often forgot to take the medication. The mother noted that the patient had been increasingly short of breath during the last 24 hours. The rescue squad obtained a blood pressure of 130/90 mm Hg, a pulse of 140 beats/min, and a respiratory rate of 30/min. She was not diaphoretic but looked pale. She was using accessory muscles to aid her breathing and had bilateral wheezing on chest examination.

At this point, the rescue squad needs to proceed rapidly and efficiently. Their transport time is estimated to be 20 minutes, and some field intervention is necessary. The patient is given 6 liters of oxygen per minute by nasal cannula, and an intravenous (IV) line of D/W 5% is started. A call is placed by radiotelemetry to the base hospital, and the emergency physician orders aerolized metaproterenol to be given.

INITIAL APPROACH IN THE EMERGENCY DEPARTMENT

If the patient is in severe distress, treatment precedes or accompanies data gathering. If the patient is in less distress, management can proceed in a more traditional sequence. All patients receive the following three interventions:

1. **Oxygen.** If the patient is in severe respiratory distress, high-flow oxygen at 8 to 10 liters/min is begun. Nasal prongs are usually used, but a Venturi or a nonrebreather mask may be used depending on patient tolerance. When there is less distress, oxygen at 2 to 4 liters/min is adequate. In COPD patients suspected of carbon dioxide retention, 1 to 2 liters/min is started and the patient is observed for hypoventilation. Sufficient

oxygen is not withheld in these patients, but the physician must be aware of the possible need for ventilatory support.

   2. **Cardiac monitoring.** Dysrhythmias are often seen in these patients. They can be caused by hypoxia, adrenergic stimulation or therapy, and underlying disease causing wheezing, e.g., myocardial infarction with secondary congestive heart failure.

   3. **Intravenous access.** An IV is placed and 5% dextrose in water is infused initially.

As the oxygen, cardiac monitor, and intravenous line are being initiated, a screening evaluation is performed.

History

   1. Does the patient have known COPD or asthma? Are there any other possible causes?
   2. What is the length of the episode?
   3. What is the patient's assessment of the severity?
   4. What are the present medications, especially the ones most recently taken?

Physical Examination

   1. What is the ability of the patient to speak, and how long are the sentences?
   2. Auscultation of the heart and lungs is performed, and the inspiratory-to-expiratory ratio of breathing is noted.
   3. The use of accessory muscles is noted.
   4. Is there jugular venous distention or peripheral edema?
   5. Is there cyanosis or diaphoresis?

Intervention

If the patient is wheezing significantly or if there is little or no air exchange, aerosolized bronchodilator therapy is begun immediately. A beta-adrenergic agonist, such as metaproterenol, is given by nebulizer or inhaler. Early pulmonary function testing is useful.

If the patient is felt to be in severe respiratory distress by clinical examination or by pulmonary function testing (see below) but not in immediate need of intubation, arterial blood gas measurements and a portable chest radiograph are obtained.

In patients with asthma, intubation and assisted ventilation are required only in 0.3% of patients. Absolute indications for immediate intubation of the wheezing patient are apnea and coma. Intubation is considered if:

   1. PO_2 is less than 50 mm Hg (with supplemental oxygen).
   2. PCO_2 is greater than 50 mm Hg with acute respiratory acidosis.
   3. PCO_2 is increasing despite maximal therapy.
   4. Patient is fatigued.
   5. Mental status is depressed.

Prior to intubation every attempt is made to reverse the bronchoconstriction with aerosolized beta-adrenergic agonists, theophylline in appropriate doses, and corticosteroids.

Orotracheal intubation is used in emergent situations. A large-bore tube is placed to aid pulmonary toilet. The nasotracheal route is better tolerated in the awake patient. Intubation is not without risks. Stimulating the pharynx, larynx, or tracheal mucous membranes with the laryngoscope or endotracheal tube may precipitate vagally induced apnea, laryngospasm, dysrhythmia, or worsening of bronchospasm.

Assisted ventilation is supplied with a volume-cycled respirator. Initial settings are inspiratory-to-expiratory ratio at 1:3 allowing for a prolonged expiratory phase, tidal volume at 10 to 12 ml/kg with 10 to 12 breaths/min, and FIO_2 set to maintain adequate tissue oxygenation. If the patient is not tolerating assisted ventilation, a long-acting intravenous paralyzing agent, e.g., pancuronium bromide, is used in combination with sedation. The risk of pneumothorax is significant in these patients. Close monitoring with serial examination and arterial blood gas measurements is necessary. Initial hypercapnia is not rapidly corrected because respiratory alkalosis can result. This increases the risk of dysrhythmia, seizures, or increased bronchospasm.

Often the wheezing associated with congestive heart failure cannot be distinguished from that of COPD and rales may be absent or scarce. A portable chest radiograph can usually resolve the issue. If not, treatment for both entities often proceeds simultaneously.

PROBLEM The rescue squad alerted the emergency department staff that the patient was in serious distress. A monitored bed and resuscitation equipment were prepared in advance. Assistance was requested from respiratory therapy. On arrival, the patient was in severe respiratory distress. She could speak only two or three words at a time, preferred to remain upright, and continued to use accessory breathing muscles. She was alert but tired. Her vital signs were 150/100 mm Hg, heart rate 140 beats/min, respiratory rate 40/min as reported by the rescue squad. Her expiratory-to-inspiratory ratio was markedly prolonged, and poorly audible wheezing was auscultated bilaterally. A peak expiratory flow rate (PEFR) was found to be 90 liters/min. The rescue squad thought that she had improved slightly after she inhaled metaproterenol. The oxygen and intravenous lines were transferred and were set at 6 to 8 liters/min and 150 cc/hr, respectively.

The most important decision to be made is whether endotracheal intubation and ventilating support are necessary. The patient is young. Although she is in severe respiratory distress, she is not apneic or somnolent. She continues to use her accessory muscles and makes a respiratory effort. Her PEFR is borderline between severe and moderate airway obstruction. She does not require immediate endotracheal intubation in this situation. Another metaproterenol treatment by aerosolized nebulizer, a portable chest radiograph, and a theophylline level are ordered. The latter is particularly important because of her history of noncompliance. Because of the severity of her condition, arterial blood gas analysis is included in the orders.

DATA GATHERING

The goal of data gathering is to confirm the origin of wheezing and to better assess the severity of the episode.

History

The history is extremely important in directing diagnosis and management of the wheezing patient. In patients with known asthma or COPD, an important goal is to detect disorders exacerbating or complicating these diseases. Important factors in the history of a wheezing asthmatic or COPD patient include:

1. The *time of onset* and *duration of symptoms*—the longer the symptoms have lasted, the more likely is the need for admission. Sudden onset may suggest aeroallergens, inhaled foreign body, acute congestive heart failure, or spontaneous pneumothorax.

2. *Events that preceded the symptoms*, e.g., exposure to allergens, preceding respiratory infections, situational stress.

3. *Elements* of this episode that are *atypical relative to previous episodes*. Is there chest pain, a productive cough or fever and chills? Ischemic heart disease, pneumothorax, and pulmonary infection are always considered in the acutely wheezing patient.

4. *Medications* the patient is taking and *level of compliance*. Data are obtained about the amount and most recent dosage of beta-adrenergic agonists, theophylline, and corticosteroids.

5. *Self-treatment* used by the patient *since* he or she became *ill*. Specifically, inhaler and over-the-counter medication use are discussed.

6. *Severity of the patient's underlying COPD or asthma*. Has hospitalization (especially ICU admission) or endotracheal intubation occurred in the past? Are corticosteroids given as part of care?

7. *Patient's assessment* of the *severity* of this episode *relative* to *prior episodes*. Patients are often the best judges of the severity of their attacks and their progress during acute intervention.

8. What is the *past medical history*—cardiopulmonary disease, hypertension, or diabetes; smoking history?

In a patient without a prior history of asthma or COPD, the history is aimed at ruling out other causes of wheezing. All of the points above are ascertained, and other questions are asked:

1. Is there *recent-onset dyspnea on exertion, orthopnea*, or *paroxysmal nocturnal dyspnea*?
2. Is there *recent weight gain* or *peripheral edema*?
3. What *nonpulmonary medications* have been taken, e.g., especially beta-adrenergic blocking agents?
4. Has there been *possible toxic gas exposure*?
5. Is there a *possibility* of *foreign body aspiration*, especially in children?

Physical Examination

Ominous findings consistent with severe bronchospasm and pulmonary insufficiency are sought immediately:

1. Excessive use of accessory muscles of respiration
2. Diaphoresis
3. Altered mental status and fatigue
4. The need to sit upright to breathe
5. An inability to speak
6. Presence of central cyanosis

In the wheezing patient who is less severely ill, the physical examination centers on:

Vital Signs. Vital signs generally have limited usefulness in assessing the severity of bronchospasm. Those with some use are heart rate, respiratory rate, and the presence of an elevated temperature. In adults a persistent heart rate over 130 beats/min despite therapy suggests serious disease. Respiratory rates of under 12 and over 40 are signs of serious problems. Fever places the patient at risk for infection and warrants a more extensive evaluation. Pulsus paradoxus can be measured, and when elevated above 20 mm Hg it indicates severe airway obstruction. An elevated pulsus is an insensitive parameter and is highly dependent on respiratory effort. It is absent in almost half of asthmatics with severe respiratory obstruction.

Neck. The neck is examined for neck vein distention, suprasternal retractions, or the use of accessory musculature, and the midline position of the trachea. The neck is auscultated to determine if the "wheezing" is upper airway stridor.

Thorax. The thorax is assessed for respiratory excursion and prolongation of the expiratory phase and palpated for subcutaneous air. A "barrel chest" with an increased anteroposterior diameter may be seen in the patient with severe chronic airway disease. The thorax is percussed for hyperresonance or dullness. The lungs are auscultated for rales, wheezing, adequate air exchange, signs of consolidation, and symmetry of breath sounds. The experienced examiner can roughly gauge severity based on the lung examination, but there can be significant errors. In patients with very severe respiratory insufficiency, inadequate air exchange may not create sufficient turbulence to produce wheezing. The "silent chest" in a patient working hard to breathe represents a serious situation.

Cardiac Examination. During the cardiac examination one determines the point of maximal cardiac impulse to estimate heart size and position. The heart is auscultated for rate and rhythm, the presence of any gallops, murmurs, or rubs, and the possible presence of a mediastinal "crackling" with the heart beat, which indicates pneumomediastinum.

Abdomen. The abdomen is assessed for hepatomegaly, hepatojugular reflux, or ascites.

Extremities. The extremities are examined for adequacy of circulation and the presence of edema.

PROBLEM As the patient was being treated, the physician questioned the mother further about the history. Her daughter developed asthma in childhood but had not had an exacerbation of the condition for 1 year. Three days prior to the present episode she developed a cough and rhinorrhea. She stayed home from school because she felt ill. She had not complained of shortness of breath until the previous night. She had a theophylline preparation at home, but it was not used because it was "too old." The mother believed that her daughter might "get by" using an OTC inhaled "mist." Further physical examination did not reveal any evidence of an infectious site in the ear, nose or throat. There was no change in the pulmonary findings. A rectal temperature was 101.6°F (38.7° C).

The history of upper respiratory symptoms, cough, and especially fever are indicative of a respiratory infection. It is likely that infection is the precipitant for this attack. The patient's use of an OTC medication may mask the true severity of her disorder. Pneumonia is the most significant complication to be identified; therefore, the chest radiograph assumes importance in her evaluation.

DECISION PRIORITIES AND PRELIMINARY DIFFERENTIAL DIAGNOSIS

At this point, three questions need to be answered.

1. *If the patient does not have known asthma or COPD, what is the cause of the wheezing?*

   Table 56–1 lists the major diseases in the preliminary differential diagnosis of the wheezing patient. Only a few of these are difficult to distinguish from bronchospasm caused by asthma or COPD.

   Congestive heart failure (CHF) is a difficult differential diagnosis in the patient with exacerbated COPD or when asthma-like symptoms appear in an elderly patient. Since management of CHF is quite different from that of asthma or COPD, it is an important consideration. Historical points indicative of left-sided heart failure include nocturnal dyspnea or orthopnea preceding the wheezing, and a prior history or symptoms consistent with ischemic heart disease. Physical findings include an S_3 or S_4 extra heart sound, rales, and peripheral right-sided CHF signs—peripheral edema, jugular venous distention, or hepatojugular reflux.

   Pulmonary embolism (PE)—"the great imitator"—occasionally presents with wheezing, but usually there is associated pleuritic chest pain, and in more than 94% of patients an associated predisposing factor will be present. It is important to note that COPD is a known predisposing condition for the development of PE. It is therefore considered in the known COPD patient who presents with acute shortness of breath and chest pain.

   Certain life-threatening disorders of the *upper airway* may be mistaken for lower airway disease if care is not taken to differentiate the high-pitched, predominantly inspiratory sound of stridor from true wheezing. Upper airway disorders include epiglottitis, croup, and laryngeal foreign body. Failure to diagnose the disorder in such cases can lead to disastrous consequences (see Chapter 37).

2. *If the patient has known asthma or COPD, what may have exacerbated the problem?*

A number of common precipitants of asthma and COPD need review. They may be short-lived or exist as significant diseases by themselves. The following precipitating causes are listed in order of decreasing relative concern:

- Pulmonary embolism
- Congestive heart failure
- Pneumothorax
- Infection
- Noncompliance with medications
- Irritant/allergic exposure

3. *What is the estimated severity of respiratory difficulty associated with the patient's wheezing?*

Table 56–2 lists the physical findings in the three categories of respiratory severity. Although occasionally spirometric results are available, the physical findings and history are usually enough to categorize the distress as mild, moderate, or severe. This information is most pertinent to patients with known asthma, because COPD is best evaluated with serial arterial blood gas analyses. This initial classification is only a first impression of severity. Reassessment after the first aerosol therapy is a more accurate time to assess the patient's true status.

PROBLEM The patient was in moderately severe to severe distress. It is important to note that she remained in this category despite undergoing a beta-adrenergic aerosol treatment. Changes in severity usually occur early in therapy, especially after the first aerosol treatment.

TABLE 56–2. Severity of Asthma as Gauged by Physical Findings

Degree of Severity	Physical Findings
Mild	Tachypnea <30/min
	Patient tolerance good when recumbent
	Accessory musculature not used
	Pulsus paradoxus not present
	Wheezing audible
Moderate	Tachypnea 20–40/min
	Patient tolerance fair with sitting
	Accessory musculature not used
	Pulsus paradoxus not present
	Wheezing diffuse, may be higher pitched
Severe	Tachypnea greater than 40/min or inappropriately "normal"
	Mental status may be confused or depressed
	Patient tolerance poor with sitting, diaphoresis
	Accessory muscles active
	Pulsus paradoxus present, >10–20 mm Hg
	Wheezing may be high pitched, of low intensity, or absent ("silent chest")
Drawbacks of assessing severity by physical examination	Assessment varies with examiner and patient
	Provides only late signs
	Accessory musculature and pulsus paradoxus related to FEV_1 <1 liter not always present

DIAGNOSTIC ADJUNCTS

Each of the following ancillary tests plays a role in the assessment of the patient with asthma or COPD. The usefulness of each measurement varies with the underlying disease.

Laboratory Studies

Arterial Blood Gas Analysis. In asthmatic patients, arterial blood gas (ABG) measurements are obtained if the patient is in severe distress, fails to respond to emergency department therapy, or has a history of complex disease. The results do not always correspond to pulmonary function test results. In severe disease, the Pco_2 level may rise to normal and even to hypercarbic levels (Pco_2 greater than 45 mm Hg). This is a truly ominous finding and indicates impending respiratory failure. The degree of hypoxemia in this setting is usually severe (Po_2 less than 50 mm Hg on room air).

In COPD patients, ABGs are obtained routinely. The physical findings and pulmonary function test results are difficult to interpret in these patients. Optimally, ABG results can be compared with the patient's previous values.

Complete Blood Count and Differential. If an infectious cause is suspected in the wheezing patient, a white blood cell count (WBC) may be helpful; it is often elevated in the presence of infection. It has limited use in the asthmatic patient since it is increased in about half of these patients, often with a left shift in the differential count because of endogenous catecholamines or administered adrenergic agonists.

Serum Electrolytes. In the asthmatic or COPD patient, serum electrolytes are generally required only when there is concern about significant dehydration.

Serum Theophylline. In any patient with exacerbated disease who is taking theophylline, a serum level of the drug is measured. The therapeutic range of serum theophylline is 10 to 20 µcg/ml. Theophylline metabolism is affected by a number of factors. This level is important if theophylline will be added to the patient's regimen. If a subtherapeutic level is found, it may explain the exacerbation of disease.

Radiologic Imaging

Chest radiographs are indicated if the cause of wheezing is in question. They are examined closely for signs of left-sided cardiac failure (cardiomegaly, cephalization of vascular flow, Kerley's lines, alveolar infiltrates), pulmonary infiltrate, pneumothorax, pneumomediastinum, interstitial lung disease, and foreign body or mass.

Chest radiography has limited usefulness in asthmatics. It influences the management in only 10% of patients. Indications for chest radiographs in asthmatics include fever, sputum production, and chest pain. In these patients the radiograph often shows hyperinflation or atelectasis due to mucous plugging.

In patients with COPD a chest radiograph is part of the assessment because infection and pneumothorax are common, and physical findings are not accurate. The patients have limited respiratory reserve and do not tolerate complications.

Electrocardiography

An ECG is indicated in the wheezing patient if there is a complaint of chest pain or a history of prior cardiac disease or dysrhythmia. ECG during acute asthma is usually performed to evaluate sinus tachycardia and premature beats. The most common abnormal findings include right ventricular strain with right axis deviation and premature ventricular contractions. These findings are reversible and resolve with therapy and improvement. The ECG is important in patients suspected of wheezing due to left-sided cardiac failure ("cardiac asthma").

Pulmonary Function Tests

Pulmonary function tests (PFT) using simple hand-held devices such as the Wright peak flow meter are helpful in determining the initial severity of airway obstruction in the wheezing patient. Repeated measurements aid in following the patient's response to therapy and are valuable in determining appropriate disposition. Parameters most often measured are the forced expiratory volume in 1 second (FEV_1) and the peak expiratory flow rate (PEFR). Each measures the velocity of air flow and estimates the degree of airway obstruction. They are effort dependent and can be altered by changes in lung volume. The results are compared with a table of normal values and the patient's historical values. Table 56–3 is a guide to interpreting PFT results in asthma.

Sputum Analysis

If the wheezing patient has a productive cough, a sputum specimen is obtained for wet mount examination and possibly Gram stain. The wet mount is examined for neutrophils and eosinophils. Eosinophils are cells with shiny green granules and represent an allergic component in the cause of bronchospasm. These studies are particularly important in COPD patients because infection is a frequent complication.

PROBLEM After the first metaproterenol treatment in the emergency department, the patient showed some clinical improvement. She remained in moderately severe respiratory distress but was able to complete short sentences and used her accessory muscles less. Her wheezing became audible. A repeat PEFR showed a value of 150 liters/min. The CBC showed a white blood cell count of 17,000 with a shift to the left as indicated by a high number of band forms. The theophylline level was zero. The chest radiograph revealed a right lower lobe infiltrate. The sputum wet mount showed sheets of neutrophils, and the Gram stain showed gram-positive diplococci.

An infiltrate and possible pneumonia is a relatively rare complication of

TABLE 56–3. Use and Interpretation of Pulmonary Function Tests in Asthma

PEFR (liters/min)	% Predicted	FEV_1 (liters)	% Predicted	Significance
Pretreatment				
<100	<20	<0.7	<20	Severe exacerbation. Early aggressive therapy required. Intubation may be required. ABGs and CXR appropriate. Most patients require admission
100–200	20–30	0.7–1.0	20–25	Moderate exacerbation. ABGs appropriate in 16 to 40 year old asthmatics (individualize in other age groups). CXR indicated if improvement is slow
200–300	30–60	1.0–2.1	25–60	Mild exacerbation
>300	>60	>2.1	>60	Goal of therapy (but must be individualized)
After initial aerosol therapy				
Improve <60	—	Improve <0.3	—	Severe exacerbation. Early aggressive therapy required. Intubation may be required. ABGs and CXR appropriate. Most patients require admission
Final value after maximal emergency department therapy				
<300	<60	<2.1	<60	Admit or schedule early follow-up. If discharged, adequate bronchodilator therapy and, if indicated, steroids are continued
>300	>60	>2.1	>60	Discharge on appropriate medications and with early follow-up arranged

asthma in this age group. It will be difficult to resolve this episode of bronchospasm during an emergency department stay. The patient shows signs of improvement, and additional therapy is expected to reduce her symptoms.

PRINCIPLES OF MANAGEMENT

The basic principles of management in the wheezing patient are to protect the airway, relieve bronchospasm and hypoxia, rehydrate the patient, and treat causes or complications, e.g., pneumothorax and pneumonia. Management proceeds following these guidelines:

1. Each patient is unique, and therapy is tailored to their needs and response.
2. Because of differences in age groups and pathophysiology, patients with asthma and COPD with wheezing are not managed in the same manner. Treatment in asthmatics emphasizes reversal of bronchospasm and hypoxemia. In patients with COPD the highest priority is reversal of hypoxemia. Bronchospasm is treated to the degree that it contributes to the problem. Since wheezing, particularly from reversible airway obstruction, is the theme of this chapter, the reversal of bronchospasm is the focus of management.
3. Initial management is based on the category of severity that applies to the patient. It is adjusted as the patient responds.
4. The best time for categorizing the severity of a patient's wheezing is after the first beta-adrenergic aerosol treatment. Inhaled aerosol is the first therapy used in patients with all categories of wheezing, except patients needing immediate intubation.

Figure 56–1 is an algorithm for management of reversible obstructive airway disease based on the broad categories of mild, moderate, and severe. It is intended as a guide to therapy and cannot replace attentive assessment, clinical judgment, and appropriate response to changes in the patient's condition. More information on the measures applied within this algorithm is supplied below. The goal is to explain where and why a specific treatment fits in.

Relief of Bronchospasm

Beta-Adrenergic Agonists. The beta-adrenergic agonists are the mainstay in managing acute exacerbations of asthma and COPD. Stimulation of beta-2 receptors in the tracheobronchial tree results in bronchial smooth muscle relaxation and decreases mediator release from mast cells, enzyme release from neutrophils, and antibody production in lymphocytes. Table 56–4 lists the route, dose, and frequency of administration of the most commonly used agents.

Subcutaneous Epinephrine. Epinephrine has a long history of use in patients with asthma. It has significant beta-1 and alpha effects causing unpleasant and sometimes dangerous side effects—muscle tremors, tachycardia, dysrhythmias, and cardiac ischemia. Recent data suggest that lengthening the timing to every 40 minutes may decrease the side effects without lessening the therapeutic response. Sus-phrine is a long-acting form of epinephrine. Theoretically it provides sustained activity, but its use is limited to time of discharge in selected patients.

"Beta-2 Selective" Agents. Beta-2 agents are the first-line therapeutic choice. Those available include terbutaline, metaproterenol, and albuterol. All have significantly fewer beta-1 effects and long durations of action. Terbutaline is given either subcutaneously (SQ) or by aerosol, the latter not currently approved in the United States. The other two agents are available in aerosol, oral, or intravenous preparations. The intravenous form is not yet approved in the United States. The aerosol produces excellent bronchodilation and reduced adverse systemic side effects. Albuterol or metaproterenol given by hand-held nebulizer is the first line of treatment in patients with exacerbations of asthma or COPD. It is given as often as every 20 to 30 minutes as needed to reverse severe wheezing episodes. New selective beta-2 agonists are currently being researched.

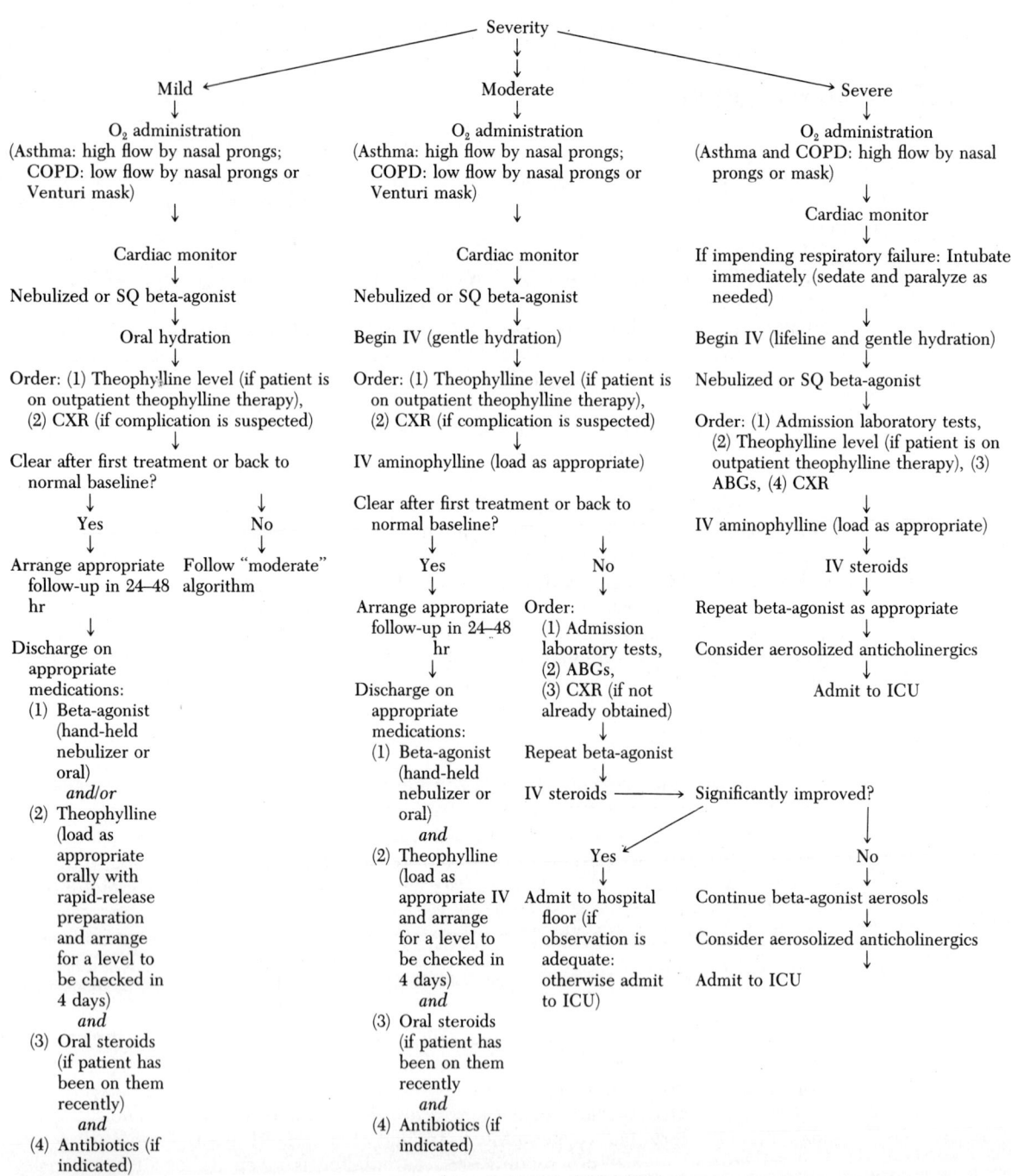

SQ = subcutaneous; ABGs = arterial blood gases; CXR = chest radiograph.
This algorithm is meant only as a management guideline. It cannot replace good clinical judgment, especially in response to changes in patient condition.

FIGURE 56–1. *Management algorithm for reversible obstructive airway disease.*

TABLE 56–4. Medications Commonly Used in Asthma and COPD

Drug	Route	Dose	Frequency	Comment
Epinephrine 1:1000	SQ	Adults: 0.3–0.4 ml	q 20 min up to three doses	Peak effect: 15–30 min Duration: up to 3 hr
		Children: 0.01 ml/kg (0.3 ml max)	q 20 min up to three doses	Do not use concurrently with terbutaline Avoid in first-trimester pregnancy, patients over 40 yr, hypertension, or coronary artery disease
Sus-Phrine (epinephrine in oil)	SQ	Adults: 0.1–0.3 ml Children: 0.005 ml/kg (0.15 ml/max)	q 6 hr q 6 hr	Peak effect: 2 hr Duration: up to 6 hr Avoid in first-trimester pregnancy, patients over 40 yr, hypertension, or coronary artery disease
Albuterol	Oral	Adults: 2–4 mg	t.i.d.–q.i.d.	Peak effect: 1–2 hr Duration: 4–6 hr
		Children: 0.10 mg/kg	t.i.d.–q.i.d.	
	Aerosol (0–0.5% soln)	Adults: 0.5–1.0 ml in 2 ml saline	q 20 min up to three doses	Peak effect: 30–60 min Duration: 4–6 hr
		Children: 0.01 ml/kg (1 ml max) in 2 ml saline	q 20 min up to three doses	
Metaproterenol	Oral	Adults: 20 mg	t.i.d.–q.i.d.	Peak effect: 30–60 min Duration: 3–6 hr
		Children: 0.3–0.5 mg/kg	t.i.d.–q.i.d.	
	Aerosol (5% soln)	Adults: 0.3 ml in 2 ml saline	q 20 min up to three doses	Peak effect: 30–60 min Duration: 4–6 hr
		Children: 0.01 ml/kg (0.3 ml max) in 2 ml saline	q 20 min up to three doses	
Terbutaline	Oral	Adults: 5 mg	t.i.d.	Peak effect: 2–3 hr Duration: 3–5 hr
		Children: 0.075 mg/kg	t.i.d.	Not currently recommended in patients <12 yr
	SQ	Adults: 0.25 ml	May repeat once in 30 min (max of 0.5 ml in 4 hr)	Peak effect: 30 min Duration: 4–6 hr Do not use concurrently with epinephrine
		Children: 0.01 ml/kg (0.25 ml max)	May repeat once in 30 min (max of 0.5 ml in 4 hr)	Not currently recommended in patients <12 yr
Aminophylline	IV	Loading dose adults and children (based on actual body weight): 5.6 mg/kg given over 20 min		Each 1 mg/kg loading dose should raise the serum level approximately 2 μg/ml Loading dosage depends on timing of last theophylline dose: a. Less than 12 hr—start maintenance dose only b. 12–24 hr—give 2.5 mg/kg loading dose c. Greater than 24 hr—full loading dose
		Maintenance dose (based on ideal body weight) Children <18 yr: 1.0 mg/kg/hr Adult nonsmoker <50 yr: 0.5 mg/kg/hr Adult smoker <50 yr: 0.8 mg/kg/hr Adult >50 yr: 0.4 mg/kg/hr COPD: 0.4 mg/kg/hr CHF or liver dysfunction: 0.2–0.3 mg/kg/hr	Continuous infusion	Optimally, the serum level is measured before administering dose. Adjustments can be made when the value returns from the laboratory

Table continued on following page

TABLE 56–4. Medications Commonly Used in Asthma and COPD *Continued*

Drug	Route	Dose	Frequency	Comment
Theophylline	Oral	Adults and children: Calculate total daily dose for IV aminophylline and multiply by 0.8 to convert to dose of theophylline. Then divide total daily dose into appropriate dosing interval for preparation chosen (q 8–12 hr for sustained release preparations; q 6 hr for rapid release preparations)		
Methylprednisolone	IV	Adults: 40–60 mg Children: 1–2 mg/kg	q 6 hr q 6 hr	After the first two doses, the dosage can be doubled until a response is noted. Tapering is done rapidly. This is inpatient therapy
Prednisone	Oral	Adults: 40–60 mg Children: 1–2 mg/kg	q day divided b.i.d.	If used for only 7–10 days, can stop without tapering. Usually for outpatient therapy
Atropine sulfate	Aerosol	Adults: 1.0–1.5 mg in 2 ml saline Children: 0.02 mg/kg (1.0 mg max) in 2 ml saline	q 4–6 hr q 4–6 hr	Duration: 3–5 hr Should be tried after other measures have failed Contraindicated in patients with glaucoma

Other Catecholamines. Other catecholamines occasionally used in asthma include isoproterenol and isoetharine. Isoproterenol has equal beta-1 and beta-2 effects and is associated with significant adverse effects. It is still used intravenously in severe status asthmaticus in children in an attempt to obviate intubation. It is used only by experienced physicians because the risk of cardiac dysrhythmias is significant. Isoetharine is an aerosol that has fewer beta-1 effects than isoproterenol. It has a short duration of action.

Theophylline Preparation. Theophylline is a basic medication in outpatient therapy of patients with chronic asthma and COPD. Its mechanism of action is thought to be inhibition of phosphodiesterase, causing decreased degradation of intracellular cAMP and resulting in bronchial smooth muscle relaxation. Recently, other mechanisms of action have been thought possible, including blockade of adenosine receptors, alterations of calcium influx into cells, or inhibition of prostaglandin production. Its mechanism is different from that of the beta agonists, and its effects are additive. Theophylline stimulates the respiratory center and strengthens contractility of the diaphragm, advantageous effects in the tiring asthmatic or COPD patient.

Serum levels at which theophylline is most effective without significant adverse effects are 10 to 20 μcg/ml. Optimally, the serum theophylline level is measured in the patient taking this preparation. An estimated loading dose is started as noted in Table 56–4 and is adjusted when results return from the laboratory.

There is serious question about the efficacy of theophylline in acute bronchospasm. Until this question is resolved, it remains part of the regimen.

Corticosteroids. The use of glucocorticoids in asthma is an area of controversy in terms of mechanism of action, indications, and dosage. Evidence points to a beneficial effect in asthma and COPD patients when the drugs are used appropriately. Proposed mechanisms of action include improved responsiveness of bronchial smooth muscle and leukocytes to beta agonists, stimulation of adenylate cyclase, stabilization of mast cell membranes, and direct anti-inflammatory effects. These drugs do not possess any direct bronchodilating effects. Corticosteroids are given to any patient with an acute exacerbation who (1) is taking steroids (including aerosolized steroids), (2) has a known history of complex or severe disease, (3) has evidence of severe airway obstruction that is not responding rapidly to other maximal therapy, (4) requires intubation, and (5) is refractory to aerosols because of overuse. These drugs are given as early as possible because their onset of action may take several hours. If the patient is to be discharged from the emergency department, a brief (7 to 10 days) tapering course of oral steroids is prescribed.

Anticholinergic Agents. Recently, interest has been revived in the use of anticholinergic agents in treating asthma and COPD. These agents decrease intracellular levels of cAMP, resulting in bronchial smooth muscle relaxation and diminished mast cell degranulation. These agents can be tried in patients with severe exacerbations of disease that are failing to respond to beta agonists and theophylline.

Atropine sulfate, administered via aerosol, is the anticholinergic agent currently available in the United States for the treatment of asthma and COPD. A newer agent, ipratroprium bromide, is currently being investigated for aerosol use. Ipratroprium is a derivative of atropine but is less lipid soluble and thus is less systemically absorbed, resulting in fewer adverse effects.

General Anesthesia

As a last resort in the wheezing asthmatic whose condition continues to deteriorate despite maximal therapy (including intubation and mechanical ventilation), general anesthesia with halothane can be tried. Halothane has a direct bronchodilating effect on airway smooth muscle. The risks of halothane include myocardial depression, vasodilation, and dysrhythmias.

General Measures

Rehydration. Most decompensated asthmatics are at least mildly dehydrated from increased insensitive fluid losses (tachypnea, fever) and decreased oral intake. Theophylline has a diuretic effect and may worsen this state. Mucous viscosity may be increased and clearance decreased by dehydration. Oral fluids may be satisfactory, but IV hydration is more often used. The average deficit is 2 to 4 liters. Overhydration is avoided because it may worsen mucosal edema and precipitate pulmonary edema. COPD patients are less likely to have concomitant dehydration than are asthmatics.

Antibiotics. Antibiotics are added to the treatment regimen if there is evidence of bacterial infection, e.g., purulent sputum with a predominance of neutrophils on wet mount. Broad-spectrum antibiotics are selected: ampicillin, erythromycin, or tetracycline. Erythromycin decreases theophylline metabolism and may lead to toxicity. Patients with pneumonia are admitted to the hospital for intravenous antibiotics unless they respond promptly to bronchodilator therapy. The choice of antibiotic is guided by the patient's history and sputum Gram stain.

Sodium Bicarbonate. Significant acidemia of metabolic origin may inhibit the effectiveness of beta-adrenergic agonists. Some authors recommend infusing small amounts of sodium bicarbonate if the arterial pH is less than 7.1 and monitoring the clinical and acid-base response. Acidemia due to respiratory acidosis is treated with improved ventilation.

PROBLEM After the second metaproterenol treatment, the patient stated that she was no better but no worse either. Her PEFR remained at 150 liters/min. Her weight was determined to be 60 kg. Because of her minimal improvement, she remained in a moderately severe category. She was given 60 mg of methylprednisolone intravenously, and a loading dose of 300 mg of aminophylline (5.0 mg/kg) plus a maintenance infusion of 30 mg/hr was started. Antibiotics were started for the pneumonia.

As anticipated, the attack in this patient is not resolving as rapidly as an attack in most uncomplicated cases of asthma. She requires multiple agents to relieve the bronchospasm. Hydration and aggressive pulmonary toilet to promote removal of secretions are important in the eventual resolution of the problem. Methods of removing secretions may include positioning and respiratory therapy.

SPECIAL CONSIDERATIONS

Pediatric Patients

Wheezing is commonly seen in infants and children under 2 years of age. It is most commonly due to viral infections and is usually diagnosed as *bronchiolitis*. This disorder is characterized by inflammatory obstruction of the small airways and its incidence peaks at approximately 6 months of age. It occurs most frequently during the winter and early spring months and can be either sporadic or epidemic. The question of asthma often arises in the course of treating these children, and there is a great deal of controversy about the possible relationship of bronchiolitis to later development of asthma. Factors that suggest a diagnosis of asthma include:

1. A family history of asthma
2. Recurrent attacks (less than 5% of recurrent attacks of wheezing are due to viral infections in this age group)
3. Sudden onset without evidence of a preceding viral infection
4. Markedly prolonged expiration
5. Eosinophilia
6. Response to bronchodilators

Once other disorders are ruled out, such as foreign body aspiration or cardiac disease, children in this age group who present with wheezing should receive a trial of bronchodilator therapy in order to judge the response. If the patient responds, further bronchodilator therapy can be instituted as outlined for asthma. If there is no response and the child is in any respiratory distress, he or she is treated with humidified oxygen and parenteral fluids and admitted for observation.

Asthma in Pregnancy

Approximately one-third of pregnant asthmatics will experience worsening of the course of their disease during their pregnancy, 33% will show improvement in their symptoms, and one-third will remain unchanged. Management of wheezing in the pregnant asthmatic can proceed as in the nonpregnant patient with the following cautions:

1. Care must be exercised in using parenteral beta-agonists in the pregnant patient near term because these drugs may decrease uterine contractility and inhibit labor. When required in this setting, beta-agonists are given as aerosols to limit systemic absorption.
2. Subcutaneous epinephrine used during the first months of gestation may be associated with increased fetal malformations and should be avoided.
3. Extra care is necessary to prevent hypoxia in the pregnant asthmatic to prevent fetal anoxia.

As a final note, the physician must be aware that the pregnant state is a predisposing factor to the development of deep venous thrombosis and subsequent pulmonary embolism. This is kept in mind in treating the wheezing, pregnant female, especially if there is associated chest pain or if there is no history of asthma.

DISPOSITION AND FOLLOW-UP

Up to 80% of patients who present with wheezing are discharged from the emergency department. The physician must use all available parameters in deciding the appropriate disposition for a wheezing patient. This decision is made generally after between 2 and 4 hours of therapy. More time is acceptable but warrants explanation.

Admission

Patients who fail to relieve their wheezing but are not in sufficient respiratory distress to warrant ICU admission are admitted to a regular hospital bed if the nursing staff is adequate to maintain close observation. This also applies to patients who are not in significant distress but who have complications such as pneumonia, dehydration, or inability to tolerate oral medications.

ICU Admission

ICU admission is necessary for the following patients:
1. Patients requiring intubation
2. Patients with severe obstruction and failure to improve after initial bronchodilator therapy
3. Patients with altered mental status
4. Patients with hypercapnia and respiratory acidosis
5. Patients with dysrhythmia other than mild sinus tachycardia
6. Patients with borderline reserve and complications such as pneumothorax, pneumomediastinum, or pneumonia
7. Any patient who is felt to have borderline indications for ICU admission when close observation is unavailable on a regular hospital unit

It is better to err on the side of ICU admission and transfer the patient to a regular unit after he or she is stable than it is to place a potentially unstable patient in a regular hospital bed.

Discharge

Patients are discharged from the emergency department when their symptoms are generally asymptomatic. Though not always possible, it is best for them to be wheeze-free. In an earlier study of asthmatics, the FEV_1 was 40% of predicted when the patient subjectively was wheeze-free, and 60% of predicted when the wheezing was gone on auscultation. This result means that significant bronchospasm is still present in the wheeze-free patient. It can serve as the basis of the next symptomatic episode. Other guidelines include a PEFR of more than 300 liters/min or an FEV_1 of more than 2 liters.

Being wheeze-free does not always correlate well with outcome. Up to 25% of patients return with a relapse within 10 days. A practical test prior to discharge is to ask the patient to walk 30 to 50 feet in the emergency department. If this brief exercise results in wheezing, the appropriateness of discharge is reconsidered.

Prior to discharge the following points are managed:
1. Patients are prescribed adequate bronchodilator therapy to carry them through this residual period.
2. If steroids have been begun in the emergency department, they are continued, e.g., oral prednisone is continued after discharge.
3. The patient's understanding of the dose and use of medication is clarified.
4. An understanding of the patient's home environment is necessary. Is an element present that may precipitate bronchospasm?
5. Patients are instructed to return promptly to the emergency department at the earliest sign of relapse.
6. All discharged patients must have appropriate follow-up arranged with their primary physician 24 to 48 hours following their emergency department visit.

PROBLEM After 3 hours of emergency department management, continuous aminophylline, rehydration, and three metaproterenol treatments, the patient was more comfortable. Clinically, her wheezing was less and her breathing was less labored. The PEFR rose to 220 liters/min.

Clearly, because of the presence of pneumonia and the slow resolution of wheezing, this patient requires hospital admission. The need for intensive care is a clinical judgment. Because of her age and steady improvement, she is not admitted to the ICU. Typically, she will improve over a 24- to 48-hour period with continued hydration, bronchodilator therapy, and antibiotics.

DOCUMENTATION

1. Onset of wheezing and patient assessment of severity.
2. Previous history of wheezing pattern of attacks.
3. Current medications, particularly bronchodilators and steroids.
4. A complete set of vital signs (including temperature).
5. General level of distress and ability to speak in sentences.
6. Chest sounds and use of accessory muscles.
7. Results of pulmonary function testing, and, if obtained, blood gas measurements and chest radiographs.
8. A complete record of all interventions used (including times, dosages, and routes).
9. A brief notation of each reassessment of the patient made by the emergency department physician to include changes in symptomatology, physical examination, and pulmonary function test results.
10. Discharge instructions given to the patient and what follow-up has been arranged for patients who leave the hospital.

SUMMARY AND FINAL POINTS

- The most common cause of wheezing is obstructive pulmonary disease, e.g., asthma, emphysema, chronic bronchitis. However, it may be the common symptom of other disorders such as congestive heart failure, anaphylaxis, and pulmonary embolism.
- The underlying pathology is severe bronchospasm resulting in hypoxemia and acidemia.
- *The only absolute indications for endotracheal intubation in the wheezing patient are apnea and coma.*
- When assessing the patient with asthma and wheezing, the complications of pneumothorax and pneumonia are always considered.
- The severity of wheezing is gauged by physical findings, pulmonary function test results, and arterial blood gas measurements. The degree of wheezing on auscultation is a weak indicator of the severity of the attack. Air flow may not be sufficient to create enough turbulence to generate the sound of wheezing. Arterial blood gases are overutilized in patients with asthma and wheezing. They are obtained only in patients with severe attacks or in those who do not respond to therapy. Pulmonary function test results can be effort dependent and often are not readily available.
- Beta-2 selective aerosols are the first-line therapy for acute wheezing from obstructive pulmonary disease.
- Theophylline has less efficacy in this setting but is a mainstay of chronic management.
- Corticosteroids are administered early in the course of moderate or severe attacks or if indicated by the history.
- Fluid replacement is important to reduce the viscosity of pulmonary secretions and to promote their clearance from the bronchial tree.
- The decision to discharge a patient after treatment of an acute attack of wheezing is not based on single clinical or laboratory parameters. Patients must feel they have returned close to their normal state. Wheezing is resolved even with limited exercise. Vital signs are near normal. Bedside pulmonary function test results are significantly improved (more than 60% of predicted).

BIBLIOGRAPHY

Texts
1. Baum JL, Wolinsky E (eds): Textbook of Pulmonology. Boston, Little, Brown, 1983.
2. Hamilton GC: Asthma. In Baines HV (ed): Clinical Medicine: Selected Problems with Pathophysiologic Correlations. Chicago, Year Book, 1987.

Journal Articles
1. Brown DL, Maddux MS, Organek HW, et al: Rapid and sustained oral theophylline loading: An alternative to intravenous aminophylline therapy. Arch Intern Med 143:794–796, 1983.
2. Brenner BE: Bronchial asthma in adults: Presentation to the emergency department. Am J Emerg Med 1(1):50–70, 1(3):306–333, 1983.
3. Carden DL, Nowak RM, Sarkar D, et al: Vital signs including pulsus paradoxus in the assessment of acute bronchial asthma. Ann Emerg Med 12:80–83, 1983.
4. Downie RL: Obstructive airway disease. Topics Emerg Med 8:13–31, 1987.
5. Fanta CH, Rossing, TH, McFadden ER: Glucocorticoids in acute asthma: A critical controlled trial. Am J Med 74:845–851, 1983.
6. Galant SP: Current status of beta-adrenergic agonists in bronchial asthma. Pediatr Clin North Am 30:931–942, 1983.
7. Nowalk RM, Tomlanovich MC, Sarkar DD, et al: Arterial blood gases and pulmonary function testing in acute bronchial asthma: Predicting patient outcomes. JAMA 249:2043–2046, 1983.
8. Reyes de la Rocha S, Brown MA: Asthma in children: Emergency management. Ann Emerg Med 16:109–119, 1987.
9. Rothstein RJ: Intravenous theophylline therapy in asthma: A clinical update. Ann Emerg Med 9:327–330, 1980.
10. Stibolt TB: Asthma. Med Clin North Am 70:909–920, 1986.

CHAPTER 57

CHEST TRAUMA

MICHAEL SPADAFORA, M.D.
ALEXANDER T. TROTT, M.D.

PROBLEM 1 A 44 year old woman was the unrestrained driver in a high-speed motor vehicle accident. There was extensive damage to the car, including a crushed steering wheel. The police arrived and called for a rescue squad.

PROBLEM 2 A 27 year old man was reportedly stabbed in the chest by two men. The police arrived and found him obtunded and breathing hard. They called the rescue squad.

QUESTIONS TO CONSIDER

1. What are the pathophysiologic mechanisms of injury in patients with blunt and penetrating thoracic trauma?
2. What are the major threats to life in the patient with thoracic trauma?
3. Which salient points of the history and physical examination lead to the diagnosis of these threats?
4. How are diagnostic adjuncts selected when evaluating the patient with chest trauma?
5. What are the clinical indications for needle thoracostomy? Tube thoracostomy? Pericardiocentesis? Emergency thoracotomy?
6. Which patients with chest trauma require early operative intervention?
7. What is the appropriate disposition of patients with chest trauma who do not require operative intervention?

INTRODUCTION

Thoracic injuries are a major contributor to mortality and morbidity in more than 60% of multiply injured patients. Blunt thoracic injuries rank second only to head injury as a cause of death and disability in these patients. In spite of these statistics, operative thoracotomy is necessary in only 10% to 15% of patients with thoracic trauma. Most are managed with advanced airway care, needle and tube thoracostomy, ventilatory support, or volume resuscitation.

Trauma to the thorax occurs by means of four basic forces: *shearing, compression, torsion,* and *acceleration/deceleration*. The simplest example of shearing is a knife wound. Tissue is divided with little force imparted and the actual damage is small. The critical factor in these injuries is the potential involvement of a major vessel, leading to exsanguination or loss of negative intrapleural pressure that causes ventilatory compromise. Compression is the main mechanism by which ribs are broken as the force delivered exceeds the elastic capacity of the bone. The bone fragment can then "shear" lung tissue, leading to a pneumothorax or hemothorax. Enough compression to the thoracic cage can cause a segment of ribs to break in at least two places. The "flail" segment, no longer a stable portion of the thoracic cage, can collapse into the chest cavity with the negative intrathoracic pressure of inspiration. This instability of the thoracic cage may contribute to ventilatory compromise. Significant compressive forces are also imparted to the underlying lung, with resultant pulmonary contusion. Shearing and compression occur with gunshot wounds. Tissue is divided by the bullet, and the area around the path is directly compressed. In wounds resulting from high-velocity missiles, the area of injury is expanded into tissue by the force of the energy released by the bullet as it decelerates in the body.

Shearing or compression can result in a rapidly fatal outcome. Shearing penetration of the heart usually results from a knife or bullet. Compression against a blood-filled chamber can cause myocardial rupture. Hemorrhage from the myocardial wound ensues, but the pericardial injury often remains closed. The accumulation of blood in the pericardium results in cardiac tamponade. As intrapericardial pressure rises, the return blood flow to the heart decreases until the right ventricular diastolic filling pressure is exceeded. In this setting, as little as 50 ml of blood may cause a pericardial tamponade. Hypotension and shock follow rapidly.

Shearing, compression, and torsion play roles in creating a tension pneumothorax (Fig. 57–1). When the pleural space or lung is penetrated, a tissue flap is created that is in effect a one-way valve, allowing air to escape into the pleural cavity but preventing its exit. Because of the one-way valve effect, positive intrapleural pressure quickly builds and begins to compress the lung. As intrapleural (and intrathoracic) pressure increases, it begins to exceed the right ventricular filling pressure and decreases blood return to the heart. The expanding pneumothorax on the affected side compresses the mediastinum and unaffected hemithorax, depending on the mobility of the mediastinum. This pressure and torsion of the mediastinal vessels may contribute to impaired cardiac venous return.

The most lethal result of acceleration-deceleration thoracic injury is transection of the aorta. The aorta is relatively fixed in the mediastinum at a point just distal to the left subclavian artery. Distally, it is more mobile until it reaches the diaphragm. In a rapid deceleration injury, such as occurs with blunt impact of the chest against a steering wheel, the aorta accelerates forward as the thorax decelerates. At the point of fixation, shearing and torsion cause tearing in the aortic intima and media. If the force is sufficient, the adventitia may tear as well, and rapid exsanguination will follow. This mechanism is the underlying cause of immediate death in most fatal motor vehicle accidents. In 10%

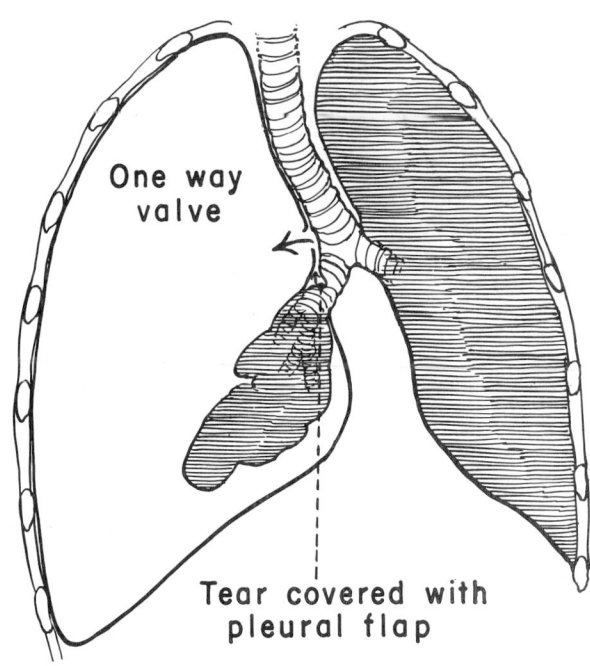

FIGURE 57–1. Tension pneumothorax. (From Zuidema GD, Rutherford RB, Ballinger WF [eds]: *The Management of Trauma*, 4th ed. Philadelphia, WB Saunders, 1985.)

to 20% of patients with this injury, the adventitia remains intact, and the patient has a chance of survival depending on the recognition and treatment of the lesion.

Although the spectrum of types of injuries occurring in thoracic trauma varies with the mechanism of injury, the underlying result is generally similar: Impairments in cardiac output, ventilatory efficiency, and gas exchange may occur with injury to the chest wall, pleura, heart, tracheobronchial tree, or pulmonary parenchyma whether caused by an ice pick or by impact with a steering wheel.

PREHOSPITAL CARE

As in most field assessments of traumatic injuries, the goal is rapid transport to the hospital. The patient is stabilized in transit if possible. Information gathered by the rescue squad includes the following:

History

1. What is the mechanism of injury and the forces involved in the trauma?
2. What are the patient's symptoms? Is chest pain present? Is dyspnea present?
3. Is the patient usually in good health?
4. Has the patient recently used ethanol or another substance of abuse?
5. If this was a motor vehicle accident, were seat belts used? Is the windshield intact or steering wheel bent?

Physical Examination

1. Is the patient's airway patent and protected? How much respiratory effort is being made? How effective is the effort? If there is breathing difficulty, prehospital diagnosis of a tension pneumothorax or open pneumothorax ("sucking" chest wound) can be lifesaving. A *tension pneumothorax* is recognized by the presence of tachypnea, marked respiratory distress, hypertympany on percussion, and decreased breath sounds on the involved side with deviation of the trachea toward the contralateral hemithorax. *Open pneumothoraces* are in direct communication through the chest wall to the pleural space. They are usually quickly recognized by the sound of rushing air.
2. A pulse rate and blood pressure are obtained. Circulation is assessed by observing for pallor, diaphoresis, cyanosis, and capillary refill time.
3. A rapid survey is done to identify other major threats to life and limb, and management actions are taken when appropriate.
4. Continued scrutiny is maintained to detect changes in the patient's condition during stabilization and transport.

Intervention

Depending on the severity of the patient's injuries and the urgency of treatment, appropriate field management includes the following measures:

Airway Management and Oxygenation. Endotracheal intubation may be necessary in critically ill patients. Otherwise, administration of supplemental oxygen at 6 to 8 liters/min by nasal cannula is appropriate.

Cardiac Monitoring. Both blunt and penetrating injuries to the chest can precipitate cardiac dysrhythmias.

Intravenous Access. Establishing intravenous (IV) access and beginning isotonic crystalloid replacement is ideal but *not* essential in prehospital management. Attempts to achieve IV access should not delay transportation of an unstable trauma patient.

Pneumatic Antishock Garment (PASG). The use of this garment is not appropriate in most patients with isolated chest trauma.

Specific Interventions

Suspected Tension Pneumothorax. Many emergency medical service (EMS) personnel are trained to decompress a tension pneumothorax by inserting a 14- to 16-gauge catheter-type intravenous needle through the second intercostal space. This procedure is best carried out under the guidance of a physician by means of radiotelemetry.

Closure of Open Pneumothoraces. Any sucking chest wound is closed by prehospital care personnel with an airtight dressing, such as Vaseline gauze, taped on three sides only to create a "one-way valve" effect. Air may leave the chest cavity during expiration but cannot return during inspiration. This prevents the development of a tension pneumothorax.

PROBLEM 1 At the scene of the accident the patient was awake and alert but pinned by the collapsed steering wheel. She complained of chest pain, difficulty in breathing, and pain from an obviously fractured left femur. A hard cervical collar and short spine board were applied, and the patient was extricated from the vehicle. Spinal immobilization with a cervical collar and a long back board was secured. The patient's vital signs were blood pressure 130/70 mm Hg, pulse 130 beats/min, respiratory rate 24/min. A 16-gauge intravenous line was started with Ringer's lactate, and the patient was placed on 8 liters of oxygen and a cardiac monitor. A traction splint was applied to the left leg.

At this point, the appropriate interventions have been accomplished. Because the patient is alert and able to protect her airway and maintain her perfusion, the rescue squad is able to complete the standard field stabilization procedures at the scene. If the patient were in shock or otherwise unstable, these actions would be performed during transport. The mechanism of injury and the forces involved are significant, and continued observation and monitoring of the patient for deterioration of status are necessary. Focusing on chest trauma, the type of injury sustained raises concerns about aortic tear, myocardial contusion, and pulmonary contusion.

PROBLEM 2 At the scene of the stabbing, the patient was found to be pale, diaphoretic, and obtunded. His pulse was palpable at a rate of 50 beats/min; the blood pressure was unobtainable. The stab wound was in the left chest at the midclavicular line at approximately the fourth intercostal space. The trachea was at midline, the neck veins were not elevated, and the left chest was not hyperresonant on percussion. The patient was ventilated and oxygenated with a bag and mask, and transport was initiated without delay. PASG was rapidly applied en route and inflated without effecting improvement. Transport time to the hospital was 7 minutes. A brief notification call was made by radiotelemetry to the receiving emergency department.

This is clearly a case where excessive field stabilization procedures could endanger the life of the patient. Endotracheal intubation and volume resuscitation are not likely to alter the patient's outcome with such a short transport time, particularly if their placement would delay transport. The physical findings do not support needle thoracostomy for a possible tension pneumothorax. Notifying the emergency department is important to allow the resuscitation team time for preparation.

INITIAL APPROACH IN THE EMERGENCY DEPARTMENT

The potential for a rapidly fatal outcome mandates that patients with thoracic injuries be rapidly triaged to the critical care area of the emergency department and seen immediately by the emergency physician.

History

1. The prehospital care history is repeated and confirmed.
2. If shortness of breath is present, the patient is asked about its severity, response to oxygen supplementation, and, if available, any positioning that offers relief.
3. If the patient has chest pain, its nature, location, and severity are explored.

Physical Examination

Airway and Breathing

Upper Airway. The upper airway is assessed for patency. Any obvious sources of obstruction, such as dentures or broken teeth, are removed. The anterior neck is palpated for signs of laryngeal trauma, including tenderness and subcutaneous air (palpable crepitance) in the area of the thyroid cartilage.

Chest Wall. The chest wall is compressed anteroposteriorly and laterally to find sites of pain or instability. Areas of pain are palpated for bony or subcutaneous crepitus. The chest is observed for asymmetry during respiration or open pneumothorax. Auscultation and percussion are completed, searching for signs of tension pneumothorax or hemothorax.

Respiratory Status. Respiratory rate, ventilatory effort, and skin color are assessed to evaluate respiratory status.

Circulation. Blood pressure, pulse rate, skin appearance (pallor, diaphoresis), and capillary refill are assessed. Hypovolemia is the most common cause of circulatory compromise in chest trauma, but cardiac tamponade and tension pneumothorax are reversible "obstructive" causes.

Other Injuries. The cervical spine is examined and immobilized as necessary. A rapid survey is performed of the abdomen, central nervous system, pelvis, and extremities. Intra-abdominal injuries, head trauma, and long bone fractures are frequently associated with thoracic injuries.

Intervention

Airway Management. Patients in extreme respiratory distress require airway management and ventilatory support (see Chap. 2). Endotracheal intubation is the preferred technique. Cricothyrotomy is the procedure of choice if there are severe injuries to the face or upper airway. Supplemental oxygen is given to all patients.

Intravenous Access and Volume Resuscitation. Stable patients with thoracic trauma require two large-bore peripheral intravenous catheters. Unstable patients may need additional IV lines. If central venous access is necessary, the internal jugular or subclavian vein on the injured side of the chest is preferred to avoid complications in the functioning hemithorax. Isotonic crystalloid is the fluid of choice; the rate depends on the initial vital signs and estimated blood loss. In patients who do not respond to crystalloid or who arrive with "agonal" vital signs, uncross-matched type O or type-specific blood is given.

Needle Thoracostomy. Any patient who has clinical evidence of a tension pneumothorax is decompressed by needle thoracostomy. Needle decompression is performed by inserting a 14- to 16-gauge catheter–covered intravenous needle into the second intercostal space at the midclavicular line. The needle is inserted just over the superior edge of the second rib to avoid possible injury to the intercostal artery. On entering the pleural space, there will be an expulsion of air with a characteristic hissing sound. The steel needle portion of the catheter is removed, and the plastic catheter is left in place. Needle thoracostomy is a temporizing measure and is followed as soon as possible by tube thoracostomy.

Tube Thoracostomy. Tube thoracostomy is used for continuous evacuation of air and fluid from the pleural space. In the patient with thoracic trauma, the indications for tube thoracostomy include pneumothorax (simple, tension, open), hemothorax, hemopneumothorax, and conditions requiring anesthesia or positive pressure ventilation in patients with penetrating chest trauma. Tube thoracostomy is done in a sterile field. A large-bore (36 to 40 Fr) chest tube is inserted over the superior edge of the rib in the fourth or fifth intercostal space in the midaxillary line, connected to a closed drainage system with a water seal, and secured in place (Fig. 57–2). Initially, suction is set at -20 cm of water pressure. A chest radiograph to assess the degree of lung reexpansion, tube placement, and presence of associated injuries is mandatory after decompression has been accomplished.

Pericardiocentesis. In the deteriorating or hypotensive patient with clinical findings and a mechanism of injury consistent with cardiac tamponade (e.g., penetrating trauma in the central chest area), subxiphoid pericardiocentesis is a potentially lifesaving procedure (Fig. 57–3). An 18-gauge spinal needle is inserted in the xiphoid process and the left costal margin and directed toward the sternal notch or left shoulder. The only test of its success is restoration of a measurable blood pressure after withdrawal of blood from the pericardial space. If there is time, placement may be aided by attaching the needle to the V_1 chest lead of an electrocardiographic machine. The limb leads are in place. The needle is advanced with intermittent attempts to aspirate blood. Contact with the myocardium is demonstrated by acute ST-segment elevation. If this distant limit is reached, the needle is withdrawn slightly and an attempt made to aspirate blood in the pericardial space.

Pericardiocentesis is a hazardous procedure with a high potential for misdiagnosis. For example, in up to 60% of patients with acute traumatic pericardial tamponades the blood is all or partly clotted. At best the procedure is a temporizing measure while preparations for surgery are made. Emergency thoracotomy is performed if deterioration in condition continues and suspicion of tamponade remains.

Emergency Thoracotomy. Emergency thoracotomy is indicated in the patient with:
1. Penetrating thoracic or abdominal injuries who had vital signs during the

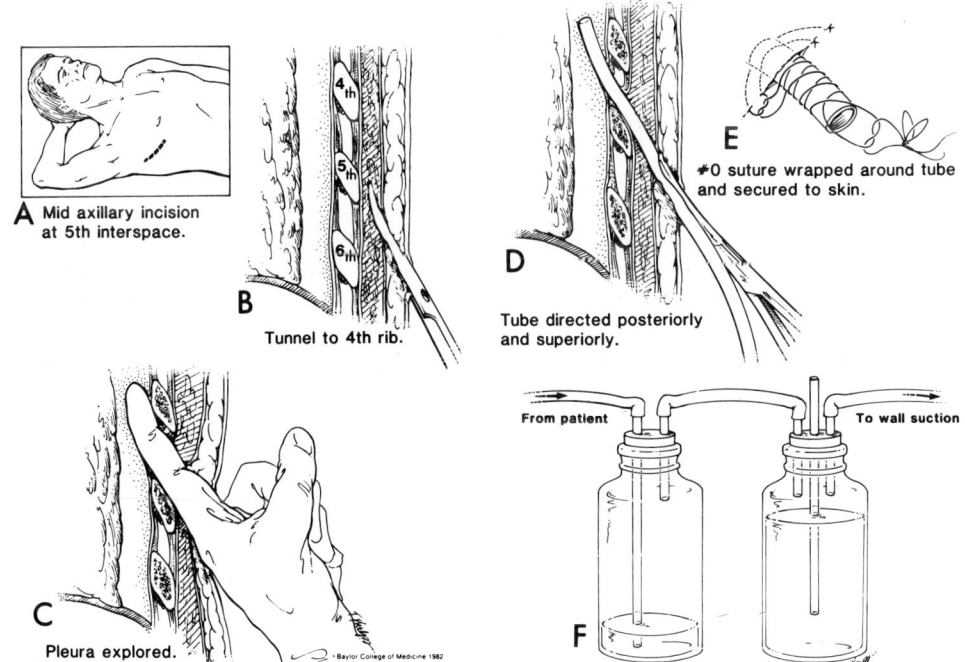

FIGURE 57–2. Technique for tube thoracostomy. Note that the pleural space is entered with the gloved finger, not a trocar or a sharp instrument. (From Emergency department treatment of chest injuries. Emerg Clin North Am 2[4]:786, 1984.)

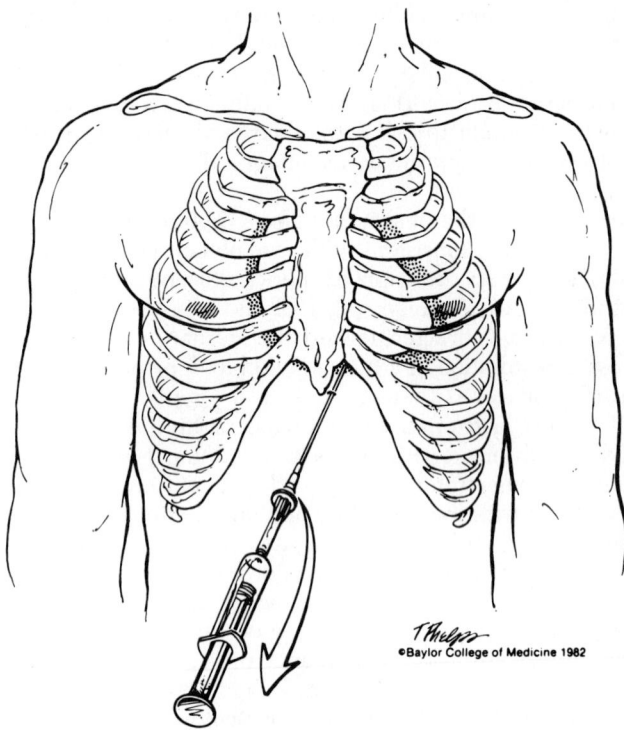

FIGURE 57-3. *Technique for pericardiocentesis. (From Emergency department treatment of chest injuries. Emerg Clin North Am 2[4]:787, 1984.)*

prehospital phase of care and who arrives at the emergency department in agonal condition or cardiac arrest.

2. Penetrating thoracic or abdominal trauma whose condition deteriorates rapidly in spite of maximal therapy.

Emergency thoracotomy, with few exceptions, has little clinical utility in victims of blunt traumatic cardiac arrest or nontraumatic cardiac arrest. Resuscitative thoracotomy (Fig. 57–4) is performed by the most experienced physician in the emergency department.

Chest Radiography. Plain chest films are important in any injured patient with thoracic trauma. They are *not* indicated prior to treatment in the unstable patient suspected of a tension pneumothorax, open pneumothorax, or cardiac tamponade. Treatment in these cases is based on clinical judgment. *Portable* chest radiographs are obtained as soon as possible after stabilization. Upright portable radiographs may be taken in clinically stable patients who are at no risk for spinal injury. Chest radiographs increase the chances of finding small pneumothoraces or hemothoraces. A clinically unstable or partially evaluated patient should not leave the emergency department for radiography.

PROBLEM 1 The patient was brought directly to the trauma area. Nursing personnel undressed her, took repeat vital signs, obtained additional IV access, and continued cardiac monitoring and supplemental oxygen. On the primary survey the patient was found to be alert, diaphoretic, and in moderate respiratory distress. Her upper airway was clear. Her vital signs were blood pressure 80 mm Hg systolic by palpation, pulse 150 beats/min, and respiratory rate 36/min. On palpation tenderness was found in the left lateral chest wall with obvious subcutaneous emphysema. Decreased breath sounds were heard in the left chest. The left hemithorax was hyperresonant to percussion.

The patient's status is now changed from that in the field. She is now

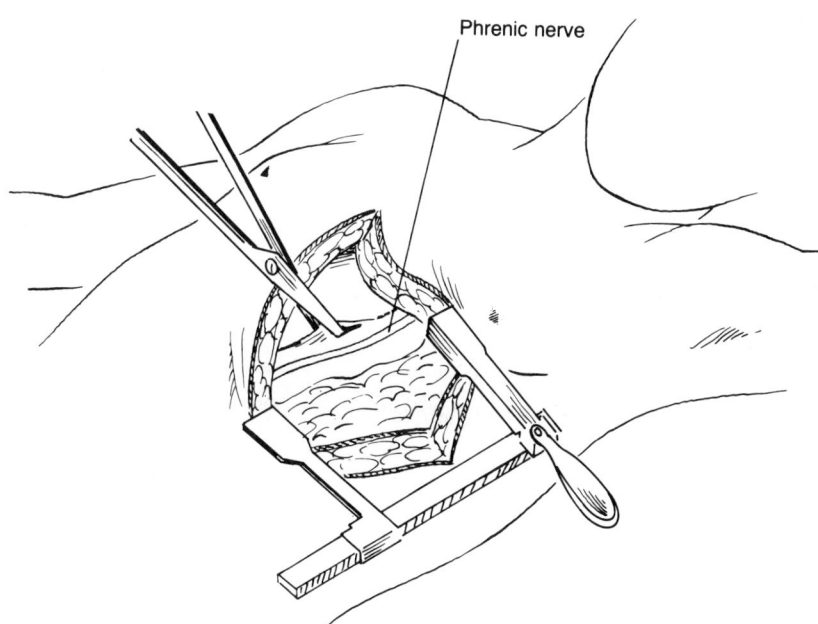

FIGURE 57-4. Left anterolateral location of resuscitative thoracotomy. (From Roberts JR, Hedges JR [eds]: Clinical Procedures in Emergency Medicine, 2nd ed. Philadelphia, WB Saunders, 1990.)

hemodynamically unstable and in respiratory distress with clinical evidence of a tension pneumothorax. Immediate decompression is indicated. A needle thoracostomy is performed, and a rush of air is heard. Her respiratory distress improves dramatically. Repeat vital signs are blood pressure 110/70 mm Hg, pulse 110 beats/min, respiratory rate 20/min. A tube thoracostomy is performed and a portable chest radiograph ordered.

PROBLEM 2 On arrival in the emergency department the patient had no spontaneous ventilations or pulse. His neck veins appeared distended. Several emergency department personnel acted simultaneously in their preassigned roles. The patient was preoxygenated rapidly by bag and mask, and endotracheal intubation was performed. After intubation, breath sounds were noted to be equal. A cardiac monitor was placed and showed electrical activity at a rate of 30 beats/min. Two 14-gauge intravenous catheters were placed, and Ringer's lactate was infused at a wide-open rate. Uncrossmatched type O blood was begun. While the thoracotomy tray was being prepared, an 18-gauge spinal needle was introduced at the xiphosternal junction and directed into the pericardium. Ten milliliters of nonclotting blood were withdrawn. Vital signs did not return. Immediately the senior physician team member performed an emergency thoracotomy. An incision was made in the fourth left intercostal space from the sternal border to the posterior axillary line. Rib retractors were placed and opened. The lung was gently retracted, exposing a bulging pericardial sac. With operative scissors, a longitudinal incision was made into the pericardium just anterior and parallel to the phrenic nerve. A large rush of blood was observed. The incision was extended, and multiple clots were gently swept from the pericardial sac. An actively bleeding 2-cm wound was encountered on the anterior aspect of the actively contracting right ventricle. A 20-Fr Foley catheter with a 30-ml balloon was inserted through the wound into the right ventricle. The balloon was gently inflated until the hemorrhage was controlled. With continued volume resuscitation, a carotid pulse of 70 beats/min and a blood pressure of 80/60 mm Hg were obtained.

After initial control of the blood loss and volume replacement are achieved, the emergency department phase of resuscitation is complete. Rapid transport to the operating suite for definitive repair then proceeds without delay. The team functioned effectively and smoothly and made rapid and appropriate critical decisions.

DATA GATHERING

After the initial assessment and necessary interventions have been performed, a more complete history and physical examination are completed.

History

1. *When did the accident occur and what was the mechanism?*
   The time of injury and onset of symptoms (if not simultaneous) and the mechanism of injury and amount of force involved are documented. The latter information is particularly important in patients with blunt trauma. It is often available only from EMS personnel. Specific mechanisms of injury require knowledge of specific information. In motor vehicle accidents the following information is helpful:
   - Type of vehicle and estimated speed at the time of the accident.
   - Victim's position in vehicle (driver or passenger).
   - Amount of damage occurring to the vehicle, particularly to the internal structures (e.g., steering wheel, windshield).
   - Where victim was found.
   - Use and type of restraints (e.g., seat belts).

   Most victims of penetrating trauma have either gunshot wounds or stab wounds. For patients with gunshot wounds it is helpful to know:
   - The type and caliber of weapon used.
   - Victim's distance from assailant.
   - Number of shots fired.

   For patients with stab wounds, useful information includes:
   - Type of weapon used.
   - Length of weapon.
   - Direction of stabbing.

2. *Is shortness of breath present?*
   The sensation of "shortness of breath" is the most common subjective complaint in patients with thoracic trauma. The sensation of dyspnea may result from a number of processes involving the airway, chest wall, lungs, other deep thoracic structures, or hemorrhage (see Chap. 55, Dyspnea).

3. *Is there chest pain?*
   Pain is a common symptom after injury to the musculoskeletal chest wall. The pain is usually described as sharp or stabbing and is made worse by deep inspiration or movement of the thorax. Aching or pressurelike pain may be related to injury to the thoracic visceral structures or referred pain from associated injuries.

4. *Are there associated symptoms?*
   Are there other areas of pain and discomfort? Were there symptoms *prior* to the accident? Chest pain or dizziness from myocardial or cerebrovascular disease may have contributed to the accident.
5. *What is the past medical history?*
   Is there a past history of cardiorespiratory disease or previous surgical procedures? When was the patient's last tetanus immunization?
6. *Is there current use of medications or other substances?*
   All medications are noted. Alcohol or drug use is questioned.
7. *Is there a history of allergies?*
   Allergies to medications, contrast materials, or anesthetics are discussed.
8. *When did the patient last eat?*
   This question helps to anticipate the potential for aspiration and is useful for the anesthesiologist and trauma surgeon.

Physical Examination

Table 57–1 summarizes the physical assessment of the patient with chest trauma. Because of the potential for clinical instability of patients with chest trauma, the examination may initially be limited. The importance of repeated evaluation can not be overstressed. The findings and evolution of response to trauma often change.

PROBLEM 1 After tube thoracostomy, the patient remained stable. A more thorough examination was completed. Palpation of the chest wall revealed bony crepitance over the left eighth and ninth ribs at the posterior axillary line. Breath sounds were equal bilaterally. There was minimal tenderness in the left upper quadrant of the abdomen. The left femur was obviously fractured, but there were good distal pulses. The traction splint remained in place. The chest tube was actively draining blood, and a total of 250 ml were measured.

In spite of the current stability of the patient's condition, there are several causes for concern. The active bleeding of the left hemithorax, although not yet sufficient to warrant surgical intervention, raises the possibility of an operative thoracotomy if it continues or increases. Fractures of the lower left ribs with their accompanying abdominal tenderness, no matter how mild at present, raise the suspicion of an intra-abdominal process such as a splenic injury. The femoral fracture is often associated with significant blood loss and complications and also represents the significant force involved in the accident.

DECISION PRIORITIES AND PRELIMINARY DIFFERENTIAL DIAGNOSIS

Throughout the early management of thoracic trauma, the clinician constantly reevaluates the condition of the patient as well as the differential diagnoses of potentially life-threatening problems. The following questions provide a framework for action.

1. *Is the patient currently unstable in spite of resuscitative efforts?*
   Circulatory impairment, massive hemorrhage, and ventilatory insufficiency are the three primary causes of continued instability. Diagnoses to be entertained in this setting include those listed in Table 57–2. Although they are considered during the initial stabilization efforts, because of the potential for rapid changes in chest trauma, each is reconsidered at this point. For example, a hemothorax may be missed because 200 to 400 ml of blood must be lost into the chest cavity before it is detectable on upright chest radiographs. It is often difficult to detect

TABLE 57-1. Physical Examination in Patients with Chest Trauma

Examination	Observation	Comments
Vital Signs		
Pulse	Pulse deficit	Suspect hypovolemia, tamponade, tension pneumothorax, arterial injury
	Tachycardia	Associated with hypovolemia, hypoxemia, increased sympathetic tone
	Bradycardia	A critical sign. May be a *preterminal event* in patients with airway or ventilatory compromise
Blood pressure	Narrow pulse pressure	Early sign of hypovolemia
	Hypertension	Secondary to increased sympathetic tone
	Hypotension	A critical sign. May be secondary to hypovolemia, tension pneumothorax, or cardiac tamponade
Respiratory rate and effort	Tachypnea	Common, insensitive for serious injury. Has multiple causes
	Bradypnea	A critical sign. May be a preterminal event
	Labored	Effort required is indicative of level of respiratory distress
Temperature	Abnormal	Hypothermia is common in trauma victims
General		
Appearance	Skin abnormal	Observe for diaphoresis, pallor, cyanosis
	Wounds	Suspect pneumothorax, cardiac tamponade, or opening to pleural space
HEENT	Upper airway obstruction	Observe for patency and protection of airway, presence of secretions, fractured larynx
	Cervical spine	Palpate for tenderness, deformity. Immobilize until cleared
Neck	Discolored, swollen	Swelling, hematoma. Check position of trachea, carotid pulsations, presence of subcutaneous emphysema, crepitance over fractured larynx
	Distended neck veins	Suspect tamponade, tension pneumothorax
Chest	Contusions, tenderness	Compress thorax gently in the anteroposterior and lateral directions to localize fractured ribs. A flail chest may not be readily apparent
	Asymmetry, hyperresonance, decreased breath sounds	Tension pneumothorax
	Hyporesonance	Hemothorax or other density in chest cavity, e.g., bowel from diaphragmatic rupture
Cardiac	Decreased heart sounds	Usually indicative of shock. Not sensitive for tamponade
	Regurgitant murmurs	Valvular damage, most often mitral or aortic
Abdomen	Tenderness, decreased bowel sounds	Associated intra-abdominal injuries
Neurologic	Decreased consciousness, neurologic deficits	Intracranial trauma and possible peripheral nerve injuries

if the patient remains supine during radiography. If the patient continues to bleed, false security in interpreting the first film may hinder discovery of the problem. Even without changes in the patient's condition, equipment failures can complicate the diagnosis, e.g., a treated tension pneumothorax can reoccur if there is a malfunction of the chest tube apparatus.

2. *What potential life-threatening problems may exist in a currently stable patient?* The injuries listed in Table 57-2 are also considered in this setting. Most patients present in a temporarily stable condition at best, which is followed by rapid deterioration. A particularly insidious injury is traumatic disruption of the aorta. Suspicion for this injury is raised if the patient has sustained a blunt deceleration

TABLE 57–2. Immediately Life-Threatening Injuries in Chest Trauma

Condition	Mechanism of Injury	Vital Signs	Physical Findings	Useful Diagnostic Tests	Initial Management	Comments
Tension pneumothorax	Blunt or penetrating trauma	Hypotension Tachycardia Tachypnea	Respiratory distress Decreased breath sounds and hyperresonance on the affected side Tracheal deviation Subcutaneous emphysema	*None* in the unstable patient Portable anteroposterior CXR—collapsed lung with deviation of mediastinal structure to the opposite side	Needle thoracostomy followed by tube thoracostomy	Chest radiograph is still most common source of diagnosis. Late formation is anticipated in all patients having positive pressure ventilation
Open pneumothorax	Blunt or penetrating trauma	Tachycardia Tachypnea	Respiratory distress Open "sucking" chest wound Decreased breath sounds Subcutaneous emphysema	None for initial diagnosis and treatment	Immediate closure of wound with an airtight or ball-valve type of dressing (e.g., Vaseline gauze) Tube thoracostomy as soon as appropriate Endotracheal intubation and positive pressure ventilation as necessary	Physiologic mechanism is that of a large functional dead space. Function of both lungs is affected
Cardiac tamponade	More common in penetrating trauma; in blunt trauma associated with cardiac rupture	Hypotension Tachycardia Tachypnea Narrow pulse pressure	Muffled heart sounds Distended neck veins Cyanosis of head, neck, upper extremities Triad of muffled heart sounds, elevated venous pressure, and hypotension seen in only 30% of patients	Elevated central venous pressure may be earliest finding None in unstable patients with penetrating trauma in the precordial region	Volume repletion Needle pericardiocentesis Emergency thoracotomy for patients who rapidly deteriorate	Occurs in <2% of chest trauma. Rare after blunt injury. Echocardiography may be useful if patient is stable and there is sufficient blood in pericardial space. Patients can deteriorate rapidly
Large hemo- or hemopneumothorax (>500 ml or continuous hemorrhage)	Blunt or penetrating trauma	Hypotension Tachycardia Tachypnea	Respiratory distress Decreased or absent breath sounds on the affected side May be dullness to percussion	Portable anteroposterior CXR—Fluid density air-fluid level involving entire hemithorax	Tube thoracostomy	Both chest wall vessels and lung parenchyma are sources of bleeding. More often bleeding results from penetrating injury. These patients are autotransfusion candidates. Chest cavity can hold 2000–3000 ml
Aortic disruption	Blunt trauma; usually rapid deceleration injury	May be normal Hypotension Tachycardia Tachypnea	Patients may have *no* signs of major trauma Mechanism of injury more important than clinically obvious chest trauma Upper extremity hypertension, attenuation of femoral pulse may be seen	Portable anteroposterior CXR—highest yield: widened superior mediastinum (>8 cm) or loss of contour of aortic knob	High index of suspicion required Patients with appropriate mechanism of injury and clinical or radiographic findings receive emergency aortic angiography or computed tomography	Only 10–20% of patients arrive alive. In one-third of these exsanguination will occur in 6 hours
Tracheobronchial disruption	Blunt trauma; usually rapid deceleration injury, less often penetrating injury	Tachypnea Tachycardia	Massive subcutaneous emphysema Pneumothorax Pneumomediastinum	Portable anteroposterior CXR; massive SQ and mediastinal air	Airway management Initial tube thoracostomy may be inadequate Bronchoscopy	Rare injury (<3% of chest trauma patients) with high mortality (>30%) Majority occur within 3 cm of carina
Flail chest and pulmonary contusion	Blunt trauma	Tachypnea Tachycardia	Paradoxically moving segment of chest wall Respiratory distress Tenderness or crepitation of chest wall Chest wall bruising	Portable or standard chest radiograph; multiple fracture of adjacent ribs. Infiltrates usually seen within 1–2 hours and always by 4–6 hours after injury Arterial blood gas measurements; hypocarbia and hypercarbia, hypoxemia	Observation Supplemental O_2 Ventilatory support Pain control Anticipation and treatment of pulmonary contusion	Usually three or more ribs fractured at two points. Derangement of chest wall expansion contributes to ventilatory compromise. Contusion characterized by edema and hemorrhage without laceration

CXR = Chest radiograph.

injury to the chest, particularly as an unrestrained driver. The most important first study is the chest radiograph, which is preferably taken in the anteroposterior upright position at a distance of 100 cm. An upper mediastinal width of 8 cm or greater, deviation of the nasogastric tube or trachea to the right of the midline, and loss of the shadow of the aortic knob are three key radiographic signs that require further immediate investigation through computed tomography or angiography. Patients with thoracic trauma can become unstable at any time. Since changes can be subtle, constant monitoring of vital signs is mandatory.

3. *Are there associated injuries or conditions?*

Because of the high association of other injuries with thoracic trauma, a complete assessment is always necessary. One injury with great potential for occult morbidity is the penetrating wound at or below the nipple line. The diaphragm rises up to the fourth intercostal space, and a penetrating injury of the peritoneal cavity may be clinically evident on examination. Other inquiries are related to the mechanism and focus of injury. The most common associated injuries are abdominal (lacerated spleen and liver), craniospinal (subdural and epidural hematomas, cervical spine), and fractures (pelvis, femur).

Patients often have complicating medical illnesses and need to be evaluated for these conditions. The question of "what caused this accident?" cannot be lost in the urgency of management. Myocardial infarction, cerebrovascular accident, hypoglycemia, or a suicide attempt may have precipitated the traumatic event.

Chest trauma often results in a combination of potentially life-threatening injuries. The emergency physician assesses and treats the physiologic derangements while anticipating the underlying pathological conditions. A reasonable rule is always to search for more than one cause of the patient's condition. At a minimum, this rule encourages repeated examination.

PROBLEM 1 The patient continued to bleed actively from the chest tube, and 700 ml had accumulated in approximately one-half hour. She looked less well and slightly pale. Her pulse was 130 beats/min and her blood pressure was 110/90 mm Hg. A chest radiograph showed a well-placed chest tube, an expanded lung, and a poorly defined left hemidiaphragm.

The patient is becoming hemodynamically unstable secondary to continued hemorrhage. She is probably an exception to the 85% of patients with hemothorax who are definitively treated without tube thoracostomy. The emergency physician continues vigorous fluid resuscitation and considers the use of blood products. A decision is then made with the surgical consultant concerning further diagnostic efforts and surgical intervention.

DIAGNOSTIC ADJUNCTS

The use of diagnostic adjuncts is always tempered by the condition of the patient. It is not uncommon for patients to receive definitive care prior to diagnostic testing.

Laboratory Studies

Standard laboratory profiles are obtained for all seriously injured patients. These include complete blood count and differential, serum electrolytes, serum glucose, blood urea nitrogen (BUN) and creatinine, blood for type and cross-match, and urinalysis. Additionally, the patient with thoracic injury usually requires the following studies.

Arterial Blood Gas Measurements. Arterial blood gas samples are obtained early in the care of chest trauma patients who have signs of airway or ventilatory compromise, hemodynamic instability, altered mental status, or a history of significant trauma to the chest. Hypoxemia (PO_2 less than 60 mm Hg on room air) is indicative of a serious derangement of oxygenation. It is often an early finding in patients with pulmonary contusion and a variety of other conditions. Hypercarbia (PCO_2 more than 40 mm Hg) reflects ventilatory insufficiency, which may have a variety of causes, e.g., major hemothorax or pneumothorax, or airway obstruction. Acidemia (pH less than 7.35) may be primarily respiratory or secondary to hypoperfusion and shock. *Pulse oximetry* may be used for continuous monitoring of oxygen levels.

Cardiac Enzyme Levels. The myocardial fraction of creatine kinase (CK-MB) is often measured in patients suspected of having sustained a myocardial contusion. The levels usually peak by 24 hours. A level greater than 5% is considered diagnostic. Unfortunately, patients with normal or minimally elevated CK-MB (less than 2%) have shown significant myocardial wall motion abnormalities consistent with a diagnosis of cardiac contusion. It remains a relatively insensitive test.

Radiologic Imaging

Chest Radiograph. A portable or standard view chest radiograph is obtained as early as possible in the evaluation of all patients with significant thoracic trauma. An upright study is preferable in patients who are not at risk for spinal injury. A pneumothorax and hemothorax may be obscured in the supine position, and the mediastinum may appear falsely widened. The need for chest radiographs should not delay the treatment of a patient with a clinically evident tension or open pneumothorax. Serial radiographs may be useful in evaluating the development or evolution of clinically unapparent pneumothorax or hemothorax. A chest film is also obtained after therapeutic interventions, such as tube thoracostomy or endotracheal intubation, to assess tube position.

Aortography. The selection of patients for contrast aortography to evaluate for traumatic aortic disruption is based on the mechanism of injury, primarily rapid deceleration (falls, motor vehicle accidents) and an abnormal chest radiograph showing:

- Widened mediastinum (more than 8 cm), a sign that is positive in 50% to 85% of patients with aortic disruptions
- Loss of definition of the aortic knob
- Presence of "paraspinal stripe" or apical pleural hematoma
- Loss of the distal aortic shadow
- Displacement of the trachea or the esophagus (nasogastric tube) to the right of the midline
- Depression of the angle of the left main stem bronchus

The first two criteria are most useful, but none is so specific that its absence precludes an aortogram if clinical suspicion is high.

Computed Tomography (CT) of the Chest. Contrast-enhanced CT of the chest has been increasingly useful in diagnosing aortic injury. It can detect the extraluminal hematoma but cannot localize the site of the internal tear. In some centers it is performed before aortography.

Gated Radionuclide Angiogram (MUGA Scan). The MUGA scan is not routinely obtained from the emergency department. It is an excellent diagnostic tool for the patient with suspected cardiac contusion. The scan has a high degree of sensitivity in detecting the segmental wall motion abnormalities characteristic of the condition.

Echocardiography. Two-dimensional and Doppler pulsed echocardiography may assist in the diagnosis of pericardial tamponade and myocardial contusion, and with valvular function abnormalities. In myocardial contusions, findings include right ventricular dilatation and segmental wall motion abnormalities. These studies are obtained relatively easily in patients with chest trauma. Their use in emergency medicine remains to be clearly defined.

Electrocardiography

A standard 12-lead electrocardiogram is obtained in all patients with significant thoracic trauma. Cardiac dysrhythmias often occur as a direct result of myocardial contusion or penetrating cardiac injury. They may be secondary to metabolic derangements such as hypoxemia or acidosis. Rarely, myocardial infarction may result from coronary vascular damage. ECG changes compatible with myocardial contusion include ST–T wave elevation or depression, conduction disturbances, and rhythm disturbances. If positive, ECG findings can support the suspicion of myocardial contusion. A normal ECG does not rule it out. Additionally, a primary myocardial event may have caused the accident, and hypotension or hypoperfusion from any cause may precipitate myocardial ischemia or infarction.

PROBLEM 1 In spite of infusion of 2 liters of isotonic crystalloid and 2 units of type-specific blood, the patient's pulse rose to 140 beats/min and her blood pressure was 100/80 mm Hg. Her original hematocrit was 32%. Arterial blood gas results were Po_2 130 mm Hg on 8 liters of oxygen, a Pco_2 of 38 mm Hg, and a pH of 7.31. She was increasingly restless, and the chest tube had drained 900 ml of blood. She began to complain of abdominal pain, and the abdomen was significantly more tender.

At this point, the patient requires surgical intervention for hemorrhage control and clearer delineation of the extent of her injuries. Although diagnostic peritoneal lavage and computed tomography of the abdomen are considered, both the emergency physician and the surgeon agree that little information is to be gained from these studies. She is rapidly prepared for transport to the operating suite.

REFINED DIFFERENTIAL DIAGNOSIS

After the immediately life-threatening disorders are managed or ruled out, a number of potentially serious injuries are considered. The diagnoses of diaphragmatic rupture, myocardial contusion, simple pneumothorax, hemothorax, sternal fracture, and rib fracture are outlined in Table 57–3. These entities can cause morbidity and even mortality for the patient if appropriate therapeutic modalities are not instituted.

PRINCIPLES OF MANAGEMENT
General Principles

Airway Management. Early, aggressive airway control and constant airway monitoring are essential to patient survival (see Chapter 2). Supplemental oxygen therapy is initially administered to all patients with thoracic injuries. Continued therapy is guided by arterial blood gas analysis results. Indications for intubation and ventilatory support include (1) Pao_2 of less than 55 mm Hg on room air; (2) $Paco_2$ greater than 50 mm Hg in previously eucapneic patients; (3) respiratory rate of greater than 40/min; (4) inability to protect airway; and (5) need for intubation to provide anesthesia for operative procedures.

Volume Resuscitation. Volume resuscitation follows the same guidelines given in Chapter 4. Close monitoring of the volume is important in lung injuries because of potential adult respiratory distress syndrome (ARDS) complications.

Monitoring and Recognition of Immediately Life-Threatening Disorders. Rapid recognition and management of respiratory and cardiovascular insufficiency from any cause are essential for patient survival. Constant vigilance is mandatory throughout the course of the patient's management.

Specific Thoracic Injuries

Tension Pneumothorax. Most of the information pertaining to tension pneumothorax is listed in Table 57–2. The absence of near-complete reexpansion of the lung on chest radiograph or a massive air leak as manifested by increasing subcutaneous emphysema and continuous air collection in the chest tube drainage system is an indicator of possible tracheal or bronchial injury. Further evaluation by flexible bronchoscopy and treatment with an additional chest tube are necessary.

Open Pneumothorax. If a tension pneumothorax develops after occlusion of the chest wall defect, immediate decompression by briefly opening the occlusive dressing is required. A chest tube is inserted at a remote site as soon as clinically feasible to ensure continued lung expansion.

Cardiac Tamponade. Patients with penetrating thoracic trauma and suspected cardiac tamponade who respond initially to pericardiocentesis and then deteriorate or who do not respond at all, are candidates for emergency thoracotomy.

Massive Hemothorax or Hemopneumothorax. Initial chest tube drainage of 1000 ml of blood or continued drainage of 200 ml of blood/hr for the first 3 hours is indicative of significant injury and warrants operative thoracotomy.

Pulmonary Contusion or Flail Chest. Partial ventilatory support using intermittent mandatory ventilation (IMV) and positive end-expiratory pressure (PEEP) is the most effective means of treatment for these patients.

Myocardial Contusion. There is no evidence that prophylactic antidysrhythmic therapy is beneficial.

Rib Fracture. Narcotic analgesia improves ventilatory effort and is the only intervention required in the majority of patients. The use of external stabilization devices such as rib belts and tape is discouraged. They may provide some measure of pain relief, but they significantly limit the expansion of the chest and may predispose the patient to atelectasis and pneumonia. If used at all, their use should be limited to young, otherwise healthy patients with isolated rib fractures.

SPECIAL CONSIDERATIONS

Pediatric Patients

The management of thoracic injuries is the same in the child as in the adult. The increased elasticity of the chest wall in the child makes injuries to the bony thorax less common, but abdominal injuries occur more often.

Geriatric Patients

As in children, the pathophysiology of thoracic injuries in the geriatric patient is not unique. The older patient has less physiologic reserve and is more likely to have significant underlying disease. Elderly patients with thoracic trauma require aggressive monitoring and are frequently admitted for further observation.

DISPOSITION AND FOLLOW-UP

Since operative intervention may be required, consultation with the appropriate surgical specialist is obtained early in the evaluation and management of the thoracic trauma patient in unstable condition. Disposition of the critically injured patient may depend on the facilities available at a particular institution. Patients requiring operative thoracotomy, cardiopulmonary bypass, or specialized critical care support are best treated at a regional trauma center.

Admission to Critical Care Facilities

Critically ill patients require skilled continuous care for an optimal outcome. Patients with the following conditions initially receive close hemodynamic and cardiorespiratory monitoring:

TABLE 57–3. Less Potentially Serious Injuries in Chest Trauma

Condition	Mechanism of Injury	Vital Signs	Physical Findings	Useful Diagnostic Tests	Initial Management	Comment
Diaphragmatic rupture	Blunt trauma	If severe, tachypnea Tachycardia	May be respiratory distress, dullness to percussion, bowel sounds in affected hemithorax. Most often no specific symptoms	Portable or standard chest radiograph—signs may vary from gastrointestinal gas pattern in hemithorax to blurred diaphragmatic margins. Diagnosis may be aided by contrast studies. Arterial blood gas measurements show hypoxemia, hypercarbia	Supplemental O_2 Ventilatory support Operative repair	Usually results from abdominal compression into chest. 95% occur on the left side. Can be very subtle and is often discovered later. Complications are bowel obstruction or strangulation
Myocardial contusion	Blunt trauma, usually deceleration injuries	Dysrhythmias including sinus tachycardia (70% of cases), premature atrial or ventricular beats. Rarely, ventricular tachycardia or fibrillation, otherwise dependent on associated injuries	Dependent on associated injury. About 75% of patients with same finding: rib fracture, pulmonary contusion, sternal fracture	ECG—Initial and serial 12-lead ECG needed to document dysrhythmias, conduction disturbance (RBBB most common), or ST-T wave changes. Often appear after 24 hr. Changes may be due to other diseases. CPK-MB—Initial and serial determination. Usually peaks in 24 hours. Level >5% significant. MUGA scan—Not available in ED. Two-dimensional echocardiogram—Excellent sensitivity	Observation Continuous cardiac monitoring Standard pharmacologic therapy for dysrhythmias	Occurs in about 10% of patients with chest trauma. Difficult clinical diagnosis. Major concerns are complications—dysrhythmias, cardiac and valve rupture, coronary vessel injury. May evolve into traumatic myocardial infarction. Most contusions do not result in clinically significant myocardial impairment
Simple pneumothorax	Blunt or penetrating trauma	Tachypnea Tachycardia	May be respiratory distress (>50% have dyspnea and chest pain) Absent or decreased breath sounds on the affected side Hyperresonance to percussion Trachea in midline (no mediastinal shift)	Portable or standard chest radiograph—shows presence of extrapleural air shadow. Note size as percentage of lung volume	Observation if less than 5% Catheter aspiration or tube thoracostomy if less than 15% Tube thoracostomy if greater than 20% or if patient in distress or requires surgery or mechanical ventilation	Occurs in 10%–30% of patients with blunt chest trauma and almost 100% (to some degree) of those with penetrating trauma

Condition	Mechanism	Signs/Symptoms	Physical/Diagnostic Findings	Management	Comments
Hemothorax	Blunt or penetrating trauma	Tachycardia Tachypnea	"Effusion" line of dullness to percussion Decreased breath sounds at base	Portable or standard chest radiograph—200 ml of blood necessary to be seen. Supine view may make diagnosis difficult. Costophrenic angle blunting is earliest finding. Repeated chest views may be useful	Volume resuscitation as necessary Tube thoracostomy in most cases	Often seen with pneumothorax, usually self-limited. Tube thoracostomy suitable for almost all cases
Sternal fracture	Significant blunt trauma, usually anterior (e.g., steering wheel)	Tachypnea	Tenderness and pain over sternum	Lateral radiograph of sternum ECG—changes characteristic of myocardial contusion	Search for associated injury Analgesia as allowable	Seen in <5% of chest trauma patients, usually due to severe trauma. Because of this, there may be mortality of up to 30% from associated injuries. High association with myocardial contusion or rupture, pulmonary contusion
Rib fracture	Blunt trauma	Tachypnea Tachycardia	Tenderness, crepitation of chest wall May be respiratory distress	Standard chest radiographs—More than 50% of simple fractures missed on initial standard view. Ordered to evaluate for complications: hemothorax, pneumothorax, pulmonary contusion. Rib views rarely necessary Arterial blood gas measurements—Ordered to check for evidence of respiratory compromise or underlying pulmonary disease (e.g., COPD)	Observation Analgesia Elderly patients and patients with significant cardiopulmonary disease are admitted and observed	Accounts for 50% of injuries in cases of blunt chest trauma. Increased morbidity associated with increasing age, number of fractures, and location of fractures. More common in adults. Fractures of the first and second ribs require significant trauma and mandate careful evaluation for associated injuries. Great vessels, lung, and bronchial plexus are at risk. High morbidity if associated with other injuries, including other rib fractures. Fractures of ribs 9–11 can cause intra-abdominal injuries, e.g., splenic puncture

1. Tension pneumothorax
2. Open pneumothorax (postoperative as necessary)
3. Cardiac tamponade
4. Postoperative thoracotomy
5. Flail chest or pulmonary contusion
6. Myocardial contusion, sternal fracture
7. First or second rib fracture
8. Hemothorax (initially more than 500 ml of blood or with continued hemorrhage)

Patients with simple pneumothoraces or small hemothoraces (500 ml or less without continued hemorrhage) who are hemodynamically stable may be safely observed in a "step-down" unit or other monitored bed.

Admission

Patients with rib fractures may require admission. Most are treated in a noncritical care setting. Patients in this category include (1) elderly or cardiorespiratory disease patients with isolated fractures, (2) those with inward displacement of jagged fragments, and (3) those with multiple (more than three) rib fractures.

Discharge

Patients with minor blunt trauma, such as isolated rib fractures in an otherwise healthy patient, who remain clinically stable after emergency department observation are discharged with follow-up arranged in 24 to 48 hours. Sufficient analgesia and an awareness of the patient's support system are important concerns when considering discharge.

PROBLEM 1 At surgery a single lacerated intercostal artery was found to be the source of the continued bleeding. The fractured ribs were the only thoracic injuries found. Abdominal laparotomy revealed a small splenic laceration that was repaired without sacrificing the spleen. The patient was transferred to the critical care unit for continued evaluation and monitoring.

In 85% of cases, reexpansion of the lung by means of tube thoracostomy stops bleeding from the pulmonary parenchyma or thoracic cage. Significant hemorrhage from an intercostal artery is not uncommon. The associated splenic injury is typical of this type of injury.

PROBLEM 2 In the operating suite the heart and major vessels were explored for other injuries. No other injuries were found. The primary cardiac wound was repaired without difficulty, and, at the time of discharge from the operating suite, the patient had a pulse of 100 beats/min and a blood pressure of 110/80 mm Hg. He recovered uneventfully and was discharged from the hospital in 8 days.

Although not a common occurrence, patients with direct myocardial trauma can be salvaged by an aggressive team effort in diagnosis and treatment.

DOCUMENTATION

1. Mechanism and forces of injury
2. Prehospital presentation and interventions
3. Specific symptoms, e.g., chest pain, dyspnea
4. Vital signs initially and throughout course of care
5. Pertinent physical examination findings
6. Radiographic, ECG, and laboratory findings

7. Patient response to interventions
8. Results of consultation with surgeon or other specialists
9. Diagnosis of extent and types of injury
10. Disposition and follow-up

SUMMARY AND FINAL POINTS

- The mechanism of trauma can be predictive of the type of injury that will be encountered.
- Only 10% to 15% of patients with thoracic trauma require thoracotomy. The remainder can be appropriately managed in the emergency department.
- Tension pneumothorax, open pneumothorax, and cardiac tamponade are the three rapidly reversible, life-threatening disorders that every emergency physician must strive to recognize and treat appropriately.
- Needle thoracostomy can be lifesaving for patients with tension pneumothorax. It is followed by tube thoracostomy.
- The only measure of success for pericardiocentesis in cardiac tamponade is the restoration of blood pressure. This procedure is frequently unsuccessful, and emergency thoracotomy is often necessary.
- A chest radiograph is obtained only after initial efforts are made to stabilize the patient with thoracic trauma. Tension pneumothorax, open pneumothorax, and cardiac tamponade are diagnosed by clinical assessment.
- Myocardial contusion is not uncommon in patients with blunt thoracic trauma. It is rarely associated with significant morbidity or mortality.
- Thoracotomy is indicated in massive hemothorax or continued hemorrhage after tube thoracostomy.
- Most patients with thoracic trauma—penetrating or blunt—are admitted to the hospital. Exceptions include single rib fractures in otherwise healthy patients or minor chest wall contusions.

BIBLIOGRAPHY

Texts

1. Hurst JM (ed): Common Problems in Trauma. Chicago, Year Book, 1987.
2. Mattox K, Moore E, Feliciano D (eds): Trauma. New York, Appleton-Century-Crofts, 1986.

Journal Articles

1. Barone JE, Pizzi WF, Nealon TF, et al: Indications for intubation in blunt chest trauma. J Trauma 26:334–338, 1986.
2. Beel T, Harwood AC: Traumatic rupture of the thoracic aorta. Ann Emerg Med 9:483–488, 1980.
3. Dubrow TJ: Myocardial contusion in the stable patient: What level of care is appropriate? Surgery 106:267–273, 1989.
4. Helling TS, Gyles NR III, Eisenstein CL, Soracco CA: Complications following blunt and penetrating injuries in 216 victims of chest trauma requiring tube thoracostomy. J Trauma 29(10):1367–1370, 1989.
5. Nakayama DK, Ramenofsky ML, Rome MI: Chest injuries in childhood. Ann Surg 210(6):770–775, 1989.
6. Richardson JD: Indications for thoracotomy in thoracic trauma. Curr Surg 42:361–364, 1985.
7. Shackford SR: Blunt chest trauma: The intensivist's perspective. J Intensive Care Med 1:125–136, 1986.
8. Sturm JT, et al: Significance of symptoms and signs in patients with traumatic aortic rupture. Ann Emerg Med 13:876–878, 1984.
9. Tenzer ML: The spectrum of myocardial contusion: A review. J Trauma 25:620–627, 1985.
10. Trinkle JK, Toon RS, Franz JL, et al: Affairs of the wounded heart: Penetrating cardiac wounds. J Trauma 19:467–472, 1979.
11. Washington B, Wilson RF, Steiger Z, et al: Emergency thoracotomy: A four year review. Ann Thorac Surg 40:188–196, 1985.

SECTION SIXTEEN

UROGENITAL DISORDERS

CHAPTER 58

DYSURIA

MICHAEL EARL, M.D.
ALEXANDER T. TROTT, M.D.

PROBLEM A 21 year old woman came to the emergency department with the complaint of 2 days of pain on urination associated with lower abdominal pain and a blood-tinged appearance of the urine.

QUESTIONS TO CONSIDER

1. What disorders can cause dysuria?
2. What factors help differentiate between upper and lower urinary tract infection (UTI)?
3. What groups of patients are at greatest risk for developing upper urinary tract infections (pyelonephritis)?
4. How can the clinical laboratory establish the diagnosis of urinary tract infection? What role does a urine culture play in the treatment of UTI in the outpatient setting?
5. Once UTI is established, what antibiotics are appropriate and for how long should they be administered?
6. Which patients with UTI are admitted to the hospital?

INTRODUCTION

Dysuria is the symptom of painful or difficult urination. The pain originates in the mucosa and is generally localized to the bladder and urethra. Dysuria is a common presenting complaint accounting for up to 5 million ambulatory care visits each year. The vast majority of these patients are female. The estimated incidence of dysuria in the adult female population is reported to be as high as 25% per year. Urinary tract infection is the most common cause of dysuria and the second most common infectious disease the emergency physician encounters. Therefore, it is the emphasis of this chapter.

The definition of what constitutes a urinary tract infection, the ability to localize this infection accurately on the basis of history or physical examination, and the optimum duration of antibiotic therapy have undergone many changes in the last 10 years. These issues remain somewhat controversial, but a rational clinical approach to this problem is available.

The urinary tract extends from the kidneys to the proximal urethra. Understanding the natural defense mechanisms that maintain its normal sterility can clarify why some individuals are more predisposed to infections causing dysuria.

A normal micturition frequency and complete bladder emptying are the most crucial mechanisms for preventing infection. Anatomic barriers to infection include the mucopolysaccharide lining of the bladder, an angled ureterocystic junction that helps prevent urinary reflux, and urethral length. Obstruction along any part of the urinary tract predisposes to infection. Its origin can be physiologic, such as a gravid uterus impeding normal ureteral flow, or pathologic, such as renal stones. Conditions that interfere with normal bladder innervation such as spinal cord injury, multiple sclerosis, tabes dorsalis, or diabetes mellitus may result in incomplete bladder emptying, urinary stasis, and increased risk of UTI.

Vesicoureteral reflux, often the result of an abnormal ureterocystic junction, is relatively common in childhood and may account for up to 50% of UTIs in this age group. Urethral length is an important barrier that separates the sterile bladder from the coliform bacteria that normally colonize the perineum. This additional length is thought to be largely responsible for the relative infrequency of UTIs in men throughout most of life. Urethral catheterization, especially indwelling catheters, circumvent these normal barriers.

Periurethral and introital colonization with coliforms of increased virulence occur in certain women. This hypervirulence is thought to be related to enhanced bacterial adherence capabilities. The absence of normal periurethral antibodies may also be a factor in women who have increased frequency of UTI.

INITIAL APPROACH IN THE EMERGENCY DEPARTMENT

The dysuric patient's evaluation starts by ensuring hemodynamic stability. The first nurse or physician evaluator should be alerted by a history that includes fever, flank pain, and vomiting. These symptoms are suggestive of a systemic and potentially serious illness, especially in the elderly or debilitated patient. Vital signs are obtained without delay in these patients. Hypotension or tachycardia suggests possible sepsis or volume depletion secondary to protracted vomiting. Mental status changes, also suggestive of sepsis, may be the only symptom in the elderly patient with UTI. For the ill or septic-appearing patient, the following initial steps are taken prior to performing a more comprehensive work-up:

1. Adequate ventilation is ensured. Supplementary oxygen is given at 4 to 6 liters/min.
2. Vital signs, including orthostatic measurements as appropriate, are obtained.
3. An intravenous line with an isotonic crystalloid infusate is started.
4. Cardiac monitoring is established.
5. Basic blood samples are collected to perform a complete blood count, electrolyte measurements, renal function profile, and a blood culture.
6. A pregnancy test is done in a woman of childbearing age.
7. A properly collected urine specimen is obtained.

When either localization of the source of dysuria or accurate identification of the offending organism is crucial, bladder catheterization or, more rarely, suprapubic aspiration is considered. Patients who are incontinent or at the extremes of age and females with vaginal discharge are all candidates for these active urine collection methods. Both straight catheterization and suprapubic bladder aspiration, although invasive, are procedures that pose minimal risk to the patient. Iatrogenic infection, introduced by straight catheterization, occurs in approximately 1% of patients. Newer and smaller diameter catheters (mini-cath), designed just to collect urine specimens, have much lower rates of infection. Suprapubic aspiration is well tolerated and is also a low-risk procedure in experienced hands with properly selected patients.

PROBLEM Initial questioning by the nurse revealed that the patient's abdominal pain was not severe and she had no vomiting. The patient affirmed that the blood was coming from the urinary tract. Her last menses was 2 weeks earlier and was normal. The patient appeared alert and in no obvious distress. Vital signs were blood pressure 120/80 mm Hg, pulse 80 beats/min, temperature 96.7°F (37°C). A clean-catch urine specimen was collected and sent to the laboratory. She was placed in a regular examination room and the chart put in order behind other charts of stable patients.

This brief evaluation was appropriately directed toward potential life-threatening processes and hemodynamic instability. Neither the history, patient appearance, nor vital signs alerted the nurse to an unstable condition. A correct decision was made to triage the patient to a regular examination room.

DATA GATHERING

In addition to determining the general condition of the patient, the history and physical examination are focused on identifying the cause of dysuria and, if in the urinary tract, the location of the problem.

History

1. *What is the character of the discomfort?*
   True "burning" on urination occurs more commonly in cystitis and urethritis and when the introitus is inflamed. Lower abdominal discomfort may be the only sign of a UTI. Localization of the symptoms is very important. Many women are able to differentiate the external irritation of urine passing over inflamed introital tissue, caused by vaginitis, from the internal discomfort of cystitis. Flank pain is the hallmark of pyelonephritis but is present in only 50% of patients.
2. *What is the duration of symptoms?*
   Symptoms lasting longer than 7 days suggest pyelonephritis, nonbacterial urethritis, or vaginitis. Most uncomplicated bacterial cystitis in women will resolve spontaneously prior to this time. Some authorities state that UTI symptoms of 48 hours or longer define a complicated UTI.
3. *Are there associated symptoms?*
   Systemic toxicity, as indicated by high fever or vomiting, increases the suspicion of pyelonephritis. Localization studies of infection have shown that over 50% of patients with pyelonephritis do not have signs of systemic toxicity. Conversely, 5% of patients with simple cystitis may have symptoms such as fever and vomiting. Vaginal discharge suggests possible vaginitis or pelvic inflammatory disease.
4. *Is the patient currently taking antibiotics?*
   Patients with dysuria often obtain antibiotics from a variety of sources and self-medicate themselves prior to their arrival. The urinalysis of a partially treated UTI may be uninterpretable, and a urine culture is almost useless in this setting. Use of broad-spectrum antibiotics may also increase the risk of candidal vaginitis, another cause of dysuria. Inquiry is also made about whether the patient has been taking chronic suppressive antibiotic therapy for frequent UTIs.
5. *Have there been similar symptoms in the past?*
   Women may relate a history of frequent prior UTIs. Discovering when the last episode occurred may help to establish whether reinfection or treatment failure has occurred. No precise definition exists as to what length of time should transpire before a subsequent infection is classified as a reinfection as opposed to a persistent infection. Less than 1% of frequent UTIs are felt to be due to persistent infection. Reinfection is the most common cause of recurrent symptoms.
6. *Is there a contributing past medical history?*
   Diabetics with bacteriuria not only have a higher incidence of pyelonephritis but also are more likely to have complications of renal invasion such as perinephric abscess and renal papillary necrosis. Patients with sickle cell disease and those with a history of nonsteroidal anti-inflammatory overuse also are predisposed to papillary necrosis and ureteral obstruction from tissue sloughing.

Physical Examination

Vital Signs. Tachycardia, hypotension, or altered mental status, as mentioned previously, suggests sepsis or volume depletion. Fever is a significant finding as well and occurs most often in patients with pyelonephritis.

Flank Examination. Costovertebral angle (CVA) tenderness and fever are often seen with pyelonephritis. These findings are, however, surprisingly insensitive and certainly not pathognomonic for pyelonephritis. Pyelonephritis may exist without CVA tenderness, and cystitis, in a small percentage of cases, may show that sign.

Abdominal Examination. The goal of the abdominal examination is to attempt to palpate the kidneys. Normally a difficult task, even in thin patients, a prominence may suggest a pathologic process, such as a polycystic kidney or severe hydronephrosis. Normally the bladder is not palpable or percussable. When 500 ml or more of urine is present, the bladder becomes an abdominal organ in adults, and percussion may reveal its presence.

Male Genitals. This examination focuses on the prostate, testes, epididymis, and urethral meatus. Tenderness, edema, erythema, or discharge is noted.

Pelvis. A pelvic examination is required if vaginal discharge, abdominal pain, or an atypical history of UTI is obtained. Pelvic pathology is sought routinely because urethritis secondary to a venereal pathogen such as *Neisseria gonorrhoeae* or *Chlamydia trachomatis* may coexist with pelvic inflammatory disease. A purulent cervical discharge or adnexal tenderness raises the suspicion that a venereal pathogen is the cause of dysuria. Cervical and periurethral cultures for *N. gonorrhoeae* and *C. trachomatis* are obtained. The vaginal introitus and canal are inspected for evidence of inflammation; a wet mount is examined microscopically for yeast, *Trichomonas*, and "clue" cells.

PROBLEM The patient reported that the pain was a dull ache that became worse when she urinated. It was accompanied by the dysuria. Although she had no nausea or vomiting, her appetite was decreased. In the past she had been treated for a bladder infection but had no other remarkable illnesses or conditions. On examination, she was slightly warm to the touch. There was no flank pain and only mild abdominal tenderness to palpation of the suprapubic area. A pelvic examination was normal.

Of particular note during this patient's examination was the fact that she felt slightly warm. This finding did not match the recorded temperature. Because of the importance of fever in deciding on the extent of infection in the urinary tract, a rectal temperature is recommended.

DECISION PRIORITIES AND PRELIMINARY DIFFERENTIAL DIAGNOSIS

Following the history and physical examination, the emergency physician addresses the following question: *Does the patient have an extraurinary cause of the dysuria?*

Dysuria can be caused by vaginitis, prostatitis, pelvic disorders, or abdominal pathology. Results of the abdominal and pelvic examinations direct the physician to specific pathology such as ectopic pregnancy, pelvic inflammatory disease, or acute appendicitis. Chapter 5 reviews the differential diagnosis of abdominal pain, whereas Chapter 59 focuses on the patient with pelvic pain. Vaginitis is a relatively common cause of dysuria. The dysuria may be perceived as an external sensation as urine passes through an inflamed labia. Such patients complain of a vaginal discharge and irritation. The diagnosis of vaginitis is reviewed in Chapter 61.

Although the history and physical examination direct attention to extraurinary causes of dysuria, the emergency physician turns to the clinical laboratory to determine whether the symptom is originating from the urinary tract.

DIAGNOSTIC ADJUNCTS

Laboratory Studies

The diagnosis of urinary tract infection in the emergency department hinges on finding evidence of inflammatory changes in the urine. The microscopic and colorimetric tests for diagnosis are all rapidly and easily performed.

Urinary Dipstick Analysis. With the emphasis on cost containment and the need for a rapid, accurate indicator of UTI, urinary dipstick analysis as a screening aid has enjoyed wide acceptance. The nitrite test is the oldest and least sensitive of the colorimetric screening tests. Bacteria reduce nitrates to nitrites, which react with the dipstick reagent. For this reaction to occur, urine must be in contact with coliform bacteria in the bladder for at least 4 hours; therefore, the early morning urine specimen is the most reliable. Reported sensitivities of this test compared to positive urine cultures range from 11% for random collected urine to 44% for first-voided morning specimens. Although this test suffers from a low sensitivity, the predictive value of a positive test result is 72%.

The leukocyte esterase test is another colorimetric dipstick study employed in the detection of UTI. This test can detect the presence of leukocytes in urine by virtue of their esterase activity. This esterase activity is not normally found in serum, urine, or kidney tissue. The leukocyte esterase strip is both qualitative and to a large extent quantitative, producing a color change with an intensity that is grossly proportional to the concentration of leukocytes present in fresh uncentrifuged urine. The commercially available strip will detect both intact and lysed leukocytes without apparent interference by medications, urine osmolarity, pH, protein, or renal function. Sensitivity in detecting leukocytes is reported to range from 74% to 96% and specificity from 94% to 98% when compared with culture results.

Urinary dipstick analysis is recommended as a rapid screening method for detecting UTI in otherwise healthy, nonpregnant dysuric women. A positive nitrite result or a positive result of the leukocyte esterase test in an uncentrifuged, uncontaminated (no epithelial cells) urine sample is highly suggestive of UTI. Vaginal contamination of the sample, as evidenced by epithelial cells, reduces the predictive value of a positive test result.

Microscopic Urinalysis. The presence of significant pyuria in a noncontaminated urine specimen is the current gold standard for the diagnosis of infection. Significant pyuria is defined as 2 to 5 white blood cells (WBCs) per high power field in centrifuged urine. The presence of pyuria correlates with bacteriuria and justifies therapy. Pyuria is found in 90% to 95% of symptomatic patients with UTIs of the lower urinary tract. Conversely, less than 1% of asymptomatic nonbacteriuric patients have pyuria. The urine is also examined microscopically for WBC casts, which indicate upper urinary tract infection or pyelonephritis.

The presence of bacteria on urinalysis is a less reliable predictor of infection. Bacteria may not be visible microscopically despite urinary culture concentrations of 10,000 to 100,000 bacteria/ml. Normal vaginal flora such as the rod-shaped lactobacilli may be misidentified as a gram-negative enteric urinary pathogen. Additionally, up to 30% of those with dysuria and bacteriuria based on microscopic examination have sterile urine cultures. With these caveats, the presence of any gram-negative rods on high power field examination of uncentrifuged urine has a sensitivity of 93% and a specificity of 88% in predicting a urine culture of greater than 100,000 bacteria/ml. The presence of both pyuria and bacteriuria has a very high predictive value for infection.

Urine Culture. The long-held threshold for diagnosing infection by culture has been 100,000 bacteria/ml. Recent investigations have found this number to be poorly sensitive. Up to one-third of symptomatic patients with coliform bacteria isolated on suprapubic aspirate will have less than 100,000 bacteria/ml. Reasons for this poor correlation may include partial obstruction below the site of infection, a dilutional effect of diuresis following large fluid intake, the inhibiting action of periurethral cleansing agents, prior antibiotic therapy, early infection, or a low urine pH. Additionally, infection with more fastidious organisms such as *Staphylococcus saprophyticus*, which can be isolated in up to 28% of sexually active young females with UTI, commonly have less than 100,000 bacteria/ml on clean-catch urine. It is important to remember that the original criteria used for differentiating infection from contamination applied to coliform bacteria only.

Routine urine culture in all patients with dysuria is not recommended. In addition to concern about accuracy, cost is a limiting factor to using urine culture as a screening method. It ranges from $35 to $60 and contributes significantly to the average cost of diagnosis and treatment of UTI, $80 to $140. From a practical standpoint, the turnaround time of 24 to 48 hours makes the routine urine culture an inefficient use of resources in an ambulatory care setting. The routine use of sensitivity testing of common antibacterials against the isolated pathogen also is of little value because therapeutic failures are uncommon and most failures are manifested by persistent symptomatology.

Patients at risk for pyelonephritis or sepsis who present with urinary symptoms such as dysuria, frequency, urgency, or suprapubic pain should always have a urine culture performed to identify the offending agent accurately.

Microscopic Examination of Discharge. In patients with a vaginal or penile discharge on examination, smears for *Trichomonas*, *Candida*, and "clue cells" are made. A Gram stain of any cervical or expressed urethral discharge in the male is examined to look for gram-negative intracellular diplococci if the diagnosis of gonorrheal urethritis needs to be confirmed. Failure to see organisms points to chlamydial or *Ureaplasma urealyticum* urethritis.

Cultures. Cultures for gonorrhea and *Chlamydia* are often useful. Chapter 61 reviews the specifics of these diagnostic adjuncts.

Complete Blood Count and Differential. A complete blood count and differential are indicated in patients who appear systemically ill with fever, flank pain, nausea, and vomiting. The presence of leukocytosis and a shift to the left can help in the evaluation of systemic infection and dictate treatment. This may be especially important in elderly and pregnant patients.

Renal Function Tests. Creatinine and blood urea nitrogen (BUN) are not routinely ordered in dysuric patients who do not have systemic symptoms consistent with sepsis. A similar statement applies to serum electrolyte measurements.

PROBLEM Urinalysis results were as follows:

Dipstick	Microscopic Examination
Leukocyte esterase, 2+	WBC, 20–25/HPF
Nitrite, negative	RBC, 25–50/HPF
Blood, 1+	Squamous epithelial cells, 1–2/HPF
Glucose, negative	Bacteria, 2+

These results clearly implicate the urinary tract as the site of infection. A key finding is the low number of squamous epithelial cells. A number of these cells (more than 5 to 10/HPF) is indicative of contamination of the specimen by the perineum or vagina. If the squamous epithelial cell count is high, a "mini-cath" catheterization for a second specimen is indicated.

REFINED DIFFERENTIAL DIAGNOSIS

The most common urinary tract cause of dysuria is infection. Infection can be divided into four separate entities: pyelonephritis, subclinical pyelonephritis, cystitis, and urethritis (see Table 58–1). A small percentage of patients present with dysuria and have no evidence of infection such as pyuria, bacteriuria, or culturable microbial pathogens. In these patients a variety of causes for dysuria are possible including chemical irritation

TABLE 58–1. Differential Diagnosis of Dysuria: Clinical and Laboratory Findings

Suspected Cause and Clinical Findings	Diagnostic Tests and Expected Results
Acute pyelonephritis Fever, rigors, nausea, vomiting, flank pain, costovertebral angle tenderness	Urinalysis: Pyuria and bacteriuria Urine culture: >100,000 bacteria/ml Urine Gram stain: Gram-negative bacilli or gram-positive cocci

Subclinical pyelonephritis
  Underlying urinary tract disease
  Diabetes mellitus
  Immunocompromised state
  Urinary infections before age 12
  Symptoms for 7 to 10 days before seeking care
  Documented relapsing infection with same organisms at any time in the past year
	Urinalysis: Pyuria and bacteriuria
	Urine culture: >100,000 bacteria/ml

Lower urinary tract (cystitis) bacterial infection None of the above clinical indicators, but presence of pyuria	Urinalysis: Pyuria and bacteriuria

Urethritis—*Chlamydia*
  Sexual partner with recent urethritis
  New sexual partner
  Stuttering onset of symptoms
  Absence of hematuria
  Mucopurulent cervical discharge with edematous exocervix
	Urinalysis: Pyuria without bacteriuria, culture for *Chlamydia*

Urethritis—Gonococcal
  Sexual partner with recent urethritis
  Recent history of documented gonorrhea in patient or sexual partner
	Urinalysis: Pyuria without bacteriuria
	Gram stain of purulent discharge from urethral or cervical os: Gram-negative intracellular diplococci
	Culture for *Neisseria gonorrhoeae*

Vaginitis Symptoms of vaginal discharge, itch, or irritation (always ask about such symptoms; patient may not volunteer)	Vaginal examination: Abnormal discharge Microscopic examination of abnormal discharge: Budding yeast and pseudohyphae, trichomonads, "clue cells"
No apparent infectious pathogen None of the above clinical indicators and absence of pyuria	Urinalysis: No pyuria, no bacteriuria

(spermacides), mechanical irritation, and psychogenic causes. In the future, specific etiologic agents may be discovered as the cause of dysuria in these patients.

Pyelonephritis

Pyelonephritis is a bacterial infection of the upper urinary tract, specifically the kidney parenchyma. In contrast to the simple lower UTI, in which infection is usually limited to the mucosa, tissue invasion has occurred that frequently results in systemic toxicity. Classically, symptoms of fever, chills, flank pain (which may radiate to the groin), myalgias, and vomiting are present. Bacteremia is infrequent in young healthy women and children but has been described in up to 50% of neonates and up to two-thirds of elderly patients during an episode of pyelonephritis.

Pyelonephritis is a serious disease in those at the extremes of age. Gram-negative sepsis in the elderly most frequently originates from the urinary tract. During infancy and early childhood the disease is most difficult to diagnose and also presents the greatest risk of renal scarring. Largely because the infection goes unrecognized, it is estimated that 20% to 30% of patients who have pyelonephritis during early childhood (under 3 years of age) eventually develop end-stage renal disease.

Subclinical Pyelonephritis

Subclinical pyelonephritis is an upper urinary tract infection with an absence of systemic toxicity. This form of upper tract disease has been shown to be relatively common. Its frequency among women presenting to a general medical clinic with only dysuria may be 30% and as high as 80% in indigent inner city women. Distinguishing subclinical pyelonephritis from lower urinary tract infection can be done through bilateral ureteral catheterizations, bladder washout techniques, or assays for antibody-coated bacteria. None of the preceding techniques is readily available or practical in the emergency department. The difficulty for the emergency physician lies in attempting to define this subset. Currently, other than demonstrating white blood cell casts in urinary sediment, there is no practical way of establishing upper tract infection conclusively in the absence of toxicity. However, there are risk factors that guide the clinician in revealing patients at risk for this form of upper tract disease. These risk factors are listed under subclinical pyelonephritis in Table 58–1. A patient with any of these risk factors who has pyuria or white blood cell casts in the urine requires a full course of 10 days of antibiotics as well as pre- and post-treatment urine cultures.

Cystitis

Cystitis is traditionally diagnosed in patients with urinary symptoms such as dysuria, frequency, and urgency without systemic toxicity and with a culture result of greater than 100,000 bacteria/ml. A series of studies done in the early 1980s challenged this definition by finding that in 46% of acutely dysuric women with "negative" urine cultures (less than 100,000 bacteria/ml) on clean-catch urine samples, uropathogens were found by suprapubic aspirate or sterile catheter specimens. The frequency of isolated bacterial pathogens was similar to that characteristic of classic cystitis (Table 58–2). This group of patients, who had what had been termed *acute urethral syndrome*, had a frequency of vaginal and urethral uropathogen colonization similar to that found in the cystitis group. Therefore, acute urethral syndrome appeared to be part of the continuum of bacterial lower urinary tract infection.

Subsequent studies established that more than 100 coliform bacteria/ml in a true clean-catch urine specimen was a sensitive and specific indicator of a true coliform bacterial infection. This threshold has been verified by suprapubic aspirate and catheter culture specimens.

Urethritis and Vaginitis

The other two main causes of dysuria, urethritis and vaginitis, are briefly summarized in Table 58–1. A more complete discussion, including diagnosis and therapy, is found in Chapter 61.

TABLE 58–2. Infectious Etiologies of Dysuria

Agent	Comments
Escherichia coli	Found in 90% of patients with UTI
Staphylococcus saprophyticus	Found in 10%–12% of sexually active females with UTI; usually $<10^5$ bacteria
Proteus sp.	Urea splitter—consider if urine pH ≥ 8.0; associated with stone formation; uncommon
Klebsiella, Enterobacter, Serratia, Pseudomonas sp.	Found in small proportion of total UTIs; *Klebsiella* also associated with stones
Chlamydia trachomatis	Associated with multiple sexual partners
Neisseria gonorrhoeae	Associated with recent change in partners; vaginal discharge
Trichomonas, Candida	Vulvovaginitis
Enterobius vermicularis (pinworms)	Periurethral irritation in girls

PROBLEM The patient's rectal temperature was 101.2°F (38°C). A complete blood cell count was ordered, which showed a hematocrit of 40% and a white blood cell count of 14,000 with 80 segmented polymorphonuclear leukocytes (PMNs), 6 bands, and 20 lymphocytes.

At this point, the physician can confidently diagnose early pyelonephritis. The initial presentation suggested a lower tract infection. However, the skin temperature alerted the physician to the possibility of fever in spite of the recorded temperature. This finding led to the ordering of a blood count, which revealed an elevated WBC, another sign of pyelonephritis. The accuracy of initial temperature readings is variable in emergency departments. Therefore, rectal temperatures are often taken to overcome that inaccuracy.

PRINCIPLES OF MANAGEMENT

General Principles

Management principles for the patient with dysuria include:
1. Cardiovascular stability. Hypotension or a resting tachycardia out of proportion to fever suggests volume depletion or sepsis. Obtaining orthostatic vital signs may also identify possible volume depletion. Intravascular volume is generally restored with intravenous crystalloid infusion.
2. Fever control. Fever control is too often overlooked by physicians. Although rarely life-threatening in itself, fever reduction with antipyretics often plays a major role in patient comfort without detracting from the careful monitoring of a patient's clinical condition. Fever that lasts more than 72 hours raises the question of a resistant organism or a complicating feature such as a perinephric or intrarenal abscess.
3. Pain relief. When dysuria is a very prominent part of the patient's complaint, phenazopyridine (Pyridium) may be given as a urinary anesthetic. It is taken orally three times daily for a maximum of 2 days and provides prompt relief from the irritative urinary symptoms characteristic of dysuria. This drug is started concurrently with antibiotic therapy to provide symptomatic relief while urinary tract sterilization takes place. The patient is warned that phenazopyridine will impart an orange tint to the urine and that if urinary symptoms have not improved following 2 days of antibiotic therapy, the patient should be reevaluated. Acetaminophen and phenazopyridine are usually adequate for pain control in the great majority of patients with UTIs. Pain not controlled by these measures implies an obstructive process that requires further assessment.

Specific Conditions

Pyelonephritis and Subclinical Pyelonephritis. Upper urinary tract infections require a full 10- to 14-day course of antibiotics. Patients without toxic symptoms who are at low risk for sepsis and who tolerate oral medications are treated as outpatients with the antibiotics listed in Table 58–3 for 10 to 14 days. Choosing an antibiotic with a low

TABLE 58–3. Oral Antibiotic Treatment for Dysuria in Adult Women

Oral Antibiotic Agents (Adults)	3–14 Day Therapy
Sulfisoxazole (Gantrisin)	1 gm PO q 6 hr
Trimethoprim	100 mg PO b.i.d.
Trimethoprim-sulfamethoxazole	1 double strength tablet b.i.d.
Amoxicillin	250–500 mg t.i.d.
Cephalexin	250–500 mg t.i.d.–q.i.d.
Tetracycline	250–500 mg b.i.d.–q.i.d.
Norfloxacin	400 mg b.i.d.
Ciprofloxacin	250–500 mg b.i.d.

likelihood of bacterial resistance such as trimethoprim-sulfamethoxazole is preferable and has the added advantage of twice daily dosing. Additionally, the practitioner may elect to initiate therapy with a single parenteral dose of ampicillin and an aminoglycoside or a third-generation cephalosporin. The third-generation cephalosporins have a favorable antibacterial action against common uropathogens, a low potential for toxicity, and the added advantage of an extended biologic half-life. This one-time parenteral dose is followed by 10 to 14 days of oral therapy.

Inpatient therapy is advised when unrelenting vomiting makes oral therapy impossible or when generalized toxicity such as significant volume depletion, high fever (more than 102°F [38.9°C]), marked costovertebral angle tenderness, and risk factors for urosepsis are present (see later section, Disposition and Follow-Up). Ampicillin and an aminoglycoside are good choices for empiric therapy of pyelonephritis (see Table 58–4). Ampicillin alone is not recommended because of the high rate of bacterial resistance (up to 30% of *Escherichia coli*) to this drug. A third-generation cephalosporin is also appropriate as initial therapy.

For patients who have urosepsis or are immunocompromised, an antipseudomonal penicillin such as ticarcillin-clavulanate (Timentin) in combination with an aminoglycoside is good initial coverage pending culture results. Alternatives to this regimen include imipenem-cilastin (Primaxin) or ciprofloxacin (Cipro), both of which provide exceptionally broad antibacterial coverage.

Parenteral therapy is continued until the patient has been afebrile for at least 24 hours, at which time oral agents are begun and continued for at least 14 days. Patients who are not afebrile after 72 hours of antibiotic therapy are considered for intravenous urography to search for an obstructive process. Computed tomography or ultrasound may be needed in the search for perirenal or intrarenal abscess.

Cystitis. A lower urinary tract infection in a patient not felt to be at risk for subclinical pyelonephritis (see Table 58–1) is usually treated with a 3-day course of antibiotic therapy. Table 58–3 gives a list of commonly used oral antibiotics in women. A 3-day regimen is used for compliant patients who have access to prompt medical follow-up. Whenever adequate follow-up is lacking, 10 days of antibiotics are prescribed on the assumption that subclinical pyelonephritis could exist.

PROBLEM After the care of the patient was discussed with her primary care physician, she was instructed to schedule a follow-up appointment in 48 hours. Because the diagnosis was acute pyelonephritis, a decision was made to treat the patient with trimethoprim-sulfamethoxazole for 10 days. A urine specimen was sent to the laboratory for culture. She was given acetaminophen for her fever and 2 days of phenazopyridine for dysuria.

SPECIAL CONSIDERATIONS

Although the overwhelming number of patients presenting with dysuria are otherwise healthy women, several other patient populations deserve special consideration. These

TABLE 58–4. Choices of Parenteral Therapy for Patients Admitted with Urinary Tract Infection

Parenteral Antibiotics for Adult Pyelonephritis	Dose
Ampicillin and an aminoglycoside, such as gentamicin or tobramycin	1–2 gm q 4 hr
Ticarcillin with clavulanate (Timentin)	3.1 gm q 4 hr
Gentamicin (Tobramycin)	2 mg/kg loading dose
Ceftriaxone (Rocephin)	1–2 gm q.d.
Cefoperazone (Cefobid)	2–4 gm b.i.d.
Ceftazidime (Fortzaz)	1–2 gm q 8–12 hr
Ceftizoxime (Cefizox)	1–2 gm q 8–12 hr
Imipenem and cilastatin (Primaxin)	0.5–1.0 gm q 6 hr

include children, elderly patients, male patients who present with a chronic indwelling urinary catheter, and patients who have asymptomatic bacteriuria. Another special consideration is the patient in whom pyuria is discovered but no clinical symptoms and signs of UTI.

Pediatric Patients

Urinary tract infections in children are challenging owing to the often nonspecific presenting signs and symptoms in this population. The fact that the pediatric age group is at greatest risk for renal scarring and possible renal failure due to prolonged unrecognized pyelonephritis makes early diagnosis crucial. The prevalence of UTI in children varies with sex and age. Following the neonatal period, UTI is noted much more frequently in girls than boys. Interestingly, the male appears to be at greatest risk for UTI at both age extremes, in neonates and in elderly men.

Obstructive abnormalities are more likely to be discovered in childhood and occur in up to 20% of children with UTI. Although the presence of these abnormalities does not necessarily predispose the patient to infection, the potential for renal damage is far greater in the presence of infection. Voiding dysfunction and vesicoureteral reflux are frequently associated with UTI in children.

The signs of UTI vary with the age of the child. Failure to thrive, fussiness, and unexplained weight loss are the most common presenting signs in neonates. Fever during infancy is variable, and symptoms may remain nonspecific before 2 years of age. Dysuria in the older child is most frequently a result of vulvovaginitis or voiding dysfunction rather than a true UTI. Physical examination may reveal a flank mass in the presence of hydronephrosis. Suprapubic distention often accompanies a neurogenic bladder. Constipation suggested by a fecal mass on abdominal or rectal examination is associated with UTI in neonates.

For urine collection, the common practice is to secure a urine collection bag to the infant's perineum. This may be an adequate practice for a screening examination for the otherwise healthy child. However, it is discouraged for the child in whom a true UTI is suspected. Suprapubic bladder aspiration is both safe and easily performed in the infant when accurate bacteriologic identification is necessary. In contrast to adults, pyuria in children does not correlate well with bacteriuria. Febrile children may have pyuria in the absence of urinary tract infection.

The neonate with UTI is treated as if sepsis were present. This age group has a high rate of bacteremia (50%) and is prone to the rapid development of overwhelming sepsis. Parenteral therapy with ampicillin and gentamicin covers the likely pathogens including group B *Streptococcus*, the coliforms, and *Enterococcus*. A minimum of 10 days of parenteral antibiotic therapy is indicated.

Elderly Patients

Elderly patients presenting with systemic toxicity and urinary tract infection are at much greater risk of bacteremia and sepsis than their younger counterparts. Admission to the hospital for parenteral antibiotic treatment is the rule in this setting. Agents similar to those mentioned earlier for the inpatient treatment of pyelonephritis are used. However, the diminished renal clearance that accompanies aging must always be considered, especially when aminoglycosides are used.

Dysuria in the Male

Dysuria in the postpubescent male has a bimodal age and etiology distribution. The most common cause of dysuria in young men is gonococcal or chlamydial urethritis. Urethral discharge in men with these sexually transmitted diseases is common and makes the diagnosis relatively straightforward. The older male with dysuria presents a more challenging problem. Most cases of dysuria in males older than 50 years of age are linked to the prostate.

Prostatitis has become an overused term to describe almost any genitourinary complaint in the older man that can in any manner be referred to the prostate. Irritative voiding symptoms, perineal aching, genital or perigenital pain, sexual dysfunction, and low back pain may be symptoms of prostatitis.

Acute prostatitis may have a dramatic presentation with high fever (up to 40°C), myalgias, arthralgias, and generalized malaise. Difficulties in micturition or acute urinary obstruction can occur, but more commonly urinary frequency, urgency, and dysuria predominate. Perineal, rectal, or low back pain is often present. Rectal examination in acute prostatitis may reveal a very tender, warm, swollen prostate. Palpation may result in a thick purulent urethral discharge. Prostatic massage in the presence of an acute infection is painful and serves little purpose, since the bacteria found in the bladder urine are usually the same organisms that infect the prostate. Prostatic massage may also post a risk of bacteremia.

The organisms responsible for acute bacterial prostatitis are predominantly the gram-negative enteric bacteria. *E. coli* is responsible for approximately 80% of all infections. *Pseudomonas* species, gram-positive staphylococci, and streptococci are also important pathogens. Viral, parasitic, tubercular, and mycotic infections are uncommon.

Acute bacterial prostatitis is a self-limited disease and is rarely a precursor of chronic prostatitis. In contrast to chronic bacterial prostatitis, response to appropriate antibacterial therapy is often quite rapid. The acutely inflamed prostate readily allows tissue penetration of most antibiotics.

In the toxic-appearing patient both blood and urine cultures are sent to the laboratory before one embarks on a 7-day hospital course of an intravenous broad-spectrum penicillin or cephalosporin in conjunction with an aminoglycoside. The less toxic patient can be treated as an outpatient with trimethoprim-sulfamethoxazole (Septra, Bactrim), ciprofloxacin (Cipro), tetracycline, or ampicillin for a full 14-day course of therapy. Irritative symptoms on micturition following bacteriologic cure are not unusual and may represent slow resolution of the inflammatory process. Several months may also lapse before the prostate regains its normal soft consistency. Acute prostatitis can lead to acute urinary retention, and urgent urologic consultation is often indicated.

Chronic bacterial prostatitis is mainly a bacteriologic diagnosis defined in the setting of recurrent urinary tract infections. Symptoms resemble simple lower UTI more than acute bacterial prostatitis. Pyuria and bacteriuria are generally seen on urinalysis. Antibiotic penetration of the nonacutely inflamed prostate is difficult owing to the highly charged prostatic epithelium. The ideal antibiotic would be a highly lipid-soluble drug, have a high percentage of unionized drug in the plasma, and be minimally protein bound. Current recommendations are one double strength tablet of trimethoprim-sulfamethoxazole twice daily for 3 months, or ciprofloxacin 500 mg orally twice daily for 2 weeks. Even with optimal therapy the cure rate is under 50%.

Patients with Chronic Indwelling Urinary Catheters

The emergency physician is frequently called on to evaluate the chronically ill patient who may have an indwelling urinary catheter to control incontinence. Unfortunately, common clues to urinary tract infection in this patient population are infrequent or are masked by underlying chronic medical conditions. The debilitated patient with a UTI may have an altered mental status, vague abdominal pain, or tachypnea, which may mislead the physician to suspect diseases such as meningitis, diverticulitis, or pneumonia.

Urine obtained from an indwelling catheter may not narrow the diagnostic possibilities. Bacteriuria is to be expected in the vast majority of asymptomatic patients who have had indwelling catheters for longer than 2 weeks. Most studies show the incidence of bacteriuria increases at least 5% per day of indwelling catheterization. Treating asymptomatic bacteriuria has not been shown to decrease morbidity or mortality in catheterized patients and may select for organisms resistant to future therapy if true infection should develop. Additionally, urine obtained from a chronic indwelling catheter does not accurately reflect the true bacterial environment of the urinary tract. Therefore, bacteriuria in catheter urine is not helpful in identifying the offending organism in UTI.

Patients with indwelling catheters are considered infected if bacteriuria is accompanied by pyuria. The presence of fever and leukocytosis alerts the clinician to infection, but bacteriuria in the absence of pyuria in a chronically catheterized patient should direct the search for infection elsewhere. When bacteriuria and pyuria are present, the existing catheter is removed, and urine is obtained for culture and sensitivity testing following insertion of the new catheter. When possible, alternative methods of controlling incontinence such as condom catheters, diapers, or intermittent straight catheterizations are used for the course of antibiotic therapy.

Patients with Asymptomatic Bacteriuria

The presence of asymptomatic bacteriuria in the absence of evidence of upper urinary tract disease does not demand treatment. In the absence of pregnancy, immunosuppression (including diabetes mellitus), upper urinary tract obstruction, or severe vesicoureteral reflux, serious morbidity is unlikely. Although asymptomatic bacteriuria in the presence of pyuria does correlate with definable urinary tract abnormalities, there is little evidence that treatment will prevent further scars or renal dysfunction. Asymptomatic bacteriuria in the elderly is correlated with increased mortality, but there is no evidence that treatment reduces this risk.

Pregnant women are a special population in which asymptomatic bacteriuria must be vigorously sought, since this group without treatment has an increased risk (up to 20% to 30%) of pyelonephritis in the third trimester of pregnancy, leading to possible prematurity and neonatal complications. Several factors are responsible for this high rate of pyelonephritis including hormonal-induced ureteral dilatation and stasis, physiologic obstruction from the gravid uterus compressing the ureters, and a change in the introital flora that favors bacterial colonization.

Other Causes of Pyuria

Pyuria may be the result of inflammatory conditions adjacent to the urinary tract. Pelvic inflammatory disease (PID) is the best example of this phenomenon. Dysuria, lower abdominal pain, and the findings of pyuria on a urinary specimen may lead the clinician mistakenly to diagnose UTI when the above symptoms are the result of PID. This is best avoided by performing a careful pelvic examination searching for cervical motion and adnexal tenderness. Urethral catheterization will help differentiate true pyuria from the purulent cervical discharge that may contaminate the urine in PID.

The inflamed cecal appendix is another organ adjacent to the urinary collecting system that may result in pyuria owing to direct irritation of these structures in the absence of UTI. Urinary frequency and urgency are not expected in this setting.

Renal tuberculosis is an uncommon, although catastrophic, cause of pyuria. Classically described as pyuria without bacteriuria, this cause is considered in immigrants from developing nations. Tuberculosis is still endemic throughout much of the developing world. Constitutional symptoms such as weight loss, night sweats, or prolonged fever are unusual but are sought in a high-risk individual with pyuria and sterile urine cultures.

DISPOSITION AND FOLLOW-UP

The great majority of patients with UTI will do well as outpatients with a short course of oral antibiotics. The following are guidelines for selecting patients requiring admission and those who are appropriate for outpatient therapy and follow-up.

Admission

Patients in the following categories are admitted.
1. Those with generalized toxicity (high fever and leukocytosis).
2. Patients with intractable vomiting.
3. Patients with diabetes mellitus, sickle cell disease, urinary obstruction, recent instrumentation or underlying carcinoma.
4. Pregnant women with pyelonephritis.
5. Patients with infection in the presence of recent urinary tract instrumentation.
6. Males with fever or other signs of toxicity such as an elevated white blood cell count.
7. All neonates.

Discharge and Outpatient Therapy

Patients in these categories can be discharged on outpatient therapy.
1. Patients with cystitis. Follow-up with primary care physician is optional.
2. Patients with uncomplicated pyelonephritis. Follow-up in 48 hours is required for examination and culture check to ensure that the proper antibiotic has been prescribed.
3. Males with uncomplicated infection. These patients all need close follow-up in 48 hours and consideration for formal urologic evaluation. Prepubescent females with their first UTI belong in the same category.

DOCUMENTATION

1. Duration of dysuria.
2. Associated signs and symptoms, e.g., presence or absence of flank or abdominal pain, vaginal discharge, vomiting.
3. Any previous UTIs.
4. Recent instrumentation or hospitalization.
5. Recent antibiotics.
6. Vital signs.
7. Flank or abdominal pain.
8. The method of obtaining the urine sample—clean-catch, straight catheterization, closed drainage system, suprapubic aspirate. Urinalysis and other laboratory results.
9. Antibiotics prescribed.
10. Follow-up recommendations.

SUMMARY AND FINAL POINTS

- Dysuria is not synonymous with UTI. A pelvic examination is necessary when symptoms of vaginitis or PID are elicited.
- Signs and symptoms of UTI are often lacking in patients at the extremes of age. Bacteremia is very common in these populations. The elderly patient with UTI and signs of systemic toxicity and all neonates with UTI are treated as if sepsis were present.
- Urethral catheterization is the preferred method of urine collection in a female with vaginal discharge and in debilitated patients who are unlikely to provide a clean-catch specimen. Catheterization, or suprapubic aspiration for patients less than 2 years of age, is the method of choice when a urine culture is crucial.
- Dipstick analysis of uncentrifuged urine for leukocyte esterase is a good screening method for establishing UTI in otherwise healthy, nonpregnant women with dysuria. Pyuria in the presence of dysuria is the best indicator of UTI in the emergency department setting.

- The previous standard (10^5 bacteria/ml by culture) used for establishing UTI is outmoded and should be discarded because much lower concentrations of bacteria (as low as 10^2 bacteria/ml) can represent true infection.
- Subclinical pyelonephritis is not uncommon, especially in inner city indigent women. The risk of subclinical pyelonephritis and the need for extended antibiotic therapy are assessed by determining whether the patient belongs to a high-risk group for this disease. Failure of short-course antibiotic therapy also implies probably subclinical pyelonephritis.
- Short-course antibiotic therapy (less than 10 days) is not appropriate for patients at risk of pyelonephritis and is considered only for patients with uncomplicated cystitis who have adequate and prompt medical follow-up.
- The pediatric age group is at greatest risk for renal scarring from prolonged, unrecognized urinary tract infections. Early diagnosis is crucial.
- Pyelonephritis is a serious disorder that requires admission to the hospital under the following conditions: generalized toxicity, vomiting, underlying debilitating illness, pregnancy, recent instrumentation, males with evidence of toxicity, and all neonates.

BIBLIOGRAPHY

Texts

1. Kunin MK (ed): Detection, Prevention, and Management of Urinary Tract Infection (4th ed). Philadelphia, Lea & Febiger, 1987.
2. Youmans GP, Patterson PY, Sommers HM (eds): Biologic and Clinical Basis of Infectious Diseases (3rd ed). Philadelphia, Saunders, 1985.

Journal Articles

1. Fowler JE: Urinary tract infections in women. Urol Clin North Am 13:673–683, 1986.
2. Kellogg JA, Manzella JP, Shaffer SN, et al: Clinical relevance of culture versus screens for the detection of microbial pathogens in urine specimens. Am J Med 83(4):739–745, 1987.
3. Komaroff AL: Acute dysuria in women. N Engl J Med 310:368–374, 1984.
4. Komaroff AL: Urinalysis and urine culture in women with dysuria. Ann Intern Med 104:212–216, 1986.
5. Latham RH: Urinary tract infections and the urethral syndrome in adult women: Pathogenesis, diagnosis and therapy in emergency medicine. Emerg Med Clin North Am 3:75–86, 1985.
6. Lipsky BA: Urinary tract infections in men. Epidemiology, pathophysiology, diagnosis and treatment. Ann Intern Med 110(2):138–150, 1989.
7. Sanford JP, Favour CB, Mao FH, et al: Evaluation of the "positive" urine culture: An approach to positive differentiation of significant bacteria from contaminants. Am J Med 20:88–93, 1956.
8. Stamm WE, Hooten TM, Johnson JR, et al: Urinary tract infections: From pathogenesis to treatment. J Infect Dis 159(3):400–406, 1989.
9. Walter FG, Knopp RK: Urine sampling in ambulatory women: Midstream clean catch versus catheterization. Ann Emerg Med 18(2):166–172, 1989.
10. Werman HA, Brown CG: Utility of urine culture in the emergency department. Ann Emerg Med 15:302–307, 1986.
11. Zhanisl GG: Single dose versus traditional therapy for uncomplicated urinary tract infections. Drug Intell Clin Pharm 22(1):21–24, 1988.

CHAPTER 59

PELVIC PAIN IN WOMEN

SAMUEL T. COLERIDGE, D.O.

PROBLEM A 24 year old woman complained of increasing lower abdominal (pelvic) pain and nausea that had persisted for 24 hours. She described the pain as a dull ache with occasional sharp spasms. Her family placed a call to the rescue squad.

QUESTIONS TO CONSIDER

1. What catastrophic illnesses can occur in patients presenting with pelvic pain?
2. How can serious pelvic disease be differentiated from a benign condition?
3. To what extent is the diagnosis of pelvic pain influenced by the patient's age, parity, and menstrual and sexual history?
4. What are the roles of pregnancy testing, ultrasonography, and culdocentesis in evaluating pelvic pain?
5. When is specialty consultation indicated?
6. When is the patient with pelvic pain considered for admission to the hospital?

INTRODUCTION

Pelvic pain is one of the most common complaints of adolescents and younger women. The reported incidence varies considerably with the population group served at a given institution. As a presenting complaint, pelvic pain occurs in 7% to 20% of all patients with abdominal pain.

Pelvic pain in women usually originates from the gastrointestinal or genitourinary tract. Visceral pain afferents that arise from the pelvic viscera also innervate the appendix, ureters, and most of the colon. The significant overlap of these fibers and their common bilateral entry through spinal segments T10 and T11 into the spinal cord make accurate location of the pain difficult for the patient. Eliciting somatic tenderness may allow the examiner to localize the anatomic region of disease.

Hemorrhagic shock resulting from a ruptured ectopic pregnancy and septic shock secondary to pelvic inflammatory disease (PID) are the two most important emergent conditions that present with pelvic pain. Severe pain can also be an emergent condition. It can result from a number of problems, including ectopic implants of endometrial tissue, mechanical torsion of the fallopian tube or ovary around its vascular pedicle, or rupture of graafian follicles or corpus luteum cysts.

Many causes of pelvic pain have potentially devastating sequelae. For example, untreated pelvic inflammatory disease may lead to an acute tubo-ovarian abscess or an increased risk of infertility and ectopic pregnancy. With a single episode of acute salpingitis the risk of infertility is 11%; it rises to 34% after two episodes and to 54% beyond three episodes of PID. In comparison, an equivalent population without salpingitis has an infertility rate of 3%. In recent years, with salpingitis as a leading risk factor, there has been a dramatic rise in the incidence of ectopic pregnancy. Between 1970 and

1980 the incidence of ectopic pregnancy rose from 4.5 to 10.5 in 1000 live births. The diagnosis is considered in any woman of childbearing age presenting to an emergency department with the complaint of lower abdominal or pelvic pain.

PREHOSPITAL CARE

Prehospital evaluation of the patient with pelvic pain is limited to the primary survey, efficient stabilization, and transport.

History

1. A description of the pain is obtained, including rate of onset, location, severity, duration, and character.
2. Associated symptoms are noted, such as dizziness, vomiting, and vaginal bleeding.
3. The relevant medical history is also obtained, including the presence of pregnancy and any medication being taken.

Physical Examination

1. Vital signs are measured.
2. Peripheral evidence of hypoperfusion, such as cool clammy skin and capillary refill, is noted.
3. Abdominal tenderness is sought.

Intervention

Field stabilization and precautions taken for the female patient with pelvic pain include the following:

Supplemental Oxygen. Oxygen is usually given at 2 to 4 liters/min by nasal cannula if the patient is diaphoretic or hypotensive. Otherwise, it probably is not indicated.

Cardiac Monitor. A cardiac monitor is usually not indicated unless the patient is diaphoretic or hypotensive, as noted above. Elderly patients and those with known cardiac disease are also monitored.

Intravenous Access. An IV line with isotonic crystalloid is preferred if clinical signs of hypoperfusion (e.g., cool, clammy skin, dizziness, or outright hypotension) are present. Additionally, severe pelvic pain without signs of hypotension also warrants an intravenous line if a life-threatening process such as ectopic pregnancy is suspected, or if transport time is prolonged (greater than 10 to 15 minutes).

Pneumatic Antishock Garment. This garment (PASG) may provide some temporary hemodynamic support and is used in patients with overt signs of hypoperfusion or hypotension.

Estimated transport time given by the rescue squad provides significant information and allows the physician to give additional orders by radiotelemetry if needed.

PROBLEM The rescue squad reported that the patient's pain was in the lower right abdomen and was described as a constant ache of moderate severity. She did not think that she was pregnant. Vital signs: Blood pressure 100/60 mm Hg, pulse 110 beats/min, respiratory rate 20/min. She was in moderate distress and lay supine on the stretcher with legs flexed. The squad gave oxygen by nasal cannula at 2 liters/min and started an intravenous (IV) line of normal saline at a minimal keep-open rate. A monitored rhythm showed sinus tachycardia. Transport time was estimated to be 12 minutes.

It is difficult to assess the severity of this patient's complaint in the prehospital care setting. However, her age, sex, description of the pain, and elevated pulse and respiratory rate raise concern about serious illness. The rescue squad precautions and transport for evaluation were appropriate, although more aggressive volume resuscitation might be warranted, e.g., two to three fluid boluses of 250 to 300 ml during transport while monitoring vital signs.

INITIAL APPROACH IN THE EMERGENCY DEPARTMENT

Because of the potential for catastrophic illness, care is taken to recognize quickly patients who require volume resuscitation, surgery, or sepsis evaluation. The following initial history, physical examination, and interventions focus on those primary concerns. Volume resuscitation is the primary goal of early therapy.

History

1. The rescue squad report is verified.
2. A brief history covering the following points is taken.
   a. Current pregnancy status
   b. Vaginal bleeding and amount
   c. Last normal menstrual period
   d. Prior pregnancies, particularly ectopic pregnancies and miscarriages
   e. Postural dizziness
   f. Vomiting, not only as a nonspecific gauge of illness, but also as a contributor to volume loss
   g. Presence of fever

Physical Examination

1. Vital signs are repeated and compared to the prehospital values. Orthostatic vital signs are taken in patients with normal supine vital signs if possible. A pulse rate rise of 20 beats/min and a drop in systolic pressure of 20 mm Hg after 1 minute in the standing position are indicative of significant hypovolemia.
2. The patient is undressed and observed for signs of shock, e.g., pallor, diaphoresis, poor capillary refill time.
3. A brief and gentle examination of the abdomen is performed. Areas of specific tenderness or peritoneal signs are noted.
4. A pelvic examination is performed at this point only if the patient is unstable and likely to need immediate consultation and operative intervention. A culdocentesis might be carried out under these conditions.

Intervention

1. Cardiac monitoring and supplemental oxygen are continued or established. The need to establish a second large-bore (16- to 18-gauge) intravenous line is assessed. Volume repletion with isotonic crystalloid is given as necessary to correct the patient's hemodynamic compromise.
2. In the hemodynamically compromised patient, the following immediate laboratory tests are ordered: urinalysis, spun hematocrit, complete blood count (CBC) and differential, blood type and cross-match or type and screen, and pregnancy test (beta subunit of human chorionic gonadotropin [beta hCG]).

PROBLEM Although the patient's pain was not severe, her borderline vital signs and childbearing potential placed her in a high-risk group. She was brought into the emergency department and seen by the physician as a high-priority patient. The patient complained that the abdominal pain continued to be moderately severe and remained in the right lower pelvic area. Although still nauseated, she denied vomiting and postural dizziness. Repeat vital signs showed blood pressure 100/60 mm Hg, pulse 110 beats/min, respiratory rate 18/min, temperature 99.8°F (37.7°C) orally. She was slightly pale. The monitor confirmed a sinus tachycardia of 110 beats/min. Orthostatic vital signs were performed and showed no significant changes in heart rate or blood pressure.

It is always valuable to glance quickly at a patient arriving by rescue squad as she is being moved to the hospital bed. How willing and able is she to move? This single observation can provide the clinician with an early valuable clue to the severity of the problem. Any questions or apparent changes from what is observed in the emergency department compared to the observations recorded in the prehospital report can be discussed with the paramedics before they depart. This patient was still of concern for serious illness, though the concern was slightly lessened by her normal orthostatic vital signs.

DATA GATHERING

The history and physical examination often provide the diagnosis or presumptive diagnosis without laboratory and other diagnostic procedures. Since the physical findings may be completely normal in early pelvic disease, a meticulous, probing history is paramount in diagnosing the cause of pelvic pain.

History

An adequate history and description of pelvic pain is often very difficult to obtain. Many patients keep poor menstrual histories. Additionally, one must ask sensitive questions regarding sexual behavior and sexual organs. Not all patients are comfortable volunteering the information necessary to diagnose their disease. Some patients are embarrassed or ashamed and the physician must maintain a sensitive demeanor while gaining the patient's confidence. Key historical points include:

1. *Pain history*
   a. *What is the character or quality of the pain?* The patient is asked to answer whether the pain is "sharp," "dull," "heavy," or "crampy" (colicky). The patient with PID or torsion of a fallopian tube or ovary may initially complain of a "dull ache" instead of the expected sharp, severe pain encountered in the later stages of torsion, ruptured ovarian cysts, or hemorrhage from a ruptured ectopic pregnancy.
   b. *When did the pain start?* This information includes the timing and rate of onset of pain. Pain first associated with exercise or coitus is consistent with a ruptured ovarian cyst. Coincidence with menses suggests endometriosis. The rupture of a follicular cyst during midcycle produces the pain of Mittelschmerz. Salpingitis is frequently associated with pelvic pain during or shortly after menstruation. Pain of very rapid onset is consistent with a ruptured viscus and occasionally an acute infectious process.
   c. *Where is the pain located and where does it radiate?* Unilateral pelvic pain that results from adnexal disease, tubal torsion, cyst rupture, or tubal inflammation may also be confused with the pain of a ureteral stone or pelvic appendicitis in the same location. Radiation to the low back can occur from retroperitoneal abscess, bladder infection, and dysmenorrhea. Radiation to an extremity has been reported with pedunculated fibroids, ectopic pregnancy, and dysmenorrhea. The generalized peritonitis resulting from benign cysts rupturing into the peritoneum may be indistinguishable from that resulting from a ruptured ectopic pregnancy.

d. *How severe is the pain?* Gauging the pain on a scale of 0 (no pain) to 10 (the worst pain in your life) can provide the examiner with a relatively "objective" assessment of the level of pain. There is no clear relationship between the severity of pain and the seriousness of the disease. It is best to initially believe the patient's assessment even if it is inconsistent with other findings.
e. *What is the duration and pattern of the pain?* The length of the episode and the variation of pain within this time frame are carefully explored. Ruptured ectopic pregnancy presents with sudden onset of severe, continuous unilateral pelvic pain that rapidly becomes diffuse, whereas PID can present with either acute or more insidious bilateral pelvic pain that becomes progressively worse over several days.
f. *Is there a previous history of pain?* Has the same type of pain been previously experienced? How does this pain compare with it?
g. *How has the pain been treated?* Use of a "friend's" antibiotic or an analgesic may alter the patient's presentation. The patient's efforts to remedy the pain offer some insight into its severity.
2. *What is the patient's sexual history?*
   a. When was the patient's last menstrual period (LMP)? Was it normal or abnormal? When was the last normal menstrual period (LNMP)?
   b. Is there a history of any sexually transmitted diseases?
   c. What is the gravida, parity, and abortus history?
   d. What method, if any, of contraceptive is or has been used?
   e. Is the patient sexually active? How often and with how many partners? When was the last sexual intercourse?
3. *Are there associated symptoms?*
   a. Fever or chills are often associated with PID.
   b. Dizziness suggests hypovolemia or septic shock.
   c. Nausea and vomiting may occur concurrently with the onset of severe genitourinary pelvic pain (e.g., torsion, imminent tubal rupture, ureterolithiasis) but generally precedes the pain of appendicitis and small bowel obstruction or perforation.
   d. Bladder or rectal pressure or fullness may result from fibroids, adjacent adnexal masses, or endometrial implants.
   e. Vaginal bleeding or spotting, breast tenderness or fullness, and weight gain may represent pregnancy (intrauterine or ectopic), premenstrual syndrome (PMS), dysmenorrhea, endometriosis, or ectopic pregnancy.
4. *Do risk factors for ectopic pregnancy and pelvic inflammatory disease exist?*
   a. Age and race. Women aged 20 to 30 demonstrate the highest rate of ectopic pregnancy, and rates are also higher for black women of all ages. However, adolescence (ages 15 to 19 years) is associated with the highest incidence of PID.
   b. Intrauterine devices. Intrauterine device (IUD) use is associated with an increased risk of developing PID. Patients using an IUD 25 months or more are 2 to 6.5 times more likely to have an ectopic pregnancy than are short-term users. There is an increased risk of spontaneous and septic abortions with both increased mortality and morbidity. IUD use is also associated with an increased incidence of uterine perforation and uterine bleeding (usually shortly after IUD insertion but occasionally occurring months later).
   c. Frequent sexual activity. Multiple sexual partners have been associated with PID. Previous PID, particularly when secondary to gonorrhea or chlamydial infection, is associated with recurrent or chronic PID as well as with tubo-ovarian abscesses, Fitz-Hugh-Curtis syndrome (gonococcal perihepatitis), ectopic pregnancy, and recurrent urinary tract infections.
   d. Previous tubal pregnancy. There is a 10% recurrence rate for ectopic pregnancy. Tubal surgery is associated with a tenfold increase in ectopic pregnancy. There is a 12% increased incidence of ectopic pregnancy after recent dilatation and curettage.

5. *Are there urinary tract or gastrointestinal tract symptoms?* These may reinforce certain pelvic disorders or change the evaluation to emphasize different organ systems.

Physical Examination

Coupled with a good history, the physical examination rapidly limits the differential of possible pain sources.

Vital Signs. Orthostatic measurements are performed if not contraindicated. A rectal temperature is indicated if infection or fever is suspected.

General Appearance. Pallor, clamminess, and restlessness are signs of hypovolemia. The degree of patient discomfort is noted. Patients with cramping pain tend to move around, whereas those with peritoneal signs lie more still.

Abdominal Examination. All quadrants are examined for specific localized tenderness, guarding, and rebound. Bowel sound changes are seldom useful in this setting. Much of the valuable information can be obtained by palpation of the abdomen during the bimanual examination.

Pelvic and Rectal Examination. The pelvic and rectal examinations are carried out gently but thoroughly. The patient's discomfort should not overrule the need for a complete examination. An attentive, caring demeanor and explanation of the process can do much to lessen the patient's pain.

External Genitalia. Inspection of the external genitalia can yield clues to the cause of pelvic pain. For example, Bartholin gland cysts are associated with gonococcal infections.

Internal Genitalia. The speculum is inserted carefully. PID and ectopic pregnancy can be so painful that minimal manipulation of the internal genitalia is intolerable. Once the speculum is inserted, an inspection is made for bleeding, inflammation of the cervix, and sources of discharge. An endocervical culture and swab for Gram stain are routinely obtained.

Bimanual Examination. The goals of the bimanual examination are to localize tenderness, define the pelvic anatomy, and reveal abnormal masses. A rectovaginal examination is also performed to better appreciate the pelvic viscera in its entirety. Tenderness in PID is usually bilateral, whereas in ectopic pregnancy it is most often localized to one adnexa.

DECISION PRIORITIES AND PRELIMINARY DIFFERENTIAL DIAGNOSIS

At this point in the evaluation of the patient with pelvic pain, preliminary impressions about the acuity of the pain and the disease process can be made. Three questions need answers:

1. *Is the patient hemodynamically unstable?*
   Obviously, this will influence the degree of evaluation and management. Early volume resuscitation and consultation may be required. Causes of pelvic abdominal pain that can cause hemodynamic instability include ectopic pregnancy, hemorrhagic rupture of a cyst, sepsis from a pelvic infection, and, in the elderly, abdominal aortic aneurysm.

2. *Is the patient pregnant?*
   Unfortunately, the history and physical examination are not sensitive for the diagnosis of early pregnancy. In recent years, the availability of rapidly performed, sensitive and specific tests for pregnancy has become essential in the management of patients with pelvic pain. A pregnancy test is invaluable in directing diagnostic efforts toward discovering ectopic pregnancy; also, pregnancy is a significant risk factor for patients who have PID. Therefore, in order to make informed decisions

about these patients, the pregnancy test has to be ordered early, often during the initial evaluation by the triage nurse.
3. *Is the pain of true pelvic origin?*
The ability to make a decision concerning the true origin of the pain, pelvic or abdominal, can significantly influence further diagnostic efforts and also the choice of a surgical as opposed to a gynecologic consultation. It also broadens the differential diagnosis to include urinary problems such as infection and gastrointestinal disorders, e.g., perirectal abscesses, appendicitis.

PROBLEM The patient had no previous pregnancy (G_0P_0) and reported that her last normal menstrual period was 6 weeks earlier. She admitted to being sexually active. Her most recent intercourse had been 4 days previously. She did not use any birth control method. She had no other risk factors except an "infection in the tube" 6 years ago. She denied having urinary or gastrointestinal tract symptoms. On physical examination she appeared to be in moderate distress. The abdomen was tender bilaterally in both lower quadrants, the right greater than the left, with involuntary guarding and mild rebound tenderness. On pelvic examination the external genitalia and vaginal vault were unremarkable. No discharge was noted. There was mild cervical tenderness to motion and marked bilateral adnexal tenderness, right side greater than left. No masses were found. Rectal examination was normal.

Because of the low-grade fever and the bilateral adnexal tenderness, suspicion is raised of an infectious etiology for this patient's complaint. However, these findings are consistent with other diagnoses such as ectopic pregnancy. Continued careful observation of the patient's vital signs and general condition is necessary until further specific diagnostic procedures are carried out.

DIAGNOSTIC ADJUNCTS

Several laboratory and other diagnostic procedures are useful in diagnosing pelvic pain. The sequence of ordering these tests can vary according to the individual clinical circumstances, availability of diagnostic modalities, and hemodynamic stability of the patient.

Laboratory Studies

Pregnancy Tests. Virtually all patients of childbearing age with pelvic pain require a screening test for pregnancy. Measurement of the beta subunit of human chorionic gonadotropin (beta hCG) is currently the best method for determining pregnancy in its earliest stages. The sensitivity of this test allows detection of pregnancy within 7 to 10 days of conception. The sensitivity of the serum beta hCG measurement in pregnancy approaches 100%, and the specificity is 96%. Urine tests for beta hCG are slightly less sensitive and specific but are clinically reliable. Current immunoassay methodology allows both serum and urine tests to be performed in 20 to 45 minutes.

Complete Blood Count and Differential. A hemoglobin and hematocrit are performed in patients in whom blood loss is suspected. These tests do not reliably distinguish between acute or chronic blood loss. In the anemic patient, the decision to transfuse a patient immediately is based on vital signs and the presence of peripheral signs of hypovolemia. An elevated or "left-shifted" white blood cell (WBC) count can be indicative of an infectious cause of pelvic pain, e.g., acute salpingitis. However, a WBC count can also be elevated secondary to the stress of blood loss.

Microbial Studies. Staining of the endocervical discharge is a rapid, easy test but lacks specificity and sensitivity for the two most common causes of mucopurulent vaginal discharge—*Neisseria gonorrhoeae* and *Chlamydia trachomatis*. In any patient for whom infection is suspected, gonococcal and chlamydial cultures are recommended to allow later analysis by the follow-up care giver.

Urinalysis. The urinalysis is useful for differentiating urinary tract infection and ureteral calculi from PID or ectopic pregnancy. It is important to be certain that the urine sample originates from the bladder and is not contaminated by material from the vagina, labial folds, or rectum. A "clean-catch" urine specimen is often difficult to obtain and cannot be relied on to make the above differentiation. Straight catheterization ("mini-cath") is suggested if serious illness is suspected and precision is required. However, be aware that one disease can coexist with another. The patient with PID can also have cystitis or pyelonephritis.

Radiologic Imaging

Plain Radiographs. Although not often useful in diagnosing the cause of pelvic pain, the acute abdominal series (AAS) is occasionally helpful. This series is ordered when the history or physical examination suggests ureteral calculus, intestinal obstruction, localized peritonitis (a result of severe PID, appendicitis, or diverticulitis), or bowel obstruction. The AAS comprises the upright posteroanterior chest, the upright abdomen, and the flat-plate abdomen and pelvis films.

Ultrasonography. Ultrasonography effectively excludes an ectopic pregnancy if it demonstrates the presence of an intrauterine pregnancy (IUP). The earliest sign of an IUP is the presence of a gestational sac that can be seen at 4 to 5 weeks' gestation with current high-resolution intravaginal and sector abdominal scanners. It is not until 7 to 8 weeks that real-time ultrasound can detect fetal heart motion. Patients with an ectopic pregnancy may show an adnexal mass, fluid in the cul-de-sac, or an extrauterine gestational sac or fetus. Also, extrauterine fetal pulsation may be a late (and rare) finding with an ectopic pregnancy.

Other Tests

Culdocentesis. Most often a culdocentesis is performed in the setting of suspected ectopic pregnancy when the beta hCG is positive but the ultrasound study does not reveal an intrauterine pregnancy. Culdocentesis may also help the clinician differentiate between the inflammatory and hemorrhagic causes of pelvic pain. In the patient with a ruptured tubal ectopic pregnancy or a ruptured ovarian cyst, nonclotting blood is obtained on aspiration. Overall, in cases of proved ectopic pregnancy, a culdocentesis is positive (nonclotting blood is present) in 70% to 95% of cases, negative in 2.4% to 10%, and nondiagnostic in 5% to 16.5%. In patients with inflammatory pelvic diseases, such as salpingitis or tubo-ovarian abscess, cul-de-sac aspiration often yields purulent material. Aspirates are sent to the laboratory for Gram stain and culture. In the patient with pelvic inflammatory disease, a high degree of correlation has been found between cultures of organisms obtained by means of culdocentesis and those obtained from laparoscopy or laparotomy. It should be noted that current ultrasound technology is rapidly decreasing the need and indications for culdocentesis.

PROBLEM The physical examination was followed by a complete blood count, a urine beta hCG, and a urinalysis. The hemoglobin was 12.6 gm, hematocrit 37%, and WBC 11,200. The beta hCG was positive. The urinalysis demonstrated 0 to 2 RBCs and 5 to 8 WBCs per high power field and showed many epithelial cells. Dipstick testing was negative for glucose, acetone, and albumin.

Because of the positive pregnancy test, further testing was needed to diagnose or definitively rule out ectopic pregnancy.

REFINED DIFFERENTIAL DIAGNOSIS

After the results of the diagnostic tests return, a more precise diagnosis is often made. An extensive listing of the potential causes of pelvic pain is contained in Table 59–1. The more common and serious causes of pain of true pelvic etiology are described in Table 59–2. Finally, the common abdominal causes of pelvic pain are listed in Table 59–3.

Gastrointestinal causes of pelvic pain such as pelvic appendicitis, diverticulitis, and bowel obstruction with or without perforation can present frequent diagnostic dilemmas as can genitourinary diseases, e.g., pyelonephritis, perinephric abscess, and ureterolithiasis. These causes of pelvic pain are discussed in Chapters 5 and 58.

PRINCIPLES OF MANAGEMENT

As noted earlier, the major concern in the early evaluation and resuscitation of patients with pelvic pain is to anticipate the worst possible problem and then institute early resuscitative measures. The final common threat to patients with a serious cause of pelvic pain is volume loss through either blood loss, intravascular volume shift, or vomiting. The single key principle in the emergency management of these patients is volume restoration. Other principles that guide management include treatment of infection and control of pain.

Specific Measures

Suspected conditions requiring specific management regimens are listed below and in Tables 59–2 and 59–3.

Ectopic Pregnancy (see Fig. 59–1). Rupture with hemodynamic collapse can be the earliest presenting clinical sign of ectopic pregnancy. Early identification of the hemodynamically unstable patient with severe abdominal or pelvic pain, peritoneal findings, and abnormal vital signs will expedite aggressive treatment for blood loss. Fluid resuscitation is initiated and continued while culdocentesis or preparations for laparoscopy or laparotomy occur concurrently. Appropriate consultation and notification of the operating room personnel are carried out at this time as well.

In clinically stable patients, ultrasonography, if available, is the next step after confirmation of pregnancy. Ultrasound results prompt additional options for culdocentesis, laparoscopy, or laparotomy. Early consultation with a gynecologist is necessary.

Pelvic Inflammatory Disease. Antibiotic-treated gonococcal salpingitis generally has a better prognosis for fertility than chlamydial salpingitis. Gonococcal salpingitis is generally identified earlier in its clinical course owing to its classic picture of high fever, leukocytosis, and purulent endocervical discharge associated with pelvic pain and tenderness. *Chlamydia* is associated with a more indolent, less acute, less severe clinical picture of PID, with greater potential for permanent tubal damage and resultant infertility. However, *N. gonorrhoeae* and *C. trachomatis* often occur simultaneously (in 30% to 40% of cases). This concurrence explains the rationale for double antibiotic or broad-spectrum treatment of PID. Until recently, all PID was thought to result from gonococcal infection. However, despite the ability to culture this organism from the cervix in 39% to 94% of PID patients, cultures of peritoneal fluid using culdocentesis or laparoscopy revealed that one-third had gonococci alone, one-third had gonococci plus anaerobes and aerobes (e.g., *Bacteroides, Peptococcus, Peptostreptococcus*), and one-third had other organisms such as *Mycoplasma, Ureaplasma,* or *Chlamydia*.

The decision to institute "ambulatory treatment" is controversial. There are no data available to evaluate the difference between hospitalization and ambulatory management of PID. For economic and logistic reasons, only 25% to 30% of all PID patients are hospitalized in the United States. Recommendations for hospitalization are noted below, but all ambulatory patients should be reevaluated within 48 hours to determine the

TABLE 59-1. Etiologic Classification of Pelvic Pain

I. True pelvic etiology
   A. Ovaries, uterus, adnexa
      1. Torsion of ovarian pedicle, cyst or tumor
      2. Polycystic ovaries
      3. Ruptured ovarian cyst
      4. Ruptured ectopic or ovarian pregnancy
      5. Pelvic inflammatory disease, salpingitis, tubo-ovarian abscess
      6. Endometriosis, adenomyosis
      7. Degeneration of uterine myoma, fibroid
      8. Mittelschmerz
      9. Puerperal infections, endometritis
     10. Incomplete septic abortion
     11. Dysmenorrhea
   B. Premenstrual syndrome (PMS)
II. Abdominal pelvic pain
   A. Gastrointestinal tract
      1. Appendicitis
      2. Diverticulitis
      3. Femoral hernia
      4. Incarcerated hernia
      5. Small bowel obstruction
      6. Volvulus
      7. Dietary indiscretion, gastroenteritis
      8. Constipation
      9. Parasites
     10. Dysentery, diarrhea
     11. Colitis
     12. Regional enteritis
     13. Carcinoma
     14. Ruptured viscus
     15. Trauma
     16. Mesenteric adenitis
   B. Urinary tract
      1. Cystitis
      2. Pyelonephritis
      3. Ureteral stone
      4. Urethral syndrome
   C. Vascular causes
      1. Aortic or iliac aneurysm
      2. Pelvic thrombophlebitis
      3. Mesenteric vein thrombosis
   D. Liver and gallbladder
      1. Hepatitis
      2. Cholecystitis, cholelithiasis
      3. Fitz-Hugh-Curtis syndrome
   E. Pancreas
      1. Acute pancreatitis
      2. Pancreatic pseudocyst
   F. Primary streptococcal or pneumococcal peritonitis
   G. Leukemia and other lymphomas
   H. Sickle cell crisis
   I. Metabolic causes
      1. Lead poisoning
      2. Diabetic acidosis
      3. Acute porphyria
      4. Hereditary angioedema
   J. Musculoskeletal causes
      1. Ankylosing spondylitis
      2. Degenerative joint disease of symphysis
      3. Osteitis pubis
      4. Prolapsed intervertebral disc
      5. Spondylolisthesis
      6. Muscular strain
   K. Psychogenic causes

TABLE 59–2. Differential Diagnosis of True Pelvic Pain

Illness	Pain History	Precipitating or Relieving Factors	Associated Signs and Symptoms	Key Laboratory or Radiologic Data	Management or Disposition
Pelvic inflammatory disease	Sudden or gradual; colicky pain usually bilateral in lower pelvis, but unilateral salpingitis can occur	Occurs 2–3 days after menstruation due to gonorrhea or *Chlamydia*; after recent D&C or IUD insertion	Fever, chills, malaise, vomiting uncommon; marked tenderness and moderate rigidity of lower abdomen with distention; tenderness or fullness on either adnexa; enlarged uterus with post abortion or puerperal sepsis; cervical motion tenderness; possible rebound tenderness	Leukocytosis; purulent urethral or cervical discharge in GC infection; uterine bleeding with infected abortion; profuse fetid discharge in puerperal sepsis; culdocentesis may reveal pus; ESR often increased	See text and Table 59–4
Ruptured corpus luteum cyst, twisted ovarian cyst	Sudden onset; initially severe, intermittent, and localized to one adnexa; becomes continuous with local then general peritonitis	Usually no apparent precipitating factor; may have history of similar episodes lasting from hours to days; corpus luteum cyst usually ruptures 6–8 weeks from LNMP	Normal menses; afebrile or tachycardia out of proportion to fever; abdomen tender, distended, rigid; pelvic mass may be palpated in abdomen; pain on cervical motion; adnexal tenderness; discrete cystic adnexal mass palpated independently from uterus	Leukocytosis; culdocentesis may yield serosanguineous fluid; ultrasound may reveal pathologic process causing torsion, but laparoscopy needed to establish diagnosis. Type and cross-match or type and screen blood	Ruptured cysts usually resolve in 2–4 hr with pain relief. Twisted cysts require further diagnostic and therapeutic interventions (ultrasound, surgery)
Ruptured ectopic pregnancy	Sudden onset, severe, continuous, unilateral pelvic pain; rapidly becomes diffuse across entire lower abdomen and pelvis; may radiate to shoulder	Occurs usually 5–8 wk after LNMP (3–6 wk after ectopic fertilization); with rupture, the sharp localized pain is replaced by generalized hypogastric pain	Nausea and vomiting are rare but may occur prior to rupture; afebrile; dizziness, pallor, tachycardia, hypotension, breast tenderness, uterus enlarged with cervical motion tenderness; adnexal mass palpated in 50% of cases (+ tender)	ESR normal; possible anemia noted; positive results on serum beta hCG; generally diagnosis is made by positive culdocentesis, ultrasound, laparoscopy, or diagnostic peritoneal lavage; type and cross-match	See text and Fig. 59–1
Endometriosis	Tends to be constant, beginning 2–7 days before onset of menses, increases in intensity until menstrual flow lessens; may radiate to back, thighs, rectum, bladder, vagina, or adnexa; usually history of repeated attacks, associated with menses, and can be very severe (due to chemical causes, i.e., blood peritonitis)	Limited to reproductive years; more frequent in whites and nulliparas; tenderness on examination; more prominent during menses; all sites of endometriomas symptomatic during menses	May palpate tender indurated nodules in cul-de-sac or on rectal examination; dyspareunia more prominent near the menses; 50% have hypermenorrhea; associated with infertility or sterility; dyschezia (painful defecation) is common	Laboratory tests of no immediate value; laparoscopy can confirm the diagnosis, but even laparotomy may fail to identify lesions	Usually can be managed with pain relief at home

TABLE 59–2. Differential Diagnosis of True Pelvic Pain *Continued*

Illness	Pain History	Precipitating or Relieving Factors	Associated Signs and Symptoms	Key Laboratory or Radiologic Data	Management or Disposition
Degeneration of uterine myomas/fibroids	Sudden, severe pain, poorly localized in the pelvis	Older females, especially blacks	Menorrhagia, intermenstrual bleeding, occasionally dysmenorrhea or urinary frequency depending on size of fibroid; bimanual examination demonstrates mobile, usually nontender, firm, smooth masses; degeneration of myomas (ischemic episode) can occur in 30%–35% of women over age 35 yr	CBC, ESR, beta hCG, ultrasound, laparoscopy, or CT needed to confirm	After diagnostic work-up, patients often require admission for volume replacement and pain relief. Surgery is considered
Mittelschmerz	Sudden onset, sharp, continuous, sometimes severe and localized to one adnexa; may radiate to ipsilateral shoulder	History of similar episodes	Afebrile; may have nausea and fever; adnexal tenderness, guarding; may have rigidity and rebound; uterus normal size and no adnexal mass	ESR normal; no leukocytosis; may have positive culdocentesis but no anemia; negative beta hCG results	Managed with pain relief at home

D&C = dilatation and curettage; IUD = intrauterine device; LNMP = last normal menstrual period; GC = gonococcal; ESR = erythrocyte sedimentation rate; beta hCG = beta human chorionic gonadotropin (pregnancy test).

effectiveness of ambulatory therapy. The Center for Disease Control recommended outpatient treatment schedule for PID is outlined in Table 59–4.

Ruptured Ovarian Cyst. Primary therapy is directed toward hemodynamic resuscitation. Diagnostic laboratory tests are performed to rule out pregnancy and assess blood loss anemia. Ultrasonography will usually support the diagnosis and direct the course of ultimate therapy. The key findings are fluid in the cul-de-sac on ultrasound and a negative pregnancy test.

In the majority of patients with simple rupture of an ovarian cyst pain will rapidly resolve, and the patients will remain hemodynamically stable. Significant pain relief will take place in less than 4 to 6 hours, and the patient can be observed in the emergency department.

> **PROBLEM** Ultrasonography was carried out and demonstrated an intrauterine pregnancy.
> The symptoms, signs, and laboratory tests now pointed to the diagnosis of PID with an incidental pregnancy. There was still the possibility of a ruptured ovarian cyst or torsion, but it was less likely than PID.

SPECIAL CONSIDERATIONS

Prepubertal Pelvic Pain

Sexual abuse and vaginal or urethral foreign bodies are the most common causes of pelvic pain in the pediatric patient. Malodorous or bloody vaginal discharge and painful urination or defecation often suggest a foreign body. Toilet paper, crayons, and tampons are the most common culprits. Rectal examinations, radiologic studies, and ultrasound may be helpful.

Sexual abuse is always considered with children who demonstrate evidence of rectal or vaginal injury, unexplained or unusual ecchymoses, or abrasions or lacerations in the

TABLE 59-3. Differential Diagnosis of Abdominal Causes of Pelvic Pain

Illness	Pain History	Precipitating or Relieving Factors	Associated Signs and Symptoms	Key Laboratory or Radiologic Data	Management or Disposition
Ureteral calculus	Intermittent, severe, comes in spasms of several minutes and then generally decreases, but can be constant; maximal in flank or lower abdomen; may radiate to iliac crest	May be precipitated by exercise, motion, dehydration	Nausea, vomiting, sweating, syncope, even shock; fever and chills if associated with infection; rigidity of abdomen with pain; soreness and tenderness to palpation may persist between attacks of pain	Generally red cells in urine; occasionally WBCs, albumin, and crystals. Radiopaque stones seen often (80%) on abdominal plain film; IVP shows filling defect (in 80%)	Most patients can be managed with pain relief and fluids at home with close follow-up. Continued obstruction requires relief
Acute pyelonephritis	Continuous, aching pain; maximally felt in flank, upper/lower abdomen, or midback	Asymptomatic bacteriuria or partially treated UTI	Shaking, chills, and fever; skin hot and dry; tachycardia; frequently nausea and vomiting; occasional dysuria; flank tenderness to palpation or percussion	Many WBCs in urine, occasional RBCs and WBC casts; leukocytosis	Can be treated with antibiotics as outpatient if not toxic or not vomiting
Acute pelvic appendicitis	Unruptured pelvic appendicitis presents tense, peristaltic pain, felt chiefly in epigastrium or periumbilical area, after rupture, epigastric pain diminishes to give rise to local right-sided pelvic peritonitis that is less severe	Pain worsened with flexion of right thigh with internal rotation	Pain in both left and iliac fossae preceded by anorexia, nausea, or vomiting; may have frequency of urination or dysuria, diarrhea or tenesmus; right pelvic wall tenderness with rectal examination or pelvic mass (abscess) in later stage	Leukocytosis, occasional mild hematuria, low-grade fever, low-lying fecalith present or ileus, ultrasound of abscess present; barium enema sometimes advocated	Requires surgical removal if suspected
Strangulated femoral hernia	Often small fluctuant sac appears suddenly; may become larger and painful, may easily escape notice in thick fat in saphenous region	History of previous unilateral pelvic fullness or pain; occasionally incarceration associated with activities precipitating increasing intra-abdominal pressure	Generalized abdominal pain and vomiting with or without a palpable hernial sac; generally a painful swelling is noted in femoral ring	Late stages may be leukocytosis; may show obstructed pattern on acute abdominal radiologic series	Requires prompt surgical intervention
Leaking or ruptured abdominal aortic (or iliac) aneurysm	Variable; may be no symptoms before rupture; main symptoms may be unbearable pain starting in thorax, gradually extending to abdomen, hip, or thigh; not relieved with narcotics; history of aneurysm	Significant arterial hypertension of long duration is usually a forerunner; with rupture, hypovolemic shock is common	Throbbing pain before rupture; steady pain after rupture; pain possible for 4–5 days before rupture and collapse; nausea and vomiting rare; pulsatile mass anywhere in abdomen but left flank most common site; back pain common; occasional unequal femoral pulses	Chest, flat-plate abdomen, or cross-table lateral plain radiograph usually demonstrates calcifications of aortic aneurysms; hematuria and elevated BUN are present if renal artery is involved; type and cross-match blood	Requires immediate surgical intervention

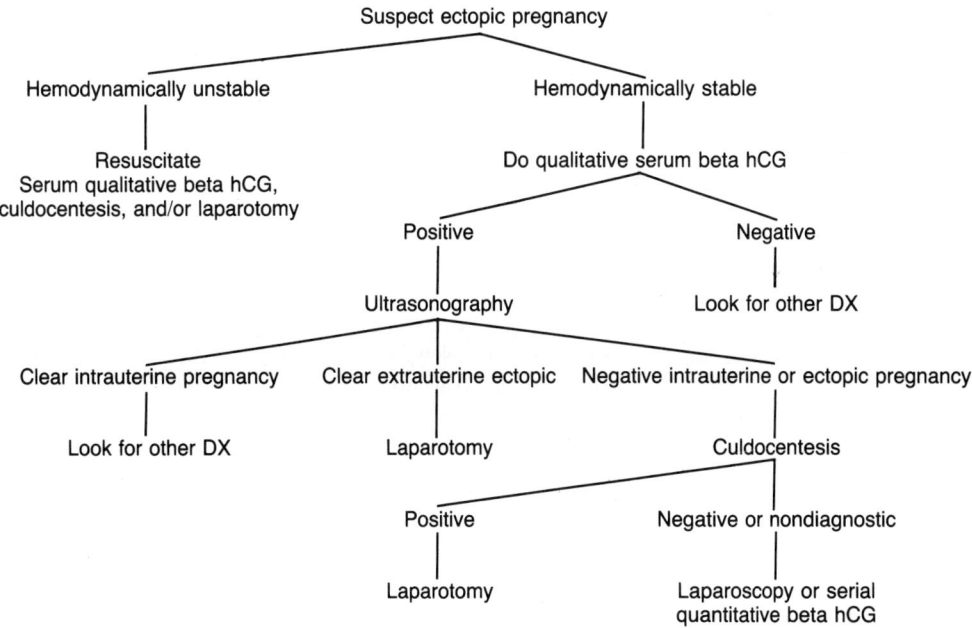

FIGURE 59–1. *Management algorithm for the patient with a suspected ectopic pregnancy.*

genital area. The pelvic examination for the young virginal patient may satisfactorily include the visual examination, rectal examination, and a moistened cotton swab for vaginal cultures and slides. Adnexal disease, such as torsion of the ovary, ruptured ovarian cyst, and acute salpingitis can account for a significant portion (nearly 50% in one series) of pelvic pathology in prepubertal patients.

Other causes of prepubertal pelvic pain include the following:

- Vulvovaginitis
- Dermatitis of the vulva
- Imperforate hymen
- Congenital anomalies of the genitourinary tract
- Appendicitis
- Pyelonephritis
- Sickle cell crisis

Geriatric and Postmenopausal Pain

Due to decreased circulating estrogen in the postmenopausal female, senile vaginitis can become an annoying if not painful condition. Additionally, uterine fibroids, cervical polyps, and endometrial hyperplasia can cause significant pelvic pain as well as vaginal

TABLE 59–4. CDC Guidelines for the Outpatient Treatment of Women with Acute Pelvic Inflammatory Disease[a]

Single dose[b] of:
    Cefoxitin, 2 gm IM
    or
    Ceftriaxone, 250 mg IM
    or
    Amoxicillin, 3 gm PO
    or
    Ampicillin, 3.5 gm PO
Followed by
    Doxycycline, 100 mg PO twice daily for 10–14 days

[a]When PPNG-associated PID is suspected, the use of cefoxitin, cefotaxime, or ceftriaxone plus doxycycline is recommended.
[b]Each single-dose agent except ceftriaxone is given with probenecid, 1 gm PO.

bleeding. During the pelvic examination, asking the patient to perform the Valsalva may also reveal uterine prolapse, cystourethrocele, or rectocele. The bimanual examination may reveal an adnexal cancer. The other causes of pelvic pain, e.g., appendicitis, can be difficult to diagnose in geriatric patients. Their response to pain, ability to provide a clear history, leukocyte response to infection or inflammation, and temperature elevations are not as obvious or as elevated as in females of childbearing age.

DISPOSITION AND FOLLOW-UP

The decision to admit or discharge the patient with pelvic pain depends on numerous criteria for each suspected condition. Ultimately, however, clinical judgment, often based on subtle findings or suspicion alone, is required to ensure the safety of the patient. The following are helpful criteria to guide the decision process.

Admission

1. Suspected ectopic pregnancy
   a. Evidence of hemodynamic instability
   b. Positive culdocentesis (nonclotting blood is present)
   c. More than 6 weeks since last normal menstrual period
   d. Severe pain
2. Pelvic inflammatory disease
   a. Suspected pelvic or tubo-ovarian abscess
   b. Pregnancy
   c. Intrauterine device in place
   d. Adolescents with salpingitis (high noncompliance rate for taking antibiotics)
   e. Temperature greater than 38°C
   f. Nausea and vomiting, precluding oral medications
   g. Significant peritoneal signs
   h. Failure to respond to outpatient oral antibiotics
   i. Uncertain diagnosis
3. Ruptured ovarian cyst
   a. Hemodynamically unstable
   b. Persistent pain

Discharge

1. Suspected ectopic pregnancy
   a. Patient is hemodynamically stable and no orthostatic changes appear on initial presentation
   b. Negative or nondiagnostic culdocentesis and/or ultrasonogram
   c. Minimal pain
   d. Last normal menstrual period less than 6 weeks ago
   e. These patients are discussed with a consultant before they are discharged, and repeat evaluation with serum quantitative hCG testing is arranged within 48 to 72 hours
2. Pelvic inflammatory disease
   a. None of the criteria for admission are met
   b. Patient is able to obtain close follow-up
3. Ruptured ovarian cyst
   a. Hemodynamically stable

    b. Marked pain relief during observation
    c. Lack of vomiting
    Follow-up arrangements are usually made with a gynecologist in 48 to 72 hours.

Pelvic Pain of Uncertain Etiology

In spite of an extensive emergency department evaluation, which may even include ultrasonography, a certain number of patients will remain without a specific diagnosis. These are often patients who have been evaluated for similar complaints in the past. As a general rule, these patients can be referred to their primary physician or gynecologist for further diagnostic efforts if they meet the following guidelines:
 1. Negative pregnancy test
 2. Hemodynamically stable, including no abnormal orthostatic vital sign changes
 3. Afebrile
 4. No peritoneal findings on abdominal examination
 5. No masses, significant pelvic tenderness, or bleeding

In sexually active females it is especially important to take both gonococcal and chlamydial cultures prior to releasing the patient. In patients who have mild or vague pelvic complaints, the etiology is often infectious, and antibiotic therapy is given if a culture is positive.

PROBLEM The patient fulfilled one of the criteria for admission because she was pregnant with suspected PID. The gynecologic consultant was called, and the patient was admitted for further evaluation and treatment.

DOCUMENTATION

 1. Character, quality, location, duration, radiation, and exacerbating or relieving factors relating to pain.
 2. Associated symptoms, e.g., fever, vomiting, shoulder pain.
 3. Age, parity, gravity, sexual history, last menstrual period, last normal menstrual period, contraceptive usage, history of sexually transmitted diseases.
 4. Vital signs.
 5. Chest, flank, abdomen, and pelvic examination results.
 6. Pregnancy test results.
 7. Diagnostic impression.
 8. Consultant recommendations.
 9. Therapeutic and follow-up plan.

SUMMARY AND FINAL POINTS

- Although pelvic pain most commonly originates in the reproductive organs, other sources of pain include the gastrointestinal, urinary, and vascular systems.
- Ectopic pregnancy and pelvic inflammatory disease are the two most important conditions to discover or rule out in the evaluation of the woman of reproductive age who presents with pelvic pain.
- Pregnancy testing is the key laboratory study that determines whether the diagnosis of ectopic pregnancy should be pursued.
- The most important use of ultrasonography is to confirm the presence of an intrauterine pregnancy in patients with suspected ectopic pregnancy.
- Although chlamydial PID often is not as clinically evident as gonococcal PID, the damage potential to the reproductive organs is the same.
- Early during the clinical course, a ruptured ovarian cyst may be clinically indistinguish-

able from an ectopic pregnancy. Rapid decrease in the level of pain and negative results on the beta hCG test confirm the diagnosis of a ruptured cyst.
- Sexual abuse and foreign bodies are the most common causes of pelvic pain in the prepubertal age group.

BIBLIOGRAPHY

Texts
1. Farrell RG (ed): OB/GYN Emergencies. Rockville, MD, Aspen, 1986.
2. Sweeet RL, Gibbs RS (eds): Infectious Diseases of the Female Genital Tract. Baltimore, Williams & Wilkins, 1985.

Journal Articles
1. Beard RW, Reginald PW, Pearce S: Pelvic pain in women. Br Med J 293:1160–1162, 1986.
2. Chapin DS: Pelvic inflammatory disease. Med Times 115:49–64, 1987.
3. Gleicher N, Giglia RV, Deppe G, et al: Direct diagnosis of unruptured ectopic pregnancy by real-time ultrasonography. Obstet Gynecol 61:425–428, 1983.
4. Hedges JR, Kalb JJ, Armao JC: Detection of ectopic pregnancy in an outpatient population: The role of the beta-hCG level. J Emerg Med 2:85–93, 1984.
5. Mansi ML: The role of the culdocentesis in evaluating pelvic pain in women. J Am Osteopath Assoc 83:576–581, 1984.
6. Spence MR: Pelvic inflammatory disease. J Reprod Med 34:605–609, 1989.
7. Steinheber FU: Medical conditions mimicking the acute surgical abdomen. Med Clin North Am 57:1559–1567, 1973.
8. Trott A: Diagnostic modalities in gynecologic and obstetrical emergencies. Emerg Med Clin North Am 5:405–423, 1987.

CHAPTER 60

VAGINAL BLEEDING

THOMAS KRISANDA, M.D.

PROBLEM A 20 year old woman was in her primary physician's office awaiting an examination for recent irregularity of her menstrual cycle. After calling her to an examining room, the nurse noted that the patient appeared pale and unsteady in her gait. The nurse obtained a pulse of 120 beats/min and a blood pressure of 90/50 mm Hg in a sitting position. After a brief assessment by the physician, a decision was made to transfer the patient to the emergency department by rescue squad.

QUESTIONS TO CONSIDER

1. What conditions can cause severe and potentially life-threatening vaginal bleeding?
2. When should a pelvic examination NOT be performed in evaluating a patient with abnormal bleeding?
3. Which ancillary tests are most helpful in emergently evaluating abnormal vaginal bleeding?
4. How reliable are current methods for pregnancy testing?
5. What is the role of ultrasonography in these patients?
6. What differential diagnostic considerations are unique to prepubertal and postmenopausal patients?
7. Can hormonal causes of abnormal vaginal bleeding be accurately diagnosed in the emergency department?
8. What factors influence the decision to admit or discharge the patient?

INTRODUCTION

Vaginal bleeding is the visible result of hemorrhage occurring anywhere along the female reproductive tract. In premenarchal and postmenopausal patients, vaginal bleeding is almost always the result of a nonhormonal cause. Women of reproductive age may exhibit physiologic vaginal bleeding that reflects cyclic endometrial stimulation orchestrated by the interplay between estrogen and progesterone. These ovarian hormones in turn are controlled by a complex endocrine system mediated by the hypothalamus and pituitary gland and incorporating multiple hormonal feedback loops. This system, although providing the hormonal integration necessary for female reproduction, also produces opportunities for dysfunction. Vaginal bleeding is one of the most common genitourinary complaints of women in the emergency department.

Vaginal bleeding is caused by one of six basic pathophysiologic mechanisms. These are pregnancy-related, neoplastic, infectious, traumatic, hormonal, and hematologic. The most potentially life-threatening mechanism is pregnancy-related. Pregnancy can cause abnormal bleeding in three ways. The ovum can fail to develop properly, in which case its growth will be terminated and it will be expelled from the uterus (spontaneous abortion). Implantation can occur in a site other than the uterus; bleeding will then occur when the fetus can no longer be accommodated by the site of implantation (ectopic pregnancy). Later in pregnancy, the placenta can bleed profusely if it is located over the os at the time of cervical dilatation and effacement or if the placenta prematurely separates from the uterine wall (placenta previa or abruptio placentae).

Neoplasms cause bleeding by invading normal pelvic structures or by necrosis of the tumor mass itself. Both benign and malignant processes can cause bleeding. For example, uterine polyps occur in 4% of women and can ulcerate and bleed. Postmenopausal bleeding always raises concern that a malignancy is present, but malignancy is proved in only 20% of cases. A neoplasm can invade any anatomic structure from the introitus to the ovary. The goal of routine screening of women with regular pelvic examinations and cervical cytology is to find early signs of cancer.

Infection can cause abnormal bleeding at one or multiple anatomic sites. It may be caused by many organisms, the most important being *Neisseria gonorrhoeae* and *Chlamydia trachomatis*. In one clinical setting, when other causes of bleeding were excluded in sexually active, reproductively capable patients, gonococcal infection (as proved by culture) was the cause of bleeding in 30% of cases. It is routine in many centers to obtain a cervical culture for *N. gonorrhoeae* in all sexually active females with vaginal bleeding. Abnormal bleeding resulting from infection can be very subtle and difficult to diagnose.

Trauma as a cause of bleeding is more common in the pediatric age group. The bleeding is usually the result of lacerations of the perineum, vulva, or vagina. In adults, traumatic bleeding can be caused by sexual intercourse.

Unless prolonged, hormonally related hemorrhage rarely poses a significant risk to the patient. It is often a diagnosis of exclusion, made after other possible mechanisms have been ruled out.

Finally, hematologic causes result from abnormalities of hemostasis. Platelet disorders more commonly present as abnormal vaginal bleeding than coagulopathies. A disorder of the pelvic organs may secondarily "unmask" a defect of the clotting mechanism.

Depending on the time course, rate, and compensatory response to bleeding, the presentation of the patient may range from a "normal" condition to overt shock. The emergency physician must work quickly to identify the patient at high risk from this hemorrhage.

PREHOSPITAL CARE

The prehospital evaluation and care of the patient with vaginal bleeding, whether pregnancy-related or not, are handled no differently from the initial resuscitation of any bleeding patient. The basic assessment includes:

History

1. What is the time of onset and estimated amount of vaginal bleeding?
2. Is abdominal pain present?
3. What are the associated symptoms—fever, vomiting, dizziness, syncope?

Physical Examination

1. Vital signs are measured.
2. The presence of active vaginal bleeding is noted.
3. A search is made for evidence of hypovolemia (pallor, clammy skin, apprehension).
4. Signs of pregnancy are noted.
5. The presence of abdominal tenderness is noted on palpation.

Intervention

Supplemental Oxygen. Oxygen is provided at 8 to 10 liters/min by nasal cannula if there is a suspicion of significant blood loss.

Intravenous Access. Isotonic crystalloid solutions are delivered through large-bore (16- or 14-gauge) intravenous (IV) lines. In hemodynamically unstable patients, fluid is administered as rapidly as possible. For patients with normal vital signs but a history or evidence of profuse bleeding, 500 to 1000 ml can be safely given over 60 minutes to replace potential volume loss.

Cardiac Monitor. Monitoring is indicated in any hemodynamically unstable patient.

Pneumatic Antishock Garment. Although controversial, the pneumatic antishock garment (PASG) is recommended as a temporary adjunct in the actively hemorrhaging, hemodynamically unstable patient. Only the leg compartments are used in the pregnant patient.

The Patient in Labor. For the patient who presents with vaginal bleeding in a later stage of pregnancy (i.e., third trimester), additional cautions are necessary. The most common cause of vaginal bleeding in late pregnancy is impending childbirth. This possibility is usually clinically obvious, and the patient is questioned about:

1. The time of onset of labor
2. Present timing and severity of contractions
3. Number and outcome of previous pregnancies
4. Any problems anticipated by the patient's obstetrician

For the patient in labor an IV line is placed (if this will not delay transport significantly), oxygen is given, and the patient is placed in the position of comfort. Pressure exerted by the gravid uterus on the inferior vena cava can lead to impairment of circulatory return to the heart. Transport in the left lateral decubitus position can alleviate this problem.

A rapid *visual* inspection of the external genitalia is carried out. Evidence of excessive hemorrhage, a prolapsed umbilical cord, or "crowning" is sought. Crowning occurs when the baby's head remains visible in the introitus between contractions. If this is noted, rescue squad crew members must prepare for emergency childbirth.

PROBLEM On arrival at the physician's office, the rescue squad found that the patient had been placed in the Trendelenburg position and that an intravenous line was infusing lactated Ringer's solution. The patient still appeared to be pale and complained of right lower quadrant pain. She was alert, cooperative, and slightly diaphoretic. Repeat vital signs revealed a pulse of 120 beats/min and blood pressure of 90/60 mm Hg. The paramedics inserted a second line and rapidly infused a total of 500 ml of lactated Ringer's solution. PASG were placed in the uninflated state.

In this case, the onset of abdominal pain and evidence of hemodynamic compromise in a young female with abnormal vaginal bleeding pointed to a potentially life-threatening problem until proved otherwise. After the initial assessment and establishment of IV access, the squad was instructed by radiotelemetry to proceed with further resuscitation and supportive care *while en route* to avoid delay in initating hospital-based definitive diagnosis and therapy. The PASG were to be inflated if the patient's hemodynamic condition deteriorated.

INITIAL APPROACH IN THE EMERGENCY DEPARTMENT

On arrival, patients with a complaint of vaginal bleeding are evaluated and managed according to the following general guidelines. Patients with supine or orthostatic vital signs indicative of hemodynamic compromise secondary to blood loss, with other evidence of hypovolemia (pallor, diaphoresis, apprehension), or with objective evidence of significant vaginal bleeding are triaged to the resuscitation area of the emergency department and seen immediately by the physician. Patients without these findings are placed in a gynecologic examination area and seen in order of their time of appearance in the emergency department.

History

The brief history as described in the section on Prehospital Care is obtained by the physician, and the rescue squad information is confirmed. The severity of symptoms and potential for pregnancy are the important points of the history.

Physical Examination

A primary survey of the airway, breathing, and circulation is combined with a rapid assessment of the level of consciousness and an abdominal examination. An initial estimate of the patient's blood loss is made according to the principles outlined in Chapter 4.

Intervention

1. Preliminary interventions for possibly unstable patients:
    a. One or more large-bore (16- or 14-gauge) intravenous lines are established, and isotonic crystalloid solution is given.
    b. Oxygen therapy at 8 to 10 liters/min is begun or continued.
    c. Cardiac monitoring is started.
    d. A blood sample is sent to the laboratory for initial hematocrit, and also for type and screen or for cross-match for four to six units.
    e. Blood or urine samples are obtained for pregnancy testing by a rapid measurement of beta hCG. Blood is saved in anticipation of additional blood tests, e.g., serum beta hCG, platelet count, coagulation studies.
2. Patients in labor who are experiencing vaginal bleeding and beyond 20 weeks of pregnancy are handled in a similar manner. As in the prehospital care setting, the possibility of emergency delivery is always considered. Once stabilization is carried out, the patient is transferred to an obstetric unit.

Patients of reproductive age who are complaining of vaginal bleeding accompanied by abdominal pain but have no evidence of significant distress, obvious bleeding, or hemodynamic instability can be triaged to a gynecology examining room and seen expeditiously by the physician. An intravenous line is established at the discretion of the nursing staff. Serum or urine pregnancy testing is carried out. The possibility of ectopic pregnancy is a foremost concern in these patients.

Patients of any age complaining of painless vaginal bleeding who have stable vital signs, appear well, and have no obvious evidence of significant hemorrhage may be triaged and seen as a lower priority in the context of other problems in the emergency department.

PROBLEM On arrival in the emergency department, the patient was assigned immediately to the resuscitation area. She was pale and complained of pain in the lower abdomen. There was blood staining on her pants. Her vital signs, taken by the nurse, were: blood pressure 80/40 mm Hg, pulse 130 beats/min, respiratory rate 24/min. She was afebrile but was restless and complaining of thirst. The nurse ensured that the intravenous lines were patent and contained isotonic crystalloid. Both lines were increased to a wide-open rate. Blood was drawn for an immediately spun hematocrit, type, and cross-match for six units of packed red cells and a rapid serum assay for beta hCG. The physician was asked to see the patient immediately and to speak briefly with the rescue squad. Five hundred milliliters of fluid had been given in the field.

This patient's condition has become worse during transport despite the initial volume resuscitation. Active bleeding is present. The patient needs rapid and aggressive volume resuscitation. In response to the physician's view of her condition, the PASG are inflated.

DATA GATHERING

The goals of the history and physical examination in the patient with vaginal bleeding are to elicit clues to the etiology of the bleeding, discover signs and symptoms of pregnancy, and determine the extent and effect of the blood loss.

History

1. *What is the reproductive status of the patient?*
   The physician determines whether the patient is reproductively capable or is either prepubertal or postmenopausal. The potential causes of the bleeding are profoundly influenced by this determination.
2. *When did the bleeding begin?*
   The time of onset of the bleeding is noted. Recent onset of abnormal bleeding is consistent with more immediately threatening problems such as ectopic pregnancy. Abnormal bleeding that has occurred over a prolonged period of time is more consistent with uterine problems such as malignancy or leiomyomas.
3. *What is the extent of the bleeding?*
   The amount of bleeding, as reported by the patient, is notoriously unreliable. As a rough gauge, the patient can be asked to measure the blood flow as more or less than her usual menses. Attempts to quantify the bleeding are less important than questioning about easy fatigability or postural dizziness, symptoms that might indicate significant blood loss.
4. *What is the menstrual history of the patient?*
   A careful menstrual history is essential to evaluate the complaint of vaginal bleeding. If the patient is menstruating, the cycle length, the number of days of menses, and any associated symptoms such as cramping or back pain are determined. There is marked individual variability in menstrual cycles. Normal menstrual cycles may vary from 18 to 40 days and, once established, plus or minus 5 days is considered normal variability. Total duration of menstrual flow is normally 3 to 7 days and is rarely constant for each woman. The most common cause of cessation of menses is pregnancy. Subtle changes in cycle length or amount of menses may be the only clinical signs of chlamydial or gonorrheal infection of the reproductive organs. Bleeding that occurs outside of the regular menstrual cycle may indicate malignancy or a blood dyscrasia.
5. *Is the passed blood clotted or nonclotted?*
   Menstrual blood usually does not clot. Clotting occurs with heavy bleeding when the blood does not remain in the uterine cavity long enough to undergo fibrinolysis.
6. *Is the patient sexually active?*
   Sexually active women are at greater risk for serious bleeding because of possible pregnancy. The method of birth control used is determined.
7. *What is the pregnancy history?*
   The number of previous pregnancies, live births, and any spontaneous or induced abortions are recorded. It is easiest to record these in annotated form, using the respective terms *gravida*, *para*, and *abortion* (or G–P–Ab). For example, a woman with four previous pregnancies, three live births, and one miscarriage is noted as $G_4P_3Ab_1$.
8. *Are there associated symptoms?*
   It is important to elicit a history of fever, abdominal or pelvic pain, and vaginal discharge if present. Pain may be caused by distention of a hollow organ, such

as a fallopian tube secondary to an ectopic pregnancy. Sudden vascular occlusion, e.g., torsion of an ovary or uterine fibroid, can cause sudden severe pain. Peritoneal irritation due to blood or pus may result in diffuse abdominal pain with rigidity and guarding. Disorders confined to the pelvis may present as pain referred to the back.

9. *Is there a pertinent past medical history?*

Inquiries are made about any previous abdominal or pelvic surgeries. Any previous episodes of pelvic inflammatory disease are noted. Both are important risk factors in ectopic pregnancy. Is there endocrine disease? Diabetes mellitus, hyper- and hypothyroidism, pituitary disease, or adrenal disease can be associated with vaginal bleeding.

10. *Does the patient have a known disorder of hemostasis?*

Platelet disorders are more common in women and present primarily as mucosal bleeding. The patient is asked whether other problems with abnormal bleeding have occurred (e.g., nosebleeds, dental extraction, menorrhagia). Use of platelet-inhibiting drugs such as aspirin is explored.

Physical Examination

Vital Signs

Heart Rate. Tachycardia may be secondary to pain, anxiety, or hypovolemia.

Blood Pressure. Hypotension (systolic blood pressure less than 80 to 90 mm Hg) is a serious sign reflecting significant blood loss. All normotensive patients with abnormal bleeding should have orthostatic vital signs measured. A drop in the systolic pressure of 20 mm Hg or a rise of 20 in the pulse rate may indicate a significant volume loss. Women in the later stages of pregnancy have a physiologic augmentation of circulating blood volume approaching 40%. Hypotension in this setting indicates major hemorrhage, presenting grave risks to mother and fetus. On the other hand, hypotension in pregnancy may be due to uterine pressure on the inferior vena cava, which can lead to decreased venous return to the heart. Placing the patient on the left side may correct this problem.

Respiratory Rate. Like tachycardia, tachypnea may reflect hypovolemia, pain, or anxiety.

Temperature. The presence of fever points to an underlying infectious etiology for the bleeding.

General Appearance. Patients with significant bleeding or a life-threatening pelvic organ disease often have signs of serious illness. They will look "uncomfortable" and are not inclined to voluntary movement on the stretcher. If hypovolemia is present, pallor, moist skin, and apprehension are observed in spite of a normal blood pressure reading. Conversely, patients with early ectopic pregnancy can appear remarkably well and in no distress. Pursuit of the diagnosis by appropriate testing must be particularly diligent in these cases.

Skin. The skin and mucosa (primarily oral) are examined for signs of abnormal bleeding, which may reveal a systemic process, e.g., petechiae, ecchymosis.

Abdomen

Inspection. The abdomen is inspected for pregnancy or abdominal distention.

Auscultation. Auscultation is carried out to assess bowel sounds or bruits if they are present.

Fetal Heart Tones. If the patient is pregnant, a Doppler stethoscope is used to detect fetal heart tones, but this test may be falsely negative at less than 8 to 10 weeks of gestation.

Palpation. All four quadrants of the abdomen are palpated. Any areas of tenderness are noted, especially if there is associated involuntary rigidity or rebound or signs of peritoneal irritation. If the uterus is palpable, the fundal height is determined. Uterine tenderness, rigidity, and contractions are assessed. The location of the uterine fundus may be used as a rough estimate of fetal gestational age as follows: top of symphysis pubis, 12 weeks; level of umbilicus, 20 weeks; tip of xiphoid, 36 weeks. After the thirty-sixth week, the uterine fundus recedes slightly as the fetal head drops into and engages the pelvis.

Pelvic Examination. Reassurance and positioning of the patient are the keys to an adequate pelvic examination. Ideally, the patient is placed in the dorsal lithotomy position; however, if the patient's condition is unstable and the work-up needs to proceed more rapidly, the examination can be performed with the patient in a frog-leg position and the buttocks elevated on a bedpan on the stretcher. Because the potential for additional harm is real, *pregnant patients with vaginal bleeding after the twentieth week should NOT receive a pelvic or rectal examination* unless provisions are made for both emergency surgical and vaginal delivery in a delivery suite.

Inspection. The external genitalia are carefully inspected. Bleeding, discharge, inflammation, and infection are noted. Particularly in the elderly, it is important to do a digital vaginal examination before inserting the speculum. This step will serve to detect foreign bodies, atrophic vaginitis with synechiae, and evidence of trauma or masses. It will also allow the position of the cervix to be located in advance of the speculum examination.

Speculum Examination. After insertion of the speculum, bleeding may be observed as originating from the external cervical os or elsewhere. The os is visually inspected, and whether it appears open is noted. This is indicative of an ongoing abortion in the pregnant patient. In the circumstance of suspected threatened abortion, the patency of the internal os is tested by a cotton-tipped applicator or ring forceps. The nonpregnant cervix is firm to the touch, with a uniform pink color. A bluish, soft cervix suggests pregnancy. If indicated, cervical cultures and specimens for microscopic examination are obtained at this time.

Bimanual Examination. A careful bimanual examination is performed. The consistency of the cervix (patulous, firm, nodular) and the presence of any cervical motion tenderness are key findings. The external cervical os is digitally palpated to reveal any dilatation or cervical effacement. The cul-de-sac is examined. Any fullness could indicate fluid, blood, or pus. The uterus is palpated for size, position, asymmetry, and tenderness. A "nodular" feel is suspicious of fibroids, malignant tumor, or endometriosis. Tenderness or masses (or both) are the important findings in the examination of the adnexae. Two important points to be remembered: The round ligaments are often mistaken for the fallopian tubes, especially in young, thin women, and the ovaries are not palpable in a postmenopausal woman. Because the ovaries are atrophic after menopause, any palpated mass is abnormal.

Rectal Examination. A rectal examination confirms the position of the uterus and the presence or absence of fluid in the cul-de-sac. If the patient has had previous infections, the cul-de-sac may be obliterated. Only positive findings have diagnostic significance.

PROBLEM A brief history revealed that the patient usually had a regular menstrual cycle with routine flow. She was $G_0P_0Ab_0$. Her last regular menstrual period had been shorter than usual, followed now, 2 weeks later, by a heavy flow with accompanying abdominal pain. She had been treated 1 year before for an infection of her "tubes" and used foam for contraception but not consistently. She denied any recent medication use, including aspirin. After two liters of lactated Ringer's had been infused, her pulse had decreased to 110 beats/min and her blood pressure had increased to 100/60 mm Hg with PASG inflated. Her skin was cool, but there was no abnormal bruising. She had mild lower abdominal tenderness on palpation. Her pelvic examination showed blood clots in the vaginal vault and active bleeding from the cervical os. She had right-sided tenderness and a sensation of "fullness" on bimanual examination. The uterus was normal, and movement did not significantly increase the pain.

DECISION PRIORITIES AND PRELIMINARY DIFFERENTIAL DIAGNOSIS

After initial stabilization and data gathering, preliminary diagnostic impressions were organized. The emergency physician seeks to answer four questions:

1. *Does the patient have severe blood loss with or without hemodynamic instability?*
   Regardless of the cause of bleeding, the initial resuscitation and stabilization of the patient are directed toward correcting the blood loss and volume depletion. A means of estimating the severity of volume loss is detailed in Chapter 4. Once appropriate resuscitative measures have been taken, a search for the source of hemorrhage is begun. If the hemorrhage has occurred over an extended time period, compensatory mechanisms may mask a significant loss of red blood cell mass.

2. *Is the patient pregnant?*
   Because the disorders of pregnancy that cause abnormal vaginal bleeding (e.g., ectopic pregnancy, placenta previa, abruptio placentae) tend to be more immediately life-threatening than non–pregnancy-related causes, determining the pregnancy status of the patient is paramount.

3. *Is the source of bleeding the reproductive tract or is it related to other anatomic areas?*
   The woman complaining of abnormal vaginal bleeding is usually accurate in localizing the site. In some cases, particularly in elderly women, the bleeding may be originating from the urinary or gastrointestinal tract. Occasionally, the bleeding originates from other anatomic sites but enters the vagina through a fistula. This finding is usually caused by malignancy.

4. *Is it systemic in origin?*
   Systemic disorders of hemostasis, especially platelet disorders, may manifest as mucosal bleeding (see Chapter 24). Most of these problems are drug-related (aspirin inhibition of platelet aggregation or thrombocytopenia due to chemotherapeutic agents) or acquired from immunologic (idiopathic thrombocytopenic purpura), infectious (disseminated intravascular coagulation), or unknown origins (thrombotic thrombocytopenic purpura).

PROBLEM The patient clearly was in hemodynamic jeopardy and remained so in spite of her improving vital signs. Based on the historical findings, the pain accompanying the bleeding, and the risk factors elicited by the history (prior infection, less than adequate birth control practices), she was likely to be pregnant. Ectopic pregnancy is the most common serious complication of pregnancy and the most likely diagnosis in this patient. The decision was made to continue with the inflated PASG, maintain rapid fluid administration, obtain additional diagnostic data, and consult with a gynecologist.

DIAGNOSTIC ADJUNCTS

The laboratory evaluation of abnormal vaginal bleeding is straightforward. Considerable information can be gained from only a few tests.

Laboratory Studies

Complete Blood Count and Differential. Patients presenting with a complaint of vaginal bleeding require a complete blood count (CBC) if there is evidence of significant blood loss by the history or physical examination (pallor or abnormal orthostatic vital signs). If the hemoglobin and hematocrit are in the normal range, the results will allow comparison at a future time to assess the degree of ongoing blood loss. Low levels represent chronic loss or acute loss of some severity. An elevated white blood cell (WBC) count and left-shifted differential suggest underlying infection or inflammation as a cause. The platelet count is diagnostic of thrombocytopenia. Interpreting the red blood cell (RBC) indices may provide evidence of iron deficiency or megaloblastosis.

Pregnancy Testing. In general, all women of reproductive capability with a complaint of vaginal bleeding should have an analysis of the beta subunit of human chorionic gonadotropin (beta hCG). A new generation of enzyme immunoassay pregnancy tests is available. These tests have a sensitivity as low as 5 to 25 mIU/liter and are greater than 96% specific for the beta subunit of hCG. These newer, more sensitive tests are important because up to 50% of women with ectopic pregnancies have serum hCG levels of less than 100 mIU at the time of discovery. A positive qualitative urinary beta-hCG analysis is just as useful as a positive serum assay. However, a negative urine test is not as reassuring as a negative serum test because of the lower inherent sensitivity (50 to 100 mIU/liter hCG serum equivalents) of the urine assays. In general, serum assays will consistently give positive results with hCG levels above 15 mIU/liter, whereas urinary assays are consistently positive only when serum levels exceed 50 to 100 mIU/liter.

Cervical Cultures. Endocervical gonococcal cultures should be performed in all sexually active women. Cultures or antigen screening for *Chlamydia trachomatis* are strongly suggested when infection is suspected as the cause of the bleeding.

Radiologic Imaging

Ultrasound. Ultrasonography is an extremely useful and versatile tool in evaluating the patient with abnormal vaginal bleeding. Currently available equipment is capable of resolving masses that are less than one centimeter in size. The accuracy of ultrasound in proved cases of ectopic pregnancy ranges from 65% to 100%, with a false-negative range of 2% to 35% and a false-positive range of 3% to 30%. Despite the acceptance of ultrasonography as a diagnostic adjunct in cases of suspected ectopic pregnancy, it remains an imprecise technique that is dependent on three variables: equipment, operator, and interpreter. Of the different sonographic findings possible in evaluating for an ectopic pregnancy, the most specific finding is the visualization of an extrauterine, extraovarian ectopic mass in which fetal heart motion or fetal parts can be detected. The best sonographic finding to *exclude* an ectopic pregnancy is the presence of an intrauterine gestational sac in which a fetal heart beat can be recognized. This finding corresponds approximately to a 42- to 45-day gestation.

Ultrasound is excellent for detecting an intrauterine pregnancy and for evaluating the position of the placenta. It is also good for detecting other adnexal abnormalities and the presence of as little as 5 to 20 ml of blood or fluid in the cul-de-sac. It is unreliable in determining the degree of placental separation in abruptio placentae and in determining the presence or extent of endometrial or cervical carcinoma.

Other Tests

Culdocentesis. The primary utility of culdocentesis is the diagnosis of ectopic pregnancy as the cause of vaginal bleeding. The procedure is a needle aspiration of the cul-de-sac. Nonclotting blood obtained in a patient with a positive pregnancy test is virtually diagnostic (95% sensitivity) of a ruptured ectopic pregnancy. A negative result on culdocentesis, on the other hand, does not rule out an ectopic pregnancy. Purulent material in the cul-de-sac is suggestive of pelvic inflammatory disease or a tubo-ovarian abscess. Chapter 59 has more information on the use of culdocentesis and ultrasonography in the detection of ectopic pregnancy.

PROBLEM The pregnancy test result was unequivocally positive. The patient's hematocrit was 28%. After 2000 ml of lactated Ringer's solution had been infused, the patient remained pale with a pulse rate of 110 and a blood pressure of 100/60 mm Hg. Packed red blood cell replacement was started. Although difficult to perform with the PASG inflated, a culdocentesis was carried out through the perineal opening of the PASG by using a vaginal speculum and an 18-gauge needle introduced into the cul-de-sac. It yielded 5 ml of nonclotting blood.

Between the culdocentesis result and the positive pregnancy test result, the diagnosis of ectopic pregnancy was virtually ensured. The gynecology consultant was on his way to the emergency department, and the operating room was prepared.

REFINED DIFFERENTIAL DIAGNOSIS

This section is organized with the various causes of vaginal bleeding grouped according to the presence or absence of pregnancy (Table 60–1).

Conditions Causing Vaginal Bleeding When the Pregnancy Test Result Is Positive

Ectopic Pregnancy

Ectopic pregnancy is a true emergency and is the most serious cause of vaginal bleeding. It is the leading cause of maternal mortality and occurs in 1:100 to 1:200 pregnancies. Ectopic pregnancy can become manifest in a variety of ways. The presentation of abdominal pain, vaginal bleeding, adnexal mass, and confirmatory laboratory evidence of pregnancy is straightforward. However, the diagnosis can be difficult in many cases. A high index of suspicion is always maintained. The symptoms and signs of ectopic pregnancy, with their approximate incidence, are listed below.

Symptoms
1. Abdominal pain (97%)
2. Symptoms of pregnancy—amenorrhea, nausea, breast tenderness (75%)
3. Vaginal bleeding (55%)
4. Syncopal or presyncopal symptoms (34%)

TABLE 60–1. Differential Diagnosis of Vaginal Bleeding

Pregnancy Status	
Positive	*Negative*
<20 weeks' gestation	*Vaginal*
Ectopic pregnancy	Trauma
Threatened abortion	Foreign body
Inevitable abortion	Infection
Incomplete abortion	Neoplasm
Completed abortion	Vascular—arteriovenous malformation
Missed abortion	Atrophic vaginitis
Infection, septic abortion	Endometriosis—cervical/vaginal
Trophoblastic disease	Immunologic—lichen sclerosis et atrophicus or lichen simplex chronicus
>20 weeks' gestation	*Uterine*
Placenta previa	Ovulatory
Abruptio placentae	Menses
Uterine rupture	Infection
Vasa previa	Neoplasms, benign or malignant
Premature labor	Hematologic
Normal labor	Iatrogenic
	Anovulatory
	Endocrine
	Psychogenic

Signs
1. Lower abdominal tenderness (83%)
2. Adnexal tenderness (72%)
3. Clinical evidence of hypovolemia (38%)
4. Blood in the cul-de-sac (30%)
5. Adnexal mass (25%)
6. Uterine enlargement (25%)

In short, any reproductively capable woman who presents with abdominal pain, abnormal vaginal bleeding, and a positive test for pregnancy is assumed to have an ectopic pregnancy until proved otherwise. The definitive diagnosis of ectopic pregnancy is by no means easy. The differential diagnosis is extensive and includes conditions of varying severity in both the pregnant and nonpregnant conditions. Table 60–2 categorizes some commonly encountered conditions often confused with ectopic pregnancy.

Spontaneous Abortion

Spontaneous abortion is commonly seen in the emergency department. Spontaneous abortion, or "miscarriage," is defined as the natural termination of a pregnancy before the fetus is capable of extrauterine life, which is approximately 20 weeks' gestation and 500 gm fetal weight.

Six subcategories of spontaneous abortion concern the emergency practitioner. *Threatened abortion* is defined as any uterine bleeding that occurs in the first half of a normal pregnancy. This definition is thus met in 20% to 25% of all pregnant women, and in half of these, the process will go on to completion. There is no dilatation of the internal cervical os at the time or at presentation to the emergency department. An *inevitable abortion* occurs when the above definition is met and the bleeding increases and pain persists. Dilatation of the internal cervical os is the major differential point. There is no possibility of fetal survival in this circumstance.

An *incomplete abortion* is the natural evolution of an inevitable abortion, but only some of the products of conception from the uterine cavity are passed. A *complete abortion* may be suspected when there is cessation of "pregnancy symptoms" (breast engorgement and tenderness, nausea) following passage of the entire conceptus.

A *missed abortion* occurs when the conceptus dies but is not passed. This condition usually is not accompanied by vaginal bleeding. *Second-trimester abortions* are rare but often are due to identifiable causes such as abruptio placentae, chorioamnionitis, uterine anomalies, cervical incompetence, and the lupus anticoagulant syndrome.

Bleeding in Late Pregnancy

Third-trimester bleeding is an unusual event, occurring in only 2% to 3% of patients. Although a trivial etiology such as vaginal condylomas, cervical polyps, or minor trauma

TABLE 60–2. Differential Findings in Conditions Mimicking Ectopic Pregnancy

Diagnosis	Amenorrhea	Beta hCG	Adnexal Mass or Tenderness	Vaginal Bleeding
Ectopic pregnancy	+	+	+	+
Corpus luteum cyst	+	−	+	+/−
Threatened abortion	+	+	−	+
Pelvic inflammatory disease	−	−	Bilateral	+/−
Appendicitis	−	−	RLQ tenderness	−
Degenerating fibroid	−	−	Uterine mass	+/−
Ovarian torsion	−	−	Adnexal mass, tenderness	−

+ = present; − = absent.
RLQ = right lower quadrant.

may be the cause, placental abnormalities and uterine rupture must be considered first. As such, pelvic and rectal examinations are avoided until provision is made for management of severe hemorrhage, including emergent delivery in an operating suite.

Placenta Previa. Placenta previa is the condition in which placental implantation has occurred in the lower uterine segment. Placenta previa is characterized by bright red, painless vaginal bleeding that is initiated by the beginnings of cervical effacement and dilatation. Complications of placenta previa are fetal distress and demise secondary to a reduction or interruption of the fetoplacental circulation. Maternal morbidity or mortality is a direct result of the degree of hemorrhage that occurs before definitive control.

Abruptio Placentae. Abruptio placentae is the complete or incomplete detachment of the normally implanted placenta at any time before the birth of the infant. Placental separation may be complete or partial, and the bleeding is either *revealed* after dissection under the membranes to the outside, or *concealed* behind the placenta or membranes. The patient classically presents with a painful, tender uterus that demonstrates variable degrees of uterine contraction with incomplete relaxation. Vaginal bleeding is usually dark red. Fetal distress or demise is usually seen. In the latter instance, fetal heart tones are unobtainable.

Conditions Causing Vaginal Bleeding When the Pregnancy Test Is Negative

When the pregnancy test is negative, abnormal vaginal bleeding may be secondary to lower genital tract (vaginal or cervical) pathology or to upper tract (uterus, fallopian tubes, ovaries) disease (Table 60–1).

Bleeding secondary to a vaginal abnormality is easily evaluated by speculum and by digital and microscopic examinations. All these examinations are easily performed in the emergency department. Many of the conditions resulting in lower genital tract bleeding can be diagnosed and treated primarily in the emergency department. Upper genital tract bleeding usually originates in the uterus. Abnormal uterine bleeding may be either *ovulatory* or *anovulatory*. Ovulatory refers to bleeding interspersed with what is otherwise regular, cyclic ovulatory uterine bleeding. Anovulatory bleeding is usually associated with an underlying endocrine disturbance.

Common causes of ovulatory abnormal uterine bleeding include neoplasms (benign and malignant), endometriosis, infections, intrauterine devices, endogenous sex steroid hormones, and blood dyscrasias. Common causes of anovulatory uterine bleeding include endocrine disturbances, most commonly physiologic immaturity of the hypothalamic-pituitary-ovarian axis, psychogenic causes including stress, athletic activity, and eating disorders, and "dysfunctional uterine bleeding" (DUB).

Dysfunctional uterine bleeding is often construed as a "catch-all" diagnosis. Actually it is defined as abnormal uterine bleeding with no organic cause, and therefore it is a diagnosis of exclusion. This exclusion often cannot be properly made in the emergency department. Causes of dysfunctional uterine bleeding may be grouped according to the age and menstrual status of the patient as follows:

1. Menarche to age 20. The usual cause of DUB in this age range is immaturity of the hypothalamic-pituitary-ovarian axis. Anovulatory cycles with irregular spotting and bleeding are the most common cause of abnormal bleeding in teenagers. Other causes include use of oral contraceptive agents or an IUD.

2. Ages 20 to 40. Anovulatory abnormal uterine bleeding is responsible for less than 20% of cases in this age group. In this group, causes are more likely to be psychogenic, i.e., stress, depression. Rapid weight changes and intense physical activity can also alter menses significantly.

3. Age over 40. As in the young perimenarchal patient, anovulation again becomes the major cause of abnormal bleeding; however, malignancy *must* be assumed until a thorough evaluation excludes it. Endometrial cancer has now superseded invasive cervical carcinoma as the most frequent gynecologic cancer.

PRINCIPLES OF MANAGEMENT

General Principles

The first principle of management of the patient with abnormal vaginal bleeding is to ensure hemodynamic stability. Volume loss must be vigorously treated with fluid or blood component therapy and oxygen, and continuously monitored. If the emergency evaluation reveals evidence of surgical disease, i.e., ruptured ectopic pregnancy or a complication of late pregnancy, then provisions for immediate transfer to the operating suite are made. The second major principle is to maintain fetal viability in women with advanced pregnancies but not at the expense of maternal safety. Early consultation with an obstetrician or gynecologist is essential in all cases in which either the mother or the fetus is endangered.

Specific Situations

Ectopic Pregnancy. Once an ectopic pregnancy is diagnosed, preparations for urgent laparotomy are made while the emergency department resuscitation is underway. The definitive surgical procedure of choice is a total salpingectomy. Refined, newer surgical techniques, including use of the operating laparoscope, make it possible to consider tubal salvage rather than removal. Systemic methotrexate therapy has shown promise as a nonsurgical therapy in some cases of unruptured ectopic pregnancy.

Spontaneous Abortion. No specific treatment regimen has proved efficacious in *threatened abortion*. Generally, patients are reassured and sent home with instructions to avoid sexual activity and to remain at bed rest for several days, although the latter has not been conclusively shown to be of benefit. The patient is instructed to return if bleeding persists or becomes worse, if pain increases, or if tissue is passed. Obstetric referral is mandatory and pelvic ultrasonography is performed within a few days to evaluate fetal viability. Doppler ultrasonographic determinations of fetal heart tones provide useful prognostic information, although it may be falsely negative before 8 to 10 weeks' gestation. A pregnancy test that reverts to negative is diagnostic of fetal demise.

The mainstay of treatment for *inevitable, incomplete, completed*, and *missed abortions* is uterine suction curettage. Curettage is necessary even after complete abortion because small tissue products can remain behind, resulting in unnecessary bleeding or infection. When the bleeding is severe, an oxytocin infusion can be initiated in the emergency department until the patient can be transferred for curettage. The final diagnosis of abortion rests on pathologic examination of the products of conception. Any tissue seen on examination is preserved for further evaluation. Finally, all patients should have an Rh determination. Rh-negative patients, who are unsensitized following an abortion or ectopic pregnancy, need $Rh_0(D)$ immune globulin. This determination is usually made by the consultant obstetrician-gynecologist, but occasionally it is the responsibility of the emergency physician.

Placenta Previa. Diagnosis and management occur simultaneously in the patient with third-trimester bleeding. When the diagnosis of placenta previa is suspected, diagnosis and management are determined by the amount of ongoing bleeding. If the bleeding is minor and the mother remains hemodynamically stable, a diagnostic ultrasound examination is performed. Blood is sent for CBC, typing, and cross-matching. Fetal heart tones are recorded. When the fetus is immature and the patient has only minimal bleeding, tocolytics and bed rest may suffice. If the bleeding is unremitting or copious, immediate Caesarean section is the treatment of choice.

Abruptio Placentae. Again, resuscitation and diagnosis must proceed simultaneously. Placental abruption may release large quantities of thromboplastin into the systemic circulation, placing the patient at risk for a coagulopathy. Therefore, coagulation studies are routinely ordered. Management consists of a vaginal examination and immediate amniotomy. An oxytocin infusion is started if labor does not ensue immediately. Caesarean delivery is performed if there is any evidence of fetal distress or delay in the establishment of effective labor.

Ovulatory Causes of Bleeding. Unless vaginal bleeding has led to hemodynamic instability, severe chronic blood loss, or anemia (hematocrit less than 30%), suspected malignancies, fibroid tumors, and endometriosis are expeditiously referred to a gynecologist for further management. Treatment for infections is initiated in the emergency department, and specific treatment guidelines are discussed in Chapters 59 and 61.

Dysfunctional Uterine Bleeding. Patients with anovulatory, or "dysfunctional," uterine bleeding are generally best served by reassurance and referral. Anovulatory bleeding in young women may be treated with medroxyprogesterone acetate (Provera) 10 mg daily for 5 to 7 days, every 60 days if necessary, or given as Depo-Provera as a single 200-mg injection. Hormonal manipulation to arrest bleeding is considered only after consultation with a gynecologist.

PROBLEM The patient was admitted to the operating suite from the emergency department. On laparotomy, the gynecologist found 1000 ml of free blood in the peritoneal cavity. The bleeding site was identified as a right-sided tubal pregnancy and controlled. Further volume resuscitation restored the patient to a normal hemodynamic status. Unfortunately, the site and extent of the ectopic mass did not allow tubal salvage, and a unilateral salpingectomy was performed. The patient recovered uneventfully.

SPECIAL CONSIDERATIONS

Premenarchal Patients

Abnormal vaginal bleeding in premenarchal girls is an uncommon problem. Seventy percent of cases are due to vulvovaginitis of either infectious or inflammatory etiology, usually from poor perineal hygiene or nonspecific irritants such as soaps, bubble baths, or clothes. "Sandbox vulvitis" is a well-known clinical entity in this category. Proven cases of sexually transmitted disease require appropriate medical therapy and a child sexual abuse evaluation.

Traumatic "straddle" injuries and foreign bodies are not uncommon. An uncooperative child may require either examination or treatment while under anesthesia if this problem is suspected. Table 60–3 lists the common and uncommon causes of vaginal bleeding seen in prepubertal girls.

Postmenopausal Patients

Bleeding in the older, postmenopausal woman immediately raises the suspicion of malignancy. Carcinomas of the endometrium and cervix are common; those of the vagina and ovary are less so, but all can result in vaginal bleeding. Invasive colorectal carcinoma is also considered. Fortunately, however, 80% of cases of postmenopausal bleeding ultimately prove to have a nonmalignant cause. Most cases of bleeding originate in the endometrium and are related to estrogenic over- and understimulation.

DISPOSITION AND FOLLOW-UP

The following are guidelines for the disposition and follow-up of patients with vaginal bleeding.

Admission

Patients requiring hospital admission have evidence of hemodynamic instability or unremitting hemorrhage. Also, patients in need of immediate surgery and most pregnant

TABLE 60–3. Causes of Vaginal Bleeding in Prepubertal Girls

Infectious, Inflammatory
Inflammatory processes
Poor hygiene
Chemical irritants (soaps, clothes, cosmetics)
Sexually transmitted diseases
Nonsexually transmitted disease (*Staphylococcus*, *Streptococcus*, gram-negative enteric organisms, molluscum contagiosum, condyloma acuminata)
Parasitic infections (amebiasis, *Enterobius vermicularis*, fungal)

Traumatic
Physical activity (bicycle riding)
Sexual abuse
Foreign bodies

Hormonal
Neonatal hormone withdrawal
Accidental hormonal ingestions—birth control pills, estrogen creams
Precocious puberty
Sex hormone–producing tumors

Urologic
Urinary tract infections (bacterial, viral, chlamydial)
Urethral prolapse
Hematuria
Neoplasm

Neoplasms
Gonadal stromal tumors (granulosa-theca cell)
Benign tumors (polyps, condyloma acuminata)
Sarcoma botryoides

Dermatologic
Lichen sclerosis et atrophicus
Lichen simplex chronicus
Atopic or irritant dermatitis

patients with the exception of threatened abortions are admitted. Patients with hemodynamic stability but with severe chronic blood loss anemia (hematocrit of less than 30%) are considered for admission.

Discharge

There is a certain subset of patients with suspected early ectopic pregnancy but are otherwise stable and reliable who are candidates for outpatient management. These patients are hemodynamically stable, have minimal abdominal pain and pelvic tenderness, and are less than 6 weeks from their last normal menstrual period. These patients may be observed with serial *quantitative* beta-hCG testing and ultrasonography. Women with ectopic and other abnormal pregnancies produce lower serum levels of hCG than those with normal pregnancies of similar gestational age. Serial serum hCG levels drawn 48 hours apart allow quantitation of this level as well as a determination of its rate of rise in the serum. Both quantitation and the rate of rise of hCG are abnormal in the setting of an ectopic pregnancy.

The patient with a threatened abortion may be safely discharged from the emergency department to receive outpatient follow-up. She is asked to return if bleeding, pain, cramping, or the suspected passage of tissue occurs.

Nonpregnant patients without evidence of hemodynamic instability generally do not require hospital admission. Patients with pelvic and vaginal infections, foreign bodies, minor genital trauma, and atrophic vaginitis are usually treated in the emergency department. Regimens for infectious causes are given in Chapters 59 and 61. Patients with suspected neoplastic disease (benign or malignant) and endometriosis are referred to a gynecologist for further evaluation.

DOCUMENTATION

1. Reproductive status of the patient: gravida, pregnancy, abortion (G–P–Ab).
2. Characteristics of the bleeding—time of onset, duration, presence of pain or cramping, estimated amount of bleeding.
3. Last normal menstrual period.
4. History of previous pregnancies.
5. Sexual activity and birth control use.
6. Previous history of gynecologic infections.
7. General physical appearance and vital signs.
8. Results of pelvic examination.
9. Laboratory results, especially the complete blood count and serum pregnancy test.
10. Final diagnosis, disposition, and follow-up arrangements.

SUMMARY AND FINAL POINTS

- The emergency evaluation of the patient complaining of vaginal bleeding should be geared to detect the few instances in which the correct diagnosis is "not to be missed." These situations include: a bleeding complication of pregnancy, sexual abuse in children, and malignant disease.
- Because bleeding in the setting of a pregnancy is a potentially life-threatening problem, a rapid qualitative pregnancy test is performed in *all* women of reproductive capability.
- Ectopic pregnancies are common, can be disastrous, and are often confused with other entities, e.g., threatened abortion.
- The resuscitation of the woman with vaginal bleeding is initially no different from the resuscitation of any hemorrhaging, hemodynamically unstable patient.
- Vaginal bleeding in the premenarchal patient is sexual abuse until proved otherwise.
- Postmenopausal bleeding is caused by malignancy until proved otherwise.
- Infection should not be forgotten as a common etiology of vaginal bleeding.
- Dysfunctional uterine bleeding is a diagnosis of exclusion and cannot be made with certainty in the emergency department.
- Always encourage a return emergency department visit for a discharged patient in whom symptoms become worse before a follow-up appointment can be kept.

BIBLIOGRAPHY

Texts

1. Jones HW, Wentz AC, Burnett LS (eds): Novak's Textbook of Gynecology (11th ed). Baltimore, Williams & Wilkins, 1988.
2. Pernoll ML, Benson RD (eds): Current Obstetric and Gynecologic Diagnosis and Treatment, 6th ed. Norwalk, CT, Appleton and Lange, 1987.
3. Wynn RM: Obstetrics and Gynecology, The Clinical Core. Philadelphia, Lea & Febiger, 1988.

Journal Articles

1. Anderson MM, et al: Abnormal vaginal bleeding in adolescents. Pediatr Ann 15(10):697–701, 704–707, 1986.
2. Fedele L, Acaia B, Parazini F, et al: Ectopic pregnancy and recurrent spontaneous abortion: Two associated reproductive failures. Obstet Gynecol 73:206–208, 1989.
3. Fletcher JL, Jr: Update on pregnancy testing. Primary Care 13(4):667–677, 1986.
4. Hochbaum SR: Vaginal bleeding. Emerg Med Clin North Am 5(3):429–442, 1987.
5. Keely MT, Santos-Ramos R, Duenhoetter JH: The value of sonography in suspected ectopic pregnancy. Obstet Gynecol 53:703, 1979.
6. Laferia JJ: Spontaneous abortion. Clin Obstet Gynecol 13(1):105–114, 1986.
7. Naryshkin S, et al: Comparison of the performance of serum and urine hCG immunoassays in the evaluation of gynecologic patients. Ann Emerg Med 14(11):1074–1076, 1985.
8. Rubin SC: Postmenopausal bleeding: Etiology, evaluation and management. Med Clin North Am 71(1):59–69, 1987.
9. Sanfilippo JS, et al: Bleeding and vulvovaginitis in the pediatric age group. Clin Obstet Gynecol 30(3):653–661, 1987.
10. Trott AT: Diagnostic modalities in gynecologic and obstetric emergencies. Emerg Med Clin North Am 5(3):405–423, 1987.

CHAPTER 61

PENILE AND VAGINAL DISCHARGE

SETH W. WRIGHT, M.D.

PROBLEM 1 A 17 year old male presented with a chief complaint of a "groin strain." Further questioning by the emergency physician revealed that the patient had a 2-day history of dysuria associated with a white penile discharge.

PROBLEM 2 A 26 year old female presented with a 3-week history of yellow-green vaginal discharge and pruritus. She denied abdominal pain, dysuria, or urgency.

QUESTIONS TO CONSIDER

1. What historical facts are important in evaluating penile and vaginal discharge?
2. Can gonococcal urethritis be accurately differentiated from nongonococcal urethritis on clinical examination?
3. What physical findings are significant in ruling out serious associated illnesses?
4. What are the common organisms found in men with penile discharge?
5. What are the common causes of vaginal discharge?
6. How is cervicitis differentiated from vaginitis?
7. What are the therapies for the common causes of vaginitis?
8. What are the current recommendations for the treatment of gonococcal infections?
9. Which patients with discharge require follow-up cultures for test of cure?

INTRODUCTION

Infections of the male and female genitourinary tract are commonly encountered in the practice of emergency medicine and often present diagnostic and therapeutic dilemmas. Treatment failures and recurrences are common despite optimal treatment.

Urethritis in males is virtually always caused by the sexually transmitted organisms *Neisseria gonorrhoeae* and *Chlamydia trachomatis*. It is well known that these two entities are not mutually exclusive and often present in the same patient. The concurrence rate of these two organisms in males is approximately 20% to 40%.

The Centers for Disease Control (CDC) estimates that three million cases of gonococcal urethritis (GCU) occur per year, although only one million are reported. *C. trachomatis* urethritis is not a reportable disease, but most health clinics report that it is two to three times more common than GCU in clinical settings.

The risk of a male acquiring gonorrhea from an infected female during a single episode of intercourse is approximately 20%, and the risk rises to virtually 100% with repeated intercourse. Gonococcal urethritis usually results from vaginal or rectal intercourse but may be acquired from the pharynx or from contact with secretions without actual penetration. When untreated, the symptoms of GCU can persist for up to 3 to 7 weeks. The patient may remain an asymptomatic carrier of the organism.

Nongonococcal urethritis (NGU) is a disorder with several causes. *Chlamydia trachomatis* and *Ureaplasma urealyticum* appear to be the primary pathogens involved in NGU, although other organisms play a minor and unproved role. As with GCU, NGU is most often seen in young men or in those of lower socioeconomic status.

Complaints of vaginal discharge are commonly seen in the emergency department, particularly in institutions serving indigent populations. Most are infectious in origin, but some cases have a noninfectious etiology. The vaginal mucosa contains no secretory cells, unlike the vulva, cervix, endometrium and fallopian tubes, all of which produce secretions in response to pathologic and physiologic stimuli. The vaginal mucosa does contribute to the normal vaginal secretion by desquamation of its epithelial cells, which increase under the influence of estrogen. Glycogen is secreted from the cells and is broken down to a variety of organic acids by the resident vaginal flora, resulting in a normal vaginal pH of 2.5 to 4.5. This low pH, in combination with the presence of normal lactobacilli, is inhibitory to most pathogens. Nevertheless, a variety of pathologic organisms may inhabit the vagina and lead to the presence of discharge. Common causes of vaginal discharge include *Candida albicans*, *Trichomonas vaginalis*, and *Gardnerella vaginalis* (formerly *Hemophilus vaginalis*) infections. In addition, *Herpes simplex* type II infections may present primarily as a vaginal discharge.

DATA GATHERING

Emergency physicians occasionally consider the presence of an abnormal discharge to be a trivial complaint. For the patient, the discomfort, social embarrassment, and concerns about infertility make this a significant problem. A complete history and physical examination will determine the likely etiologic factors in the majority of cases.

Evaluation of Penile Discharge

History
1. *How long has the discharge been present?*
   A sudden onset of symptoms is suggestive of a gonococcal origin.
2. *What does the discharge look like?*
   Does it drain spontaneously from the penis, or is it only present with stripping of the urethra? The discharge caused by gonorrhea is usually yellow and copious and drains spontaneously from the penis.
3. *Is there a new sexual partner?*
   Have any sexual partners been treated recently for a sexually transmitted disease, or do they have signs or symptoms suggestive of one?
4. *Is there associated testicular, abdominal, or rectal pain?*
   Does the patient have fever, rash, or joint pain? Epididymitis, prostatitis, proctitis, and disseminated gonococcal infections occasionally occur.
5. *Does the patient have any allergies?*
   This question is particularly important because of the numerous antimicrobials that are considered for the treatment of this problem.

Physical Examination
1. *Is the patient febrile?*
   The presence of fever suggests the possibility of epididymitis, acute prostatitis, pyelonephritis, or disseminated gonococcal infection.
2. *Is there other evidence of systemic illness?*
   A rash or joint pain is suggestive of disseminated gonorrhea, secondary syphilis, or Reiter's syndrome. Conjunctivitis is also seen with Reiter's syndrome.
3. *What are the findings on the genital, perirectal, and rectal examination?*
   What does the discharge look like? The discharge in GCU is usually whitish-yellow and copious. In NGU, it tends to be thin and watery. (The penis may

need to be massaged or "stripped" from the base to the glans to obtain discharge material.) What does the discharge look like? Are there lesions such as ulcers, warts, or rash? Is there inguinal adenopathy? Are the testes, epididymis, or prostate tender?

PROBLEM 1 The patient denied complaints other than dysuria and discharge. He admitted to having a new sexual partner in the past several weeks. The examination revealed a pleasant teenager who was afebrile. Results of the general physical examination are normal. He had a small amount of white discharge with stripping of the penis. There were no lesions present, and the testes and epididymis were in their normal position and nontender. The prostate was normal.

One of the primary goals of the physical examination of the patient with penile discharge is to exclude other, more serious illnesses such as epididymitis, prostatitis, or testicular torsion. Patients with genitourinary complaints are frequently embarrassed and may neglect to tell the physician about other physical problems they may be having. Thus, a thorough genitourinary examination, including a digital rectal examination, is always indicated.

Evaluation of Vaginal Discharge

History
1. *How long has the discharge been present?*
2. *What is the quality and quantity of the discharge?*
   The color, odor, and amount of the discharge may help to determine the etiology. Greenish, frothy discharge is often seen with *Trichomonas* infection. Copious yellow-white drainage is consistent with gonococcal or *Gardnerella* infection. A "fishy" odor, especially during the potassium hydroxide (KOH) preparations, is typical of *Gardnerella*.
3. *What is the obstetric and menstrual history of the patient?*
   Is she sexually active? Does she use any form of birth control? A complete gynecologic and obstetric history is obtained from all patients.
4. *Is there any correlation between the discharge and the menstrual cycle?*
   Many women have a normal physiologic variation of their normally clear vaginal secretions.
5. *Are there associated symptoms such as abdominal pain, dyspareunia, pruritus, dysuria, or frequency?*
   Pain points to extension of the infection beyond the vaginal vault. Urinary symptoms are common in vaginitis from inflammation of the urethral meatus and concomitant urinary tract infection.
6. *Are there risk factors for Candida infection, e.g., diabetes, antibiotic use, immunosuppression, pregnancy?*

Physical Examination
1. *Is fever present?*
   Fever suggests the presence of pelvic inflammatory disease, pyelonephritis, disseminated gonococcal infection, or other systemic infection.
2. *Is the general physical examination normal?*
   Specifically, one looks for associated pharyngitis, costovertebral angle tenderness, abdominal tenderness, and adenopathy.
3. *What are the findings on the pelvic examination?*
   The external genitalia and urethra are inspected for lesions, erythema, edema, and secretions. A speculum is inserted, and the volume, odor, color, and consistency of the discharge is noted. The upper vagina and cervix are inspected

for lesions or signs of inflammation. A bimanual examination is then performed. The patient is examined for cervical motion tenderness, adnexal masses or tenderness, and uterine size. A rectal examination is routinely performed. During the examination, specimens are collected for *Neisseria gonorrhoeae* culture, KOH examination for *Candida albicans*, and saline for examination for *Trichomonas vaginalis*. Some authorities strongly recommend also making cultures for *Chlamydia trachomatis* at this time.

PROBLEM 2 A review of the patient's medical record revealed that she had a prior emergency department visit for pelvic inflammatory disease and vaginitis. She was currently sexually active but did not use any birth control method. On examination, she was afebrile, and her general physical examination results were unremarkable. The speculum examination showed copious yellow frothy discharge with a fishy odor. The adnexa were nontender, and the uterine size was normal.

This patient's history of previous visits for sexually transmitted diseases is relatively common in urban emergency departments. Many patients have a poor understanding of these diseases, and as a result, there is a high incidence of treatment failures, reinfections, and noncompliance with medications.

DECISION PRIORITIES AND PRELIMINARY DIFFERENTIAL DIAGNOSIS

After the history and physical examination are completed, there are only two questions to answer:

1. *Has the infection extended beyond the urethra in the male or beyond the vagina in the female?*
   Extension of the infection into additional anatomic sites in the genitourinary tract represents a complication. Complications need a more detailed evaluation, potentially more potent antibiotics given over a longer time period, possible hospital admission, and close follow-up with referral. Extension of the infection places the patient in a category of a patient who requires careful assessment and aggressive therapy. This is also the time to consider the presence of syphilis as a systemic concomitant disease with penile or vaginal discharge.
2. *Is the infection gonococcal or nongonococcal?*
   The question is asked only to point out that the clinical diagnosis of gonococcal infection without the use of the laboratory in both penile and vaginal discharge is notoriously poor. Diagnostic adjuncts have a routine role in the assessment and care of these patients.

DIAGNOSTIC ADJUNCTS

The use of laboratory testing in patients with genital discharge is straightforward and results in a definitive diagnosis in the majority of cases. A more complex microbiologic evaluation is occasionally required in patients in whom the diagnosis is not obvious and for treatment failures.

Laboratory Studies for Penile Discharge

Gram Stain. Gram staining of a discharge specimen, when done properly, has a specificity approaching 99% and a sensitivity of 95% for *N. gonorrhoeae*. A smear is positive if two or more gram-negative intracellular diplococci (GNID) are found in two or more leukocytes. Even when the pathognomonic gram-negative diplococci are demonstrated on Gram stain, a culture is sent to the laboratory to determine antibiotic sensitivities.

The Gram stain of a discharge specimen from a patient with NGU will show five or more leukocytes per high power field without the presence of GNID.

Culture. Definitive diagnosis of GCU is obtained by culture of the organism. Proper technique is essential to reduce the number of false-negative cultures. First, it is important to ensure that the patient has not voided for at least 1 hour prior to collection of the specimen. Calcium alginate swabs are preferable because the fatty acids in cotton fibers are known to be bactericidal. The swab is inserted 2 to 4 cm into the urethra, gently rotated, and then directly inoculated onto the culture medium. Culture of expressed discharge may lead to false-negative results and should be avoided.

Culture of *C. trachomatis* or *U. urealyticum* is diagnostic of NGU but is not often performed in males. There is a high concurrence of *N. gonorrhea* and *C. trachomatis* in males with penile discharge.

Serologic Tests for Syphilis. Many authorities recommend sending specimens for serologic studies for syphilis in all males with a penile discharge to rule out coexistent disease. The recent rise in cases of syphilis makes this recommendation more compelling.

PROBLEM 1 A Gram stain was performed on a specimen of the patient's discharge and showed many leukocytes but no gram-negative diplococci. A swab from the urethra was plated on a chocolate agar plate and sent to the laboratory for a gonorrhea culture. A serologic sample to test for syphilis was also sent.

Although the Gram stain does not show any gram-negative diplococci, it does not provide a secure diagnosis for the cause of the discharge. The stain is consistent, however, with a diagnosis of NGU, *C. trachomatis* being the most likely organism.

Laboratory Studies for Vaginal Discharge

Wet Mount. The saline wet mount is the single most important study in evaluating vaginal discharge. Proper collection and examination of the wet mount are crucial to increase the number of positive findings. A sample of vaginal fluid is obtained and immediately placed in 0.2 ml of physiologic saline. The swab is gently agitated, and a drop is placed on a microscope slide with a cover slip and examined under oil emersion at high power. The saline wet mount is useful in the diagnosis of several common causes of vaginitis:

Candidiasis. Candidal infections can be diagnosed with a sensitivity ranging from 40% to 80% with the wet mount technique.

Trichomoniasis. The wet mount is the most practical method of diagnosing *Trichomonas* infections in the emergency department. Trichomonads are pear-shaped, motile, flagellated organisms slightly larger than white blood cells. They are easy to detect in fresh specimens but are difficult to differentiate from leukocytes when they die. The wet mount has recently been found to be relatively insensitive in diagnosing *Trichomonas*, revealing only 60% of cases compared with cultures. However, there are no other practical methods currently available.

Gardnerella Vaginitis. Specimens from patients with *Gardnerella* vaginitis have large numbers of small coccobacilli organisms on wet mount. The presence of "clue cells" is considered to be highly suggestive of *Gardnerella* infections. Clue cells are vaginal epithelial cells that are covered with small coccobacilli bacteria that are identified by the typical salt and pepper appearance.

Potassium Hydroxide Preparation. A drop of 10% KOH solution added to a drop of vaginal discharge and then gently heated, will lyse all cellular elements except *Candida* organisms. The characteristic hyphae and spores are best demonstrated with this technique. Trichomonads and clue cells are not visible with this method.

Cultures. Cultures for *N. gonorrhoeae* are indicated in all patients with vaginal discharge. The culture is obtained from the endocervix and plated on the appropriate media. Cultures for *Candida, Trichomonas,* and *Gardnerella* are rarely indicated but may be of use when other studies do not reveal the organism. Some authorities recommend routine culture for *C. trachomatis.* Newer, rapid reagent kits (MicroTrak and Chlamydiazume systems) that are sensitive and specific for this organism may be of use in the emergency department.

Testing for Herpes Simplex. The Tzanck smear is used to identify the multinucleated giant cells and intranuclear inclusion bodies that are characteristic of *Herpes simplex* infections. The roof of a blister is gently removed, and the base is scraped with a blade and plated on a glass slide. The slide is immersed in alcohol, air dried, stained with Giemsa or Wright's stain, and examined for the typical cells. A positive Tzanck smear is highly suggestive of a herpes infection, but a negative test result does not rule it out. A viral culture taken from a suspicious lesion may be performed to confirm a suspected diagnosis.

Serologic Test for Syphilis. Women with one sexually transmitted disease are at risk for others. A serologic test for syphilis is recommended for patients with vaginal discharge.

PROBLEM 2 Two swabs were taken from the woman with vaginal discharge. An endocervical sample was sent to the laboratory for gonorrhea culture, and a wet mount was performed on a sample of vaginal fluid. The wet mount showed many *Trichomonas* organisms. No clue cells or yeast were seen. KOH preparation was negative for hyphae. A pregnancy test was done and was negative.

The findings were typical of *Trichomonas* infection, which is often seen in association with other infective organisms. It is important to take a thorough menstrual history. Menstrual histories are often inaccurate; therefore, if there is any doubt at all, a pregnancy test is performed. Many medications commonly used to treat vaginal discharge are contraindicated during pregnancy, e.g., tetracycline, doxycycline, metronidazole.

REFINED DIFFERENTIAL DIAGNOSIS

Penile Discharge

As mentioned previously, urethritis is divided into two general classifications: gonococcal urethritis and nongonococcal urethritis. The signs and symptoms of these two infections overlap considerably, and a mixed organism infection is common.

Gonococcal Urethritis. Gonorrhea is the most common reportable communicable disease in the United States, and as such represents a major public health concern. The causative organism, *Neisseria gonorrhoeae*, is a gram-negative diplococcus with an average incubation period of 3 to 10 days. Patients with GCU usually present with complaints of dysuria and penile discharge. The discharge is usually copious, spontaneous, and purulent but can be mucoid or mucopurulent. Complications of gonococcal infections in men include the development of epididymitis, prostatitis, and urethral strictures. Disseminated gonococcal infections will occur in 1% to 3% of patients with mucosal infections.

Nongonococcal Urethritis. NGU is a sexually transmitted disorder that has seen a dramatic rise in incidence during the past several decades. The incubation period for NGU is usually 2 to 3 weeks. The presenting symptoms are generally less acute than those of GCU. The symptoms consist of a penile discharge, dysuria, and penile discomfort. The discharge is usually less purulent than that seen with GCU and is often present only in the morning or with stripping of the urethra. About 25% of patients are asymptomatic, and others have only minimal penile discomfort. NGU may be caused by several infectious agents. *Chlamydia trachomatis* is the most important pathogen resulting in NGU. It is cultured from the urethra in 25% to 60% of patients. *Ureaplasma urealyticum* accounts for 30% to 40% of NGU infections.

In approximately 10% to 20% of cases, neither *C. trachomatis* nor *U. urealyticum* is isolated from the urethra. Several other organisms may play a role in these cases. The *Herpes simplex* virus can cause urethritis in about 30% of men with primary genital infection. *Trichomonas vaginalis* and *Gardnerella vaginalis* are both sexually transmitted but do not usually cause penile discharge. They do not appear to be significant pathogens in men and generally cause no symptoms when present in the urethra. *Candida albicans* does not have a major role in male urethritis. Occasionally a patient will come to the emergency department with the complaint of dysuria after intercourse. The history may determine an exposure to a spermicidal agent. These gels and creams can cause urethral irritation.

Vaginal Discharge

There are numerous causes of vaginal discharge (Table 61–1). An accurate diagnosis can usually be made with a thorough history, physical examination, and appropriate laboratory studies. The majority of cases of vaginal discharge seen in the emergency department are caused by the following entities:

Vaginal Candidiasis. Vaginal infections with *Candida albicans* usually result from contamination by the patients' own flora from the gastrointestinal tract. The cardinal symptom of candidiasis is vulvar and vaginal pruritus, often accompanied by a thick white odorless discharge. Characteristic "cottage cheese" plaques adherent to the vaginal mucosa are usually present. The diagnosis is confirmed by the KOH preparation or wet mount. Patients with vaginal candidiasis usually have a predisposing condition such as antibiotic or steroid use, pregnancy, diabetes mellitus, or immunosuppression. Oral contraceptive use does not increase the susceptibility to candidiasis but does make it more difficult to treat.

***Gardnerella* Vaginitis.** The organism *Gardnerella vaginalis* is responsible for the majority of cases of "nonspecific or bacterial" vaginitis. *Gardnerella* vaginitis is now known to be sexually transmitted and is characterized by a fishy odor, particularly after intercourse, a thin discharge, and lack of itching and burning. The presence of a thin white discharge, vaginal fluid with a pH greater than 4.5, a positive "whiff" test (a fishy

TABLE 61–1. Causes of Vaginal Discharge

Physiologic	*Infectious*
Ovulation	Vaginal
Coitus	*Candida*
Oral contraceptive use	*Trichomonas*
Pregnancy	*Gardnerella*
Premenstrual	Toxic shock syndrome
Premenarchal	Vulvar
Intrauterine device	Herpes
Noninfectious	Condylomata acuminata
Atrophic (senile) vaginitis	Syphilis
Vaginal foreign body	Bartholinitis
Vaginal adenosis	Lymphogranuloma venereum
Allergic or irritant vulvovaginitis	Chancroid
Vulvar, vaginal carcinoma	Granuloma inguinale
Cervical polyps	Urethritis
Cervical carcinoma	Pyoderma
Endometrial myoma	Cervical
Vesicovaginal fistula	Gonorrhea
Enterovaginal fistula	Chlamydial or bacterial cervicitis
	Chronic cervicitis
	Pelvic inflammatory disease

From Reilly BM: Practical Strategies in Outpatient Medicine. Philadelphia, WB Saunders, 1984.

odor with 10% KOH), and the presence of clue cells on the wet mount are very suggestive of *Gardnerella* infection.

Trichomoniasis. *Trichomonas vaginalis,* a unicellular protozoan, is a common cause of vaginitis. Infection is sexually transmitted with highly variable clinical features. The manifestations range from asymptomatic colonization to profuse, malodorous, frothy, yellow-green discharge accompanied by severe pruritus. The vagina is frequently erythematous, and speckling of the cervix (strawberry cervix) may occur. Diagnosis is usually made by demonstrating the organism on a wet mount, although culture is more sensitive.

Cervicitis. Many women complaining of a vaginal discharge do not have a vaginal infection. They have a discharge from an infected endocervical mucosa, known as cervicitis. It is usually caused by *N. gonorrhoeae, C. trachomatis,* or the *Herpes simplex* virus. Cervicitis is differentiated from vaginitis by the presence of a nonodorous, yellow, mucopurulent endocervical discharge on speculum examination. The discharge does not irritate the vagina or vulva, so patients usually do not have symptoms of pruritus and burning. Pelvic discomfort is common. The wet mount shows many leukocytes but no apparent pathogen. Patients with active *Herpes simplex* infections have the characteristic grouped vesicles or ulcers on the cervix.

PRINCIPLES OF MANAGEMENT

Most causes of genital discharge are curable if appropriate therapy is instituted; however, successful therapy depends on an accurate diagnosis.

Penile Discharge

Ideally, antibiotic therapy for patients with penile discharge specifically treats the causative organism. Because of the frequency of combined gonorrhea and *Chlamydia* infections in men with discharge, the Centers for Disease Control and most other authorities recommend that these entities be treated in concert.

Antibiotics effective against gonorrhea are listed in Table 61–2. The choice of antibiotic used will depend on:
1. The local prevalence of penicillin-resistant gonorrhea organisms.
2. The potential of concurrent pharyngeal or anorectal infections.
3. The likelihood of patient compliance with an oral regimen.

Treatment for gonorrhea is always followed by coverage for *Chlamydia,* either tetracycline 500 mg PO q.i.d. for 7 days or doxycycline 100 mg PO b.i.d. for 7 days. Strains resistant to these regimens have not been reported. Tetracycline-resistant *U. urealyticum* is well known; therefore, treatment failures are treated with a course of erythromycin.

PROBLEM 1 The patient was treated with amoxicillin 3.0 gm PO and probenecid 1.0 gm PO in the emergency department. He was given a prescription for doxycycline 100 mg PO b.i.d. for 7 days. A referral was given to a family physician for follow-up, and he was instructed to refrain from sexual intercourse for 1 week.

He returned to the emergency department in 3 weeks with a continued discharge and was upset that the medication had not worked. He insisted adamantly that he had not had intercourse since the treatment was given and had completed the full course of antibiotics. He did not follow up with the family physician. A repeat examination led to results similar to those of the previous episode. Another culture was made, and he was treated with erythromycin 500 mg PO q.i.d. for 10 days for a presumed diagnosis of *U. urealyticum* infection. A follow-up phone call in 1 week found that he was free of symptoms.

TABLE 61-2. Antibiotic Therapy for Gonorrhea

Antibiotic	Effective Against PPNG	Comment
Ceftriaxone 125–250 mg IM	Yes	Considered first-line therapy by some authorities. Current CDC recommendations limit use to PPNG endemic areas and for outpatient treatment of PID
Cefoxitin 2.0 gm IM with probenecid 1.0 gm PO	Yes	Painful injection
Aqueous procaine penicillin G 4.8 million units IM with probenecid 1.0 gm PO	No	Painful injection. Possible procaine reaction
Ampicillin 3.5 gm PO or amoxicillin 3.0 gm PO with probenecid 1.0 gm PO	No	Ineffective against anorectal or pharyngeal infections
Tetracycline 500 mg PO b.i.d. for 7 days or doxycycline 100 mg PO q.i.d. for 7 days	No	Increasing tetracycline resistance has been reported. Compliance is a problem. Ineffective against anorectal infections. Contraindicated in pregnancy and in children
Spectinomycin 2.0 gm IM	Yes	Useful in penicillin-allergic patients. Ineffective for pharyngeal infections.
Trimethoprim-sulfamethoxazole 80/400, 9 tabs PO q.d. for 5 days	Yes	Not approved for this purpose. Particularly useful for treating pharyngeal infections. Has some coverage for *Chlamydia*. Compliance is a problem
Ciprofloxacin 750 mg PO b.i.d. for 7 days	Yes	Not recommended for this purpose. Effective against *Chlamydia*. Compliance is a problem

PPNG = Penicillinase-producing *Neisseria gonorrhoeae*; PID = pelvic inflammatory disease.

Vaginal Discharge

Vaginal Candidiasis. Vaginitis caused by *Candida* is effectively treated with a variety of antifungal preparations:

1. Miconazole (Monistat) 200 mg vaginal tablets qHS for 3 days or 2% cream qHS for 7 to 14 days.
2. Clotrimazole (Lotrimin) 100 mg vaginal tablets qHS for 3 days or 1% cream for 7 to 14 days.
3. Nystatin vaginal tablets 1 q.d. for 14 days.
4. Butoconazole (Femstat) 2% cream qHS for 3 days.

Trichomonas Vaginitis. Metronidazole (Flagyl) 2.0 gm as a single dose is usually adequate treatment for trichomoniasis. A longer regimen of metronidazole, 500 mg PO b.i.d. for 5 days or 250 mg PO t.i.d. for 7 days, may lead to a slightly higher cure rate, but patient compliance is lower. Metronidazole is contraindicated during the first trimester of pregnancy and should be avoided throughout pregnancy, if possible. Alternative treatment during pregnancy consists of symptomatic relief with 20% saline douches or clotrimazole suppositories. Treatment of the sexual partner is recommended to prevent recurrent infection. The patient is warned about the disulfiram (Antabuse)-like reaction that occurs when ethanol is ingested during a course of therapy with metronidazole.

***Gardnerella* Vaginitis.** Metronidazole is the drug of choice for *Gardnerella* infections. A dosage of 500 mg PO b.i.d. for 7 days is effective in eradicating the infection. Ampicillin 500 mg PO q.i.d. for 7 days is the alternative drug, but it is less efficacious.

Cervicitis. Mucopurulent cervicitis is treated with an agent effective for gonorrhea (Table 61-2) followed by either tetracycline or doxycycline.

Herpes. The primary infection of herpes can be treated with acyclovir 200 mg orally five times a day for 7 to 10 days. This regimen must be instituted within 6 days of the onset of symptoms to shorten the duration of the outbreak and reduce the systemic symptoms.

PROBLEM 2 The diagnosis of *Trichomonas* was confirmed with the wet mount. The patient was treated with a single dose of metronidazole 2.0 gm orally. She was referred to the local Public Health Department for follow-up and advised of the need for her partner(s) to be treated to prevent a recurrence.

It is important to tell the patient to have her sexual partner obtain medical examination. Treating the woman without treating the partner is useless and contributes to the spread of the infection. Some physicians send a prescription home for the partner, but this is generally not recommended because of potential problems with allergies or toxic reactions. All patients should be given the benefit of an evaluation before any therapy is instituted.

SPECIAL CONSIDERATIONS

Pediatric Patients

Emergency physicians are occasionally called on to evaluate pediatric patients with vaginal discharge. The presence of a discharge in a prepubertal girl is strongly suggestive of sexual abuse, but other causes such as foreign bodies should be ruled out. The evaluation of the child with alleged sexual abuse is discussed in Chapters 38 and 54. A thorough examination of the vagina and rectum is performed, and specimens for cultures for gonorrhea and *Chlamydia* are obtained from the pharynx, rectum, and vagina.

Postmenopausal Women

Women of any age are susceptible to any of the sexually transmitted causes of vaginitis, but the cause of discharge in the postmenopausal woman is usually secondary to either *Candida* or atrophic vaginitis. Atrophic vaginitis results from a deficiency of estrogen and is characterized by scant discharge, vaginal irritation, and the presence of many leukocytes on the wet mount. Treatment is with topical estrogen cream.

DISPOSITION AND FOLLOW-UP

Patients with penile and vaginal discharge rarely require admission to the hospital. Follow-up is arranged with their personal physician or the Public Health Department.

Penile Discharge

Follow-up with repeat cultures of *N. gonorrhoeae*-positive sites is recommended in 7 days. Sexual partners are contacted and treated with antibiotics as indicated.

Vaginal Discharge

Vaginal Candidiasis. Patients are instructed to follow up in 7 to 14 days as needed if symptoms do not resolve. Male partners generally do not require treatment.

Trichomoniasis. A follow-up appointment in 7 to 10 days is recommended for test cure. Sexual partners are treated simultaneously to prevent recurrent infection.

***Gardnerella* Vaginitis.** Follow-up is arranged as needed if symptoms do not respond to treatment. Treatment of sexual partners has not been shown to reduce the rate of recurrent disease. Nevertheless, many authorities recommend treatment of sexual partners.

Cervicitis. Patients are given follow-up in 7 days for a reexamination and repeat cultures. Sexual partners are treated.

Herpes Simplex. Patients with primary herpes infections are counseled on the episodic nature of genital herpes. They are advised to avoid intercourse while lesions are present.

DOCUMENTATION

In addition to thorough documentation of the history, vital signs, and physical examination, the following data are included on the medical records:
1. Laboratory data (including Gram stain and wet mount results)
2. Treatment plans
3. Instructions given to the patient
4. Follow-up arrangements

SUMMARY AND FINAL POINTS

- Although it rarely constitutes a true emergency, the presence of discharge from the penis or vagina leads many patients to seek care in the emergency department.
- In most cases, the causative organism is sexually transmitted and, if not treated properly, may lead to continued spread of the organism and significant morbidity.
- Common causes of penile discharge include *N. gonorrhoeae* and *C. trachomatis* with other organisms playing a smaller role.
- Vaginal discharge in women is caused by a wide variety of physiologic factors and organisms. *Candida albicans, N. gonorrhoeae, T. vaginalis,* and *G. vaginalis* are the most common organisms.
- The high concurrence rate of *N. gonorrhoeae* and *C. trachomatis* necessitates treatment for both in males who present with penile discharge and females with cervicitis.
- Clear follow-up instructions, including the importance of notifying partners and obtaining tests for cure, are important to ensure a good outcome.

BIBLIOGRAPHY

Texts

1. Barker LR, Burton JR, Zieve PD (eds): Principles of Ambulatory Medicine. Baltimore, Williams & Wilkins, 1986.
2. Mandell GL, Douglas RG, Bennett JE (eds): Principles and Practice of Infectious Diseases (2nd ed). New York, John Wiley and Sons, 1985.

Journal Articles

1. Bardin E, Berger RE: Sexually transmitted disease in men. Primary Care 12:761–785, 1985.
2. Bowie WR: Nongonococcal urethritis. Urol Clin North Am 11:55–64, 1984.
3. Centers for Disease Control: 1989 Sexually Transmitted Diseases Treatment Guidelines. MMWR 38 (No. 5–8):1–43, 1989.
4. Felman YM, Nikitas JA: Nongonococcal urethritis: A clinical review. JAMA 245:381–386, 1981.
5. Fleury FJ: Adult vaginitis. Clin Obstet Gynecol 24:407–438, 1981.
6. Fouts AC, Kraus SJ: Trichomonas vaginalis: Re-evaluation of its clinical and laboratory presentation. J Infect Dis 141:137–143, 1980.
7. Friedrich EG. Vaginitis. Am Fam Phys 28:238–242, 1983.
8. Krieger JN, Tam MR, Stevens CE, et al: Diagnosis of trichomoniasis: Comparison of conventional wet-mount examination with cytologic studies, cultures, and monoclonal antibody staining of direct specimens. JAMA 259:1223–1227, 1988.
9. Lucas LM, Smith DL: Nongonococcal urethritis: Diagnosis and management. J Gen Intern Med 2:199–203, 1987.
10. Wasserheit JN, Holmes KK: Sexually transmitted diseases in women: Approach to common syndromes in emergency medicine. Emerg Clin North Am 3:47–74, 1985.

SECTION SEVENTEEN

ADMINISTRATION

CHAPTER 62

MEDICOLEGAL

RICHARD FELDMAN, M.D.

PROBLEM 1 A 15 year old girl with a history of an irregular menstrual cycle and vaginal discharge presented to the emergency department but refused to give the name or telephone number of her parents, saying she would be seen only if they were not called.

PROBLEM 2 A 40 year old man was involved in a motor vehicle accident and complained of neck pain. He had an odor of alcohol on his breath and was obnoxious and uncooperative.

PROBLEM 3 An 80 year old woman was brought in by ambulance from a nursing home because she had had a fever for 2 days. The patient responded incoherently. There was no family or legal guardian.

PROBLEM 4 A 50 year old male presented with a history of vomiting blood. He said he was a devout Jehovah's Witness and refused to receive blood or blood products.

PROBLEM 5 A 5 year old boy was brought in by the rescue squad following a bicycle accident. The parents or legal guardian could not be reached.

PROBLEM 6 A 50 year old man with chest pain at work was brought in by his coworkers. After the coworkers left, he refused admission to the hospital.

QUESTIONS TO CONSIDER

1. How do legal concerns affect patient care in the emergency department?
2. How does one determine whether patients are competent to make decisions about their own health care?
3. Which patients do not have the legal right to give consent for their medical care?
4. Under what circumstances may patients be involuntarily restrained in the emergency department?
5. What is the liability of emergency department personnel for patients who refuse care against medical advice?
6. What is the appropriate documentation when there are legal concerns in the treatment of a patient in the emergency department?

INTRODUCTION

The emergency department is a unique environment. Unlike in private offices, clinics, and inpatient settings, the patient is unknown to the staff and is rarely the sole focus of the physician's attention. The luxury of time is usually absent. Under these stressful circumstances, there is a significant potential for legal problems. Working with a limited data base, the emergency care team opens itself to errors of omission or commission. Without proper patient consent, the physician may be charged with assault and battery or depriving a patient of his or her civil liberties. On the other hand, the physician who fails to restrain or treat an uncooperative, hostile patient who may be under the influence of alcohol, drugs, or acute injury can be charged with malpractice.

Laws exist to protect the rights of patients. In order to practice emergency medicine, we need to be aware of the legal boundaries our society has set on this practice. These include a variety of medicolegal questions:

1. When can we evaluate and treat patients, and when is such treatment a violation of the rights of the patient?

2. What are our duties and obligations to the patient when we enter a physician-patient relationship? What is privileged communication and confidentiality of records?

3. What are our duties and obligations to society? What cases do we report to health authorities, police, or hospital administration?

The answers to these questions are deeply rooted in case law. The treatment of individual patients depends on a balance of medical, legal, and ethical concerns for the patient. This chapter will review the general obligations of the emergency department and discuss the concepts of consent, competence, involuntary restraints, patients leaving against medical advice, reporting requirements, and appropriate documentation.

GENERAL OBLIGATIONS OF THE EMERGENCY DEPARTMENT

A patient presenting for medical care engenders a duty on the emergency department staff to provide service according to need and to use due care to ensure that no harm comes to the patient. Case law has firmly established that hospitals holding themselves out to the public as providing emergency medical services must evaluate any patient requesting care regardless of the complaint or ability to pay. After assessment, if no emergency treatment is warranted, there is no definitive obligation to treat or render ongoing care. Every patient discharged from the emergency department must receive written discharge instructions, which include direction to a health care provider for medical follow-up if necessary or desired. If the patient reappears for emergency department care, reevaluation must be undertaken to ensure that the patient was appropriately treated and that nothing new or serious has occurred.

CONSENT

Consent can be defined as a voluntary agreement by a person to a proposal by another. It is a free rational act that presupposes knowledge of the thing to which consent is given. The concept of consent in the medical setting is predicated on the principle that every human being of adult years and sound mind is "competent" and has the right to determine what shall be done with his or her own body.

The key elements of consent are as follows:

1. A person is competent to make the decision.

2. There must be disclosure of information, including significant risks based on the magnitude of harm for each risk and the probability that it will occur.

3. There is comprehension of relevant information by the person.

4. There is voluntary granting of consent without coercion or duress.

There are two basic types of consent, expressed and implied, pertinent to the practice of medicine. *Expressed consent* is given directly, either verbally or in writing. The person is stating that he agrees to certain actions on his behalf. Ambulatory patients in no obvious distress sign a general consent form at the time of registration (Fig. 62–1).

1. THE PATIENT OR HIS REPRESENTATIVE, RECOGNIZING THE NEED FOR HOSPITAL CARE, CONSENTS TO THE HOSPITAL SERVICES AS ORDERED BY THE ATTENDING PHYSICIAN INCLUDING LOCAL OR REGIONAL ANESTHESIA, LABORATORY PROCEDURES, MEDICAL TREATMENT, MINOR OR EMERGENCY SURGICAL TREATMENT, EXAMINATION IN THE RADIOLOGY DEPARTMENT, OR OTHER HOSPITAL SERVICES RENDERED UNDER THE GENERAL AND SPECIFIC INSTRUCTIONS OF THE PHYSICIAN.

   I, ALSO, UNDERSTAND THAT INFORMATION CONCERNING MY MEDICAL CONDITION AND RECORDS MAY BE OF BENEFIT FOR MEDICAL RESEARCH AND EDUCATION. I AGREE THAT INFORMATION FROM MY MEDICAL RECORDS MAY BE USED FOR RESEARCH, EDUCATIONAL, AND SCIENTIFIC PURPOSES, INCLUDING PUBLICATION, PROVIDED MY NAME IS NOT REVEALED.

   I, ALSO, UNDERSTAND AND AGREE THAT INFORMATION FROM MY MEDICAL RECORDS MAY BE RELEASED TO OTHER MEDICAL SERVICE ORGANIZATIONS FOR CONTINUITY OF CARE AFTER DISCHARGE.

   I, ALSO, CONSENT TO THE PERFORMANCE OF DIAGNOSTIC TESTING, INCLUDING THE DRAWING OF BLOOD, IN THE EVENT OF HOSPITAL EMPLOYEE AND/OR PHYSICIAN EXPOSURE TO ANY OF MY BODY FLUIDS.

2. THE PATIENT OR HIS REPRESENTATIVE HEREBY CONSENTS TO THE HOSPITAL SEARCHING HIS PERSON AND/OR HIS BELONGINGS SHOULD THERE BE REASONABLE GROUNDS TO BELIEVE HE IS CONCEALING ANY WEAPONS OR UNAUTHORIZED DRUGS OR MEDICATIONS.

3. THE PATIENT OR HIS REPRESENTATIVE RELIEVES THE HOSPITAL OF ANY AND ALL LIABILITY FOR THE LOSS OF ANY VALUABLES NOT DEPOSITED IN THE HOSPITAL SAFE.

FINANCIAL AUTHORIZATION

1. GUARANTEE OF ACCOUNT-FOR AND IN CONSIDERATION OF SERVICES RENDERED BY _____ HOSPITAL AND HEALTH CENTER AND/OR THE ATTENDING PHYSICIANS OR THEIR DESIGNATES, I HEREBY GUARANTEE PAYMENT OF ALL CHARGES INCURRED.

2. ASSIGNMENT OF INSURANCE BENEFITS-I HEREBY ASSIGN PAYMENT DIRECTLY TO _____ HOSPITAL AND HEALTH CENTER AND/OR THE ATTENDING PHYSICIANS OR THEIR DESIGNATES OF THE BENEFITS HEREIN SPECIFIED AND OTHERWISE PAYABLE TO ME BUT NOT TO EXCEED THE REGULAR CHARGES. I UNDERSTAND I AM RESPONSIBLE FOR ALL CHARGES (HOSPITAL AND/OR PHYSICIAN) UNTIL THE BILLS ARE PAID IN FULL.

3. AUTHORIZATION TO RELEASE INFORMATION-I HEREBY AUTHORIZE _____ HOSPITAL AND HEALTH CENTER AND/OR THE ATTENDING PHYSICIANS OR THEIR DESIGNATES TO RELEASE GENERAL DIAGNOSTIC AND MEDICAL RECORD INFORMATION RELATIVE TO MY CARE TO THE PRIMARY AND SECONDARY PAYORS LISTED BELOW FOR THE PURPOSE OF PROCESSING MY HOSPITAL AND/OR PHYSICIAN BILLS FOR PAYMENT. THIS AUTHORIZATION INCLUDES, BUT IS NOT LIMITED TO, INFORMATION RELATIVE TO TREATMENT FOR PSYCHIATRIC CONDITIONS, IF KNOWN AT TIME OF REGISTRATION.

4. MEDICARE PATIENTS ONLY-I CERTIFY THAT THE INFORMATION GIVEN BY ME IN APPLYING FOR PAYMENT UNDER TITLE XVIII OF THE SOCIAL SECURITY ACT IS CORRECT. I AUTHORIZE ANY HOLDER, INCLUDING THE ATTENDING PHYSICIANS AND/OR THEIR DESIGNATES, OF MEDICAL OR OTHER INFORMATION ABOUT ME TO RELEASE THE SOCIAL SECURITY ADMINISTRATION AND/OR THE MEDICARE PROGRAM OR ITS INTERMEDIARIES OR CARRIERS OR TO THE PROFESSIONAL STANDARDS REVIEW ORGANIZATION ANY INFORMATION NEEDED FOR THIS OR A RELATED MEDICARE CLAIM. I REQUEST THAT PAYMENT OF AUTHORIZED BENEFITS BE MADE ON MY BEHALF, TO THE HOSPITAL AND/OR THE ATTENDING PHYSICIANS OR THEIR DESIGNATES.

FIGURE 62-1. Expressed consent form.

A financial authorization is usually included under the patient's signature. This form gives the emergency department staff written approval to perform a routine history and physical examination, and, if necessary, limited tests and procedures such as routine radiographs, blood tests, and cardiac monitoring. Expressed consent is automatically expanded in situations in which an urgent, critical problem is discovered that requires immediate intervention to prevent morbidity or mortality, e.g., intubation, cardioversion, or defibrillation.

Implied consent is given by deduction from the circumstances or the conduct of the parties involved. Implied consent is manifested by signs, actions, or facts, or by inaction or silence; all raise a presumption that consent has been given. When a nurse approaches a patient to perform a phlebotomy, the patient usually spontaneously rolls up their sleeve and extends an arm to allow the procedure. Implied consent for the procedure is given without a word exchanged. The law assumes that the competent patient understands what is going to occur and grants permission for the procedure to be done.

When an invasive procedure such as a laparotomy or angiography is indicated, the legal community recommends obtaining separate written informed consent. The patient is informed about the need for the test and the risks and alternatives of undergoing or not allowing the procedure recommended. The competent patient or guardian, under most circumstances, has the right to comply with or refuse any and all testing and treatment offered. There are a number of "needle-related" procedures such as central venous catheterization, lumbar puncture, and culdocentesis that remain controversial in terms of a separate consent form. Some authorities recommend this be documented only by a note in the chart. Following the standard in the area is a reasonable course to choose.

In the truly emergent situation, consent is always implied. The privilege to proceed in emergencies without consent is afforded the physician because inaction at that time would be contrary to good medical practice and to the health and welfare of the patient. In such circumstances the emergency department staff is obligated to pursue all necessary care without delay. The circumstances surrounding the need for emergency intervention without consent need to be thoroughly and clearly documented in the emergency medical record. Consent from the patient or guardian may be obtained as soon as possible but should not delay evaluation and treatment.

PROBLEM 3 The 80 year old patient's vital signs were blood pressure 80/40 mm Hg, heart rate 116/min and thready, respiratory rate 28/min and labored, temperature 103.5°F (39.7°C) rectally. The patient moaned to verbal stimuli. This patient was unable to give consent for treatment and a guardian was not immediately available. In her shock state, delaying care would result in a worsened morbidity or mortality. The emergency department is obligated to begin evaluation and treatment immediately.

Consent in Minors

Special consent laws apply to minors. Minors are defined in most states as individuals under the age of 18 years and in general are not considered competent to make decisions regarding their own health care. Exceptions have been created to provide the opportunity for some minors to make decisions regarding their health care needs. Consent can be given by minors in the following circumstances:

1. The minor is emancipated—either married or living alone and managing his own financial affairs.
2. The minor seeks health services for his child.
3. The minor seeks treatment for venereal disease, alcohol and drug abuse, and pregnancy-related problems.
4. The minor is considered sufficiently mature in some states to make the decision in question.

PROBLEM 1 The 15 year old girl was found to have recurrent salpingitis. She feared severe punishment if her parents learned that she was sexually active. Outpatient treatment was provided. If evaluation and treatment were denied this patient, there was a high likelihood that she would not actively pursue timely alternative medical care, resulting in a significant risk of both short- and long-term morbidity.

Most states have laws similar to the law in Minnesota that states that "any minor regardless of residence may give effective consent for health services to determine presence of or to treat pregnancy, venereal disease and alcohol or other drug abuse." The law is not specific about the lowest applicable age, but many states include children from the age of 12 to 18 in this category. Most states strongly recommend that contact with parents be encouraged, especially after evaluation is completed.

When a minor presents to the emergency department without a parent or guardian, the staff must quickly assess the circumstances and decide on the extent of intervention required. The following points may guide the decision:

1. Consent for intervention is implied in any true emergency.
2. Nonurgent problems require consent by a responsible adult.
3. The court system has established mechanisms for reasonably rapid appointment of a guardian should there be none available. This guardian has the right and responsibility to make all necessary medical decisions for the minor until a parent or previously appointed guardian is available.
4. If the parent or guardian refuses to give consent when the child is in imminent danger, care is provided, and the case is reported to the Child Protection Agency.
5. Standard school or camp presigned consent forms allow initiation of routine evaluation and treatment.

PROBLEM 5 On evaluation, the 5 year old child who fell off his bike was found to have a scalp laceration and deformed wrist. The responsibility of the emergency staff in this case is initially the same as with any other patient who has experienced a traumatic event and presents for evaluation and treatment. The evaluation should include all testing necessary to rule out a life or limb threat, and treatment should include all interventions required to reverse these threats. A hypotensive child with a provisional diagnosis of a lacerated liver must be taken expeditiously to the operating room. The physician is on firm medical and legal ground if he operates because inaction at such time may result in greater injury to the patient and is contrary to good medical practice. No physician has been successfully sued for undertaking such a course of action under emergency circumstances. In this case, the scalp wound was sutured and the wrist reduced and splinted. Simultaneously with these medical activities, the support staff must actively pursue contact with a parent or guardian and document each and every attempt, including time, telephone number called, and persons spoken to; each entry is signed.

COMPETENCE

We function under the societal assumption that every person has the right to determine what happens to their body provided they are competent to make that decision. The whole issue of consent is predicated on the presumed competence of the person giving consent. The person who gives or refuses consent for medical care for himself or another person must be competent for the consent to be valid. Competence for medical decision making depends on the ability of the individual to understand the risks, benefits, and consequences of his decision. Key elements of competence are the following:

1. The ability to understand the options.
2. The ability to understand relevant consequences of acting on the various options.
3. The ability to evaluate the risks and benefits of these consequences and relate them to a stable set of personal values and priorities.
4. The ability to communicate the choice.

In the emergency department, competence is presumed and not specifically assessed unless mental impairment is suspected. The need to provide care for the acutely or chronically incompetent patient is a frequent occurrence in emergency departments.

Intoxicants, infections, metabolic disorders, and trauma may all contribute to acute incompetence.

PROBLEM 2 Per paramedic history, the obnoxious auto accident victim's windshield was shattered, he had a transient loss of consciousness, and had been combative since they arrived on the scene. He insisted that he was "just fine" and threatened to sue if he was not immediately released. Attempts to reason with him were to no avail. Is this patient competent to make decisions regarding his medical care?

The need to determine and document competence to make decisions is most critical when there is concern that the patient is making a serious judgment error by choosing a potentially harmful alternative to necessary medical evaluation and care. In this situation, when mental incapacity is presumed to be secondary to intoxicants or acute brain injury, physically restraining the patient and proceeding with the evaluation is the appropriate course of action (see section below on involuntary restraints).

When an otherwise cooperative patient is not willing to accept recommendations for his care and his reasons appear not to be in his best interest, the decision of how to proceed must be undertaken with respect for his right of self-determination. Determining if the patient is competent is critical at this juncture. The most direct method available to decide this issue is the mental status examination (see Chap. 52). Speech patterns, general appearance, and a focused physical examination lend additional data in determining whether an organic brain syndrome is present. Complete documentation of all details of the evaluation are mandatory, no matter what final action is taken. The competent person has the right to decide how he is or is not to be treated, regardless of what we feel is medically "right."

If a patient is thought to be incompetent, treatment may proceed and consent is sought from a relative or legal guardian. If this option is not available, advice is obtained from the hospital attorney, risk management department, or a hospital administrator. In some municipalities, a designated person may assume legal temporary guardianship and give consent to proceed with medical intervention.

INVOLUNTARY RESTRAINTS

Uncooperative, intoxicated patients are frequently seen in emergency departments. The consequences of making an erroneous decision can be significant, and the options available to the physician are few. Staff response ranges from the inappropriate "get out of my emergency department," to shackling the patient under the weight of six large security guards. Although a significant show of force may occasionally be necessary, releasing a temporarily incompetent patient without adequate evaluation is incorrect and can have disastrous consequences.

Faced with an uncooperative and belligerent patient, the physician should attempt to reason with him in as nonthreatening a manner and setting as possible. The physician must quickly assess the patient's level of understanding of his condition. If the patient is judged to be incompetent, he cannot give valid consent for treatment nor refuse treatment offered. If the patient's lack of cooperation presents a danger to himself or others, the only option left is to use restraints adequate to keep him from leaving or striking out at the staff without being so excessive as to harm the patient.

Staff are often concerned that a charge of battery could be brought against them. Simply stated, "battery" consists of the unlawful touching of another person that is considered to be without justification or excuse. This concern is understandable but unjustified. The courts have found invariably in favor of the physician who has used reasonable and appropriate force to restrain a combative "incompetent" patient. The reverse is also true. Failure to use restraints adequately has resulted in a number of successful suits against the doctor and hospital for harm that subsequently befell the patient or innocent third parties.

As soon as the patient is restrained, a thorough physical evaluation is mandatory to rule out any obvious threats to the patient. Any and all testing and interventions dictated by the clinical evaluation must be undertaken with the understanding that a valid consent may never be signed, nor is it necessary if proper medical decisions have been made. If the patient is intoxicated, he or she should remain under restraint until the acute effects of the intoxicant have worn off. (See Chapter 52.)

AGAINST MEDICAL ADVICE (AMA)

Approximately one out of every 100 patients attempts to leave the emergency department against medical advice. Patients who have altered decision-making capacity can be detained for further evaluation and treatment, as discussed previously. Some competent patients have valid reasons for refusing recommended medical care. Personal priorities may intervene and warrant their immediate attention.

Faced with a competent patient who wants to leave the hospital with a life-threatening illness, the physician must maintain an objective and professional attitude toward the patient. The physician should attempt to ascertain the underlying reasons for the patient's refusal. If there are social or monetary factors involved, social service or hospital administration may allay some of these fears. Enlisting the assistance of the patient's primary physician or family members may convince the patient to accept medical care. If all attempts to persuade the patient to stay fail, the patient is given thorough discharge instructions, including the reassurance that he is welcome and is encouraged to return at any time to the emergency department. Medication for the treatment of his most obvious illnesses is not withheld. This is inappropriate medically and may be seen by a future jury as malintent on the part of the physician. Last, an Against Medical Advice (AMA) form is signed by the patient and witnessed by two staff persons along with anyone accompanying the patient. If the patient refuses to sign the form, this fact is documented and witnessed in the same manner. If at all possible, a safe means of getting the patient home is arranged.

PROBLEM 6 The provisional diagnosis after evaluation of this patient was chest pain with a high suspicion for acute myocardial infarction. Admission was recommended and refused. Further evaluation demonstrated that the patient was competent and otherwise stable.

If all attempts to persuade but not coerce the patient have been tried, the patient may be released after he has signed an AMA form. The patient's competence and reasoning must be carefully documented in the chart.

Case law in the United States has set precedents for the treatment of patients who have deeply held religious beliefs. For example, the devout Jehovah's Witness who refuses blood products is a potential medical, legal, and ethical dilemma. The courts generally uphold the principle that a person is the master of his own body and has the right to prohibit expressly the performance of lifesaving medical or surgical treatment as long as suicide is not the intent.

The courts have not supplied a clear approach to deciding when to transfuse a Jehovah's Witness and when to abide by the wishes of the patient or his family. Table 62-1 illustrates general guidelines that incorporate the concepts of competency, minors, dependents, and pregnancy when applied to a Jehovah's Witness patient who needs a transfusion. Individual hospitals may develop guidelines and protocols in consultation with legal counsel to guide the treatment of patients with deeply held religious beliefs.

TABLE 62–1. Guidelines for Dealing with the Jehovah's Witness Needing a Transfusion

1. Minor
    a. Transfuse if patient will die without it, then obtain a court order.
    b. Apply for court order if not a life or death decision.
2. Incompetent adult, with family refusing to allow transfusion: Follow 1a and b.
3. Competent adult, without dependents: Abide by his wishes.
4. Competent adult with dependents
    a. Abide by wishes if dependents have an alternative means of support, i.e., spouse or relatives willing to raise the dependents. A court order is still sought.
    b. Transfuse if dependents will otherwise become wards of the state: Considered an overriding state interest, wherein the state can limit the right of religious beliefs.
5. Pregnant woman
    a. Transfuse if fetus will die without it.
    b. Transfuse if criteria in 4b apply.
    c. Do not transfuse if life of fetus is not at risk.

PROBLEM 4 The 50 year old man refused blood transfusions and continued to bleed from his gastrointestinal tract. One hour later he was hypotensive and unresponsive. Is it appropriate to administer blood at this point to save his life? Once the patient had made his intentions known and standard therapies were unsuccessful in stopping the hemorrhage, his subsequent shock state does not void his prior refusal of consent for transfusion, and the physician is legally in jeopardy only if he intervenes with blood or blood products.

REPORTING REQUIREMENTS

Most states have statutes that require hospitals to disclose specific information from the patient's medical records without the consent of the patient. Adhering to this statute, the hospital is not liable for disclosure, even if done against the wishes of the patient. The reportable conditions vary from state to state, but in most areas include the following:

1. *Child abuse* is reported to the appropriate public agency when there is reasonable cause to suspect it.
2. *Communicable diseases* can include venereal disease, acquired immune deficiency syndrome (AIDS), suspected rabies, and certain childhood infections, e.g., measles, diphtheria.
3. *Victims of violence* may include elderly abuse, sexual assault, gunshot wounds, and stabbings.
4. *Other disclosures* can include suicide attempts, drug abuse, animal bites, unexplained death, and poisoning.

It is important for the emergency physician to be aware of these requirements, as civil and criminal liability issues are involved.

DOCUMENTATION

The medical record is permanent proof of what transpired during the patient-physician interaction and serves two critical functions. In the short term, it enables the patient's primary care physician or the next emergency physician to determine what transpired during the emergency department encounter. In the long run, a well-documented record may serve as the physician's best ally, or, if poorly documented, his worst enemy should litigation ensue. The medical record, to be most useful, must contain a legible, thorough, and well-organized patient evaluation. In addition, all orders, discharge instructions, and follow-up arrangements must be clearly recorded.

Full documentation is particularly important whenever legal questions such as consent, competence, and use of restraints are being considered, or refusal of necessary care occurs. An accurate description of what transpired must be recorded in objective professional language. In addition, any discussions with other physicians, family or friends, social workers, or hospital administration should be spelled out in detail.

Occasionally information is recorded that is in error and needs correction. Erasures or complete obliteration is inappropriate and leads to questions of possible cover-up. The standard technique is to put a single dark line through the erroneous words, date and time the change, and initial it. The corrections are written in next to the errors. If on review of the chart, additions or changes need to be made, an addendum sheet is added to the medical record with a write-up and explanation of the additions or changes. The original medical record, once the secretarial staff has separated the various sections for billing and other purposes, must never be manipulated. Evidence of chart tampering is the plaintiff's best friend in court.

SUMMARY AND FINAL POINTS

- Consent, to be valid, requires the consentor to comprehend what is being proposed as well as the risks involved and the available alternatives, and to do so without coercion or duress.
- Consent is implied in the truly emergent situation.
- Minors presenting without valid consent must be evaluated to the extent necessary to rule out an emergent situation.
- Parental consent is not necessary if the minor is emancipated, seeks treatment for venereal disease, alcohol, or drug abuse, and pregnancy related problems, or seeks health services for his child.
- The competent person generally has the right to refuse necessary medical care, even if the refusal is not in his best interest.
- Restraining patients against their desire is warranted when they are acutely or chronically incompetent and they choose a course of action potentially harmful to themselves or others.
- A knowledge of reporting requirements to government agencies is essential. The physician is liable for civil or criminal penalties.
- Thorough, focused, and legible documentation is essential both for ongoing medical care and for providing the best defense in possible litigation.

BIBLIOGRAPHY

Texts

1. Iserson KV, Sanders AB, Mathieu DR, et al: Ethics in Emergency Medicine. Baltimore, Williams & Wilkins, 1986.
2. Rozovsky FA: Consent to Treatment: A Practical Guide. Boston, Little, Brown, 1984.
3. Lewis SM, McCutchen JR: Emergency Medicine Malpractice. New York, Wiley Law Publications, 1987.

Journal Articles

1. Griglak MJ, et al: Medicolegal management of the organically impaired patient in the emergency department. Ann Emerg Med 14:685–689, 1985.
2. Kolber JL: Malpractice law and emergency department medicine. Emerg Med Clin North Am (3):625–635, 1985.
3. Purdie FRJ, et al: Prudent handling of patients signing out against medical advice. Prac J Primary Care Phys 3:73–78, 1982.
4. Rogers JT, et al: Medical record documentation. ACEP Foresight Issue 8, 1988.
5. Schlauch RW, et al: Leaving the hospital against medical advice. N Eng J Med 300:22–24, 1979.
6. Selbst SM: Leaving against medical advice. Pediatr Emerg Care 2:266–268, 1986.
7. Zun L, et al: The mental status evaluation: Application in the emergency department. Am J Emerg Med 6:165–171, 1988.

SECTION EIGHTEEN

EMERGENCY MEDICAL SERVICES

CHAPTER 63

EMERGENCY MEDICAL SERVICES AND PREHOSPITAL PERSONNEL

JON R. KROHMER, M.D.
RICHARD HUNT, M.D.

PROBLEM Emergency medical technicians (EMTs) reported by radio that they were in an alley with an unkempt male who had been transported numerous times for acute alcohol intoxication. The patient was unconscious with a blood pressure of 140 by palpation, a radial pulse rate of 96, and respirations of 20. There was a small abrasion on the patient's forehead and a laceration on the back of the head. Physical signs were otherwise normal. It was snowing with an ambient temperature of 25°F. The EMTs had administered oxygen by nasal cannula at 6 liters/min and were requesting further orders.

QUESTIONS TO CONSIDER

1. What levels of care can the different categories of prehospital personnel deliver?
2. How do the prehospital personnel in the field communicate with the emergency department?
3. Who is responsible for the care provided by prehospital personnel?
4. How do physicians provide prehospital personnel with permission to perform the necessary procedures to care for the patient appropriately?
5. How do emergency physicians assess the quality of care provided to patients before they arrive at the hospital?

INTRODUCTION

Origin and Funding of Emergency Medical Services

The history of prehospital care dates back to the Napoleonic Wars, when treatment of injuries was at or near the battlefield. Soldiers were "triaged" (French for "sorted" or "selected") to allow the least injured to be treated rapidly and return to battle. Although this concept of triage continues in the military, civilian-based triage "sorts" injuries according to severity. The most care is directed toward the most ill, and the most good is done for the largest number of victims with the resources that are available.

Most of the developments in prehospital emergency care have arisen from military medical experiences. Since 1917, each war fought by our country has improved our ability to recognize and treat field injuries. The result has been to decrease the time from injury to definitive care from 12 to 18 hours during World War I to 1 to 2 hours in the Vietnam War, and to decrease field mortality from 10% to 12% in World War I to approximately 1% in Vietnam.

The quality of prehospital emergency care in the civilian community was first evaluated in 1966 when the National Academy of Sciences–National Research Council

TABLE 63–1. Fifteen Components of EMS Systems Outlined in the Emergency Medical Services Act of 1973

1. Provision of manpower	9. Accessibility of care
2. Training of personnel	10. Transfer of patients
3. Communications	11. Standard record keeping
4. Transportation	12. Consumer information and education
5. Facilities	13. Independent review and evaluation
6. Critical care units	14. Disaster linkage
7. Use of public safety agencies	15. Mutual aid agreements
8. Consumer participation	

published a report entitled *Accidental Death and Disability: The Neglected Disease of Modern Society*. This report pointed out the poor quality of civilian prehospital and hospital care in the United States. Many ambulances at that time were hearses, ambulance attendants often lacked any first-aid training, and emergency departments were poorly equipped and were staffed primarily by interns without supervision.

In response to this publication, the National Highway Safety Act of 1966 became law. It gave the United States Department of Transportation (DOT) the legislative and financial authority to work toward improving emergency care. The DOT developed programs and standards for improving ambulance services and providing training for prehospital personnel. The Emergency Medical Services (EMS) Act of 1973 provided federal funds ($185 million) for establishment and expansion of regional EMS programs and for EMS research. It dictated that federally funded programs plan for a "systems" approach to emergency medical services and address 15 areas of concern in establishing these systems (see Table 63–1). Each of these components was considered critical toward providing emergency medical services in a coordinated manner. The act targeted seven patient groups who had unique needs to be addressed by the system (Table 63–2). States receiving federal support for EMS activities were required to provide matching funds.

The provisions of this act and the funds provided allowed many areas of the United States to train and equip qualified emergency care providers. The Act was renewed in 1976 and in 1979, but in 1981 the EMS division of the federal government was dissolved, and federal EMS programs were integrated into the Health Prevention Block Grants administered by the Centers for Disease Control (CDC). These grants could be dispersed for programs such as rodent control, water fluoridation, sexual assault crisis centers, home health care, hypertension screening, and EMS. Much of the support went for non-EMS programs, significantly limiting the federal funds available for EMS activities. Financial support for EMS is now primarily a local and state responsibility, although the federal government is again considering designating specific funding.

Each state has a lead governmental EMS agency that oversees and coordinates EMS activities in that state. Many of these lead agencies are part of the Department of Public Health, although some states have created separate EMS departments or placed responsibility in other state agencies, e.g., Department of Education. Many regions have agencies, EMS councils, or medical control authorities that regulate or coordinate EMS activities. The reader is encouraged to investigate the specific state and local EMS structure of his or her own area.

EMS PERSONNEL

As EMS developed, a number of different EMS provider levels evolved. Each has different levels of training and expertise (Table 63–3). An understanding of their

TABLE 63–2. Seven Emergency Patient Target Groups Outlined in the Emergency Medical Services Act of 1973

1. Major accidental trauma	5. Poisonings
2. Burn injuries	6. High-risk infants and mothers
3. Spinal cord injuries	7. Behavioral or psychiatric emergencies
4. Acute coronary or heart attacks	

TABLE 63–3. Prehospital Care Providers in the United States: Major Classes, Training Hours, Estimated Numbers, Capabilities

Level	Hours of Training	Total Numbers of Providers[a] (% Total Known)	Capabilities
First responders	40–50	Unknown	CPR, first aid, patient stabilization
EMT-A	120	434,498 (83.3%)	BLS = basic life support, patient extrication and stabilization, oxygen, splinting, MAST?[b], EOA?[b]
EMT-D	4–40 (additional)	Unknown	Automatic defibrillator
EMT-1[b]	12–85 (additional)	35,971 (6.9%)	EOA = esophageal obturator airway, intubation, IV, medications, automatic defibrillator[b]
EMT-P	500–1500	51,265 (9.8%)	Advanced airway management, medications, manual defibrillation, chest decompression, cricothyrotomy
EMD (Dispatch)	25		Priority dispatching, prearrival instructions

[a]Based on 1989 figures, The National EMS Clearinghouse.
[b]State variations.

capabilities is necessary to ensure their proper use and guidance. The levels described are generally found in each state, although specific designations may vary. For example, Paramedic, EMT-P, Advanced EMT-A, and EMT-III or IV identify the same training level in different states.

All EMS providers are taught anatomy, physiology, and the principles of initial patient assessment and stabilization. These include ABC (airway, breathing, and circulation) assessment, CPR (cardiopulmonary resuscitation), vital signs measurement, hemorrhage control, fracture stabilization, oxygen administration, and care of common emergency situations, e.g., diabetic problems, seizures, and normal deliveries. The length and depth of training in each of these areas increases with each care provider level.

First responders are trained to assess and care for patients prior to the arrival of other EMS care providers. Generally, they are police or fire personnel who have received 40 to 50 hours of training in initiating patient stabilization.

Basic emergency medical technicians (EMT-A) are the largest group of prehospital care providers. They receive 120 to 150 hours of education in patient assessment, basic life support, extrication, and stabilization (Table 63–4). They can use oxygen, extrication equipment, splinting and bandaging equipment, and, in some states, pneumatic antishock garments (PASG) and esophageal obturator airways (EOA).

Prehospital studies of sudden cardiac death have shown that early defibrillation is

TABLE 63–4. Basic EMT Curriculum

Topic	Hours	Topic	Hours
Introduction to emergency care training	3	Injuries to the chest, abdomen, and genitalia	3
Anatomy and physiology and patient assessment	3	Medical emergencies	6
		Emergency childbirth	3
Airway obstruction and respiratory arrest	3	Burns and hazardous materials	3
Cardiac arrest	3	Environmental emergencies	3
CPR practice and certification	4	Psychological aspects of emergency care	3
Practical use of airway adjuncts	3	Lifting and moving patients	3
Bleeding and shock	3	Principles of extrication	3
Review of shock and MAST	4	Ambulance operations	6
Soft tissue injuries	3	Situational review	3
Principles of musculoskeletal care and fractures of the upper extremities	3	Practical sessions	12–17
		Testing sessions	8
Fractures of the pelvis, hip, and lower extremity	3		
Injuries of the head, face, eye, neck, and spine	3		

TABLE 63–5. EMT-Intermediate Curriculum—In Addition to EMT-A Training

Topic	Hours
Roles and responsibilities	2–3
EMS systems/medical control	2–3
Medical/legal considerations	2–3
Medical terminology	1–2
EMS communications	2–4
General patient assessment and management	18–26
Airway management and ventilation	3–4
Assessment and management of shock	6–10
Defibrillation (optional)	

the most important factor that positively affects survival from sudden cardiac death. Thus, a new provider level has been created: the *EMT-Defibrillator (EMT-D)*. This person is usually a basic EMT who has been given 8 to 40 hours of additional training to allow the use of either a manual or an automatic defibrillator in the field. Automatic external defibrillators (AEDs) sense the underlying cardiac rhythm and discharge an electrical charge if the rhythm is ventricular fibrillation (VF) or pulseless ventricular tachycardia (VT). The use of automated defibrillators by first responders and the lay public may allow even more rapid defibrillation in the prehospital setting.

EMT-Intermediate has a variety of designations in different states. In 1987 there were at least 22 designations, e.g., EMT-I, EMT-Specialist, and Cardiology Tech, with 30 to 35 different levels of care provided by EMT-Intermediates. Their capabilities include intravenous (IV) access, endotracheal intubation, and possibly administering IV medications such as epinephrine, dextrose, naloxone, or sodium bicarbonate. They receive 12 to 85 hours of additional instruction beyond the basic EMT level (Table 63–5).

The *Paramedic (EMT-P)* receives from 500 to 1500 hours of didactic and practical instruction in preparation for providing advanced life support (Table 63–6). This training adds manual defibrillation, cardioversion, and the use of medications to the basic EMT-A skills. The types of invasive procedures that paramedics are permitted to perform include needle decompression for tension pneumothorax, percutaneous transtracheal jet ventilation, and cricothyrotomy.

The value of obtaining adequate information about the need for medical assistance led to the formalized training of *Emergency Medical Dispatchers (EMDs)*. This training provides the dispatcher with the knowledge and skills to dispatch the appropriate personnel and equipment, and if necessary, to provide medical assistance instructions to the caller while EMS units are responding. Pre-arrival instructions have facilitated successful resuscitations from cardiac arrest. EMDs receive approximately 25 hours of training (Table 63–7).

TABLE 63–6. EMT-Paramedic Curriculum (500–1500 hours)

Module I	The emergency medical technician, his role, responsibilities, and training
Module II	Human systems and patient assessment
Module III	Shock and fluid therapy
Module IV	General pharmacology
Module V	Respiratory system
Module VI	Cardiovascular system
Module VII	Central nervous system
Module VIII	Soft tissue injuries
Module IX	Musculoskeletal system
Module X	Medical emergencies
Module XI	Obstetric and gynecologic emergencies
Module XII	Pediatric and neonatal transport
Module XIII	Emergency care of the emotionally disturbed
Module XIV	Extrication and rescue techniques
Module XV	Telemetry and communications

TABLE 63–7. EMT-Dispatcher Curriculum

Topic	Hours
Introduction to EMS dispatcher roles and responsibilities	1
Basic EMS telecommunications equipment and operating procedures	2–3
Emergency care and cardiopulmonary resuscitation	4–6
Obtaining information from callers	2–3
Providing emergency care instructions	4–6
Allocation of resources and EMS dispatching	2–3
Disaster procedure	2–3
Practical	5–6
Written and practical testing	2

PROBLEM The request for an ambulance was received from a passerby who told the dispatcher that there was a "drunk lying in the alley." The emergency medical dispatcher found out that the patient was breathing and moving a little but was unconscious and bleeding from the head. Because of that information, an advanced life-support unit was sent to the scene. The dispatcher also called the police to assist the EMS personnel and to ensure their safety. The passerby refused to stay at the scene.

The paramedics arrived on the scene after the police. They questioned whether the patient had fallen from a height or sustained a possible neck injury from an assault. They carefully "log-rolled" the patient while maintaining cervical spine stability. They immobilized the patient, initiated oxygen therapy and an intravenous (IV) line, and administered naloxone, dextrose, and thiamine. They then carefully but expeditiously transported the patient to the hospital.

Had the passerby remained at the scene, the EMD could have instructed him in bleeding control. In the event of a cardiac arrest, the EMS dispatcher could have talked the passerby through the technique of basic CPR. Of course, it would help to have the victim close by the telephone! As an advanced life-support unit, paramedics have the knowledge and equipment to treat an unconscious patient aggressively. This treatment includes endotracheal intubation if there is concern about the stability of the airway, cardiac monitoring, establishing an IV line, and administering medications. The other basic elements of care for this patient are available from all levels of care providers.

COMMUNICATIONS

There are two purposes of communication between prehospital care providers and emergency department personnel:

1. To allow the EMTs to inform the hospital of the patient's condition and the care already given to allow them to prepare for his arrival.

2. To permit medical control personnel to give the EMTs further guidance and orders.

There are several communications devices available. The telephone has been used in the past but was limited to use from a home or office. With the advent of cellular technology, more ambulances are using cellular telephones for that communication. Usage of this mode may expand because technology currently exists to transmit 3- or 12-lead electrocardiograms by cellular telephones.

Most communication between the field and the emergency department occurs via radio. The radio system can be structured in one of two ways: simplex or duplex. The simplex mode uses the same frequency for transmitting and receiving, allowing only one-way communication. When one person is talking, the other person cannot speak. The duplex mode uses two frequencies. The field unit transmits on frequency A and receives on frequency B; the hospital unit transmits on frequency B and receives on frequency A. This establishes a two-way communication that is similar to talking on the telephone. Understanding the type of equipment existing in the emergency department is necessary to communicate effectively with the providers in the field.

Telemetry radios convert electrical impulses into a modulated radio signal to transmit an electrocardiographic (ECG) tracing to the emergency department. Telemetry radios are used in systems in which most advanced life support orders are provided by on-line medical control. Problems with the quality of the ECG tracing received in the emergency department are common, and many areas have phased out the use of telemetry transmission except in situations in which the paramedics have specific questions. Cellular technology may supplant the need for telemetry radios.

The extent to which EMS personnel contact the emergency department by radio is individualized to the EMS system and its hospitals. Some institutions request extensive information about every patient coming to their facility. Others focus on certain types of patients, such as critically ill patients, multiple trauma patients, or pediatric patients. Some EMS systems have established protocols based on scoring systems that outline when the hospital should be contacted.

Regardless of the mechanism established, the report from the EMS personnel should be well organized and provide specific information (Table 63–8). This organization allows consistent exchange of information in a rapid manner. Further orders or interventions can then be appropriately initiated.

When the emergency physician talks with EMS personnel via radio or telephone, it is necessary to identify himself clearly, speak in a calm voice, and give concise orders. Proper terminology is used, and slang terms are avoided, e.g., "10–4, good buddy." When providing specific orders, they are repeated to ensure understanding. Many systems request that the EMTs repeat the orders as a form of acknowledgment. Above all else, familiarity with the local EMS protocols is mandatory before transmitting orders or information on the radio.

Radio communication between prehospital providers and the emergency department is documented in some manner. Many systems tape record the conversation for future review and reference. Most emergency departments also manually record the information received and the orders given on a radio log (Table 63–9). Both the tape and the radio log can be used for incident review and medical control functions.

Another important method of communication is the EMS Run Report (Fig. 63–1). This written record documents the prehospital providers' history, physical examination, and care provided. It is the only permanent record of the prehospital component of the patient interaction. It becomes part of the patient's medical record and should be appropriately completed. It also is used for the quality assurance review of the case.

PROBLEM The radio communication in the case was as follows:
        EMT-P: This is Medic 101, Paramedic Jones. We are on scene with a late

TABLE 63–8. Format for EMS Radio Communications

EMT	Medical control
Identify unit/self	Acknowledge
Age and sex of patient	Further questions
Priority status	Orders
Estimated time of arrival and destination	EMT
Chief complaint	Acknowledge
Appropriate history	Repeat orders
Vital signs (blood pressure, pulse, respiratory rate, level of consciousness)	Further questions or comments
Appropriate physical examination	
Interventions or treatments	

TABLE 63-9. Emergency Medical Services Hospital Communications Form

```
                                          Date _____
                                          Time _____
Telemetry _____   HEAR _____   Telephone _____
Agency: _____
Patient Info:  Age _____   M   F
    Name _____
    Physician _____
    Priority Status _____                              ETA _____
    Prehospital Index _____
Chief Complaint: _____
_____
_____

PMHx: _____
Meds: _____ Allergies: _____
Assessment:  LOC: A/O _____ Confused _____ Resp to pain _____ Unresp _____
             GCS _____
             Pupils: PERRL _____ unequal _____ nonrx _____
Vital Signs:
    Time:     _____   _____   _____
    BP:       _____   _____   _____
    Pulse:    _____   _____   _____
    Resp:     _____   _____   _____
Head: AT _____ Lac _____
Chest: clear _____ wheezes _____ rales _____
Abdomen: soft _____ tender _____ distended _____ trauma _____

Ext: _____ NV: Intact _____ Other _____
Skin: W/D _____ cool _____ moist _____ diaphoretic _____
Treatment: O₂ _____ IV: LR _____ NS _____ D₅W _____ Rate: TKO _____ WO _____
Other _____
    Meds: D₅W _____ Narcan _____ Lasix _____ Lido _____ NTG _____
    Other: _____
    Immobilization: Spine _____ Ext _____ Other _____
    Monitor: RSR _____ ST _____ PVCs _____ PACs _____ Rate: _____
Orders: _____
_____
_____
_____

Physician: _____ Nurse: _____
```

Reprinted with permission of Jon R. Krohmer, MD.

20s male. Patient found unconscious by bystanders. Have treated this patient previously with known ETOH abuse. No other history available. Vital signs: blood pressure 180/100, pulse 96, respiratory rate 20. Not responsive to verbal or painful stimuli. Has small abrasion on forehead and bleeding from back of head. Patient is immobilized. On oxygen. Request IV and unconscious patient protocol. ETA 15 minutes.

Base Station Physician (BSP): Understand, Medic 101. Gag reflex present?

EMT-P: Negative.

BSP: Understand. Any nearby bottles, drugs, or weapons?

EMT-P: Several bottles. No weapons.

BSP: Could the patient be hypothermic?

EMT-P: Affirmative. Wearing only light jacket. Skin is cold.

BSP: Okay, Medic 101. Because of level of consciousness and gag absent, go ahead and intubate patient nasotracheally, continue immobilization, and go ahead with unconscious patient protocol, warm blankets, and transport. Please hyperventilate, also.

EMT-P: Understand NT intubation, immobilization, blankets, and unconscious protocol. Will see you in about 15 minutes.

BSP: Okay, Medic 101. Notify of any changes. ED clear.

EMT-P: Medic 101 clear.

DEPT. DIST./OFFICE

AGENCY(S) INVOLVED

EMS RUN MEDICAL FORM

MEDCOM OR HOSPITAL NUMBER

COUNTY / TOWNSHIP OR CITY

NAME		ADDRESS		DATE	DAY
PATIENT PHONE	AGE	D.O.B.	SEX M ☐ F ☐	RACE	UNIT NO.
INCIDENT LOCATION		NEXT OF KIN			
DISPATCH / "CHIEF COMPLAINT"		REPORTING POLICE DEPARTMENT		EST. TIME—INCIDENT	
MED. HX.		ALLERGIES			
CURRENT MEDS.					
PT. PHYSICIAN		HOSPITAL			

COMPLAINT NO.

ONF NO.

AMB. RESPONSE ______

Dispatch ______

Arr. Scene ______

Dep. Scene ______

Arr. Hosp. ______

PHYSIOLOGIC STATUS

TIME	BLOOD PRES	PULSE		RESP.		PUPILS		GLASGOW COMA SCALE				SKIN
		RATE	QUAL.	RATE	QUAL.	RIGHT	LEFT	EYE	MOTOR	VERBAL	TOTAL	

W-Weak, T-Thready, B-Bounding, A-Absent, I-Irregular, R-Regular, S-Shallow, L-Labored, E-Equal, C-Constricted, D-Dilated, O-Reactive, U-Unreactive, M-Moist, DR-Dry, G-Warm, H-Cool, P-Pale, FL-Flushed, CY-Cynotic

PRIOR AID		GIVEN BY	
☐ Artificial Respiration	☐ Other	☐ Dr.	☐ Nurse
☐ First Aid	☐ None	☐ EMS	☐ Citizen
☐ CPR		☐ Fire	☐ Other
		☐ Police	______

AIRWAY PROCEDURE # ATTEMPTS BY # EST. BY # O_2 FLOW TIME OTHER

I.V. SITE GAUGE FLUID # ATTEMPTS BY # EST. BY # RATE FLUID GIVEN CC TIME

DRUG TIMES

DRUGS	TIME	DOSE	ROUTE	BY NO.	TIME	DOSE	ROUTE	BY NO.	TIME	DOSE	ROUTE	BY NO.	TIME	DOSE	ROUTE	BY NO.

DEFIBRILLATION

TIME	WATT/S	ECG	BY NO.

MONITORED? Yes ☐ No ☐ INTERPRETATION

Sample EKG Attached Yes ☐ No ☐

DESTINATION

Hospital ______

City ______

By ______

CHOSEN BY

☐ Patient ☐ MEDCOM ☐ Relation ☐ Hospital ☐ EMT ☐ Physician ☐ Other______

PROTOCOL___REQUESTED

Granted Yes ☐ No ☐

Amended Yes ☐ No ☐

Denied Yes ☐ No ☐

Physician ______

Hospital ______

CPR INITIATED

Yes ☐ No ☐

Time ______

By ______

MAST	CHAMBER	PRESSURE	TIME	BY NO.
Yes ☐ No ☐ In Place	Right Leg			
	Left Leg			
	Abdomen			

EQUIPMENT USED

NARRATIVE

☐ FORM COMPLETED BY: #

SIGNATURE

PRINTED NAME OF DOCTOR

DEA NUMBER

LEVELS Adv. EMT (P) EMT Specialist (S) Basic EMT (A) Other (O)

AMBULANCE PERSONNEL	No./Level	OTHER AGENCY PERSONNEL	No./Level
1. ______		1. ______	
2. ______		2. ______	
3. ______		3. ______	

OTHER AGENCY RESPONSE

Dispatch ______

Arr. Scene ______

Dep. Scene ______

Arr. Hosp. ______

White - Patient Chart • Green - Agency • Canary - Pharmacy • Pink - EMS Coord. • Gold-Supporting Unit

FIGURE 63–1. EMS run report.

The above interaction assumes that the paramedic and the physician both understand the unconscious patient protocol. If not, then the physician should specify intravenous naloxone, 2 mg; thiamine, 100 mg; and 50% dextrose, 25 gm.

INTERACTION WITH EMS PERSONNEL

Communication between EMS personnel and emergency department staff continues when the patient arrives in the emergency department. EMS personnel can provide a more complete history and physical examination report as well as an update about the care provided and the patient's condition. It is very important that emergency department personnel make themselves available to receive that information. To facilitate the exchange, there are a number of "Rules of the Road."

1. *Know your EMS system and the personnel.*
    It is critical for physicians to be familiar with the capabilities of the individual care providers. Asking an EMT-A or an EMT-I to start a dopamine infusion will only frustrate both the EMT and the physician because it cannot be done. By personally knowing the providers, one understands their individual abilities.
2. *Know the standing orders and the equipment available.*
    It is important for the physician to be familiar with the standing orders and protocols under which the EMTs operate and the medications they carry. Physicians need not ask paramedics to give an unconscious patient naloxone, dextrose, and thiamine if that is part of the standing orders. One should not request dopamine if it is not carried in the drug boxes.
3. *Be supportive and understanding.*
    EMTs often work under adverse conditions. The patients and families that EMS personnel encounter are not always cooperative, patient, or understanding. Patients may be injured, intoxicated, or both. They may be in physically difficult and emotionally hostile settings. EMS personnel do not have the luxury of working in a warm, well-lighted, well-equipped emergency department. It helps to be cognizant of these factors when talking with EMTs.
4. *Ride on the ambulance.*
    A medical control physician's request on the radio for an immediate IV line while the paramedics at the scene of an automobile accident are managing the fully dressed driver's airway and cervical spine from the back seat of the car in 15° weather is not conducive to good physician-paramedic relations. The only way to understand the prehospital environment is to experience it. It is an excellent learning experience for the physician, and it allows the EMTs an opportunity to work with the physician in a setting outside the emergency department. State laws and liability insurance rules must be checked, but if possible, the opportunity is well worth the effort.
5. *Meet them at the door.*
    As time permits, take time to talk with the EMTs about their patient. Try to meet them as they bring the patient into the emergency department. The EMTs are intimately involved in the patient's care, and that extends to providing the emergency department staff with further information about the case, including any changes that have occurred since the original report. In addition, the EMTs may be the only ones able to provide a reliable history of the event, including information about the scene of injury or illness.
6. *Talk with EMS personnel.*
    When problems arise concerning the prehospital care of patients, talk with the providers as soon as possible to clarify the issue. Often they will have questions or concerns as well. When they do a good job, don't hesitate to commend them;

patients don't often thank them. Remember the old adage, "Praise in public, criticize in private."

7. *EMS coordinators are there for a reason.*

Many hospitals employ EMS coordinators who facilitate the interaction with EMS personnel. Often they are either paramedics or nurses with extensive EMS experience. They are often the interface with the medical control agency and routinely review run sheets and radiotelemetry tapes. They should be made aware of any problems that arise. They can do follow-up investigations in a more complete manner when the situation is more relaxed than when the patient was brought into the hospital. EMS coordinators can also provide EMS crews with feedback on the patient's course after arriving in the emergency department. They are a valuable resource for EMS education as well.

MEDICAL CONTROL

Prehospital care providers function as extenders of the physicians who supervise their activities. Physicians serving in this role are legally responsible for the activities of these providers. Historically, the concept of medical control has applied only to intermediate and advanced EMTs. Many physicians believe that basic EMTs should also operate under some form of medical control.

There are two types of medical control: on-line and off-line. On-line medical control involves the direct supervision or communication between the EMT and the physician. It allows each case to be discussed while care is being given. This generally occurs via communications devices such as radio, telemetry, or telephone. It can also occur with the medical control physician at the scene.

On-line medical control at the scene should not be confused with the physician intervenor, a nonmedical control physician who stops at the scene of an accident to offer assistance. In many situations, these physicians can offer valuable assistance. In some cases, they may interfere because they are not familiar with the EMS system, its protocols, and the capabilities of prehospital personnel. Most EMS systems have developed policies to address the issue of the physician intervenor (Table 63–10).

Off-line medical control involves all the other aspects of directing an EMS system. This includes the establishment of standing orders and protocols, training, continuing education and recertification of personnel, and performance review by audits and run reviews. Off-line medical control is often conducted by physicians, nurses, or paramedics under the supervision of the medical director of the system.

Generally, EMTs deliver care either after direct communication with the emergency department or by means of standing orders or protocols (Table 63–11). Standing orders allow EMTs to perform procedures and administer medications under defined circumstances without contacting the physician, e.g., advanced cardiac life support (ACLS) protocols for cardiac arrest. In other situations, EMTs must contact medical control before performing an intervention, e.g., administering certain medications or performing needle chest decompression for tension pneumothorax. The extent to which standing orders are used is a function of the particular EMS system.

TABLE 63–10. On-Scene Physician Intervention Policy

Thank you for your offer of assistance. Be advised that these paramedics are operating under the authority of Michigan law. No physician or other person may intercede in patient care without the Medical Control physician on duty relinquishing responsibility of the scene via radio or telephone. If responsibility is given to a physician on the scene, that physician is responsible for any and all care given at the scene of the incident and should accompany patient enroute to the hospital, and upon arrival, sign the Medical Record. Thank you.

Reference: Public Act 368 of 1978, amended by Public Act 79 of 1981.
Reprinted with permission of Kent County Emergency Medical Services, Grand Rapids, MI, 1986.

TABLE 63–11. Acute Pulmonary Edema Protocol

B	D	S	P		
B	D	S	P	I.	Signs of acute pulmonary edema
					A. Distended neck veins
					B. Peripheral edema
					C. Rales
					D. Respiratory distress
					E. History
B	D	S	P	II.	Reassurance is mandatory
B	D	S	P	III.	**Support ventilations:** Administer 6 liters/min oxygen via nasal cannula or 10 liters/min oxygen by mask
		S	P		Consider intubation now or later if needed
		S	P	IV.	**Start IV of D_5W**—250 ml
					A. Run TKO
					B. Maximum of four tries, two per EMT and 20 minutes total maximum time
			P	V.	**Sublingual nitroglycerine,** 0.4 mg (1/150 gr) if patient is having chest pain
					A. Do not give if blood pressure is less than 100 systolic
					B. May repeat every 5 minutes (limit three doses)
			P	VI.	**May give Lasix 40 mg IVP**
					CONTACT MEDICAL CONTROL
				VII.	*Possible orders post-radio contact*
			P		A. Morphine sulfate 2–5 mg IV slowly over 1 min if systolic pressure is greater than 100 mm Hg
			P		B. May give nitroglycerine, 0.4 mg (1/150 gr) SL if systolic pressure is greater than 100 mm Hg

Note: Blood pressure should be monitored before and after administering these medications.
Reprinted with permission of Kent County Emergency Medical Services, Grand Rapids, MI, 1986.
B, D, S, and P are levels of training in this system.

A critical component of medical control is the EMS Medical Director of the system. This physician should be involved in daily supervision of EMS activities and should have intimate knowledge of and experience in the practice of prehospital care. Training in emergency medicine is desirable. The medical director is involved in all aspects of medical control and is ultimately responsible for the quality of care provided within the system.

PROBLEM In this case, the paramedics were allowed by standing orders to initiate oxygen therapy and cardiac monitoring and establish an IV line. The standing orders also required the paramedics to draw a blood sample while the IV line was started. They had already immobilized the cervical spine.

After contact with the medical control hospital, the paramedics were advised to intubate the patient (to protect the airway) and to hyperventilate the patient (in case of a closed head injury). The physician also requested that the paramedics administer 2 mg of naloxone, 100 mg of thiamine, and 25 gm of glucose IV. The paramedics were then encouraged to transport the patient as quickly as possible.

Had the medical control system provided standing orders for the unconscious patient, the paramedics could have administered the dextrose, naloxone, and thiamine prior to contact with the physician.

Once the paramedics arrive at the hospital, the physician or nurse will talk with them further to obtain more information about the patient and the scene and determine whether there was any change in the patient's condition during transport. The physician or nurse can try to answer any questions the paramedics may have about the patient or the care provided at that time.

As part of the off-line medical control function, the EMS Medical Director or his designee will review the completed EMS run form (Fig. 63–2), the EMS hospital communications form, and perhaps the radio tape to ensure that the appropriate standing orders were followed and that medical control

FIGURE 63–2.

was provided in an appropriate manner. Problems or exceptional performances can be noted at that time with the appropriate recognition or reprimand.

IMPACT OF EMERGENCY MEDICAL SERVICES

In examining the impact that emergency medical services have had on the public, the discussion revolves around two main patient groups: those with cardiovascular disease and trauma patients.

There is general agreement that improved EMS services have made a significant impact on the mortality associated with sudden cardiac death. If a victim can be found quickly, CPR initiated within 4 minutes, and defibrillation accomplished within 4 to 8 minutes, the likelihood of survival to hospital discharge may approach 30% to 40%. These findings have provided support for the development of EMT-D programs throughout the country. There is some interest in providing automatic defibrillators to family members of patients at risk of sudden cardiac death to allow more rapid defibrillation.

The utility of EMS systems in treating acute myocardial infarction patients is undergoing reassessment. The early usefulness of paramedics' prolonged stabilization efforts in the field with IV therapy and administration of multiple medications is being questioned. With the advent of early thrombolytic therapy, some are advocating rapid transport to the hospital for such therapy. There are those, however, who support the use of thrombolytic agents in the field to allow earlier initiation of therapy. This will continue to be an area of intense interest and investigation.

The impact of EMS systems on multiple trauma patients has been less impressive. Early in the development of prehospital care, the goal was early stabilization of the patient, often using IV therapy, pneumatic antishock garment (PASG), and spinal immobilization. Much of the research in trauma patient care outcome has been conflicting, but most physicians advocate rapid extrication, immobilization, and transport to the hospital, with other advanced life support procedures being performed en route. Optimally, patients are transported to the facility most appropriate to care for the injuries incurred. Multiple trauma patients should be transported to trauma centers capable of rapidly stabilizing and operating on these patients.

Another factor that has affected prehospital care and the rapid transport of patients has been the growth of rotary-wing air ambulance programs throughout the country. There are now over 300 programs in the United States. Although there are also conflicting reports about the usefulness of this expensive mode of transportation, air ambulances have been found useful in transporting victims of cardiac disease and trauma from smaller institutions to tertiary referral centers where more advanced therapy is available. Rotary-wing aircraft have also been useful in transporting trauma victims from rural scenes to facilities capable of providing definitive care.

SUMMARY AND FINAL POINTS

The EMS team is composed of the prehospital providers and the emergency department staff. Physicians who interact with EMS personnel must

- Be familiar with the level of training and the capabilities of the personnel.
- Know the specific standing orders and protocols under which they function.
- Understand the communications equipment and the proper way of communicating patient reports.
- Understand the uniqueness of the prehospital setting of patient care.
- Be actively involved in the education, administration, and critique of the EMS system.

BIBLIOGRAPHY

Texts

1. Boyd DR, Edlich RF, Micik S: Systems Approach to Emergency Medical Care. East Norwalk, CT, Appleton-Century-Crofts, 1983.
2. Caroline NL: Emergency Care in the Streets. 3rd Ed. Boston, Little, Brown and Co., 1987.
3. Cleary VL, Wilson P, Super G: Prehospital Care: Administrative and Clinical Management. Rockville, MD, Aspen Publishers, 1987.
4. Kuehl AE: EMS Medical Director's Handbook (National Association of EMS Physicians). St. Louis, MO, CV Mosby Co, 1989.
5. Roush WR: Principles of EMS Systems. A Comprehensive Text for Physicians. American College of Emergency Physicians. Dallas, TX, 1989.

Journal Articles

1. American College of Emergency Physicians: Medical control of prehospital emergency medical services (position paper). Ann Emerg Med 11(7):387, 1982.
2. Boyd DR: The conceptual development of EMS systems in the United States, Part I. Emerg Med Serv 11(1):19–23, 1982.
3. Boyd DR: The conceptual development of EMS systems in the United States, Part II. Emerg Med Serv 11(2):26–35, 1982.
4. Clawson JJ: Regulations and standards for emergency medical dispatchers: A model for state or region. Emerg Med Serv 13(4):25–29, 1984.
5. Holroyd BR, Knopp R, Kallsen G: Medical control–quality assurance in prehospital care. JAMA 256:1027–1031, 1986.
6. Hunt RC, McCabe JB, Hamilton GC, Krohmer JR: Influence of Emergency Medical Services systems and prehospital defibrillation on survival from sudden cardiac death. Am J Emerg Med 7:68–82, 1989.
7. Mhyre N: The enhanced 911 program. Emerg Med Serv 13:32–37, 1984.
8. Mustalish AC: Emergency Medical Services: Twenty years of growth and development. NY State J Med 8:414–420, 1986.
9. National Academy of Sciences–National Research Council, Division of Medical Sciences: Accidental death and disability: A neglected disease of modern society. Washington DC, 1966.
10. Pepe PE, Stewart RD: The role of the physician in the prehospital setting. Ann Emerg Med 15(12):1480–1484, 1986.
11. Stewart RD: Medical direction in Emergency Medical Services: The role of the physician. Emerg Med Clin North Am 5:1:119–132, 1987.
12. United States Department of Transportation: Department of Transportation (DOT) Training Guidelines. Emerg Med Serv 18(11):196–200, 1989.

SECTION NINETEEN

PHYSICIAN INTERPERSONAL SKILLS

CHAPTER 64

THE PROBLEM PATIENT

KENNETH V. ISERSON, M.D., M.B.A.

PROBLEM 1 A 30 year old asthmatic arrived at the emergency department with an acute exacerbation of his disease. He had been on a course of oral steroids intermittently in the past. After two albuterol inhalation treatments there was very little improvement. He demanded a steroid injection, which he claimed always "cures me within 15 minutes."

PROBLEM 2 A 32 year old woman with known significant cardiomyopathy was brought in by her sister. Her complaint, delivered in a "whining manner," was that "she is just not feeling well." After examining the patient and reviewing her old chart, there was no discernible difference from her normal state of poor health. She wanted to be admitted to the hospital but could not contact her regular physician.

PROBLEM 3 A 3 year old was brought in after tripping and hitting his head against a table at a family picnic. There was no loss of consciousness and the neurologic examination by the emergency physician was normal. The physician explained head injury precautions to the parents and was ready to discharge the child when they asked, "Doctor, aren't you going to get an x-ray?"

PROBLEM 4 A 35 year old man was brought into the emergency department supine, with his eyes open and tracking activity, but not responding to verbal stimuli. Suddenly he screamed out and became violent.

QUESTIONS TO CONSIDER

1. What expectations do physicians have that may cause them to view some patients as "problems"?
2. Why is emergency medicine particularly vulnerable to receiving "problem patients"?
3. How are manipulative patients handled? Should a patient's manipulation of the medical system always be seen as a problem?
4. How do physicians deal with patients who insist on dictating or bargaining their medical care?
5. How are dissatisfied patients or family managed? Can some problems be avoided at the onset?
6. What problems do hostile or violent patients present to the physician?

INTRODUCTION

The emergency physician usually has had no previous contact with the patients he or she treats. Neither the patient nor the physician has chosen each other. On presenting to the emergency department, patients are often under stress because they perceive an acute change in their health and feel an urgent need for medical evaluation. Whether or not this perception ultimately proves to be true, it may lead to anxiety, fear, and anger.

The clinician's response to the patient, rather than the patient himself, is often the root of many problems. Derogatory terms may be used to describe problem patients. These terms may be used when there are difficulties in interpersonal communication between the physician and patient. Physicians and emergency department staff may have trouble dealing with certain types of patients or complaints. Many clinicians have difficulty in dealing with broad categories of patients, such as alcoholics, drug abusers, children, homosexuals, or the very old. Some patients elicit feelings of aversion, fear, frustration, or even malice in their doctors. Problem patients often represent for the physician a fear of not being in control and of intensely disliking the experience of losing control. These feelings must be recognized to determine how they are interfering with optimal patient care.

As physicians mature as clinicians they are able to recognize those patients they find personally distasteful. Once physicians recognize the traits, behaviors, and personalities that they have difficulty with, they will recognize that their evoked feelings rather than the patient is the "problem."

The clinician has options in dealing with a patient he finds personally distasteful. First, just by recognizing his own dislikes, the clinician may be able to repress these feelings consciously while evaluating and treating the patient. Alternatively, he can ask a colleague to see the patient. Even in the smaller private emergency department, this is more easily done than imagined. By contacting the patient's private physician, another clinician can be used to evaluate the patient's condition and ensure objective management. The patient's primary physician may be able to put the complaint and behavior in the perspective of a long-term relationship. If this is not possible, colleagues can be asked to consult, giving a second opinion about the case. If physicians are free to ask for help without any type of overt or covert censure, many problem patients can be successfully managed.

This chapter will review the characteristics of the manipulative, dissatisfied, hostile, and violent patient.

MANIPULATIVE PATIENT

The manipulative patient wants something and may use indirect means to achieve that goal. Most manipulative patients are perceived as dictating their medical care to the physician. These patients often know something about their disease and have preconceived views about how they should be managed. Their information may or may not be medically accurate. These patients are labeled problem patients because the clinician senses a loss of control and an alteration of the traditional physician–"obedient" patient relationship.

Patient advocate groups and many health care professionals recommend that, whenever possible, the clinician and patient work together to treat a disease process. Information and respect should flow in both directions. The patient's ideas and wishes, when not in conflict with the physician's personal and medical ethics, good medical judgment, and the law, should be respected.

In the emergency department there are many opportunities to involve patients in health care decisions. It is important, when possible, to respect the patient's autonomy, allowing him as much say as possible in the direction of the care given. There are multiple constraints on what the clinician can do medically, ethically, and legally. The patient may request services that are simply beyond the physician's capabilities. More frequently, he may ask for treatment that diverges from accepted medical practice or might pose a danger to himself.

The emergency physician can approach the manipulative patient from several directions.

1. Understand the patient's need to be "in control." Explain important decision points and allow him to choose between medically accepted alternatives.

2. If possible, involve a third party the patient trusts in the discussion (e.g., family member, primary physician, or friend).

3. Determine whether there are other problems that are causing the demand for a specific treatment. Are there financial, social, or drug-related concerns that need to be addressed?

4. Educate the patient calmly and rationally. Use general terms. Avoid "you" and "I" or confrontational language. Do not let your "feelings" dictate the conversation.

5. Try to satisfy the patient whenever it is medically, legally, and ethically acceptable. It will help heal the illness.

6. If the demand is medically, legally, or ethically unacceptable, try to educate the patient. Document the request and response. Make sure the patient is competent to understand the consequences of his actions (see Chap. 62).

PROBLEM 1 The 30 year old asthmatic requested a steroid injection. He claimed that this cures him within 15 minutes. Pharmacologically, this is impossible, yet he seemed rational as he claimed this response.

Because steroids are probably indicated as part of the treatment for the patient's asthma, the emergency physician ordered parenteral Solu-Medrol. He reasoned that any psychogenic component of the patient's asthma would be considerably helped. The patient felt in control of his health care.

PROBLEM 2 The physician attending the 32 year old woman with cardiomyopathy had a strong aversion to dealing with this type of patient personality. She described the woman as speaking in a "whining manner" and noted that she was "beginning to annoy" her. This description is certainly pejorative and may signify that a major problem in this case is the clinician's dislike of these mannerisms. The clinician may describe the patient's attitude as annoying when in fact anger toward the patient has developed. This is a dangerous situation.

In the actual case, this patient was sent home and died within 24 hours. It is unknown whether hospital admission would have made a difference in the patient's outcome. However, the clinician's clinical judgment may have been influenced by her attitude toward the patient.

DISSATISFIED PATIENT

The dissatisfied patient may not be recognized as such until the emergency physician receives a letter, often forwarded from the hospital administrator, that the family was not pleased with the treatment, or another physician calls to ask why the family was so upset about their care.

Each patient or family comes to the emergency department with certain expectations. Most are related to rapidity of care, communication, sense of caring, and alleviation of concerns about treatment of a problem. It is common for emergency department patients to assume that specific activities will take place during evaluation and treatment. Expectation of these actions may originate from prior experience, experiences of friends or relatives, extensive reading, television shows, or cultural beliefs. In some cases, the expectations may be medically accurate. A physician orders an electrocardiogram (ECG) to evaluate chest pain, gives medication to relieve an exacerbation of asthma, and "x-rays" a deformed extremity. However, a patient arriving in the emergency department with abdominal pain may not receive medication for pain relief until the evaluation is completed, and a patient with a 2-day-old laceration to the hand may not receive suturing.

These patient expectations do not match their standards of medical care, and patients do not always understand why.

Frustration is a form of anger. In the emergency department, frustration about the seeming inability of the physician or staff to meet the patient's expectations is commonplace. If these expectations are not addressed, they will result in a dissatisfied patient. The emergency physician can take steps both to prevent and to address the dissatisfied patient.

1. Try to find out and address the expectations of the patient and the family.
2. If the patient is dissatisfied with the entire emergency department visit, consider writing off the emergency department bill if possible.
3. If the patient is dissatisfied, offer to make arrangements for him to be seen by another physician at an appropriate time.
4. Document the specific reasons for the patient's dissatisfaction and the reasons why the emergency department was unable to meet these expectations.

Once a complaint has been filed

1. Personally call the patient to determine what the problem is. It may be related to a simple misunderstanding that can be addressed by the physician.
2. Don't be defensive.
3. Don't confront the patient because of a difference in point of view. Listen to the argument even if it is not medically sound. Calmly educate the patient as to why the emergency department was unable to meet his or her expectations.

PROBLEM 3 The family of the 3 year old who was brought in after hitting his head against a table was ready to leave the emergency department in a highly dissatisfied state. The neurologic examination was normal, and the emergency physician was satisfied that the child had suffered no significant injury. The family, however, requested skull radiographs.

By talking further with the family about the request for a specific test, the emergency physician discovered that a sibling had had a severe skull fracture following a fall and is now disabled. They felt that if they had brought the sibling in for medical care earlier, the disability might have been prevented. If the parents still insist on the radiographs after hearing an explanation of the utility and limitations of skull radiographs, it is prudent to order the radiographs to reassure the parents.

HOSTILE PATIENT

Alcoholics and other drug abusers are the most common types of hostile "problem patients" seen in the emergency department. They are frequently traumatized and cannot be relied on to feel the pain or notice other bodily abnormalities associated with injury. Therefore, they pose a major diagnostic dilemma. To compound this, they are often uncooperative and may become hostile or violent.

Many clinicians have difficulty in dealing with intoxicated patients. Substance abusers are often seen by the emergency department staff as being disruptive to the hospital routine. Many are chronic emergency department patients and make one or more visits per month. They often have chronic psychiatric diseases, are older, poorer, and more socially isolated than other patients. They become the responsibility of the emergency department by default, because their underlying disease often prevents them from complying with any therapeutic regimen. This familiarity on the part of the staff may lead to careless evaluation. Because of their loss of sensibility and uncooperativeness, many alcoholics have the potential of being discharged from the emergency department without a complete evaluation.

Some patients may react with hostility for reasons other than drugs. Fear, discomfort, pain, frustration, or loss of control may become manifest as hostility. The patient's anger is not meant personally and should not be interpreted as such by the emergency department staff.

How should emergency physicians deal with the hostile alcoholic or substance abuser?

1. The emergency physician, nursing personnel, and the social worker all contribute to a successful interaction with these patients. Nearly all patients will respond positively to kindness, food, and the promise of a warm bed.

2. With time and metabolism of ethanol or drugs, the hostility usually abates.

3. Although physical restraint is a possibility, it should be used only as a last resort. Restraints may be necessary if the patient is thought to be incompetent to make decisions about the consequences of his or her injuries (see Chaps. 52 and 62). Restraining an inebriated individual to care for a small laceration is inappropriate; however, restraining the same patient to treat an open femoral fracture would be very reasonable.

4. The limitations of the system must be acknowledged. There are occasions when "discharge to jail" is the correct disposition.

VIOLENT PATIENT

Patients who become physically threatening in the emergency department fit into one of three general classes: (1) they have fear leading to anger, (2) they have grief leading to anger, or (3) they are delirious or intoxicated. About 90% of these patients belong in the last category (see Chap. 52).

The major principle of dealing with violent patients is protection—protection of oneself, the emergency department staff, and the patient. This is not a vacant concept. Violent patients can and have seriously injured emergency department staff. They must be rendered harmless without harming them.

If an individual being treated by the clinician becomes hostile, it is important to recognize the danger signals of potential violence. If the clinician is uncomfortable in an examining room with the patient, the interview can be conducted in the hall, and the security personnel can be asked to wait down the hall while the assessment is performed. Some of the danger signs to look for include:

1. Is the anger directed at the physician?

2. Does the physician feel uneasy or threatened? One should rely on one's gut reaction in answering this question.

3. Does the individual feel that he or she is still in control? The physician asks him.

4. Has the individual expressed anger violently in the past? If so, it is likely to happen again.

There are usually protocols in each emergency department dealing with just this situation. One thing to keep in mind is that during this entire process, although it is sometimes difficult, it is important to maintain a professional attitude toward the patient. The physician should avoid being involved in any physical struggle with the patient. This only arouses feelings in both the patient and the doctor that cause barriers to later communication.

Hostile patients may be dealt with by assessing the reasons for their hostility and their level of rationality.

1. Avoid confrontation. Many patients are not initially overtly violent but have poor control of their feelings of anger. Aggressive behavior in these individuals represents a defensive stance against overwhelming feelings of helplessness and fragility. By avoiding unnecessary provocation of a potentially hostile, angry individual in borderline control, you can reduce the likelihood and frequency of physical confrontations in the emergency department.

2. Show of force. If the individual is mentally competent, a show of force is sometimes useful. This is the demonstration of enough people with enough physical force to obviously overpower the individual. These people are normally security personnel. If

the individual is cognizant of his or her surroundings, and does not have a self-destructive bent, this demonstration will often be enough to calm him. Violent patients are very much afraid of their own impulses; assuring them and demonstrating to them that they will not be allowed to act on these feelings often has a calming effect.

3. Physical restraints. Physical restraints may need to be used until it is clear that all danger is past. Once the patient is willing to communicate rationally, an inquiry should be made about whether he or she would desire medications.

If the patient is violent because of drugs or paranoid delusions, a show of force will be useless. However, the same amount of force, or more, may be necessary to place the patient under physical restraint. Pharmacologic agents are then often helpful (see Chap. 52).

PROBLEM 4 The 35 year old man was brought into the emergency department supine, eyes open and tracking actively, but not responding to verbal stimuli. He appeared to be a quiet, nonviolent individual. The initial impression might be akinetic mutism. However, he quickly became violent. Not responding to a show of force, he was restrained and sedated. But because of this lack of prior psychiatric history, his age, and some physical findings, he had a rapid work-up for organic disease. He was diagnosed as having encephalitis.

DOCUMENTATION AND THE PROBLEM PATIENT

There are several key points to be made in the emergency department charting for the problem patient.

If the patient participates in the decision, this is noted in the chart: "Treatment options discussed with patient. Patient opts (not) to get XXX at this time." This is especially important when a common diagnostic or treatment option is being omitted, such as a radiograph of an injured ankle without major deformity.

If the care of a patient is turned over to another clinician, for whatever reason, it should be documented. If a patient refuses treatment and leaves against medical advice (AMA), he should sign an AMA form (see Chap. 62). In addition, it is important to document the options given the patient. It is often helpful for two observers to document independently on the chart the patient's attitude or behavior when refusal of treatment (AMA) or restraints are necessary. If a patient needs to be restrained, documentation is made of why and how it was done, and whether there was fear for the safety of self, staff, or patient.

SUMMARY AND FINAL POINTS

- Clinicians often regard patients as problems when they themselves fear that they are no longer in control and are beyond their depth.
- In general, patients in an emergency department have experienced an event that makes them think that there is an urgent need for medical evaluation. This concern heightens their feelings of anxiety, fear, and often anger.
- The clinician's response to the patient rather than the patient himself is often the root of many problems.
- With the manipulative patient, unreasonable bargaining, demands, and preconditions for therapy comprise a power struggle. The physician runs the danger of being pushed into errors of either commission or omission.
- In the physician-patient relationship, information should flow in both directions; the patient's wishes and ideas, when not in conflict with the physician's personal and medical ethics, good medical judgment, and the law, are respected. Patients should be involved, when possible, in their own health care decisions.

- The options the physician has in dealing with a patient he finds personally distasteful are either to consciously repress these feelings or to ask a colleague to see the patient instead.
- Each patient or family comes to the emergency department with certain expectations based on prior similar experiences, the experiences of friends or relatives, extensive reading, television programs, or cultural beliefs. These expectations must be discovered and addressed, when possible.
- Substance abusers are often seen by the emergency department staff as disruptive to the hospital routine; their behavior increases the great danger that serious illness or injury will be overlooked.
- The major consideration in dealing with violent patients is protection of oneself, the staff, and the patient.

BIBLIOGRAPHY

Texts

1. Howell JB, Schroeder DP: Physician Stress: A Handbook for Coping. Baltimore, University Park Press, 1984.
2. Lion JR: Evaluation and Management of the Violent Patient. Springfield, IL, Charles C Thomas, 1972.

Journal Articles

1. Groves JE: Taking care of the hateful patient. N Engl J Med 298:883–887, 1978.
2. Makadon HJ, Gerson S, Ryback R: Managing the care of the difficult patient in the emergency unit. JAMA 252:2585–2588, 1984.
3. Weissberg MP, Heitner M, Lowenstein SR, et al: Patients who leave without being seen. Ann Emerg Med 15:813–817, 1986.

INDEX

Note: Page numbers in *italics* refer to illustrations; page numbers followed by t refer to tables.

AAPCC. See *American Association of Poison Control Centers.*
Abdomen, examination of, acute diarrhea and, 125
  acute gastrointestinal bleeding and, 110
  multiple trauma and, 74–75
 pain in, 83–102
  abdominal aortic aneurysm and, 93t
  acute diarrhea and, 125
  acute gastrointestinal bleeding and, 109
  antiemetics in, 99
  associated symptoms and, 89–90
  common causes of, 84t, 94t–95t
  data gathering in, 89–92
  decision priorities in, 92–94, 93t–96t
  diagnostic adjuncts in, 96–98
  differential diagnosis in, 83, 84t, 85, 86
   preliminary, 93, 93t–94t, 95t–96t
  discharge in, 101–102
  disposition and follow-up in, 101–102
  documentation in, 102
  electrocardiogram in, 98
  gastric emptying and, 99
  general considerations for, 83, 102
  geriatric patient and, 100, 101t
  history in, 85–86, 89
  initial emergency department approach in, 87–88
  intervention in, prehospital care and, 86–87
  laboratory studies in, 96–97
  life-threatening causes of, 93t–94t
  low back pain and, 786, 787, 793, 793t
  management principles in, 98–100
  neuroanatomy of pain transmission and, 84–85, *85*
  nonspecific, 83, 92t
  observation in, 101
  pediatric patient and, 100
  pelvic pain and, in women, 1070t
  physical examination in, 90–92
   prehospital care and, 86
  pneumatic antishock garment in, 86
  prehospital care in, 85–87
  radiographic imaging in, 97–98

Abdomen *(Continued)*
  risk factors in, 87
  surgical consultation in, 101
  volume repletion and, 99
 sepsis in, 325, 329t
 trauma to, 152–169
  admission in, 168
  angiography in, 162
  antibiotics in, 166
  blunt, 152, 153t
   management principles in, 163, 166, *166*
  bony pelvis and, 159
  data gathering in, 157–159
  death due to, 154
  decision priorities in, 159–160
  definition of, 152, *153*
  diagnostic adjuncts in, 160–163
  diagnostic peritoneal lavage in, 162, 162t
  differential diagnosis in, preliminary, 159–160
   refined, 163
  discharge in, 168–169
  disposition in, 168–169
  documentation in, 169
  follow-up in, 168–169
  gender differences in, 152
  general considerations for, 152–154, 169
  geriatric patient and, 168
  gunshot wound and, 153–154, 154t, 166
  history in, 157–158
   initial emergency department approach and, 155
   prehospital care and, 154
  incidence of, 152
  initial emergency department approach in, 155–157
  injury site in, 160
  intervention in, initial emergency department approach and, 156–157
   prehospital care and, 154–155
  intravenous pyelogram in, 161
  laboratory studies in, 160–161
  management principles in, 163, 164t–165t, *166*, 166–167, *167*
  multiple trauma and, 152
  neck and, 158

Abdomen *(Continued)*
  neurologic disorders in, 159
  organ injury and, 152, 153t
  pediatric patient and, 167
  penetrating, 152–154, 153t, 154t
   in major organs, 164t–165t
   management principles in, 166, *167*
  pregnancy and, 167–168
  physical examination in, 158–159
   initial emergency department approach and, 155–156
   prehospital care and, 154
  pneumatic antishock garment in, 155
  prehospital care in, 154–155
  radiologic imaging in, 161–162
  stab wound and, 153–154, 154t, *166*, *167*
  surgery in, 159–160
  tetanus prophylaxis in, 166
Abdominal aortic aneurysm, abdominal pain and, 93t. See also *Abdomen, pain in.*
 pelvic pain and, 1070t. See also *Pelvis, female, pain in.*
Abortion, spontaneous, vaginal bleeding and, 1085, 1087
Abrasion, 272
Abruptio placentae, vaginal bleeding and, 1087–1088
Abscess, cerebral, meningitis and, 854
 corneal, 584t, 585, 587
 peritonsillar, 555, *555*
 retropharyngeal, 643t, 648
  management principles in, 649
  meningitis and, 855
  radiographic imaging in, 645
  sore throat and, 550, 551, 555–556
Acetaminophen, for febrile infant, 622, 631
 in earache, 562
 toxicity due to, 364–365
Acid-base disorder(s), 516–534
 acid-base physiology and, 517
 anion gap and, 523
 bicarbonate reabsorption and, 517–518, *518*
 blood pH and, 516, 523
 critical care unit admission in, 532
 data gathering in, 519–520, 521t

1141

1142 — INDEX

Acid-base disorder(s) *(Continued)*
  decision priorities in, 522
  diagnostic adjuncts in, 521–522
  differential diagnosis in, preliminary, 522–525, *524*
    refined, 525–530, 526t–528t
  discharge in, 532–533
  disposition in, 532–533
  documentation in, 533
  dyspnea and, 992t
  electrocardiogram in, 522
  ethylene glycol ingestion in, 528
  exogenous toxins in, 527t, 528
  follow-up in, 532–533
  general considerations for, 516–517, 533–534
  history in, 519–520
    metabolic acidosis and, 519–520
    metabolic alkalosis and, 520
  initial emergency department approach in, 519
  ketoacidosis as, differential diagnosis of, 526t, 526–527, 527t
  laboratory studies in, 521–522
  lactic acidosis as, differential diagnosis of, 527, 527t, 528t
  management principles in, 530–531
  metabolic acidosis as, 516, 518. See also *Metabolic acidosis*.
  metabolic alkalosis as, 516, 518. See also *Metabolic alkalosis*.
  methanol ingestion in, 528
  mixed, 517
  pathophysiology of, 518
  physical examination in, 520, 521t
  potassium level in, 523
  radiologic imaging in, 522
  renal insufficiency and, 527–528
  respiratory, 516
  simple, 516–517
Acneiform dermatitis, 264
Acoustic neuroma, dizziness and, 932t
Acquired immune deficiency syndrome, pediatric patient and, 633
  sepsis and, 330
Acromioclavicular separation, 710t, 712. See also *Orthopedic injury(ies), upper extremity*.
Activated charcoal therapy, in poisoning, 361, 363
Adenovirus, sore throat and, 548t, 556
Adnexa, red and painful eye and, 580
Adolescent, suicide potential in, 951, 960
Adrenal insufficiency, hyponatremia and, 493t
Adult respiratory distress syndrome, dyspnea and, 993t
Advanced life support, in hypothermia, 419
Aerotitis, in earache, 570t
Against Medical Advice form, 1111–1112, *1112*
Air ambulance service, 1129
  statistical and historical profile of, 4t
Airway management, 19–38
  adult vs. pediatric, 36t
  airway anatomy and, *20*, 20–21

Airway management *(Continued)*
  airway devices in, 22, 24, *24*
  assessment in, 21–22, *23*
  blind nasotracheal intubation in, 29–31, 30t
  decision making in, *23*, 27
  definitive, 26–35
  diagnostic adjuncts in, 35–36
  differential diagnosis in, 35, 35t
  disposition in, 37
  documentation in, 37–38
  drugs used in, 21, 32–33
  endotracheal tube placement in, confirmation of, 31, 43
    supplemental techniques in, 31–32
  esophageal obturator airway in, 25–26, *26*
  general considerations for, 19–20, 38
  in acute gastrointestinal bleeding, 105
  in anaphylaxis, 303
  in cardiopulmonary cerebral resuscitation, 41–42, 42t, 43
  in multiple trauma, 67
  in stroke, 880
  in trauma, 36
  indications for, 21
  manual airway opening maneuvers in, 22, 24, *24*
  orotracheal intubation in, 28t, 28–29, *29*, 43
  oxygen delivery in, 24–25, 25t
  pediatric patient and, 36t, 36–37
  prehospital care in, 21–26
  preparation in, 27–28
  suction in, 22
  surgery in, 33, *34*, 35
  temporizing vs. definitive, 27t
  ventilation in, 25
Airway opening maneuver, manual, 22, 24, *24*
Albuterol, in wheezing, 1011, 1013t
Alcohol intoxication, 378–393. See also *Alcoholism*.
  admission in, 392
  agents in etiology of, 390
  alcohol withdrawal seizure and, 391
  alcoholic hallucinosis and, 391
  anion-gap and, 386, 386t
  benzodiazepines in, 391
  beta-adrenergic blocking agents in, 391
  data gathering in, 382–383
  decision priorities in, 383–384, 384t
  diagnostic adjuncts in, 384–388, 385t, 386t
  differential diagnosis in, preliminary, 383–384, 384t
    refined, 388
  discharge in, 392–393
  disposition in, 392–393
  documentation in, 393
  electrocardiogram in, 387–388
  ethanol metabolism and, 379
  ethanol withdrawal and, 391–392
  ethylene glycol intoxication as, 390
  follow-up in, 392–393

Alcohol intoxication *(Continued)*
  general considerations for, 378–379, 393
  haloperidol in, 391
  history in, 382
    prehospital care and, 379–380
  hyperthermia and, 406
  initial emergency department approach in, 380–381
  intensive care unit admission in, 392
  intervention in, prehospital care and, 380
  isopropanol intoxication as, 390
  laboratory studies in, 385, 385t
  management principles in, 388–389
  metabolic acidosis and, 386, 386t
  methanol intoxication as, 390
  naloxone in, 381
  observation in, 389
  pediatric patient and, 389
  physical examination in, 382–383
    prehospital care and, 380
  physical restraints in, 389
  prehospital care in, 379–380
  radiologic imaging in, 387
  referral in, 392
  serum ethanol determination in, 385t, 385–386
  thiamine in, 381
Alcoholic hallucinosis, 391
Alcoholism, 378–379, 379t. See also *Alcohol intoxication*.
  acute abdominal pain and, 90
  definition of, 378
  delirium and, 808–809. See also *Mental status, altered*.
  incidence of, 378
  sepsis and, 329
  systemic effects of, 379t
Aldosteronism, in hypertension, 241
ALS. See *Advanced life support*.
Alzheimer's disease, delirium and, 809. See also *Mental status, altered*.
Ambu bag and mask, 42
American Association of Poison Control Centers, 347–348
American College of Emergency Physicians, formation of, 3
American College of Surgeons Committee on Trauma, criteria for trauma centers, 60–61
American Heart Association, Standards for Advanced Cardiac Life Support, 39, 58
American Medical Association, definition of emergency medicine, 4–5
Aminoglycoside, in dysuria, 1052t
Aminophylline, in anaphylaxis, 308–309
  in wheezing, *1012*, 1013t
Ammonia level, in acute gastrointestinal bleeding, 113
Amnesia, 809. See also *Mental status, altered*.
Amoxicillin, in earache, 569, 572t
  in gonorrhea, 1099t
Amphetamine poisoning, 355, 372–373
Ampicillin, in dysuria, 1052, 1052t

Ampicillin (Continued)
  in earache, 569, 572t
  in gonorrhea, 1099t
  in meningitis, 850t, 859
Amputation, hand and wrist, 742, 744
Amrinone, in congestive heart failure, 996
Amylase level, in acute abdominal pain, 97
Analgesia, in acute abdominal pain, 86, 88, 99
  in acute chest pain, 175
  in closed upper extremity injury, 708
  in earache, 570
  in hand and wrist injury, 728
  in sickle cell crisis, 463
Anaphylaxis, 299–311
  admission in, 310
  airway management in, 303
  aminophylline in, 308–309
  anesthetic in, 307t
  angioedema and, 305, 305t
  antibiotic in, 307t
  antihistamine in, 301, 308
  aspirin in, 307t
  bee sting and, 307t
  beta-adrenergic agent in, 308
  beta blocker in, 309
  bronchospasm and, 305t
  cardiac patient and, 309
  catecholamines in, 308
  cimetidine in, 308
  complete proteins in, 307t
  conjunctivitis and, 305t
  crystalloid administration in, 303
  data gathering in, 304–306, 305t
  decision priorities in, 305–306
  diagnostic adjuncts in, 307–308
  differential diagnosis in, preliminary, 305t, 305–306, 307t
  diphenhydramine in, 310
  discharge in, 310
  disposition in, 310
  documentation in, 310–311
  dopamine infusion in, 303
  drugs used in, 300–301
  electrocardiogram in, 308
  epinephrine in, 301, 302–303, 308, 309
  follow-up in, 310
  food additives and, 307t
  food and, 307t
  gastroenteritis and, 305t
  general considerations for, 299–301
  geriatric patient and, 309
  glucagon in, 309
  history in, 305
    initial emergency department approach and, 302
    prehospital care and, 301
  hydrocortisone in, 308
  hypotension and, 302
  infection and, 306
  initial emergency department approach in, 302–304
  intervention in, initial emergency department approach and, 302–304

Anaphylaxis (Continued)
    prehospital care and, 301
  iodinated contrast media and, 307t
  laboratory studies in, 307
  laryngeal edema and, 302, 305t
  management principles in, 308–309
  MAST suit in, 303, 309
  mechanisms in, 299–301, 300
  methylprednisolone in, 308
  Munchausen's syndrome and, 306
  nonsteroidal anti-inflammatory drugs in, 307t
  physical examination in, 304–305, 305t
    initial emergency department approach and, 302
    prehospital care and, 301
  prednisone in, 308, 310
  prehospital care in, 301
  prevalence of, 301
  radiologic imaging in, 307–308
  ranitidine in, 308
  rescue squad in, 301
  rhinitis and, 305t
  scombroid fish poisoning and, 306
  self-treatment in, 301
  steroids in, 301, 308
  Trendelenburg position in, 303
  urticaria and, 302, 305t
  vasodilation in, 305t
Anemia, sickle cell, 455–468. See also *Sickle cell disease.*
Anesthetic, in anaphylaxis, 307t
  in closed upper extremity injury, 708
  in dysuria, 1051
  in eye trauma, 603, 610
  in rash, 264–265
  in red and painful eye, 588, 588t
  in wheezing, 1015
  in wound care, 278–280, 279t
Aneurysm, aortic, abdominal, pain and, 93t
  pelvic pain and, 1070t. See also *Pelvis, female, pain in.*
Angina, unstable, 181t
Angiodysplasia, acute gastrointestinal bleeding and, 116
Angioedema, anaphylaxis and, 305, 305t
  hereditary, anaphylaxis and, 306
Angioscopy, in acute gastrointestinal bleeding, 113–114
Animal bite, wound care and, 290, 291t
Anion gap, acid-base disorder and, 523
  alcohol intoxication and, 386, 386t
  poisoning and, 357, 357t
Ankle and foot injury(ies), 767–769, 771–775. See also *Orthopedic injury(ies), lower extremity.*
  anatomy and, 755–756, 756–768
  calcaneal fracture as, 772, 772–773
  eversion injury as, 767, 770
  external rotation injury as, 767
  fracture-dislocation as, 771–772
  inversion injury as, 767, 769
  maisonneuve fracture as, 769, 771, 771
  malleolar fracture as, 769
  march fracture as, 774–775
  mechanisms in, 767, 767t, 769, 770

Ankle and foot injury(ies) (Continued)
  metatarsal fracture as, 774
  metatarsophalangeal dislocation as, 775
  phalangeal dislocation as, 775
  phalangeal fracture as, 775
  physical examination in, 756–758
  proximal fifth metatarsal fracture as, 775, 776
  sprain as, 767t, 767–769
  stress fracture as, 774–775
  talar dislocation as, 773
  talar fracture as, 773
  tarsal fracture as, 773–774
  tarsometatarsal fracture-dislocation as, 774
Anorexia, acute abdominal pain and, 90
Antibacterial, in rash, 266
Antibiotic, in abdominal trauma, 166
  in anaphylaxis, 307t
  in earache, 569–570, 572, 572t
  in eye trauma, 610
  in fever, infant and, 631–632
  in gonorrhea, 1099t
  in joint pain and swelling, 698, 698t
  in red and painful eye, 592t
  in sepsis, 327–328
  in wheezing, 1015
  in wound care, 292
Anticholinergic agent, in wheezing, 1014–1015
Anticoagulant, in pulmonary embolus, 995
Anticonvulsant, in seizure, 864, 870, 872
Antiemetic, in acute abdominal pain, 99
  in acute diarrhea, 131
  in nausea and vomiting, 147
Antifungal agent, in rash, 266
Antigen testing, sepsis and, 322–323
Antihistamine, in acute gastrointestinal bleeding, 117
  in anaphylaxis, 301, 308
  in nausea and vomiting, 147
  in rash, 265
Antihypertensive, in hypertension, 243
Anti-inflammatory agent, in joint pain and swelling, 698, 699
Antimicrobial, in pneumonia, 995
Antiperistaltic agent, in acute diarrhea, 131–132
Antiplatelet agent, in stroke, 890
Anus, as source of gastrointestinal bleeding, 115
Anxiety, 945t. See also *Behavioral disorder(s).*
Aorta, injury to, 165t
Aortic aneurysm, abdominal, pain and, 93t
Aortic dissection, acute chest pain and, 182t, 190
  hypertension and, 238–239, 244
  management principles in, 190
Appendicitis. See also *Abdomen, pain in.*
  abdominal pain and, 95t
  pelvic pain and, 1070t. See also *Pelvis, female, pain in.*
Arthritis. See also *Joint pain and swelling in.*

1144 — INDEX

Arthritis *(Continued)*
  degenerative, 697
    management principles in, 700
    intra-articular injection in, 700
  polyarticular, 697
    management principles in, 700
  septic, 695t, 695–696, 696t
    antibiotic in, pediatric patient and, 632t
    bacterial agent in, 695, 696t
    detection of, 692t, 692–695, *694*
    management principles in, 698, 698t
Arthrocentesis, in joint pain and swelling, 692t, 692–693
  in lower extremity injury, 760
Aspirin, in anaphylaxis, 307t
  in joint pain and swelling, 699, 700
  poisoning due to, 365, 367
Asplenia, sepsis and, 632
Asthma, corticosteroid in, 995
  definition of, 1000
  diagnostic adjuncts in, 1009–1011
  differential diagnosis in, 1001t, 1008
  dyspnea and, 990t, 993
    disposition in, 998
  electrocardiogram in, 1009
  history in, 1005–1006
  incidence and prevalence of, 1000
  intubation in, 1004
  laboratory studies in, 1009
  management principles in, 1011, *1012*, 1013t–1014t, 1014–1015
  pathophysiology of, 1000–1002
  pregnancy and, 998
  pulmonary function test in, 1010, 1010t
  radiologic imaging in, 1009
  sputum analysis in, 1010, 1011
  theophylline in, 994–995
  wheezing and. See *Wheezing.*
Asystole, 49, *52*. See also *Cardiopulmonary cerebral resuscitation.*
Atrial fibrillation, 202–203, *203*. See also *Palpitation.*
  management principles in, 207
Atrial flutter, 203, *203*. See also *Palpitation.*
  management principles in, 207
Atrioventricular block, syncope and, 223–224, *224*, 225
Atropine, in pediatric CPR, 55, 55t
Atropine sulfate, in red and painful eye, 589t
  in wheezing, 1014t
Audiometry, in dizziness, 931
  in earache, 569
Aureomycin. See *Tetracycline.*
Aztreonam, in sepsis, 327

Bacillus cereus, in acute diarrhea, 120t, 127t
Bacitracin, in eye trauma, 610
  in red and painful eye, 592t
Back, pain in. See *Low back pain.*

Bacteremia, antibiotic in, pediatric patient and, 632t
  occult, febrile infant and, 629–630, 630t
  pneumococcal, 630
Bacterial infection, in diarrhea, acute, 127t
  in sore throat, 548t, 556
Bacterial meningitis. See *Meningitis, bacterial.*
Bacteriuria, asymptomatic, dysuria and, 1055
  indwelling urinary catheter and, 1054–1055
BAER. See *Brain stem auditory evoked responses.*
Bag-valve-mask, in oxygen delivery, 25t
Bandaging, in wound care, 291–292
Barany's test, *928*, *928*
Bee sting, and anaphylaxis, 307t
Behavioral disorder(s), 937–950
  admission in, 948
  affective, 945t
  anxiety and, 945t
  benzodiazepine in, 946–947
  borderline personality and, 945t
  butyrophenone in, 946–947
  data gathering in, 939–942
  decision priorities in, 942–943
  depression and, 945t
  diagnostic adjuncts in, 943–944
  diazepam in, 947
  differential diagnosis in, preliminary, 942–943
    refined, 944, 945t, 946
  discharge in, 949
  disposition in, 947–949
  documentation in, 949
  drug abuse and, 945t
  electrocardiogram in, 944
  financial considerations in, 937
  follow-up in, 947–949
  functional etiology of, 942, 942t, 945t
  general considerations for, 937–938, 949–950
  geriatric patient and, 947
  haloperidol in, 946–947
  history in, 939–940
    prehospital care and, 938
  incidence of, 937
  initial emergency department approach in, 939
  involuntary commitment in, 948
  laboratory studies in, 943–944
  management principles in, 946–947
  mania and, 945t
  medical illness and, 938, 945t
  medication in, 946–947
  mental status examination in, 940–942
  organic etiology of, 942, 942t, 945t
  pediatric patient and, 947
  personality disorder and, 945t
  pharmaceutical use and, 945t
  physical examination in, 941
    prehospital care and, 938
  prehospital care in, 938–939
  psychiatric consultation in, 948

Behavioral disorder(s) *(Continued)*
  radiologic imaging in, 944
  rapport in, 946
  schizophrenia and, 945t
  state laws and, 948
Bell's reflex, 597
Benoxinate hydrochloride, in red and painful eye, 588t
Benzodiazepine, in alcohol intoxication, 391
  in behavioral disorder, 946–947
  in orotracheal intubation, 32
Beta blocker, in alcohol intoxication, 391
  in anaphylaxis, 308, 309
  in syncope, 225
  in wheezing, 1011, *1012*
Betamethasone, in skin disorder, 265, 265t
Bicarbonate, reabsorption of, 517, *518*
  defects in, 517. See also *Acid-base disorder(s).*
Bicarbonate therapy, in hyperkalemia, 505
Biliary tract disease, 95t
  sepsis and, 329
Biologic agent, accidental exposure to, 333–343
  data gathering in, 334–335
  diagnostic adjuncts in, 338t, 338–342
  differential diagnosis in, 336–338
  documentation in, 342
  general considerations for, 333–334, 342–343
  hepatitis A virus in, 334, 340
  hepatitis B virus in, 334, 336
    testing and management for, 339–340, 340t
  herpes virus in, 334, 337
    testing and management for, 341–342
  history in, 335
  human immunodeficiency virus in, 334, 336
    testing and management for, 338–339
  initial emergency department approach in, 334
  meningitis and, 334, 337
    testing and management for, 340–341, 341t
  physical examination in, 335–336
  serologic testing in, 338t, 338–342
  tetanus and, 340
  universal precautions for, 334–335, 335t
  varicella-zoster virus in, 334
    testing and management for, 341
Bismuth subsalicylate, in acute diarrhea, 132
Bite, wound care and, 290
Bleeding disorder(s), 439–454
  blood component therapy in, 451–452
  coagulation and, 440, *440*
  coagulation disorder as, 440–441, 445t, 445–446, 447t

Bleeding disorder(s) *(Continued)*
  combined platelet and coagulation disorder as, 445t, 445–446, 447t, 450
    disposition in, 453
  congenital disorder as, 440–441
  cryoprecipitate in, 451–452
  data gathering in, 444–445
  differential diagnosis in, preliminary, 445t, 445–446
    refined, 447–450, 451t
  disposition in, 452–453
  disseminated intravascular coagulation as, 447t, 450, 451t
  documentation in, 453
  factor VIII-ahf in, 452
  follow-up in, 452–453
  fresh frozen plasma in, 451–452
  general considerations for, 439–441, 453–454
  geriatric patient and, 452
  hemophilia A as, 448–449, 449t
  hemostasis and, 439–440, *440*
  history in, 444
    initial emergency department approach and, 442
    prehospital care and, 441
  idiopathic thrombocytopenic purpura as, 447t, 448
  initial emergency department approach in, 442, 443t, 444
  intervention in, initial emergency department approach and, 442, 443t, 444
  prehospital care and, 441–442
  laboratory studies in, 442, 443t, 446–447, 447t
  management principles in, 451–452
  packed red blood cells in, 451
  pediatric patient and, 452
  physical examination in, 444–445
    initial emergency department approach and, 442
    prehospital care and, 441
  platelet disorder as, 440, 445t, 445–446, 447t
    acquired, 450
    disposition in, 453
    specific, 448–450, 449t
  prehospital care in, 441–442
  thrombocytopenia as, 447t, 447–448
  thrombotic thrombocytopenic purpura as, 447t, 448
  vascular disorder as, 440
  von Willebrand's disease as, 447t, 449–450
Bleph 10. See *Sulfacetamide*.
Blood component therapy, in bleeding disorder, 451–452
Blood loss, in multiple trauma, 68t, 68–69
Blood sample, in multiple trauma, 69
Blood transfusion, in epistaxis, 542
  in gastrointestinal bleeding, 107–108
  in multiple trauma, 69
Blowout fracture of orbit, eye trauma and, 606t, 607–608
Boerhaave's syndrome, 115

Boerhaave's syndrome *(Continued)*
  vomiting and, 137
Borderline personality, 945t. See also *Behavioral disorder(s)*.
Bowel movement, acute abdominal pain and, 90
Bradycardia, intoxication and, 352, 353t
  management principles in, 227
  syncope and, 223
Bradydysrhythmia, 49. See also *Cardiopulmonary cerebral resuscitation*.
Brain injury, 896t, 896–897. See also *Head and neck trauma*.
Brain stem auditory evoked responses, in dizziness, 931
Brain tumor, seizure and, 867
Breathing, assessment of, 21–22
Bronchitis, chronic, 1002
  dyspnea and, 990t
  wheezing and. See *Wheezing*.
Bronchodilator, in congestive heart failure, 996
  in dyspnea, 983
Bronchospasm, anaphylaxis and, 305t
Brudzinski's sign, 853
Bruise, child abuse and, 656, 656t, 657
Bulbar conjunctiva, 575, 577
Bullous myringitis, earache and, 570t
Bupivacaine, in wound care, 279, 279t
Burn(s), admission in, 290t
  chemical, red and painful eye and, 578
  child abuse and, 656–657, *658*
  general considerations for, 272
  multiple trauma and, 77
  sore throat and, 556
Burow's solution, 264
Bursitis, joint pain and swelling and, 697
Butyrophenone, in behavioral disorder, 946–947

Calamine lotion, 264, 265
Calcitonin, in hypercalcemia, 513
Calcium, function of, 508–509
  hypercalcemia and, 508–515. See also *Hypercalcemia*.
  regulation of, 508–509, *509*
Calcium channel blocker, as cause of syncope, 225
Calcium chloride, in pediatric CPR, 55t
Calcium therapy, in hyperkalemia, 505
Calculus, ureteral, pelvic pain and, 1070t. See also *Pelvis, female, pain in*.
Caloric testing, in dizziness, 931
Campylobacter, in acute diarrhea, 120t, 127t, 133t. See also *Diarrhea, acute*.
Cancer, acute gastrointestinal bleeding and, 116
  hypercalcemia and, 512–513
  pediatric patient and, 632–633
  sore throat and, 556
  vaginal bleeding and, 1076, 1086

Candida, in vaginal infection, 1097, 1097t
  follow-up in, 1100
  laboratory studies in, 1095
  management principles in, 1199
Captopril, in hypertension, 235t
Carbon monoxide poisoning, 354t, 368–369
Cardiac arrest. See also *Cardiopulmonary cerebral resuscitation*.
  causes of, 40, 45, 46t, 48t
  cocaine abuse and, 433–434
  multiple trauma and, 77
  prognosis in, 40, 40t
Cardiac patient, anaphylaxis and, 309
Cardiac tamponade, chest trauma and, 1031t, 1035
Cardiopulmonary cerebral resuscitation, 35–59
  arterial blood gases in, 47
  bicarbonate vs. alveolar ventilation in, 50, 52–53
  cardiac arrest rhythm and, 49, 49t, *50, 51*, 51–52
  cardiac monitoring in, 47
  cardiac rhythm changes and, 53
  cerebral stabilization in, 54, 55t
  crash cart airway equipment in, 42, 42t
  death and, 57t, 57–58
  diagnostic adjuncts in, 47–48
  differential diagnosis in, preliminary, 45–47, 46t
    refined, 48t, 48–49, 49t
  disposition in, 56–57
  do not resuscitate orders and, 56
  documentation in, 58
  drugs used in, 42, 42t
  electrocardiogram in, 47
  electrocution and, 56
  general considerations for, 39–40, 58–59
  history in, 44
  initial emergency department approach in, 41–43, 42t
  laboratory studies in, 47
  management principles in, 49, 51–55
  pediatric patient and, 55, 55t
  perfusion and, 53
  physical examination in, 44–45, 45t
  postresuscitative period in, 53–54, 55t
  pregnancy and, 56
  prehospital care in, 40–41
  prognosis in, 40, 40t
  radiographic imaging in, 47–48
  reperfusion injury and, 54
  serum electrolytes in, 47
  trauma and, 56
Cardiopulmonary disorder, acute abdominal pain and, 90
Cardiovascular disorder, hypertension and, 238–239
  low back pain and, 786–788
Cardioversion, in palpitation, 207
Cataplexy, seizure and, 868
Catecholamine, in anaphylaxis, 308

Cathartic, in poisoning, 361–362
Cauda equina syndrome, low back pain and, 788t, 792–793
Caustic poisoning, 369–370
Cautery, in epistaxis, 543
Cefaclor, in earache, 569, 572t
  in sepsis, 327–328
Cefizox. See *Ceftizoxime.*
Cefobid. See *Cefoperazone.*
Cefoperazone, in dysuria, 1052t
Cefotaxime, in meningitis, 850t, 859
Cefoxitin, in gonorrhea, 1099t
Ceftazidime, in dysuria, 1052t
  in sepsis, 327–328
Ceftizoxime, in dysuria, 1052t
Ceftriaxone, in dysuria, 1052t
  in gonorrhea, 1099t
  in meningitis, 850t, 859
  in sepsis, 327–328
Cefuroxime, in sepsis, 327–328
Cellulitis, antibiotic in, pediatric patient and, 632t
  rash and, 257t, 261
Centers for Disease Control, universal precautions from, 335t
Central nervous system, in hypertension, 238
  infection in, neonate and, 324
    pediatric patient and, 324
    sepsis and, 324–325, 329t
Cephalosporin, in dysuria, 1052
  in sepsis, 327
Cerebral abscess, meningitis and, 854
Cerebral edema, stroke and, 880
Cerebral resuscitation, 54, 55t. See also *Cardiopulmonary cerebral resuscitation.*
Cerebrospinal fluid analysis, for febrile infant, 628
Cerumen, impacted, in earache, 570t
Cervical spine trauma, 67. See also *Head and neck trauma; Trauma.*
Cervicitis, 1097t, 1098
  follow-up in, 1100
  management principles in, 1099
Cetamide. See *Sulfacetamide.*
Charcoal, activated, in poisoning, 361, 363
Chelation, in hypercalcemia, 514
Chemical injury, eye trauma and, 599–600, 606t, 608. See also *Eye, trauma to.*
  management principles in, 612
  red and painful eye and, 578
Chest, pain in, analgesia in, 175
  aortic dissection and, 182t, 190
  bedside tests in, 179–180
  cardiac, nonischemic, 188t
  characteristics of, 176–178
  data gathering in, 176–178
  decision priorities in, 180, 184, 184t
  diabetic patient and, 191
  diagnostic adjuncts in, 185–186
  differential diagnosis in, preliminary, 180, 181t–183t, 184, 184t
    refined, 186–187, 188t–189t
  disposition in, 191–193

Chest *(Continued)*
  documentation in, 193–194
  electrocardiogram in, 176, 185–185t, 192
  esophageal rupture and, 183t, 190
  follow-up in, 193
  gastrointestinal system and, 188t
  general considerations for, 173–174, 194
  geriatric patient and, 191
  history in, 176–178
    initial emergency department approach and, 175
    prehospital care and, 174
  initial emergency department approach in, 175–176
  intervention in, initial emergency department approach and, 176
    prehospital care and, 175–176
  laboratory studies in, 186
  management principles in, 187, 190
  musculoskeletal system and, 189t
  myocardial infarction and, 181t, 190, 192
  neurogenic, 189t
  organ systems and, 188t–189t
  pediatric patient and, 190–191
  physical examination in, 178, 179t
    initial emergency department approach and, 175
    prehospital care and, 174
  pneumothorax and, 183t, 190
  prehospital care in, 174–175
  psychogenic, 189t
  pulmonary embolism and, 182t, 190
  pulmonary system and, 188t
  radiologic imaging in, 185–186
  risk factors in, 177
  unstable angina and, 181t
  trauma to, 1020–1039. See also *Multiple trauma; Trauma.*
    acceleration-deceleration in, 1021–1022
    admission in, 1037–1038
    airway management in, 1024, 1034
    cardiac tamponade and, 1031t, 1035
    compression in, 1020–1021
    critical care facility for, 1035, 1038
    data gathering in, 1028–1029
    decision priorities in, 1029–1030, 1031t, 1032
    diagnostic adjuncts in, 1032–1034
    diaphragmatic rupture and, 1036t
    differential diagnosis in, preliminary, 1029–1030, 1031t, 1032
      refined, 1034, 1036t–1037t
    discharge in, 1038
    disposition in, 1035, 1038
    documentation in, 1038–1039
    electrocardiogram in, 1033–1034
    flail chest and, 1031t, 1035
    follow-up in, 1035, 1038
    general considerations for, 1020–1022, *1021*, 1039
    geriatric patient and, 1035
    hemothorax and, 1037t
      massive, 1031t, 1035

Chest *(Continued)*
  history in, 1028–1029
    initial emergency department approach and, 1024
    prehospital care and, 1022
  initial emergency department approach in, 1023–1028, *1025–1027*
  intervention in, initial emergency department approach and, 1024–1028, *1025–1027*
    prehospital care and, 1022–1023
  laboratory studies in, 1032–1033
  life-threatening injuries in, 1030, 1031t, 1032, 1034
  massive hemopneumothorax and, 1031t, 1035
  myocardial contusion and, 1035, 1036t
  open pneumothorax and, 1031t, 1035
    intervention in, 1023
    management principles in, 1035
    physical examination in, 1022
  pediatric patient and, 1035
  pericardiocentesis in, 1025, *1026*
  physical examination in, 1029, 1030t
    initial emergency department approach and, 1024
    prehospital care and, 1022
  prehospital care in, 1022–1023
  pulmonary contusion and, 1031t, 1035
  radiologic imaging in, 1033
  rib fracture and, 1035, 1037t
  shearing in, 1020–1021
  simple pneumothorax and, 1036t
  sternal fracture and, 1037t
  tension pneumothorax and, 1021, *1021*, 1031t, 1034–1035
    intervention in, 1023
    management principles in, 1035
    physical examination in, 1022, 1030t
  thoracostomy in, emergency, 1025–1026, *1027*
    needle, 1024
    tube, 1024–1025, *1025*
  torsion in, 1021
  tracheo-bronchial disruption and, 1031t
Child abuse, 652–668
  abdominal examination in, 659
  bruise as sign of, 656, 656t, *657*
  burn as sign of, 656–657, *658*
  child abuse law and, 663, 664t
  data gathering in, 655–656
  diagnostic adjuncts in, 660–662
  differential diagnosis in, preliminary, 660, 660t, 661t
  disposition in, 666–667
  documentation in, 668
  emotional abuse as, 666
  failure to thrive as sign of, 666, *667*
  family observation in, 655–656
  follow-up in, 666–667

Child abuse (Continued)
  general considerations for, 652–653, 668
  genitourinary-perineal examination in, 659
  history in, 655
    prehospital care and, 653–654
  incidence of, 652–653
  initial emergency department approach in, 654
  intervention in, prehospital care and, 654
  laboratory studies in, 662
  legal implications in, 663, 664t
  management principles in, 662–663
  medical management in, 662
  neglect as, 666, 667
  neurologic examination in, 657, 659
  physical examination in, 656–657, 657–659, 659–660
    prehospital care and, 654
  prehospital care in, 653–654
  psychosocial management in, 662–663
  radiologic imaging in, 660–662, 661
  risk factors in, 653, 653, 661t
  sexual abuse as, 663, 665t, 665–666, 975. See also *Sexual assault*.
    incidence of, 964–965
    sexually transmitted disease and, 973–974, 974t
  skeletal injury as sign of, 657
  stress factors in, 653, 653
  team approach in, 663
  trauma and, 660, 660t
Chinese restaurant syndrome, 306
Chlamydia, in conjunctivitis, 584
  in penile discharge, 1091–1092. See also *Penis, discharge from*.
  in sore throat, 548t, 556
  sexual assault and transmission of, 974, 974t
Chloramphenicol, in eye trauma, 610
  in meningitis, 850t, 859
  in red and painful eye, 592t
Chloromycetin. See *Chloramphenicol*.
Chloroptic. See *Chloramphenicol*.
Cholesteotoma, in earache, 570t
Chondrocalcinosis, joint pain and swelling in, 691, 692
Chronic bronchitis, 1002
Chronic obstructive pulmonary disease (COPD), diagnostic adjuncts in, 1009–1011
  differential diagnosis in, 1001t, 1008
  dyspnea and, disposition in, 998
    management principles in, 994–995
  electrocardiogram in, 1009
  general considerations for, 1002
  history in, 1005–1006
  laboratory studies in, 1009
  oxygen therapy in, 1003–1004
  pulmonary embolism and, 1007
  pulmonary function test in, 1010, 1010t
  radiologic imaging in, 1009
  sepsis and, 329
  sputum analysis in, 1010, 1011
  wheezing and. See *Wheezing*.

CIE. See *Counterimmune electrophoresis*.
Cilastatin, in sepsis, 327
Cimetidine, in anaphylaxis, 308
Cipro. See *Ciprofloxacin*.
Ciprofloxacin, in dysuria, 1052, 1054
  in gonorrhea, 1099t
  in sepsis, 327
Clavicular fracture, 710t, 712–713. See also *Orthopedic injury(ies), upper extremity*.
Clinical problem solving, process of, 8–10
Clonidine, in hypertension, 235t, 243
Clostridium, in acute diarrhea, 120t, 127t, 133t
Clotrimazole, in skin disorder, 266
Coagulation, process of, 440, 440
Coagulation disorder. See also *Bleeding disorder(s)*.
  acquired, 450
  disposition in, 453
  platelet disorder and, 445t, 445–446, 447t, 450. See also *Bleeding disorder(s)*.
    disposition in, 453
  primary, 448–450, 449t
Cocaine abuse, 424–436. See also *Substance abuse*.
  admission in, 434
  "body packers" and, 432–433
  cardiovascular effects of, 433t
  central nervous system effects of, 433t
  clinical manifestations of, 426, 428, 428t
  confidentiality and, 435
  crystalloids in, 433t
  dantrolene in, 433t
  data gathering in, 427–429
  decision priorities in, 429–430
  diagnostic adjuncts in, 430–431
  diazepam in, 433t
  differential diagnosis in, preliminary, 429t, 429–430
    refined, 431
  discharge in, 435
  disposition in, 434–435
  diuretics in, 433t
  documentation in, 435–436
  electrocardiogram in, 431
  follow-up in, 435
  general considerations for, 424–425, 436
  haloperidol in, 433t
  history in, 427
    initial emergency department approach and, 425–426
  initial emergency department approach in, 425–426
  intervention in, initial emergency department approach and, 426
  labetalol in, 433t
  laboratory studies in, 430
  lidocaine in, 433t
  management principles in, 431–432, 433t
  nitrate in, 433t

Cocaine abuse (Continued)
  organ system complications and, 432t
  pathophysiologic effects of, 425, 425t
  phenytoin in, 433t
  physical examination in, 427–429, 428t
    initial emergency department approach and, 426
  prehospital care in, 425
  prevalence of, 424
  propranolol in, 433t
  psychological effects of, 428, 428t, 429t
  radiologic imaging in, 431
  red and painful eye and, 588t
  renal effects of, 433t
  sudden cardiac death and, 433–434
  urine toxicology screen in, 430
Colchicine, in joint pain and swelling, 699
Colic, ureteral, 95t
Colles' fracture, 717–718. See also *Orthopedic injury(ies), upper extremity*.
Colonic cancer, acute gastrointestinal bleeding in, 116
Coma, 808
  Glasgow Coma Scale and, 810, 810t
Community-acquired pulmonary infection, 324
Compartment syndrome, 777–779, 780. See also *Orthopedic injury(ies), lower extremity*.
Compazine. See *Prochlorperazine*.
Competence, clinical definition of, 1109–1110
Confusional state, 808. See also *Mental status, altered*.
Congestive heart failure, amrinone in, 996
  bronchodilator in, 996
  diuretic in, 996
  dobutamine in, 996
  dyspnea and, 992t
    disposition in, 998
    management principles in, 996
  hyponatremia and, 494t
  inotropic agent in, 996
  morphine sulfate in, 996
  nifedipine in, 996
  nitrate in, 996
  nitroprusside, 996
  wheezing and, 1005, 1007
Conjunctiva, anatomy of, 595, 596
Conjunctivitis. See also *Eye, red and painful*.
  allergic, 585, 586
  anaphylaxis and, 305t
  chlamydial, 584, 585–586
  infective, 584t, 584–586, 585
  management principles in, 590, 591t, 592t
Consent, 1106–1108
  expressed, 1106–1107, 1107
  implied, 1107–1108
  pediatric patient and, 1108–1109
Constipation, acute diarrhea and, 125
Contact dermatitis, rash and, 257t, 263

Contact lens, eye trauma and, 600, 607t, 608–609
Cooperative Needlestick Surveillance Group, 336
COPD. See *Chronic obstructive pulmonary disease (COPD)*.
Cornea, anatomy of, 595, 596
  chemical injury to, 606t, 608
  examination of, 580–581, 581
  infection in, 584t, 585, 587
    management principles in, 591t
  trauma to, 591t
    abrasion and, 606t, 609
    foreign body and, 606t, 608
    management principles in, 591t, 612
Coronary artery disease, incidence of, 173
Coronavirus, sore throat and, 548t
Corticosteroid, in asthma, 995
  in hypercalcemia, 513
  in wheezing, 1014
Corynebacterium, in sore throat, 548t
Counterimmune electrophoresis, 856–857
CPCR. See *Cardiopulmonary cerebral resuscitation*.
Crack, 424–425. See also *Cocaine abuse*.
CRAMS, 64, 64t, 65t
Crash cart airway equipment, 42, 42t
Cricoid ring, pediatric, 637, 637
Cricothyroidotomy, 33, 34
Cricothyrotomy, pediatric patient and, 637
Criminal Sexual Conduct Act, 977
Crotamiton, in skin disorder, 266
Croup. See *Viral laryngotracheobronchitis*.
Crutches, 781
Cryoprecipitate, in bleeding disorder, 451–452
Cryptosporidium, in acute diarrhea, 127t, 130t, 133t
Crystal-induced arthritides, 695t, 696
  management principles in, 699
Crystalloid administration, in anaphylaxis, 303
  in cocaine abuse, 433t
  in nausea and vomiting, 147
Culdocentesis, in ectopic pregnancy, 1065, 1083
  in pelvic pain, 1065
  in vaginal bleeding, 1083
Cutaneous disorders, 249–295. See also *Rash; Wound care*.
  joint pain and swelling and, 689
Cyclic antidepressant poisoning, 355, 367–368
Cyclogel. See *Cyclopentolate hydrochloride*.
Cyclopentolate hydrochloride, in red and painful eye, 589t
Cycloplegic, in red and painful eye, 583, 588, 589t
Cystitis. See also *Urinary tract infection*.
  dysuria and, 1049t, 1050
  management principles in, 1051t, 1052

Cytomegalovirus, sore throat and, 548t, 556

Dantrolene, in cocaine abuse, 433t
Decision priorities, 11–12. See also names of specific conditions.
Decongestant, in earache, 570
Defibrillation, 40. See also *Cardiopulmonary cerebral resuscitation*.
  preparation for, 42
Dehydration, admission in, 682
  body weight and, 673, 674t, 676
  causes of, 675, 675t
  data gathering in, 672–674
  decision priorities in, 674–676
  diagnostic adjuncts in, 676–677
  diarrhea and, 672, 678, 678t
  differential diagnosis in, preliminary, 674–676, 675t
    refined, 677–678
  discharge in, 682–683
  disposition in, 682–683
  documentation in, 683
  endocrine causes of, 675t
  estimated degree of, 674t, 674–675
  fluid and electrolyte therapy in, 678–682. See also *Fluid and electrolyte therapy*.
  follow-up in, 682–683
  gastrointestinal causes of, 675t, 678
  general considerations for, 669–670, 683
  history in, 672–673
    prehospital care and, 670
  hypertonic, 670, 671–672
  hypotonic, 670
  iatrogenic causes of, 675t
  in adolescent, causes of, 675t
  in infant, causes of, 675t
  in pediatric patient, causes of, 675t
  initial emergency department approach in, 671–672
  intervention in, initial emergency department approach and, 671–672
    prehospital care and, 670–671
  isotonic, 669–670
  isotonic crystalloid solution in, 670, 671
  laboratory studies in, 676–677
  management principles in, 678–682
  mild, 674, 674t
  moderate, 674t, 674–675
  physical examination in, 673–674
    initial emergency department approach and, 671
    prehospital care and, 670
  prehospital care in, 670–671
  renal causes of, 675t
  seizure and, 671–672
  severe, 674t, 675
  vomiting and, 672
Delirium, 808–809. See also *Mental status, altered*.

Dementia, 809. See also *Mental status, altered*.
Demerol. See *Meperidine*.
Dendritic keratitis, 585, 587
Depression, 945t. See also *Behavioral disorder(s)*.
Dermatitis, acneiform, 264
Desonide, in skin disorders, 265, 265t
Dexamethasone, in skin disorders, 265, 265t
Dextrose, in hypothermia, 413
  in metabolic complications of diabetes mellitus, 474, 481
Diabetes mellitus, acute chest pain and, 191
  earache and, 562–563
  incidence of, 471
  metabolic complications of, 471–485
    altered mentation in, 471
    assessment in, 474–475
    data gathering in, 476–478
    decision priorities in, 478, 478–479
    diabetic ketoacidosis in, 472, 472, 481–482
    diagnostic adjuncts in, 479–481
    differential diagnosis in, preliminary, 478–479
    documentation in, 485
    electrocardiogram in, 475
    general considerations for, 471–472
    geriatric patient and, 484
    history in, 475–476
      prehospital care and, 472
    hyperglycemia in, 484–485
    hyperosmolar nonketotic coma in, 482–483
    hypoglycemia in, 471, 481, 484
    initial emergency department approach in, 474–476
    intervention in, prehospital care and, 473
    laboratory studies in, 479–480
    management principles in, 481–483
    pediatric patient and, 483–484
    physical examination in, 477–478
    prehospital care and, 473
    radiologic imaging in, 480–481
  red and painful eye and, 582
  sepsis and, 329
  type I, 471
  type II, 471
Diabetic ketoacidosis, 472, 472, 481–482. See also *Diabetes mellitus, metabolic complications of*.
Dialysis, in hyperkalemia, 506
Diaphragm, injury to, 165t, 1036t. See also *Abdomen, trauma to*.
Diarrhea, acute, 122–135
  admission in, 133
  antiemetic in, 131
  antimicrobial therapy in, 132, 133t
  antiperistaltic agent in, 131–132
  Bacillus cereus in, 120t, 127t
  bacteria in, 127t
  bismuth subsalicylate in, 132
  Campylobacter in, 120t, 127t, 133t

Diarrhea *(Continued)*
    causes of, 122–123
    Clostridium in, 120t, 127t, 133t
    Cryptosporidium in, 127t, 130t, 133t
    data gathering in, 124–126
    decision priorities in, 126–127
    dehydration and, 672, 678, 678t. See also *Dehydration.*
    diagnostic adjuncts in, 127–129, *128*
    differential diagnosis in, preliminary, 126–127, 127t
        refined, 129, 130t
    disposition in, 132–133
    documentation in, 134
    Entamoeba in, 127t, 130t, 133t
    Escherichia coli in, 120t, 127t
    evaluation of, *128*
    exogenous factors in, 124–125
    fecal leukocyte stain in, 128, *128*
    follow-up in, 133–134
    general considerations for, 122–123, 135
    Giardia lamblia in, 127t, 130t, 133t
    history in, 124–125
        initial emergency department approach and, 123
    infectious, 123, 130t
        acute gastrointestinal bleeding and, 116
        clinical categorization of, 127t
        discharge instructions in, 134t
        management principles in, 132, 133t
        prevention in, 132
    inflammatory bowel disease and, 132
    initial emergency department approach in, 123–124
    intervention in, 124
    irritable bowel syndrome and, 123
    kaolin-pectins in, 131
    laboratory studies in, 127–129, *128*
    management principles in, 129–131
    meperidine in, 131
    microbial studies in, 128–129
    Norwalk agent in, 127t, 130t
    outpatient management in, 133–134, 134t
    parasitic disease and, 127t, 129, 130t
    pathophysiologic mechanisms in, 122–123
    physical examination in, 125–126
        initial emergency department approach and, 123
    prochlorperazine in, 131
    promethazine in, 131
    radiologic imaging in, 129
    rehydration in, 130–131, 131t
    rotavirus and, 130t
    Salmonella in, 120t, 127t, 132, 133t
    scombroid fish poisoning and, 127t
    serum electrolytes and, 128
    Shigella in, 120t, 127t, 133t
    solvent drag and, 130
    Staphylococcus in, 120t, 127t
    stool culture in, 128–129
    symptomatic therapy in, 131–132

Diarrhea *(Continued)*
    symptoms associated with, 125
    toxin-induced, 123–124, 126, 127t
    Vibrio in, 120t, 127t
    virus in, 120t, 127t
    Yersinia in, 120t, 127t, 133t
Diascopy, rash and, 259
Diazepam, in behavioral disorder, 947
    in cocaine abuse, 433t
    in orotracheal intubation, 32
    in seizure, 850, 864, 865, 872
Diazoxide, in hypertension, 235t, 243
DIC. See *Disseminated intravascular coagulation.*
Dicloxacillin, in skin disorder, 266
    in wound care, 292
Diethylstilbestrol, as postcoital therapy, 974
Differential diagnosis, 11–12. See also names of specific conditions.
Digoxin, 207, 208
    as cause of syncope, 225
Diphenhydramine, in anaphylaxis, 310
Diphosphonate, in hypercalcemia, 513
Diphtheria, sore throat and, 553, 556
Disc herniation, 788t, 797, 798t, 799
Discharge, from emergency department, 12, 14–15. See also names of specific conditions.
Disseminated intravascular coagulation, 447t, 450, 451t
Diuretic, hyponatremia and, 493t
    in congestive heart failure, 996
    in dyspnea, 983
    in hypercalcemia, 513
    in hyperkalemia, 506
    in poisoning, 363
Diverticulitis, 95t
Diverticulosis, acute gastrointestinal bleeding and, 115
Diverticulum, Meckel's, acute gastrointestinal bleeding and, 119
Dizziness, 924–934
    acoustic neuroma and, 932t
    admission in, 933
    audiometry in, 931
    brain stem auditory evoked responses in, 931
    caloric testing in, 931
    data gathering in, 926t, 926–929
    decision priorities in, 929–930
    diagnostic adjuncts in, 930–931
    differential diagnosis in, preliminary, 929–930
        refined, 931, 932t
    discharge in, 933
    disposition in, 933
    documentation in, 933–934
    dysrhythmias and, 932t
    electrocardiogram in, 930
    electronystagmography in, 931
    follow-up in, 933
    general considerations for, 924–925, 934
    history in, 926t, 926–927
    hyperventilation and, 932t
    incidence of, 924, 934

Dizziness *(Continued)*
    initial emergency department approach in, 925–926
    laboratory studies in, 930
    lightheadedness as, 924–925
    management principles in, 931–932
    medications associated with, 926, 926t, 934
    neck hyperextension and, 929
    orthostatic hypotension and, 932t
    otolaryngology test in, 931
    pediatric patient and, 932
    physical examination in, 927–929, *928*
    radiologic imaging in, 930
    vertigo as, 924, 925t
    vestibular neuritis and, 932t
Do not resuscitate order, cardiopulmonary cerebral resuscitation and, 56
Dobutamine, in congestive heart failure, 996
    in sepsis, 327
Documentation, 15. See also names of specific conditions.
Dopamine, in anaphylaxis, 303
    in pediatric CPR, 55t
    in sepsis, 327
Dorsacaine. See *Benoxinate hydrochloride.*
Doxycycline, in gonorrhea, 1099t
Dressing, in hand and wrist injury, 739
Drowning, hypothermia and, 421
Duodenal ulcer, acute gastrointestinal bleeding and, 114–115
Dyspnea, acid-base disorders and, 992t
    adult respiratory distress syndrome and, 993t
    asthma and, 990t, 993
        disposition in, 998
        management principles in, 994–995
    bronchodilator in, 983
    chronic bronchitis and, 990t
    congestive heart failure and, 992t
        disposition in, 998
        management principles in, 996
    data gathering in, 985–987
    decision priorities in, 987–989
    diagnostic adjuncts in, 989, 993t, 993–994
    differential diagnosis in, preliminary, 987–989, 988t, 989t
    disposition in, 998–999
    diuretic in, 983
    documentation in, 999
    electrocardiogram in, 994
    emphysema and, 990t, 993
    follow-up in, 998–999
    general considerations for, 981–982, 999
    history in, 985
    prehospital care and, 982
    hyperventilation syndrome and, 992t
        disposition in, 998
        management principles in, 996
    initial emergency department approach in, 984–985

Dyspnea (Continued)
  intervention in, prehospital care and, 982–984
  laboratory studies in, 989, 993
  management principles in, 994–997
  morphine in, 983
  myocardial infarction and, 998
  myocardial ischemia and, 992t
  needle decompression in, 983, 995
  nitrate in, 983
  nonpulmonary causes of, 988, 989t, 992t
  of unknown cause, 997, 998
  oxygen therapy in, 984–983
  pathophysiology of, 981–982
  pediatric patient and, 997
  physical examination in, 985–987
    prehospital care and, 982
  pneumonia and, 991t, 993t
    disposition in, 998
    management principles in, 995
  pneumothorax and, 991t, 993t
    disposition in, 998
    management principles in, 995
  pregnancy and, 997–998
  prehospital care in, 982–984
  pulmonary causes of, 988, 988t, 990t–991t
  pulmonary edema and, 993t
    disposition in, 998
    management principles in, 996
  pulmonary embolus and, 991t, 993t
    disposition in, 998
    management principles in, 995–996
  pulmonary function testing in, 994
  pulse oximetry in, 994
  radiologic imaging in, 993, 993t
  terminology in, 982
Dysrhythmia. See also names of specific dysrhythmias; Palpitation.
  dizziness and, 925, 932t
  seizure and, 865t, 866t
Dysuria, 1043–1057
  admission in, 1056
  aminoglycoside in, 1052t
  ampicillin in, 1052, 1052t
  anesthetic in, 1051
  antibiotic in, 1045, 1051t, 1052–1053
  asymptomatic bacteriuria and, 1055
  cefoperazone in, 1052t
  ceftazidime in, 1052t
  ceftizoxime in, 1052t
  ceftriaxone in, 1052t
  cephalosporin in, 1052
  ciprofloxacin in, 1052, 1054
  cystitis and, 1049t, 1050
    management principles in, 1051t, 1052
  data gathering in, 1045–1046
  decision priorities in, 1046
  diagnostic adjuncts in, 1047–1048
  differential diagnosis in, preliminary, 1046
    refined, 1048–1051, 1049t–1051t
  discharge in, 1056
  disposition in, 1056–1057
  documentation in, 1056

Dysuria (Continued)
  extraurinary causes of, 1046
  follow-up in, 1056–1057
  general considerations for, 1056–1057
  gentamicin in, 1052t
  geriatric patient and, 1053
  history in, 1045
  imipenem-cilastatin in, 1052t
  in female patient, 1043
  in male patient, 1046, 1053–1056
  in neonate, 1053
  indwelling urinary catheter and, 1054–1055
  infectious etiologies of, 1050t
  initial emergency department approach in, 1044–1045
  laboratory studies in, 1047–1048
  management principles in, 1051–1052
  outpatient therapy in, 1056
  pediatric patient and, 1053
  pelvic inflammatory disease and, 1055
  phenazopyridine in, 1051
  physical examination in, 1046
  predisposing factors in, 1043–1044
  pregnancy and, 1055
  prostatitis and, 1054
  pyelonephritis and, 1049t, 1049–1051
    management principles in, 1051t, 1051–1052, 1052t
  renal tuberculosis and, 1055
  ticarcillin-clavulanate in, 1052, 1052t
  trimethoprim-sulfamethoxazole in, 1054
  urethritis and, 1048, 1049t
  urinalysis in, 1047
  urinary dipstick analysis in, 1047
  urine collection in, 1053
  urine culture in, 1047–1048
  vaginitis and, 1048, 1049t

Ear, laceration of, wound care and, 289
Earache, 561–574
  acetaminophen in, 562
  aerotitis in, 570t
  amoxicillin in, 569, 572t
  ampicillin in, 569, 572t
  analgesia in, 570
  antibiotics in, 569–570, 572, 572t
  audiometric testing in, 569
  bullous myringitis and, 570t
  cefaclor in, 569, 572t
  cholesteatoma and, 570t
  consultation in, 573
  data gathering in, 563–566
  decision priorities in, 566–568
  decongestant in, 570
  diabetes mellitus and, 562–563
  diagnostic adjuncts in, 568–569
  differential diagnosis in, preliminary, 566–568, 567t
    refined, 567t, 569, 570t, 571t
  discharge in, 573
  disposition in, 573
  documentation in, 573–574
  erythromycin in, 569, 572t

Earache (Continued)
  extraotic examination in, 565–566
  follow-up in, 573
  foreign body and, 567t
    management principles in, 572–573
  general considerations for, 574
  hearing acuity and, 565
  herpes zoster and, 570t
  history in, 563–564
    initial emergency department approach and, 562
  impacted cerumen and, 570t
  initial emergency department approach in, 562–563
  intervention in, initial emergency department approach and, 562–563
  laboratory studies in, 568
  management principles in, 569–573
  otic drops in, 572, 572t
  otitis externa and, 562, 567t
    management principles in, 571–572, 572t
  otitis media and, 562, 567t
    diabetes mellitus and, 562–563
    management principles in, 569–571, 572t
  otoscope in, 565, 565
  pain in, 563
  physical examination in, 564–566
    initial emergency department approach and, 562
  radiologic imaging in, 568
  steroids in, 572, 572t
  sulfisoxazole in, 569, 572t
  trauma in, 570t
  trimethoprim-sulfamethoxazole in, 569, 572t
Eclampsia, 245–246
  seizure and, 865t, 866t
Econochlor. See Chloramphenicol.
Ectopic pregnancy, culdocentesis in, 1065, 1083
  low back pain and, 791, 792t
  management principles in, 1066, 1071, 1087
  pelvic pain and, 1058, 1062–1063. See also Pelvis, female, pain in.
  ruptured, 1068t
  salpingitis and, 1058–1059
  vaginal bleeding and, 1084t, 1084–1085, 1085t. See also Vagina, bleeding from.
Eczematous disease, in rash, 257t, 263
Edema, cerebral, stroke and, 880
  in hand and wrist injury, 728
  pulmonary, dyspnea and, 993t
    disposition in, 998
    pregnancy and, 998
  hypertension and, 238, 243–244
    pregnancy and, 998
    protocol in, 1127t
  tonsillar, 550, 551
  uvular, 550, 551
Elbow injury, 710t, 714–717, 716. See also Orthopedic injury(ies), upper extremity.
  olecranon process fracture as, 716

INDEX — 1151

Elbow injury *(Continued)*
  radial head fracture as, 715
  radial head subluxation as, 716–717
Electrocardiogram, in acid-base disorders, 522
  in acute abdominal pain, 98
  in acute chest pain, 176, 192
  in acute gastrointestinal bleeding, 113
  in alcohol intoxication, 387–388
  in altered mental status, 820
  in behavioral disorder, 944
  in cocaine abuse, 431
  in diabetic ketoacidosis, 475
  in dizziness, 930
  in dyspnea, 994
  in hypercalcemia, 511–512
  in hyperkalemia, 500, 500–503, *501*
  in hyponatremia, 491
  in multiple trauma, 74
  in palpitation, 201, *202*
  in stroke, 888
  in vomiting, 145
  in wheezing, 1009
Electrocardiography, in anaphylaxis, 308
  in heat illness, 403–404
  in hypothermia, 418
  in poisoning, 359
Electrocution, cardiopulmonary cerebral resuscitation and, 56
Electroencephalography, in seizure, 871
Electromechanical dissociation, 49, 49t, 51–52
Electronystagmography, in dizziness, 931
ELISA. See *Enzyme-linked immunoassay.*
Embolism, pulmonary. See *Pulmonary embolism.*
Embolus, pulmonary, dyspnea and, 991t, 993t
  disposition in, 998
  management principles in, 995–996
  pregnancy and, 997
  wheezing and, 1007
Emergency, definition of, 5
Emergency medical services, 1117–1129. See also names of specific conditions.
  air transport and, 1129
  statistical and historical profile of, 4t
  definition of, 4–5
  Emergency Medical Services Act and, 1118, 1118t
  financial considerations in, 13t–14t
  funding of, 1118, 1118t
  general considerations for, 1117, 1129
  Health Prevention Block Grants and, 1118
  history of, 1117–1118
  impact of, 1129
  medical control and, 1126, 1126t, 1129
  multiple trauma and, 1129
  myocardial infarction and, 1129
  National Highway Safety Act and, 1118
  personnel in, 1118–1121, 1119t
    basic emergency medical technician as, 1119, 1119t

Emergency medical services *(Continued)*
  communication between, 1121–1123, 1122t, 1125
    radio, 1122, 1122t, 1123t, 1125
    Run Report in, 1122, *1124*
  emergency medical dispatcher as, 1119t, 1120, 1120t
  emergency medical technician-defibrillator as, 1119t, 1119–1120, 1120t
  first responder as, 1119, 1119t
  interaction between, 1125–1126
  paramedic as, 1119t, 1120
  training for, 1119–1121, 1119t–1121t
  principles in, 5–8, 16–18
  sudden cardiac death and, 1129
Emergency Medical Services Act of 1973, 1118, 1118t
Emergency medical technician, statistical and historical profile of, 4t
Emergency medicine, statistical and historical profile of, 4t
Emergency nurse, statistical and historical profile of, 4t
EMIT. See *Enzyme-mediated immunoassay for toxins.*
Emotional abuse, 666. See also *Child abuse.*
Emphysema, definition of, 1002
  dyspnea and, 990t, 993
  wheezing and. See *Wheezing.*
Encephalitis, 851, 854
Encephalopathy, hypertensive, 243, 837t, 841
Endocrine disorder, seizure and, 866
Endometriosis, pelvic pain and, 1068t. See also *Pelvis, female, pain in.*
Endoscopy, in acute gastrointestinal bleeding, 114
Endotoxin, definition of, 315
  gram-negative, 316
Endotracheal intubation, 26
  confirmation of, 31, 43
  general preparation in, 27–28
  in cardiac arrest, 43
  nasotracheal approach in, 30t, 30–31
  orotracheal approach in, 28t, 28–29, *29*
  supplemental techniques in, 31–32
Enophthalmos, eye trauma and, 596. See also *Eye, trauma to.*
Entamoeba, in acute diarrhea, 127t, 130t, 133t
Environmental disorder(s), 394–423. See also specific disorder, e.g., *Heat illness; Hypothermia.*
Enzyme-linked immunoassay, 339
Enzyme-mediated immunoassay for toxins, in poisoning, 358, 358t
Epiglottitis, 643t, 646–647
  management principles in, 648
  pediatric, 636, *636*
  sore throat and, 550–551, 553, 555
  thumb sign in, 644, *644*
Epilepsy, 862. See also *Seizure(s).*
Epinephrine, in anaphylaxis, 301, 302–303, 308, 309

Epinephrine *(Continued)*
  in pediatric CPR, 55t
  in wheezing, 1011, 1013t
Epiphysis, femoral, 777, 778. See also *Orthopedic injury(ies), lower extremity.*
Epistat balloon, 539, *539*
Epistaxis, 537–546
  balloon tamponade device in, 539, *539*
  causes of, 541, 542t
  cautery in, 543
  consultation in, 545
  data gathering in, 539–541
  decision priorities in, 541–542, 542t
  diagnostic adjuncts in, 542
  differential diagnosis in, preliminary, 541–542, 542t
  discharge in, 545
  disposition in, 545
  documentation in, 546
  follow-up in, 545
  general considerations for, 537–538, 538, 546
  hematologic disorder and, 542, 542t
  history in, 539–540
  hospitalization in, 545
  incidence of, 537
  initial emergency department approach in, 538–539, *539*
  laboratory studies in, 542
  management principles in, 542–544, *543*
  nasal examination in, 540–541
  nasal pack in, *543*, 543–544
  pediatric patient and, 544
  physical examination in, 540–541
  prehospital care in, 538
  radiologic imaging in, 542
  refractory, 544
  septal hematoma in, 544
  vascular anatomy and, 537–538, *538*
  vascular disorder and, 542t
Epstein-Barr virus, sore throat and, 548t, 556
Erosive gastritis, acute gastrointestinal bleeding and, 114–115
Erythema infectiosum, 267t. See also *Rash.*
Erythema multiforme, 257t, 263
Erythema multiforme bullosum, 257t, 260, 263
Erythromycin, in earache, 569, 572t
  in red and painful eye, 592t
  in sepsis, 328
  in skin disorder, 266
Escherichia coli, 315. See also *Sepsis.*
  antibiotic in, pediatric patient and, 632t
  in acute diarrhea, 120t, 127t
Esmolol, in hypertension, 235t
Esophageal obturator airway, 25–26, *26*
  in cardiac arrest, 43
Esophageal tracheal airway, in cardiac arrest, 43
Esophageal varices, acute gastrointestinal bleeding and, 115

Esophagogastroduodenoscopy, acute gastrointestinal bleeding and, 117
Esophagus, rupture of, acute chest pain and, 183t, 190
  management principles in, 190
  tamponade of, in acute gastrointestinal bleeding, 117
Estradiol, as postcoital therapy, 973
Estrogen, as postcoital therapy, 973
Ethanol. See also *Alcohol intoxication; Alcoholism.*
  withdrawal from, 391–392
Ethylene glycol ingestion, 390. See also *Alcohol intoxication.*
  in acid-base disorders, 528
Exanthem, 263, 268t. See also *Rash.*
Exercise, in low back pain, 801
Exfoliative dermatitis, 264
Exotoxin, definition of, 315
Eye, acute glaucoma in, 584t, 585, 587–588
  management principles in, 590, 591t
  anatomy of, 575–576, 577, 595–597, 596, 597
  chemical burn in, 578
  conjunctivitis in, allergic, 585, 586, 590
    chlamydial, 584, 585–586
    infective, 584t, 584–586, 590
    management principles in, 590, 591t, 592t
  corneal infection in, 584t, 585, 587, 591t
  corneal trauma in, 591t
  dendritic keratitis in, 585, 587
  herpetic infection in, 585, 587
  iritis in, 581, *581*, 585, 586
    management principles in, 590, 591t, 592t
  keratitis in, 575, 586–587
    dendritic, 585, 587
    management principles in, 590, 591t, 592, 592t
  red and painful, 575–594
    adnexa examination in, 580
    anatomy and, 575–576, 577
    anesthetic in, 588, 588t
    anterior chamber examination in, 581, *581*
    atropine sulfate in, 589t
    bacitracin in, 592t
    benoxinate hydrochloride in, 588t
    chloramphenicol in, 592t
    cocaine abuse and, 588t
    cornea examination in, 580–581, *581*. See also *Cornea.*
    cyclopentolate hydrochloride in, 589t
    cycloplegic in, 588, 589t
    data gathering in, 578–582
    decision priorities in, 583
    diabetes mellitus and, 582
    diagnostic adjuncts in, 583–584
    differential diagnosis in, external signs in, *585*
      preliminary, 583
      refined, 584–588, *585*

Eye *(Continued)*
  disposition in, 592–593
  documentation in, 593
  erythrocyte sedimentation rate in, 584
  erythromycin in, 592t
  eyelid examination in, 580
  follow-up in, 592–593
  general considerations for, 575–576, 593
  gentamicin sulfate in, 592t
  geriatric patient and, 592
  history in, 578–580
  homatropine hydrobromide in, 589t
  inflammation relief in, 589
  initial emergency department approach in, 576, 578
  laboratory studies in, 583–584
  lens examination in, 581
  management principles in, 588t, 588–592, 589t, 591t, 592t
  mydriatic in, 588, 589t
  neomycin in, 592t
  pain management in, 588t, 588–589, 589t
  pediatric patient and, 592
  phenylephrine hydrochloride in, 589t
  physical examination in, 580–582, *581*, *582*
  proparacaine hydrochloride in, 588t
  pupil examination in, 580
  radiologic imaging in, 584
  retina examination in, 576, *577*, 581–582
  scopolamine hydrobromide in, 589t
  special tests in, 582–583
  sulfacetamide in, 592t
  sulfisoxazole in, 592t
  tetracaine hydrochloride in, 588t
  tetracycline in, 592t
  tobramycin in, 592t
  tonometry in, 583
  topical ophthalmic antibiotic in, 592t
  trauma and, 578, 579
  tropicamide in, 589t
  visual acuity testing and, 578
  visual loss and, 576
  vitreous examination in, 581
  trauma to, 595–614
    anatomy and, 595–597, 596, 597
    anesthetic in, 603, 610
    antibiotic in, 610
    bacitracin in, 610
    blowout fracture of orbit and, 606t, 607–608
    chemical injury and, 599–600, 606t, 608
      management principles in, 612
    chloramphenicol in, 610
    contact lens and, 600, 607t, 608–609
    corneal abrasion and, 606t, 609
      management principles in, 612
    cycloplegic in, 610
    data gathering in, 599–601
    decision priorities in, 604–605
    diagnostic adjuncts in, 605

Eye *(Continued)*
  differential diagnosis in, preliminary, 604–605
    refined, 605, 606t–607t, 607–609
  disposition in, 613–614
  documentation in, 614
  enophthalmos and, 596
  extraocular muscle testing in, 603
  eye irrigation in, 610
  eye patch in, 610–611, *611*
  fluorescein staining in, 603
  follow-up, 613–614
  foreign body and, 606t, 608
    management principles in, 612
  funduscopic examination in, 603
  gaze disturbances and, 596
  general considerations for, 595
  gentamicin in, 610
  geriatric patient and, 613
  gray line laceration and, 597
  history in, 599–600
    initial emergency department approach and, 598
    prehospital care and, 598
  hyphema and, 605, 606t, 607
    management principles in, 611
  incidence of, 595
  initial emergency department approach in, 598–599
  intervention in, prehospital care and, 598
  laboratory studies in, 605
  lid eversion in, *601*, 601–602
  limbic flush and, 596
  management principles in, 609–613
  mydriatic in, 610
  neomycin in, 610
  orbital blowout fracture and, management principles in, 611–612
  pain and, 600
  pediatric patient and, 613
  peripheral visual field testing, 603
  physical examination in, *601*, 601–604, *602*
    prehospital care and, 598
  polymyxin in, 610
  prehospital care in, 597–598
  prevention of, 613
  proparacaine in, 610
  pupillary dilation in, 602, *602*
  radiologic imaging in, 605
  red and painful eye and, 578, 579
  slit lamp examination in, 603
  Snellen eye chart and, 599
  steroid in, 610
  sulfacetamide in, 610
  sulfisoxazole in, 610
  tetracaine in, 610
  tetracycline in, 610
  tobramycin in, 610
  tonometry in, 603–604
  visual acuity and, 599, 600, 604
  uveitis in, 581
Eye patch, 610–611, *611*
Eyelid, examination of, 580

Face, wound care for, 288–289
Factor VIII-ahf, in bleeding disorder, 452
Factorate, 452
Failure to thrive. See also *Child abuse.*
  nonorganic, 666, *667*
Family, unexpected death and, 57t, 57–58
Fascicular block, syncope and, 224–225
Felon, in hand and wrist injury, 741
Fever, acetaminophen in, 631
  definition of, 619–620
  in acute diarrhea, 125
  management principles in, 631
  pediatric patient and, 619–634. See also *Infant, febrile.*
Fibular fracture, 766. See also *Orthopedic injury(ies), lower extremity.*
Flail chest, chest trauma and, 1031t, 1035
Flatulence, in acute diarrhea, 125
Fluid and electrolyte therapy, bolus fluid for, 680–681
  fluid loss estimate in, 679–680
  in acute diarrhea, 129–131, 131t
  in dehydration, 669–683. See also *Dehydration.*
  in heat illness, 404–405
  in nausea and vomiting, 147–148
  maintenance levels in, 679, 679–680
  oral vs. parenteral, 680
  refined estimates in, 681–682
Fluocinonide, in skin disorders, 265, 265t
Fluorescein staining, in eye trauma, 603
Fluoroquinolone, in sepsis, 327
Foley catheter, in head and neck trauma, 919
Food, anaphylaxis and, 307t
  as cause of acute diarrhea, 124
Food additive, anaphylaxis and, 307t
Forearm fracture, 710t, 717. See also *Orthopedic injury(ies), upper extremity.*
Foreign body, airway obstruction and, 647–648
  management principles in, 649
  eye trauma and, 606t, 608
  nasal, 544
  radiographic imaging in, 645, *645*
  wound care and, 289
Fortaz. See *Ceftazidime.*
Fracture, prehospital care in, 275
Fresh frozen plasma, in bleeding disorder, 451–452
Frostbite, 272, 421–422
Funding, of emergency medical services, 1118, 1118t
Funduscopy, 815–816
Furosemide, in hypertension, 235t
  in hyponatremia, 495

Gamma aminobutyric acid (GABA), in ethanol withdrawal, 391

Gangrene, 325–326
Gantrisin. See *Sulfisoxazole.*
Garamycin. See *Gentamicin sulfate.*
Gardnerella, in vaginal infection, 1097t, 1097–1098
  infection by, follow-up in, 1000
  laboratory studies in, 1095
  management principles in, 1099
Gas gangrene, 325–326
Gastric emptying, in poisoning, 360t, 360–361
Gastric intubation, in acute gastrointestinal bleeding, 108
Gastric lavage, in acute gastrointestinal bleeding, 117
  in poisoning, 360–361
Gastritis, erosive, acute gastrointestinal bleeding and, 114–115
Gastroccult test, in acute gastrointestinal bleeding, 108, 110
  in nausea and vomiting, 139
Gastroenteritis, acute diarrhea and, 124
  anaphylaxis and, 305t
Gastrointestinal bleeding, acute, 104–120
  admission in, 119
  airway management in, 105
  ammonia level in, 113
  angiodysplasia and, 116
  anorectal sources of, 115
  blood transfusion in, 107–108
  cancer and, 116
  coagulation studies in, 113
  data gathering in, 109–110
  decision priorities in, 111–112
  diagnostic adjuncts in, 112–114
  differential diagnosis in, 111t, 111–112, 112t
    refined, 114–116
  discharge in, 120
  disposition in, 119
  diverticulosis and, 115
  documentation in, 120
  duodenal ulcer and, 114–115
  electrocardiogram in, 113
  electrolytes in, 113
  endoscopy in, 114
  erosive gastritis and, 114–115
  esophageal tamponade in, 117
  esophageal varices and, 115
  esophagogastroduodenoscopy in, 117
  fluid and blood requirements for, 107, 107t
  gastric intubation in, 108
  gastric lavage in, 117
  Gastroccult test in, 108, 110
  general considerations for, 104–105, 120
  Hemoccult card in, 110
  hemorrhoid and, 115
  histamine antagonist in, 117
  history in, 109
    initial emergency department approach and, 106
    prehospital care and, 105
  infectious diarrhea and, 116
  inflammatory bowel disease and, 116

Gastrointestinal bleeding *(Continued)*
  initial emergency department approach in, 106–109
  laboratory studies in, 108, 112–113
  liver function test in, 113
  lower, 115–116
  Mallory-Weiss tear and, 115
  management principles in, 116–118
    lower gastrointestinal bleeding and, 117–118
    upper gastrointestinal bleeding and, 117–118
  Meckel's diverticulum and, 119
  mesenteric ischemia and, 116
  nasogastric intubation in, 108
  neonate and, 119
  occult, 110
  patient comfort in, 106
  pediatric patient and, 119
  peptic ulceration and, 114–115
  physical examination in, 109–110
    initial emergency department approach and, 106–107
    prehospital care and, 105
  platelet count in, 113
  pneumatic antishock garment in, 106
  prehospital care in, 105–106
  radiologic imaging in, 113
  sigmoidoscopy in, 114
  surgery in, 118
  upper, 114–115
    causes of, 112t
    therapy for, 117–118
  vasopressin in, 117, 118
  volume resuscitation in, 107
  vomiting and, 119
Gastrointestinal disorder(s), dehydration and, 675t, 678. See also *Dehydration.*
Gastrointestinal tract, injury to, 164t. See also *Abdomen, trauma to.*
Gaze disturbance, eye trauma and, 596. See also *Eye, trauma to.*
Genitourinary disorder, acute abdominal pain and, 90
Genitourinary tract, injury to, 165t. See also *Abdomen, trauma to.*
Genoptic. See *Gentamicin sulfate.*
Gentamicin, in dysuria, 1052t
  in eye trauma, 610
  in meningitis, 850t, 859
Gentamicin sulfate, in red and painful eye, 592t
Geriatric patient. See also names of specific conditions.
  abdominal pain in, 100, 101t
  abdominal trauma in, 168
  anaphylaxis in, 309
  behavioral disorder in, 947
  bleeding disorder in, 452
  chest pain in, 191
  chest trauma in, 1035
  closed upper extremity injury in, 724
  dizziness in, 924, 932–933, 934
  dysuria in, 1053
  eye trauma in, 613

Geriatric patient *(Continued)*
  headache in, 844
  heat illness in, 406
  metabolic complications of diabetes mellitus in, 484
  nausea and vomiting in, 149
  orthostatic hypotension in, 228
  palpitation in, 211
  red and painful eye in, 592
  stroke in, 891
  suicide potential in, 960
  syncope in, 228
  urinary tract infection in, 324
Giant cell arteritis, headache and, 839t, 841–842
  management principles in, 843
Giardia lamblia, in acute diarrhea, 127t, 130t, 133t
Glasgow Coma Scale, 64, 64t, 65t
  in head and neck trauma, 899, 899t, 904
Glaucoma, acute, 584t, 585, 587–588
  headache and, 843
  management principles in, 590, 591t
Glossopharyngeal neuralgia, sore throat and, 556
Glucagon, in anaphylaxis, 309
Glucocorticoid, in wheezing, 1014
Glucose level, metabolic complications of diabetes mellitus and, 472, 473
  normalization of, 483
  reagent strips and, 474–475, 480
Gonococcemia, in rash, 260
Gonococcus, in pelvic inflammatory disease, 1066
  in sore throat, 553, 556
Gonorrhea, 1091, 1096. See also *Penis, discharge from*.
  management principles in, 1098, 1099t
  sexual assault and, 973–974
Gout, 695t, 696
  management principles in, 699
Gram's stain, 259
Gray line laceration, 597. See also *Eye, trauma to*.
Griseofulvin, in skin disorder, 266
Gunshot wound, abdominal trauma and, 153–154, 154t, 166

Haemophilus infection, antibiotics in, in meningitis, 849, 850t
  pediatric patient and, 632t
Hallucinosis, alcoholic, 391
Haloperidol, in alcohol intoxication, 391
  in behavioral disorder, 946–947
  in cocaine abuse, 433t
  in suicide potential, 959
Hand and wrist injury(ies), closed, 710t, 717–722, 719, 720
  open, 727–743
    analgesia in, 728
    anatomy and, 729–732, 730, 733–735, 734t
    circulation and, 731, 733
    data gathering in, 729–736

Hand and wrist injury(ies) *(Continued)*
    diagnostic adjuncts in, 736–737
    disposition in, 744–746
    documentation in, 746
    dressing in, 739
    edema in, 728
    elevation in, 739
    extensor tendon laceration as, amputation and, 742, 744
      infection and, 740–741, 741–743
      management principles in, 740
      nailbed injury and, 741–742
      nerve injury and, 740
      vascular injury and, 740
    felon in, 741
    flexor tendon laceration as, management principles in, 739–740
    general considerations for, 727, 746–747
    high-pressure injection injury as, 744, 745
    history in, prehospital care and, 728
    immobilization in, 739
    initial emergency department approach in, 728
    intervention in, prehospital care and, 728
    management principles in, 737–740
      general, 737–739, 738t
      specific, 739–740
    neurologic examination in, 731–732, 734, 734t
    palpation in, 730–731
    paronychia in, 740–741, 741
    physical examination in, 729–732, 733–735, 734, 736
    prehospital care and, 728
    prehospital care in, 727–728
    radiologic imaging in, 736–737, 737, 738
    replantation in, 742, 744
    resting position and, 730, 731, 732
    suppurative flexor tenosynovitis as, 741, 742, 743
    tendon anatomy in, 732, 734, 735, 736, 737, 738t
    wound care in, 738–739
Hand, foot, mouth disease, 268t. See also *Rash*.
Hand injury, 710t, 718–722, 719, 720. See also *Hand and wrist injury(ies)*; *Orthopedic injury(ies), upper extremity*.
  dislocation as, 710, 719–722
  mallet finger as, 721–722
  metacarpal fracture as, 718–719
Hare traction splint, 749, 750. See also *Orthopedic injury(ies), lower extremity*.
HBIG, 340, 340t
Head, anatomy of, 895, 895, 896
  trauma to. See also *Head and neck trauma*.
    anatomy and, 895, 895, 896
    blunt, 914, 914–915
    classification of, 896t
    general considerations for, 894

Head *(Continued)*
    headache and, 831, 840t
    pathophysiology of, 896–897
    pediatric patient and, 920
    penetrating, 915
    prevalence of, 894
Head and neck trauma, 894–923
  admission in, 920–921
  anatomy and, 895, 895, 896, 911, 912
  classification of, 896t
  data gathering in, 902–906
  decision priorities in, 907–908
  diagnostic adjuncts in, 909–913
  differential diagnosis in, preliminary, 907–908
    refined, 913–918
  discharge in, 921–922
  disposition in, 920–922
  documentation in, 922–923
  Foley catheter in, 919
  follow-up in, 921–922
  general considerations for, 894, 923
  Glasgow Coma Scale in, 899, 899t, 904
  glucose therapy in, 900
  history in, 902–903
  immobilization in, 919
  initial emergency department approach in, 901–902
  intracranial pressure and, 900, 919
  ischemia and, 908
  laboratory studies in, 913
  life-threatening, 908, 910t
  management principles in, 918–919
  mass lesion and, 907
  metabolic rate in, 907–908
  metabolic substrate replacement in, 907
  methylprednisolone in, 919
  motor deficit and, 905t
  naloxone in, 900
  nasogastric tube in, 919
  pathophysiology of, 895–897
  pediatric patient and, 919–920
  physical examination in, 903–906, 905t, 906
  prehospital care in, 897, 899–901
  prevalence of, 894
  radiologic imaging in, 909–913, 910t, 911, 912
    arteriography and, 912
    cervical spine series and, 909–912, 911, 912
    head, 909
    skull, 909
  scalp laceration in, 919
  sensory dermatomes and, 904, 906
  steroid in, 919
  tissue edema and, 908
  toxins and, 907
Headache, 830–846
  acute glaucoma and, 843
  admission in, 845
  cerebrovascular accident and, 839t, 841
  cluster, 838t, 841
    management principles in, 843
  common causes of, 836t, 842

Headache *(Continued)*
    management principles in, 844
    data gathering in, 832–834
    decision priorities in, 835–837
    definition of, 830–831
    diagnostic adjuncts in, 837–840
    differential diagnosis in, preliminary, 835–837, 836t–838t
        refined, 841–842
    discharge in, 845–846
    disposition in, 844–846
    documentation in, 846
    emergent causes of, 836, 837t, 841
        management principles in, 843
    general considerations for, 830–831, 846
    geriatric patient and, 844
    giant cell arteritis and, 839t, 841–842
        management principles in, 843
    head trauma and, 831, 840t
    history in, 832–834
        initial emergency department approach and, 831
    hypertensive encephalopathy and, 837t, 841
    incidence of, 830
    initial emergency department approach in, 831–832
    intervention in, initial emergency department approach and, 832
    laboratory studies in, 838
    lumbar puncture in, 839–840
    management principles in, 842–844
    meningitis and, 837t, 841, 851
    migraine, 838t, 841
        management principles in, 843
    muscle contraction and, 840t, 842
        management principles in, 844
    neurologic examination in, 834–835
    pediatric patient and, 844
    physical examination in, 834–835
        initial emergency department approach and, 831
    prehospital care in, 831
    radiologic imaging and, 838–839
    sinusitis and, 840t, 842
        management principles in, 844
    stress and, 840t, 842
    subarachnoid hemorrhage and, 837t, 841
        management principles in, 843
    toxic exposure and, 833
    urgent causes of, 836, 838t, 841–842
        management principles in, 843
Health Prevention Block Grant, 1118
Heat cramp, 400t, 400–401, 407. See also *Heat illness.*
Heat exhaustion, 400, 400t, 401t, 407. See also *Heat illness.*
Heat illness, 394–407. See also *Hyperthermia.*
    acclimatization and, 395
    agitation and, 406
    data gathering in, 397–398, 398t
    decision priorities in, 399–401
    diagnostic adjuncts in, 402–404

Heat illness *(Continued)*
    differential diagnosis in, preliminary, 399–401, 399t–402t
    disposition in, 407
    documentation in, 407
    electrocardiogram in, 403–404
    elimination of excess heat in, 404
    fluid and electrolyte replacement in, 404–405
    follow-up in, 407
    general considerations for, 394–395, 407
    geriatric patient and, 406
    heat cramp and, 400t, 400–401, 407
    heat exhaustion and, 400, 400t, 401t, 407
    heat loss and, 395
    heat stroke and, 400t, 400–401, 402t, 407
        management principles in, 405–406
    history in, 397–398
        prehospital care and, 395
    incidence of, 394
    initial emergency department approach in, 396–397
    intervention in, prehospital care and, 395–396
    intoxicated patient and, 406
    laboratory studies in, 403, 404t
    management principles in, 404–406
    mechanisms in, 394–395
    pediatric patient and, 406
    physical examination in, 398–399
        prehospital care and, 395
    prehospital care in, 395–396
    primary, 399t, 399–401
    radiologic studies in, 403
    risk factors in, 398t
    vital signs in, 398–399
Heat stroke, 400t, 400–401, 402t, 407. See also *Heat illness.*
    management principles in, 404–406
Hemarthrosis, 696
    management principles in, 699–700
Hematemesis, 104–105. See also *Gastrointestinal bleeding, acute.*
Hematochezia, 105. See also *Gastrointestinal bleeding, acute.*
Hematocrit, in acute gastrointestinal bleeding, 112
    in multiple trauma, 69
Hematologic disorder(s), 437–468. See also *Bleeding disorder(s); Sickle cell disease.*
    and epistaxis, 542, 542t
Hematoma, subdural, meningitis and, 854
Hemoccult card, in acute gastrointestinal bleeding, 110
Hemodialysis, in hypercalcemia, 513
    in poisoning, 362, 362t
Hemoperfusion, in poisoning, 362–363
Hemopneumothorax, chest trauma and, 1031t, 1035
Hemorrhage, in wound care, 274
    intracerebral, 885t, 887, 887
        management principles in, 890

Hemorrhage *(Continued)*
    intracranial, seizure and, 865
    subarachnoid, 885t, 887, 887
        headache and, 837t, 841
            management principles in, 843
        management principles in, 890
        meningitis and, 854
Hemorrhagic shock, 62–63
    pelvic pain and, 1058. See also *Pelvis, female, pain in.*
Hemorrhoid, acute gastrointestinal bleeding and, 115
Hemostatic disorder. See *Bleeding disorder(s).*
Hemothorax, chest trauma and, 1031t, 1035
Heparin, in pulmonary embolus, 995–996
Heparinization, in stroke, 890
Hepatic failure, hyponatremia and, 494t
Hepatitis, accidental exposure to, 336–337. See also *Biologic agent, accidental exposure to.*
    prevalence of, 334
Hepatitis B immune globulin, 340, 340t
Hepatitis B vaccine, 340, 340t
Hepatitis B virus, exposure to, 334, 336. See also *Biologic agent, accidental exposure to.*
    testing and management for, 339–340, 340t
Hereditary angioedema, anaphylaxis and, 306
Hernia, femoral, strangulated, pelvic pain and, 1070t. See also *Pelvis, female, pain in.*
Herniation, disc, 788t, 797, 798t, 799
Herniation syndrome, stroke and, 880
Herpes simplex, in rash, 257t, 261–262
    in red and painful eye, 585, 587
    in sore throat, 548t
    in vaginal infection, 1097t, 1099
        follow-up in, 1101
        laboratory studies in, 1096
        management principles in, 1099, 1099t
Herpes virus, accidental exposure to, 334, 337. See also *Biologic agent, accidental exposure to.*
Herpes zoster, in earache, 570t
High-pressure injection injury, hand and wrist, 744, 745
Hip injury, 761–764. See also *Orthopedic injury(ies), lower extremity.*
    anatomy and, 752, 752–753
    physical examination in, 753
History, patient, 11. See also names of specific conditions.
HIV infection, accidental exposure to, 334, 336. See also *Biologic agent, accidental exposure to.*
    prevalence of, 333–334
Holter monitor, 201–202
Homatropine hydrobromide, in red and painful eye, 589t

Human immunodeficiency virus, exposure to, testing and management in, 338t, 338–339
Humeral fracture, 712, 713–714, 714, 715. See also *Orthopedic injury(ies), upper extremity.*
Hydralazine, in hypertension, 235t
Hydration, febrile infant and, 631
  in sickle cell crisis, 463–464
Hydrocortisone, in anaphylaxis, 308
  in skin disorder, 265, 265t
Hydroxyzine, in acute abdominal pain, 99
  in nausea and vomiting, 147
Hyoscine. See *Scopolamine hydrobromide.*
Hypercalcemia, 508–515
  admission in, 514
  calcitonin in, 513
  calcium homeostasis and, 508–509, 509
  calcium removal in, 513
  cancer and, 512–513
  cardiac symptoms in, 509, 510
  causes of, 512t
  chelation in, 514
  corticosteroid in, 513
  data gathering in, 509–510
  decision priorities in, 512–513
  definitive care in, 514
  diagnostic adjuncts in, 511–512
  differential diagnosis in, 512t, 512–513
  diphosphonate in, 513
  discharge in, 514
  disease processes and, 509
  disposition in, 514
  diuresis in, 513
  documentation in, 514
  electrocardiogram in, 511–512
  follow-up in, 514
  gastrointestinal symptoms in, 509, 510
  general considerations for, 508–509, 514–515
  hemodialysis in, 513
  history in, 510
  hyperparathyroidism and, 512
  laboratory studies in, 511
  management principles in, 513–516
  mild, 514
  mithramycin in, 513
  neurologic symptoms and, 509, 510
  organ system changes in, 509
  phosphate in, 513–514
  physical examination in, 510
  radiologic tests in, 511
  rehydration in, 513
  renal symptoms and, 509, 510
  sodium-EDTA in, 514
  total body calcium and, 508
Hyperglycemia, diabetes mellitus and, 484–485. See also *Diabetes mellitus, metabolic complications of.*
  hypothermia and, 417
Hyperkalemia, 499–507
  antagonizing potassium in, 505
  bicarbonate therapy in, 505
  calcium therapy in, 505

Hyperkalemia *(Continued)*
  causes of, 504t
  data gathering in, 501–502
  decision priorities in, 503–505
  diagnostic adjuncts in, 502–503
  dialysis in, 506
  differential diagnosis in, 503–505, 504t
  disposition in, 506–507
  diuretic in, 506
  documentation in, 507
  electrocardiogram in, 500, 500–501, 501, 502–503
  exogenous potassium sources and, 500
  follow-up in, 506–507
  general considerations for, 499–500, 507
  glucose therapy in, 505
  history in, 501–502
  initial emergency department approach in, 500, 500–501, 501
  insulin therapy in, 505
  kayexalate in, 506
  laboratory studies in, 502–503
  management principles in, 505–506
  physical examination in, 502
  potassium homeostasis and, 499–500
  pseudohyperkalemia and, 503
  reducing total body potassium in, 505–506
Hyperosmolar nonketotic coma, 482–484. See also *Diabetes mellitus, metabolic complications of.*
Hyperparathyroidism, hypercalcemia and, 512
Hypertension, 231–247
  admission in, 246
  aldosteronism in, 241
  antihypertensive in, 235, 235t, 243
    withdrawal from, 244
  aortic dissection in, 238–239, 244
  aortography in, 240
  blood pressure and, 232t, 236–237
  captopril in, 235t
  cardiovascular system and, 238–239
  central nervous system and, 238
  chest pain and, 234–235
  clonidine in, 235t, 243
  congestive heart failure and, 235
  data gathering in, 234–238
  decision priorities in, 238–239
  diagnostic adjuncts in, 239–240
  diazoxide in, 235t, 243
  differential diagnosis in, preliminary, 238–239
    refined, 240–242
  discharge in, 246–247
  disposition in, 246–247
  dizziness and, 925
  documentation in, 247
  drug-induced, 242, 244–236
  electrocardiogram in, 239–240
  emergencies, 243–244
  encephalopathy and, 243
  esmolol in, 235t
  follow-up in, 246–247
  furosemide in, 235t

Hypertension *(Continued)*
  general considerations for, 231–232, 247
  hematuria and, 235–236
  history in, 234
    prehospital care and, 233
  hydralazine in, 235t
  initial emergency department approach in, 234
  intervention in, prehospital care and, 233–234
  intoxication and, 352, 353t
  intracranial, 243
  labetalol in, 235t, 243
  laboratory studies in, 239
  low back pain and, 685–686
  magnesium sulfate in, 235t
  malignant, 237
  management principles in, 242–245
  moderate, 245
  morphine sulfate in, 243–244
  neurologic signs and, 234
  nifedipine in, 235t, 243
  nitroglycerin in, 235t, 243
  nitroprusside in, 235t, 243
  pediatric patient and, 246
  pheochromocytoma and, 241–242
  physical examination in, 236–238
    prehospital care and, 233
  pregnancy and, 236, 245–246
  prehospital care in, 232–234
  propranolol in, 235t
  pulmonary edema and, 238, 243–244
  radiologic imaging in, 240
  renal artery stenosis and, 241
  renal disease and, 241
  renal failure and, 239, 244
  stroke and, 880
  trimethaphan in, 235t
  urgency, 243, 244–245
  with encephalopathy, headache and, 837t, 841
Hypertensive encephalopathy, 243, 837t, 841
Hyperthermia. See also *Heat illness.*
  intoxication and, 352, 353t
Hyperventilation, dizziness and, 932t
  intoxication and, 352, 353t
  seizure and, 869
Hyperventilation syndrome, dyspnea and, 992t
  disposition in, 998
  management principles in, 996
  hydroxyzine in, 996
Hyphema, 605, 606t, 607
  management principles in, 611
Hypoglycemia, acute confusion and, 808. See also *Mental status, altered.*
  diabetes mellitus and, 471, 481, 484. See also *Diabetes mellitus, metabolic complications of.*
  hypothermia and, 417
  poisoning and, 349
  seizure and, 865t, 866t
Hyponatremia, 486–498
  admission in, 497
  altered mental status in, 487

Hyponatremia *(Continued)*
  central nervous system and, 487
  consultation in, 497
  data gathering in, 488–489
  decision priorities in, 489–490
  diagnostic adjuncts in, 490–491
  differential diagnosis in, preliminary, 489–490
    refined, 491–492, *492*, 493t, 494t, 494–495
  discharge in, 497
  disposition in, 497
  documentation in, 497–498
  drug-induced, 489
  electrocardiogram in, 491
  euvolemic, 492, 494
    management principles in, 495–496
  follow-up in, 497
  furosemide in, 495
  general considerations for, 486–487, 498
  history in, 488–489
  hypervolemic, 494t, 494–495
    management principles in, 496
  hypovolemic, 492, *492*, 493t
  initial emergency department approach in, 487–488
  laboratory studies in, 490–491
  loop diuretic in, 495
  management principles in, *492*, 495–497
  normal saline in, 495–496
  pediatric patient and, 497
  physical examination in, 489
  radiologic imaging in, 491
  seizure and, 487–488
  signs and symptoms of, 488t, 488–489
  volume deficit in, 487
    management principles in, 495
Hypotension, anaphylaxis and, 302
  dizziness and, 925
  heat stroke and, 405
  intoxication and, 352, 353t
  orthostatic, dizziness and, 932t
Hypothermia, 409–423
  active core rewarming in, 420–421
  active external rewarming in, 420, 420t
  admission in, 422
  advanced life support in, 419
  core rewarming options in, 413, 413t, 420–421
  data gathering in, 414–416
  decision priorities in, 416
  definition of, 409
  dextrose in, 413
  diagnostic adjuncts in, 416–418, *417*
  differential diagnosis in, preliminary, 416
  discharge in, 422
  disposition in, 422
  documentation in, 422–423
  drowning and, 421
  electrocardiogram in, 418
  extracorporeal rewarming in, 420
  follow-up in, 422
  frostbite and, 421–422

Hypothermia *(Continued)*
  general considerations for, 409–410, 423
  heat loss prevention in, 419
  history in, 414
    initial emergency department approach and, 413
    prehospital care and, 411
  hyperglycemia and, 417
  hypoglycemia and, 417
  initial emergency department approach in, 412–414
  intervention in, initial emergency department approach in, 413t, 413–414
    prehospital care and, 412
  intoxication and, 352, 353t
  laboratory studies in, 416–418
  localized, 421–422
  management principles in, 418–421
  naloxone in, 413
  passive external rewarming and, 419, 420t
  pathophysiology of, *410*, 410–411, *411*
  pediatric patient and, 421
  physical examination in, 414–416
    initial emergency department approach and, 413
    prehospital care and, 412
  predisposing factors in, 415t
  prehospital care in, 411–412
  radiologic imaging in, 418
  rewarming techniques in, 419t, 419–421
  thiamine in, 413
Hypoventilation, intoxication and, 352, 353t
Hypoxia, acute confusion and, 808. See also *Mental status, altered.*
  seizure and, 865t, 866t

Idiopathic thrombocytopenic purpura, 447t, 448
Ilotycin. See *Erythromycin.*
Imipenem-cilastatin, in dysuria, 1052t
Immobilization, in closed upper extremity injury, 709–710, 710t
  in head and neck trauma, 919
Immune globulin, 340
Immune system compromise, meningitis and, 860
  pediatric patient and, 632–633
  seizure and, 867
  sore throat and, 558
Immune therapy, in sepsis, 328
Immunization, fever and, 623–624
Impetigo, 268t. See also *Rash.*
Infant. See also *Neonate; Pediatric patient.*
  airway management for, 36t, 37
  febrile, 619–634
    acquired immune deficiency syndrome and, 633
    admission for, 633
    antibiotic for, 631–632, 632t

Infant *(Continued)*
    asplenia and, 632
    cancer and, 632–633
    cerebrospinal fluid analysis for, 628
    chronic illness and, 633
    data gathering for, 622–626
    decision priorities for, 626–627
    definition of, 619–620
    dehydration and, 678. See also *Dehydration.*
    diagnostic adjuncts for, 627–629
    differential diagnosis for, preliminary, 626–627
      refined, 629–631, 630t
    discharge for, 633–634
    disposition for, 633–634
    documentation for, 634
    follow-up for, 633–634
    general considerations for, 619–620, 634
    history for, 622–624
      prehospital care and, 620
    hydration and, 631
    immune system compromise and, 632–633
    immunization and, 623–624
    implications of, 620
    incidence of, 619
    infection and, 620, 624–627, 627t
    initial emergency department approach for, 621–622
    intensive care unit admission for, 633
    intervention for, prehospital care and, 620–621
    joint aspiration for, 629
    laboratory studies for, 628
    leukemia and, 632–633
    lumbar puncture for, 628
    management principles for, 631–632, 632t
    occult bacteremia and, 629–630, 630t
    physical examination for, 624–626, 625t
    prehospital care and, 620
    prehospital care for, 620–621, 621t
    radiologic imaging for, 628
    sepsis and, 630–631
    sickle cell disease and, 632
    steroid therapy and, 633
    synovial fluid analysis for, 629
    vital signs and, 625t, 625–626
    Yale Observation Scale for, 621, 621t
Infection, anaphylaxis and, 306
  bacterial, in acute diarrhea, 127t
    in sore throat, 548t, 556
  in febrile infant, 620, 624–627, 627t. See also *Infant, febrile.*
    occult bacteremia and, 629–630, 630t
  in hand and wrist injury, 740–741, *741–743*
  in sickle cell crisis, 459
  pediatric, common, 627t
  pulmonary, community-acquired, 324

Infection (Continued)
    in neonate, 324
        sepsis and, 324, 329t
    vaginal bleeding and, 1076
    wound healing and, 273, 274t
Infectious disorder, 313–343. See also *Biologic agent, accidental exposure to; names of specific infectious disorders; Sepsis.*
Inferior vena cava, injury to, 164t. See also *Abdomen, trauma to.*
Infertility, salpingitis and, 1058
Inflammatory bowel disease, acute gastrointestinal bleeding and, 116
    diarrhea and, 132
Influenza viruses A and B, sore throat and, 548t
Inotropic agent, in congestive heart failure, 996
Insulin therapy, in hyperkalemia, 505
Intestinal obstruction. See also *Abdomen, pain in.*
    abdominal pain and, 93t
Intracerebral hemorrhage, 885t, 887, 887
    management principles in, 890
Intracranial hemorrhage, seizure and, 865t, 866t
Intracranial pressure, increased, altered mental status and, 812
    head and neck injury and, 900, 919
Intubation, endotracheal. See *Endotracheal intubation.*
    nasogastric, in acute gastrointestinal bleeding, 108
    orotracheal, 28t, 28–29, 29
        in cardiac arrest, 43
        in wheezing, 1004
Iris, 575, 576, 577
Iritis, 581, *581*
    differential diagnosis in, 585, 586
    management principles in, 590, 591t, 592t
Iron poisoning, 370–371
Irritable bowel syndrome, acute diarrhea and, 123
Isoetharine, in wheezing, 1014
Isopropanol intoxication, 390. See also *Alcohol intoxication.*
Isoproterenol, in pediatric CPR, 55t
    in wheezing, 1014
Isotonic crystalloid solution, in dehydration, 670, 671

Janeway lesion, 320
Jehovah's Witness, 1111, *1112*
Joint, aspiration of, for febrile infant, 629
    pain and swelling in, 687–702. See also *Arthritis.*
        analgesia in, 698, 699
        anti-inflammatory agent in, 698, 699
        antibiotic in, 698, 698t
        arthrocentesis in, 692t, 692–693
        aspiration in, 699
        aspirin in, 699, 700
        bursitis and, 697

Joint (Continued)
    chondrocalcinosis and, 691, *692*
    colchicine in, 699
    common causes of, 690, 690t
    crystal-induced arthritides and, 695t, 696
        management principles in, 699
    data gathering in, 688–689
    decision priorities in, 690–691
    degenerative joint disease and, 697
        management principles in, 700
    diagnostic adjuncts in, 691–695
    differential diagnosis in, preliminary, 690t, 690–691
        refined, 695t, 695–697, 696t
    discharge in, 701
    disposition in, 701
    disseminated gonococcal infection and, 695t, 695–696
    documentation in, 701
    drainage in, 698
    follow-up in, 701
    general considerations for, 687–688, 702
    gout and, 695t, 696
        management principles in, 699
    hemarthrosis and, 696
        management principles in, 699–700
    history in, 688–689
    initial emergency department approach in, 688
    intra-articular injections in, 700
    joint drainage in, 698
    laboratory studies in, 691, 692t, 692–695
    management principles in, 697–700
    nonsteroidal anti-inflammatory agent in, 699
    osteomyelitis and, 697
    periarticular syndromes and, 697
    physical examination in, 689
    polyarticular arthritides and, 697
        management principles in, 700
    prehospital care in, 688
    pseudogout and, 696
    radiographic imaging in, 691, *692*
    referral in, 701
    septic arthritis and, 695t, 695–696, 696t
        bacterial agents in, 695, 696t
        detection of, 692t, 692–695, *694*
        management principles in, 698, 698t
    synovial fluid analysis in, 692t, 692–695, *694*
    synovitis and, 696
    tendinitis and, 697
    trauma and, 696
        management principles in, 699–700
    trauma to, 710t, 718–722, *719, 720*. See also *Orthopedic injury(ies), upper extremity.*

Kaolin-pectins, in acute diarrhea, 131

Kawasaki's syndrome, 268t. See also *Rash.*
Kayexalate, in hyperkalemia, 506
Keratitis, 575
    dendritic, 585, 587
    differential diagnosis in, 586–587
    management principles in, 590, 591t, 592, 592t
Kernig's sign, 853
Ketaconazole, in skin disorder, 266
Ketoacidosis, 526t, 526–527, 527t
Klebsiella, in sepsis, 315. See also *Sepsis.*
Knee injury, 764–766, *765*. See also *Orthopedic injury(ies), lower extremity.*
    anatomy and, 753, *754*
    classification of, 765
    incidence of, 765
    physical examination in, 755
KOH. See *Potassium hydroxide solution.*

Labetalol, in cocaine abuse, 433t
    in hypertension, 235t, 243
Labor, vaginal bleeding and, 1077
Laboratory study(ies). See also names of specific conditions.
    cost range for, 13t
Lactic acidosis, 527, 528t. See also *Acid-base disorder(s).*
    seizure and, 874
Laminectomy, in low back pain, 801
Laryngeal edema, anaphylaxis and, 302, 305t
Laryngotracheobronchitis, viral, 643t, 647, 647t
    management principles in, 649
    radiographic imaging in, 644–645
Larynx, pediatric, 636, *636*
Latex particle agglutination, 857
Laxative abuse, acute abdominal pain and, 90
Leg injury, 764–766, *765*. See also *Orthopedic injury(ies), lower extremity.*
    anatomy and, 755, *756*
    physical examination in, 755
Legal considerations. See *Medicolegal considerations.*
Legg-Calvé-Perthes disease, 775–777. See also *Orthopedic injury(ies), lower extremity.*
Lens, examination of, 581
Leukemia, pediatric patient and, 632–633
Lidocaine, in cocaine abuse, 433t
    in orotracheal intubation, 32
    in pediatric CPR, 55t
    in ventricular premature beats, 207
    in wound care, 279, 279t
Lightheadedness, 924, 925. See also *Dizziness.*
Limbic flush, eye trauma and, 596
Lindane, in skin disorders, 266
Lip, wound care for, 289

Lipopolysaccharide, 316
Liver, injury to, 164t. See also *Abdomen, trauma to.*
Liver function test, in acute abdominal pain, 97
 in acute gastrointestinal bleeding, 113
Living will, 56
Loop diuretic, in hyponatremia, 495
Low back pain, 783–803
 abdominal aneurysm and, 791
 abdominal pain and, 786, 787, 793, 793t
 admission in, 801–802
 bed rest in, 800
 cardiovascular problems and, 786–788
 cauda equina syndrome and, 788t, 792–793
 data gathering in, 787–791
 decision priorities in, 791
 decompression in, 801
 diagnostic adjuncts in, 794–796
 differential diagnosis in, preliminary, 791–794, 792t–793t
  refined, 796–798, 797t–799t, 799, 800
 disc herniation and, 788t, 797, 798t, 799
 discharge in, 802
 disposition in, 801–802
 documentation in, 802–803
 ectopic pregnancy and, 791, 792t
 exercise in, 801
 financial considerations in, 783
 follow-up in, 801–802
 general considerations for, 783–785, 803
 history in, 787–789
  prehospital care and, 785
 hypertension and, 685–786
 initial emergency department approach in, 786–787
 intervention in, prehospital care and, 785–786
 laboratory studies in, 795–796
 laminectomy in, 801
 lumbar spine anatomy and, 784, *784*
 malingering and, 783, 793t
 management potential principles in, 800–801
 microdiscectomy in, 801
 muscle relaxation in, 800–801
 nerve root compression in, 787–788
  examination for, 788t
  management principles in, 801
 overexertion and, 800
 pain relief in, 801
 physical examination in, 789–791
  prehospital care and, 785
  prone, 790
  sitting, 790
  standing, 789
  supine, 789–790
 prehospital care in, 785–786
 primary causes of, 797t–799t
 psychosomatic, 793
 radiologic imaging in, 794t, 794–795

Low back pain *(Continued)*
 secondary causes of, 791–792, 792t–793t
 spinal stenosis and, 793, 794t, 798, 799t, 800
 surgery in, 801
 traction in, 800
Lower extremity injury, 748–782. See also *Orthopedic injury(ies), lower extremity.*
Lumbar puncture, for febrile infant, 628
 in altered mental status, 820
 in headache, 839–840
 in seizure, 870
 in sepsis, 322
 in stroke, 888
Lynch algorithm, rash and, 256, 257t

Magill forceps, in endotracheal intubation, 31–32
Magnesium citrate, in poisoning, 362
Magnesium sulfate, in hypertension, 235t
 in poisoning, 362
Mallory-Weiss tear, acute gastrointestinal bleeding and, 115
 vomiting and, 137
Mania, 945t. See also *Behavioral disorder(s).*
Marcus-Gunn pupil, 602
MAST suit, in anaphylaxis, 303, 309
McMurray's test, 755
Meckel's diverticulum, acute gastrointestinal bleeding and, 119
Medicolegal considerations, 17, 1105–1113
 Against Medical Advice form and, 1111–1112, *1112*
 competence and, 1109–1110
 consent and, 1106–1108, *1107*
 documentation and, 1112–1113
 emergency department obligations and, 1106
 general, 1105–1106, 1113
 involuntary restraint and, 1110–1111
 reporting requirements and, 1112
Ménière's disease, 932t
Meningitis, 848–861. See also *Biologic agent, accidental exposure to.*
 accidental exposure to, 334, 337
 age factor and, 850t, 856t
 altered mental status and, 812
 antibiotic in, 329t, 850t, 850–851, 859
  pediatric patient and, 632t
 bacterial, accidental exposure to, 334, 337
  testing and management for, 340–341, 341t
 admission in, 860
 clinical findings in, 855t
 differential diagnosis of, 858
 headache and, 837t, 841
 incidence of, 848
 mortality in, 849
 pathogens in, 849, 850t

Meningitis *(Continued)*
 cerebrospinal fluid analysis in, 855t, 855–857, 856t
 data gathering in, 851–854
 decision priorities in, 854–855
 diagnostic adjuncts in, 855–857
 diagnostic triad of, 324–325
 differential diagnosis in, preliminary, 854–855
  refined, 858–859
 disposition in, 860–861
 documentation in, 861
 follow-up in, 860–861
 general considerations for, 848–849, 861
 Haemophilus in, 849, 850t
 headache and, 837t, 841, 851
 history in, 851–852
 immunocompromised patient and, 860
 incidence of, 848
 initial emergency department approach in, 849–851
 laboratory studies in, 855t, 855–857, 856t
 lumbar puncture in, 850, 855t, 855–857, 856t
 management principles in, 859
 meningococcal, 858
 Neisseria in, 849, 850t
 neurologic examination in, 853
 nonbacterial, 858, 860–861
 physical examination in, 852–853
 pneumococcal, 858
 prevalence of, 848
 radiologic imaging in, 857
 rash and, 260–261
 seizure and, 850, 865t, 866t
 Streptococcus in, 849, 850t
 viral, admission in, 860–861
  clinical findings in, 855t
  differential diagnosis of, 858
  incidence of, 848
Meningococcemia, rash and, 257t, 261
Menstruation, acute abdominal pain and, 90
Mental status, altered, 807–829
 admission in, 827–828
 amnesia and, 809
 coma and, 808
 confusional state and, 808
 decision priorities in, 817–818
 delirium and, 808–809
 dementia and, 809
 diagnostic adjuncts in, 818–820
 differential diagnosis in, preliminary, 817–818, 818t, 819t
  refined, 821t–822t, 821–824
 discharge in, 828
 disposition in, 827
 documentation in, 828–829
 electrocardiogram in, 820
 follow-up in, 827
 general considerations for, 807, 829
 geriatric patient and, 827
 Glasgow Coma Scale and, 810, 810t
 history in, 813–814

Mental status *(Continued)*
  initial emergency department approach and, 812–813
  prehospital care and, 809–810
 hyponatremia and, 487
 increased intracranial pressure and, 812
 intervention in, initial emergency department approach and, 812–813
  prehospital care and, 810–811
 laboratory studies in, 818–819
 level of consciousness and, 807
 lumbar puncture in, 820
 management principles in, 824, 825, 826, 827
 meningitis and, 812
 metabolic complications of diabetes mellitus and, 471. See also *Diabetes mellitus, metabolic complications of.*
 naloxone in, 811, 812
 pediatric patient and, 827
 physical examination in, 814–817, 956
  extraocular movements and, 815, *816*
  eye examination and, 814–816, *815, 816*
  funduscopic examination and, 815–816
  initial emergency department approach and, 812–813
  mental status examination and, 816–817, 817t
  prehospital care and, 810
 prehospital care in, 809–811
 radiologic imaging in, 819–820
 seizure and, precautions for, 812
 syncope vs., 217
 thiamine in, 812
Meperidine, in acute diarrhea, 131
Mepivacaine, in wound care, 279, 279t
Mesenteric ischemia, abdominal pain and, 94t. See also *Abdomen, pain in.*
 acute gastrointestinal bleeding and, 116
Metabolic acidosis. See also *Acid-base disorder(s).*
 alcohol intoxication and, 386, 386t
 differential diagnosis in, preliminary, 522–525, *524*
  refined, 525–530, 526t–528t
 management principles in, 530–531
 poisoning and, 357, 357t
Metabolic alkalosis. See also *Acid-base disorder(s).*
 classification of, 529t
 differential diagnosis in, preliminary, 522–525, 524, *524*
  refined, 525–530, 526t–528t, 528–530, 529t
  saline-resistant, 529t, 529–530
  saline-responsive, 528–529, 529t
 general considerations for, 516, 518
 history in, 519–520, *520*

Metabolic alkalosis *(Continued)*
 management principles in, 530–531, 531–532
 pathophysiology of, 518
 physical examination in, 520, 521t
 saline-resistant, 529t, 529–530
 saline-responsive, 528–529, 529t
Metabolic disorder. See also names of specific disorders.
 acute confusion and, 808. See also *Mental status, altered.*
 diabetes mellitus and, 471–485. See also *Diabetes mellitus, metabolic complications of.*
 nausea and vomiting and, 146, 146t
Metaproterenol, in wheezing, 1011, 1013t
Methanol ingestion, in acid-base disorder, 528
Methanol intoxication, 390. See also *Alcohol intoxication.*
Methylprednisolone, in anaphylaxis, 308
 in head and neck trauma, 919
 in wheezing, 1014t
Metoclopramide, in nausea and vomiting, 148
Michigan Comprehensive Reform Law, 977
Miconazole, in skin disorder, 266
Microdiscectomy, in low back pain, 801
Midazolam, in orotracheal intubation, 32
Migraine headache, 838t, 841. See also *Headache.*
 management principles in, 843
Military, medical experiences in, 1117
Mithramycin, in hypercalcemia, 513
Mittelschmerz, pelvic pain and, 1069t. See also *Pelvis, female, pain in.*
Morphine, in dyspnea, 983
Morphine sulfate, in congestive heart failure, 996
 in hypertension, 243–244
Motor vehicle accident, 62t. See also *Multiple trauma; Trauma.*
Mouth, acute gastrointestinal bleeding and, 110
 nausea and vomiting and, 141, 142
Mouthwash, in ulceration and erosion, 265
Multifocal atrial tachycardia, 203. See also *Palpitation.*
 management principles in, 207
Multiple trauma, 60–79. See also *Trauma.*
 burn and, 77
 cardiac arrest and, 77
 data gathering in, 70–71
 decision priorities in, 71
 diagnostic adjuncts in, 71–75
  electrocardiogram as, 74
  evaluation of abdomen as, 74–75
  Foley catheter as, 74
  laboratory studies as, 73, 73t
  nasogastric tube as, 74
  radiologic imaging as, 71, 73
 differential diagnosis in, 71
 disposition in, 78

Multiple trauma *(Continued)*
 documentation in, 78
 emergency medical services for, 1129
 Foley catheter in, 74
 general considerations for, 60–61, 78–79
 hemorrhagic shock and, 62–63
 initial emergency department approach in, 66–70
  primary resuscitation in, 68t, 68–70
 management principles in, 75–76
 mechanism of injury in, 61t, 61–62, 62t
 pediatric patient and, 76t, 76–77
 physical examination in, 71, 72t
 prehospital care in, 63–64
 shock and, 62–63
 tetanus prophylaxis in, 75
 trauma scores in, 64, 65t, 66, 66t
  pediatric, 76t
Münchausen's syndrome, anaphylaxis and, 306
Mupirocin, in skin disorder, 266
Murphy's sign, in acute abdominal pain, 92
Muscular disorder, in acute abdominal pain, 92
Mycoplasma infection, antibiotic in, pediatric patient and, 632t
 in sore throat, 548t, 556
Mydriacil. See *Tropicamide.*
Mydriatic, in eye trauma, 610
 in red and painful eye, 583, 588, 589t
Myocardial contusion, in chest trauma, 1035, 1036t
Myocardial infarction. See also *Chest, pain in; Palpitation.*
 acute chest pain and, 181t, 190
 disposition in, 192–193
 dyspnea and, 992t
  disposition in, 998
 emergency medical services and, 1129
 management principles in, 190
 syncope and, 223
Myocardial ischemia, dyspnea and, 992t

N-acetylcysteine, in acetaminophen poisoning, 365, *366*
NAC. See *N-acetylcysteine.*
Nailbed injury, hand, 741–742
Naloxone, in alcohol intoxication, 381
 in head and neck trauma, 900
 in hypothermia, 413
 in sepsis, 317, 328
Naltrexone, in sepsis, 328
Narcotic antagonist, in sepsis, 328
Narcotic overdose poisoning, 349
Nasal cannula, in oxygen delivery, 25t
Nasogastric intubation, acute gastrointestinal bleeding and, 108
Nasogastric tube, acute abdominal pain and, 88
 head and neck trauma and, 919
 multiple trauma and, 74

Nasopharyngeal airway device, 22, 24, *24*
Nasotracheal intubation, 29–31, 30t
National Highway Safety Act of 1966, 1118
Nausea and vomiting, 136–151. See also *Vomiting*.
  abdominal pain and, 89–90
  abdominal radiographs in, 144
  acute diarrhea and, 125
  acute gastrointestinal bleeding and, 119
  admission in, 149
  alimentary system and, 145–146, 146t
  amylase level and, 144
  antiemetic in, 147
  antihistamine in, 147
  cardiovascular system and, 146, 146t
  catastrophic disorder and, 143
  central nervous system and, 145, 146t
  common causes of, 137
  crystalloid solution in, 147
  data-gathering in, 140–142
  decision priorities in, 142–144
  diagnostic adjuncts in, 144–145
  differential diagnosis in, preliminary, 142–143
    refined, 145–147, 146t
  discharge in, 149–150, 150t
  disposition in, 149–150, 150t
  documentation in, 150
  drug-related, 146t, 146–147
  electrocardiogram in, 145
  emesis control in, 148
  endoscopy in, 144
  fluid resuscitation in, 139
  follow-up in, 149–150, 150t
  Gastroccult test in, 139
  gastroenteritis and, 143
  general considerations for, 136–137, 150–151
  geriatric patient and, 149
  history in, 140–141
    initial emergency department approach in, 139
    prehospital care and, 138
  hydroxyzine in, 147
  initial emergency department approach in, 139–140
  intervention in, 139
  laboratory studies in, 144
  management principles in, 147–148
  mechanisms in, 136–137, *138*
  metabolic disorder and, 146, 146t
  metoclopramide in, 147
  neurologic disorder in, 142
  pediatric patient and, 148
  physical examination in, 141–142
    initial emergency department approach in, 139
    prehospital care and, 138
  pregnancy test in, 144
  prehospital care in, 137–139
  prochlorperazine in, 147
  promethazine in, 147
  psychological system in, 146t, 147

Nausea and vomiting *(Continued)*
  radiologic imaging in, 144
  serious consequences of, 137
  serum electrolytes and, 144
  skin disorder in, 141
  stool examination in, 145
  symptoms associated with, 141, 141t
  underlying disease in, 146t, 148
  volume restoration in, 147–148
  vomiting center and, 136–137, *137*
Neck, anatomy of, 895, *895*, *896*
  hyperextension of, dizziness and, 929
  trauma to, 915–918. See also *Head and neck trauma*.
    common fracture as, 915, *916*, *917*
    ligament and muscle strain as, 916
    pediatric patient and, 919–920, *920*, *921*
    penetrating, 917–918
Needle decompression, in dyspnea, 983, 995
Neglect, 666, *667*. See also *Child abuse*.
Neisseria infection, antibiotic in, pediatric patient and, 632t
  in meningitis, 849, 850t
  in meningococcemia, 261
  in skin disorder, 320
  in sore throat, 548t
Neo-Synephrine. See *Phenylephrine hydrochloride*.
Neomycin, in eye trauma, 610
  in red and painful eye, 592t
Neonate. See also *Infant*; *Pediatric patient*.
  acute gastrointestinal bleeding and, 119
  central nervous system infection and, 324
  febrile, 633
  meningitis in, antibiotic in, 850t
  premature, airway management for, 37
  pulmonary infection and, 324
  sepsis and, 330–331
  urinary infection and, 323–324, 1053
Neosporin. See *Neomycin*.
Nephrotic syndrome, hyponatremia and, 494t
Nerve block, in wound care, 279–280, *281*
Nerve injury, hand and wrist, 740
Neuroanatomy, pain transmission and, 84–85
Neurologic disorder, acute chest pain and, 179
  nausea and vomiting and, 142
  syncope and, 226
Neuroma, acoustic, dizziness and, 932t
Nifedipine, in congestive heart failure, 996
  in hypertension, 235t, 243
Nitrate, in cocaine abuse, 433t
  in congestive heart failure, 996
  in dyspnea, 983
Nitroglycerin, in hypertension, 235t, 243
Nitroprusside, in congestive heart failure, 996
  in hypertension, 235t, 243

Nitroprusside *(Continued)*
  in sepsis, 327
Nonsteroidal anti-inflammatory agent, in anaphylaxis, 307t
  in joint pain and swelling, 699
  in sepsis, 328
Norfloxacin, in sepsis, 327
Norgestrel, as postcoital therapy, 973
Normal saline, in hyponatremia, 495–496
Norwalk agent, in acute diarrhea, 130t
Nose, acute gastrointestinal bleeding and, 110
  wound care for, 289
Nosebleed, 537–546. See also *Epistaxis*.
Nurse, emergency, statistical and historical profile of, 4t

Obturator sign, in acute abdominal pain, 92
Ocular disorder. See *Eye, red and painful*; names of specific disorders.
Ophthaine. See *Proparacaine*.
Ophthetic. See *Proparacaine*.
Ophthochlor. See *Chloramphenicol*.
Opioid, in orotracheal intubation, 32–33
Orbit, blowout fracture of, 606t, 607–608. See also *Eye, trauma to*.
  management principles in, 611–612
Oropharyngeal airway device, 22, 24, *24*
Orotracheal intubation, 28t, 28–29, *29*
  in cardiac arrest, 43
  in wheezing, 1004
Orthopedic injury(ies), lower extremity, 748–782
  admission in, 779–780
  ankle and foot injury as, 767–769, 771–775. See also *Ankle and foot injury(ies)*.
  arthrocentesis in, 760
  compartment syndromes and, 777–779, *780*
  crutches in, 781
  data gathering in, 751
  decision priorities in, 758
  diagnostic adjuncts in, 758–760
  differential diagnosis in, preliminary, 758
  disposition in, 779–781
  documentation in, 781–782
  femoral shaft-injury as, 752, 764
  fibular fracture as, 766
  general considerations for, 748–749, 782
  Hare traction splint in, 749, *750*
  hemorrhage and, 750
  hip injury as, 761–764
    anatomy and, *752*, 752–753
    physical examination in, 753
  immobilization in, 761
  initial emergency department approach in, 749–751
  knee injury as, 764–766, *765*
    anatomy and, 753, *754*
    classification of, *765*

Orthopedic injury(ies) *(Continued)*
  incidence of, 765
  physical examination in, 753, 755
  laboratory studies in, 760
  leg injury as, 764–766, *765*
    anatomy and, 755, *756*
    physical examination in, 755
  Legg-Calvé-Perthes disease and, 775–777
  ligamentous laxity in, 755, 757
  management principles in, 760–775
    general, 760–761
    specific, 761–775
  McMurray's test in, 755
  neurovascular injury in, 750–751
  Osgood-Schlatter disease and, 777
  outpatient management in, 780–781
  physical examination in, 751–753, *754*, 755–758, *756*, *757*
  prehospital care in, 749, *750*
  radiographic imaging in, 758–760
  slipped capital femoral epiphysis and, 777, *778*
  surgery in, 779
  thigh injury as, 761–764
    anatomy and, *752*, *753*
    physical examination in, 753
  tibial shaft fracture as, 766–767
  upper extremity, closed, 703–725
    acromioclavicular separation as, 710t, 712
    admission in, 724–725
    analgesia in, 708
    anesthesia in, 708
    clavicular fracture as, 710t, 712–713
    consultation in, 724–725
    data gathering in, 705–706
    decision priorities in, 706–707
    diagnostic adjuncts in, 707–708
    differential diagnosis in, preliminary, 706–707
    discharge in, 725
    disposition in, 724–725
    documentation in, 725
    elbow injury as, 710t, 714–717, *716*
    follow-up in, 724–725
    forearm fracture as, 710t, 717
    general considerations for, 703–704, 725
    geriatric patient and, 724
    hand fracture as, 710t, 718–722, *719*, *720*
    history in, 705–706
      prehospital care and, 704
    humeral fracture as, 712, 713–714, *714*, *715*
    immobilization in, 709–710, 710t
    initial emergency department approach and, 705
    intervention in, prehospital care and, 704–705
    joint fracture as, 710t, 718–722, *719*, *720*
    laboratory studies in, 708

Orthopedic injury(ies) *(Continued)*
    management principles in, 708–709
    pediatric patient and, 722–724, *723*, *724*
    physical examination in, 706
      prehospital care and, 704
    prehospital care in, 704–705
    radiologic imaging in, 707–708
    shoulder injury as, 710t, 711–712, *712*
    specific, 711–722
    wrist fracture as, 710t, 717–718
  hand and wrist injury as. See also *Hand and wrist injury(ies)*.
    closed, 710t, 717–722, *719*, *720*
    open, 727–743
Orthostatic hypotension, dizziness and, 932t
  in geriatric patient, 228
  syncope and, 226, 227, 228, 229
Osgood-Schlatter disease, 777. See also *Orthopedic injury(ies), lower extremity*.
Osler's node, 320
Osmotic diuresis, in hyponatremia, 493t
Osteomyelitis, joint pain and swelling and, 697
Otic drops, in earache, 572, 572t
Otitis media, antibiotic in, pediatric patient and, 632t
Otolaryngologist, referral to, 573
Otolaryngology test, in dizziness, 931
Otoscopy, pneumatic, 565, *565*
Ovary, cystic, culdocentesis in, 1065
  pelvic pain and, 1061, 1067t, 1073–1074. See also *Pelvis, female, pain in*.
  rupture of, 1068t, 1069
  injury to, 165t. See also *Abdomen, trauma to*.
Oxygen therapy, in airway management, 24–25, 25t

Packed red blood cells, in bleeding disorders, 451
Pain, abdominal, 83–102. See also *Abdomen, pain in*.
  chest, acute, 173–194. See also *Chest, pain in*.
  eye trauma and, 600
  in earache, 563
  ocular, 588t, 588–589, 589t
  pelvic, in women, 1058–1074. See also *Pelvis, female, pain in*.
  red and painful eye and, 579
Palpable purpura, 264
Palpitation, 196–213
  abdominal signs in, 199
  cardiovascular system in, 199
  cardioversion in, 207
  data gathering in, 198
  decision priorities in, 199–201
  definition of, 196
  diagnostic adjuncts in, 201–202, *202*

Palpitation *(Continued)*
  differential diagnosis in, preliminary, 199–201, 200t
    refined, 202–207
  disposition in, 211–212
  documentation in, 212
  electrocardiogram in, 201, *202*
  etiology of, 200t
  extremities in, 199
  follow-up in, 212
  general considerations for, 196, 212–213
  geriatric patient and, 211
  history in, initial emergency department approach and, 198–199
    prehospital care and, 197
  holter monitoring in, 201–202
  in atrial fibrillation, 202–203, *203*
    management principles in, 207
  in atrial flutter, 203, *203*
    management principles in, 207
  in multifocal atrial tachycardia, 203
    management principles in, 207
  in paroxysmal supraventricular tachycardia, 203, *204*
    management principles in, 208
  in premature atrial contraction, 203
    management principles in, 207
  in serious dysrhythmia, 198t
  in ventricular premature beats, 203–204
    management principles in, 207
  in ventricular tachycardia, 203, *204*
    management principles in, 207–208, *208*
  in wide-complex tachycardia, 202, 204–207, *205*, 205t
    management principles in, 209, *209*, *209*
  in Wolff-Parkinson-White syndrome, 203, 210, *211*
  initial emergency department approach in, 198, 198t
  intervention in, immediate, 207
    prehospital care and, 197
  laboratory studies in, 201
  management principles in, 207–210
  neurologic signs in, 199
  noncardiac causes of, 210
  pediatric patient and, 210
  physical examination in, initial emergency department approach and, 199
  prehospital care in, 196–198
  pulmonary system in, 199
  radiologic imaging in, 201
  without dysrhythmia, 210
Pancreas, injury to, 164t. See also *Abdomen, trauma to*.
Pancreatitis, 93t. See also *Abdomen, pain in*.
Papilledema, 854
Papulosquamous diseases, 257t, 262
Parainfluenza virus, sore throat and, 548t
Parasitic disease, acute diarrhea and, 127t, 129, 130t

Paronychia, in hand and wrist injury, 740–741, *741*
Paroxysmal supraventricular tachycardia, 203, *204*
 management principles in, 208
 pediatric patient and, 210
PASG. See *MAST garment; Pneumatic antishock garment.*
Patient, problem, 1137–1138. See also *Problem patient.*
Patient satisfaction, general considerations for, 16
PCP. See *Phencyclidine poisoning.*
Pediatric patient. See also *Adolescent; Infant; Neonate.*
 abdominal pain and, 100. See also *Abdomen, pain in.*
 abdominal trauma and, 167
 acquired immune deficiency syndrome and, 633
 acute chest pain and, 190–191
 acute gastrointestinal bleeding and, 119
 airway anatomy and, 36t
 airway management and, 36t, 36–37, 37t
 asthma and, medication in, 1013t–1014t
 behavioral disorders and, 947
 bleeding disorders and, 452
 cancer and, 632–633
 cardiopulmonary cerebral resuscitation and, 55, 55t
 central nervous system infection and, 324
 chest trauma and, 1035
 closed upper extremity injury and, 722–724, 723, 724. See also *Orthopedic injury(ies), upper extremity.*
  epiphyseal injury as, 722–724, 724
  greenstick fracture as, 722
  Salter-Harris fracture as, 722–724, 724
  torus fracture as, 722, 723
 consent and, 1108–1109
 cricothyrotomy and, 637
 dyspnea and, 997
 epiglottis in, 553, 555
 epistaxis and, 544
 eye trauma and, 613
 fever and, 619–634. See also *Infant, febrile.*
 general considerations for, 17
 head and neck trauma and, 919–920
 headache and, 844
 heat illness and, 406
 hypertension and, 246
 hyponatremia and, 497
 hypothermia and, 421
 immune system compromise and, 632–633
 leukemia and, 632–633
 metabolic complications of diabetes mellitus and, 483–484
 multiple trauma and, 76t, 76–77
 nausea and vomiting and, 148

Pediatric patient *(Continued)*
 neck injury and, 919–920, *920*, *921*
 normal respiratory rates in, 639t
 palpitation and, 210
 pelvic pain and, 1069, 1071
 red and painful eye and, 592
 seizure and, 869t, 874
 sepsis and, 632
 sexual assault and, 975. See also *Sexual assault, child victim of.*
 sickle cell disease and, 466
 steroid therapy and, 633
 strep throat and, 551, 551t, 552t
 stridor and, 636–651. See also *Stridor.*
 stroke and, 891
 suicide potential and, 960
 syncope and, 227–228
 trauma score for, 76, 76t
 urinary tract infection in, 323–324, 1053
 wheezing and, 1016
Pelvic appendicitis, 1070t
Pelvic examination, in women, 1063
Pelvic inflammatory disease, 1055
 culdocentesis in, 1065
 differential diagnosis in, 1068t
 dysuria and, 1055
 management principles in, 1066, 1069, 1071t
  outpatient, *1071*
 pelvic pain and, 1058, 1062–1063. See also *Pelvis, female, pain in.*
Pelvis, female, pain in, 1058–1074
 abdominal aortic aneurysm and, 1070t
 abdominal causes of, 1070t
 admission in, 1072
 culdocentesis in, 1065
 data gathering in, 1061–1063
 decision priorities in, 1063–1064
 diagnostic adjuncts in, 1064–1065
 differential diagnosis in, preliminary, 1063–1064
  refined, 1066, 1068t–1069t, 1069, 1070t
 discharge in, 1072–1073
 disposition in, 1072–1073
 documentation in, 1073
 endometriosis and, 1068t
 etiologic classification of, 1067t
 follow-up in, 1072–1073
 general considerations for, 1058–1059, 1073–1074
 geriatric patient and, 1071–1072
 hemorrhagic shock and, 1058
 history in, 1061–1063
  initial emergency department approach and, 1060–1061
 prehospital care and, 1059
 incidence of, 1058
 initial emergency department approach in, 1060–1061
 intervention in, initial emergency department approach and, 1060–1061
 prehospital care and, 1059

Pelvis *(Continued)*
 laboratory studies in, 1060, 1064–1065
 Mittelschmerz and, 1069t
 of uncertain etiology, 1073
 ovarian cyst and, 1061, 1067t, 1073–1074
  culdocentesis in, 1065
  rupture of, 1068t, 1069
 pediatric patient and, 1069, 1071
 pelvic appendicitis and, 1070t
 physical examination in, 1063
  initial emergency department approach and, 1060
 prehospital care and, 1059
 pneumatic antishock garment in, 1059
 postmenopausal, 1071–1072
 pregnancy and, 1063–1064
  ectopic, 1058, 1062–1063
  culdocentesis in, 1065
  management principles in, 1066, 1068t, *1071*
 prehospital care in, 1059–1060
 prepubertal, 1069, 1071
 pyelonephritis and, 1070t
 radiologic imaging in, 1065
 salpingitis and, 1066, 1069, 1071t
 septic shock and, 1058
 strangulated femoral hernia and, 1070t
 ureteral calculus and, 1070t
 uterine myomas and fibroids and, 1069t
 fractured, 165t. See also *Abdomen, trauma to.*
Penicillin, in meningitis, 850t, 859
 in skin disorders, 266
Penicillin-allergic patient, 292
 spectinomycin for, 1099t
Penicillin G, in gonorrhea, 1099t
Penis, discharge from, 1091–1101
 data gathering in, 1092–1093
 decision priorities in, 1094
 diagnostic adjuncts in, 1094–1095
 differential diagnosis in, preliminary, 1094
  refined, 1096–1097
 disposition in, 1100
 documentation in, 1100
 dysuria and. See *Dysuria.*
 follow-up in, 1100
 general considerations for, 1091–1092
 laboratory studies in, 1094–1095
 management principles in, 1098, 1099t
 microscopic examination in, 1048
Peptic ulcer, abdominal pain and, 96t. See also *Abdomen, pain in.*
 acute gastrointestinal bleeding and, 114–115
Pepto Bismol. See *Bismuth subsalicylate.*
Percutaneous transcricothyroid catheter ventilation, 33, *34*, *35*
Pericardiocentesis, in chest trauma, 1025, *1026*

Peritoneal lavage, in multiple trauma, 74
Peritonsillar abscess, sore throat and, 555, 555
Personality disorder, 945t. See also *Behavioral disorder(s)*.
Petroleum distillate poisoning, 373–374
Pharyngitis. See *Sore throat*.
   antibiotic in, pediatric patient and, 632t
Phenazopyridine, in dysuria, 1051
Phencyclidine poisoning, 355, 373
Phenergan. See *Promethazine*.
Phenobarbital, in seizure, 850, 873
Phentolamine, in sepsis, 327
Phenylephrine hydrochloride, in red and painful eye, 589t
Phenytoin, in cocaine abuse, 433t
   in seizure, 850, 873
Pheochromocytoma, in hypertension, 241–242
Phosphate, in hypercalcemia, 513–514
Photosensitivity, rash and, 264
Physician, as patient advocate, 16
   interaction with emergency medical services personnel, 1122, 1125–1126
   medical control and, 1126, 1126t, 1129
   mental health of, 17
   on-scene intervention policy for, 1126t
PID. See *Pelvic inflammatory disease*.
Pityriasis rosea, 257t, 262
Placenta previa, vaginal bleeding and, 1087
Platelet disorder(s). See also *Bleeding disorder(s)*.
   coagulation disorders and, 445t, 445–446, 447t, 450
      disposition in, 453
   disposition in, 452–458
   specific, 447–448
   vaginal bleeding and, 1076
Platelet transfusion, 451
Pneumatic antishock garment, 69–70
   abdominal trauma and, 155
   acute abdominal pain and, 86
   acute gastrointestinal bleeding and, 106
   pelvic pain in women and, 1059
   sepsis and, 318
   vaginal bleeding and, 1077
Pneumonia, antibiotic in, pediatric patient and, 632t
   antimicrobial therapy in, 995
   dyspnea and, 991t, 993t
      management principles in, 995
   sepsis and, 329
Pneumothorax, acute chest pain and, 183t, 190
   chest trauma and, 1021, *1021*, 1031t, 1035, 1036t
      intervention in, 1023
      physical examination in, 1022, 1023t
   dyspnea and, 991t, 993t
      management principles in, 995
   management principles in, 190
   thoracostomy in, 995
Poisindex, 359

Poisoning, absorption minimization in, 360–362
   accidental, 375
   acetaminophen, 364–365
   activated charcoal in, 361, 363
   altered mental status in, 350
   amphetamine, 355, 372–373
   anion gap and, 357, 357t
   anticholinergic, 355, 367–368
   aspirin, 365, 367
   blood levels and, 358, 358t
   butyrophenone, 356
   carbon monoxide, 354t, 368–369
   cathartic in, 361–362
   caustic, 369–370
   cholinergic, 355
   cyclic antidepressant, 355, 367–368
   data gathering in, 351–354, 353t
   decision priorities in, 354–356
   decontamination in, 349, 350, 360
   diagnostic adjuncts in, 356–359, 357t, 358t
   differential diagnosis in, 354t, 354–356
   dilution in, 349, 350
   disposition in, 374–376
   diuresis in, 363
   documentation in, 376–377
   electrocardiogram in, 359
   elimination in, 349
      maximization of, 362t, 362–363
   emergency stabilization in, 350, 360
   enzyme-mediated immunoassay in, 358, 358t
   follow-up in, 376
   gastric emptying in, 360t, 360–361
   gastric lavage in, 360–361
   general considerations for, 347–348, 377
   hemodialysis in, 362, 362t
   hemoperfusion in, 362–363
   history in, 351–352
      initial emergency department approach and, 349–350
      prehospital care and, 348
   hypoglycemia screening in, 349
   incidence of, 347–348
   initial emergency department approach in, 349–351
   intervention in, initial emergency department approach and, 350–351
      prehospital care and, 349
   iron, 370–371
   laboratory studies in, 357t, 357–358
   magnesium citrate in, 362
   magnesium sulfate in, 362
   management principles in, 359–374
   Matthew-Rumack nomogram in, 365, 366
   medical considerations in, 374
   metabolic acidosis and, 357, 357t
   narcotic overdose and, 349
   neurologic system in, 353, 353t
   nontoxic ingestion in, 374, 375t
   odors associated with, 354, 354t
   opiate, 354, 373
   petroleum distillate, 373–374
   phencyclidine, 355, 373

Poisoning (Continued)
   phenothiazine, 356
   physical examination in, 352–354, 353t
      prehospital care and, 348
   physiologic antagonists in, 363–364, 364t
   Poisindex in, 359
   prehospital care in, 348–349
   primary survey in, 349–350
   psychosocial considerations in, 374–376
   pupillary abnormalities in, 353, 353t
   salicylate, 356, 365, 367
   sedative-hypnotic, 355–356, 373
   seizure and, 865
   skin disorders and, 353–354
   sorbitol in, 362
   substance abuser and, 375–376
   suicide attempt and, 375
   sympathomimetic, 355, 372–373
   syrup of ipecac in, 360–360t
   theophylline, 371–372
   toxicology screens in, 357–358, 358t
   vital signs in, 352, 353t
   whole bowel irrigation in, 362
Polydipsia, hyponatremia and, 494t
Polymyxin, in eye trauma, 610
Polysporin. See *Bacitracin*.
Pontocaine. See *Tetracaine*.
Positive pressure ventilation, 25
Post-traumatic stress disorder, sexual assault and, 965
Potassium, 499–500. See also *Hyperkalemia*.
   endogenous sources of, 500
   exogenous sources of, 500
   in acidosis, 500
   in alkalosis, 500
   in hyperkalemia, 500
   transcellular shifts of, 500
Potassium hydroxide solution, in diagnosis of rash, 259
Prednisone, in anaphylaxis, 308, 310
   in skin disorders, 266
   in wheezing, 1014t
Preeclampsia, 245–246
Pregnancy. See also *Ectopic pregnancy*.
   asthma and, 998
   cardiopulmonary cerebral resuscitation and, 56
   dyspnea and, 997–998
   dysuria and, 1055
   hypertension and, 236, 245–246
   in acute abdominal pain, 97
   pulmonary edema and, 998
   pulmonary embolism and, 997
   syncope and, 220t, 221
   testing for, 1064, 1083
   urinary tract infection and, 324
   vaginal bleeding and, 1075–1076, 1084t, 1085–1086
      ectopic pregnancy and, 1084t, 1084–1085, 1085t
      labor and, 1077
   wheezing and, 1016
Prehospital care, 10–11. See also names of specific conditions.

Premature atrial contraction, 203. See also *Palpitation.*
  management principles in, 207
Primaxin. See *Imipenem-cilastatin.*
Probenecid, in gonorrhea, 1099t
Problem patient, 1133–1139
  dissatisfied, 1135–1136
  documentation and, 1138
  general considerations for, 1133–1134, 1138–1139
  hostile, 1136–1137
  manipulative, 1134–1135
  physician's attitude toward, 1134
  violent, 1137–1138
Problem solving, clinical, 8–10
  process of, 8–10
Procainamide, 208, 209
Prochlorperazine, in acute diarrhea, 131
  in nausea and vomiting, 147
Promethazine, in acute diarrhea, 131
  in nausea and vomiting, 147
Proparacaine, in eye trauma, 610
  in red and painful eye, 588t
Propranolol, 207, 208
  in cocaine abuse, 433t
  in hypertension, 235t
Prostatitis, dysuria and, 1054
Pseudogout, 696
Pseudohyperkalemia, 503
Pseudomonas, in sepsis, 315. See also *Sepsis.*
Psoas, in acute abdominal pain, 92
Psychiatric consultation, for suicidal patient, 961
Psychiatric disturbance, seizure and, 869
Pulmonary contusion, chest trauma and, 1031t, 1035
Pulmonary edema, dyspnea and, 993t
  disposition in, 998
  pregnancy and, 998
  hypertension and, 238, 243–244
  pregnancy and, 998
  protocol in, 1127t
Pulmonary embolism, acute chest pain and, 182t, 190
  chronic obstructive pulmonary disease and, 1007
  dyspnea and, 991t, 993t
    disposition in, 998
    management principles in, 996
  heparin in, 995–996
  management principles in, 190
  pregnancy and, 997
  vena cava interruption in, 996
Pulmonary function test, in dyspnea, 994
  in wheezing, 1010, 1010t
Pulmonary infection, community-acquired, 324
  in neonate, 324
  sepsis and, 324, 329t
Pulse oximetry, in dyspnea, 994
  in stridor, 646
Pulseless ventricular tachycardia, 50. See also *Palpitation.*
Puncture wound, 272
Pupil, examination of, 580
  dilation in, 602, *602*

Pupil (*Continued*)
  in red and painful eye, 580
  Marcus-Gunn, 602
Pustular disease, rash and, 257t, 260
Pyelonephritis, 1057
  dysuria and, 1049t, 1049–1051
  management principles in, 1051t, 1051–1052, 1052t
  pelvic pain in women and, 1070t
  subclinical, 1057
Pyridium. See *Phenazopyridine.*
Pyuria, 1055
  dysuria and. See *Dysuria.*

Quinidine, 208, 218
  as cause of syncope, 225

Rabies, prophylactic treatment in, 290, 290t
Radiologic imaging. See also names of specific conditions.
  cost range for, 13t–14t
Rantidine, in anaphylaxis, 308
Rape, 964. See also *Sexual assault.*
Rash, 251–270
  acneiform dermatitis in, 264
  admission in, 269
  anesthetic in, 264–265
  antibacterial in, 266
  antifungal agent in, 266
  antihistamine in, 265
  cellulitis and, 257t, 261
  common, 261–264
  contact dermatitis and, 257t, 263
  data gathering in, 254–255
  decision priorities in, 256, *256*, 258
  diagnostic adjuncts in, 258–260
  diascopy in, 259
  differential diagnosis in, preliminary, 256, 257, 257t, 258
    refined, 260–264
  discharge in, 269
  disposition in, 269
  documentation in, 269
  drug eruption as, 263–264
  eczematous disease and, 257t, 263
  erythema multiforme and, 257t, 263
  erythema multiforme bullosum and, 257t, 260, 263
  exanthems and, 263
  exfoliative dermatitis and, 264
  follow-up in, 269
  general considerations for, 251–252, 270
  gonococcemia in, 260
  Gram's stain in, 259
  herpes simplex in, 257t, 261–262
  history in, 254–255
  initial emergency department approach in, 252–254
  interventions in, 254
  joint pain and swelling and, 689
  life-threatening, 260–261

Rash (*Continued*)
  lubricant in, 264
  Lynch algorithm in, 256, 257t
  management principles in, 264–266
  meningitis and, 853
  meningococcemia and, 257t, 261
  observation in, 269
  palpable purpura and, 264
  papulosquamous disease and, 257t, 262
  pediatric patient and, 266, 267t–268t
  photosensitivity and, 264
  physical examination in, 255–256
    initial emergency department approach and, 253–254
  pityriasis rosea and, 257t, 262
  potassium hydroxide preparation in, 259
  pustular disease and, 257t, 260
  Rocky Mountain spotted fever and, 257t, 261
  scabicide in, 266
  scabies and, 257t, 262
  skin anatomy and, 251–252, *252*
  steroid in, 265t, 265–266
  Stevens-Johnson syndrome and, 257t, 260
  terminology in, 252, 253t
  tinea and, 257t, 262
  topical medication in, 264
  toxic epidermal necrolysis and, 260
  Tzanck smear in, 259
  urticaria and, 257t, 261, 263
  vascular reaction and, 257t, 261
  vasculitis and, 264
  Venereal Disease Research Laboratories rapid protein reagin in, 260
  vesiculobullous disease and, 257t, 260, 261–262
  wet dressing in, 264
  Wood's lamp examination in, 259
Rebreather mask, in oxygen delivery, 25t
Rectum, acute diarrhea and, 125
  acute gastrointestinal bleeding and, 110
  as source of gastrointestinal bleeding, 115
  examination of, for women, 1063
Red and painful eye, 575–594. See also *Eye, red and painful.*
Reglan. See *Metoclopramide.*
Regurgitation, 136. See also *Nausea and vomiting.*
Renal artery stenosis, in hypertension, 241
Renal disease, in hypertension, 241
  seizure and, 866
Renal failure, heat stroke and, 405
  hypertension and, 239, 244
  hyponatremia and, 494t
Renal insufficiency. See also *Acid-base disorder(s).*
  hyponatremia and, 493t
  metabolic acidosis and, 527t, 527–528
Renal tuberculosis, dysuria and, 1055
Reperfusion injury, 54
Replantation, hand and wrist, 742, 744

Reporting requirements, 1112
Research, on health care services, 5
Residency program, statistical and historical profile of, 4t
Respiratory failure, pediatric, 639
  stridor and. See *Stridor*.
Restraint, involuntary, 1110–1111
Retching, 136. See also *Nausea and vomiting*.
Retina, red and painful eye and, 576, 577, 581–582
Retropharyngeal abscess, 643t, 648
  management principles in, 649
  meningitis and, 855
  radiologic imaging in, 645
  sore throat and, 550, 551, 555–556
Reye's syndrome, meningitis and, 855
Rhabdomyolysis, heat stroke and, 405
Rheumatic fever, sore throat and, 559
Rhinitis, anaphylaxis and, 305t
Rhinovirus, sore throat and, 548t
Rib fracture, chest trauma and, 1035, 1037t
Rifampin, prophylactic, 341
Rocephin. See *Ceftriaxone*.
Rocky Mountain spotted fever, 257t, 261
Roseola, 267t. See also *Rash*.
Roseola infantum, 268t. See also *Rash*.
Rotator cuff tear, 710t, 711–712, 712. See also *Orthopedic injury(ies), upper extremity*.
Rotavirus, acute diarrhea and, 130t
Rubella, 267t. See also *Rash*.
Rumination, 136. See also *Nausea and vomiting*.

Sad Person's Scale, suicide potential and, 958, 958t
Salmonella, antibiotic in, pediatric patient and, 632t
  in acute diarrhea, 120t, 127t, 132, 133t. See also *Diarrhea, acute*.
Salpingitis, ectopic pregnancy and, 1058–1059
  infertility and, 1058
  management principles in, 1066, 1069, 1071t
  pelvic pain and, 1065, 1067t. See also *Pelvis, female, pain in*.
Salt-wasting nephropathy, hyponatremia and, 493t
Scabicide, 266
Scabies, 257t, 262
  management principles in, 266
Scalp, laceration of, 919
  wound care for, 288
Scar, formation of, wound care and, 273–274
Scarlet fever, 267t. See also *Rash*.
Schiötz tonometry, 603
Schizophrenia, 945t. See also *Behavioral disorder(s)*.
Sclera, 575, 577
Scombroid fish poisoning, 306
  acute diarrhea and, 127t

Scopolamine hydrobromide, in red and painful eye, 589t
Seizure(s), 862–876
  admission in, 874–875
  age factor and, 869t
  alcohol withdrawal and, 391
  anticonvulsant in, 864, 870, 872
  aspiration and, 873
  brain tumor and, 867
  cardiac disorders and, 865t, 866, 866t, 868
  cataplexy and, 868
  causal factors of, 872
  classification of, 871t
  complications of, 873–874
  data gathering in, 865–868
  decision priorities in, 868–869
  dehydration and, 671–672
  diagnostic adjuncts in, 869–871
  diazepam in, 850, 864, 865, 872
  differential diagnosis in, preliminary, 868–869, 869t
    refined, 871t, 871–872
  discharge in, 875
  disposition in, 874–875
  documentation in, 875
  eclampsia and, 865t, 866t
  electroencephalography in, 871
  endocrine disorder and, 866
  etiology of, 867t
  factitious, 869
  follow-up in, 875
  general considerations for, 862–863
  grand mal, 871t, 873
  heredity and, 867
  history in, 866t, 866–867
    prehospital care and, 863
  hyperventilation and, 869
  hypoglycemia and, 865t, 866t
  hyponatremia and, 487–488
  hypoxia and, 865t, 866t
  immunocompromised patient and, 867
  incidence of, 863
  initial emergency department approach in, 864–865
  intervention in, prehospital care and, 864
  intracranial hemorrhage and, 865t, 866t
  laboratory studies in, 870
  lactic acidosis and, 874
  lumbar puncture in, 870
  management principles in, 872–874, 873t
  meningitis and, 865t, 866t
  musculoskeletal injury and, 874
  neurologic examination in, 867
  neurology consultation in, 875
  pediatric patient and, 874
  pharmacologic control of, 872
  phenobarbital in, 850, 873
  phenytoin in, 850, 873
  physical examination in, 867–868
    prehospital care and, 863
  poisoning and, 865
  precautions against, 812
  prehospital care in, 863–864

Seizure(s) (*Continued*)
  prevention of, 872–873
  psychiatric disturbance and, 869
  radiologic imaging in, 870
  renal disorder and, 866
  status epilepticus and, 872, 873t
  syncope and, 868
  tonic-clonic, 871t, 873
Sepsis, 315–332
  abdominal infection and, 325, 329t
  acquired immune deficiency syndrome and, 330
  adjunctive therapies in, 328
  airway and ventilatory support in, 326
  antibiotic in, 327–328, 329t
    pediatric patient and, 632t
  antigen testing in, 322–323
  arthritis and, 695t, 695–696, 696t
    antibiotic in, pediatric patient and, 632t
    bacterial agent in, 695, 696t
    detection of, 692t, 692–695, *694*
    management principles in, 698, 698t
  aztreonam in, 327
  cefaclor in, 327–328
  ceftazidime in, 327–328
  ceftriaxone in, 327–328
  cefuroxime in, 327–328
  central nervous system infection and, 324–325, 329t
  cephalosporin in, 327
  cilastatin in, 327
  ciprofloxacin in, 327
  cold shock and, 316, *316*
  continuum in, 316, *316*
  data gathering in, 319–321
  decision priorities in, 321–322
  definition of, 315
  dextrose in, 317
  diagnostic adjuncts in, 322–323
  differential diagnosis in, preliminary, 321–322
    refined, 323–326
  disposition in, 331
  disseminated intravascular coagulation and, 320
  dobutamine in, 327
  documentation in, 331
  dopamine in, 327
  erythromycin in, 328
  febrile infant and, 630–631
  fluid therapy in, 326
  fluoroquinolone in, 327
  follow-up in, 331
  from unknown sources, 326
  general considerations for, 315–316, 331–332
  hemodynamic support in, 326–327
  history in, 319
    initial emergency department approach and, 318
    prehospital care and, 317
  immune therapy in, 328
  initial emergency department approach in, 317–319
  intervention in, initial emergency department approach and, 318–319

Sepsis (Continued)
  prehospital care and, 317
  invasive monitoring in, 327
  laboratory studies in, 318, 322–323
  lumbar puncture and, 322
  management principles in, 326–328
  naloxone in, 317, 328
  naltrexone in, 328
  narcotic antagonist in, 328
  neonatal, 330–331
  nitroprusside in, 327
  nonsteroidal anti-inflammatory drugs in, 328
  norfloxacin in, 327
  pediatric patient and, 632
  phentolamine in, 327
  physical examination in, 319–321
  pneumatic antishock garment in, 318
  prehospital care in, 316–317
  pulmonary infection and, 324, 329t
  radiologic imaging in, 323
  shock and, pelvic pain and, 1058
    sickle cell disease and, 457
  skin infection and, 325–326, 329t
  standard therapies in, 326–328
  steroid in, 328
  thiamine in, 317
  toxic shock syndrome and, 320, 328, 330
  trimethoprim/sulfamethoxazole in, 328
  urinary tract infection and, 323–324, 329t
  vasoactive drug in, 327
  vital signs in, 320
  warm shock and, 316, *316*
Sexual assault, 964–977
  age factor in, 965
  child victim of, 663, 665t, 665–666, 975
    incidence of, 964–965
    sexually transmitted disease and, 973–974, 974t
  confidentiality in, 976–977
  conviction rate in, 965
  data gathering in, 966, *967–971*
  diagnostic adjuncts in, 973
  differential diagnosis in, 973
  disposition in, 976
  documentation in, 976–977
  elderly female victim of, 975–976
  follow-up in, 976
  general considerations for, 964–965, 977
  history in, 966, *967–971*
  HIV infection and, 976
  incidence of, 964–965
  informed consent in, 965
  initial emergency department approach in, 965–966
  laboratory studies in, *971*, 973
  legislation on, 977
  male victim of, 975
  management principles in, 973–974
  medical report in, *967–971*
  physical examination in, *969–971, 972*
  poistcoital therapy in, 973
  post-traumatic stress disorder and, 965

Sexual assault (Continued)
  pregnancy and, 973
  prehospital care in, 965
  sexually transmitted disease and, 973–974, 974t
  terminology in, 964
Sexually transmitted disease, sexual assault and, 973–974, 974t
Shigella, in acute diarrhea, 120t, 127t, 133t. See also *Diarrhea, acute.*
Shock, management principles in, 68t, 68–69
  multiple trauma and, 62–63
  septic, pelvic pain and, 1058
  sickle cell disease and, 457
Shoulder injury, 710t, 711–712, *712*. See also *Orthopedic injury(ies), upper extremity.*
SIADH. See *Syndrome of inappropriate antidiuretic hormone secretion.*
Sickle cell disease, 455–468
  crisis in, 456–468
    abdominal, 464, 464t
    analgesia in, 463
    aplastic, 459, 466
    appearance in, 458
    bone and joint swelling in, 464, 464t
    data gathering in, 458–459
    decision priorities in, 459–461
    diagnostic adjuncts in, 461–463
    differential diagnosis in, preliminary, 459–461
      refined, 463, 464
    disposition in, 467
    documentation in, 467–468
    follow-up in, 467
    history in, 456, 458–459, 460t
    infection and, 459
    initial emergency department approach in, 457–458
    intervention in, 456–457
    laboratory studies in, 461–462, 462t
    management principles in, 463–465, 465–466
    neurologic, 458, 465t, 466
    organ system damage in, 460t
    oxygen administration in, 464–465
    pain and, 458
    pediatric patient and, 466
    physical examination in, 456, 459, 460t
    precipitating factors in, 458
    prehospital care in, 456–457
    priapism and, 465t, 466
    pulmonary, 465t, 466
    radiologic imaging in, 462–463
    splenic sequestration and, 459
    vaso-occlusive, 459–460
      subsets of, 464t–465t
  general considerations for, 455–456, 468
  hemoglobin S in, 455–456
  pediatric patient and, 466
  sepsis and, 632
  sickle cell trait and, 456
Sickle cell trait, 456

Sigmoidoscopy, acute gastrointestinal bleeding and, 114
Sinusitis, headache and, 840t, 842
  management principles in, 844
Skeletal injury, child abuse and, 657
Skin, anatomy of, 251–252, *252*, 271–272
Skin disorders, poisoning and, 353–354
  sepsis and, 320, 325–326, 329t
Slit lamp examination, eye trauma and, 603
Snellen eye chart, 599
Sodium bicarbonate, in cardiopulmonary cerebral resuscitation, *50*, 52–53
  in pediatric CPR, 55t
  in wheezing, 1015
Sodium-EDTA, in hypercalcemia, 514
Solvent drag, acute diarrhea and, 130
Sorbitol, in poisoning, 362
Sore throat, 547–560
  adenovirus in, 548t, 556
  admission in, 559
  age factor in, 558
  bacterial infection in, 548t, 556
  burn and, 556
  cancer and, 556
  Chlamydia in, 548t, 556
  consultation in, 559
  coronavirus in, 548t
  Corynebacterium in, 548t
  cytomegalovirus in, 548t, 556
  data gathering in, 548–550
  decision priorities in, 550–552, 551t
  diagnostic adjuncts in, 552–553
  differential diagnosis in, 550–552, 551t
    refined, 553, 555, 555–557
  diphtheria and, 553, 556
  discharge in, 559
  disposition and, 559
  documentation in, 559
  epiglottitis and, 550–551, 553, 555
  Epstein-Barr virus in, 548t, 556
  follow-up in, 559
  general considerations for, 547–548
  glossopharyngeal neuralgia in, 556
  Gonococcus in, 553, 556
  herpes simplex in, 548t
  history in, 549
  immune status and, 558
  infectious agent in, 547–548, 548t, 556
  influenza virus A and B in, 548t
  initial emergency department approach in, 548, 556
  laboratory studies in, 552–553
  life-threatening disease and, 553, 555–556
  management principles in, 557–558
  Mycoplasma in, 548t, 556
  Neisseria in, 548t
  noninfectious cause of, 551–552, 556–557
  parainfluenza virus in, 548t
  peritonsillar abscess and, 555, *555*
  physical examination in, 549–560
  psychogenic, 557
  radiologic imaging in, 553
  retropharyngeal abscess and, 550, 551, 555–556

Sore throat (Continued)
  rheumatic fever and, 559
  rhinovirus in, 548t
  Streptococcus in. See Streptococcus, in sore throat.
  subacute thyroiditis in, 556
  throat culture in, 553, 554
  thrush and, 556
  tonsillar edema and, 550, 551
  trauma and, 556
  uvular edema and, 550, 551
  viral infection in, 548t, 556
Spectinomycin, in gonorrhea, 1099t
Spinal cord injury. See also Head and neck trauma.
  anatomy and, 895, 895, 896
  cord syndrome and, 918
  diagnosis in, 907
  pathophysiology of, 895–896
Spinal stenosis, low back pain and, 793, 794t, 798, 799t, 800
Spleen, injury to, 164t. See also Abdomen, trauma to.
Stab wound, abdominal trauma and, 153–154, 154t, 166, 167
  general considerations for, 272
Staphylococcus, antibiotic in, pediatric patient and, 632t
  in acute diarrhea, 120t, 127t. See also Diarrhea, acute.
  in sepsis, 315. See also Sepsis.
  wound care and, 292
Status epilepticus, 872, 873t
Statutory rape, 964. See also Sexual assault.
Sternal fracture, chest trauma and, 1037t
Steroid therapy, in anaphylaxis, 301, 308
  in earache, 572, 572t
  in eye trauma, 610
  in head and neck trauma, 919
  in rash, 265t, 265–266
  in sepsis, 328
  pediatric patient and, 633
Stevens-Johnson syndrome, rash and, 257t, 260
Stool, blood in. See also Gastrointestinal bleeding.
  test for, 110
  culture of, acute diarrhea and, 128–129
  in acute diarrhea, 124
  vomiting and, 145
Strangulated femoral hernia, pelvic pain in women and, 1070t
Strep throat. See Streptococcus, in sore throat.
Streptococcus, antibiotic in, pediatric patient and, 632t
  febrile infant and, 628, 629
  in cellulitis, 261
  in meningitis, 849, 850t
  in sepsis, 315. See also Sepsis.
  in skin disorder, 320
  in sore throat, age factor and, 558
    differential diagnosis of, 551, 551t
    disposition in, 559
    follow-up in, 559

Streptococcus (Continued)
  general considerations for, 548, 548t
  history in, 549
  immune status and, 558
  laboratory studies in, 552–553, 554
  management principles in, 558
  pediatric patient and, 552t
  rheumatic fever and, 559
Stress, headache and, 840t, 842
Stridor, 636–651
  airway anatomy and, 636–637, 637
  data gathering in, 640–642
  decision priorities in, 642–644, 643t
  definition of, 636
  diagnostic adjuncts in, 644, 644–646, 645
  differential diagnosis in, preliminary, 642–644, 643t
    refined, 646t, 646–648
  epiglottitis and, 643t, 646–647
    management principles in, 648
    radiographic imaging in, 644, 644
  etiology of, 643t
  foreign body and, 643t, 647–648
    management principles in, 649
    radiographic imaging in, 645, 645
  general considerations for, 636–637, 651
  history in, 641
    initial emergency department approach and, 639
    prehospital care and, 638
  initial emergency department approach in, 638–640
  intervention in, initial emergency department approach and, 639–640
    prehospital care and, 638
  laboratory studies in, 646
  management principles in, 643t, 648–650
  physical examination in, 641–642
    initial emergency department approach and, 639, 639t
    prehospital care and, 638
  prehospital care in, 637–638
  pulse oximetry in, 646
  radiologic imaging in, 644, 644–645, 645
  retropharyngeal abscess and, 643t, 648
    radiographic imaging in, 645
  viral laryngotracheobronchitis and, 643t, 647, 647t
    management principles in, 649
    radiographic imaging in, 644–645
Stroke, 877–893
  admission in, 892
  airway management and, 880
  anatomy and, 877, 878
  anterior cerebral artery syndrome and, 889
  anticoagulation therapy in, 890
  antiplatelet agent in, 890
  carotid bruit and, 882t, 888
  carotid syndrome and, 889
  cerebral artery syndrome and, 889
  cerebral edema and, 880
  clinical manifestations of, 878

Stroke (Continued)
  complete, 878, 884t, 886
    management principles in, 890
  data gathering in, 880–883
  decision priorities in, 883, 886
  definition of, 877
  diagnostic adjuncts in, 886
  differential diagnosis in, preliminary, 883, 886, 884t–885t
  discharge in, 892
  disposition in, 892
  documentation in, 893
  electrocardiogram in, 888
  embolic, 885t
    management principles in, 890
  follow-up in, 892
  general considerations for, 877–878, 893
  geriatric patient and, 891
  heat illness and, 400t, 400–401, 402t, 407
    management principles in, 405–406
  heparinization in, 890
  herniation syndrome and, 880
  history in, prehospital care and, 878–879, 881t
  hypertension and, 880
  in evolution, 878, 884t, 886
    management principles in, 890
  incidence of, 878
  initial emergency department approach in, 879–880
  intervention in, prehospital care and, 879
  intracerebral hemorrhage and, 885t, 887, 887
    management principles in, 890
  laboratory studies in, 886
  lacunar infarct syndrome and, 889
  lumbar puncture in, 888
  management principles in, 889–890
  neurologic examination in, 882t
  pediatric patient and, 891
  physical examination in, prehospital care and, 879, 882t
    refined, 889
  prehospital care in, 878
  previously impaired patient and, 891–892
  radiologic imaging in, 886–888, 887
  risk factors for, 881, 881t
  subarachnoid hemorrhage and, 885t, 887, 887
    management principles in, 890
  thrombolytic, 890
  transient ischemic attack and, 877, 883, 884t
    management principles in, 890
  vascular syndrome and, 889
  vertebral basilar syndrome and, 889
  Wallenberg syndrome and, 889
Substance abuse. See also Alcoholism; Cocaine abuse.
  acute confusion and, 808. See also Mental status, altered.
  drug toxicity and, 375–376

INDEX — 1169

Succinylcholine, in orotracheal intubation, 32
Sudden cardiac death, emergency medical services and, 1129
Suicide potential, 951–963
  adolescent and, 951, 960
  age factor in, 951
  data gathering in, 954–957
  decision priorities in, 957–959, 958t
  diagnostic adjuncts in, 959
  differential diagnosis in, preliminary, 957–959, 958t
  disposition in, 960–962
  documentation in, 962
  follow-up in, 960–962
  gender factor in, 951
  general considerations for, 951–952, 962–963
  geriatric patient and, 960
  haloperidol in, 959
  history in, 954–955
    prehospital care and, 952, 952t
  initial emergency department approach in, 953–954
  management principles in, 959–960
  medical illness and, 957
  pediatric patient and, 960
  physical examination in, 956–957
    prehospital care and, 952–953
  planning and, 955
  prehospital care in, 952–953
  psychiatric consultation and, 961
  risk assessment in, 961
  risk factors in, 952t, 957–958
  Sad Person's Scale in, 958, 958t
Sulamide. See Sulfacetamide.
Sulfacetamide, in eye trauma, 610
  in red and painful eye, 592t
Sulfisoxazole, in earache, 569, 572t
  in eye trauma, 610
  in red and painful eye, 592t
Surgical consultation, in acute abdominal pain, 101
Suture, closure technique and, 283–284, 283–287, 288
  material and equipment for, 280, 282, 282t
  removal of, 293, 293t
Syncope, 214–230
  altered mental status vs., 217
  arterial pressure in, 215, 215
  atrioventricular block and, 223–224, 224, 225
  cardiac dysrhythmia and, 222t, 223–225, 224, 225, 228
    management principles in, 227
  cardiac medication as cause of, 224–225, 228
  cardiovascular system in, 220t
  common causes of, 222t
  data gathering in, 217–219
  decision priorities in, 219–220
  definition of, 214
  diagnostic adjuncts in, 220–222
  differential diagnosis in, preliminary, 219–220
    refined, 222t, 222–226

Syncope (Continued)
  disposition in, 228–229
  documentation in, 229–230
  electrocardiogram in, 221
  electroencephalogram in, 221
  etiology of, 220t
  extremities in, 217
  follow-up in, 229
  general considerations for, 214–215, 230
  geriatric patient and, 228
  history in, 217–218
    prehospital care and, 216
  holter monitor and, 221
  initial emergency department approach in, 217
  intervention in, prehospital care and, 216
  laboratory studies in, 221
  management principles in, 226–227
  medications as cause of, 218
  metabolic abnormalities and, 220t, 226
  neurologic disease and, 219t, 220t, 226
  of uncertain etiology, 229
  orthostatic hypotension and, 226, 227, 228, 229
  pediatric patient and, 227–228
  physical examination in, 218–219, 219t
    prehospital care and, 216
  pregnancy and, 220t, 221
  prehospital care in, 215–216
  psychological, 220t
  radiologic imaging in, 221
  seizure and, 868
  situational, 220t, 226, 228, 229
  special tests in, 221–222
  vasovagal faint and, 222t, 222–223, 229
    management principles in, 226
Syndrome of inappropriate antidiuretic hormone secretion, 494
Synovial fluid analysis, in febrile infant, 629
  in joint pain and swelling, 692t, 692–695, 694
Syphilis, serologic test for, 1096
  sexual assault and, 973
Syrup of ipecac, contraindications in, 360, 360t
  in poisoning, 360–360t

Tachycardia. See also specific tachycardias.
  intoxication and, 352, 353t
  management principles in, 227
  syncope and, 223
TEN. See Toxic epidermal necrolysis.
Tendinitis, joint pain and swelling and, 697
Tendon(s), hand and wrist. See also Hand and wrist injury(ies).
  anatomy of, 732, 734, 735, 736, 737
  laceration of, 739–740
Tenosynovitis, flexor, suppurative, 741, 742, 743

Terbutaline, in wheezing, 1011, 1013t
Tetanus, accidental exposure to, 340, 341t. See also Biologic agent, accidental exposure to.
  prophylactic, in abdominal trauma, 166
  in multiple trauma, 75
  in wound care, 290–291, 291t
Tetracaine, in eye trauma, 610
  in red and painful eye, 588t
Tetracycline, in eye trauma, 610
  in gonorrhea, 1099t
  in red and painful eye, 592t
  in skin disorders, 266
Theophylline, in asthma, 994–995
  in poisoning, 371–372
  in wheezing, 1012, 1014, 1014t
Thiamine, in alcohol intoxication, 381
  in hypothermia, 413
  in sepsis, 317
Thigh injury, 761–764. See also Orthopedic injury(ies), lower extremity.
  anatomy and, 752, 753
  physical examination in, 753
Third-space loss, hyponatremia and, 493t
Thoracostomy, in pneumothorax, 995
Thoracotomy, emergency, 77
  in chest trauma, 1020
Thorax, trauma to, 1020–1039. See also Chest, trauma to.
Thrombocytopenia, 447t, 447–448
Thrombolytic, in pulmonary embolus, 995
  in stroke, 890
Thrombotic thrombocytopenic purpura, 447t, 448
Thrush, 556
Thyroiditis, subacute, sore throat and, 556
TIA. See Transient ischemic attack.
Tibial shaft fracture, 766–767. See also Orthopedic injury(ies), lower extremity.
Ticarcillin-clavulanate, in dysuria, 1052, 1052t
Timentin. See Ticarcillin-clavulanate.
Tinea, in rash, 257t, 262
Tobex. See Tobramycin.
Tobramycin. See also Gentamicin.
  in eye trauma, 610
  in red and painful eye, 592t
Tonometry, in eye trauma, 603–604
  in red and painful eye, 583
Tonsillar edema, sore throat and, 550, 551
Topical ophthalmic antibiotic, in red and painful eye, 592t
Toxic epidermal necrolysis, rash and, 260
Toxic exposure, headache and, 833
Toxic ingestion, delirium and, 808–809. See also Mental status, altered.
Toxic shock syndrome, sepsis and, 320, 328, 330
Toxologic disorder, 345–393. See also Alcohol intoxication; Cocaine abuse; Poisoning.

Trachea, pediatric, 637, 637
Tracheal airway, esophageal, in cardiac arrest, 43
Tracheobronchial disruption, chest trauma and, 1031t
Tracheostomy, in airway management, 33
Traction, in low back pain, 800
Transient ischemic attack, management principles in, 890
Trauma. See also *Multiple trauma*; names of specific types of trauma.
  abdominal, 152–169. See also *Abdomen, trauma to*.
  airway management in, 36
  cardiopulmonary cerebral resuscitation and, 56
  cervical spine, 67
  child abuse and, 660, 660t
  corneal, 591t
  earache and, 570t
  head and neck, 894–923. See also *Head and neck trauma*.
  joint pain and swelling and, 696
  orthopedic, lower extremity, 748–782. See also *Orthopedic injury(ies), lower extremity*.
    upper extremity, 703–747. See also *Hand and wrist injury(ies); Orthopedic injury(ies), upper extremity*.
  red and painful eye due to, 578, 579
  sore throat and, 556
  to eye, 595–614. See also *Eye, trauma to*.
  vaginal bleeding and, 1076
Trauma center, criteria for, 60–61
Trauma score, 64, 65t, 66, 66t
  pediatric, 76t
Travel, as cause of acute diarrhea, 124
Trendelenburg position, in anaphylaxis, 303
Triamcinolone, in skin disorder, 265, 265t
Trichomonas, in vaginal infection, 1097t, 1098
  follow-up in, 1100
  laboratory studies in, 1095, 1096
  management principles in, 1199
Trimethaphan, in hypertension, 235t
Trimethoprim-sulfamethoxazole, in dysuria, 1054
  in earache, 569, 572t
  in gonorrhea, 1099t
  in sepsis, 328
Tropicamide, in red and painful eye, 589t
Tuberculosis, renal, pyuria and, 1055
Tympanic membrane, 562
  examination of, 564–565
Tzanck smear, 1096
  in rash, 259

Ulcer, acute gastrointestinal bleeding and, 114–115

Ulcer (*Continued*)
  duodenal, acute gastrointestinal bleeding and, 114–115
  peptic, abdominal pain and, 96t. See also *Abdomen, pain in*.
    acute gastrointestinal bleeding and, 114–115
  sepsis and, 325, 329t
Upper airway obstruction, causes of, 35, 35t
  pediatric, uncommon causes of, 646t
  stridor and, 636–651. See also *Stridor*.
Upper extremity injury, 703–743. See also *Orthopedic injury(ies), upper extremity*.
Ureaplasma, penile discharge and. See also *Penis, discharge from*.
Ureteral calculus, pelvic pain in women and, 1070t
Ureteral colic, 95t. See also *Abdomen, pain in*.
Urethritis, dysuria and, 1048, 1049t
  gonococcal, 1091, 1096, 1099t
  nongonococcal, 1096–1097
  penile discharge and, 1091–1092. See also *Penis, discharge from*.
Urinalysis, in acute abdominal pain, 97
  in dysuria, 1047
  in pelvic pain, 1065
Urinary catheter, indwelling, dysuria and, 1054–1055
Urinary dipstick analysis, in dysuria, 1047
Urinary tract infection, dysuria and. See *Dysuria*.
  geriatric patient and, 324
  neonate and, 1053
  pediatric patient and, 323–324
  pregnancy and, 324
  sepsis and, 323–324, 329t
Urination, painful. See *Dysuria*.
Urine culture, in dysuria, 1047–1048
Urticaria, 257t, 261, 263
  in anaphylaxis, 302, 305t
Uterus, injury to, 165t. See also *Abdomen, trauma to*.
  myoma and fibroid in, pelvic pain and, 1069t. See also *Pelvis, female, pain in*.
Uveitis, 581
  management principles in, 591t, 592t
Uvular edema, sore throat and, 550, 551

Vagina, bleeding from, 1075–1090
  abruptio placentae and, 1087–1088
  admission in, 1088–1089
  age factor in, 1086, 1088
  cervical culture in, 1083
  culdocentesis in, 1083
  data gathering in, 1079–1081
  diagnostic adjuncts in, 1082–1084
  differential diagnosis in, preliminary, 1082
    refined, 1084t, 1084–1086, 1085t
  discharge in, 1089

Vagina (*Continued*)
  disposition in, 1088–1089
  documentation in, 1090
  general considerations for, 1075–1076, 1090
  hematologic causes of, 1076
  history in, 1079–1080
    initial emergency department approach and, 1078
    prehospital care and, 1076
  infection and, 1076
  initial emergency department approach in, 1077–1078
  intervention in, prehospital care and, 1076–1077
  laboratory studies in, 1082–1083
  malignancy and, 1076, 1086
  management principles in, 1087–1088
  negative pregnancy test and, 1086
  pathophysiology of, 1075–1076
  physical examination in, 1080–1081
    initial emergency department approach and, 1078
    prehospital care and, 1076
  placenta previa and, 1087
  platelet disorder and, 1076
  pneumatic antishock garment and, 1077
  postmenopausal patient and, 1088
  pregnancy and, 1075–1076, 1084t, 1085–1086
    culdocentesis in, 1083
    ectopic, 1084t, 1084–1085, 1085t
    labor and, 1077
    pregnancy testing and, 1083
  prehospital care in, 1076–1077
  premenarchal patient and, 1088, 1089t
  spontaneous abortion and, 1085, 1087
  trauma and, 1076
discharge from, 1091–1101
  antibiotic in, 1099
  antifungal preparation in, 1099
  candidiasis and, 1097, 1097t
    follow-up in, 1100
    laboratory studies in, 1095
    management principles in, 1199
  causes of, 1097t
  cervicitis and, 1097t, 1098
    follow-up in, 1100
    management principles in, 1099
  culture in, 1095, 1196
  data gathering in, 1092, 1093–1094
  decision priorities in, 1094
  diagnostic adjuncts in, 1094, 1095–1096
  differential diagnosis in, preliminary, 1094
    refined, 1097t, 1097–1098
  disposition in, 1100–1101
  documentation in, 1101
  follow-up in, 1100–1101
  Gardnerella vaginitis and, 1097t, 1097–1098
    follow-up in, 1100

Vagina (Continued)
    laboratory studies in, 1095
    management principles in, 1199
    general considerations for, 1091–1092, 1101
    herpes simplex and, 1097t, 1099
        follow-up in, 1101
        laboratory studies in, 1096
        management principles in, 1099, 1099t
    infectious causes of, 1097t, 1097–1098
    laboratory studies in, 1094–1095
    management principles in, 1099t, 1099–1100
    noninfectious causes of, 1097t
    pediatric patient and, 1100
    physiologic causes of, 1097t
    postmenopausal patient and, 1100
    potassium hydroxide preparation in, 1095
    trichomoniasis and, 1097t, 1098
        follow-up in, 1100
        laboratory studies in, 1095, 1096
        management principles in, 1099
Vaginitis, 1049t
    candidiasis, 1097, 1097t
        follow-up in, 1100
        laboratory studies in, 1095
        management principles in, 1099
    dysuria and. See Dysuria.
    Gardnerella, 1097t, 1097–1098
        follow-up in, 1100
        laboratory studies in, 1095
        management principles in, 1199
    herpes simplex, 1097t, 1099
        follow-up in, 1101
        laboratory studies in, 1096
        management principles in, 1099, 1099t
    microscopic examination of, 1048
    trichomoniasis, 1097t, 1098
        follow-up in, 1100
        laboratory studies in, 1095, 1096
        management principles in, 1099
    vaginal discharge and. See Vagina, discharge from.
Valsalva maneuver, 929
Varicella, 267t. See also Rash.
Varicella zoster virus, accidental exposure to, 334, 337. See also Biologic agent, accidental exposure to.
Varices, esophageal, acute gastrointestinal bleeding in, 115
Vascular injury, in hand and wrist, 740
Vasculitis, rash and, 264
Vaso-occlusive crisis, in sickle cell crisis, 459–460
    subsets of, 464t–465t
Vasoactive drug, in sepsis, 327
Vasodilation, in anaphylaxis, 305t
Vasopressin, acute gastrointestinal bleeding and, 117, 118
Vasosulf. See Sulfacetamide.
Vasovagal faint, management principles in, 226

Vasovagal faint (Continued)
    syncope and, 222t, 222–223, 229
VDRL/RPR. See Venereal Disease Research Laboratories/rapid protein reagin.
Vena cava interruption, in pulmonary embolism, 996
Venereal Disease Research Laboratories/rapid protein reagin, in rash, 260
Ventilatory support, in wheezing, 1004–1005
Ventimask, in oxygen delivery, 25t
Ventricular fibrillation, 49, 50. See also Cardiopulmonary cerebral resuscitation.
Ventricular premature beat, 203–204. See also Palpitation.
    management principles in, 207
Ventricular tachycardia, 49, 51, 203, 204. See also Palpitation.
    management principles in, 207–208, 208
Venturi mask, in oxygen delivery, 25t
Verapamil, 207, 208, 209
Vertigo, 924, 925t. See also Dizziness.
    classification of, 925t
    differential diagnosis in, 929–930, 932t
    Ménière's disease and, 932t
    positional, 925t, 932t
    test for, 928, 928–929
Vesicoureteral reflux, 1044
Vesiculobullous disease, rash and, 257t, 260, 261–262
Vestibular neutitis, dizziness and, 932t
Vibrio, in acute diarrhea, 120t, 127t
Violent patient, 1137–1138. See also Problem patient.
Viral laryngotracheobronchitis, 643t, 647, 647t
Vistaril. See Hydroxyzine.
    in hyperventilation syndrome, 996
Visual acuity, eye trauma and, 599, 600, 604
    red and painful eye and, 576, 578
Vomiting. See also Nausea and vomiting.
    abdominal pain and, 89–90
    acute gastrointestinal bleeding and, 119
    dehydration and, 672
VZ (varicella zoster) immune globulin, 341

Wallenberg syndrome, stroke and, 889
Warm shock, sepsis and, 316, 316
Waterhouse-Friderichsen syndrome, 858
Weight loss, in acute diarrhea, 125
Western blot, 339
Wheezing, 639, 1000–1018. See also Stridor.
    admission in, 1016–1017
    albuterol in, 1011, 1013t
    aminophylline in, 1012, 1013t
    anesthesia in, 1015
    antibiotic in, 1015
    anticholinergic agent in, 1014–1015

Wheezing (Continued)
    atropine sulfate in, 1014t
    beta-agonist in, 1011, 1012
    bronchospasm and, 1011, 1012–1013, 1014t, 1014–1015
    congestive heart failure and, 1005, 1007
    corticosteroid in, 1014
    data gathering in, 1005–1007
    diagnostic adjuncts in, 1009–1011
    differential diagnosis in, 1001t
        preliminary, 1007–1008
    discharge in, 1017–1018
    disposition in, 1016–1018
    documentation in, 1018
    electrocardiogram in, 1009
    epinephrine in, 1011, 1013t
    follow-up in, 1016–1018
    general considerations for, 1000–1002
    glucocorticoid in, 1014
    history in, 1005–1006
        initial emergency department approach and, 1004
        prehospital care and, 1002
    initial emergency department approach in, 1003–1005
    intensive care unit admission in, 1017
    intervention in, prehospital care and, 1003
    intubation in, 1018
    isoetharine in, 1014
    isoproterenol in, 1014
    laboratory studies in, 1009
    management principles in, 1011, 1012–1013, 1014t, 1014–1015
    metaproterenol in, 1011, 1013t
    methylprednisolone in, 1014t
    orotracheal intubation in, 1004
    pediatric patient and, 1016
    physical examination in, 1006–1007
        initial emergency department approach and, 1004
        prehospital care and, 1003
    prednisone in, 1014t
    pregnancy and, 1016
    prehospital care in, 1002–1003
    pulmonary function test in, 1010, 1010t
    radiologic imaging in, 1009
    rehydration in, 1015
    sodium bicarbonate in, 1015
    sputum analysis in, 1010–1011
    terbutaline in, 1011, 1013t
    theophylline in, 1012, 1014, 1014t
    ventilatory support in, 1004–1005
Whole bowel irrigation, in poisoning, 362
Wide-complex tachycardia, 202, 204–207, 205, 205t. See also Palpitation.
    management principles in, 208–209, 209
Wolff-Parkinson-White syndrome, 203, 210, 211
Wood's lamp examination, in rash, 259
World Health Organization Solution, rehydration and, 131, 131t

Wound care, 271–295
    aftercare in, 290–294, 293t
    anesthesia in, 278–280, 279t
    antibiotic in, 292
    assessment in, 282–283
    bandaging in, 291–292
    bupivacaine in, 279, 279t
    cleansing in, 280
    closure technique in, 283, 283–284, 283–287, 285–287, 288
    computed tomography in, 278
    corner suture in, 284, 287, 288
    data gathering in, 276–277
    debridement in, 282–283
    decision priorities in, 277–278
    deep closure in, 284, 285
    diagnostic adjuncts in, 278
    dicloxacillin in, 292
    differential diagnosis in, preliminary, 277–278
    disposition in, 292–294
    documentation in, 294
    dressings in, 739
    flap suture in, 284, 287, 288
    follow-up in, 292–293
    fracture and, 275
    general considerations for, 271, 294–295

Wound care *(Continued)*
    hemorrhage in, 274
    hemostasis in, 280
    history in, 276
        prehospital care and, 274
    impaired healing and, 274t
    in animal bite, 290, 291t
    in bite, 290
    in burn, 289–290, 290t
    in ear laceration, 289
    in eyelid laceration, 288
    in facial wound, 288–289
    in foreign body, 289
    in hand and wrist injury, 738–739
    in intraoral laceration, 289
    in lip laceration, 289
    in nasal injury, 289
    in scalp wound, 288
    infection and, 273, 274t
    initial emergency department approach in, 275
    inpatient management in, 293–294
    intervention in, 274–275
    laboratory studies in, 278
    lidocaine in, 279, 279t
    management principles in, 278–288
    mattress technique in, 284, 286

Wound care *(Continued)*
    mechanisms of injury and, 272
    mepivacaine in, 279, 279t
    nerve block in, 279–280, *281*
    outpatient management in, 292–293
    percutaneous closure in, 283, *283, 284*
    physical examination in, 276–277
        prehospital care and, 274
    prehospital care in, 274–275
    radiologic imaging in, 278
    running technique in, 284, 287
    scar formation and, 273–274
    skin anatomy and, 271–272
    stages of, 273–274
    Staphylococcus in, 292
    suture materials and equipment in, 280, 282, 282t
    tetanus prophylaxis in, 290–291, 291t
    wound preparation in, 278–280, 279t, *281*, 282t, 282–283
Wrist fracture, 710t, 717–718. See also *Orthopedic injury(ies), upper extremity.*

Yale Observation Scale, 621, 621t
Yersinia, in acute diarrhea, 120t, 127t, 133t. See also *Diarrhea, acute.*